Supplements and New Media

for INSTRUCTORS

Instructor's Resource Manual

ISBN: 0-13-049426-7

This manual contains a wealth of material to help faculty plan and manage the medical-surgical nursing course. It includes chapter overviews, detailed lecture suggestions and outlines, learning objectives, a complete test bank, teaching tips, and more for each chapter. The IRM also guides faculty how to assign and use the text-specific Companion Website, www.prenhall.com/burke, and the CD-ROM that accompany the textbook.

Instructor's Resource CD-ROM

ISBN: 0-13-049428-3

This cross-platform CD-ROM provides illustrations in PowerPoint from this textbook for use in classroom lectures. It also contains an electronic test bank. This supplement is available to faculty free upon adoption of the textbook. (For a printed test bank, e-mail your request to nursing@prenhall.com.)

Companion Website Syllabus Manager

www.prenhall.com/burke

Faculty adopting this textbook have free access to the online Syllabus Manager feature of the Companion Website, www.prenhall.com/burke. Syllabus Manager offers a whole host of features that facilitate the students' use of the Companion Website, and allows faculty to post syllabi and course information online for their students. For more information or a demonstration of Syllabus Manager, please contact a Prentice Hall Sales Representative.

also AVAILABLE

Wilson, Nurses Drug Guide

ISBN: 0-13-097872-8

The most complete source for drug administration information and the only source to identify prototype drugs.

Smith, Sandra Smith's Review for the NCLEX-PN 7E

ISBN: 0-13-028673-7

Nursing content review including thousands of questions to help students prepare for the NCLEX-PN.

Brief Table of Contents

Part I Medical-Surgical Nursing Practice *1*

UNIT I ➤ Introduction to Medical-Surgical Nursing *1*
1. The Medical-Surgical Nurse *1*
2. The Adult Client in Health and Illness *15*
3. Community-Based and Home Care of the Adult Client *31*
4. Guidelines for Health Assessment *45*

UNIT II ➤ Alterations in Health Patterns *63*
5. Caring for Clients with Altered Fluid, Electrolyte, or Acid–Base Balance *63*
6. Caring for Clients in Pain *101*
7. Caring for Clients Having Surgery *125*
8. Caring for Clients with Cancer *155*
9. Loss, Grief, and End-of-Life Care *183*

Part II Health Perception–Health Management Pattern *199*

UNIT III ➤ Altered Health Management *199*
10. Caring for Clients Experiencing Shock, Trauma, or Critical Illness *199*
11. Caring for the Client with Substance Abuse or Dependency *221*

UNIT IV ➤ Altered Immune System Responses *237*
12. Caring for Clients with Inflammation and Infection *237*
13. Caring for Clients with Altered Immunity *265*

Part III Nutritional–Metabolic Pattern *297*

UNIT V ➤ Altered Integumentary System Responses *297*
14. Caring for Clients with Skin Disorders *297*
15. Caring for the Client with Burns *325*

UNIT VI ➤ Altered Endocrine Responses *341*
16. Caring for Clients with Endocrine Disorders *341*
17. Caring for Clients with Diabetes Mellitus *365*

UNIT VII ➤ Altered Nutritional Responses *393*
18. Caring for Clients with Nutritional and Upper GI Disorders *393*
19. Caring for Clients with Gallbladder, Liver, and Pancreatic Disorders *425*

Part IV Elimination Pattern *453*

UNIT VIII ➤ Altered Elimination Responses *453*
20. Caring for Clients with Bowel Disorders *453*
21. Caring for Clients with Renal and Urinary Tract Disorders *493*

Part V Activity–Exercise Pattern *537*

UNIT IX ➤ Altered Cardiovascular System Responses *537*
22. Caring for Clients with Cardiac Disorders *537*
23. Caring for Clients with Peripheral Vascular Disorders *595*
24. Caring for Clients with Hematologic and Lymphatic Disorders *623*

UNIT X ➤ Altered Respiratory System Responses *655*
25. Caring for Clients with Upper Respiratory Disorders *655*
26. Caring for Clients with Lower Respiratory Disorders *679*

UNIT XI ➤ Altered Musculoskeletal System Responses *731*
27. Caring for Clients with Musculoskeletal Trauma *731*
28. Caring for Clients with Musculoskeletal Disorders *757*

Part VI Cognitive–Perceptual Pattern *789*

UNIT XII ➤ Altered Neurologic System Responses *789*
29. Caring for Clients with Intracranial Disorders *789*
30. Caring for Clients with Degenerative Neurologic and Spinal Cord Disorders *827*

UNIT XIII ➤ Altered Sensory Responses *855*
31. Caring for Clients with Eye and Ear Disorders *855*

Part VII Sexuality–Reproductive Pattern *885*

UNIT XIV ➤ Altered Reproductive System Responses *885*
32. Caring for Male Clients with Reproductive System Disorders *885*
33. Caring for Female Clients with Reproductive System Disorders *907*
34. Caring for Clients with Sexually Transmitted Diseases *947*

Appendices *963*
I. Standard Precautions *963*
II. NANDA-Approved Nursing Diagnoses 2001–2002 *965*
III. Common Laboratory Values *967*
IV. Glossary *968*
V. NCLEX-PN Answers; Hints for Critical Thinking *978*

Bibliography *1000*

Credits *1012*

Index *1013*

Medical-Surgical Nursing Care

Karen M. Burke, RN, MS
Director of Health Occupations
Clatsop Community College
Astoria, Oregon

Priscilla LeMone, RN, DSN, FAAN
Associate Professor
Director of Undergraduate Studies
Sinclair School of Nursing
University of Missouri
Columbia, Missouri

Elaine L. Mohn-Brown, RN, EdD
Faculty
ADN Nursing Program
Chemeketa Community College
Salem, Oregon

Prentice
Hall

Upper Saddle River, New Jersey 07458

Library of Congress Cataloging-in-Publication Data

Burke, Karen M.
    Medical surgical nursing care/Karen Burke, Priscilla LeMone, Elaine Mohn-Brown.—1st ed.
        p.;cm.
    Includes bibliographical references and index.
    ISBN 0-13-028162-X
    1. Surgical nursing. 2. Nursing. I. LeMone, Priscilla. II. Mohn-Brown, Elaine. III. Title.
    [DNLM: 1. Perioperative Nursing—methods. 2. Nursing Care—methods. 3. Nursing Process. WY 161 B959m 2003]
    RT41 .B89 2003
    610.73'677—dc21

                                                    2002025244

Publisher: Julie Levin Alexander
Assistant to Publisher: Regina Bruno
Executive Editor: Maura Connor
Acquisitions Editor: Barbara Krawiec
Managing Development Editor: Marilyn Meserve
Development Editor: Rachel Bedard
Assistant Editor: Yesenia Kopperman
Editorial Assistant: Sheba Jalaluddin
Director of Manufacturing and Production: Bruce Johnson
Managing Production Editor: Patrick Walsh
Production Liaison: Mary C. Treacy
Production Editor: Linda Begley, Rainbow Graphics
Manufacturing Manager: Ilene Sanford
Manufacturing Buyer: Pat Brown
Design Director: Cheryl Asherman
Senior Design Coordinator: Maria Guglielmo Walsh
Manager of Media Production: Amy Peltier
New Media Project Manager: Stephen Hartner
New Media Production: Jack Yensen, Synergy
Senior Marketing Manager: Nicole Benson
Marketing Coordinator: Janet Ryerson
Product Information Manager: Rachele Strober
Composition: Rainbow Graphics
Cover Printer: Phoenix Color
Printer/Binder: Von Hoffman Press

Pearson Education LTD.
Pearson Education Australia PTY, Limited
Pearson Education Singapore, Pte. Ltd
Pearson Education North Asia Ltd
Pearson Education Canada, Ltd.
Pearson Educación de Mexico, S.A. de C.V.
Pearson Education–Japan
Pearson Education Malaysia, Pte. Ltd
Pearson Education, Upper Saddle River

10 9 8 7 6 5 4 3
ISBN 0-13-028162-X

The end is just the beginning...

Student practical and vocational nurses from around the country told us that they start their chapter reading from the end of the chapter. So, to ensure students' success, in the classroom, on the NCLEX-PN exam, and in the workplace, we put dynamite preview/review materials in a three-page Chapter Review at the end of each chapter, right where students will benefit most from them!

Key Terms by Topic provides an overview for organizing study

Key Points provide a quick highlight of lifelong need-to-know items

MediaLink provides multimodal reinforcement for different learners

For Further Study provides references to related chapters to broaden understanding

Critical Thinking Care Map
prepares students step by step for much needed on-the-job critical thinking leading to clinical success. Includes:

- NCLEX-PN exam focus area
- Case Study
- Nursing Diagnosis
- Data Collection
- Reporting
- Nursing Care
- Documentation

NCLEX-PN Exam Preparation includes:

- Test-Taking Tip that provides a focused study hint to help promote NCLEX-PN success
- NCLEX-PN style questions that provide content preview/review, as well as invaluable practice for taking the test.

Student success is built-in from the start...

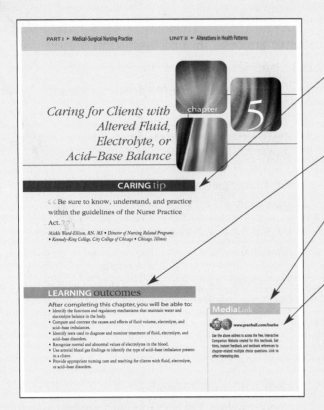

Caring Tip words of wisdom from dedicated practical and vocational nurse educators and practicing LPN's and LVN's from around the country support, encourage, and teach students to think and to behave as competent caring nurses.

Learning Outcomes identify key skills and concepts.

MediaLink calls student attention to two key complementary learning tools. These tools foster preview, review, reinforcement, and enrichment and can be used more than once, at multiple stages in the learning process.

CD-ROM with chapter-specific features, including:

- **Audio Glossary**
- "Test Your Thinking on Assessment and Interventions" critical thinking questions that relate to the Nursing Care discussions
- NCLEX-PN style multiple choice questions
- Case Studies that foster critical thinking skills

www.prenhall.com/burke, a free Website provides chapter-specific online resources for students and educators!

Objectives—presents the learning outcomes

Chapter Outline—provides the content outline for student reference

Audio Glossary—provides key terms, definitions, and correct pronunciations

NCLEX Review Style Questions—provides practice and immediate feedback for NCLEX-PN style questions

Case Study—provides a brief client scenario followed by critical thinking questions

Study Tip—provides helpful suggestions for learning challenging skills and concepts

Message Board—presents a question that stimulates nation-wide community discussion among students and instructors

Web Links—presents hyperlinks

Faculty Office—provides lecture notes for your convenience

Syllabus Manager—allows faculty and students the convenience of creating and easily updating an electronic syllabus

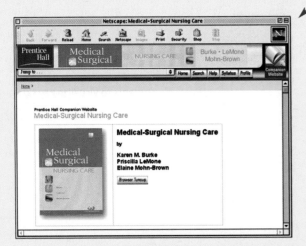

Need-to-know concepts and skills are readily accessible and easily memorable...

BOX 5-8
TEACHING FOR DISCHARGE

TEACHING CLIENTS ABOUT A LOW-SODIUM DIET

- The body needs less than 1 teaspoon (about 500 mg) of salt per day. About one third of sodium intake comes from adding salt during cooking and at the table; one fourth to one third comes from processed foods; and the rest comes from food and fluids naturally high in sodium.
- In place of salt or salt substitutes, use herbs, spices, lemon juice, vinegar, and wine as flavoring when cooking. The taste for salt will eventually diminish.
- Use salt substitutes sparingly; they often taste bitter instead of salty in large amounts.
- Low-sodium salt substitutes may contain half the sodium of regular salt.
- Read labels. Salt, monosodium glutamate, baking soda, and baking powder contain significant amounts of sodium. Processed foods list the sodium content. Some nonprescription drugs (such as laxatives and antacids) co...

BOX 5-1
population FOCUS

Fluid Volume Deficit in Older Adults

The older adult is at risk for fluid volume deficit from a variety of factors:

- Decreased thirst perception
- Decreased total body water
- Age-related changes renal function and the ability to regulate body temperature
- Self-limiting of fluids due to fear of incontinence
- Self-care deficits or disabilities that limit access to fluids
- Cognitive impairments (confusion, dementia, depression)
- Medications such as diuretics, sedatives

BOX 5-12
NURSING CARE CHECKLIST

INTERPRETING ARTERIAL BLOOD GASES

1. Look at the pH.
   - ☐ pH < 7.35 = acidosis
   - ☐ pH > 7.45 = alkalosis
2. Look at the $PaCO_2$.
   - ☐ $PaCO_2$ < 35 mm Hg = hypocapnia; more carbon dioxide is being exhaled than normal.
   - ☐ $PaCO_2$ > 45 mm Hg = hypercapnia; carbon dioxide is being retained.
3. Evaluate the pH–$PaCO_2$ relationship for a possible respiratory problem.
   - ☐ If the pH is < 7.35 (acidosis) and the $PaCO_2$ is > 45 mm Hg (hypercapnia), retained carbon dioxide is causing *respiratory acidosis*.
   - ☐ If the pH is > 7.45 (alkalosis) and the $PaCO_2$ is < 35 mm Hg (hypocapnia), low carbon dioxide levels are causing *respiratory alkalosis*.
4. Look at the bicarbonate.
   - ☐ If the HCO_3^- is < 22 mEq/L, bicarbonate levels are lower than normal.
   - ☐ If the HCO_3^- is > 26 mEq/L, bicarbonate levels are higher than normal.
5. Evaluate the pH, HCO_3^-, and base excess (BE) for a possible metabolic problem.
   - ☐ If the pH is < 7.35 (acidosis), the HCO_3^- is < 22 mEq/L, and the BE is < −3 mEq/L, low bicarbonate levels are causing *metabolic acidosis*.
   - ☐ If the pH is > 7.45 (alkalosis), the HCO_3^- is > 26 mEq/L, and the BE is > +3 mEq/L, high bicarbonate levels are causing *metabolic alkalosis*.
6. Look for compensation.
   - *Renal compensation:*
     - ☐ In respiratory acidosis (pH < 7.35, $PaCO_2$ > 45 mm Hg), the kidneys retain HCO_3^- to buffer the excess acid, so the HCO_3^- is > 26 mEq/L.
     - ☐ In respiratory alkalosis (pH > 7.45, $PaCO_2$ < 35 mm Hg), the kidneys excrete HCO_3^- to minimize the alkalosis, so the HCO_3^- is < 22 mEq/L.
   - *Respiratory compensation:*
     - ☐ In metabolic acidosis (pH < 7.35, HCO_3^- < 22 mEq/L), the rate and depth of respirations increase, increasing carbon dioxide elimination, so the $PaCO_2$ is < 35 mm Hg.
     - ☐ In metabolic alkalosis (pH > 7.45, HCO_3^- > 26 mEq/L), respirations slow, and carbon dioxide is retained, so the $PaCO_2$ is > 45 mm Hg.

BOX 5-4
ASSESSING FOR DISCHARGE

FLUID VOLUME IMBALANCE
Client

- Self-care: Ability to perform activities of daily living (ADLs), access fluids
- Knowledge:
  - Risks for fluid deficit (e.g., vomiting, diarrhea, strenuous exercise during ho... apy, chronic diseases like dia... tive measures; early manifest...
  - Risks for fluid excess (e.g., h... failure; medications); preven... manifestations; low-sodium...
- Home environment: Appropria... access to clean water and other...

Family

- Availability and knowledge of... ADLs, monitor fluid intake, as... restrictions as ordered

Community

- Resources for aged, debilitated...
- Access to health care resources

BOX 5-7
ASSESSING FOR FLUID VOLUME EXCESS

SUBJECTIVE DATA

- Complaints of cough, shortness of breath, difficulty sleeping or breathing when lying down
- Recent changes in fluid intake, output, or weight
- Risk factors such as renal failure, heart failure, cirrhosis of the liver, or an endocrine disorder; medications such as corticosteroid drugs (e.g., prednisone), nonsteroidal anti-inflammatory drugs (NSAIDs)

OBJECTIVE DATA

- Vital signs, peripheral pulses, and weight
- Mental status, level of consciousness
- Presence of peripheral or facial edema; color and moisture of skin and mucous membranes
- Observe for distended jugular or distal veins
- Auscultate breath sounds for crackles, wheezes; heart sounds for S_3 (heard immediately after S_2) and/or S_4 (heard immediately before S_1)

Client Teaching boxes (identifiable in orange) help students to prepare for and practice client instruction

Nursing Care and Procedure Checklist boxes, with sample documentation, (identifiable in blue) provide students with a ready-reference summary of important nursing interventions

Nutrition and Population Focus boxes (identifiable in green) help students to meet the age-specific and other special needs of different groups of clients

Assessment boxes (identifiable in red) help students to see what type of data to collect during assessment and assist students in planning the client's discharge needs

Full-color Visuals enable students to visualize key skills and concepts

Pharmacology tables highlight the nursing implications and client teaching for primary drugs and drug groups

Figure 5-12. ❖ Metabolic acid–base imbalances. (A) Metabolic acidosis. (B) Metabolic alkalosis.

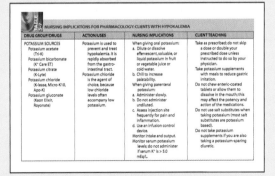

	NURSING IMPLICATIONS FOR PHARMACOLOGY: CLIENTS WITH HYPOKALEMIA			
DRUG GROUP/DRUGS	**ACTION/USES**	**NURSING IMPLICATIONS**	**CLIENT TEACHING**
POTASSIUM SOURCES Potassium acetate (Tri-K) Potassium bicarbonate (K+ Care ET) Potassium citrate (K-Lyte) Potassium chloride (K-lease, Micro-K10, Apo-K) Potassium gluconate (Kaon Elixir, Royonate)	Potassium is used to prevent and treat hypokalemia. It is rapidly absorbed from the gastrointestinal tract. Potassium chloride is the agent of choice, because low chloride levels often accompany low potassium.	When giving oral potassium: a. Dilute or dissolve effervescent, soluble, or liquid potassium in fruit or vegetable juice or cold water. b. Chill to increase palatability. When giving parenteral potassium: a. Administer slowly. b. Do not administer undiluted. c. Assess injection site frequently for pain and inflammation. d. Use an infusion control device. Monitor intake and output. Monitor serum potassium levels; do not administer if serum K+ is > 5.0 mEq/L.	Take as prescribed; do not skip a dose or double your prescribed dose unless instructed to do so by your physician. Take potassium supplements with meals to reduce gastric irritation. Do not chew enteric-coated tablets or allow them to dissolve in the mouth; this may affect the potency and action of the medications. Do not use salt substitutes when taking potassium (most salt substitutes are potassium based). Do not take potassium supplements if you are also taking a potassium-sparing diuretic.

Students learn to deliver safe, effective nursing care as team members in different care environments...

NURSING CARE

ASSESSING

Nursing care focuses on early identification and reporting of abnormal serum potassium levels and monitoring cardiac status. Ask about potassium-wasting diuretics (such as loop and thiazide diuretics; see Table 5-4) and other drugs associated with potassium loss (e.g., corticosteroids). Question the client about compliance with prescribed potassium supplements and dietary intake of foods and fluids.

DIAGNOSING, PLANNING, AND IMPLEMENTING

RISK FOR INJURY

- Carefully monitor serum potassium levels in clients at risk for imbalances, and not... abnormal levels (< 3.5 ... cation of a potassium imba... reduces the risk for injury levels.
- Monitor for manifestati... muscle weakness, naus... ing, or decreased bowel... tions of potassium imbala... or aspiration of vomitus.
- Closely monitor clients... sodium polystyrene sulf... excess. *Increased sodium ...*
- Closely monitor the EC... conate, particularly if t... *Digitalis toxicity may de... talis are given concurrentl...*

DECREASED CAR...

- Monitor vital signs, inc... report any irregularities... *easily detected by listening... peripheral pulses.*
- Place on a cardiac moni... rhythm or pattern (e.g... ment and T wave chan... (See Chapter 22 for mo...

Notify the physician of changes. *A monitor allows early iden-tification and intervention for life-threatening dysrhythmias.*
- Monitor clients taking digitalis for signs of digitalis toxic-ity (see Chapter 22). *Hypokalemia increases the risk for dig-italis toxicity.*
- Monitor intravenous potassium infusions closely. Dilute intravenous potassium as recommended, and administer using an electronic infusion device. *A rate above 40 mEq of potassium per hour is not safe.*

CLINICAL alert

Do not administer undiluted potassium directly into the vein. Potassium usually is mixed to a concentration of 20 to 40 mEq/L of solution and should not exceed 60 mEq/L. The rate of infusion should not exceed 20 to 40 mEq of potassium per hour. Evaluate the serum potassium level during therapy. In clients requiring rapid potassium replacement, monitor the ECG. Too rapid administration of intravenous potassium may cause cardiac dysrhythmias and death.

- Promote comfort by slowing the intravenous infusion rate or applying an ice pack to the IV site if necessary. *Potassium may cause local irritation to the vein wall.*

EVALUATING

Collect data related to the client's serum potassium level, safety, and cardiovascular status to evaluate the effectiveness of nursing interventions for clients with potassium imbalances.

Discharge Considerations

Discharge planning for clients with potassium imbalances focuses on teaching about prescribed medications (potassium supplements or diuretics), diet, and the importance of regular follow-up assessments. Include the family, a significant other, or a caregiver in teaching as indicated. Provide both written and verbal instructions. Provide a list of salt substitutes and foods high in potassium, with instructions for their use (see Box 5-9). Instruct clients taking supplemental forms of potas-sium and potassium-sparing diuretics to avoid salt substitutes that contain potassium. Instruct clients with chronic renal failure to avoid foods high in potassium. Discuss measures to make potassium supplements more palatable: Dilute liquid potassium supplements with water or juices, or mix with sher-bet or gelatin. Emphasize the importance of regular laboratory tests as ordered by the physician. Teach the client taking digi-talis to count the pulse before taking the medication. Report a rate of less than 60 to the primary health care provider.

Nursing Process Case Study
■ CLIENT WITH HYPOKALEMIA

Rose Ortiz is a 72-year-old woman who is being treated for mild heart failure with digoxin (Lanoxin) 0.125 mg, hydrochlorothiazide (Oretic) 75 mg orally (PO) daily and a mildly sodium-restricted diet (2 g daily). For the last several weeks, Ms. Ortiz has been feeling weak and sometimes faint, light-headed, and dizzy. Her physician ordered serum elec-trolytes drawn, which showed a potassium level of 2.4 mEq/L. Potassium chloride solution (Kaochlor, 20 mEq/15 mL) PO twice daily is prescribed, and the clinic nurse does a nursing assessment prior to teaching Ms. Ortiz about her care.

Assessment Ms. Ortiz has adhered to her sodium-restricted diet and has been taking her prescribed medications. She occa-sionally takes an additional "water pill" when her ankles swell. She says she is reluctant to take the potassium the doctor has ordered because her neighbor says it causes "heartburn." Physical assessment findings include T 98.4, P 70, R 20, and BP 138/84.

Diagnosis The following nursing diagnosis is identified for Ms Ortiz:
- *Risk for Ineffective Health Maintenance* related to lack of knowledge of side effects of diuretic therapy and of foods high in potassium

Expected Outcomes The expected outcomes specify that Ms. Ortiz will:
- Have a potassium level within normal limits (3.5 to 5.0 mEq/L).
- Verbalize understanding of the side effects of diuretic ther-apy.
- State measures to avoid gastrointestinal irritation when taking oral potassium.
- Identify potassium-rich foods.

Planning and Implementation The following nursing inter-ventions are planned and implemented:
- Discuss the side effects of diuretic therapy, and explain how taking additional diuretics may have contributed to her hypokalemia.
- Explain the need for the prescribed potassium and its role in reversing her muscle weakness.
- Instruct her to take the potassium supplement after breakfast and supper, diluted in 4 oz of juice or water, and sipped slowly over a 5- to 10-minute period. Instruct her to call if gastric irritation occurs.
- Discuss dietary sources of potassium, and provide a list of potassium-rich foods (see Box 5-9).

Evaluation On a follow-up visit 1 week later, Ms. Ortiz says

Critical Thinking in the Nursing Process

1. What did Ms. Ortiz do that contributed to her hypokalemia?
2. What additional teaching at the time that digitalis and hydrochlorothiazide were prescribed might have prevented Ms. Ortiz from developing hypokalemia? How could the nurse reinforce this teaching?

Collaborative Care

The *total serum calcium* will be less than 8.5 mg/d, and ionized calcium (the active form) generally is about 50% of that. *Serum magnesium* is measured because hypocalcemia is often associ-ated with hypomagnesemia. *Serum phosphate* is measured because there is a relationship between phosphorus and cal-cium levels (i.e., the serum level of one often rises as the other falls, and vice versa). *Parathyroid hormone (PTH)* is measured to

---

Nursing Care related to diseases and disorders is presented in the five-step nursing process format, applicable to the practical/vocational nurse's scope of practice. Nursing interventions are supported by rationales.

Case Studies that conclude the discussion of many major disorders bring the disorder into "real life." The case studies in this text emphasize the holistic aspects of nursing care.

Clinical Alerts call attention to clinical roles and responsibilities for heightened awareness, monitoring, and/or reporting.

Discharge Considerations focus student attention on their role to provide family and client teaching for helping clients achieve and maintain health promotion and wellness subsequent to discharge.

Critical Thinking Questions that conclude each case study allow students to apply their newfound learning.

Collaborative Care encourages students to recognize themselves as key members of a health care team.

Cultural Care Strategies prepare students to deliver more culturally sensitive adult nursing care...

Cultural Care STRATEGIES

Responding to Pain as a Cross-Cultural Variable

Mr. Chu, a 48-year old Chinese client, refused pain medication following surgery. When asked by the nurse about whether he needed pain medication, he said his discomfort was bearable and he could survive without any medication. Later, the nurse noticed he was restless and perspiring. Again, the nurse offered pain medication. Again, he refused, saying her responsibilities were far more important than his discomfort and he did not want to impose. The nurse knew that many Chinese are taught self-restraint and that some Chinese view the needs of the group as more important than individual needs. She also knew that some Chinese individuals have been taught it is polite to say no the first time an offer is extended. The nurse said, "Mr. Chu, it will help you recover sooner if you are able to relax. I have time to get it for you and would like to do that. If I bring you some medication, will you take it?" Mr. Chu smiled, look relieved, and said, "Yes, you are very kind."

Pain is a universal experience of human existence, but it is not a concrete entity. McCaffery and Thorpe (1988) stated: "Pain is whatever the experiencing person says it is, existing whenever the experiencing person says it does." Today, this phrase is often quoted when holistic pain management is discussed.

Holistic pain management involves consideration of the physical, emotional, social, and spiritual components of pain. It also includes consideration of the client in the context of family, culture, past experiences, and the meaning of the event being experienced (Davidhizar, Shearer, & Giger, 1997). Culture shapes beliefs and behaviors related to pain and influences the way pain is expressed.

Affective Response to Pain

Cultural responses to pain have been divided into two categories: stoic and emotive. Stoic clients are those who tend to "grin and bear it." Emotive people are more likely to verbalize their feelings of pain. A child raised in a Jewish home may react to a physical injury stoically, saying, "It does not hurt much," while a child raised in a Hispanic home may react to the same injury very demonstratively.

Communication of Pain

Words used to describe symptoms differ among cultures. A nurse may understand what is said by a client from the same cultural background, but have less understanding of a client from another culture who uses different terms, is less fluent in English, or speaks another language.

Nonverbal communication also differs among cultures. A client may feel that he or she is communicating the level of pain nonverbally and does not need to describe it. However, the nurse may not recognize culturally unique communications of pain (Giger & Davidhizar, 1999).

Biological Variations and Cultural Reaction to Pain

People within cultural groups may differ biologically in their reaction to pain and to pain medication. For example, when white clients and Chinese clients were compared for reactions to morphine, white clients reported less pain but greater incidence of drug-induced gastrointestinal effects (Levy, 1993).

Nursing Implications

- **Assess individuals in pain from a holistic and cultural perspective.** A "meaning-centered" approach must be used when assessing the client in pain. This approach includes an assessment not only of what the client is saying verbally and nonverbally, but also of personal meanings that pain may have for that person.
- **Avoid reacting judgmentally to the client who is demonstrative about pain.** When a client's reaction to pain appears excessive, the nurse should appreciate that the behavior may be customary in the client's culture and that any other behavior would be considered abnormal. The nurse should react with sensitivity and provide emotional support.
- **Provide appropriate care to promote health in a client who may have a stoic reaction to pain.** When the client is stoic, the nurse may need to be more directive in controlling pain. The nurse should assess for physiological symptoms of pain and tell the client why intervention will help recovery.
- **Recognize differences in responses to pain among health team members.** If team members are stoic themselves, they may be less responsive to complaints of pain by clients.

Self-Reflection Questions

1. What is your attitude toward pain—your own and others?
2. How do you think your family has shaped your attitude toward pain?
3. How do you react when you are around people who have different reactions to pain than yours?

Each strategy includes five key elements:

- **Introductory Scenario** humanizes the cultural considerations by providing a real-world nursing care situation
- **Discussion of the Cultural Phenomenon** provides students with an informational context
- **Nursing Implications** help students apply what they have learned to their scope of practice
- **Self-Reflection Questions** provide opportunities for students to get in touch with their own cultural beliefs and experiences
- **References**

Ten strategies are the focus:

1. Assessing Communication Variables from a Cultural Perspective
2. Appreciating Variations in Nonverbal Communication in Relating to the Client from Another Culture
3. Integrating Cultural Diversity in Client Education
4. Assessing the Client from Another Culture in a Social Context
5. Responding to Beliefs Related to Death, Dying, and Grief from a Cultural Perspective
6. Considering Cultural Variations Related to Time
7. Considering Cultural Variations Related to Space
8. Considering Cultural Variations Related to Environmental Control
9. Recognizing Biological Variations Between Cultures
10. Responding to Pain as a Cross-Cultural Variable

Preface

The need for nurses is greater than ever before. There are no short-term solutions to this problem: as currently practicing nurses age and retire, so does the population as a whole, further increasing the need for health care services. Today, more than ever before, we need you, the nursing student, to succeed in your studies. Today, more than ever before, we need you, the nursing student, to enter the nursing profession. Today, more than ever before, we need you, the nursing student, to see nursing as a career, not just a job.

This book is dedicated to your success as a student and as a practicing nurse. We believe a strong foundation in understanding the common diseases and disorders that affect adult clients is necessary to provide effective nursing care. We believe that understanding the basis for nursing care activities is vital to providing individualized care for clients. We believe that client teaching is a vital nursing role at all levels and in all settings. *Medical-Surgical Nursing Care* provides a strong foundation for caring through its emphasis on pathophysiology, nursing care, and client teaching.

Understanding comes not through memorization, but through practice and integration of new material into your thinking. *Medical-Surgical Nursing Care* promotes understanding in several ways. The writing style is clear, with a focus on readability. Its content is streamlined but thorough, focusing on what you ***need to know and to be able to do.***

Organization

Medical-Surgical Nursing Care is organized to promote learning. Part One, Medical-Surgical Nursing Practice, focuses on concepts, issues, and nursing care applicable to caring for adults in many different situations and settings. Parts Two through Seven focus on diseases and disorders affecting adults. These disorders are organized by functional health patterns (for example, nutritional–metabolic, activity–exercise) and by affected body systems under each functional health pattern (for example, common skin problems, bowel disorders, cardiac disorders).

Each chapter begins with a **Caring Tip** that provides words of wisdom from the lived experience of a practicing nursing or nurse educator. You will be able to use these tips as you move into and through your career in nursing. **Learning Outcomes** help focus and define your learning as you read and study the material.

The structure and function of the affected body system is reviewed at the beginning of the chapter. Disorders affecting that body system are presented in a consistent format: the disorder is defined; its **Pathophysiology,** signs and symptoms,

and complications are explained; and **Collaborative Care** (including diagnostic tests, pharmacology, surgery, and other treatments) for the disorder is outlined. **Nursing Care** related to the disorder is presented in a nursing process format. When a disorder is major, very complex, or very common, all of the **Nursing Process** steps are provided. When it is not, the text provides an abbreviated, more focused discussion, similar to the focused assessment nurses perform. Because teaching is a vital nursing role, discussion of each disorder concludes with **Discharge Considerations** and teaching for the client and family.

Case Studies following many major disorders bring the disorders to life. Clients rarely arrive in a health care setting as a pure medical diagnosis. As humans, clients bring all their roles and responsibilities as individuals, spouses, parents, children, workers, students, friends, and volunteers. They arrive as unique individuals influenced by their ethnicity, culture, and background. They arrive with psychosocial issues such as fear, guilt, or difficulty meeting financial responsibilities. They often arrive with other diseases and disorders complicating the current problem. The case studies in this text emphasize the holistic aspects of nursing care.

Critical Thinking Questions conclude each case study. These questions allow you to practice your new found learning and to expand your thinking beyond the immediate focus of the disease or disorder presented. Additional **Critical Thinking Self-Check Questions** are provided on the CD-ROM throughout nursing care chapters. They provide more case scenarios for you to use to test your knowledge and thinking skills. These self-check questions focus on the nursing roles of collecting assessment data and implementing nursing care. Each case is matched with hints to guide your critical thinking. They will help you learn to individualize your nursing care.

Each chapter concludes with features to reinforce and enhance your learning. **Key Terms by Topic** list the boldfaced key terms in the text by the topic under which they were defined. **Key Points** provide a summary of chapter content with reminders that you can use throughout your nursing career. **For Further Study** is a handy listing of cross-references within the chapter and the topics to which they apply. An interactive **Critical Thinking Care Map** provides a brief case study, assessment data, and a nursing diagnosis for a specific client. We then ask you, the student, to sort the data and sample interventions, evaluate the results, and chart your findings. Finally, **NCLEX-PN Review Questions** and a **Test-Taking Tip** help you review the chapter material and practice your test-taking skills.

Features

Throughout each chapter, you will find consistent features to facilitate and reinforce your learning.

- To avoid interrupting your reading by reaching for your medical dictionary, **Key Terms** are presented in boldface type. They are defined in the text and the glossary at the end of the book. Other important or unfamiliar terms are italicized and defined in the text.
- **Clinical Alerts** within the text emphasize information critical to providing effective, safe clinical nursing care.
- **Cultural Care Strategies,** including nursing implications and self-reflection questions, prepare students to deliver culturally sensitive adult nursing care.
- **Color-coded boxes** organize highlighted information for quick retrieval: red **Data Collection** boxes for manifestations and risk factors of a disorder; blue **Nursing Care** boxes for nursing care related to specific tests or procedures; orange boxes highlighting **Client Teaching;** and green boxes focusing on specific **Population Groups** and **Nutrition** information.
- **Nursing Care Checklists** quickly summarize nursing care activities for particular procedures or surgeries.
- **Procedure Checklists** review key steps in performing previously learned nursing care procedures and provide **Sample Documentation.**
- **Pharmacology Tables** highlight nursing implications and client teaching for drugs used to treat particular disorders.

Acknowledgments

A project such as *Medical-Surgical Nursing Care* would not come into being without the contributions of many people.

First of all, we thank you, our students, past, present, and future, from whom we learn so much. It is your quest for learning and your enthusiasm for the profession you have chosen that stimulates us, invigorates us, and always keeps us honest and humble. You are the future of our profession.

Many nursing professionals provided invaluable expertise and input into this book. Our contributors provided their knowledge, skills, and time to this project, writing selected chapters and features of this book. Reviewers provide quality assurance for the book. They validate content, attend to details,

and challenge our ways of thinking and expressing ourselves. Contributors and reviews for *Medical-Surgical Nursing Care* are listed with their current affiliations following this preface.

A project such as this one requires the support, skills, and expertise of many people. We especially want to thank Julie Alexander, our publisher, for having the vision to create a line of books specifically for you, the practical/vocational nursing student. We also owe a debt of gratitude to Nancy Anselment, who encouraged us to take on this project. Maura Connor, executive editor for nursing, has provided unflagging support as *Medical-Surgical Nursing Care* grew from an idea into the book you are holding.

Throughout its development, our champions have been Barbara Krawiec, our editor, and Rachel Bedard, our developmental editor. We thank Barbara for her vision and support of this book. She provided endless energy to research and develop the features and create a design that promotes your interest and learning. We thank Rachel for keeping us honest, keeping us on track, attending to details and consistency, and for forever encouraging us to stay with the vision: *What do you, the student, need to know and be able to do?*

Special thanks are also due to many others. Marilyn Meserve, managing editor, guided important aspects of the editorial process from behind the scenes. Yesenia Kopperman, assistant editor, coordinated the supplements. Michael Sirinides and Sheba Jalaluddin, editorial assistants, attended to many details throughout this project (most of which happen without our knowledge or attention). Mary Treacy, production editor, moved parts in all directions, problem-solved and monitored quality. Patrick Walsh, managing production editor, and Ilene Sanford and Pat Brown, manufacturing managers, guided the scheduling, production, and manufacturing process. Linda Begley and her good staff at Rainbow Graphics did copy editing and production. Cheryl Asherman, art director, and Maria Guglielmo Walsh created a visually clear and inviting format. Bridget McDermott, research analyst, brought to life the voices of educators and students. Sarah Hayday, Amy Peltier, and Steve Hartner made all the media components happen. Nicole Benson, marketing manager, Rachele Strober, and Janet Ryerson enthusiastically worked to convey the features and benefits of these materials. To all of you we are most grateful!

Karen M. Burke, RN, MS

Karen M. Burke is the Director of Health Occupations and the Nursing Program at Clatsop Community College in Astoria, Oregon. She obtained her initial nursing education at Emanuel Hospital School of Nursing in Portland, Oregon, later completing baccalaureate studies at Oregon Health & Sciences University, and a master's degree at University of Portland. Ms. Burke has extensive clinical nursing experience in acute care and community-based settings.

At Clatsop Community College since the inception of the Associate Degree Nursing program, Ms. Burke is known as a leader and an innovator. She led the nursing faculty in developing an online program to deliver nursing education to a distant rural community. Ms. Burke is actively involved in nursing education in Oregon. She is a member of the Oregon Council of Associate Degree Nursing Programs (OCAP) and is currently on the planning committee for the 2002 Oregon Health & Science University Nursing Education Institute. She has served on Board of Nursing task forces to develop guidelines for practical nursing practice related to intravenous fluid maintenance and medication administration, and to update administrative rules for nursing education. Ms. Burke has presented workshops on using interactive learning in the classroom.

Ms. Burke is co-author of several other nursing texts: *Medical Surgical Nursing: Critical Thinking in Client Care* (3rd ed.), with Priscilla LeMone; a clinical handbook to accompany the above text; and *Fundamentals of Nursing: Concepts, Process, and Practice* (6th ed.), with Barbara Kozier, Glenora Erb, and Audrey Berman.

Priscilla LeMone, RN, DSN, FAAN

Priscilla LeMone has spent most of her career as a nurse educator, teaching medical-surgical nursing and pathophysiology at all levels from diploma to doctoral students. She has a diploma in nursing from Deaconess College of Nursing (St. Louis, Missouri), baccalaureate and master's degrees from Southeast Missouri State University, and a doctorate in nursing from the University of Alabama-Birmingham. She is currently an Associate Professor and Director of Undergraduate Studies, Sinclair School of Nursing, University of Missouri-Columbia.

Dr. LeMone has had numerous awards for scholarship and teaching during her over 30 years as a nurse educator. She is most honored for receiving the Kemper Fellowship for Teaching Excellence from the University of Missouri-Columbia and the Unique Contribution Award from the North American Nursing Diagnosis Association, and for being selected as a Fellow in the American Academy of Nursing.

She believes that her education gave her solid and everlasting roots in nursing. Her work with students has given her the wings that allow her love of nursing and teaching to continue through the years.

A widow, Dr. LeMone lives with her dog and shares time with her two children and her granddaughter. When she has time, she enjoys growing flowers and reading fiction.

Elaine L. Mohn-Brown, RN, EdD

Elaine L. Mohn-Brown received her diploma in nursing from Akron General Medical Center School of Nursing in Akron, Ohio. She has baccalaureate and master's degrees in nursing and health education from Metropolitan State College and University of Northern Colorado, and an EdD in higher education administration from Brigham Young University. She has worked in critical care units in Ohio and Colorado.

Her first teaching position was as a practical nursing instructor at Larimer County Vocational-Technical Center in Colorado. For the past 23 years, she has been on the faculty of the ADN Program at Chemeketa Community College in Salem, Oregon. Through thought-provoking classroom presentations and hands-on acute care medical-surgical experiences, she has encouraged students to question and understand the rationale for their nursing care.

Dr. Mohn-Brown serves as a member of the Editorial Advisory Board for *Nurse Educator.* She has served on two Oregon State Board of Nursing task forces. She has published nationally and conducts workshops at the national level. Her love of nursing and teaching has taken her to numerous international and national conferences.

When not working, she and her husband, Gene, spend time traveling and she enjoys flower gardening.

Contributor Team

Chapter Contributors

Linda Eby, RN, MN
Instructor of Nursing
Portland Community College
Portland, Oregon

Roxanne W. McDaniel, PhD, RN
Associate Professor
Director of Graduate Studies/MS Program
Sinclair School of Nursing
University of Missouri-Columbia
Columbia, Missouri

Frances M. Warrick, MS, RN
Program Coordinator, Vocational Nursing
El Centro College
Dallas, Texas

Cultural Care Strategies

Ruth Davidhizar, RN, DNS, CS, FAAN
Professor and Dean of Nursing
Bethel College
Mishwaka, Indiana

Joyce Newman Giger, EdD, RN, CS, FAAN
Professor, Graduate Studies, School of Nursing
University of Alabama at Birmingham
Birmingham, Alabama

Student CD-Rom

Doris A. Clark , RN, BC, BSN
Instructor
Prince George's Community College
Largo, Maryland

Betty Kehl Richardson, PhD, APRN, BC, CNAA,
LPC, LMFT
Professor Emeritus
Austin Community College
Austin, Texas

CW:
www.prenhall.com/burke

Doris A. Clark, RN, BC, BSN
Instructor
Prince George's Community College
Largo, Maryland

Betty Kehl Richardson, PhD, APRN, BC, CNAA,
LPC, LMFT
Professor Emeritus
Austin Community College
Austin, Texas

Student Study Guide

Author

Deborah Stevenson, RN, BSN
Nursing Instructor
Midlands Technical College
Columbia, South Carolina

Contributors

Paige Fletcher, RN, MSN
Associate Professor
Austin Community College
Austin, Texas

Elizabeth P. Martin, RN, BSN
VN Nursing Instructor
El Centro College
Dallas, Texas

Stephanie Randall, RN
Vocational Nursing Coordinator
Extended Health Education
Arlington, Texas

Deborah Smith, RN, MS
VN Faculty
El Centro College
Dallas, Texas

##
Frances Warrick, MS, RN
Program Coordinator, Vocational Nursing
El Centro College
Dallas, Texas

Instructor Guide

Author

Doris A. Clark, RN, BC, BSN
Instructor
Prince George's Community College
Largo, Maryland

Instructor Test Bank

Author

Mary B. Sitterley, RN, MN, MEd
PN Program Faculty
North Seattle Community College
Seattle, Washington

Contributors

Jacqueline B. Arnett, RN, BSN, CPN
Associate Faculty
College of the Redwoods
Eureka, California

Ellen R. Hoist, MSN, RN
Director LPN Program
Bronx Community College
Bronx, New York

Patty Leary, MS, ED
Allied Health Instructor
MOCC
Big Rapids, Michigan

Kathleen Baker, RN, BSN
Coordinator Health Careers
Western Suffolk BOCES
Northport, NY

Rebecca Cappo, RN, MSN
Program Coordinator
Lenape AVTS PN Program
Ford City, PA

Linda Cater, RN, MSN
Division Chair for Health and Service Careers
Director of Continuing Education
Ayers State Technical College
Anniston, AL

Mary Eggert, RN, BSN, FNP
Adjunct Faculty
Waubonsee Community College
Aurora, IL

Susan Ferguson, APRN, MSN
Allied Health Director
Snow College South
Richfield, UT

Denise Fowler, RN, BSN, MSA
Practical Nursing Instructor
Augusta Technical Instructor
Thomson, GA

Anita A. Garman, RN, MSN
Assistant Director
Emanuel Turlock Vocational Nursing Program
Turlock, CA

Teresa Jo Grooms, RN, BSN
Nursing Instructor
Southern State Community College
Hillsboro, OH

Carol Healy, MS, RN, CS
Assistant Professor of Nursing
Union County College
Elizabeth, NJ

Marilyn K. Jones, BSN, RN
Southern State Community College
Hillsboro, OH

Renee Vellucci Jones, RN, C, MSN
Nursing Instructor/Assistant Director LVN Program
Los Reos Community College District
Sacramento, CA

Geneva Lamm, RN, MSN
Chairperson
Ivy Tech State College
Columbus, IN

Debbie Lannom, MSN, RN, BC
Nursing Instructor
Sacramento City College
Sacramento, CA

Patty K. Leary, MS, ED
Allied Health Instructor
MOCC
Big Rapids, MI

Shirley A. LeDane, RN, MA
Program Coordinator
Hanover Practical Nursing Program
Hanover, PA

Annitta Love, MSN, RN
Director of Practical Nursing
H. Council Trenholm State Technical College
Montgomery, AL

Marilyn J. Lynch, RN, MED, BSN
Assistant Instructor
Waukesha County Technical College
Pewaukee, WI

Victoria L. Meyers, RN, MSN
Nursing Faculty
Grand Rapids Community College
Grand Rapids, MI

Dorothy Linau Mirkil, RN
Adjunct Faculty
Lansing Community College
Lansing, MI

Diane Neville, RN, BS
Executive Director of Nursing
American Career College
Anaheim, CA

Dee Niedringhaus, RN
Director
Vocational Nursing Orange County Regional Occupational
Program
Anaheim, CA

Diane L. Okeson, RN, MN, ARNP-CNS
Dean of Nursing and Allied Health
Pratt Community College
Pratt, KS

Connie Price, RN
Clinical Instructor
Center for Technical Studies
Plymouth, PA

Mary R. Price, RN, MSN
Chair, Nursing Program
Vincennes University Jasper Campus
Jasper, IN

Pamela Primus, BSN, RN
H.E. Struckenhoff Department of Nursing
Casper College
Casper, WY

Roberta Ramont, RN, MS
Instructor
Vocational Nursing Orange County Regional Occupational
Program
Anaheim, CA

Betty Kehl Richardson, PhD, APRN, BC, CNAA, LPC, LMFT
Professor Emeritus
Austin Community College
Austin, Texas

Sharon Romain, RN, MSN
Professor of Nursing
Bessemer State College
Bessemer, AL

Sharron Rust, RN
VN Program Director
Clarendon College
Clarendon, TX

Joanna Scalabrini, MS, RNC
Nursing Dept. Chair
Westchester Community College
Valhalla, NY

Joan M. Scribner, RN, BSN
Affiliate Faculty
Metropolitan Community College
Independence, MO

Nettie Seale, RN
Instructor of Practical Nursing
Kiamichi Technology Center
Stigler, OK

Deborah L. Stevenson, RN, BSN
Nursing Instructor
Midlands Technical College
Columbia, SC

Stephanie Valdes, RN, BSN, MS
Associate Professor of Nursing
Black Hawk College
Moline, AL

Bonnie Watts, RN, MSN
Instructor
Minneapolis Community Tech College
Minneapolis, MN

Detailed Table of Contents

Part I Medical-Surgical Nursing Practice *1*

UNIT I ➤ Introduction to Medical-Surgical Nursing *1*

CHAPTER 1

The Medical-Surgical Nurse *1*
Roles of the Nurse in Medical-Surgical Practice *2*
Framework for Practice: The Nursing Process *3*
Process of Critical Thinking *7*
Guidelines for Nursing Practice *7*
CRITICAL THINKING CARE MAP: Introduction *8*
Legal and Ethical Dilemmas in Nursing *10*

CHAPTER 2

The Adult Client in Health and Illness *15*
The Adult Client *16*
The Family of the Adult Client *19*
Health in the Adult Client *22*
Illness in the Adult Client *23*
CRITICAL THINKING CARE MAP: Caring for a Client with Early-
    Onset Diabetes *28*
Cultural Care Strategies: Assessing Communication Variables
    from a Cultural Perspective *30*

CHAPTER 3

Community-Based and Home Care of the Adult Client *31*
Community-Based Nursing Care *32*
Types of Community-Based Health Care Services *32*
Home Health Care *33*
Rehabilitation *40*
CRITICAL THINKING CARE MAP: Caring for a Client with a
    Handicap *43*

CHAPTER 4

Guidelines for Health Assessment *45*
Purposes of a Health Assessment *46*
Types of Assessment *46*
Sources and Accuracy of Assessment Data *46*
Obtaining a Health History *47*
Methods of Physical Examination *48*
Preparation for a Physical Examination *49*
The Physical Examination *50*
Documentation *57*
CRITICAL THINKING CARE MAP: Caring for a Client with Risk for
    Excess Fluid Volume *60*

Cultural Care Strategies: Appreciating Variations in Facial
    Expression when Relating to the Client from Another
    Culture *62*

UNIT II ➤ Alterations in Health Patterns *63*

CHAPTER 5

Caring for Clients with Altered Fluid, Electrolyte, or Acid–Base Balance *63*
Fluid and Electrolyte Balance *64*
Structure and Function *64*
Fluid Volume Deficit *68*
Fluid Volume Excess *72*
NURSING PROCESS CASE STUDY: Client with Excess Fluid Volume *75*
Sodium Imbalance *76*
Potassium Imbalance *78*
NURSING PROCESS CASE STUDY: Client with Hypokalemia *81*
Calcium Imbalance *82*
Magnesium Imbalance *85*
Phosphorus Imbalance *87*
Acid–Base Disorders *88*
Acid–Base Regulation *88*
Types of Acid–Base Imbalances *89*
Metabolic Acidosis *91*
Metabolic Alkalosis *93*
Respiratory Acidosis *95*
Respiratory Alkalosis *96*
CRITICAL THINKING CARE MAP: Caring for a Client with Acute
    Respiratory Acidosis *99*

CHAPTER 6

Caring for Clients in Pain *101*
Pain—the "Fifth Vital Sign" *102*
  ■ Physiology of Pain *102*
  ■ Types of Pain *104*
  ■ Collaborative Care *107*
  ■ Nursing Care *112*
NURSING PROCESS CASE STUDY: Client with Pain *119*
CRITICAL THINKING CARE MAP: Caring for a Client with Pain *122*
Cultural Care Strategies: Responding to Pain as a Cross-Cultural
    Variable *124*

CHAPTER 7

Caring for Clients Having Surgery *125*
Preoperative Phase *126*
NURSING PROCESS CASE STUDY: Preoperative Care for Client
    Having Inpatient Surgery *135*
Intraoperative Phase *137*

Postoperative Phase *142*
Outpatient Surgery *148*
CRITICAL THINKING CARE MAP: Caring for a Client After
    Surgery *152*

CHAPTER 8

Caring for Clients with Cancer *155*
Cancer, the Nurse, and the Health Care Team *156*
Cancer Incidence and Trends *156*
Physiologic and Psychological Effects of Cancer *160*
NURSING PROCESS CASE STUDY: Client with Cancer *175*
Nursing Interventions for Oncologic Emergencies *177*
CRITICAL THINKING CARE MAP: Caring for a Client Undergoing
    Chemotherapy for Cancer *180*
Cultural Care Strategies: Responding to Beliefs Related to
    Death, Dying, and Grief from a Cultural Perspective *182*

CHAPTER 9

Loss, Grief, and End-of-Life Care *183*
Loss, Grief, and Death *184*
End-of-Life Considerations *186*
End-of-Life Care *188*
NURSING PROCESS CASE STUDY: Client Experiencing Loss *193*
CRITICAL THINKING CARE MAP: Caring for a Client Experiencing a
    Loss *197*

Part II Health Perception–Health Management Pattern *199*

UNIT III ➤ Altered Health Management *199*

CHAPTER 10

Caring for Clients Experiencing Shock, Trauma,
or Critical Illness *199*
The Client in Shock *200*
NURSING PROCESS CASE STUDY: Client with Septic Shock *209*
The Client Experiencing Trauma *210*
NURSING PROCESS CASE STUDY: Client with Multiple Injuries *214*
The Client Experiencing a Critical Illness *216*
CRITICAL THINKING CARE MAP: Care for a Client at an Accident
    Scene *219*

CHAPTER 11

Caring for the Client with Substance Abuse
or Dependency *221*
Problem of Substance Abuse *222*
Commonly Abused Substances *222*

NURSING PROCESS CASE STUDY: Client with Ineffective Individual
    Coping *232*
CRITICAL THINKING CARE MAP: Care for a Client with Substance
    Dependency *235*

UNIT IV ➤ Altered Immune System Responses *237*

CHAPTER 12

Caring for Clients with Inflammation
and Infection *237*
Inflammation *238*
Infection *244*
NURSING PROCESS CASE STUDY: Client with MRSA Infection *259*
CRITICAL THINKING CARE MAP: Caring for a Client Exposed to
    Staphylococcus aureus *262*
Cultural Care Strategies: Considering Cultural Variations Related
    to Environmental Control *264*

CHAPTER 13

Caring for Clients with Altered Immunity *265*
Overview of the Immune System *266*
Natural and Acquired Immunity *269*
Altered Immune Responses *273*
Autoimmune Disorder *276*
Organ/Tissue Transplant *277*
Impaired Immune Responses and the Client with HIV *281*
NURSING PROCESS CASE STUDY: Client with HIV Infection *292*
CRITICAL THINKING CARE MAP: Caring for a Client with
    Pneumocystis carinii Pneumonia *295*

Part III Nutritional–Metabolic Pattern *297*

UNIT V ➤ Altered Integumentary System Reponses *297*

CHAPTER 14

Caring for Clients with Skin Disorders *297*
Structure and Function of the Integumentary System *298*
Common Skin Disorders *301*
Infections and Infestations of the Skin *306*
Malignant Skin Disorders *311*
NURSING PROCESS CASE STUDY: Client with Melanoma *316*
Pressure Ulcers *317*
CRITICAL THINKING CARE MAP: Caring for a Client with Herpes
    Zoster *323*

CHAPTER 15

Caring for the Client with Burns *325*

Types of Burn Injury *326*
- Stages of Burn Injury Treatment *327*
- Pathophysiology of a Major Burn *328*
- Collaborative Care *330*
- Wound Management *331*
- Nursing Care *332*

NURSING PROCESS CASE STUDY: Client with a Major Burn *335*

CRITICAL THINKING CARE MAP: Caring for a Client with Major Burns *338*

Cultural Care Strategies: Assessing the Client from Another Culture in a Social Context *340*

UNIT VI ➤ Altered Endocrine Responses *341*

CHAPTER 16

Caring for Clients with Endocrine Disorders *341*

Structure and Function of the Endocrine System *342*

Disorders of the Pituitary Gland *344*

Disorders of the Anterior Pituitary Gland *344*

Disorders of the Posterior Pituitary Gland *344*

Disorders of the Thyroid Gland *346*

Hyperthyroidism *346*

NURSING PROCESS CASE STUDY: Client with Graves' Disease *350*

Hypothyroidism *351*

Cancer of the Thyroid *354*

Disorders of the Parathyroid Glands *354*

Hyperparathyroidism *354*

Hypoparathyroidism *355*

Disorders of the Adrenal Gland *356*

Cushing's Syndrome *356*

Addison's Disease *359*

Disorder of the Adrenal Medulla *361*

CRITICAL THINKING CARE MAP: Caring for a Client with Hypothyroidism *363*

CHAPTER 17

Caring for Clients with Diabetes Mellitus *365*

Structure and Function of the Pancreas *366*

Overview of Diabetes Mellitus *366*

NURSING PROCESS CASE STUDY: Client with Type 1 DM *387*

CRITICAL THINKING CARE MAP: Caring for a Client with Diabetes Mellitus *391*

UNIT VII ➤ Altered Nutritional Responses *393*

CHAPTER 18

Caring for Clients with Nutritional and Upper GI Disorders *393*

Structure and Function of the Upper Gastrointestinal Tract *394*

Nutritional Disorders *396*

Obesity *396*

Undernutrition *400*

Upper GI Disorders *404*

Disorders of the Mouth *404*

Disorders of the Esophagus *406*

Disorders of the Stomach and Upper Intestinal Tract *407*

Peptic Ulcer Disease *412*

NURSING PROCESS CASE STUDY: Client with Peptic Ulcer Disease *418*

Cancer of the Stomach *418*

CRITICAL THINKING CARE MAP: Caring for a Client with Altered Nutrition *422*

Cultural Care Strategies: Integrating Cultural Diversity in Client Education *424*

CHAPTER 19

Caring for Clients with Gallbladder, Liver, and Pancreatic Disorders *425*

Structure and Function of the Accessory Digestive Organs *426*

Gallbladder Disorders *427*

Cholelithiasis and Cholecystitis *427*

NURSING PROCESS CASE STUDY: Client with Cholelithiasis *430*

Liver Disorders *431*

Hepatitis *431*

Cirrhosis *436*

NURSING PROCESS CASE STUDY: Client with Alcoholic Cirrhosis *442*

Cancer of the Liver *443*

Liver Trauma *443*

Exocrine Pancreatic Disorders *444*

Pancreatitis *444*

Pancreatic Cancer *447*

CRITICAL THINKING CARE MAP: Caring for a Client with Pancreatitis *450*

Part IV Elimination Patterns *453*

UNIT VIII ➤ Altered Elimination Responses *453*

CHAPTER 20

Caring for Clients with Bowel Disorders *453*
Structure and Function of the Intestines *454*
Disorders of Intestinal Motility and of Absorption *455*
Diarrhea *455*
Constipation *458*
Irritable Bowel Syndrome *462*
Fecal Incontinence *463*
Malabsorption *464*
Inflammatory and Infectious Disorders *464*
Appendicitis *465*
Peritonitis *466*
NURSING PROCESS CASE STUDY: Client with a Perforated
    Appendix *469*
Gastroenteritis *469*
Inflammatory Bowel Disease *471*
NURSING PROCESS CASE STUDY: Client with Ulcerative Colitis *477*
Structural and Obstructive Disorders *477*
Colorectal Cancer *477*
Bowel Obstruction *482*
Hernia *484*
Diverticular Disease *485*
Anorectal Disorders *486*
Hemorrhoids *486*
Anorectal Lesions *487*
CRITICAL THINKING CARE MAP: Caring for a Client with Colorectal
    Cancer *490*

CHAPTER 21

Caring for Clients with Renal and Urinary Tract
Disorders *493*
Structure and Function of the Urinary System *494*
Voiding Disorders *497*
Urinary Retention *497*
Urinary Incontinence *498*
Infectious and Inflammatory Disorders *502*
Urinary Tract Infection *502*
Glomerulonephritis *507*
NURSING PROCESS CASE STUDY: Client with Acute
    Glomerulonephritis *511*
Nephrotic Syndrome *511*
Obstructive Disorders *512*
Urinary Calculi *512*

Hydronephrosis *515*
Polycystic Kidney Disease *516*
Kidney Trauma *517*
Tumors of the Kidney and Urinary Tract *517*
Bladder Cancer *517*
NURSING PROCESS CASE STUDY: Client with Bladder Cancer *520*
Kidney Tumors *521*
Renal Failure *522*
Acute Renal Failure *522*
Chronic Renal Failure *523*
NURSING PROCESS CASE STUDY: Client with Chronic Renal
    Failure *531*
CRITICAL THINKING CARE MAP: Caring for a Client with Urinary
    Incontinence *534*
Cultural Care Strategies: Considering Cultural Variations Related
    to Time *536*

Part V Activity–Exercise Pattern *537*

UNIT IX ➤ Altered Cardiovascular System Responses *537*

CHAPTER 22

Caring for Clients with Cardiac Disorders *537*
Structure and Function of the Heart *538*
Cardiac Rhythm Disorders *542*
Cardiac Dysrhythmias *542*
Sudden Cardiac Death *551*
Coronary Heart Disease *553*
Atherosclerosis *553*
Angina Pectoris *555*
Acute Myocardial Infarction *562*
NURSING PROCESS CASE STUDY: Client with Acute Myocardial
    Infarction *569*
Disorders of Cardiac Function *570*
Heart Failure *570*
NURSING PROCESS CASE STUDY: Client with Heart Failure *577*
Cardiomyopathy *578*
Inflammatory Cardiac Disorders *580*
Rheumatic Fever and Rheumatic Heart Disease *580*
Infective Endocarditis *581*
Myocarditis *583*
Pericarditis *584*
Disorders of Cardiac Structure *586*
Valvular Heart Disease *586*
CRITICAL THINKING CARE MAP: Caring for a Client after Coronary
    Artery Bypass Surgery *593*

CHAPTER 23

Caring for Clients with Peripheral Vascular Disorders *595*

Structure and Function of the Peripheral Vascular System *596*

Hypertension *597*

NURSING PROCESS CASE STUDY: Client with Hypertension *603*

Arterial Disorders *604*

Peripheral Arteriosclerosis *604*

Arterial Thrombus or Embolism *605*

Buerger's Disease *605*

Raynaud's Phenomenon *605*

Older Adults and PVD *608*

Aneurysm *608*

Venous Disorders *612*

Venous Thrombosis *612*

Venous Insufficiency *613*

NURSING PROCESS CASE STUDY: Client with Deep Vein Thrombosis *617*

Varicose Veins *618*

CRITICAL THINKING CARE MAP: Caring for a Client with Buerger's Disease *621*

CHAPTER 24

Caring for Clients with Hematologic and Lymphatic Disorders *623*

Red Blood Cell Disorders *624*

Anemia *624*

NURSING PROCESS CASE STUDY: Client with Folic Acid Deficiency Anemia *633*

Polycythemia *634*

Platelet and Coagulation Disorders *635*

Hemostasis *635*

Thrombocytopenia *635*

Disseminated Intravascular Coagulopathy *636*

Hemophilia *637*

White Blood Cell Disorders *639*

Agranulocytosis *639*

Leukemia *640*

Multiple Myeloma *645*

Lymphatic System Disorders *647*

Lymphangitis and Lymphedema *647*

Infectious Mononucleosis *648*

Malignant Lymphoma *648*

NURSING PROCESS CASE STUDY: Client with Hodgkin's Disease *650*

CRITICAL THINKING CARE MAP: Caring for a Client with Acute Myelocytic Leukemia *653*

UNIT X ➤ Altered Respiratory System Responses *655*

CHAPTER 25

Caring for Clients with Upper Respiratory Disorders *655*

Structure and Function of the Upper Respiratory System *656*

Upper Respiratory Infections and Inflammations *656*

NURSING PROCESS CASE STUDY: Client with Upper Respiratory Infection *663*

Upper Respiratory Trauma or Obstruction *664*

Epistaxis *664*

Nasal Trauma or Deviated Septum *665*

Laryngeal Obstruction or Trauma *667*

Sleep Apnea *668*

Upper Respiratory Tumors *668*

Benign Laryngeal Tumors *668*

Laryngeal Cancer *669*

CRITICAL THINKING CARE MAP: Caring for a Client with Total Laryngectomy *677*

CHAPTER 26

Caring for Clients with Lower Respiratory Disorders *679*

Structure and Function of the Lower Respiratory System *680*

Infectious and Inflammatory Disorders *682*

Acute Bronchitis *682*

Pneumonia *683*

Pleuritis *689*

Pleural Effusion *689*

Lung Abscess and Empyema *689*

Tuberculosis *690*

Obstructive Airway Disorders *696*

Asthma *696*

Chronic Obstructive Pulmonary Disease *700*

NURSING PROCESS CASE STUDY: Client with COPD *704*

Cystic Fibrosis *705*

Atelectasis *705*

Bronchiectasis *706*

Interstitial Lung Disorders *706*

Occupational Lung Disease *706*

Sarcoidosis *707*

Lung Cancer *707*

NURSING PROCESS CASE STUDY: Client with Lung Cancer *712*

Pulmonary Vascular Disorders *712*

Pulmonary Embolism *713*

Pulmonary Hypertension *715*

Pneumothorax and Hemothorax *715*
Pneumothorax *715*
Hemothorax *718*
Chest and Lung Trauma *719*
Rib Fracture *719*
Pulmonary Contusion *719*
Smoke Inhalation *719*
Near-Drowning *719*
Respiratory Failure *721*
Acute Respiratory Distress Syndrome *722*
CRITICAL THINKING CARE MAP: Caring for a Client with
    Tuberculosis *729*

UNIT XI ➤ Altered Musculoskeletal System Responses *731*

CHAPTER 27

Caring for Clients with Musculoskeletal Trauma *731*

Structure and Function of the Musculoskeletal System *732*
Musculoskeletal Trauma *733*
Soft Tissue Trauma *734*
Fractures *735*
Hip Fracture *744*
NURSING PROCESS CASE STUDY: Client with Hip Fracture *746*
Joint Dislocation or Subluxation *747*
Repetitive Use Injuries *747*
Amputation *748*
CRITICAL THINKING CARE MAP: Caring for a Client with Below-
    Knee Amputation *754*
Cultural Care Strategies: Considering Cultural Variations Related
    to Space *756*

CHAPTER 28

Caring for Clients with Musculoskeletal Disorders *757*

Structural and Bone Disorders *758*
Scoliosis and Kyphosis *758*
Osteoporosis *759*
NURSING PROCESS CASE STUDY: Client with Osteoporosis *762*
Osteomalacia and Paget's Disease *763*
Osteomyelitis *764*
Bone Tumors *766*
Common Foot Disorders *768*
Joint and Connective Tissue Disorders *769*
Osteoarthritis *769*
Rheumatoid Arthritis *772*

NURSING PROCESS CASE STUDY: Client with Rheumatoid
    Arthritis *777*
Systemic Lupus Erythematosus *778*
Gout *780*
Lyme Disease *783*
Ankylosing Spondylitis *783*
Fibromyalgia *784*
Low Back Pain *784*
Muscular Dystrophy *785*
CRITICAL THINKING CARE MAP: Caring for a Client with
    Osteoarthritis and Total Hip Replacement *787*

Part VI Cognitive–Perceptual Pattern *789*

UNIT XII ➤ Altered Neurologic System Responses *789*

CHAPTER 29

Caring for Clients with Intracranial Disorders *789*

Structure and Function of the Nervous System *790*
Altered Intracranial Function *794*
NURSING PROCESS CASE STUDY: Client with Increased
    Intracranial Pressure and Altered Level of
    Consciousness *801*
Brain Tumor *802*
Cerebrovascular Accident *805*
Aneurysm *812*
Seizure Disorder *813*
Intracranial Infections *817*
Headaches *820*
CRITICAL THINKING CARE MAP: Caring for the Client with a
    Cerebrovascular Accident *824*

CHAPTER 30

Caring for Clients with Degenerative Neurologic and Spinal Cord Disorders *827*

Degenerative Neurologic Disorders *828*
Alzheimer's Disease *828*
NURSING PROCESS CASE STUDY: Client with Alzheimer's
    Disease *831*
Multiple Sclerosis *832*
Parkinson's Disease *834*
Myasthenia Gravis *837*
Huntington's Disease *838*
Amyotrophic Lateral Sclerosis *839*
Guillain–Barré Syndrome *839*
Trigeminal Neuralgia *840*
Bell's Palsy *840*

Rabies *841*

Tetanus *841*

Creutzfeldt–Jakob Disease *841*

Spinal Cord Disorders *842*

Spinal Cord Injury *842*

Herniated Intervertebral Disk *847*

Spinal Cord Tumor *850*

CRITICAL THINKING CARE MAP: Caring for the Client with Herniated Intervertebral Disk *852*

UNIT XIII ➤ Altered Sensory Responses *855*

CHAPTER 31

Caring for Clients with Eye and Ear Disorders *855*

Eye Structure, Function, and Disorders *856*

Infectious or Inflammatory Eye Disorders *858*

Eye Trauma *860*

Refractive Errors *862*

Cataracts *863*

Glaucoma *864*

NURSING PROCESS CASE STUDY: Client with Glaucoma and Cataracts *869*

Detached Retina *869*

Macular Degeneration *870*

Diabetic Retinopathy *871*

Enucleation *871*

Blindness *871*

Ear Structure, Function, and Disorders *872*

External Otitis *873*

Impacted Cerumen and Foreign Bodies *874*

Otitis Media *874*

Otosclerosis *876*

Inner Ear Disorders *877*

Hearing Loss *878*

CRITICAL THINKING CARE MAP: Caring for a Client with Age-Related Hearing Loss *883*

Part VII Sexuality–Reproductive Pattern *885*

UNIT XIV ➤ Altered Reproductive System Responses *885*

CHAPTER 32

Caring for Male Clients with Reproductive System Disorders *885*

Structure and Function of the Male Reproductive System *886*

Prostate Disorders *887*

Benign Prostatic Hyperplasia *887*

Prostatitis *889*

Cancer of the Prostate *890*

Disorders of the Testes and Scrotum *895*

Structural and Inflammatory Disorders *895*

Infertility *895*

Scrotal Masses and Trauma *896*

Testicular Cancer *897*

Disorders of the Penis *898*

Phimosis *898*

Priapism *899*

Cancer of the Penis *899*

Erectile Dysfunction *899*

NURSING PROCESS CASE STUDY: Client with Erectile Dysfunction *901*

Ejaculatory Dysfunction *902*

CRITICAL THINKING CARE MAP: Caring for a Client with Prostate Cancer *904*

CHAPTER 33

Caring for Female Clients with Reproductive System Disorders *907*

Structure and Function of the Female Reproductive System *908*

Breast Disorders *910*

Fibrocystic Breast Changes *910*

Mastitis *911*

Disorders Associated with Breast Augmentation *911*

Breast Cancer *911*

NURSING PROCESS CASE STUDY: Client with Breast Cancer *919*

Disorders of Menstruation *921*

Premenstrual Syndrome *921*

Dysmenorrhea *923*

Dysfunctional Uterine Bleeding *923*

Menopause *926*

Structural Disorders of the Female Reproductive System *929*

Uterine Displacement *929*

Pelvic Organ Prolapse *930*

Vaginal Fistula *931*

Disorders of Female Reproductive Tissue *931*

Endometriosis *931*

Ovarian Cysts *932*

Uterine Fibroid Tumor *933*

Malignant Tumors *933*

Cervical Cancer *933*

NURSING PROCESS CASE STUDY: Client with Cervical Cancer *935*

Endometrial Cancer *936*

Ovarian Cancer *937*

Cancer of the Vulva *938*

Infections of the Female Reproductive System *939*

Vaginitis *939*

Pelvic Inflammatory Disease *941*

Toxic Shock Syndrome *942*

CRITICAL THINKING CARE MAP: Caring for a Client Experiencing Menopause *945*

CHAPTER 34

Caring for Clients with Sexually Transmitted Diseases *947*

Chlamydia *948*

Genital Herpes *953*

Genital Warts *954*

Gonorrhea *955*

NURSING PROCESS CASE STUDY: Client with Gonorrhea *955*

Syphilis *956*

CRITICAL THINKING CARE MAP: Caring for a Client with Syphilis *959*

Cultural Care Strategies: Recognizing Biological Variations Among Cultures *961*

Appendices *963*

I. Standard Precautions *963*

II. NANDA-Approved Nursing Diagnoses 2001–2002 *965*

III. Common Laboratory Values *967*

IV. Glossary *968*

V. NCLEX-PN Answers; Hints for Critical Thinking *978*

Bibliography *1000*

Credits *1012*

Index *1014*

chapter 1

The Medical-Surgical Nurse

CARING tip

❝Set your expectations for yourself high and then strive daily to meet them. Learn to be flexible and adaptable to be employable in today's changing health care environment.❞

Bonnie Boroski, RN, MSN • Coordinator, LPN Program • Greater Johnstown Area Vocational Technical School • Johnstown, Pennsylvania

LEARNING outcomes

After completing this chapter, you will be able to:
- Describe the nurse as caregiver, teacher, client advocate, and manager of care.
- Discuss the steps of the nursing process—assessment, diagnosis, planning, implementation, and evaluation—and explain why the nursing process is used in clinical practice.
- Describe critical thinking and discuss how it contributes to nursing care.
- Describe the importance of codes for nursing and nursing standards in medical–surgical nursing care.
- Discuss some of the legal and ethical dilemmas in client care.

MediaLink

 www.prenhall.com/burke

Use the above address to access the free, interactive Companion Website created for this textbook. Get hints, instant feedback, and textbook references to chapter-related multiple choice questions. Link to other interesting sites.

Medical-surgical nursing is the health care and illness care of adults. It is based on knowledge from the arts and sciences and is shaped by knowledge from nursing. The focus of medical-surgical nursing is the adult client's response to actual or potential alterations in health. The adult requiring health care services is the *client*.

Medical-surgical nurses must address many issues simultaneously. The human responses for which nurses plan and implement care do not just result from changes in the structure and function of body systems. They also result from related changes in the client's social, cultural, economic, and personal life. Beyond this, medical-surgical nurses provide care for people from their late teens to early 100s; their stages of development can vary widely. The variety of individual health care needs and the wide range of clients' ages make medical-surgical nursing a changing and challenging area of nursing practice.

This chapter serves as a broad overview of medical-surgical nursing practice. Topics include the roles of the nurse, the need for cultural sensitivity, the steps of the nursing process, critical thinking, and legal and ethical guidelines in providing care.

Roles of the Nurse in Medical-Surgical Practice

Health care today is a vast and complex system. It reflects changes in society, changes in the populations that require nursing care, and an emphasis on health promotion as well as illness care. The roles of the medical-surgical nurse have broadened in response to these changes. Medical-surgical nurses are not only caregivers but also teachers, client advocates, and managers of care. The nurse assumes these roles to promote and maintain health, to prevent illness, and to help clients cope with disability or death in any setting.

THE NURSE AS CAREGIVER

Nurses have always been **caregivers** (people who provide personal, individual assistance), but the activities carried out within the caregiver role have changed tremendously. From 1900 to the 1960s, the nurse was almost always female; the primary definition of her caregiver role was to give personal care to the client and to carry out physicians' orders. The caregiver role for the nurse today is both independent and collaborative. Nurses may independently make assessments, plan, and implement client care based on nursing knowledge and skills (Figure 1-1 ◆). They also *collaborate* (work cooperatively) with other members of the health care team to implement and evaluate care.

As a caregiver, the nurse practices both the science and the art of nursing. Using the nursing process as the framework for care, the nurse provides **interventions** (purposeful actions) to meet the physical, psychosocial, spiritual, environmental, and cultural needs of clients and families. Cultural awareness has become an increasingly important area in recent years. Box 1-1 discusses culturally sensitive care in nursing.

Figure 1-1. ◆ In the role of caregiver, the nurse provides comprehensive, individualized care to the adult client.

The science (the knowledge base) of nursing is translated into the art of nursing through caring. *Caring* is the means by which the nurse is connected with and concerned for the client. The nurse as caregiver is knowledgeable, skilled, understanding, and caring.

Nurses have always identified problems in client care and developed interventions to meet specific needs. Until recently, though, these activities were not conducted scientifically or communicated to other nurses through nursing literature. To develop the science of nursing, nursing knowledge must be established through clinical research and then published, so that the findings based on clinical evidence can be used by all nurses to improve client care. The nurse's role as a caregiver is increasingly based on evidence-based practice.

THE NURSE AS TEACHER

The teaching role of the nurse is essential for many reasons. First, individuals, as well as all levels of government, are placing greater emphasis on health promotion and illness prevention. Second, hospital stays are becoming shorter, so the client and family must provide continuing care at home. Third, the number of chronically ill in our society is rising as the overall population ages. All these factors make the nurse's role as a teacher increasingly important.

The framework for the role of teacher is the teaching–learning process. Within this framework, the nurse must assess learning needs, plan and implement teaching to meet those needs, and evaluate the effectiveness of the teaching. The nurse must have good interpersonal skills and be familiar with adult learning principles (Figure 1-2 ◆).

A major part of the nurse–teacher role today is preparing clients and families to provide care in the home. Teaching is a major part of discharge planning. Because client and family education is such an important aspect of medical-surgical nursing, we include discharge considerations throughout this textbook.

BOX 1-1
CULTURALLY SENSITIVE NURSING

Culture is a set of socially inherited characteristics of a human group. People learn these beliefs, practices, habits, likes, dislikes, customs, and rituals from their families and pass them on to their children. A person's *ethnic identity* includes belonging to a social group within a culture and a social system, and sharing a common religion, language, ancestry, and physical characteristics. (For example, a person's ethnic identity may be Irish Catholic; the person's culture might be American.) Culture gives shape and personal meaning to health or illness events. It also affects how the client relates to others within the health care environment.

The health care system serves clients who are culturally diverse in country of origin, health beliefs, sexual orientation, race, socioeconomic level, and age. However, nursing has been slow to address the need for culturally sensitive care. This is partly because the health care system is itself a culture, and still is primarily made up of white middle-class people. Prejudice and *ethnocentrism* (people's belief that their own cultural group's beliefs and values are the only acceptable ones) have often created barriers to culturally sensitive care.

Culturally sensitive care is important for nurses for the following reasons:

- The demographic and ethnic composition of the world, and the United States in particular, has changed markedly, but ethnic groups are not well represented among health care professionals.
- There is a growing awareness and acceptance of diversity and an increased willingness to maintain and support ethnic and cultural heritage.
- People of color and immigrants face increasing unemployment, decreasing opportunity, and limited access to health care.
- Nurses make up the largest force in health care delivery and therefore have tremendous potential to push for fairness and accessibility.
- Consumers are becoming increasingly aware of what is competent and sensitive health care.

People of every culture have the right to have their cultural values known, respected, and addressed appropriately in nursing and other health care services. To provide nursing care that is culturally aware, nurses must develop a sensitivity to personal fundamental values about health and illness. They must accept the existence of differing values. They must be respectful of, interested in, and understanding of other cultures without being judgmental.

THE NURSE AS CLIENT ADVOCATE

The client who enters the health care system is often unprepared to make independent decisions. The nurse as client **advocate** (defined as one who speaks for another) actively promotes the client's rights to make decisions and choices. The nurse speaks for the client when necessary, mediates between the client and other persons, and protects the patient's right to self-determination (even when the nurse disagrees with the client's decision). As a client advocate, the nurse:

- Communicates with other health care team members
- Provides client and family teaching
- Assists and supports client decision making
- Makes referrals
- Identifies community and personal resources

THE NURSE AS MANAGER OF CARE

All nurses must learn to practice leadership. Their jobs may require them to manage time, resources, the environment in which they provide care, and other people (such as support staff). Nurses develop the skills to direct, delegate, and coordinate activities and to evaluate the quality of care provided. In the role of leader and manager, the nurse takes responsibility for the quality of client care through a process called quality assurance. **Quality assurance** includes the quality-control activities of evaluating, monitoring, or regulating the standard of services provided to the consumer. Clients are assured of quality care through professional and technical licensure of individual care providers; through accreditation of hospitals (e.g., by the Joint Commission on Accreditation of Healthcare Organizations, or JCAHO); through licensure of hospitals, pharmacies, and nursing homes; and through certification in specialty areas.

Quality-assurance methods are used to evaluate the care of individual clients against established standards of care. In this process, documentation is reviewed, client surveys are conducted, nurses are interviewed, and nurse or client performance is directly observed. The data are then used to identify differences between actual practice and established standards and to develop a plan of action to resolve the differences. Later, the actions are assessed to determine whether they were effective in improving practice.

Framework for Practice: The Nursing Process

The **nursing process** is the series of activities nurses perform as they provide care to clients. The nursing process is a model of care that differentiates nursing from other helping professions. It can be used in any setting in which the nurse provides care, from promoting wellness to coping with disability or death. Regardless of the situation, the nursing process includes activities that are specific, individualized, and *holistic* (concerned with the whole person—physical, emotional, and spiritual).

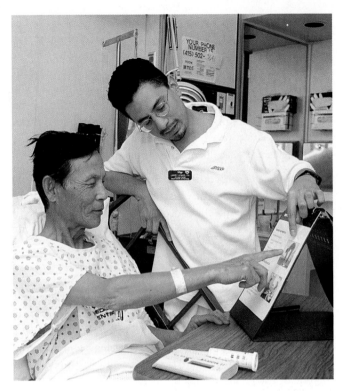

Figure 1-2. ◆ The nurse's role as teacher is an essential component of care. As part of the discharge planning process, this nurse is providing teaching for self-care at home.

STEPS OF THE NURSING PROCESS

There are five interdependent steps in the nursing process: assessment, diagnosis, planning, implementation, and evaluation. They are most often used in a cyclic manner (Figure 1-3 ◆).

The steps have been legitimized by the American Nurses Association Standards of Practice and by state nursing practice

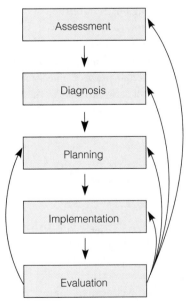

Figure 1-3. ◆ Steps of the nursing process. Notice that the steps are interrelated and interdependent. For example, evaluation of the client might reveal the need for further assessment, additional nursing diagnoses, and/or a revision of the plan of care.

acts. Licensing examinations, including the NCLEX-PN, base their structure on this model of nursing care. Entire books have been written about the nursing process. This discussion is intended only as an overview. In addition, we provide case studies that illustrate the nursing process throughout this textbook.

Assessment

Assessment, the first step of the nursing process, is a nursing activity that begins when the client first encounters the health care system and continues as long as the client requires care. During assessment, the nurse collects *data* (pieces of information) about the client's health status; these data are validated, organized, clustered into patterns, and communicated either verbally or in written form. Accurate assessments are the basis for deriving accurate nursing diagnoses, for planning and implementing individualized care, and for evaluating the care that is given. (See guidelines for collecting assessment data in Chapter 4.)

Nurses assess clients in two ways:

1. The *initial assessment* includes a thorough history and physical assessment. It provides comprehensive data about health responses. It identifies factors that contribute to these responses in a specific individual. It begins the joint process of establishing goals and outcomes of care with the client.
2. *Focused* (or *ongoing*) *assessments* are continuous assessments that occur whenever the nurse interacts with the client. They enable the nurse to evaluate nursing actions and to determine whether interventions should continue or change to meet outcomes. They provide structure for documenting nursing care. They allow the nurse to identify responses to a disease process or treatment that was not present during the initial assessment, or to monitor the status of an actual or potential problem that was previously identified (Alfaro, 1998).

To make accurate and holistic assessments, nurses must have a wide range of knowledge and skills. They must be able to assess the physical status of the client and to use effective communication techniques. Nurses must be knowledgeable in pathophysiology and pharmacology. Finally, nurses must have a solid foundation of nursing knowledge and skill to provide holistic, individualized care.

Diagnosis

The American Nurses Association (ANA) has defined nursing as "the diagnosis and treatment of human responses to actual or potential health problems" (1980, p. 9). The registered nurse identifies such a response as a **nursing diagnosis,** defined by the North American Nursing Diagnosis Association (NANDA) as "a clinical judgment about individual, family, or community responses to actual or potential health problems/life processes. Nursing diagnoses provide the basis for selection of nursing interventions to achieve outcomes for which the nurse is accountable" (NANDA, 1990, p. 5). Gordon provides a somewhat more concrete definition of a nursing diagnosis, as "a clinical diagnosis made by a professional nurse that describes actual or potential health problems which the nurse, by virtue of her [or his] education and experience, is capable and licensed to treat" (Gordon, 1994). The practical or vocational nurse does not establish the nursing diagnosis. However, the LPN or LVN collects assessment data that are the basis for nursing diagnoses, and LPN/VNs often contribute to the diagnoses that are made.

To establish appropriate nursing diagnoses, the nurse analyzes data collected during the assessment step, clustering it into categories of information that can be used to identify actual or potential alterations in health. Many different frameworks exist for identifying patterns of human behavior (Wilkinson, 2000). Some commonly used methods are: basic human needs, body systems, human response patterns, and functional health patterns (Gordon, 1982).

The broad organizational structure used in this book is based on Gordon's 11 **functional health patterns:** Functional health patterns are a system for grouping human functions (such as nutrition and elimination). This allows the nurse to collect data within that pattern to determine if the client's health function is positive, at risk, or altered. In this book, those functional health patterns that specifically relate to medical-surgical nursing are used to group disorders. These are patterns of function in the areas of health perception–health management, nutrition–metabolic, elimination, activity–exercise, cognitive perceptual, and sexuality–reproductive. However, information from the other patterns (sleep–rest, self-perception/self-concept, role–relationship, coping/stress-tolerance, and value–belief) are integrated in the discussions of nursing care.

Making a diagnosis is a complex process that always involves uncertainty. Therefore, the nurse uses diagnostic reasoning to choose nursing diagnoses that best define the individual's health problems. Critical thinking, described in the next section, is used to make decisions about which label (or diagnosis) best describes the patterns of data.

Although no one list of nursing diagnoses is universally accepted, the work of NANDA is widely used. Their *taxonomy* (system of classification) groups nursing diagnoses into classes and subclasses based on patterns and relationships. In 1988, the ANA accepted the NANDA system as the official system of diagnosis for the United States. Nursing diagnoses within the NANDA taxonomy are used in this book.

A diagnosis is written in two parts joined by the phrase *related to.* The first part of the statement is the particular human response that has been identified from the analysis of data. It identifies what needs to change in a specific client as a result of nursing interventions, and it also identifies the client outcomes that measure the change. The part of the statement that follows the *related to* phrase identifies the physical, psychosocial, cultural, spiritual, or environmental factors (etiologies) that cause or contribute to the response.

Nursing diagnoses identify two types of human responses: *actual* human responses and *potential* human responses. Nurses develop and implement a plan of care for actual responses; they also plan interventions to support health and prevent illness for potential human responses. Examples of nursing diagnoses are found throughout this textbook. (See also Appendix II, NANDA Diagnoses.)

The PES method of writing a nursing diagnosis is frequently used in nursing practice (Gordon, 1994). Diagnoses written according to this method consist of three components:

1. The problem (P), which is the NANDA label
2. The etiology (E) of the problem, which names the related factors and is indicated by the phrase *related to*
3. The signs and symptoms (S), which are the defining characteristics and are indicated by the phrase *as manifested by*

The following are examples of nursing diagnoses that are written using the PES method:

- *Anxiety* related to hospitalization as manifested by statements of nervousness and by crying
- *Bowel incontinence* related to loss of sphincter control as manifested by involuntary passage of stool
- *Fatigue* related to the side effects of chemotherapy as manifested by the inability to carry out normal daily routines and statements of overwhelming exhaustion

Planning

During the **planning** step, the nurse develops a list of nursing interventions and client **outcomes** (time-specific, achievable goals) to promote healthy responses and prevent, reverse, or decrease unhealthy responses. Outcomes, which are established by the client and nurse together, identify what the client will be able to do as a result of the nursing interventions. Both outcomes and nursing interventions are documented in a written plan of care that directs nursing activities, nursing documentation, and appropriate evaluation (Alfaro, 1998).

Nurses plan interventions for two types of client problems: those that require nursing management (stated as nursing diagnoses) and those that require collaborative management (collaborative or clinical problems). In *nursing management,* the nurse is guided by the diagnosis, initiates selected interventions, and is accountable for achieving outcomes (NANDA, 1990). In *collaborative management* (pathophysiologic, treatment-related, personal, environmental, and maturational situations), nurses monitor for onset or changes in status, and both physician-initiated and nurse-initiated interventions are used to minimize complications (Carpenito, 1995).

Expected Outcomes

Expected outcomes for nursing interventions are client centered, time specific, and measurable (e.g., "The client will demonstrate the ability to self-administer insulin injections by discharge."). Outcomes are classified into three domains:

cognitive ("knowing"), affective ("feeling"), and psychomotor ("doing"). The nurse considers all three domains to ensure holistic care.

In contrast, expected outcomes for collaborative problems are goals for the nurse, usually written as statements that begin with "to detect and report early signs and symptoms of potential complications of . . ." and "to implement preventive and corrective nursing interventions ordered by . . ." (Alfaro, 1998). In many instances, these goals are not written down as part of the plan of care. Nursing interventions for collaborative problems may be ordered by the physician or by institutional policy, procedures, protocols, or standards.

The nursing plan consists of specific, individualized interventions. If, for example, the nurse identifies that a client is at risk for Fluid Volume Deficit, it is not enough for the nurse simply to encourage the client to drink more fluids. Together, the nurse and client must identify liquids the client prefers, times that will be best for drinking them, and the amount of fluid (in ounces or milliliters). The nurse must document this information on the written care plan. Only then does care truly become a part of the plan of care.

Implementation

The **implementation** step is the "doing" phase of the nursing process, during which the nurse carries out planned interventions. Ongoing assessment of the client before, during, and after the intervention is essential. Although a plan may be appropriate, there are many variables that may make a change of plan necessary. For example, the nurse is not able to force fluids if the client is nauseated or vomiting.

When implementing the planned interventions, the nurse follows several important principles:

1. *Set daily priorities,* based on initial assessments and on the client's condition, as reported during the change of shift report or as documented in the client's chart. Critical assessments take first priority. These include the status of invasive lines and fluids infusing or changes in health status during the preceding shift.
2. *Be aware of how nursing interventions interrelate.* For example, while giving a bath, the nurse can also assess physical and psychologic status, use therapeutic communication, teach the client, do range-of-motion exercises, and provide skin care.
3. *Determine the most appropriate level of interventions* for each client, based on health status and illness treatment:
   a. Directly perform the activity for the client.
   b. Assist the client to perform the activity.
   c. Supervise the client/family while they are performing the activity.
   d. Teach the client/family about health care.
   e. Monitor the client at risk for potential complications or problems.
4. *Use available resources* to provide interventions that are realistic and practical. This depends on the equipment available, financial status of the client, and resources (including staff, agency, family, and community resources).
5. *Document nursing interventions.* This is the final part of implementation, and *it is a legal requirement.* There are many different ways of documenting care. Traditional narrative source-oriented and problem-oriented charting methods are often used. Other methods are focused charting, charting by exception, and computer-assisted documentation.

Evaluation

The **evaluation** step of the nursing process allows the nurse to determine whether the plan was effective and to continue, revise, or terminate the plan. Evaluation is based on the outcome criteria that were established during the planning step. Although evaluation is listed as the last part of the nursing process, it actually takes place continuously throughout client care.

To evaluate a plan, the nurse collects data from the client, reviews the chart, and observes the client. The nurse then compares the status of the client with the expected outcomes. If the outcomes have been accomplished, the nurse may continue or terminate the plan. If the outcomes have not been accomplished, the nurse must continue to collect data and evaluate interventions.

BENEFITS OF THE NURSING PROCESS

The nursing process benefits all those involved in the health care setting. It helps nurses identify their special areas of practice. The nursing process provides a common reference system and common terminology to serve as a base for improving clinical practice. It also provides a framework for evaluating quality of care.

The nursing process benefits clients. The nursing process creates a structure for planned, individualized interventions. It involves the client in all steps of the process. It assures continuity of care through the written care plan. The nursing process also benefits the health care institution through better resource utilization, increased client satisfaction, and improved documentation of care. As the twenty-first century progresses, increased research and theory development will continue to refine the nursing process.

THE NURSING PROCESS IN CLINICAL PRACTICE

With experience, the nursing process becomes an integral part of providing care and the nurse does not consciously stop and consider each step. For example, when caring for a client who is hemorrhaging, the nurse uses all five steps simultaneously to meet critical, life-threatening needs. In contrast, when considering the long-term needs of a client with a chronic illness or disability, the nurse makes in-depth assessments, determines goals jointly with the client, and documents care through a written plan that is revised as necessary by all nurses providing care.

Process of Critical Thinking

Critical thinking is, most basically, thinking about your thinking. It is self-directed thinking that is focused on what to believe or do in a specific situation. It involves both attitudes and skills. In nursing, critical thinking occurs when the nurse uses knowledge to consider a client care situation and uses the nursing process to make judgments and decisions about what to do in that situation. As you practice critical thinking, you must consider:

- The purpose of the thinking (e.g., is it to collect more data or is it to report your data to someone else)
- How much knowledge you have
- What prejudices may influence your thinking (e.g., believing that all poor people are dirty or all old people are incapable of learning how to care for themselves) or letting your emotions affect your decision
- What information you need from others, such as your faculty, skilled clinical nurses, a textbook or a journal article, or the policies of the health care agency
- The ability to identify other possible options, evaluate the alternatives, and reach a conclusion

It takes practice to integrate critical thinking into your attitudes and skills. Critical thinking exercises, titled *Critical Thinking Care Maps,* are included throughout this book to provide that practice. This chapter provides a sample Critical Thinking Care Map, plus suggestions for critical thinking and completing the exercise. In Appendix V, *Hints for Critical Thinking* are provided to assist you in developing your critical thinking skills.

ATTITUDES AND MENTAL HABITS NECESSARY FOR CRITICAL THINKING

Thinking critically involves more than just cognitive (knowledge) skills. It is strongly influenced by the attitudes and mental habits one has. To think critically, you must focus your attention on your attitudes and how they affect your thinking. These attitudes and mental habits are:

- Being able to *think independently* so that you make clinical decisions based on sound thinking and judgment. This means, for example, you are not influenced by negative comments from other health care providers about a client.
- Being willing to listen to and be fair in your evaluation of others ideas and beliefs by having *intellectual courage.* This involves listening carefully to other ideas and thoughts and making a decision based on what you learn instead of how you feel.
- Having *intellectual empathy* by being able to put yourself in the place of another to understand that other person better. For example, if you put yourself in the place of the person with severe pain, you are better able to understand why he or she is so upset when pain medications are late.

- Being fair-minded and considering all viewpoints before making a decision through an *intellectual sense of justice* and being *intellectually humble.* This means you consider the viewpoints of others that may be different from yours before reaching a conclusion. You also realize that you are constantly learning from others. You are not afraid to say, "I don't know the answer to that question, but I will find out and let you know."
- Being *disciplined* so that you do not stop at easy answers, but continue to consider alternatives.
- Being *creative* and *confident in self.* Nurses often need to consider different ways of providing care and constantly look for better, more cost-effective methods. Confidence in one's decisions is gained through critical thinking.

CRITICAL THINKING SKILLS

Critical thinking skills are the mental abilities that are used. The major critical thinking skills are:

- The ability to have *divergent thinking.* This means that when you collect data from a client, you can sort out the relevant data from the data that are not relevant and explore possibilities to draw a conclusion. You must consider, for example, what data are most relevant to the care of your client. Abnormal data are usually considered relevant, and normal data are helpful but may not change the care you provide.
- *Reasoning*—having the ability to discriminate between facts and guesses. By using known facts, problems are solved and decisions are made in a systematic, logical way. For example, when you take a pulse you must know the facts of normal pulse rate for a person of this age, types of medications the client is taking that may alter the pulse rate, and the emotional and physical state of the client. Based on these facts, you are able to decide if the pulse rate is normal or abnormal.
- *Clarifying*—defining terms and noting similarities and differences. For example, when caring for a client with chronic pain, you must know the definition of chronic pain, and also know the similarities and differences between acute pain and chronic pain.
- *Reflection*—taking time to think about something. It cannot take place in an emergency situation. However, as you reflect on your experiences in nursing, many of those experiences may in turn become alternatives when caring for a different client.

Critical thinking is an expected ability of all nurses. Using critical thinking to provide care that is structured by the nursing process allows the nurse to provide safe, effective, holistic, and individualized care.

Guidelines for Nursing Practice

Nursing codes of ethics and standards guide nursing practice and protect the public. These guidelines are especially impor-

This line provides an appropriate nursing diagnosis

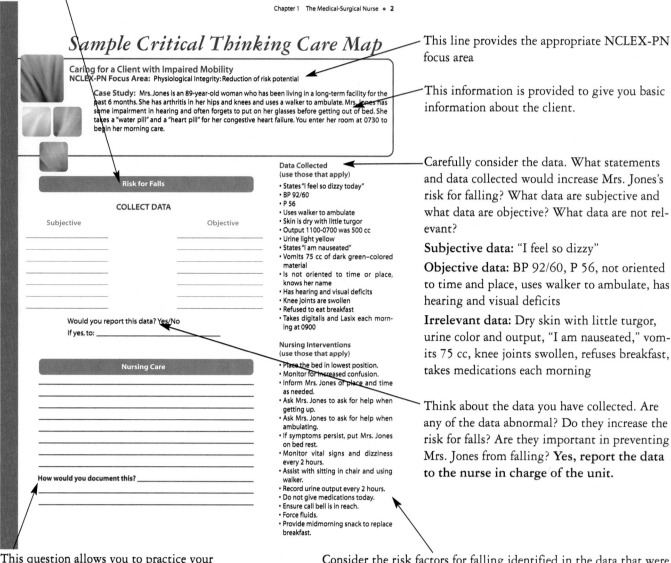

Sample Critical Thinking Care Map

Caring for a Client with Impaired Mobility
NCLEX-PN Focus Area: Physiological Integrity: Reduction of risk potential

Case Study: Mrs. Jones is an 89-year-old woman who has been living in a long-term facility for the past 6 months. She has arthritis in her hips and knees and uses a walker to ambulate. Mrs. Jones has some impairment in hearing and often forgets to put on her glasses before getting out of bed. She takes a "water pill" and a "heart pill" for her congestive heart failure. You enter her room at 0730 to begin her morning care.

Risk for Falls

COLLECT DATA

Subjective   Objective

Would you report this data? Yes/No
If yes, to: _____

Nursing Care

How would you document this? _____

Data Collected
(use those that apply)
- States "I feel so dizzy today"
- BP 92/60
- P 56
- Uses walker to ambulate
- Skin is dry with little turgor
- Output 1100-0700 was 500 cc
- Urine light yellow
- States "I am nauseated"
- Vomits 75 cc of dark green–colored material
- Is not oriented to time or place, knows her name
- Has hearing and visual deficits
- Knee joints are swollen
- Refused to eat breakfast
- Takes digitalis and Lasix each morning at 0900

Nursing Interventions
(use those that apply)
- Place the bed in lowest position.
- Monitor for increased confusion.
- Inform Mrs. Jones of place and time as needed.
- Ask Mrs. Jones to ask for help when getting up.
- Ask Mrs. Jones to ask for help when ambulating.
- If symptoms persist, put Mrs. Jones on bed rest.
- Monitor vital signs and dizziness every 2 hours.
- Assist with sitting in chair and using walker.
- Record urine output every 2 hours.
- Do not give medications today.
- Ensure call bell is in reach.
- Force fluids.
- Provide midmorning snack to replace breakfast.

This line provides the appropriate NCLEX-PN focus area

This information is provided to give you basic information about the client.

Carefully consider the data. What statements and data collected would increase Mrs. Jones's risk for falling? What data are subjective and what data are objective? What data are not relevant?

Subjective data: "I feel so dizzy"

Objective data: BP 92/60, P 56, not oriented to time and place, uses walker to ambulate, has hearing and visual deficits

Irrelevant data: Dry skin with little turgor, urine color and output, "I am nauseated," vomits 75 cc, knee joints swollen, refuses breakfast, takes medications each morning

Think about the data you have collected. Are any of the data abnormal? Do they increase the risk for falls? Are they important in preventing Mrs. Jones from falling? **Yes, report the data to the nurse in charge of the unit.**

This question allows you to practice your documentation. It is not necessary to document all the data or interventions for this exercise. For example, the assessment documentation might be:

730 States "I am dizzy". BP 92/60, P 56. Is not oriented to time and place, is oriented to person. Mr. James, nurse manager notified.

                                    J. Gomez, LVN

Consider the risk factors for falling identified in the data that were collected. Review the effect of dizziness, confusion, and hypotension on the ability to safely get out of bed and ambulate. Review the policy on fall-prevention programs in your health care clinical setting or in a current journal article. Made a decision about which interventions are relevant and which are not relevant.

Relevant interventions: Place bed in lowest position, monitor for increased confusion, inform client of place and time, ask client to ask for help when getting up and ambulating, put client on bed rest if symptoms persist, monitor vital signs and dizziness, assist with sitting in chair and using walker, ensure call bell is in reach.

Irrelevant interventions: Record urine output every 2 hours, do not give medications, force fluids, provide midmorning snack.

Note:

This sample is provided for the beginning student in medical-surgical nursing. As you learn more about pathophysiology, medications, and nursing care you will find there are more alternatives for consideration in this sample. For example, the medications Mrs. Jones is taking may cause dehydration and loss of potassium. These conditions may cause nausea, vomiting, and confusion. In turn, there would be an increased risk for falls. These data should be reported to the nurse in charge, who would report the data to the physician. The physician may order the medications to be held. The nurse would not omit the medications without a physician's order.

tant because nurses encounter legal and ethical problems almost daily.

CODES FOR NURSES

An established code of ethics is one means of defining a profession. **Ethics** are principles of conduct. Ethical behavior is concerned with moral duty, values, obligations, and the distinction between right and wrong. Nursing codes of ethics provide a frame of reference for "professionally valued and ideal nursing behaviors that are congruent with the principles expressed in the Code for Nurses" (Ketefian, 1987, p. 13). Not only do they state ideal behaviors when making moral and ethical decisions; they also help define the roles of nurses. The codes of ethics presented here were developed by the International Council of Nurses and the American Nurses Association.

The International Council of Nurses Code

The International Council of Nurses (ICN) Code for Nurses was developed in 1953 and most recently revised in 1973 (Box 1-2). This code helps guide nurses in setting priorities, making judgments, and taking action when they face ethical dilemmas in clinical practice.

Code of Ethics

The American Nurses Association (ANA) Code for Nurses states principles of ethical concern. First published in 1950, the Code was most recently revised in 2001. It guides the behavior of nurses and also defines nursing for the general public. Examples of the ANA code for nurses are:

- The nurse's primary commitment is to the patient, whether an individual, family, group, or community.
- The nurse promotes, advocates for, and strives to protect the health, safety, and rights of the patient.
- The nurse owes the same duties to self as to others, including the responsibility to preserve integrity and safety, to maintain competence, and to continue personal and professional growth.

STANDARDS OF NURSING PRACTICE

A **standard** is a statement or criterion that can be used by a profession and by the general public to measure quality of practice. Established standards make each individual nurse accountable for practice. This means that each nurse who provides care has the responsibility or obligation to account for his or her own behaviors within that role. Professional nursing organizations develop and implement standards of practice to identify clearly the nurse's responsibilities to society.

The standards of the National Association for Practical Nurse Education and Service (NAPNES) (1997) set a foundation for providing safe and competent nursing practice, guided by a commitment to ethical/legal principles (Box 1-3). The ANA standards of clinical nursing practice (1998) outline standards for care (based on the nursing process) and professional performance, including quality of care, education, ethics, collaboration, and use of resources.

BOX 1-2
THE INTERNATIONAL COUNCIL OF NURSES CODE FOR NURSES

The fundamental responsibility of the nurse is fourfold: to promote health, to prevent illness, to restore health, and to alleviate suffering. The need for nursing is universal. Inherent in nursing is respect for life, dignity, and the rights of man. It is unrestricted by considerations of nationality, race, creed, color, age, sex, politics, or social status. Nurses render health services to the individual, the family, and the community and coordinate their services with those of related groups.

Nurses and People

The nurse's primary responsibility is to those people who require nursing care. The nurse, in providing care, promotes an environment in which the values, customs, and spiritual beliefs of the individual are respected. The nurse holds in confidence personal information and uses judgment in sharing this information.

Nurses and Practice

The nurse carries responsibility for nursing practice and for maintaining competence by continual learning. The nurse maintains the highest standards of nursing care possible within the reality of a specific situation. The nurse uses judgment in relation to individual competence when accepting and delegating responsibilities. The nurse when acting in a professional capacity should at all times maintain standards of personal conduct that reflect credit upon the profession.

Nurses and Society

The nurse shares with other citizens the responsibility for initiating and supporting action to meet the health and social needs of the public.

Nurses and Coworkers

The nurse sustains a cooperative relationship with coworkers in nursing and other fields. The nurse takes appropriate action to safeguard the individual when his care is endangered by a coworker or any other person.

Nurses and the Profession

The nurse plays the major role in determining and implementing desirable standards of nursing practice and nursing education. The nurse is active in developing a core of professional knowledge. The nurse, acting through the professional organization, participates in establishing and maintaining equitable social and economic working conditions in nursing.

Source: ICN Code for Nurses: Ethical Concepts Applied to Nursing by International Council of Nurses, 1973, Geneva: Imprimeries Populaires.

BOX 1-3
NAPNES STANDARDS FOR NURSING PRACTICE OF LP/VNS

1. The LP/VN provides individual and family-centered nursing care by:
   a. Utilizing appropriate knowledge, skills, and abilities
   b. Utilizing principles of the nursing process in meeting specific client needs in diversified health care settings
   c. Maintaining appropriate written documentation and utilizing effective communication skills with clients, family, significant others, and members of the health team
   d. Executing principles of crisis intervention to maintain safety
   e. Providing appropriate education to clients, family, and significant others to promote health, facilitate rehabilitation, and maintain wellness
   f. Serving as a client advocate to protect client rights
   g. Serving as a client advocate to protect client rights
2. The LP/VN fulfills the professional responsibilities of the practical/vocational nurse by:
   a. Applying the ethical principles underlying the professions
   b. Following legal requirements
   c. Following the policies and procedures of the employing facility
   d. Cooperating and collaborating with all members of the health care team to meet the needs of family-centered nursing care
   e. Assuming accountability for his or her nursing actions
   f. Seeking educational opportunities to improve knowledge and skills
   g. Building skills to assure and increase postlicensure competence

Source: National Association for Practical Nurse Education and Service. (1999). *NAPNES standards of practice for licensed practical/vocational nurses.* Silver Spring, MD: NAPNES.

Legal and Ethical Dilemmas in Nursing

A **dilemma** is a choice between two unpleasant alternatives. Nurses providing medical–surgical nursing care face dilemmas almost daily. Some common ones are discussed here briefly.

CLIENT RIGHTS

Nurses respect the right to confidentiality of client information obtained from interviews or from the client's record. Most state nursing practice acts legally require nurses to uphold this right. However, the right to privacy and confidentiality becomes a dilemma when the nurse does not have access to information concerning the presence of acquired immune deficiency syndrome (AIDS) or human immunodeficiency virus (HIV) in clients under their care. Most states currently mandate that HIV test results can be given to another person only if the client provides written consent for the release of that information. Many health care providers believe that this law violates their own right to personal safety and so are actively working to change the law.

The client's right to refuse treatment (including surgery, medication, medical therapy, and food/fluids) is another difficult area. As client advocate, the nurse must first establish that the client is mentally competent. The nurse then carefully explains the situation, the alternatives, and the potential harm from refusing treatment. Legally, the client must establish an *advance directive* on admission to a health care agency, stating the client's choice about preserving or prolonging life. (An advance directive, or *living will,* is a document in which a client formally states preferences for health care in the event that he or she later becomes mentally incapacitated. The client also names a person who has *durable power of attorney* to serve as a substitute decision maker to implement the client's stated preferences.) Documented advance directives become a part of the client's hospital record and are honored even if the client becomes incompetent during the period of treatment. However, several states assert that artificial feeding cannot be rejected under living will statutes. The nurse must take responsibility for remaining informed about current laws in this area of practice.

ISSUES OF DYING AND DEATH

Questions about who lives, who dies, and who decides often arise in the health care setting. These issues have become increasingly pressing as advances in technology extend the lives of people with chronic debilitating illness and major trauma. These changes have changed our ideas about living and dying. They have raised ethical conflicts about quality of life and death with dignity versus technologic methods of preserving life in any form. (See Chapter 9 for further information about end-of-life care.)

CARING FOR THE CLIENT WITH AIDS

Despite great progress in controlling the course of the disease, the number of cases of HIV and AIDS continues to increase, and there is still no cure. AIDS occurs in heterosexual and homosexual men and women of all ages and at all socioeconomic levels. The disease inspires great fear and inflicts great physical, emotional, financial, and social havoc.

For nurses, AIDS poses a moral and ethical dilemma because of possible infection with the virus. According to the ANA, the nurse has a moral obligation to provide care for the client with AIDS unless the risk exceeds the responsibility. The nurse is morally obligated to provide care to the client with AIDS when all four of these criteria are met, and in most cases, they are. Most health care agencies have a written policy requiring nurses to provide care to clients with AIDS, except in certain circumstances, such as the nurse's pregnancy.

(*Note:* The bibliography listings for this and all chapters have been compiled at the back of the book.)

Chapter Review

key terms by topic

Use the CD-ROM disk enclosed with your textbook to hear the pronunciation of the key terms in the chapter.

Medical-surgical nurse
medical-surgical nursing

Roles of the nurse
caregivers, interventions, advocate, quality assurance

Framework for practice
nursing process, assessment, nursing diagnosis, functional health patterns, planning, outcomes, implementation, evaluation

Process of critical thinking
critical thinking

Guidelines for nursing practice
ethics, standards, dilemma

---

key points

- Medical-surgical nurses promote health and provide care during illness or injury to adult clients. The roles of the medical-surgical nurse include caregiver, teacher, client advocate, and manager of care.

- The nursing process is a model of care that differentiates nursing from other health care providers. The five interdependent and cyclic steps of the nursing process are assessment, diagnosis, planning, implementation, and evaluation.

- Critical thinking is self-directed thinking that is focused on what to believe or do in a specific situation. It involves both attitudes and skills. Critical thinking and the nursing process are essential in nursing practice.

- Nursing codes of ethics (principles of conduct) and standards guide nursing practice and protect the public.

- Nurses often face dilemmas—a choice between two unpleasant alternatives—in clinical practice. Some dilemmas arise in the areas of client rights, issues of death and dying, and caring for clients with AIDS.

Medialink

Additional interactive resources for this chapter can be found on the Companion Website at www.prenhall.com/burke. Click on Chapter 1 and "Begin" to select the activities for this chapter.

For NCLEX review questions and an audio glossary, access the accompanying CD-ROM in this book.

for further study

For more guidelines for collecting assessment data, see Chapter 4.
For NANDA Diagnoses, see Appendix II.
For further information about end-of-life care, see Chapter 9.

NCLEX-PN Exam Preparation

TEST-TAKING TIP

Data collection is the first step in the nursing process. Select answers that address this step when answering a question about your *initial* nursing action.

1. The nurse independently plans and implements client care based on:
   a. the physician's orders
   b. the findings of other members of the health care team
   c. nursing knowledge and skills
   d. the wishes of the family

2. The role of the nurse which is most evident when the nurse is protecting the client's rights is:
   a. caregiver
   b. advocate
   c. educator
   d. manager

3. The nurse is responsible for the quality of client care through a process called:
   a. quality assurance
   b. delegation
   c. nursing diagnosis
   d. implementation

4. The step of the nursing process in which the nurse collects data initially and through ongoing interactions with clients is:
   a. evaluation
   b. diagnosis
   c. implementation
   d. assessment

5. The step of the nursing process which is complex, involves uncertainty, and requires the nurse to use reasoning and critical thinking is:
   a. diagnosis
   b. evaluation
   c. assessment
   d. planning

6. Planned nursing interventions must be:
   a. collaborative and concise
   b. specific and individualized
   c. initiated by the physician
   d. based on medical problems

7. The nurse's role during the implementation phase of the nursing process is to:
   a. carry out planned interventions
   b. establish outcome criteria
   c. identify client problems
   d. evaluate the care given

8. The final component of implementation that the nurse is legally required to complete is:
   a. setting priorities
   b. assessing the client's condition
   c. documenting interventions
   d. teaching the client

9. The public is protected and nursing practice is guided by:
   a. the nursing process
   b. physicians
   c. policies of health care facilities
   d. standards and codes of ethics

10. According to the ANA, the nurse has a moral obligation to provide care for the client with AIDS:
    a. when the client agrees to HIV testing
    b. unless the risk exceeds the responsibility
    c. only if a release of information is obtained
    d. in all situations

Answers for Review Questions, as well as discussion of Case Study Critical Thinking questions, appear in Appendix V.

chapter

2

The Adult Client in Health and Illness

LEARNING outcomes

After completing this chapter, you will be able to:

- Describe the physical status, risks for alterations in health, and health behaviors of the young adult, middle adult, and older adult.
- Discuss the definitions, functions, and developmental stages and tasks of the family.
- Define health, the health–illness continuum, and the concept of high-level wellness.
- Identify factors affecting health status, health promotion, and health maintenance.
- Compare and contrast disease and illness.
- Describe the sequence of acute illness behaviors.
- Discuss chronic illness, including characteristics, needs of the chronically ill, and the effects of chronic illness on the family.

Gordon Hight, a 21-year-old college student, is admitted to the emergency room with multiple injuries and head trauma following a motorcycle accident. Mary Green, a 38-year-old homemaker, arrives at same-day surgery for biopsy of a tumor in her left breast. Sam Rosengarten, a 55-year-old attorney, is in the intensive care unit for treatment of a myocardial infarction. Margarite Schlefer, age 82, is receiving home health care following a fall that fractured her right hip. These examples demonstrate the striking variety among adult clients—the focus of care in medical-surgical nursing.

 # The Adult Client

Although growth and development are continuous processes throughout life, the adult years commonly are divided into three stages: the young adult (age 18 to 40), the middle adult (age 40 to 65), and the older adult (over age 65). With aging, specific changes occur in intellectual, psychosocial, and spiritual development, as well as in physical structures and functions.

DEVELOPMENTAL TASKS OF THE ADULT

The developmental tasks of adults, as described by Havighurst (1972) are divided into the young, middle, and adult years. From ages 18 to 35, young adults select and learn to live with a mate, have and raise children, have a job, manage a home, and take on civic responsibility. From ages 36 to 60, middle adults establish and maintain an economic standard of living, help adolescent children learn to become responsible adults, develop leisure activities, accept and adjust to the physical changes of middle age, and adjust to aging parents. Adults age 60 and over establish a social network with others of similar age, establish satisfactory living arrangements, and adjust to retirement. The older adult must also adjust to such losses as physical strength, health, reduced income, and the death of a spouse.

The Young Adult

From age 18 to 25, the healthy young adult is at the peak of physical development. All body systems function at maximum efficiency. Then, during the 30s, some normal physiologic changes begin to occur. (A comparison of physical status for young adults during their 20s and 30s is shown in Table 2-1 ◆.)

The nurse promotes health in the young adult by teaching the behaviors listed in Box 2-1. Information about health for the young adult is primarily provided in community settings.

The young adult is at risk for **alterations in health** (a change from the normal health state) from accidents, sexually transmitted diseases, substance abuse, and physical or psychosocial stressors. These risk factors may be interrelated.

Accidents are the leading cause of injury and death in people between ages 15 and 24 (Centers for Disease Control and Prevention [CDC], 1999). Most injuries and fatalities occur as the result of motor vehicle crashes, but injuries and death also result from drowning, fire, use of firearms, occupational accidents, and exposure to environmental hazards. Accidental injury or death is often associated with the use of alcohol or other chemical substances, or with psychologic stress.

Sexually transmitted diseases include genital herpes, chlamydia, gonorrhea, syphilis, and acquired immune deficiency syndrome (AIDS). The young adult who is sexually active with a variety of partners and who does not use condoms is at greatest risk for development of these diseases.

Substance abuse is a major cause for concern in the young adult population. (See also Chapter 11.) Although alcohol abuse occurs at all ages, it is greater in the 20s than during any other decade of the life span. Alcohol contributes to motor vehicle crashes and physical violence, and it is damaging to the developing fetus in pregnant women. It can also cause liver disease and nutritional deficits. Other substances that are commonly abused include nicotine, marijuana, ampheta-

TABLE 2-1	PHYSICAL STATUS AND CHANGES IN THE YOUNG ADULT YEARS	
ASSESSMENT	**STATUS DURING THE 20S**	**STATUS DURING THE 30S**
Skin	Smooth, even temperature	Wrinkles begin to appear
Hair	Slightly oily, shiny Balding may begin	Graying may begin Balding may begin
Vision	Snellen 20/20	Some loss of visual acuity and accommodation
Musculoskeletal	Strong, coordinated	Some loss of strength and muscle mass
Cardiovascular	Maximum cardiac output 60–90 beats/min Mean BP: 120/80	Slight decline in cardiac output 60–90 beats/min Mean BP: 120/80
Respiratory	Rate: 12–20 Full vital capacity	Rate: 12–20 Decline in vital capacity

BOX 2-1
HEALTHY BEHAVIORS
IN THE YOUNG ADULT

- Choose foods from all food groups, and eat a variety of foods.
- Choose a diet low in fat (30% or less of total calories), saturated fat (less than 10% of calories), and cholesterol (less than 300 mg daily).
- Choose a diet that each day includes at least three servings of vegetables, two servings of fruits, and six servings of grains.
- Use sugar, salt, and sodium in moderation.
- For females, increase to or maintain 18 mg of iron daily in the diet.
- Make exercise a regular part of life, carrying out activities that increase the heart rate to a set target, and maintain that rate for 30 to 60 minutes three or four times a week.
- Include exercise as part of any weight-reduction program.
- Have regular physical examinations, including assessment for cancer of the thyroid, ovaries, lymph nodes, and skin (every 3 years).
- Have a vision examination every 2 to 4 years.
- Have an annual dental checkup.
- For females, have a baseline mammogram between ages 35 and 39 and a breast examination every 3 years.
- For females, have Pap tests as recommended by a physician: annually until three or more consecutive normal results, and then at physician's discretion.
- For males, have testicular and prostate examinations every 5 years.
- Conduct breast or testicular self-examination monthly.

mines, cocaine, and crack. Smoking increases the risk of respiratory and cardiovascular diseases. Cocaine and crack can cause death from cardiovascular effects and can lead to addiction and health problems in the baby born to an addicted mother.

The young adult is subjected to a wide variety of physical and psychosocial stressors. Physical stressors that increase the risk of illness include environmental pollutants and work-related risks (e.g., electrical hazards, mechanical injuries, or exposure to toxins or infectious agents). Other physical stressors include exposure to the sun, ingestion of chemical substances (e.g., caffeine, alcohol, nicotine), and pregnancy.

Many different and individualized psychosocial stressors may affect the young adult. Choices must be made about education, occupation, relationships, independence, and lifestyle. The young adult without adequate education or job skills may face unemployment, poverty, homelessness, and limited access to health care. Also, divorces in the United States are increas-

ing. Three out of every five marriages end in divorce, and this number is even higher among young adults. Divorce often results in loneliness, feelings of failure, financial difficulties, domestic violence, and child abuse. The inability of the young adult to cope with these stressors may result in suicide, which ranks next to accidents as a major cause of death in this age group. Although difficult to prove, it is believed that some accidental deaths, especially when associated with substance abuse, are actually suicides.

The Middle Adult

The middle adult, age 40 to 65, has physical status and function similar to that of adults in their 20s and 30s. However, many changes take place between ages 40 and 65 (Table 2-2 ◆). The middle adult is at risk for alterations in health from obesity, cardiovascular disease, cancer, substance abuse, and psychosocial stressors. These factors may be interrelated.

The nurse promotes health in the middle adult by teaching the behaviors listed in Box 2-2. Information about health for the middle adult may be provided in a variety of community settings, including outpatient clinics, occupational health clinics, and health care provider offices.

The middle adult often has a problem maintaining a healthy weight. Weight gain in middle adulthood is usually the result of continuing to consume the same number of calories while physical activity and basal metabolic rate decrease. Obesity affects all the major organ systems of the body, increasing the risk of atherosclerosis, hypertension, elevated cholesterol and triglyceride levels, and diabetes. Obesity is also associated with heart disease, osteoarthritis, and gallbladder disease.

The major cardiovascular risk factors, especially for coronary artery disease, include age, male gender, cigarette smoking, hypertension, elevated blood cholesterol levels, and diabetes. Other contributing factors include obesity, stress, and lack of exercise. The middle adult is at risk for disorders of peripheral vascular, cerebrovascular, and cardiovascular disease.

Cancer is the third leading cause of death in adults between ages 25 and 64 in the United States, with one third of cases occurring between ages 35 and 64. Cancers of the breast, colon, lung, and reproductive system are common in the middle years. The middle adult is at risk for cancer from environmental toxins as a result of increased length of exposure, and is also at risk from alcohol and nicotine use.

Although the middle adult may abuse a variety of substances, the most commonly abused are alcohol, nicotine, and prescription drugs. Excess alcohol use in the middle adult contributes to an increased risk of liver cancer, cirrhosis, pancreatitis, hyperlipidemia, and anemia. Alcoholism also increases the risk of accidental injury or death and disrupts careers and relationships. Cigarette smoking increases the risk of cancer, of chronic obstructive pulmonary disorders, and of cardiovascular disorders of the larynx, lung, mouth, pharynx, bladder, pancreas, esophagus, and kidney. The most commonly abused class of prescription drugs is tranquilizers.

	TABLE 2-2 PHYSICAL CHANGES IN THE MIDDLE ADULT YEARS
ASSESSMENT	**CHANGES**
Skin	Decreased turgor, moisture, and subcutaneous fat result in wrinkles. Fat is deposited in the abdominal and hip areas.
Hair	Loss of melanin in hair shaft causes graying. Hairline recedes in males.
Sensory	Visual acuity for near vision decreases (presbyopia) during the 40s. Auditory acuity for high-frequency sounds decreases (presbycusis); more common in men. Sense of taste diminishes.
Musculoskeletal	Skeletal muscle mass decreases by about age 60. Thinning of intervertebral discs results in loss of height (about 1 inch [2.5 cm]). Postmenopausal women may have loss of calcium and develop osteoporosis.
Cardiovascular	Blood vessels lose elasticity. Systolic blood pressure may increase.
Respiratory	Loss of vital capacity (about 1 L from age 20 to 60) occurs.
Gastrointestinal	Large intestine gradually loses muscle tone; constipation may result. Gastric secretions are decreased.
Genitourinary	Hormonal changes occur: menopause, women ($\downarrow$ estrogen); andropause, men ($\downarrow$ testosterone).
Endocrine	Gradual decrease in glucose tolerance occurs.

The middle adult years are ones of change and transition, frequently resulting in stress. Both men and women must adapt to changes in physical appearance and function and accept their own mortality. Children may leave home or, as is becoming more common, choose to remain at home. Parents are aging, with illness and death probable. The middle adult thus becomes what has been called "the sandwich generation," caught between the need to care for both children and aging parents. Both men and women may make career changes, and approaching retirement becomes a reality. Divorce in the middle years is a major emotional, social, and financial stressor.

The Older Adult

The older adult period begins at age 65, but it can be further divided into three periods: the "young-old" (age 65 to 74), the "middle-old" (age 75 to 84), and the "old-old" (age 85 and over). With increasing age, a number of normal physiologic changes occur (Table 2-3 ◆).

Older adults get the same benefits from health teaching that young adults and middle adults do. They should never be viewed as being "too old" to learn healthy living practices. However, nurses should adapt teaching methods to this age group, such as by using charts and literature with large print. Hospitals, long-term care facilities, retirement centers, outpatient clinics, senior citizen centers, and other community settings all provide health education for the older adult. The nurse promotes health in the older adult by teaching the behaviors listed in Box 2-3.

The older adult population is increasing more rapidly than any other age group, accounting for more than 34 million people. During the twentieth century, the number of adults in the United States living to age 65 or older more than tripled. That percentage is projected to be slightly more than 20% by the year 2030, with the largest increase occurring in adults over the age of 75. Currently, the life expectancy in North America is 76.7 years, with the white population living 6 years longer than African Americans (American Association of Retired Persons [AARP], 2000).

The increase in numbers of older adults has important implications for nursing. Clients needing health care in all settings will be older. They will require nursing interventions and teaching designed specifically to meet their needs. Although *gerontologic nursing* (care of the older adult) is a nursing specialty area, it is also an integral component of medical-surgical nursing (Figure 2-1 ◆).

The older adult is at risk for altered health from a variety of causes. Approximately 90% of all older adults have at least one chronic illness. The most frequent conditions in the older adult are arthritis, hypertension, hearing impairments, heart disease, cataracts, sinusitis, orthopedic disorders, visual impairments, and diabetes (AARP, 1999). The leading causes of death are heart disease, cancer, and stroke.

Like the middle adult, the older adult is at risk for alterations in health from obesity, cardiovascular disease, and cancer. Other risk factors specific to this age group include injuries and pharmacologic therapy.

Injuries in the older adult cause many different problems: illness, financial burden, hospitalization, self-care deficits, loss of independence, and even death. The risk of injury is increased by normal physical changes that accompany

BOX 2-2
HEALTHY BEHAVIORS IN THE MIDDLE ADULT

- Choose foods from all food groups, and eat a variety of foods.
- Choose a diet low in fat (30% or less of total calories), saturated fat (less than 10% of calories), and cholesterol (less than 300 mg daily). Adjust daily calorie intake to maintain healthy weight.
- Choose a diet that each day includes at least three servings of vegetables, two servings of fruits, and six servings of grains.
- Use sugar, salt, and sodium in moderation.
- Increase calcium intake (in perimenopausal women) to 800 mg daily.
- Consume high-fiber foods.
- Make exercise a part of life, carrying out regular exercise that is moderately strenuous, is consistent, and avoids overexertion; exercise for 30 minutes at least three times a week.
- Include exercise as part of any weight-reduction program.
- Have an annual vision examination.
- Have an annual dental checkup.
- Have a physical examination annually, including assessment for cancer of the thyroid, testes, prostate, mouth, ovaries, skin, colon, and lymph nodes.
- For females, have a mammogram every year from age 40 on. Have a breast examination annually.
- For females, have a Pap test as recommended for the young adult (see Box 2-1).
- Have an annual stool blood test; a digital rectal examination and a flexible sigmoidoscopy every 5 years; and a colonoscopy and digital rectal examination every 10 years or a double-contrast barium enema and a digital examination every 5 to 10 years.
- For males, have testicular and prostate examinations annually, including a prostate-specific antigen blood test (PSA), after age 50.
- Conduct breast or testicular self-examination every month. (The perimenopausal woman should set a specific date each month for the exam, as menstrual periods may be irregular or absent.)

aging, by changes in health, by environmental hazards, and by lack of support systems. The three major causes of injury in the older adult are falls, fires, and motor vehicle crashes. Of these causes, falls that result in hip fractures are the most significant in terms of long-term disability and death.

The average older adult in the community has 11 prescriptions filled each year. Although older adults constitute 13% of the total population, they consume 32% of all prescriptions (Eliopoulos, 1997). While these medications do make life more comfortable for the older adult, they carry a risk of adverse drug reactions and interactions. Other factors contributing to drug therapy problems in this age group include decreased metabolism, nutritional problems, visual deficits, memory changes, cost, and noncompliance.

In the older adult, the accumulation of years of exposure to environmental hazards such as sun and noise may be manifested by skin cancer or impaired hearing. The older adult (especially the older male) may develop respiratory disorders, from years of smoking or from exposure to pollutants in the work environment. The older adult with limited income may live in substandard housing and may suffer heat- or cold-related illness and even death.

CLINICAL alert
Elder abuse and neglect further increase the risk of injury or illness.

Psychosocial stressors for the older adult include the illness or death of a spouse, decreased or limited income, retirement, isolation from friends and family because of lack of transportation or distance, return to the home of a child, or relocation to a long-term health care facility. A further stressor may be role loss or reversal, for example, when the wife becomes the caretaker of her chronically ill husband.

The Family of the Adult Client

Although some clients are totally alone in the world, most have one or more people who are significant in their lives. These significant others may be related or bonded to the client by birth, adoption, marriage, or friendship. Although not always meeting traditional definitions, people (or even pets) significant to the client are the client's family. The nurse includes the family as an integral component of care in all health care settings.

FAMILY DEFINITIONS AND FUNCTIONS

What is a family? The definitions of a family are changing as society changes. According to one definition, a **family** is a unit of people related by marriage, birth, or adoption (Duvall, 1977). An expanded definition states that a family is two or more people who are emotionally involved with each other and live close to each other. In a global society, it may not be possible for family members to live nearby, but they do remain emotionally involved.

Although every family is unique, all families have certain structural and functional features in common. *Family structure* (family roles and relationships) and *family function* (interactions among family members and with the community) provide support, guidance, and stability. The family carries out the tasks that are necessary for its survival and continuity:

- Providing shelter, food, clothing, and health care
- Sharing money, time, and space according to each member's needs

TABLE 2-3 PHYSICAL CHANGES IN THE OLDER ADULT YEARS

ASSESSMENT	CHANGES
Skin	Decreased turgor and sebaceous gland activity result in dry, wrinkled skin. Melanocytes cluster, causing "age spots" or "liver spots."
Hair and nails	Scalp, axillary, and pubic hair thins; nose and ear hair thickens. Women may develop facial hair. Nails grow more slowly; may become thick and brittle.
Sensory	Visual field narrows, and depth perception is distorted. Pupils are smaller, reducing night vision. Lenses yellow and become opaque, resulting in distortion of green, blue, and violet tones and increased sensitivity to glare. Production of tears decreases. Sense of smell decreases. Age-related hearing loss progresses, involving middle- and low-frequency sounds. Threshold for pain and touch increases. Alterations in proprioception (sense of physical position) may occur.
Musculoskeletal	Loss of overall mass, strength, and movement of muscles occurs; tremors may occur. Loss of bone structure and deterioration of cartilage in joints result in increased risk of fractures and in limitation of range of motion.
Cardiovascular	Systolic blood pressure rises. Cardiac output decreases. Peripheral resistance increases, and capillary walls thicken.
Respiratory	Continued loss of vital capacity occurs as the lungs become less elastic and more rigid. Anteroposterior chest diameter increases; kyphosis. Although blood carbon dioxide levels remain relatively constant, blood oxygen levels decrease by 10% to 15%.
Gastrointestinal	Production of saliva decreases, and decreased number of taste buds decrease accurate receptors for salt and sweet. Gag reflex is decreased, and stomach motility and emptying are reduced. Both large and small intestines have some atrophy, with decreased peristalsis. The liver decreases in weight and storage capacity; gallstones increase; pancreatic enzymes decrease.
Genitourinary	Kidneys lose mass, and the glomerular filtration rate is reduced (by nearly 50% from young adulthood to old age). Bladder capacity decreases, and the micturition reflex is delayed. Urinary retention is more common. Women may have stress incontinence; men may have an enlarged prostate gland. Reproductive changes in men occur: ▪ Testosterone decreases. ▪ Sperm count decreases. ▪ Testes become smaller. ▪ Length of time to achieve an erection increases; erection is less full. Reproductive changes in women occur: ▪ Estrogen levels decrease. ▪ Breast tissue decreases. ▪ Vagina, uterus, ovaries, and urethra atrophy. ▪ Vaginal lubrication decreases. ▪ Vaginal secretions become alkaline.
Endocrine	Pituitary gland loses weight and vascularity. Thyroid gland becomes more fibrous, and plasma T_3 decreases. Pancreas releases insulin more slowly; increased blood glucose levels are common. Adrenal glands produce less cortisol.

- Determining the roles and responsibilities of each member for the support, management, and care of the home and other family members
- Ensuring the socialization of members by raising them to take on increasingly responsible roles in the family and in society
- Establishing socially acceptable ways to interact with others through communication and the expression of feelings in areas such as love, anger, and sexuality
- Rearing and releasing children appropriately
- Relating to the community (neighborhood, school, church, work) and establishing rules for relatives, guests, and friends

BOX 2-3
HEALTHY BEHAVIORS IN THE OLDER ADULT

- Choose foods from all food groups, and eat a variety of foods. Include some high-quality protein at each meal, such as low-fat milk and cheese, peanut butter, meat, fish, or poultry.
- Choose a diet low in fat (30% or less of total calories), saturated fat (less than 10% of calories), and cholesterol (less than 300 mg daily). Adjust daily caloric intake to balance energy expenditure and maintain healthy weight. A daily caloric intake of 1,200 kcal is recommended, but it may vary according to body build and activity level.
- Choose a diet that each day includes at least three servings of vegetables, two servings of fruits, and six servings of grains. Increased amounts of high-fiber foods may be necessary; if so, fluid intake should also be increased.
- Use sugar, salt, and sodium in moderation.
- Increase calcium intake to at least 800 mg per day (1,000 to 1,500 mg per day may be recommended).
- Make exercise a part of life, following a regular program of moderate exercise, such as walking or swimming. Avoid overexertion.
- Have an annual vision examination.
- Have an annual dental checkup.
- Have an annual physical examination that includes urinalysis and assessment for cancer of the thyroid, testes, prostate, mouth, ovaries, skin, colon, and lymph nodes.
- For females, have a breast examination and a mammogram annually.
- For females, have Pap tests as recommended by health care provider.

- For males, have an annual testicular and prostate examination including a PSA.
- Have a digital rectal examination and stool blood test annually. Have examinations as recommended for the middle adult (see Box 2-2).
- Conduct breast or testicular self-examination every month.
- Maintain immunizations for diphtheria and tetanus by having boosters every 10 years.
- Obtain annual immunization against influenza, especially with a history of chronic cardiovascular or respiratory illness.
- Practice the following to avoid injury:
  a. Have adequate lighting in all rooms of the house including stairs, basements, and bedrooms.
  b. Avoid sitting or standing rapidly; if dizziness occurs, remain in one position until dizziness is gone.
  c. Have handrails installed by the toilet and in the shower or bathtub.
  d. Do not use throw rugs.
  e. Install smoke alarms.
  f. Never step into a tub or shower without checking the temperature of the water.
  g. Always wear corrective lenses and/or hearing aids when driving.
  h. Do not drive a car after taking medications that cause drowsiness or dizziness.

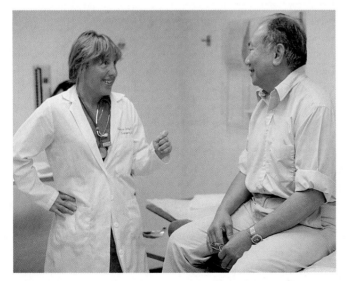

Figure 2-1. ◆ The older adult population is increasing more rapidly than any other age group, making gerontologic nursing a major part of medical-surgical nursing.

■ Maintaining morale and motivation, rewarding achievement, dealing with personal and family crises, setting attainable goals, and developing family loyalties and values

DEVELOPMENTAL STAGES AND TASKS OF THE FAMILY

The family, just like the individual, has developmental stages and tasks. Each stage brings change and requires adaptation. Each new stage also brings family-related risk factors for alterations in health. The nurse must consider both the needs of the client at a specific developmental stage and the needs of the client within a family with specific developmental tasks:

1. *A couple*—Two people, living together with or without being married, are in a period of establishing themselves as a couple. Their tasks are to adjust to living together as a couple, establish a mutually satisfying relationship, relate to kin, and decide whether or not to have children.

2. *The family with infants and preschoolers*—The young family must adjust to being more than a couple. They must support the needs and economic costs of more than two members. They must develop an attachment between parents and children, cope with lack of energy and privacy, and carry out activities that promote growth and development of the children.

3. *Family with school-age children*—The family with school-age children must adjust to the expanded world of children in school, encourage educational achievement, and promote joint decision making between children and parents.

4. *Family with adolescents and young adults*—The developmental tasks of this family unit focus on transition. Parents must provide a supportive home base and maintain open communications. They must balance freedom with responsibility and encourage adult children to become independent.

5. *Family with middle adults*—When the parents are middle-aged and children are no longer at home, their tasks are to maintain ties with older and younger generations, to plan for retirement, to reestablish their relationship, and (if necessary) to acquire the role of grandparents.

6. *Family with older adults*—The older adult family must adjust to retirement and aging. If a spouse dies, the surviving spouse must cope with the loss, adjust to living alone, or close the family home.

Health in the Adult Client

The World Health Organization (WHO) defines **health** as "a state of complete physical, mental, and social well-being, and not merely the absence of disease or infirmity" (WHO, 1974, p. 1). This definition is used as the classic definition of health. Even so, it does not take into account the many different levels of health a person may experience, or the fact that a person may be clinically described as ill and still define himself or herself as well. These additional factors, which greatly influence nursing care, include the health–illness continuum and high-level wellness.

THE HEALTH–ILLNESS CONTINUUM AND HIGH-LEVEL WELLNESS

The **health–illness continuum** represents health as a dynamic process, with high-level wellness at one extreme of the continuum and death at the opposite extreme (Figure 2-2 ◆). Individuals place themselves at different locations on the continuum at specific points in time.

Dunn (1959) expanded the concept of a continuum of health and illness in his description of high-level wellness. Dunn described wellness as an active process influenced by the environment. He distinguished good health from wellness. Good health can be passive, a state of freedom from illness in which the individual is at peace with the environment. High-level **wellness,** on the other hand, is a way of functioning to

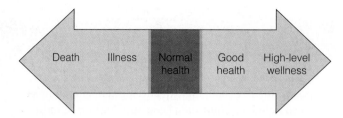

Figure 2-2. ◆ The health–illness continuum.

reach one's maximum potential at a particular point in time (Dunn, 1959, p. 4).

A person's self-concept, environment, culture, and spiritual values all influence wellness. Care based on a framework of wellness encourages active involvement by both the nurse and the client to promote, maintain, or restore health. It also supports the philosophy of *holistic health care,* in which all aspects of a person (physical, psychosocial, cultural, spiritual, and intellectual) are considered as essential components of individualized care.

FACTORS AFFECTING HEALTH

Many different factors affect a person's health or level of wellness. These factors often interact to promote health or to become risk factors for alterations in health. Major factors affecting health are listed below.

Genetic Makeup

Each person's genetic makeup influences health status throughout life. Genetic makeup affects personality, temperament, body structure, intellectual potential, and susceptibility to hereditary alterations in health. Chronic illnesses associated with genetic makeup include sickle-cell disease, hemophilia, diabetes mellitus, and cancer.

Cognitive Abilities and Educational Level

Cognitive abilities are determined prior to adulthood. The level of cognitive development (education) affects whether people view themselves as healthy or ill and may also affect health practices. Cognitive abilities may be lessened by injuries to the brain and illnesses affecting the brain. Educational level affects the ability to understand and follow health guidelines. For example, if a person cannot read, written information about healthy behaviors and health resources is worthless.

Race, Ethnicity, and Cultural Background

Certain diseases occur at a higher rate in some races and ethnic groups than in others. For example, in the United States, hypertension is more common in African Americans, tuberculosis and diabetes mellitus are among the leading causes of illness in Native Americans, and eye disorders are more prevalent in Chinese Americans. A person's ethnic and cultural background also influences health values and behaviors, lifestyle, and illness behaviors. Every culture defines health and illness in a unique way. In addition, each culture has its own health beliefs and illness treatment practices.

Age, Gender, and Developmental Level

Age, gender, and developmental level are factors in health and illness. Cardiovascular disorders are uncommon in young adults, but their incidence increases after the age of 40. Heart attacks are more common in men than women until women are past menopause. Some diseases occur only in one gender or the other, for example, prostate cancer in men and cervical cancer in women. The older adult has increased incidence of chronic illness and increased potential for serious illness or death from infectious illnesses (such as influenza and pneumonia).

Lifestyle and Environment

The components of a person's lifestyle that affect health status include patterns of eating, use of chemical substances (alcohol, nicotine, caffeine, legal and illegal drugs), exercise and rest patterns, and coping methods. Examples of altered responses are the relationship of obesity to hypertension, cigarette smoking to chronic obstructive pulmonary disease, a sedentary lifestyle to heart disease, and a high-stress career to alcoholism. The environment has a major influence on health. Occupational exposure to toxic substances (such as asbestos and coal dust) increases the risk of pulmonary disorders. Air, water, and food pollution increases the risk of respiratory disorders, infectious diseases, and cancer. Seasonal temperature variations can result in hypothermia or hyperthermia, especially in the older adult.

Socioeconomic Background

Both lifestyle and environmental influences are affected by one's income level. The culture of poverty, which crosses all racial and ethnic boundaries, negatively influences health status. Living at or below the poverty level often results in crowded, unsanitary living conditions or homelessness. Housing is often overcrowded, lacks adequate heating or cooling, and is infested with insects and rats. Crowded living conditions increase the risk of transferring communicable diseases. Other problems include lack of infant and child care, lack of medical care for injuries or illness, inadequate nutrition, use of addictive substances, and violence.

Geographic Area

The geographic area in which one lives influences health status. Illnesses like malaria are more common in tropical areas of North America. Multiple sclerosis occurs with greater frequency in the northern United States and Canada. There are more cases of skin cancers in people living in sunny, hot areas, and more sinus infections among people living in areas with high humidity.

HEALTH PROMOTION AND MAINTENANCE

For many years, nursing care focused on the acutely ill client in the hospital setting. With changes in society and in health care, this emphasis is shifting toward prevention and community-based care. The focus of this book is not community health nursing. However, teaching health maintenance and providing continuity of care as a client moves among health care settings are two essential aspects of medical-surgical nursing.

Certain practices are known to promote health and wellness:

- Eating three balanced meals a day and including foods according to the Food Guide Pyramid (see Figure 18-4, page 398)
- Eating moderately to maintain a healthy weight
- Exercising moderately, following a regular routine
- Sleeping 7 to 8 hours each day
- Limiting alcohol consumption to a moderate amount
- Eliminating smoking
- Keeping sun exposure to a minimum

The nurse promotes health by teaching the activities that maintain wellness, by providing information about the characteristics and consequences of diseases when risk factors have been identified, and by supplying specific information about decreasing risk factors. The nurse also promotes health by following healthy practices and serving as a role model.

Illness in the Adult Client

DISEASE

Disease (literal meaning, "without ease") is a medical term describing alterations in structure and function of the body or mind. Diseases may have mechanical causes, biologic causes, or normative causes. *Mechanical causes* of disease damage the structure of the body; they are the result of trauma or extremes of temperature. *Biologic causes* of disease affect body function; they are the result of genetic defects, aging, infestation and infection, changes in the immune system, and alterations in normal organ secretions. *Normative causes* are psychological but involve a mind–body interaction, so physical manifestations occur in response to the emotional disturbance (e.g., hives).

The 10 leading causes of death in the United States are heart disease, cancer, stroke, chronic obstructive pulmonary disease, accidents, pneumonia/influenza, diabetes, suicide, kidney disease, and chronic liver disease. The cause of many diseases is still unknown. The following are generally accepted as common causes of disease:

- Genetic defects
- Developmental defects resulting from exposure to viruses, chemicals, or drugs that affect the developing fetus
- Biologic agents or toxins (including viruses, bacteria, rickettsia, fungi, protozoa, and helminths)
- Physical agents, such as temperature extremes, radiation, and electricity
- Chemical agents, such as alcohol, drugs, strong acids or bases, and heavy metals
- Generalized response of tissues to injury or irritation
- Alterations in the production of antibodies, resulting in allergies or hypersensitivities

■ Faulty metabolic processes (e.g., a production of hormones or enzymes above or below normal)
■ Continued, unabated stress

In all types of disease, alterations in structure or function cause **manifestations** (signs and symptoms) that prompt a person to seek treatment. Although both subjective symptoms and objective signs commonly appear with disease, objective signs often predominate. Examples include bleeding, vomiting, diarrhea, limitation of movement, swelling, visual disturbances, or changes in elimination. However, pain (a subjective symptom) is often the main reason a person seeks health care. (Disease classifications are provided in Table 2-4 ◆.)

ILLNESS

Illness is the response a person has to a disease. This response is highly individualized, as the person responds not only to his or her own perceptions of the disease but also to the perceptions of others. Illness integrates pathophysiologic alterations; psychologic effects of those alterations; effects on roles, relationships, and values; and cultural and spiritual beliefs. A person may have a disease and not categorize himself or herself as ill, or may validate feelings of illness through the comments of others ("You don't look as though you feel well today").

Acute Illness

An **acute illness** occurs rapidly, lasts for a relatively short period of time, and is self-limiting. The condition responds to self-treatment or to medical-surgical intervention. Clients with uncomplicated acute illnesses usually have full recovery and return to normal preillness functioning.

The experience of being acutely ill is described as a sequence of behaviors for coping with the alterations in health and function caused by disease. Illness behaviors are highly individual, but the general stages were described by Suchman (1972):

1. In the first stage of an acute illness, a person experiences one or more manifestations that signal that a change in normal health. The most significant of these is pain. Others are bleeding, difficulty breathing, swelling, or fever. When manifestations are mild or are familiar (such as symptoms of the common cold or influenza), the person usually uses over-the-counter medications or a traditional remedy for self-treatment. If the symptoms are relieved, no further action is taken. However, if the symptoms are severe or become worse, the person moves to the next stage.

2. In the second stage, the person assumes the sick role, accepting the symptoms as proof that an illness is present. The person usually discusses the symptoms with others and seeks support in deciding whether to get professional treatment or to stay home from school or work. People are self-preoccupied at this stage, focusing on alterations in function that result from the illness. If the illness is resolved, the person confirms health status with others and resumes normal activities. However, if manifestations remain or increase and others agree that no improvement has occurred, the person moves to the next stage.

3. The third stage is seeking medical care. In our society, a physician most often provides validation of illness. People who believe themselves to be ill (and who are encouraged by others to contact a health care provider) make the medical contact for diagnosis, prognosis, and treatment of the illness. If the medical diagnosis is of an illness, the person moves to the next stage. If the medical diagnosis does not support illness, the client may return to normal

TABLE 2-4	DISEASE CLASSIFICATION DEFINITIONS
CLASSIFICATION	**DEFINITION**
Acute	A disease that has a rapid onset, lasts a relatively short period of time, and is self-limiting.
Chronic	A disease that has one or more of these characteristics: (1) is permanent, (2) leaves permanent disability, (3) causes nonreversible pathophysiology, (4) requires special training of the client for rehabilitation, (5) requires a long period of care
Communicable	A disease that can spread from one person to another
Congenital	A disease or disorder that exists at or before birth
Degenerative	A disease that results from deterioration or impairment of organs or tissues
Functional	A disease that affects function or performance but does not have manifestations of organic illness
Malignant	A disease that tends to become worse and cause death
Psychosomatic	A psychological disease that is manifested by physiologic symptoms
Idiopathic	A disease that has an unknown cause
Iatrogenic	A disease that is caused by medical therapy

functioning or may seek a second opinion from a different health care provider.

4. The stage of assuming a dependent role begins when a person accepts the diagnosis and planned treatment of the illness. As the severity of the illness increases, so does the dependent role. During this stage, the person may enter the hospital for treatment and care. The person's responses to care depend on many different variables: the severity of the illness, the degree of anxiety or fear about the outcome, the loss of roles, the support systems available, individualized reactions to stress, and previous experiences with illness care.

5. The final stage of an acute illness is recovery and rehabilitation. The person now gives up the dependent role and resumes normal roles and responsibilities. As a result of education during treatment and care, the person may be at a higher level of wellness after recovery is complete. There is no set timetable for recovery from an illness; each person responds differently. Both the severity of the illness and the method of treatment affect the length of time required, as does the person's compliance with treatment plans and motivation to return to normal health.

Institutional health care focuses on the acute care needs of the ill client. Recovery begins in the hospital and is completed at home. This focus makes client education and continuity of care a major goal for nursing. It has also contributed to a shift in care settings. Increasing numbers of nurses now provide care in community settings and the home.

Chronic Illness

The term **chronic illness** describes many different lifelong pathologic and psychological alterations in health. Chronic illness is the leading health problem in the world today, and it is estimated that the number of persons with chronic illnesses will triple by the year 2040. Current trends affecting an increased incidence of chronic illnesses include diseases of aging, diseases of lifestyle and behavior, the AIDS epidemic, and environmental factors.

The National Commission on Chronic Illness states that a **chronic illness** is any impairment or deviation from normal functioning that has one or more of the following characteristics:

- It is permanent.
- It leaves permanent disability.
- It is caused by nonreversible pathologic alterations.
- It requires special teaching of the client for rehabilitation.
- It may require a long period of care.

Chronic illness is also characterized by impaired function in more than one body system. Responses to the impaired function may occur in sensory perception, self-care abilities, mobility, cognition, and social skills. The demands on the individual and family as a result of these responses are often lifelong (Miller, 1983).

The intensity of a chronic illness and its related symptoms ranges from mild to severe, and the illness is usually characterized by periods of remission and exacerbation. During periods of **remission,** the person does not experience symptoms, even though the disease is still clinically present. During periods of **exacerbation,** the symptoms reappear. These periods of change do not appear in all chronic diseases.

Each person with a chronic illness has a unique set of responses and needs. The response of the person to the illness is influenced by many different factors:

- The point in the life cycle at which the onset of the illness occurs
- The type and degree of limitations caused by the illness
- The visibility of impairment or disfigurement
- The stigma attached to the impairment or disfigurement
- The pathophysiology causing the illness
- The relationship between the impairment and functioning in social roles
- Pain and fear

These factors are highly complex. They are interrelated within each person, resulting in individualized illness behaviors and needs. Because there are so many different chronic diseases and because the experience of each person with the illness is a mix of individualized responses, it is difficult to generalize about needs. However, almost all people with a chronic illness will need to do the following:

- Live as normally as possible, despite the symptoms and treatment that make them feel alienated, lonely, and different from others without the illness
- Learn to adapt activities of daily living and self-care activities
- Grieve over the loss of physical function and structure, income, status, roles, and dignity
- Learn to live with chronic pain
- Comply with a medical treatment plan
- Maintain a positive self-concept
- Maintain a sense of hope
- Maintain a feeling of being in control
- Confront the inevitability of death (Miller, 1983; Pollock, 1986)

Some people with chronic illness successfully meet health-related needs; others do not. Research indicates that adaptation is influenced by variables such as anger, depression, denial, self-concept, locus of control, hardiness, and disability. Nursing interventions for the person with a chronic illness focus on education to promote independent functioning, reduce health care costs, and improve well-being and quality of life.

The client with a chronic illness may be hospitalized for diagnosis and treatment of acute exacerbations, but the care of the client is primarily provided at home. "Although it is the individual who is diagnosed with the chronic disease, the entire family experiences life with the illness" (Woods et al., 1989, p. 46). Chronic illness in a family member is a major stressor that may cause changes in family structure and function, as well as changes in performing family developmental tasks.

Many different factors affect family responses to chronic illness. Family responses in turn affect the client's response to and perception of the illness. Factors influencing response to chronic illness include personal, social, and economic resources; the nature and course of the disease; and demands of the illness as perceived by family members.

Client and family considerations for home care are integrated throughout this book. It is important to remember that standardized teaching plans may not be effective. Chronically ill clients and families should be given the freedom to choose appropriate literature, self-help or support groups, and interactions with others with the same illness. Information provided by the nurse must be tailored to specific, current needs.

(*Note:* The bibliography listings for this and all chapters have been compiled at the back of the book.)

Chapter Review

key terms by topic

Use the CD-ROM disk enclosed with your textbook to hear the pronunciation of the key terms in the chapter.

Adult client
alterations in health

Family of the adult client
family

Health in the adult client
health, health–illness continuum, high-level wellness

Illness in the adult client
disease, manifestations, illness, acute illness, chronic illness, remission, exacerbation

key points

■ The young adult is at the peak of physical development. Risks for alterations in health include accidents, sexually transmitted diseases, substance abuse, and physical or psychosocial stressors.

■ The middle adult, although physically similar to the young adult, does have age-related changes. Risks for alterations in health include obesity, cardiovascular disease, cancer, substance abuse, and psychosocial stressors.

■ The older adult has many normal age-related physical changes. Risk factors for alterations in health include obesity, cardiovascular disease, cancer, injuries, visual and hearing deficits, and psychosocial stressors.

■ All families have structure (family roles and relationships) and function (interactions with other family members and the community). The nurse must consider the needs of the client and the needs of the client's family when providing care.

■ Health and illness are affected by many different factors. Nursing interventions to promote health are essential, no matter the degree of illness or the setting in which care is provided.

Medialink

Additional interactive resources for this chapter can be found on the Companion Website at www.prenhall.com/burke. Click on Chapter 2 and "Begin" to select the activities for this chapter.

For NCLEX review questions and an audio glossary, access the accompanying CD-ROM in this book.

for further study

For more about nursing care for clients with substance abuse problems, see Chapter 11.

For more about teaching healthy food choices, see Figure 18-4, the Food Guide Pyramid.

Critical Thinking Care Map

Caring for a Client with Early-Onset Diabetes
NCLEX-PN Focus Area: Psychosocial Adaptation

Case Study: Alexis Burd has had the chronic illness diabetes mellitus (requiring daily insulin injections) since she was 4 years old. She is now 36 years old, is married, and has two teen-age children. While you are weighing Alexis during her regular appointment at the diabetes clinic, she begins to cry and says, "I think this disease controls me more than I control it."

Nursing Diagnosis: Powerlessness

COLLECT DATA

Subjective	Objective
_____	_____
_____	_____
_____	_____
_____	_____
_____	_____
_____	_____

Would you report this data? Yes/No

If yes, to: _____

Data Collected
(use those that apply)

• Height: 5'3"
• Weight: 156 lbs.
• Blood pressure: 126/64
• Fasting blood glucose: 180 (normal 110–130)
• States, "I'm not a good mother anymore."
• States, "I have done everything I was told to do."
• States, "I think I will just stop taking my insulin."

Nursing Care

_____
_____
_____
_____
_____
_____
_____
_____
_____

How would you document this? _____
_____
_____

Nursing Interventions
(use those that apply)

• Discuss weight-reduction diet.
• Discuss exercise plan.
• Listen carefully to Alexis's concerns.
• State "Tell me more about how you think diabetes controls you."
• Suggest that Alexis join a diabetes support group.
• Ask Alexis to keep a daily diary of self-management activities.

NCLEX-PN Exam Preparation

TEST-TAKING TIP

Do not read into the questions. When answering a question, remember that the only client you are considering is the one in the question.

1. The young adult is at risk for alterations in health from:
   a. accidents, STDs, and substance abuse
   b. obesity, cardiovascular disease, and cancer
   c. chronic illness, stroke, and substance abuse
   d. injuries, pharmacologic therapy, and obesity

2. The middle adult often has a problem with weight gain as a result of having:
   a. the same calorie intake with decreased physical activity
   b. physical and psychosocial stressors
   c. chronic illness such as arthritis and hypertension
   d. normal physiologic changes of aging

3. Health promotion behaviors in the older adult include:
   a. males having prostate examinations every 5 years
   b. having a vision examinations every 2 to 4 years
   c. obtaining annual immunizations against influenza
   d. carrying out regular exercise that is strenuous

4. Significant others related or bonded to the client by birth, adoption, marriage, or friendship are the client's family, and the nurse should:
   a. ask them to step out when giving nursing care
   b. expect them to assist with care of the client
   c. speak with them regarding confidential client matters
   d. include them as an integral component of health care

5. An active process that maximizes the potential capability of a person within the environment where he or she is functioning is known as:
   a. health
   b. wellness
   c. continuum
   d. integration

6. Factors that affect a client's ability to understand and follow guidelines for health are:
   a. race and ethnicity
   b. cognitive abilities and educational level
   c. lifestyle and environment
   d. socioeconomic background and geographic area

7. The nurse, by following healthy practices, serves as a role model, which is one way to:
   a. provide continuity of care
   b. provide acute care
   c. promote health
   d. identify risk factors

8. The response a person has to disease is called:
   a. illness
   b. biologic
   c. normative
   d. developmental

9. An illness that occurs rapidly, lasts for a short period, and is self-limiting is known as:
   a. remission
   b. chronic
   c. exacerbation
   d. acute

10. Nearly all people with a chronic illness need:
    a. to live as normally as possible
    b. to live in a health care facility
    c. to be assisted with activities of daily living
    d. large doses of pain relief medication

Answers for Review Questions, as well as discussion of Case Study Critical Thinking questions, appear in Appendix V.

Cultural Care STRATEGIES

Assessing Communication Variables from a Cultural Perspective

Mrs. Kin-Lee, a 25-year-old Vietnamese woman, arrived in the emergency room in transition with very strong and closely spaced contractions. Despite her imminent delivery she did not initiate conversation or communicate urgency about getting attention from the staff. She answered questions politely, nodding and smiling respectfully at the staff between occasional grimaces during the contractions. The only other sign of pain was her white knuckles as she grasped the armrests on the wheelchair in which she was placed. Many Vietnamese, as most Asians, believe that a woman must experience pain as part of childbirth, and that expressing these feelings will bring on shame.

Verbal and nonverbal methods of communication vary significantly among persons in different cultures. Communication presents the most significant challenge in working with clients from diverse cultural backgrounds, since the meaning of communication may vary by culture. The nurse who is aware of communication variables can be more attentive to nuances and different meanings of communication across cultures.

Communication

Communication embraces the entire world of human interaction and behavior. Communication provides the means by which people connect, and it is also the means by which culture is transmitted and preserved. Regardless of culture, individuals learn to think feel, believe, and strive for what their culture considers proper. Both verbal and nonverbal communications are learned within one's culture (Giger & Davidhizar, 1999). The nurse should be aware of these communication variables:

Dialect. Dialect largely depends on geographic location. For example, clients from Appalachia, Australia, and England speak English quite differently from one another.

Language style. Words may have *different meanings* in different cultures. For example, the word "bad" may have a positive meaning to a teenager and have a more typical, negative meaning to an adult (Giger & Davidhizar, 1999).

Volume of speech. Volume of speech may be culturally determined. Irish people, for example, frequently raise their voices. In contrast, others (such as the Japanese) tend to keep their voices low.

Touch. Use of touch varies widely among cultures. Because nurses use touch to reassure, provide affirmation, and decrease loneliness, we must be aware of how it is perceived. Depending on the situation and the culture of the person, touch can also be perceived as threatening, intrusive, or seductive.

Context of speech or emotional tone. Context of speech refers to the use *of emotion* when communicating. The Black American, Jewish, or German client is less likely to use an emotional tone than one who is Italian, Irish, or Mexican (Giger & Davidhizar, 1999). Arabs may express their emotions openly through nonverbal cues and voice, but may withhold some feelings from strangers. Arabs may express agreement in front of strangers that does not reflect their true meanings (Meleis, 1996). An Arab may tend to protect others from disagreements or indicate disagreement by simply raising an eyebrow rather than responding verbally.

Kinesics. Kinesics refers to the use of stances, gestures, and eye behavior when communicating with others. Vietnamese individuals typically nod and smile to indicate respect when interacting with a health care professional (Giger & Davidhizar, 1999). However, they may or may not be agreeing with what is being said.

Nursing Implications

• **Assess verbal and nonverbal communication for cultural variations in meaning.** The nurse should be attentive to variations between and within cultures in relation to dialect, language style, volume of speech, touch, context of speech, and kinesics. A misinterpretation of communication due to cultural differences can create misunderstanding and deficits in meaning a client's needs.

• **Determine how respect can be communicated within a particular culture.** In some cultures a client will not confide information until a relationship with the caregiver has developed. Thus, use of "small talk" may be essential to develop a therapeutic relationship. In other cases, calling clients by their last names or greeting them by name is important. It may be helpful to greet an individual by title and first name, to approach and shake hands or to smile with direct eye contact. In every case, it is important to assess the response of the individual, to determine the client's comfort level, and to adapt communication strategies depending on the response of the individual.

Self-Reflection Questions

1. What personal communication techniques do you use when approaching individuals for the first time?
2. What communication techniques do you observe among other cultures during your initial greeting?
3. What generally accepted communication techniques can you use to communicate respect to persons from another culture?

chapter **3**

Community-Based and Home Care of the Adult Client

LEARNING outcomes

After completing this chapter, you will be able to:

- Define community-based nursing care.
- Identify types of community-based health care services.
- Discuss the components of home health and the roles of the home health nurse.
- Describe nursing care provided in the client's home.
- Apply the nursing process to care of the client in the home.
- Describe the philosophy of and nursing care to facilitate rehabilitation.

MediaLink

 www.prenhall.com/burke

Use the above address to access the free, interactive Companion Website created for this textbook. Get hints, instant feedback, and textbook references to chapter-related multiple choice questions. Link to other interesting sites.

As recently as two decades ago, clients went to the hospital for almost all health care services, including diagnostic tests and minor surgery. Now, hospitals have become primarily acute-care centers with services focused on high-technology care for severely ill or injured people or for people having major surgery. Even these clients rarely remain in the hospital for long periods of time. They are moved as rapidly as possible to less acute-care settings within the hospital and then to community-based care. Health care has changed from a pay-for-service inpatient method of delivery to a managed-care, community-based system. This shift in health care settings has changed the way nurses provide interventions to promote and restore health. Although many nurses are still employed in hospitals, nursing care is increasingly provided outside the hospital setting.

Community-Based Nursing Care

A community is many things. Encompassing a specific geographic area, a *community* may be a small neighborhood in a major urban city or a large area of rural residents. Communities have in common the characteristics of people, area, social interaction, and common ties. However, each community is unique. People who live in a community may share a culture, history, or heritage. Although a community is where people live, have homes, raise families, and carry on daily activities, people within a community may cross community boundaries to work or to seek health care. Nurses who provide care within a community need to know the composition and characteristics of the clients with which they will work. For example, urban residents may not know or speak to their neighbors, whereas rural residents are usually closely knit and have strong patterns of communication.

In contrast to community health nursing, which focuses on the health of the community, *community-based nursing* focuses on culturally competent individual and family health care needs. The nurse practicing community-based care provides direct services to individuals to manage acute or chronic health problems and to promote self-care. Nursing care is based on a philosophy that directs nursing care for clients wherever they are, including where they live, work, play, worship, and go to school (Zotti, Brown, & Stotts, 1996).

Nurses provide community-based care in many different settings. They do activities that range from leading support groups in a hospital (for individuals and family members diagnosed with illnesses like cancer or diabetes) to managing a free-standing clinic, to providing care in the client's home. Box 3-1 illustrates the varied settings within the community in which a nurse may provide care.

Types of Community-Based Health Care Services

There are many different types of community-based health care services.

BOX 3-1
COMMUNITY-BASED NURSING CARE SETTINGS

- Hospitals
  Inpatient care
  Outpatient (ambulatory) surgery
  Outpatient diagnostics and treatments
  Cardiac rehabilitation
  Support groups
  Education groups
- County health departments
- Senior centers
- Long-term care
- Parish nursing
- Adult day care centers
- Homeless shelters
- Mobile vans
- Mental health centers
- Schools
- Crisis intervention centers
- Ambulatory surgery centers
- Alcohol/drug rehabilitation
- Health care provider offices
- Health care clinics
- Free clinics
- Urgent care centers
- Rural health centers
- Home care
- Hospice care
- Industry
- Jails and prisons

COMMUNITY CENTERS AND CLINICS

Community centers and clinics may be directed by physicians, advanced practice nurses in collaboration with physicians, or advanced practice nurses who work independently (depending on state regulations). These health care settings may be located within a hospital, be part of a hospital but located in another area, or be independent of a hospital base. Health care centers and clinics provide a wide range of services and often meet the health needs of clients who are unable to get care elsewhere. This group includes the homeless, the poor, those with substance abuse problems, those with sexually transmitted diseases, and the victims of violent or abusive behavior.

DAY CARE PROGRAMS

Day care programs, such as senior centers, are usually located in a location where people gather for social, nutritional, and recreational purposes. These programs vary from community to community. Meals may be provided at low cost.

LONG-TERM CARE FACILITIES

People who are mentally or physically unable to care for themselves independently may require health care and help with activities of daily living in a **long-term care** facility. The care may be for only a few days, or it may last for years. Many different types of long-term care facilities are available, including skilled care, intermediate and long-term care, transitional (from acute care) care, nursing homes, retirement centers, and residential institutions for disabled persons of all ages.

The number of long-term care facilities has increased for several reasons. Care of clients at home after increasingly short hospital stays is often beyond the abilities of the client and family. Such clients are often transferred to a long-term facility for care until they can use home care. In addition, many older adults do not have any family available to provide care but can no longer safely care for themselves. More and more older adults are moving to retirement centers, where they remain independent as long as they can, and then have nursing care and other services (such as meals) readily available.

Nursing homes are long-term facilities that provide care primarily for older adults. The focus is on maintaining client function and independence. Concern for the clients' well-being, and increased knowledge of the importance of the environment, has resulted in more homelike surroundings that include plants, birds, and pets. Legislation to maintain standards of quality assurance in the nursing home industry was mandated by the 1987 Omnibus Budget Reconciliation Act (OBRA).

The roles of the nurse in long-term care include providing direct care, serving as a unit manager and teaching and supervising other health care providers. Almost all long-term care facilities require that care given to residents be performed only by or under the direct supervision of a licensed nurse.

PARISH NURSING AND BLOCK NURSING

Parish nursing and block nursing are nontraditional ways of providing health promotion and health restoration nursing interventions to specific groups of people. Both of these types of care are community based and meet the needs of people often underserved by the traditional health care system.

A nurse who practices **parish nursing** works with the pastor and staff of a faith community to promote health and healing through counseling, referrals, teaching, and assessment of health care needs. A parish nurse may be employed by a hospital and contracted by a church, employed directly by a church, or work as a volunteer with the congregation of a church. The parish nurse helps bridge gaps between members of the church and the health care system.

Block nursing is care provided by the nurse to people who live on the same block as the nurse. Services are administered based on need rather than on eligibility for reimbursement. Other residents of the block often provide volunteer services to assist the nurse, with funding for care often coming from grants and demonstration projects.

MEALS ON WHEELS

Many communities have a food service, usually called Meals on Wheels, for older people who do not have assistance in the home for food preparation. A hot, nutritionally balanced meal is delivered once a day, usually at noon. Volunteers often deliver the meals, providing not only nutrition but also a friendly, caring visit each day.

HOME HEALTH AGENCIES

Home health agencies are either public or private organizations that provide skilled nursing and other therapeutic services in the client's home. All home health agencies must meet uniform standards for licensing, certification, and accreditation. Home health agencies include the following:

- *Official or public agencies.* These are agencies operated by state or local governments, financed primarily by tax funds. Most official agencies offer home care, health education, and disease-prevention programs in the community.
- *Voluntary or private not-for-profit agencies.* These agencies are supported by donations, endowments, charities such as the United Way, and third-party reimbursement. They are governed by a volunteer board of directors, which usually represent the community they serve.
- *Private, proprietary agencies.* Most of these agencies are for-profit organizations and are governed by either individual owners or national corporations. Although some of these agencies participate in third-party reimbursement, others rely on "private-pay" sources.
- *Institution-based agencies.* These agencies operate under a parent organization, such as a hospital. The home health agency is governed by the sponsoring organization, and the mission of both is similar. Often, most of the home health referrals come from the parent organization.

Home Health Care

Home health care includes health and social services, provided to the chronically ill, disabled, or recovering person in his or her own home. Home care is usually provided when a person needs help that cannot be provided by a family member or friend on an ongoing basis for a period of time. Among clients who benefit from home health care services are those who:

- Cannot live independently at home because of age, illness, or disability
- Have illnesses such as congestive heart failure, heart disease, kidney disease, respiratory diseases, diabetes mellitus, or muscle–nerve disorders
- Are terminally ill and want to die with comfort and dignity at home (see Chapter 9).
- Do not need inpatient hospital or nursing home care but require additional assistance
- Need short-term help at home because of outpatient surgery

Services provided within the home include professional nursing care, home health care assistance, physical therapy, speech therapy, occupational therapy, medical social worker services, and nutritional services. Clients receiving home health care services are usually under the care of a physician, with the focus of care being treatment or rehabilitation. Nursing care is provided by registered nurses or licensed practical nurses based on physician orders. These nurses give direct care, supervise other health care providers, coordinate client care with the physician, advocate for the client and family, and teach family members and friends how to care for the client.

HISTORY OF HOME CARE

The concept of nurses meeting health care needs in the home and community is not new. Although many sources say the birth of home care in the United States occurred when the Boston Dispensary's first home care program opened in 1796, it wasn't until visiting nursing associations were established in the late 1800s that care of the sick in their own homes took hold.

At that time, few hospitals were available to handle the health and illness problems of a nation experiencing both rapid growth in its cities and a large influx of immigrants. Illness and hygiene problems resulted from substandard living and working conditions. In response, several philanthropic individuals and organizations sponsored nurses to visit the sick poor in their homes.

The role of the nurse then, as today, was to advocate for the client, provide direct care, and educate the client. Both illness care and health promotion were the nurse's principal focus.

Home care nursing services continued to develop and grow in the twentieth century. Home care benefits to policyholders were provided by the Metropolitan Life Insurance Company. The American Red Cross introduced visiting nursing services. The Frontier Nursing Service was established. Physician home visits declined during World War II. In 1946, the "hospital without walls" was introduced, which was a posthospitalization home care program developed by Montefiore Hospital in New York City.

The passage of Medicare in 1965, Medicaid in 1970, the addition of hospice benefits in 1973, and the introduction of diagnosis-related groups in 1983 have dramatically affected home care. In 1965, Medicare legislation entitled the nation's elderly to home care services, primarily skilled nursing and other therapies of a curative or restorative nature. This same benefit was extended to certain disabled younger Americans in 1973. As a result, between 1967 and 1980, the number of Medicare-certified home health agencies nearly doubled.

This number doubled again when diagnosis-related groups were introduced. Diagnosis-related groups (DRGs) are categories for reimbursement of inpatient services. The DRG system pays a predetermined amount of money for the care of different persons with the same medical diagnosis. DRGs were introduced in an effort to control the rapidly increasing cost of health care. Prior to their introduction, Medicare reimbursed hospitals on a cost-plus basis, paying for the actual cost of caring for an individual plus other allowable expenses, such as depreciation of facilities and administrative costs. Many changes in the health care system have been attributed to the introduction of DRGs, including earlier discharge from hospitals and the increased need for home care services.

Nurses who practice home care do so within a system where clients, referral sources, physicians, and reimbursement sources interact. Like any other system, it functions best when its members communicate and cooperate.

This discussion provides basic information about the requirements and standards for home care nursing in general. Rules and regulations for home care and for nursing licensure mandate at what level of education the nurse must be to carry out activities.

HOME CARE CLIENTS

The *client* in home health is both the person receiving care and the person's family. As mentioned, the client's family is not limited to persons related by birth, adoption, or marriage. It may include lovers, colleagues, other significant people, and even animals.

Even though home care is provided to clients of all ages, age and functional disability are the main predictors of need for home care services. A national survey by the Agency for Health Care Policy and Research found that (a) about half of all home care clients are over the age of 65, and (b) the number of home care services that are needed seems to increase with the client's age (National Association for Home Care, 2000).

REFERRALS

A *referral source* is a person who recommends home health services and supplies the agency with details about the client's needs. A referral source can be a physician, nurse, social worker, therapist, or discharge planner. Families sometimes generate their own referrals, either by approaching one of the sources already mentioned or by calling a home health agency directly. When the family seeks a referral and the agency feels that the client qualifies for services, the agency contacts the client's physician and requests a referral on the client's behalf.

HOME CARE ORDER AND INITIAL VISIT

Home care cannot begin without a physician's order and cannot proceed without a physician-approved treatment plan.

CLINICAL alert

The physician-approved treatment plan is a legal and reimbursement requirement.

Once a referral is made and an initial set of physician orders is obtained, a nursing assessment visit is scheduled to identify the client's needs. If the input of another provider, such as a physical therapist, is necessary to complete the initial assessment, the nurse arranges for this visit. Data may be collected and the treatment plan formulated through collaboration of the LPN and RN.

At the nursing assessment visit, the nurse identifies client needs and begins to formulate the plan of care. Box 3-2 lists Medicare's required data for the nursing plan of care. The plan of care is sent back to the physician for review and approval. The physician's signature on the plan of care authorizes the home health agency's providers to continue with services and also serves as a contract indicating agreement to participate in the care of the client on an ongoing basis.

REIMBURSEMENT SOURCES

A *reimbursement source* is a party that pays for home health services. Medicare is home care's largest single reimbursement source. Other reimbursement sources include Medicaid, public funding, private insurance, public donation, and self-pay.

The treatment (or care) plan formulated by the home health agency providers and authorized by the physician is used by the reimbursement source. Only interventions identified on the treatment plan are paid for. The reimbursement source evaluates each treatment plan to determine whether the goals and plans set forth by the professional providers match the needs assessed. Periodically, the reimbursement source may ask for the home health provider's notes to substantiate what is being done in the home. Therefore, accurate documentation is critical.

Medicare's regulations for reimbursement are the model for many other third-party payers. Medicare has specifically defined what skilled services will be reimbursed in home health. Medicare does not reimburse visits made to support general health maintenance, health promotion, or clients' emotional or socioeconomic needs. There are very specific criteria that both client and nurse must meet in order to secure Medicare reimbursement. The client must meet all of the following criteria:

- The client must be in need of "reasonable and necessary" home care with a "skilled need."
- The client must be essentially homebound.
- The client must have a plan of care that meets the necessary Medicare criteria.
- The client must require intervention on an intermittent basis only.

Medicare will reimburse only when the skilled provider performs at least one of the following tasks:

- Teaching about a new or acute situation
- Assessing an acute process or a change in the client's condition
- Performing a skilled procedure or a hands-on service requiring the skill, knowledge, ability, and judgment of a licensed nurse

ROLES OF THE HOME HEALTH NURSE

The roles of the home health nurse are similar to those of nurses in any setting: advocate, care provider, and educator.

Advocate

As client advocate, the nurse explores, informs, supports, and affirms the choices of clients. As a protector of client rights, the nurse discusses advance medical directives, living wills, durable power of attorney for health care, and the home health agency's bill of rights. Box 3-3 provides an example of a home health agency's bill of rights.

During the course of care, clients may need help negotiating the complex medical system (especially in regard to medical insurance), accessing community resources, recognizing and coping with required changes in lifestyle, and making informed decisions. When the family's desires differ from those of the client, advocacy can be a challenge. It is impossible for the nurse to please everyone. If a conflict arises, the nurse must remain the primary client's advocate, regardless of any negative response from the family.

Provider of Care

Home health nurses usually are not involved in providing personal care for clients (bathing, changing linens, etc.). Routine personal care usually is provided by the family or by a home health aide arranged for by the nurse. If a personal care need arises during the course of the skilled visit (e.g., if a client has an incontinent episode), the nurse typically either bathes and changes the client or assists the caregiver to do so before moving on to the skilled activities planned for the visit.

The nurse uses the nursing process to collect data, diagnose, plan and implement care, and evaluate client needs. During the course of this process, home health nurses frequently perform specific procedures and treatments, such as physical assessments, care of intravenous lines, ostomy care, wound care, and pain management.

BOX 3-2
MEDICARE'S REQUIRED DATA FOR THE PLAN OF CARE

1. All pertinent diagnoses
2. A notation of the beneficiary's mental status
3. Types of services, supplies, and equipment ordered
4. Frequency of visits to be made
5. Client's prognosis
6. Client's rehabilitation potential
7. Client's functional limitations
8. Activities permitted
9. Client's nutritional requirements
10. Client's medications and treatments
11. Safety measures to protect against injuries
12. Discharge plans
13. Any other items the home health agency or physician wishes to include

Source: Medicare Health Insurance Manual-11, Section 204.2.

BOX 3-3
A HOME HEALTH AGENCY'S BILL OF RIGHTS

The agency acknowledges the client's rights and encourages the client and family to participate in their plan of care through informed decision making. In accordance with this belief, each client/family member will receive, prior to admission, the following bill of rights and responsibilities.

1. The client and the client's property will be treated with respect by the program's staff.
2. The client will receive care without regard to race, color, creed, age, sex, religion, national origin, or mental or physical handicap.
3. The client has the right to be free from mental and physical abuse.
4. The client's medical record and related information is maintained in a confidential manner by the program.
5. The client will receive a written statement of the program's objectives, scope of services, and grievance process prior to admission.
6. The client, family, or guardian has the right to file a complaint regarding the services provided by the program without fear of disruption of service, coercion, or discrimination.
7. The client will be advised of the following in advance of service:
   a. Description of services and proposed visit frequency
   b. Overview of the anticipated plan of care and its likely outcome
   c. Options that may be available
8. The client/family is encouraged to participate in the plan of care. The client will receive the necessary information concerning the client's condition and will be encouraged to participate in changes that may arise in care.
9. The program shall provide for the right of the client to refuse any portion of planned treatment to the extent permitted by law without relinquishing other portions of the treatment plan, except where medical contraindications exist. The client will be informed of the expected consequences of such action.
10. The client has a right to continuity of care:
    a. Services provided within a reasonable time frame
    b. A program that is capable of providing the level of care required by the client
    c. Timely referral to alternative services, as needed
    d. Information regarding impending discharge, continuing care requirements, and other services, as needed
11. The client will be informed of the extent to which payment will be expected for items or services to be furnished to clients by Medicare, Medicaid, and any other program that is funded partially or fully with federal funds. Upon admission, the client will be informed orally and in writing of any charges for items and services that the program expects will not be covered upon admission. The client will be informed of any change in this amount as soon as possible, but no later than within 25 days after the program is made aware of the change.
12. Upon request, the client may obtain
    a. An itemized bill.
    b. The program's policy for uncompensated care.
    c. The program's policy for disclosure of the medical record.
    d. Identify of health care providers with which the program has contractual agreements, insofar as the client's care is concerned.
    e. The name of the responsible person supervising the client's care and how to contact this person during regular business hours.
13. The client has the right to obtain medical equipment and other health-related items from the company of the client's choice and assumes financial responsibility for such. The program's staff will assist in obtaining supplies and physician approvals as needed.
14. The client/family is responsible for
    a. Giving the program accurate, necessary information.
    b. Being available and cooperative during scheduled visits.
    c. Assisting, as much as possible, in the plan of care.
    d. Alerting the staff to any problems as soon as possible.

Source: Adapted from the Patient Bill of Rights and Responsibilities, Bon Secours Home Health and Hospice. Baltimore, MD.

Teacher

Most of the home health nurse's time is spent teaching about illness care and disease prevention (Figure 3-1 ◆). Often, the greatest educational challenge is to motivate the client. Even the most dedicated nurses can have trouble discovering what will make the client want to learn and how to focus the client on what is most important. Despite the work involved, the nurse's reward is knowing that clients have learned to manage independently. Because the nurse's role as educator is increasingly important, discharge considerations are included in the discussion of every major disorder in this text.

Figure 3-1. ◆ The home health nurse often provides client education. This nurse is teaching the client and family member how to apply dressings.

NURSING CARE IN THE HOME
ANA Standards
Home health nurses are responsible for adhering to the same codes and standards that guide all other nurses. These codes and standards (see Chapter 1) guide nursing practice and protect the public. The American Nurses Association (ANA) has established Standards for Home Health Nursing Practice and ANA Standards of Community Health Nursing as a basis for the practice of nursing in the home. The standards reflect the current state of knowledge in the field of home and community health nursing and should be the criteria for evaluating quality care.

National Association for Home Care Bill of Rights
Another source of guidance regarding home care is the National Association for Home Care (NAHC) Bill of Rights. The Home Care Bill of Rights grew out of a comprehensive code of ethics the NAHC adopted in 1982. In 1987, Congress made it a requirement for all home health agencies to use this Bill of Rights. Although home health agencies may make additions to the NAHC's original Bill of Rights, they are required by law to review it with all home health clients on the initial visit.

ANA Position Statements
The ANA has also published position statements addressing moral, ethical, and legal issues faced by home and community health nurses. These include the following:

■ A Statement on the Scope of Home Health Nursing Practice
■ Nursing Care and Do Not Resuscitate Decisions
■ Foregoing Artificial Nutrition and Hydration

LEGAL CONSIDERATIONS
The legal issues in home health center on privacy and confidentiality, client access to health information, freedom from unreasonable restraint, witnessing of documents, informed consent, and negligence or malpractice. Nurses can best avoid lawsuits by familiarizing themselves with the standards of practice, providing care that is consistent with standards and with their agency's policies, and documenting all care fully and accurately according to agency guidelines.

DISCHARGE CONSIDERATIONS
The old saying that discharge plans begin at admission makes more sense today than ever before. With shorter hospital stays, it is crucial that all clients be evaluated for their ability to manage at home. Nurses preparing to send clients home need to consider many of the following questions:

■ Does the client need follow-up therapy, treatments, or education?
■ What equipment, supplies, and information about community resources seem necessary?
■ Is printed information written at an acceptable reading level? Is it written in the appropriate language?
■ What cognitive abilities do the client and the caregiver seem to possess? Are there any sensory problems that interfere with learning?
■ Was the caregiver present during and included in instruction? How have the client and caregiver responded to health teaching? Have they understood what has been taught? Was their stress level too high for them to listen?
■ Who will be the principal caregiver in the home? Is there one? Are all caregivers comfortable in doing what needs to be done? If not, what support do they need to become comfortable?
■ Has a devastating diagnosis or prognosis just been determined?
■ Is high-technology intervention needed?

The answers to these questions suggest two equally important nursing interventions: initiating a client referral and teaching the client and family.

Initiating Referrals
The nurse considers making a referral to a home health agency, a hospice, or a community resource if the client has a need for formal follow-up beyond the present clinical setting. Hospital discharge planners, social workers, organizations for the aged, and local nonprofit agencies usually have a good command of the services and support groups available in their communities.

The nurse must talk to clients and their caregivers about their concerns related to home management. It is quite common for family members to disagree about whether additional help is necessary. Among the steps the nurse can take are: to lead an informal family meeting in which everyone shares concerns and to ask about the family's insurance coverage for home health care. Suggesting services when families have no funds to pay for them only adds to the problem. For clients with limited means, the nurse can identify staff who are knowledgeable about funding and consult with them. It is always important for the nurse to avoid making assumptions. Intelligent, well-educated, and financially secure clients can be just as overwhelmed by illness as the less educated and the poor. Everyone is a referral candidate.

If the family feels that no help is necessary and the nurse feels otherwise, the nurse may suggest an evaluation visit, explaining that the situation may look different once the client is home. If family members continue to refuse, the nurse lets them know that the door is never closed and gives them contacts in the community to call independently if their needs change.

Teaching the Client and Family

Clients need help understanding their situations, making health care decisions, and changing health behaviors. It is unrealistic to believe that clients can be taught everything they need to know during a short hospital stay. The nurse should recommend a home health referral for anyone who needs follow-up teaching.

When preparing clients for discharge, the nurse focuses on safety and survival first. Even if health education is to continue with home care, a day or two may elapse before the nurse arrives. The nurse must not discharge clients without giving them the right information and supplies to get them through the first few days at home.

Also, before discharge, clients must have complete information about their medications. They must be given a list of manifestations of complications they should report to their doctor. Finally, they must be able to manage any necessary treatments at least minimally. This means not only performing procedures safely but also knowing how to obtain necessary supplies in the community.

SPECIAL CHARACTERISTICS OF THE HOME SETTING

Nursing care in the home differs in many ways from nursing care in a hospital setting. First, nurses are invited into homes as guests; they cannot assume entry as they do in formal clinical settings. The environment belongs to the client, who retains control. Every nursing action must communicate respect for these boundaries. Nurses must establish trust and rapport quickly, because most home health nurses are with each client for only 1 hour a few times a week.

A second unique aspect of home health nursing is that it is solitary. There are no colleagues to consult, to assist, or to rely on for support.

Third, family dynamics are more visible in the home. As the nurse becomes a familiar presence and the family's behavior relaxes, the nurse can gain a clearer and more complete picture of family issues and relationships, lifestyle choices, and coping patterns.

Fourth, "families of one" are a worrisome reality for home health nurses. Today, more older adults are living alone. Some may have current or potential caregivers nearby; others have no one. These people often require considerable nursing support to remain strong, independent, and resourceful. Caring for "families of one" can take a toll on even the strongest home health nurse. Some nurses have reported calling between visits, keeping in touch after discharge, and driving by on days off because they have such difficulty "letting go" of their concerns about these clients.

Finally, caregiver burden is not easily hidden in the home. Millions of Americans are taking care of disabled relatives and friends, and many of the caregivers are themselves older adults. Health care planners picture the home as a place where all kinds of medical services can occur, but they may give little thought to how people manage. Few ever ask whether families can cope with the level of care they are expected to assume. Caregiving is now recognized as a complex activity that requires adjustment in family living patterns, relationships, and finances. For some families, the crisis of caregiving is short lived, but for others it lasts for years. As a result, caregivers are at great risk for both physical and emotional illness. The success of home care heavily depends on the supports in place, so it is crucial to address the needs of the support network.

PRACTICAL SUGGESTIONS FOR HOME CARE NURSES

A study of practicing home health nurses (Stulginsky, 1993a, 1993b) provides practical suggestions for home health nurses:

■ To establish trust and rapport, nurses must try to find common ground. They must communicate an understanding that they are guests: offer suggestions in a way that acknowledges the client's right to say no; sense "where people are" and honor that; maintain a respectful distance; and notice and honor family customs.

■ The nurse must be aware that the first contact is important. On the first nursing visit, the nurse might suggest that clients have someone else present "to help them listen." To avoid overwhelming clients, the nurse stresses essential information and repeats it on later visits. When making suggestions, the nurse offers clients the pluses and minuses of each alternative. The nurse speaks slowly, directly, and within the client's range of vision (he or she may have to lip-read) and does not shout at hearing-impaired clients. The nurse allows time for families to process the information they receive.

■ The nurse surveys the overall home environment, using common sense, intuition, and imagination. Among the things to note are sights, sounds, smells, dress, tone of voice, body language, and the use of touch; visiting patterns among family members; significant relationships; what is sacred and what is not; the appearance of the house, yard, sidewalk, and neighborhood; and the effect of illness on the family. The nurse asks questions and listens carefully to stories and offhand remarks.

■ It is important that nurses be flexible and realize they cannot tackle everything. The nurse should enter the home with a plan but be prepared to modify the plan according to conditions he or she encounters there. Safety issues, issues that concern the client, and problems that can most easily be solved should be addressed first. Alternatively, the nurse can focus on safety first, then short-term and long-term goals. If the priorities set are the nurse's, not the client's, they may not be met.

- Instead of just teaching the client, the nurse tries to promote the client's ability to learn. For example, the nurse can identify what is most important to the client and teach that. Survival takes first priority; the nurse teaches the information people need to ensure their safety until the next visit. The nurse prioritizes material on a need-to-know, want-to-know, ought-to-know basis, assessing and responding to learner readiness. Whenever possible, the nurse teaches while providing care.

- Homes are full of events or circumstances that pull a person's attention from the job at hand. Such distractions as children, animals, noise, clutter, or controlling, aggressive mannerisms can try even the most experienced nurse. Distractions should be limited as much as possible. For example, the nurse might ask a client, "May I please turn off your television while we visit?" or, "I'd like to schedule my next visit for a time when the children are in school. Is that all right with you?" The nurse must be truthful about allergies, fear of a client's pet, or difficulty hearing in a particular room, but should not debate the priority of the visit over the distraction (such as a favorite television show).

SPECIAL ISSUES IN HOME CARE
Safety
Safety assessment in the home is a nursing responsibility and a legal requirement. Nurses cannot close their eyes to an unsafe environment. On the first and later visits, the nurse must alert the family to unsafe and hazardous conditions, suggest remedies, and document the family's response to the nurse's suggestions. In particular, nurses must remain alert to the following conditions:

- How clients handle stairs
- How they manage their own care if they are alone
- The presence of a smoke detector in the home (the fire department will often install one free if notified)
- The presence of bathroom safety equipment
- Electrical hazards
- Slippery throw rugs, clutter, or furniture arrangements that may cause a fall
- Expired medications
- Inappropriate clothing or shoes
- Cooking or smoking habits that may start a fire
- An inadequate food supply
- Poorly functioning utilities
- Signs of abusive behavior

Obviously, nurses cannot go into homes and change the family's living space and lifestyle, but they can register their concern and reactions if the situation could lead to an injury or

if they suspect abuse or neglect. Within the home and community setting, ignoring an unsafe environment is considered nursing negligence. Documentation should address what information the nurse has covered, the family's response to the teaching, and assessment of their ongoing practice of safety precautions.

Infection Control
Infection control in the home centers on protecting clients, caregivers, and the community from the spread of disease. Within the home, nurses may encounter clients with infectious or communicable diseases, clients who are immunocompromised, or clients with multiple access devices, drainage tubes, or draining wounds. The home presents a challenging environment for infection control. Nurses must teach the importance of effective handwashing, the use of gloves, the disposal of wastes and soiled dressings, the handling of linens, and the practice of standard precautions.

NURSING PROCESS IN HOME CARE NURSING
The nursing process is the same for home care as for any other setting. Differences lie in assessing how the home's unique environment affects the need or problem and in using outcome criteria and mutual participation to plan goals and interventions.

Assessing
Assessment begins when the nurse calls the client to arrange a visit. That telephone call can yield much information. How alert, oriented, and stressed does the client (or family) seem to be? Does the client know the reason for the home health referral? How open to intervention do the client and family seem to be? Have they encountered any difficulties since discharge from the prior setting? Are there any supplies they need on the first visit? Because most agencies require submission of a plan of care within 48 hours of the first home visit, careful and complete data collection is essential. Nurses also collect information on an ongoing basis.

The nurse must collect the information requested on the tools and forms contained in the agency's admission packet. Many packets include a physical and psychosocial database; a medication sheet; forms for pain assessment, spiritual assessment, and financial assessment; and a family roster. Through interviewing, direct observation, and physical assessment, the nurse gains as clear and accurate a picture of the client as possible.

Diagnosing
After the initial assessment is completed, the actual or potential client problems are identified. The label of the problem (the nursing diagnosis) varies from agency to agency. No matter which method is used, meaningful statements describing the client's issues must be part of the home health record. These statements, based on data collection, are used to organize care and to justify reimbursement. Although it is the RN (not the LPN or LVN) who makes the nursing diagnosis, LPNs and LVNs contribute greatly to this process.

Planning

Planning includes setting priorities, establishing goals, and deciding on interventions to meet the needs of the client. The greatest level of success occurs when clients feel ownership of the plan. For this reason, planned interventions and expected outcomes should be client centered, realistic, achievable, and mutually agreed upon. Goals and expected outcomes should be documented clearly, in timed, measurable, and observable terms. These measures help clients and care providers focus their work together and evaluate the effectiveness of care. The expected outcomes are a way for the reimbursement source to judge the appropriateness of the plan of care.

Implementing

The home health nurse implements the plan of care that was mutually developed with the client. Some interventions may be carried out by another agency provider, by a paraprofessional brought in by the nurse case manager, or by the client.

Evaluating

Evaluation involves (a) comparing the plan of care with the goals that are achieved from visit to visit, and (b) reviewing the client's progress toward goals in order to determine the client's eligibility for discharge. Because reimbursement sources require that all skilled services be justified, many home health agency charts include space to evaluate the client's response to interventions and to document a plan of care for the next scheduled visit.

Rehabilitation

Rehabilitation is the process of learning to live to one's maximum potential with a chronic impairment and the resulting functional disability. Rehabilitation nursing is based on a philosophy that each person has a unique set of strengths and abilities that can enable him or her to live with dignity, self-worth, and independence. This philosophy applies to clients with both acute and chronic illnesses. Many rehabilitative services are provided in community-based settings.

The terms *impairment, disability,* and *handicap* are often used as synonyms, but they have different meanings. An **impairment** is a disturbance in structure or function resulting from physiologic or psychological abnormalities. A **disability** is the degree of observable and measurable impairment. A **handicap** is the total adjustment to disability that limits functioning at a normal level. For example, following a motorcycle accident, Kim Rushin had damage to her left leg that resulted in an impairment in the ability to flex her knee. This resulted in a 50% disability of that leg and caused a handicap because Kim was a school bus driver and could no longer operate the bus safely. See the Critical Thinking Care Map on health promotion for Kim at the end of this chapter.

TEAM APPROACH TO CARE

Rehabilitation promotes reintegration into the client's family and community through a team approach. The plan of care includes many different aspects of the client's life: physical function, mental health, interpersonal relationships, social interactions, and vocational status. This comprehensive consideration of the client requires the expertise of a team of health care providers. The rehabilitation team usually meets weekly to discuss the achievement of client goals (Figure 3-2 ◆). As a part of this comprehensive plan of care, the following points are included:

- Assessing the level of function
- Developing an individualized and holistic plan of care, with ongoing evaluation of outcomes
- Including the family in the plan of care
- Implementing discharge planning to ensure a smooth transition to home

NURSING CARE IN REHABILITATION

The nurse provides care for the chronically ill client of all ages and with many types of disability. The 20-year-old man with quadriplegia from a spinal cord injury has needs that are different from the 75-year-old woman who has had a stroke and is unable to move her left arm or speak. However, the plan of care developed for each of these clients considers common factors in assessing and planning individualized interventions.

Assessment of the client's needs begins with the first contact and continues throughout care. Assessment includes functional level and self-care abilities, educational needs, psychosocial needs, and the home environment. It is critical to determine the client's and family's priorities before establishing any plan of care. Questions for assessment include the following:

- What is the client's present level of physical function (mobility, self-care, communication, skin integrity, bowel and bladder function)?
- What are the client and family goals (short-term and long-term)?
- Are goals realistic and attainable?
- What concerns are verbalized by the client and family (financial, work, housing, school, transportation, sexual activities, social activities, relationships)?

Figure 3-2. ◆ The rehabilitation team discusses the client's plan of care.

■ What stage of grief and loss is present (denial, anger, bargaining, acceptance)?
■ To what home environment will the client be going?
■ What resources are available to assist reintegration (personal, support, community, federal)?

Nursing interventions to assist rehabilitation are revised to meet client and family needs as the client progresses toward reintegration. In the acute-care stage, the nurse focuses on interventions that will prevent complications. As recovery progresses, the nurse develops and implements individualized teaching plans for the client and family. General areas of interventions include the following:

■ Preventing infection
■ Maintaining correct body alignment, position, and range of motion
■ Preventing skin breakdown
■ Providing adequate nutrition and fluids
■ Providing care as necessary and appropriate, with the goal of achieving a level of independence realistic for the client
■ Referrals to community agencies (nursing care, special equipment or supplies, support groups, counseling, physical therapy, occupational therapy, respiratory therapy, vocational guidance, house cleaning, meals)

To ensure continuity of care during rehabilitation, the home health nurse is often involved in the plan of care during the acute-care stage. Continued education and support of the client and family are essential. The achievement of self-care and mobility does not guarantee that the client can function independently in all areas.

(*Note:* The bibliography listings for this and all chapters have been compiled at the back of the book.)

Chapter Review

 key terms by topic

Use the CD-ROM disk enclosed with your textbook to hear the pronunciation of the key items in the chapter.

Community-based nursing care
community-based nursing

Types of community-based health care services
long-term care, parish nursing, block nursing

Home health care
home health care, diagnosis-related groups (DRGs), rehabilitation, impairment, disability, handicap

key points

- Community-based nursing care focuses on individual and family health care needs, with the nurse providing care in a variety of community settings, including community centers and clinics, day care programs, churches, long-term care facilities, and homes.

- Long-term care facilities provide health care and activities of daily living for people who are mentally or physically unable to care for themselves.

- Home health agencies are organizations that provide skilled nursing and other therapeutic services in the client's home. Nurses make the initial visit and collect data to develop a plan of care. The plan of care is implemented and evaluated within the special characteristics of the home as a nursing care setting.

- Rehabilitation nursing care is often provided in community-based settings. The goal of rehabilitation nurses is to assist clients to again become a part of their family and community.

 Medialink

Additional interactive resources for this chapter can be found on the Companion Website at www.prenhall.com/burke. Click on Chapter 3 and "Begin" to select the activities for this chapter.

For NCLEX review questions and an audio glossary, access the accompanying CD-ROM in this book.

for further study

For further information about caring for clients who are terminally ill and want to die with comfort and dignity at home, see Chapter 9.

For more information about nursing codes and standards, see Chapter 1.

Critical Thinking Care Map

Caring for a Client with a Handicap
NCLEX-PN Focus Area: Coping and Adaptation

Case Study: After seriously damaging her left leg in a motorcycle accident six months ago, Kim Rushin is no longer able to drive a school bus safely. As part of the rehabilitation team that is caring for Kim, what data would you collect and what interventions would you suggest?

Nursing Diagnosis: Deficient Knowledge: Overcoming handicap from knee injury

COLLECT DATA

Subjective
_____
_____
_____
_____
_____

Objective
_____
_____
_____
_____
_____

Would you report this data? Yes/No

If yes, to: _____

Nursing Care
_____
_____
_____
_____
_____
_____
_____
_____

How would you document this? _____
_____
_____

Data collected
(use those that apply)

- Age 28
- Unmarried
- Height 5′6″
- Weight 140 lbs.
- BP 120/72
- Unable to bend left leg more than 15 degrees
- States, "I can't keep my present job"
- States, "I don't know where to go for help"

Nursing Interventions
(use those that apply)

- Teach crutch-walking techniques.
- Perform passive range of motion exercises on Kim's left leg.
- Suggest career counseling.
- Ask Kim if she has ever considered other types of employment.
- Recommend that Kim join Weight Watchers or similar group.
- Refer Kim to vocational rehabilitation services.
- Suggest that Kim take more time to adjust.

NCLEX-PN Exam Preparation

TEST-TAKING TIP

Evaluate each question for safety needs and *always* remember the importance of handwashing.

1. Nursing care provided directly to clients wherever they are, including where they live, work, play, worship, and go to school, is known as:
   a. home health nursing
   b. community health nursing
   c. community based nursing
   d. parish nursing

2. Community-based health care services may include:
   a. hospitals
   b. day cares
   c. emergency departments
   d. surgery units

3. When the family desires differ from those of the client, the home care nurse must:
   a. remain the primary client's advocate
   b. try to please everyone
   c. avoid negative responses from the family
   d. call the physician to resolve the conflict

4. In order for home care to receive Medicare reimbursement, certain criteria that must be met include:
   a. the client must need help with cooking and cleaning
   b. the client must live alone
   c. the client must have an income below poverty level
   d. the client must be essentially homebound

5. Clients cannot realistically be taught everything they need to know during today's shortened hospital stays. Therefore, a client needing follow-up teaching should:
   a. have a home health referral
   b. have more frequent physician appointments
   c. have the option to increase their hospital stay
   d. rely on family for continued care

6. In the home, one nursing responsibility and legal requirement is:
   a. identifying caregiver burden
   b. respecting client boundaries
   c. completing a safety assessment
   d. honoring family customs

7. Nursing interventions for unsafe and hazardous conditions in the home would include:
   a. changing the unsafe home environment regardless of client wishes
   b. ignoring the unsafe environment, allowing the client freedom to choose his or her own lifestyle
   c. threatening to discontinue home care if the environment is not made safe
   d. alerting the client/family, suggesting remedies, and documenting the response

8. The process of learning to live to one's maximum potential with a chronic impairment/functional disability is:
   a. long-term care
   b. rehabilitation
   c. reintegration
   d. infection control

9. Rehabilitation includes many different aspects of the client's life such as physical, mental, social, and vocational status. This comprehensive consideration of the client requires:
   a. a team approach to care
   b. primarily nursing care
   c. focusing on the physical disability
   d. short-term care

10. Before establishing any plan of care in rehabilitation, it is important to:
    a. guarantee the client independence in all areas of functioning
    b. determine the priorities of needs from the client's and family's perspective
    c. establish a rapport with the family
    d. complete all physical exercises

Guidelines for Health Assessment

LEARNING outcomes

After completing this chapter, you will be able to:

- Discuss the purposes of a health assessment.
- Describe the types of health assessment made by nurses.
- Identify sources and accuracy of assessment data.
- Identify components of the health history.
- Describe the methods of physical examination.
- Prepare a client for a physical examination.
- Describe the body systems and characteristics assessed in a physical examination.
- Discuss guidelines for documenting a health assessment.

One of the most important aspects of nursing care is assessment. **Assessment** is the collection of data that provides information about the client's individualized health care needs. It is the first step in the nursing process, providing the base for the planning, implementation, and evaluation of client care. Assessment by nurses is mandated by nursing standards, nurse practice acts, accrediting bodies, and institutional policies. The preamble to the standards of the Joint Commission on Accreditation of Healthcare Organizations (JCAHO) (1997) emphasizes the importance of assessment as follows:

. . . care provided to each patient is based on a determination of the patient's needs. This determination is based on an assessment of the patient's relevant physical, psychological, and social status needs. The assessment includes the collection and analysis of data about the patient to determine the need for any additional data, the patient's care needs, and the care to be provided.

Purposes of a Health Assessment

The purposes of a health assessment are to:

- Collect objective data about the client. **Objective data** (also called *signs*) are observable or measurable pieces of information. Objective data can be seen, heard, touched, or smelled. Examples of objective data are the color of urine, vital signs, moisture on skin, and breath odor. Laboratory results are also objective data.
- Collect subjective data from the client. **Subjective data** (also called *symptoms*) are experiences only the client can describe. Examples of subjective data are nausea, pain, and itching.
- Collect information about the client's family, community, culture, ethnicity, and religion.
- Identify past and present health behaviors that support health or increase the risk of illness.
- Identify data that suggest potential or actual health problems. (The RN will label these problems as *nursing diagnoses.*)

This chapter provides guidelines for conducting the two components of a health assessment: a health history and physical examination. Information about health assessments is included in each chapter of the book that discusses alterations in functional health patterns. The term **manifestations** is used throughout this book to refer to objective and subjective data that are associated with specific illnesses. It is important to remember that documenting (recording) the health assessment is as important as conducting it.

Types of Assessment

The type of assessment varies depending on the setting, the situation, and the needs of the client. The types of assessment are an initial comprehensive assessment, an ongoing partial assessment, and a focused assessment.

COMPREHENSIVE ASSESSMENT

When a client first enters a health care setting, a comprehensive assessment of the client's health history and physical status is conducted. This provides a baseline for comparing any later assessments. The comprehensive assessment may be the responsibility of one health care professional or of different members of the health care team. For example, when a client enters the hospital setting for inpatient care and receives a *comprehensive assessment,* a nurse may collect data about the client's health history, the physician may perform a complete physical examination, and a nursing technician may take vital signs and weight. In a community or home setting, the nurse usually collects all of the assessment data.

PARTIAL ASSESSMENT

An ongoing *partial assessment* is one that is conducted on a regular basis throughout the client's care. It usually reviews any problems that have been identified to determine if changes have occurred or if new problems are present. A partial assessment is conducted in any type of setting, although the timing may differ. In the hospital, the nurse conducts a partial assessment at the beginning of each shift. In the home, a partial assessment is conducted at each visit (which may vary from daily to once a week).

FOCUSED ASSESSMENT

A *focused assessment* (through both a focused interview and a focused physical examination) is one that is conducted to assess a specific client problem. For example, assessment for a client who has abdominal pain includes assessing body temperature; frequency of bowel movements; pain with urination; any associated trauma; menstrual history (for women); and the location, duration, and type of pain experienced. It does not include assessment of musculoskeletal function or visual acuity. A focused assessment is also a part of other nursing responsibilities, such as when the nurse takes an apical pulse before administering a drug that affects the heart rate. An *emergency assessment* is a special type of focused assessment. It is a very rapid assessment to determine life-threatening situations. The practice of assessing the ABCs (*A*irway, *B*reathing, *C*irculation) before beginning cardiopulmonary resuscitation is an example of an emergency assessment.

Sources and Accuracy of Assessment Data

Data may be collected from primary or secondary sources. The client is the best source of data and is the primary source. However, if the client is very young, very ill, unconscious, or confused, data may be collected from secondary sources. Secondary sources include the client's family or friends, the client records (such as medical records and laboratory data), and other health care professionals.

Data that are collected must be *accurate* and *factual.* General guidelines for ensuring this include:

■ Compare subjective and objective data. If the client says "I feel like I have a fever," compare the statement to an actual measurement of body temperature.

■ Consider factors that may interfere with accurate measurements. The client who has just walked up three flights of stairs may have an increased pulse rate that is unrelated to a disease process.

■ Clarify statements made by the client. If the client says, "I have this terrible pain in my stomach," ask the client to point to the area of pain (which may be abdominal rather than gastric).

■ Double-check data that are very high or low, such as a pulse of 120 or a blood pressure of 60/20.

■ Don't jump to conclusions. The older adult client's dry skin with decreased turgor may be a result of aging; it may not mean the client is dehydrated.

Obtaining a Health History

The health history is a collection of subjective and objective data that provide an overall picture of the client's health status (Table 4-1 ◆). The data are collected through an interview with the client. Many health care institutions and agencies have specific forms with standardized questions to use in conducting the health history. Although these may vary, most contain the data listed in Table 4-1.

During the health history, principles of therapeutic communication help you collect accurate data. Most importantly, use words the client can understand, and listen carefully. Sit in a relaxed posture and maintain eye contact. This open body language tells the client that you are interested in what is being said. Barriers to collecting accurate data include offering advice, acting disgusted or defensive, disagreeing, offering false assurance, and jumping to conclusions.

Open-ended questions ("Tell me about what brought you to the clinic today") give the client the chance to provide more information than closed-ended questions ("Did you come here today because of your back pain?"). Avoid "why" questions ("Why didn't you come last week when you first noticed this problem?"). "Why" questions often make the client feel threatened or foolish. Closed-ended questions are appropriate in emergency situations, when specific information must be collected quickly.

It is very important to be sensitive to cultural differences between yourself and the client. Cultural differences influence how both verbal and nonverbal communications are inter-

TABLE 4-1	INFORMATION INCLUDED IN A HEALTH HISTORY
COMPONENT	**INFORMATION**
Biographical data	Name, address, age, gender, marital status, occupation, religious preference, health care financing, usual source of medical care (primary health care provider)
Reason for health care visit (chief complaint)	Documented in client's own words
History of present illness	When symptoms began Whether onset was sudden or gradual Exact location of the problem Character of the problem (such as type of discharge or intensity of pain) Other associated symptoms Type of self-treatment
Past medical history	Childhood illnesses Childhood immunizations Allergies Accidents and injuries Hospitalizations All current prescribed and over-the-counter medications
Family history of health and illness	Ages of brothers/sisters, parents, grandparents Health status of living relatives and cause of death if no longer living
Lifestyle	Use, amount, and frequency of use of tobacco, alcohol, and street drugs Type and amount of foods eaten each day Sleep patterns Any difficulty with activities of daily living Type and amount of exercise Education and occupation Support systems (family, friends, community) Expectations of treatment and care

preted. Culture and ethnicity, as well as the family in which one grew up and the community in which one lives, also influence health beliefs, health behaviors, and health treatments.

If the client does not speak the same language as the nurse, a translator is necessary to assist with the interview. The room should be arranged so the client can see both the nurse and the translator at the same time. Look at the client, not the translator, and ask questions one at a time in clear, concise terms.

Methods of Physical Examination

Physical examination is a skill that takes practice. There are four basic methods of physical examination: inspection, palpation, percussion, and auscultation. The methods of physical examination used by nurses depends on the nurse's level of education, knowledge and skill acquired through clinical practice, and on institutional or agency policy. Basic methods of physical examination are included here as an introduction.

INSPECTION

Inspection is the method of observing the client in a careful and deliberate manner, using the senses of seeing, smelling, and hearing to observe abnormal findings. Some body systems are inspected with special equipment; for example, an otoscope is used to inspect the ear canal and tympanic membrane. Inspection is the first method used in an assessment of the whole body or of each body system. The guidelines for inspection are:

- The room temperature should be comfortable. If the room is too hot or too cold, it may alter the appearance of the client's skin and change his or her behavior.
- Use good lighting. Dim light can obscure abnormalities, and flourescent lights can change the perception of skin color.
- Look before touching.
- Completely expose the body part being inspected.
- Compare symmetric (matching) parts (e.g., eyes, ears, arms, legs).
- Inspect for these characteristics: color, size, symmetry, patterns, location, consistency of tissue, movement, behavior, odors, sounds.

PALPATION

Palpation is the method of using the hands to touch and feel. Light and moderate palpation are used most often by nurses. Light palpation is performed by placing your hand lightly on the surface to palpate for pulses, tenderness, skin texture, skin temperature, and skin moisture (Figure 4-1 ◆). To perform moderate palpation, the hand is placed on the skin surface and the surface is depressed 1 to 2 cm (½ to ¾ inch). A circular motion is used to feel for the size, shape, or mobility of underlying structures such as masses or body organs (Table 4-2 ◆). A

Figure 4-1. ◆ The position of the hand for light palpation.

distended urinary bladder may be assessed with moderate palpation. The guidelines for palpation are:

- Make sure hands are clean and warm and fingernails are short.
- Follow standard precautions as appropriate.
- Use the pads of the fingers to palpate pulses, texture, size, shape, and crepitus (air in subcutaneous tissue).
- Assess for the characteristics listed in Table 4-2.

PERCUSSION

Percussion is the method of tapping the body to produce sound waves. The sounds produced are used to assess underlying structures. Although percussion can be used to assess the density of tissue and the size and shape of organs, it is used most often to assess abdominal structures. *Tympany* is a characteristic loud, drumlike sound heard over an organ that is filled with air, such as the intestines.

The guidelines for percussion are:

- Make sure hands are clean and warm and fingernails are short.

TABLE 4-2	CHARACTERISTICS ASSESSED BY PALPATION
CHARACTERISTIC	**DESCRIPTORS**
Consistency	Soft, hard, filled with fluid
Mobility	Movable, fixed
Moisture	Wet, dry
Pulse strength	Strong, weak, full, bounding, thready
Shape	Regular, irregular
Size	Small, medium, large
Temperature	Warm, cold
Texture	Rough, smooth

Figure 4-2. ◆ Indirect percussion. Use the finger of one hand to tap the finger of the other.

- Follow standard precautions as appropriate.
- To use direct percussion, use one or more fingertips to tap over the area being assessed.
- To use indirect percussion (Figure 4-2 ◆):
  - Place the middle finger of your nondominant hand over the area to be percussed.
  - Use the pad of the middle finger of your dominant hand to strike the area between the knuckle and the fingernail of the hand over the body part.
  - Deliver two quick taps by flexing your wrist and listen to the tone.

AUSCULTATION

Auscultation is the method that uses a stethoscope to listen for body sounds, including those of the heart, moving blood, bowel, and lungs. Sounds are described in a variety of ways, depending on the body part being assessed. The general ways of classifying sounds are: intensity (loud/soft), pitch (high/low), duration, and quality (crackles, wheezes, etc). Auscultation is also used to assess the apical pulse.

General guidelines for auscultation are:

- Make sure hands are clean and warm and fingernails are short.
- Follow standard precautions as appropriate.
- Make the environment as quiet as possible.
- Auscultate over bare skin.
- Press the diaphragm of the stethoscope firmly on the body part being assessed to listen to normal heart sounds, breath sounds, and bowel sounds (all of which are high-pitched).
- Hold the bell of the stethoscope lightly on the body part being assessed to listen to low-pitched sounds, such as abnormal heart sounds and vascular sounds.

Preparation for a Physical Examination

Before beginning the examination, the nurse should ensure that the room temperature is comfortable, that the area is quiet, and that adequate lighting is available. All equipment that will be used should be clean and in good working order. The nurse should wash his or her hands before and after the assessment. Gloves should be worn and standard precautions followed if either the nurse or the client has an open cut or abrasion, if the client has drainage from a cut or wound, if body fluids or excretions are being collected, and for any examination of the mucous membranes, genitalia, or rectum. If there is any possibility of being splashed with fluids or secretions, the nurse should wear a mask and protective eye goggles.

The purpose and techniques of the physical examination should be explained to the client to decrease anxiety and feelings of embarrassment. Although the examination is not

---

BOX 4-1
NORMAL ASSESSMENT FINDINGS IN THE OLDER ADULT

SKIN, HAIR, AND NAILS
- Dry and wrinkled skin
- Thin scalp and body hair (men may be bald)
- Facial hair in women
- Loss of hair pigment
- Areas of pigmentation and moles
- Thickened and yellowed nails

EYES AND EARS
- Cataracts (opacity of the lens)
- Decreased visual acuity (*presbyopia*)
- Decreased hearing acuity (*presbycusis*)

MOUTH
- Loss of teeth
- Presence of dentures

HEART AND LUNGS
- Increased respiratory rate
- Increased blood pressure
- Increased, but weaker, heart rate

ABDOMEN
- Decreased frequency of bowel sounds
- More frequent voiding, including at night

EXTREMITIES
- Blood vessels more prominent and less straight
- Peripheral pulses sometimes more difficult to palpate
- Decreased muscle mass and strength
- Decreased range of motion
- Stooped posture

MENTAL STATUS
- Slower response to questions
- Occasional confusion in unfamiliar surroundings

painful, it may be difficult for some clients to sit or lie in a position necessary for a specific assessment, especially if the client is in pain or is older. The length of the examination should be adjusted to the physical condition and age of each client. It is important to know normal changes in structure and function that occur with aging because they can affect client tolerance and the data that are collected. Normal changes in the older adult are outlined in Box 4-1.

If at all possible, the nurse should conduct the physical examination in a private location at a time agreeable to the client. For a complete physical examination, the nurse should (if needed) assist the client in removing clothing and putting on a gown. The client should empty the bladder before the examination to facilitate abdominal assessment. A drape should be placed over the client so that only the body part being assessed is exposed. The nurse should also determine if any positions are contraindicated during the examination.

The Physical Examination

A comprehensive physical examination (Table 4-3 ◆) may be conducted in a system-by-system or head-to-toe sequence. Some parts of the examination, such as a rectal examination, male and female genitalia with a pelvic examination, internal eye examination and external ear canal examination are most often conducted by an advanced practice nurse or physician and are not included here. The following discussion of a basic physical examination provides structure for a head-to-toe assessment.

GENERAL SURVEY

The general survey provides the nurse with information about the client's overall appearance and behavior, as well as vital signs and height and weight. Data for the general survey are collected from the first meeting with the client and continue through the physical examination or during nursing care. The following information is assessed:

- Facial expressions, mood, speech patterns
- Hygiene, grooming, odors
- Posture, physical deformities, ability to move and walk
- Manifestations of illness, such as difficulty breathing, pain, swelling
- Vital signs (temperature, pulse, respirations, blood pressure)
- Height and weight

SKIN, HAIR, AND NAILS

The skin, hair, and nails make up the *integument* and often provide a general indication of the client's overall health. These structures are assessed by inspection and palpation in conjunction with other body parts during a head-to-toe physical examination.

The skin varies in color from pale white to dark brown, depending on race and individual characteristics. It is normally warm, smooth, dry, and intact. Various diseases and injuries or environmental exposure may change the color, moisture, or continuity of the client's skin (see Chapters 14 and 15). Changes in color are more difficult to assess in dark-skinned people (such as Native Americans, African Americans, Hispanics, those of Mediterranean descent, and Caucasians who are deeply suntanned). Abnormal assessments are described below:

- *Cyanosis.* Cyanosis is a blue or gray discoloration of the skin that is the result of a decreased level of oxygen in the blood. Cyanosis in people with dark skin is often seen as a dullness in color.

TABLE 4-3 GUIDELINES FOR A PHYSICAL EXAMINATION

COMPONENT	METHODS AND AREAS OF ASSESSMENT
General survey	Inspection, Auscultation - General appearance, posture, gait, thought processes, speech patterns - Vital signs - Height and weight
Integument	Inspection, Palpation - Skin: Color, moisture, temperature, turgor, lesions (color, size, shape) - Hair: Distribution, texture, infection, infestation - Nails: Shape, angle at nail bed, color, texture
Eyes	Inspection, Palpation - Eyebrows: Hair distribution, alignment, movement - Eyelashes: Distribution, direction of curl - Eyelids: Skin texture, symmetrical closure, ability to blink - Conjunctiva: Color, texture, lesions - Lacrimal glands: Pain, infection, edema, tearing - Cornea: Transparency, reflex - Pupils: Color, shape, symmetrical size, reaction to light, accommodation, convergence - Extraocular muscles: Coordination - Visual acuity: Near and distance vision

TABLE 4-3 **GUIDELINES FOR A PHYSICAL EXAMINATION (CONTINUED)**

COMPONENT	METHODS AND AREAS OF ASSESSMENT
Ears	Inspection, Palpation ■ Auricles: Color, symmetrical size, position, texture, pain ■ External ear: Cerumen (wax), infection, blood ■ Hearing acuity: Voice tones, watch tick
Nose/Sinuses	Inspection, Palpation ■ External nose: Shape, size, color, discharge, pain ■ Nasal cavities: Patency, mucosa, discharge, lesions, location of septum ■ Sinuses: Pain
Mouth/Oropharynx	Inspection, Palpation ■ Lips/buccal mucosa: Symmetrical, color, moisture, lesions ■ Teeth/gums: Number of teeth; dental care, caries; gum color, adherence ■ Tongue: Position: color, texture, movement, moisture, swelling, ulceration, masses, lesions ■ Palate/uvula: Color, shape, bony growth, lesions; position of uvula ■ Oropharynx/tonsils: Color, size, discharge
Neck	Inspection, Palpation, Auscultation ■ Neck muscles: Movement, range of motion, pain, swelling, masses ■ Lymph nodes: Size, pain ■ Carotid arteries, thyroid: Presence of *bruits* (soft rushing sound heard through bell of stethoscope)
Breasts/Axilla	Inspection, Palpation ■ Breasts: Size, shape, symmetrical, retraction, color, swelling, pain, masses, lesions ■ Areola: Size, shape, symmetrical, color, masses, lesions ■ Nipples: Size, shape, position, color, discharge, lesions, masses ■ Axillary lymph nodes: Size, pain, nodules
Thorax/Lungs	Inspection, Palpation, Auscultation ■ Thorax: Shape, symmetrical, spinal curves, skin lesions, pain, masses, expansion ■ Lungs: Breath sounds, respiratory patterns
Cardiovascular	Inspection, Palpation, Auscultation ■ Precordium: Location of point of maximum impulse, pulsations ■ Heart: Heart sounds, rate and rhythm of contractions ■ Peripheral pulses: Strength, symmetrical, volume ■ Peripheral veins: Visibility, symmetrical, pain ■ Circulation: Skin color, temperature, skin changes, nail changes, lesions, edema, capillary refill
Abdomen	Inspection, Auscultation, Percussion, Palpation ■ Skin: Lesions, color ■ Abdomen: Contour, distention, movements ■ Bowel sounds: Audible, timing ■ Bladder: Size, pain
Musculoskeletal	Inspection, Palpation ■ Muscles: Symmetrical, size, tone, movement, contractures, pain, masses ■ Bones: Symmetrical, alignment, pain ■ Spine: Curves
Neurologic	Inspection, Palpation, Percussion ■ Motor function/balance: Gait, ability to stand on one foot and walk heel to toe ■ Fine motor movement: Ability to repeatedly touch nose with hand, pat knees with palms and backs of ■ hands, run heel down opposite shin ■ Sensory/light touch: Ability to distinguish between sharp and dull touch ■ Cranial nerves: Ability to smell, see, clench teeth, move eyes, have facial expressions, hear, taste, feel ■ touch, swallow, shrug shoulders against resistance, protrude tongue ■ Reflexes: Type of response (using percussion hammer)

- *Pallor.* Pallor, or paleness of the skin, is most often the result of a loss of blood. Pallor may be assessed over the entire body, or only in the lips, nail beds, and conjunctiva (white area) of the eyes. People with dark skin often are ashen gray or appear slightly yellowish.
- *Jaundice.* Jaundice is a yellow color of the skin and mucous membranes. It is caused by liver or gallbladder disease, or by an excessive breakdown of red blood cells. Jaundice is usually seen first in the eyes, and then in the skin and mucous membranes. Darker skin does not show jaundice, but it can be seen in the eyes, oral mucous membranes, and palms and soles.
- *Erythema.* Erythema is redness of the skin. It may appear during a fever, in response to inflammation or allergy, or from a sunburn.
- *Ecchymosis.* Ecchymosis is a purple discoloration resulting from a collection of blood in the subcutaneous tissues. *Petechiae* are small red spots caused by capillary bleeding. The location and size of the discolorations should be documented.
- *Lesions.* Lesions are alterations in the surface of the skin. *Wounds* may be the result of an injury or a surgical incision. A *scar* is a healed wound. Other types of lesions are bites, scratches, blisters, warts, moles, acne, burns, and rashes. When assessing lesions, document the size, shape, location, drainage, odors, and associated pain.

Turgor is the fullness or elasticity of the skin. With normal turgor, skin can be pinched up in a fold, and when released it immediately returns to its shape. *Dehydration* decreases the skin's turgor, so that skin folds remain elevated (like a tent) or return to shape very slowly. *Edema,* or excess fluid in tissues, is manifested by swelling covered by tight, shiny skin. Edema may be caused by trauma, heart disease, peripheral vascular disease, kidney disease, or overhydration. Edema is often measured by palpating with the fingers; if the skin remains indented, the term *pitting edema* is used. The scale used to describe pitting edema is: 0 = none, +1 = trace (2 mm), +2 = moderate (4 mm), +3 = deep (6 mm), and +4 = very deep (8 mm) (Figure 4-3 ◆).

The nails are inspected for shape, color, and consistency. The hair is inspected for color, texture, and distribution. *Alopecia* (loss of hair on the head or all of the body), may result from hereditary factors (specific to the hair on the head in men), infection, inadequate nutrition, or treatment of cancer with chemotherapy or radiation therapy. *Hirsutism* (excessive hair) is often caused by hormone disorders.

HEAD AND NECK

A basic physical examination of the head and neck includes assessing the skull, face, eyes, ears, nose and sinuses, mouth, and lymph nodes. These structures are assessed by inspection and palpation. More advanced physical assessment techniques, not discussed here, are uses of the ophthalmoscope to examine the internal eye and the otoscope to examine the tympanic membrane and internal nasal structures.

A

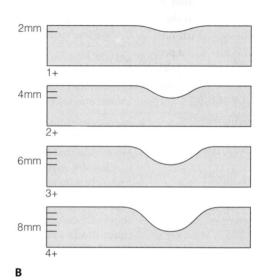

B

Figure 4-3. ◆ Assessing edema. (A) Palpating for edema over the tibia. (B) Four-point scale for grading edema.

Skull and Face

The skull and face are inspected for shape and proportion and should be symmetrical. If the skull appears abnormally large, its circumference should be measured with a tape-measure. The face is inspected for color, symmetry, and distribution of hair. The facial muscles and nerves are assessed by asking the client to raise the eyebrows, puff out the cheeks, smile, and show the teeth. Abnormal findings that should be documented are edema around the eyes (*periorbital edema*), inability to move a part of the face, and any abnormal movements such as tremors or tics.

Eyes

The external structures of the eyes (including the eyebrows, eyelids, eyelashes, and lacrimal glands) are inspected. The eyes and eyebrows should be in alignment, the eyelashes should curl outward, and the eyelids should cover the eyes equally. The lacrimal gland is palpated for tenderness. The conjunctiva should be white. The pupils are normally black and round. When a client has a cataract, the pupil appears white or cloudy. Other abnormal findings are dilation (*mydriasis*) or constriction (*miosis*) of one or both pupils (see Figure 4-4 ◆). The pupils are also assessed for reaction to light, accommodation, and convergence. The procedures for these assessments are outlined in Box 4-2.

Visual acuity is often measured with a Snellen's chart (Figure 4-5 ◆) and can be done with or without corrective lenses (eyeglasses or contact lenses). The client is placed 20 feet from the chart and asked to cover one eye. The client is asked to read the smallest possible line of letters with the uncovered eye. This procedure is repeated with the other eye. Each line on the chart has a fraction on the side, with the top number always being 20 (the distance the person with normal vision can read the line of letters). The bottom number indicates the vision of the person being tested and larger numbers represent poorer vision. Visual acuity is documented as the smallest line of letters that can be read with only two errors. For example, normal vision is 20/20, while a person with visual problems may have a visual acuity of 20/100. The visual acuity for each eye is documented, and use of corrective lenses is noted. (See Chapter 31 for disorders of the ear and eye.)

Ears

Inspect the external ears for location, symmetry, lesions, redness, and drainage. Gently palpate the external ears for tenderness and swelling. An estimate of hearing may be made by asking the client to cover one ear as you whisper a word while standing about 1 to 2 feet away out of the client's line of vision (to prevent lip-reading). Repeat with the other ear.

Nose and Sinuses

To test the patency of the client's nostrils, have the client occlude one side at a time and then inhale and exhale. A penlight can be used to assess the mucous membranes in the lower nasal passages. Abnormal findings include swelling, bleeding, discharge, and a crooked (deviated) septum. The sinuses are assessed by gentle palpation over the frontal and maxillary sinuses, noting any tenderness or pain.

Mouth

Ask the client to open the mouth widely. Inspect the lips, the oral mucous membranes, the tongue, the teeth, and the gums. The lips, mucous membranes, gums, and tongue should be pink, smooth, and moist. The teeth should be in good repair. There should be no bad odors. Abnormal findings are swelling, redness, pallor, drainage, lesions, or poor dental hygiene.

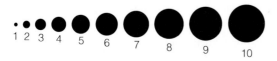

Figure 4-4. ◆ Size of pupil in millimeters.

BOX 4-2
ASSESSING THE PUPILS

REACTION TO LIGHT
- Ask the client to look straight ahead.
- Using a penlight, bring the light from the side of the client's face and briefly shine the light on one pupil. Observe the response of the pupil (it should normally constrict).
- Repeat the procedure with the other eye.

ACCOMMODATION
- Hold your finger about 10 to 15 cm (4 to 6 inches) from the bridge of the client's nose.
- Ask the client to look at your finger, then at a distant object, and then back at your finger. Observe the response of the pupils (they should normally constrict when looking at your finger (a near object) and dilate when looking at the distant object.

CONVERGENCE
- Move your finger toward the client's nose from a distance of about 15 cm (6 inches) and observe the eyes. Normally, the pupils move toward the nose, assuming a cross-eyed appearance (convergence).

Lymph Nodes

Palpate the lymph nodes of the head and neck (Figure 4-6 ◆). The lymph nodes normally are not palpable. If they are palpable, assess for size, location, consistency, and tenderness.

THORAX

Assessment of the thorax in a head-to-toe examination includes the chest and back, the lungs, the heart, and the

Figure 4-5. ◆ Types of eye charts: The preschool children's chart (left), Snellen's standard chart (center), and the Snellen E chart for clients unable to read (right).

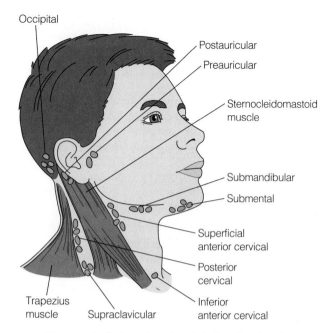

Occipital

Postauricular

Preauricular

Sternocleidomastoid muscle

Submandibular

Submental

Superficial anterior cervical

Posterior cervical

Trapezius muscle

Supraclavicular

Inferior anterior cervical

Figure 4-6. ◆ Lymph nodes of the head and neck.

breasts. The assessment techniques most often used are inspection and auscultation, with palpation also used to assess the breasts and lymph nodes in the axilla.

Chest and Back

The color, size, shape, muscles, and breathing movements of the chest and back are inspected. The color should be the same as the face and neck. Bilateral sides of the chest and back should be symmetrical, with equal expansion and relaxation during respirations. The thorax should have a greater transverse (side-to-side) diameter than anteroposterior (front-to-back) diameter. The reverse (referred to as a *barrel chest*) is seen in clients with chronic obstructive pulmonary diseases. The scapulae should be equal in height, and the spine should be aligned midline with normal curves (concave cervical and convex thoracic). Abnormal findings of the thoracic spine include *kyphosis* (increased thoracic curve) and *scoliosis* (lateral deviation). In clients with respiratory difficulty, the intercostal and upper thoracic muscles may *retract* (pull in) on inhalation.

Lungs

The lungs are assessed by inspection of the external thorax and by auscultation with a stethoscope. Inspection can be used to determine respiratory rate, depth, and rhythm. The rate is normally 12 to 20 regular breaths per minute (known as *eupnea*) in the adult. Respiratory rates may increase to more than 24 breaths per minute (*tachypnea*) in response to exercise, to fever, and to illnesses that cause an increase in the amount of carbon dioxide or a decrease of oxygen in the blood. Respiratory rates may decrease to less than 10 breaths per minute (*bradypnea*) in a client with an increase in intracranial pressure or in response to certain narcotic drugs.

The normal depth and rhythm of respirations is about equal during inspiration and expiration, but may abnormally be very deep or shallow. A client may also have increased respiratory rate and depth (*hyperventilation*) or decreased respiratory rate and depth (*hypoventilation*) in response to factors such as respiratory disorders, metabolic disorders, fear, and drug overdose. *Cheyne–Stokes respirations,* a response to organ failure, drug overdose, or increased intracranial pressure, are manifested by regular periods of alternating deep and rapid respirations followed by apnea. Other abnormal respiratory findings are *dyspnea* (difficulty breathing), *orthopnea* (breathing more easily in an upright position), and *apnea* (periods in which there is no breathing).

Auscultation is used to assess normal and abnormal (or *adventitious*) breath sounds. To auscultate the chest, have the client in a sitting position. Warm the stethoscope diaphragm before placing it on the client's chest and ask the client to breathe slowly and deeply through the mouth. A regular pattern of auscultation should be used, beginning above the clavicle or scapula and moving the diaphragm down at regular intervals to the bottom of the ribs. Compare and document sounds for both the right and left lungs.

There are several different types of abnormal breath sounds. Noisy respirations are often labeled *stertorous. Crackles,* heard most often during inspiration, are crackling sounds made as air moves through secretions in the airways. *Wheezes* are high-pitched continuous sounds heard on both inspiration and expiration. Wheezes are heard when secretions, swelling, or tumors narrow the small airways. A grating sound indicates a *pleural friction rub,* resulting from an inflamed pleura rubbing against the chest wall.

While assessing the lungs, it is important to note if the client has a cough, and to ask if and when sputum is coughed up. If the cough is productive of sputum, note the color, amount, and consistency. Depending on the cause, sputum may be clear, yellow, green, or blood tinged and may be thin or thick. Additional documentation is necessary if the client is receiving oxygen. Record how it is administered (i.e., by mask or nasal cannula) and at what rate (in L/minute). (See also Chapters 25 and 26.)

Heart

The heart is assessed by auscultation for heart sounds to take an apical pulse. The equipment used is a stethoscope with a diaphragm. The diaphragm should be warmed before placement on the client's chest, and the room should be quiet so sounds may be heard without difficulty. The nurse assesses the rate and rhythm of the heart and the normal heart sounds. Assessing abnormal heart sounds is an advanced assessment technique.

The point of maximum impulse (PMI) is used as a landmark for taking an apical pulse. This landmark is located at the fourth or fifth left intercostal space in the midclavicular line (Figure 4-7 ◆). It may often be palpated as a slight tap against the fingers. The apical pulse is the most accurate pulse

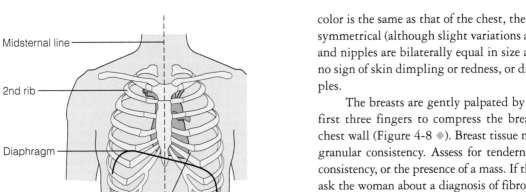

Figure 4-7. ◆ Location of the PMI (point of maximum impulse) of the heart.

Midsternal line

2nd rib

Diaphragm

Point of maximal intensity (PMI)

measurement. It should be taken if there is any question about the peripheral pulse or if the client is taking a medication that affects heart rate. The apical pulse is taken for 1 full minute; the normal rate for adults ranges from 60 to 100 beats per minute.

The first heart sound heard (S_1) is the "lub" of "lub-dub." This is a low pitched sound that occurs as the mitral and tricuspid valves close. The second heart sound (S_2) is the "dub" of "lub-dub." This sound is not as low pitched and is shorter than the first heart sound. It occurs as the aortic and pulmonic valves close. Both sounds normally occur within 1 second or less, and are counted together to determine the heart rate.

CLINICAL alert

Remember to count only once for each two sounds that are heard, and to count for 1 full minute when taking an apical pulse. It is helpful always to begin counting when the second hand of your watch is on 12 (to avoid forgetting when you began counting).

While assessing the heart rate, it is important also to note whether the rhythm is regular or irregular, and whether the sounds are strong or weak. An irregular pattern of heartbeats is called a *dysrhythmia* (see Chapter 23). The client should also be asked about any other symptoms that might indicate heart disease, such as swelling of the feet, pain in the chest, difficulty breathing, fatigue, and dizziness. During an assessment for a client who complains of chest pain, also assess skin color for cyanosis or pallor; pulse, blood pressure, and respirations; location, duration, and intensity of the pain, and any other accompanying manifestations such as nausea or loss of consciousness.

Breasts and Axillary Lymph Nodes

The breasts of both men and women are assessed by inspection and palpation. The breasts are inspected for size, symmetry, skin condition, nipple condition, and discharge. Normally, the

color is the same as that of the chest, the breasts are bilaterally symmetrical (although slight variations are normal), the areola and nipples are bilaterally equal in size and color, and there is no sign of skin dimpling or redness, or discharge from the nipples.

The breasts are gently palpated by using the pads of the first three fingers to compress the breast tissue against the chest wall (Figure 4-8 ◆). Breast tissue normally is firm with a granular consistency. Assess for tenderness or pain, abnormal consistency, or the presence of a mass. If the breasts feel nodular, ask the woman about a diagnosis of fibrocystic breast disease as well as the time of her last period. While palpating the breasts, also palpate well into the axilla for the presence of pain and enlarged lymph nodes. If present, document size and consistency. Any abnormal findings are documented by quadrant (upper inner, upper outer, lower inner, lower outer). Ask women about a history of breast cancer, self-breast examinations, and mammograms (if age appropriate). (See Chapter 33.)

ABDOMEN

Abdominal assessment includes inspecting the exterior abdomen, auscultating bowel sounds to determine intestinal function, and palpating the urinary bladder when a client has not been voiding. Because palpation may alter bowel sounds, the sequence of examination is inspection, auscultation, and palpation. Percussion and moderate to deep palpation of the abdomen are more advanced assessments and are not discussed here. Before beginning an abdominal assessment, be sure your hands are warm. For documentation purposes, mentally divide the abdomen into four quadrants (right upper, right lower, left upper, left lower) and know the underlying organs of each quadrant (Figure 4-9 ◆).

Exterior Abdomen

The abdomen is normally slightly rounded, with the umbilicus midline. Fine white or silver-colored lines (*striae*) may be

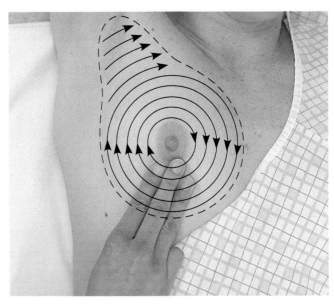

Figure 4-8. ◆ Possible pattern for palpation of the breast.

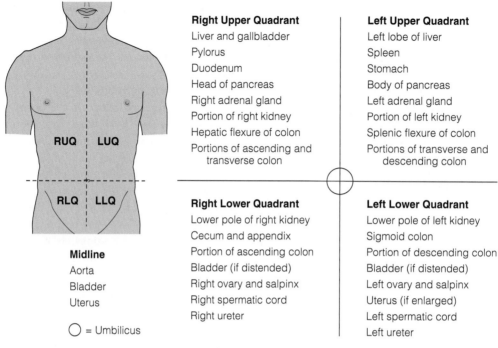

Right Upper Quadrant
Liver and gallbladder
Pylorus
Duodenum
Head of pancreas
Right adrenal gland
Portion of right kidney
Hepatic flexure of colon
Portions of ascending and
   transverse colon

Left Upper Quadrant
Left lobe of liver
Spleen
Stomach
Body of pancreas
Left adrenal gland
Portion of left kidney
Splenic flexure of colon
Portions of transverse and
   descending colon

Midline
Aorta
Bladder
Uterus

○ = Umbilicus

Right Lower Quadrant
Lower pole of right kidney
Cecum and appendix
Portion of ascending colon
Bladder (if distended)
Right ovary and salpinx
Right spermatic cord
Right ureter

Left Lower Quadrant
Lower pole of left kidney
Sigmoid colon
Portion of descending colon
Bladder (if distended)
Left ovary and salpinx
Uterus (if enlarged)
Left spermatic cord
Left ureter

Figure 4-9. ◆ The four quadrants of the abdomen, with anatomic location of organs within each quadrant.

visible; they result from skin being stretched by weight gain or pregnancy. There should be no visible masses. If the abdomen is distended, ask questions about any changes in usual patterns of bowel movements and urination.

Bowel Sounds

Bowel sounds are auscultated to assess intestinal function. Warm the diaphragm of the stethoscope and gently place it on the abdominal skin, listening in all four quadrants. Bowel sounds are clicks and gurgles made as intestinal contents move through bowel and should always be present. They normally occur every 5 to 20 seconds. Bowel sounds that occur less often are referred to as *hypoactive,* and those that occur more often are referred to as *hyperactive.* Hypoactive or absent bowel sounds may result from abdominal surgery, paralysis of the intestinal wall *(paralytic ileus),* or advanced intestinal obstruction. Hyperactive bowel sounds are heard during diarrhea and in the early stage of intestinal obstruction (see Chapter 20).

Urinary Bladder

The urinary bladder, if distended with urine, may be gently palpated in the midline of the abdomen above the symphy-sis pubis. If a client has not voided for 8 to 10 hours, or if the voidings are frequent and in small amounts, palpating a distended urinary bladder is essential to identify the need for further interventions to empty the bladder (see Chapter 21).

EXTREMITIES

The extremities are assessed for color, temperature, lesions, condition of hair and nails, peripheral circulation, and muscle strength. Skin color and temperature should be similar to that of the face. Hair distribution is normally symmetrical on arms

and legs, and nails should be intact. Clients with peripheral vascular disease often have abnormal assessments, including decreased or absent pulses; cool, pale, shiny skin; absence of hair, and thickened nails (see Chapter 24).

Peripheral Circulation

Peripheral pulses are assessed by noting the rate, rhythm, and strength of the pulse at various locations, including the temporal, carotid, brachial, radial, femoral, popliteal, posterior tibial, and dorsalis pedis arteries (Figure 4-10 ◆). The pulse is taken by gently compressing the artery against an underlying bone with the tips of the middle three fingers. During a physical examination, or if abnormalities are assessed, bilateral pulses should be palpated and compared (although both carotid arteries should never be palpated at the same time). If peripheral pulses are abnormal or cannot be palpated, a Doppler ultrasound can be used to determine the rate.

The normal pulse rate in an adult is from 60 to 100 beats per minute. A rapid heart rate (ranging from 100 to 180 beats per minute) is labeled *tachycardia.* Tachycardia may be caused by many different factors, including pain, anxiety, fever, and heart disease. A slow heart rate (< 60 beats per minute) is labeled *bradycardia.* Bradycardia may be caused by medications, increasing age, or disorders of the cardiac conduction system. The rhythm of the heartbeat (the pattern of pulsations and pauses) should be regular. An abnormal rhythm should be reported. The *amplitude* is normally strong. The amplitude may be documented as:

■ 0 or absent—no pulsation is felt

■ 1+ or thready—pulsations are not easily palpated and disappear with slight pressure

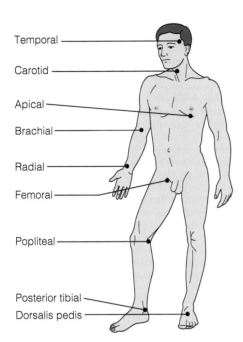

Figure 4-10. ◆ Body sites at which peripheral pulses are most easily palpated.

- 2+ or weak—although stronger than a thready pulse, disappears with light pressure
- 3+ or normal—pulsations are palpated easily and only disappear with moderate pressure
- 4+ or bounding—pulsations are strong and do not disappear with moderate pressure

If the radial pulse is irregular, an apical–radial pulse may be taken. This procedure requires two nurses who simultaneously count the apical pulse and the radial pulse for one minute. A difference in the rate is called a *pulse deficit,* and is caused by heartbeats that are weak or are not all reaching the peripheral arteries.

Capillary refill also provides information about peripheral circulation. To assess capillary refill, the nurse squeezes the client's fingernail or toenail until it turns white, then releases the pressure and observes the time for normal color to return. The return is normally immediate.

Musculoskeletal

Musculoskeletal function is initially assessed by observing the client's posture, ability to move, walk, and carry out activities of daily living. Range of motion of joints may be observed during the physical examination. Muscle strength is often assessed through hand grips and feet pushes. The nurse asks the client to grasp the nurse's index and middle finger and squeeze, and to push the soles of the feet against the nurse's hands. Muscle strength should be bilaterally equal.

MENTAL STATUS

Mental status is most often assessed by determining the client's level of awareness *(orientation)* and degree of wakefulness or ability to be aroused *(level of consciousness).* These are not the same conditions; a client may be conscious but disoriented.

The client's level of awareness is assessed by orientation to time, place, and person. When awareness is lost, the usual sequence of loss is time orientation, followed by place orientation, and then person orientation. It is important to remember that pain, trauma, illness, and a change in surroundings may make it difficult for clients to know the exact day and date. The following questions may be used to assess orientation:

- **Time**—What is the date today? What day of the week is today? What was our last holiday?
- **Place**—Where are you now? What state do we live in?
- **Person**—What is your name? How old are you?

Level of consciousness may be assessed and labeled as follows:

- *Awake and alert:* Client is fully awake, responds to verbal requests, and is oriented to time, place, and person.
- *Lethargic:* Client appears drowsy or asleep but can be awakened by calling his or her name and gently shaking.
- *Stuporous:* Client is deeply asleep most of the time and can be awakened only by shouting and shaking, responds to painful stimuli by making purposeful movements, and verbally responds but may make inappropriate responses.
- *Comatose:* Client cannot be aroused, even with painful stimuli; some reflexes (such as the gag reflex) may still be present.

Documentation

Data from the initial comprehensive assessment provides a foundation for the development and application of the nursing process. Documentation of ongoing focused assessments identifies improvement or worsening of identified health problems, provides information to help diagnose new problems, and serves as a means of communication among all members of the health care team. In addition, documentation of assessments provides the base for evaluation of health care outcomes, provides evidence to support health care cost reimbursements, and is legal evidence of the health status of the client at that point in time.

Each institution or agency has its own requirements for the timing and method of documentation. The types seen most often are the traditional narrative form; the checklist or standardized form (ranging from an initial admission record to a flow sheet for vital signs); and the nursing minimum data set (used in long-term care facilities). Increasingly, documentation is entered into a computer, where it becomes part of a database that is shared within and between health care settings. With this method, for example, a nurse caring for a client in the home would have access to previous assessment data and would not have to repeat the entire procedure, nor would the client have to repeat all the information.

To document factually and accurately, follow these principles:

Temporal
Carotid
Apical
Brachial
Radial
Femoral
Popliteal
Posterior tibial
Dorsalis pedis

■ *Document as soon as possible.* It is difficult to remember information accurately for long periods of time.

■ *Document legibly or make computer entries accurately.* Errors in documentation must legally be corrected in the format approved by the health care institution or agency. Check the policy of your institution.

■ *Organize the data in a logical way.* The health history is generally documented before the physical examination. If the health care setting uses a specific framework for organizing the data (such as Functional Health Patterns), data are documented within this framework. When documenting the health history, present health problems are described beginning with onset of the problem.

■ *Avoid inferences and judgments.* An inference is a statement about something unknown based on observation. For example, the nurse should not write "Obesity and body odor indicate little knowledge of nutrition and hygiene" or "Requests pain medication although obviously is not in pain."

■ *Record findings rather than methods of assessment.* A detailed description of the method of assessment is unnecessary. For example, when recording a blood pressure, the nurse writes "BP 120/70," not "The diaphragm of the stethoscope was placed over the brachial artery and the sounds were auscultated."

■ *Write concisely, using approved abbreviations and grammar.* It is not necessary to use entire sentences or to begin the narrative with the words "the client." Group phrases, such as "Bowel sounds heard in all four quadrants," rather than "The client has bowel sounds in the right upper and lower quadrants and left upper and lower quadrants." Use only those abbreviations approved by policy in the setting. Avoid jargon and slang words unless they are direct quotes.

■ *Do not use the word "normal" for normal findings.* It is better to write what was assessed, such as "Breath sounds clear in both lower lungs," rather than "Breath sounds normal."

■ If the agency uses documents called "charting by exception," document only abnormal findings.

(*Note:* The bibliography listings for this and all chapters have been compiled at the back of the book.)

Chapter Review

key terms by topic

Use the CD-ROM disk enclosed with your textbook to hear the pronunciation of the key terms in the chapter.

Purposes of a health assessment
assessment, objective data, subjective data, manifestations

Methods of physical examination
inspection, palpation, percussion, auscultation

key points

- Assessment is the collection of data that provides information about the client's individualized health care needs. Nurses collect this data through the health assessment, comprised of a health history and a physical examination.

- The primary source of data is the client.

- The health history, collected through an interview of the client, provides subjective and objective data.

- The four methods of physical examination are inspection, palpation, percussion, and auscultation. The skills of physical examination take practice.

- A comprehensive physical examination is conducted in a head-to-toe sequence. If a focused or emergency assessment is being conducted, the nurse assesses only the specific client problem.

- Documenting assessments factually and accurately provides the base for evaluation of health care outcomes, provides evidence to support healthcare cost reimbursement, and is legal evidence of the health status of the client at that point in time.

Medialink

Additional interactive resources for this chapter can be found on the Companion Website at www.prenhall.com/burke. Click on Chapter 4 and "Begin" to select the activities for this chapter.

For NCLEX review questions and an audio glossary, access the accompanying CD-ROM in this book.

for further study

For more information about normal skin and skin disorders, see Chapters 14 and 15.

For more information about intestinal disorders, see Chapter 20.

For more information about urinary disorders, see Chapter 21.

For more information about dysrhythmias, see Chapter 23.

For more information about assessing peripheral circulatory disorders, see Chapter 24.

For more information about respiratory disorders, see Chapters 25 and 26.

For more information about ear and eye disorders, see Chapter 31.

For more information about female reproductive and breast disorders, see Chapter 33.

Critical Thinking Care Map

Caring for a Client with Risk for Excess Fluid Volume
NCLEX-PN Focus Area: Coordinated Care

Case Study: Cath Cole, age 62, has a long history of congestive heart failure. She lives in a small apartment with her cat, Tom. She states, "You know, I have had many problems with water in my lungs and my legs swell something awful." Cath is supposed to take her "heart pill" and "water pill" every day, but she ran out of money and couldn't buy any this month. Although a low-sodium diet has been prescribed, Cath eats anything she wants.

Nursing Diagnosis: Risk for Imbalanced Fluid Volume

COLLECT DATA

Subjective

_____

_____

_____

_____

_____

Objective

_____

_____

_____

_____

_____

Would you report this data? Yes/No

If yes, to: _____

Nursing Care

_____

_____

_____

_____

_____

_____

_____

How would you document this? _____

_____

_____

Data collected
(use those that apply)

- Height: 5′5″
- Weight: 125 lbs.
- Blood pressure: 180/96
- Pupils cloudy, conjunctiva red
- States she has chronic infection in her sinuses
- Kyphosis present
- R = 30, crackles and wheezes present
- Apical pulse = 108, irregular
- Bowel sounds present in all four quadrants
- 4+ edema from toes to knees in both legs
- Has not taken medications for more than a week
- Does not follow prescribed diet

Nursing Interventions
(use those that apply)

- State "Why didn't you ask for help with your medicines?"
- Ask Cath if she would consider being seen by a social worker.
- Monitor vital signs on a regular basis.
- State "You need to follow your diet."
- Monitor breath sounds, apical pulse, and peripheral pulses.
- Measure circumference of lower legs.

NCLEX-PN Exam Preparation

TEST-TAKING TIP

Focus on key words such as *immediately, first, best, early, late, most likely, least likely,* or *on the day of.* These words are critical in selecting the correct answer.

1. When the nurse collects a urine specimen and notes the color of the urine, this assessment data is referred to as:
   a. comprehensive
   b. objective
   c. subjective
   d. secondary

2. A focused assessment for a client complaining of abdominal pain would include assessing the client's:
   a. legs
   b. vision
   c. bowel movements
   d. blood pressure

3. It is preferable to collect assessment data from secondary sources instead of directly from the client when the:
   a. client is irritable or agitated
   b. client is very young, unconscious, or confused
   c. client's family prefers to speak for him or her
   d. client's medical records are available

4. The health history data are collected through an interview with the client. Questions that give the client a chance to provide more information are called:
   a. yes or no
   b. why
   c. closed-ended
   d. open-ended

5. A basic method of physical examination that uses the hands to touch and feel is called:
   a. inspection
   b. auscultation
   c. palpation
   d. percussion

6. The first thing that the nurse should do in preparing for a physical examination is:
   a. wash his or her hands
   b. don gloves and mask
   c. set up the equipment
   d. position the client

7. The most accurate pulse measurement is the:
   a. radial pulse taken for 15 seconds
   b. radial pulse taken for 1 full minute
   c. apical pulse taken for 15 seconds
   d. apical pulse taken for 1 full minute

8. Mrs. Haynes developed a bowel obstruction following abdominal surgery 3 days ago. To monitor peristalsis, the nurse would:
   a. inspect the abdomen
   b. auscultate the abdomen
   c. percuss the abdomen
   d. palpate the abdomen

9. Mr. Scott has a history of alcohol abuse and has developed cirrhosis of the liver. The nurse might expect to observe this change in skin color:
   a. mottling
   b. erythema
   c. jaundice
   d. cyanosis

10. Documenting the health assessment is as important as the actual assessment. Identify the documentation that is most correctly stated.
    a. Breath sounds normal.
    b. The client had bowel sounds in the right upper and lower quadrants and the left upper and lower quadrants.
    c. BP 120/70.
    d. Client obese, indicating lack of knowledge about nutrition.

Answers for Review Questions, as well as discussion of Case Study Critical Thinking questions, appear in Appendix V.

Cultural Care STRATEGIES

Appreciating Variations in Facial Expression when Relating to the Client from Another Culture

The home health care supervisor received an angry call from Mrs. Espanito, a Mexican-American woman who had been the recipient of a home health care visit that day by a nurse. Mrs. Espanito explained that her infant was crying and feverish today, and it was undoubtedly because the nurse had complimented the baby but had not touched the infant during the compliment. Mrs. Espanito felt the nurse had given the infant the evil eye. Mrs. Espanito explained that in Mexican culture, babies are considered very weak and susceptible to the power of an envious glance. A simple compliment without touching a child can bring on the evil eye. While touching a child during a compliment can neutralize the power of the evil eye, no touch had occurred, and therefore she felt her child had become sick from the glance of the nurse.

Throughout the world, facial expression and eye contact are considered an important part of the communication message (Giger & Davidhizar, 1999). From birth, individuals learn how to communicate nonverbally and how to interpret different facial expressions and eye behaviors. Since nursing occurs in an interpersonal arena, nurses need to be aware of facial expression and eye behavior and the meaning that different cultures may associate with facial expressions.

Facial Expression

Facial expression is commonly used as a guide to a person's feelings. A constant stare with immobile facial muscles is generally an indication of coldness. However, it can also be an indication of shock, guardedness, or fear. In an individual with schizophrenia or Parkinson's disease it may be a symptom of the disease process. Facial expression is usually only one part of the total verbal and nonverbal communication that an individual provides. It is important to use facial expression in conjunction with other information to draw conclusions about another's feelings.

The meanings of facial expression vary between persons from different cultures. For example, Italian, Jewish, African-American, and Hispanic persons tend to smile readily and use many facial expressions, gestures, and words to communicate feelings. Persons in other cultures (including the Irish, the English, and northern Europeans) tend to use less facial expression and to be less responsive. Facial expression can also convey the opposite meaning from the one that is felt; for example, Oriental people may conceal negative emotions with a smile (Sue & Sue, 1990).

Eye Behavior

Eye contact is a valuable source of information. Typically, individuals look at each other for three to ten seconds in a glance. For many people, longer contact arouses anxiety (Argyle & Dean, 1965). Most Caucasians value eye contact. They may equate avoidance of eye contact with rudeness, disrespect, or lack of attention. Fleeting eye contact may suggest insecurity, shyness, anxiety, or, in some cases, rejection. Embarrassment, guilt, fear, or anger may be interpreted from eye contact.

Since eye contact is learned in a family and cultural context, patterns of eye behavior can sometimes be related to cultural groups. For example, most Mexican-American and African-American people are comfortable with eye contact (Giger & Davidhizar, 1999). Oriental people and some Native Americans tend to have difficulty with eye contact; they may relate eye contact to impoliteness and an invasion of privacy. Some Filipinos may interpret eye contact that is diverted as a sign of a witch. Some cultures may associate eye contact with the "evil eye" (Henderson & Primeaux, 1981).

Nursing Implications

- **Assess facial expression for possible cultural significance.** Most individuals use facial expression to reveal feelings. However, since facial expression is learned in a cultural context, the nurse should use an understanding of the individual's culture when interpreting of the meaning of a facial expression.
- **Assess eye behavior for possible cultural significance.** Since individuals are unique, nurses should interpret eye behavior in the context of other available interpersonal information. Since eye behavior is learned in a cultural context, the cultural significance of eye behavior should also be considered.
- **Be aware that your health care team members may use culturally oriented communication behaviors that make others uncomfortable.** When the communication of a co-worker makes you uncomfortable, it is important to assess whether the communication difference is related to cultural behavior.

Self-Reflection Questions

1. What facial and eye behavior do you use in communicating with others?
2. What eye behavior of others makes you uncomfortable?
3. What facial and eye behavior in clients or staff would you interpret as negative or hostile?

Caring for Clients with Altered Fluid, Electrolyte, or Acid–Base Balance

chapter 5

CARING tip

❝Be sure to know, understand, and practice within the guidelines of the Nurse Practice Act.❞

Mickle Ward-Ellison, RN, MS • Director of Nursing Related Programs • Kennedy-King College, City College of Chicago • Chicago, Illinois

LEARNING outcomes

After completing this chapter, you will be able to:

- Identify the functions and regulatory mechanisms that maintain water and electrolyte balance in the body.
- Compare and contrast the causes and effects of fluid volume, electrolyte, and acid–base imbalances.
- Identify tests used to diagnose and monitor treatment of fluid, electrolyte, and acid–base disorders.
- Recognize normal and abnormal values of electrolytes in the blood.
- Use arterial blood gas findings to identify the type of acid–base imbalance present in a client.
- Provide appropriate nursing care and teaching for clients with fluid, electrolyte, or acid–base disorders.

MediaLink

www.prenhall.com/burke

Use the above address to access the free, interactive Companion Website created for this textbook. Get hints, instant feedback, and textbook references to chapter-related multiple choice questions. Link to other interesting sites.

Normal life processes depend on a relatively stable state within the body. **Homeostasis** is the body's tendency to maintain a state of physiologic balance in constantly changing conditions. For the body to function and survive, the volume of fluids, the electrolyte balance, and the pH of body fluids all must remain within a relatively narrow and constant range.

Disorders in fluid volumes, electrolyte concentrations, and hydrogen ion concentration (pH) often occur in response to illness and trauma. Nursing care related to homeostasis focuses on assessing clients who are likely to develop imbalances, monitoring for early manifestations of imbalances, and implementing care to prevent or correct imbalances.

Fluid and Electrolyte Balance

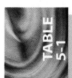

Structure and Function

BODY FLUID COMPOSITION

Water is the primary component of body fluids. Water has a number of vital functions in the body:

- It transports nutrients and oxygen to the cells, and waste products such as carbon dioxide away from the cells.
- It provides a medium for metabolic reactions within cells.
- It insulates and helps regulate and maintain body temperature.
- It provides form for body structure and acts as a shock absorber.
- It is a lubricant.

About 60% of the total body weight is water, but this amount varies with age, gender, and body fat. In people over age 65, body water may decrease to 45% to 50% of total body weight. The obese person has a smaller proportion of water to total body weight, because fat cells contain comparatively little water. Adult females have a higher percentage of body fat and a lower percentage of body water than males.

To maintain normal fluid balance, water intake and output should be approximately equal. The average daily fluid intake and output usually is about 2,500 mL. Water enters the body through ingested fluids and foods. It also is produced by the cells during metabolism. Water is lost in urine, feces, sweat, and when we exhale air from the lungs.

Besides water, body fluids contain solutes such as oxygen, dissolved nutrients, waste products of metabolism such as carbon dioxide, and electrolytes.

Electrolytes are substances that *dissociate* (separate) in solution to form *ions* (charged particles). *Cations* are positively charged electrolytes; *anions* are negatively charged electrolytes. Electrolytes have many functions:

- They help regulate water and acid–base balance.
- They contribute to enzyme reactions.
- They are essential to neuromuscular activity.

The concentration of most electrolytes in body fluids is measured in milliequivalents per liter of water (mEq/L). A *milliequivalent* is a measure of the combining power of the ion. For example, 100 mEq of sodium (Na^+) can combine with 100 mEq of chloride (Cl^-) to form sodium chloride (NaCl), or table salt. Some electrolytes (e.g., calcium) may be measured by weight, in milligrams per deciliter of water (mg/dL). (Table 5-1 ◆ lists normal laboratory values for electrolytes.)

BODY FLUID DISTRIBUTION

Body fluid is classified by its location. **Intracellular fluid (ICF)** is within the cells; it accounts for about 40% of total body weight (Figure 5-1 ◆). ICF contains solutes such as electrolytes, glucose, and oxygen. ICF is essential for normal cell function.

Extracellular fluid (ECF) is outside of cells; it accounts for about 20% of total body weight. ECF is found in three compartments:

- *Interstitial fluid* is in the spaces between most of the cells of the body (about 15% of total body weight).

TABLE 5-1	NORMAL LABORATORY VALUES FOR ELECTROLYTES, OSMOLALITY, AND URINE SPECIFIC GRAVITY	
Electrolytes	
Sodium (Na^+)	135–145 mEq/L
Potassium (K^+)	3.5–5.0 mEq/L
Calcium (Ca^{2+})	8.5–10 mg/dL
Magnesium (Mg^{2+})	1.3–2.1 mEq/L or 1.6–2.6 mg/dL
Chloride (Cl^-)	98–106 mEq/L
Bicarbonate (HCO_3^-)	22–26 mEq/L
Phosphate/phosphorus (PO_4^{2-})	2.5–4.5 mg/dL
Serum osmolality	275–295 mOsm/kg
Urine specific gravity	1.010–1.035 mEq/L

bon dioxide are carried away from the tissues to the lungs and the kidneys for elimination.

Electrolytes are found in both fluid compartments, but the electrolyte composition of ICF and ECF differs (Figure 5-2 ◆). Sodium (Na^+), chloride (Cl^-), and bicarbonate (HCO_3^-) are the principal extracellular electrolytes. The principal intracellular electrolytes are potassium (K^+), magnesium (Mg^{2+}), and phosphate (HPO_4^{2-}).

BODY FLUID MOVEMENT

Membranes such as the cell membrane and capillary walls separate the body fluid compartments. These membranes are *selectively permeable;* that is, they allow water and some solutes (e.g., oxygen, carbon dioxide, electrolytes, and glucose) to cross, but block proteins and other large molecules. Water and solutes move across these membranes by the processes of osmosis, diffusion, filtration, and active transport.

Osmosis

In the process of **osmosis,** water moves across a membrane from an area of lower solute concentration to an area of higher solute concentration (Figure 5-3 ◆). Osmosis continues until the solute concentration on both sides of the membrane is equal. For example, if a selectively permeable membrane separates pure water from a salt solution, water moves into the salt solution. Osmosis is responsible for water movement between the ICF and ECF compartments.

Osmolality is the concentration of all solutes within a body fluid compartment. It is measured in milliosmoles per kilogram (mOsm/kg). The normal osmolality of both ICF and ECF ranges between 275 and 295 mOsm/kg (see Table 5-1).

The power of a solution to draw water across a membrane is known as the *osmotic pressure* of the solution. All solutes in a solution contribute to its osmotic pressure. In the blood, plasma proteins, especially albumin, exert osmotic pressure, helping to hold water within the blood vessels.

Tonicity refers to the effect of the osmotic pressure of a solution on cells within that solution. *Isotonic* solutions (like normal saline, 0.9% sodium chloride solution) have the same

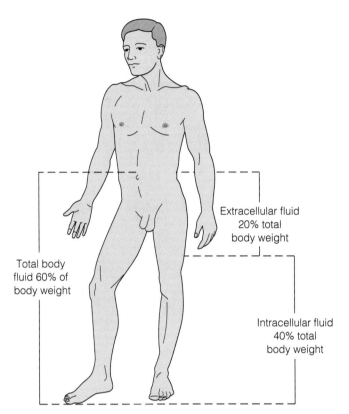

Figure 5-1. ◆ A comparison of the major fluid compartments of the body.

Total body fluid 60% of body weight

Extracellular fluid 20% total body weight

Intracellular fluid 40% total body weight

■ *Intravascular fluid* or *plasma* is in the arteries, veins, and capillaries (about 5% of total body weight).
■ *Transcellular fluid* includes cerebrospinal fluid, urine, digestive secretions, perspiration, and small amounts of fluid found within organs and joints (< 1% of total body weight).

ECF transports oxygen and nutrients to cells, and waste products away from the cells. For example, plasma transports oxygen from the lungs and glucose from the gastrointestinal tract to the tissues. Waste products of metabolism such as car-

	Na+	K+	Cl−	HCO₃−
A	142	4	102	24

	Na+	K+	Mg²⁺	PO₄
B	10	140	27	100

Figure 5-2. ◆ The principle electrolytes (in milliequivalents) of (A) extracellular fluid and (B) intracellular fluid.

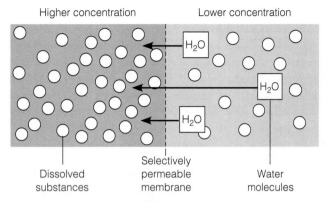

Higher concentration   Lower concentration

Dissolved
substances

Selectively
permeable
membrane

Water
molecules

Figure 5-3. ◆ Osmosis. Water moves across a selectively permeable membrane from an area of lower solute concentration to an area of high solute concentration.

A Isotonic solution

B Hypertonic solution

C Hypotonic solution

Figure 5-4. ◆ The effect of changes in the concentration of solutions on red blood cells. (A) Cells neither gain nor lose water, size, or shape in isotonic solutions. (B) Cells lose water and shrink in hypertonic solutions. (C) Cells absorb water, swell, and burst in hypotonic solutions.

concentration of solutes as plasma. Cells placed in an isotonic solution do not gain or lose water (Figure 5-4 ◆). *Hypertonic* solutions (e.g., 3% sodium chloride solution) have a greater concentration of solutes than plasma. A cell placed in a hypertonic solution shrinks as water is drawn out of it into the solution. *Hypotonic* solutions (such as 0.45% sodium chloride) have a lower solute concentration than plasma. A cell placed in a hypotonic solution swells as water moves into it. The cell may burst.

Diffusion

Diffusion is the process in which solutes move from an area of high solute concentration to an area of low concentration to become evenly distributed (Figure 5-5 ◆). There are two types of diffusion. *Simple diffusion* occurs by the random movement of solutes. Solutes such as oxygen and carbon dioxide move from plasma to the interstitial space and into cells by simple diffusion. Large water-soluble molecules such as glucose move into cells by a process of *facilitated diffusion.* Proteins within the cell membrane act as carriers to help large molecules cross the membrane.

Filtration

Filtration is the process in which water and solutes move across capillary membranes driven by fluid pressure. Fluid (or *hydrostatic*) pressure is created by the pumping action of the heart and by gravity. At the arterial end of capillaries, this pressure pushes water and solutes into the interstitial space, an area of lower fluid pressure. At the venous end of the capillary, the osmotic force of plasma proteins draws fluid back into the capillary. A balance of filtration and osmosis regulates the movement of water between the intravascular and interstitial spaces in the capillary beds of the body.

Active Transport

Active transport allows molecules to move across cell membranes into an area of higher solute concentration. This movement requires cellular energy (adenosine triphosphate or ATP) and a carrier mechanism. The sodium–potassium pump is an important example of active transport (Figure 5-6 ◆). High concentrations of potassium within cells are maintained because cells actively move potassium from interstitial fluid (where the potassium concentration is about 5 mEq/L) into intracellular fluid (K^+ concentration about 150 mEq/L). Sodium is "pumped" from ICF into ECF.

BODY FLUID REGULATION

Homeostasis depends on a number of mechanisms and processes that regulate the balance between fluid intake, output, and distribution. These regulatory mechanisms include thirst, the kidneys, the renin–angiotensin–aldosterone mechanism, antidiuretic hormone, and atrial natriuretic factor.

Thirst

Thirst is the primary regulator of water intake. It plays an important role in maintaining fluid balance and preventing dehydration. The thirst center in the brain is stimulated when

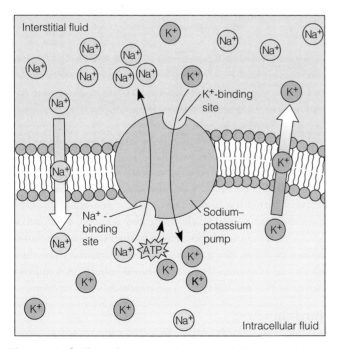

Figure 5-5. ◆ In diffusion, molecules move across a semiperme-able membrane from an area of higher solute concentration to an area of lower concentration.

the blood volume drops because of water losses or when solute content (osmolality) of body fluids increases (Figure 5-7 ◆). The thirst mechanism declines with age, so older adults are more vulnerable to dehydration. Clients with an altered level of consciousness or who are unable to respond to thirst also are at risk.

Kidneys

The kidneys are primarily responsible for regulating fluid vol-ume and electrolyte balance in the body. In adults, about 170 liters of plasma are filtered by the kidneys every day. About 99% of this filtrate is reabsorbed, and only about 1,500 mL of urine is produced. By selectively reabsorbing water and elec-trolytes, the kidneys maintain the volume and osmolality of body fluids.

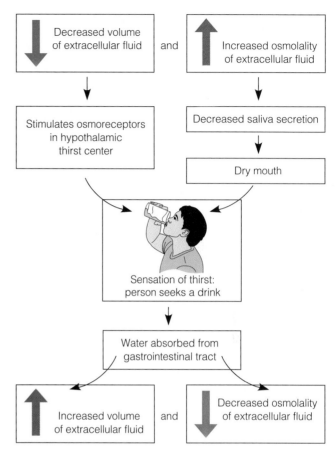

Figure 5-7. ◆ Factors stimulating water intake through the thirst mechanism.

Renin–Angiotensin–Aldosterone System

The *renin–angiotensin–aldosterone system* helps maintain in-travascular fluid balance and blood pressure. A fall in blood flow to the kidneys stimulates specialized receptors in the kid-ney to produce renin (an enzyme). Renin converts angio-tensinogen (a plasma protein) in the blood into angiotensin I. In the lungs, angiotensin I is converted to angiotensin II by angiotensin-converting enzyme (ACE). Angiotensin II con-stricts blood vessels, which raises blood pressure. It also stim-ulates thirst, releases aldosterone (a hormone) from the adrenal cortex, and acts directly on the kidneys, causing them to retain sodium and water. Aldosterone also promotes sodium and water retention by the kidneys, restoring blood volume (Figure 5-8 ◆).

Antidiuretic Hormone

Antidiuretic hormone (ADH) regulates water excretion from the kidneys. Receptors in the hypothalamus detect changes in osmolality and blood volume, stimulating ADH production and release as needed. When ADH is present, more water is reabsorbed in the kidney. Urine output falls, blood volume is restored, and serum osmolality drops as the water dilutes body fluids (Figure 5-9 ◆).

Disorders of ADH production affect urine output. In *diabetes insipidus,* ADH is not produced. The lack of ADH

Figure 5-6. ◆ The sodium–potassium pump. Active transport moves sodium and potassium ions across cell membranes against their concentration gradients.

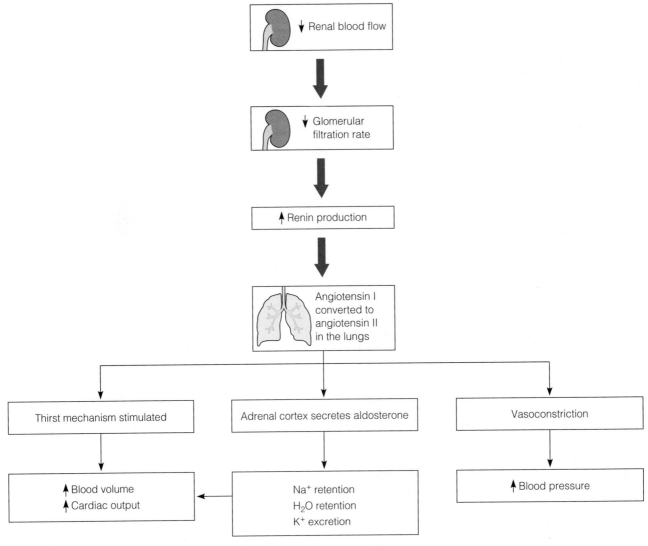

Figure 5-8. ❖ The renin–angiotensin–aldosterone system.

impairs water reabsorption in the kidney, resulting in copious, very dilute urine output. The thirst mechanism is stimulated and the client drinks additional fluids, maintaining high urine output. In the *syndrome of inappropriate ADH secretion (SIADH),* excess ADH is released. More water is reabsorbed, fluid volume increases, and urine output is scant and concentrated. (See Chapter 16 for discussion.)

Atrial Natriuretic Factor

Atrial natriuretic factor (ANF) is a hormone released by cells in the atria of the heart in response to stretching from fluid overload. ANF inhibits renin secretion and blocks the secretion and effects of aldosterone. In doing so, it promotes sodium and water loss, and causes blood vessels to dilate.

 Fluid Volume Deficit

Fluid volume deficits may be due to excessive fluid losses, insufficient fluid intake, or both. The most common causes are vomiting, diarrhea, or gastrointestinal suctioning. Other common causes are listed in Table 5-2 ❖. Inadequate fluid

intake may result from decreased thirst sensation, limited access to fluids, difficulty swallowing, or lack of awareness of the need to replace fluids. Older adults are at particular risk for fluid volume deficits (Box 5-1).

PATHOPHYSIOLOGY

Fluid volume deficit is characterized by a decrease in extracellular fluids. Usually, both water and electrolytes are lost from the body. Initial manifestations are related to *hypovolemia,* or decreased circulating blood volume. Manifestations of fluid volume deficit are related to the cause and severity of the imbalance. With rapid fluid losses, manifestations may be seen within minutes or hours. With gradual losses, interstitial fluid shifts into the vascular space to maintain blood volume. A significant amount of ECF may be lost by the time symptoms develop.

Third-Spacing

Third-spacing is a shift of fluid from the vascular space into an area where it is not available for physiologic processes (e.g., the bowel or the peritoneal cavity). Fluid may also become trapped within soft tissues following trauma or burns. Fluid

Figure 5-9. ◆ The effect of antidiuretic hormone (ADH) release.

loss due to third-spacing can be difficult to detect, because the weight may remain stable, and intake and output records may not show the loss.

population
FOCUS

BOX 5-1

Fluid Volume Deficit in Older Adults

The older adult is at risk for fluid volume deficit from a variety of factors:

- Decreased thirst perception
- Decreased total body water
- Age-related changes renal function and the ability to regulate body temperature
- Self-limiting of fluids due to fear of incontinence
- Self-care deficits or disabilities that limit access to fluids
- Cognitive impairments (confusion, dementia, depression)
- Medications such as diuretics, sedatives

COLLABORATIVE CARE

In addition to the history and physical examination, the *central venous pressure (CVP)* (pressure in the right atrium or vena cava) may be measured to help determine fluid status. The normal CVP (measured by manometer) ranges from 2 to 8 cm water. A low CVP indicates inadequate fluid volume; a high CVP occurs in fluid overload, heart failure, and some lung disorders. The procedure for measuring CVP is outlined in Box 5-2.

Depending on the severity of the deficit, fluids and electrolytes may be replaced orally, enterally, or intravenously. Whenever possible, oral or enteral (nasogastric or gastrostomy tube) fluid replacement is preferred. In acute

TABLE 5-2 **FLUID IMBALANCES**		
	FLUID VOLUME DEFICIT	**FLUID VOLUME EXCESS**
CAUSES	GI fluid losses Excess urine output: diuretics, diabetes Hemorrhage Sweating Fever Draining wounds, burns Fluid shifts (third-spacing) Inadequate fluid intake	Renal failure Heart failure Cirrhosis of the liver Medications Excess fluid intake Excess sodium intake
MANIFESTATIONS	Hypotension Postural hypotension Tachycardia Weak, thready peripheral pulses Weight loss Flat neck veins, ↓ CVP Poor skin turgor Decreased urine output	Hypertension Tachycardia Full, bounding peripheral pulses ↑ Respiratory rate Moist crackles, wheezes Weight gain Distended neck veins, ↑ CVP Dependent edema
Lab values	↑ Serum osmolality ↑ Hematocrit ↑ Urine-specific gravity	↓ Serum osmolality ↓ Hematocrit ↓ Urine specific gravity

MEASURING CENTRAL VENOUS PRESSURE (CVP) WITH A MANOMETER

CVP is used to evaluate fluid volume status. The CVP catheter is inserted by a physician, most often at the client's bedside, into the right atrium or vena cava through a large vein. Nursing responsibilities related to CVP include explaining the procedure to the client and family and monitoring the pressure at regular intervals. The steps in measuring CVP are as follows:

1. Explain what is being done.
2. Mark the level of the right atrium on the chest. This is usually at the fourth intercostal space, midaxillary line on the lateral chest wall. This mark is the reference point for all measurements.
3. Place the client in the same position for each reading, usually supine with the head of the bed flat.
4. Use a carpenter's level to make sure the 0 on the manometer is level with the mark on the client's chest for each measurement (see figure).

IV solution
Manometer
Drip chamber
Right atrium
Zero-leveling point
Three-way stopcock

5. Remove any air bubbles in the line.
6. Turn the stopcock to allow fluid to flow into the manometer, filling it a few centimeters above the expected reading. Then turn the stopcock to open the line between the manometer and the client. The fluid level will fall and then reach a point at which it fluctuates with the client's breathing. This point is recorded as the CVP.
7. After the measurement is taken, turn the stopcock so that the fluid again flows from the fluid source to the client.
8. Document the reading on the vital sign or CVP flow sheet.

situations, intravenous fluid administration is necessary. Isotonic electrolyte solutions (0.9% NaCl or Ringer's solution) are used to expand plasma volume or to replace abnormal losses (e.g., loss of gastric fluid via nasogastric suction). Five percent dextrose in water (D_5W) is used to treat total

body water deficits. Hypotonic saline solution (0.45% NaCl) or mixed solutions are used as maintenance solutions to provide electrolytes and water. (See Table 5-3 ◆.) A fluid challenge may be ordered to evaluate fluid status when a fluid volume deficit is suspected.

NURSING CARE

ASSESSING

Nursing assessment of the client with an actual or potential fluid volume deficit is outlined in Box 5-3. (Also review signs and symptoms of fluid deficit and fluid excess in Table 5-2.)

CLINICAL alert

Assess skin turgor over the sternum in older adults. Loss of subcutaneous tissue in aging makes the skin of the arms a less reliable indicator of fluid status.

BOX 5-3
ASSESSING FOR FLUID VOLUME DEFICIT

SUBJECTIVE DATA
- Complaints of weakness, thirst
- Recent weight loss
- Risk factors: Strenuous exercise (particularly in warm weather); acute illness (e.g., fever, nausea, vomiting, diarrhea); chronic diseases such as diabetes

OBJECTIVE DATA
- Vital signs, including peripheral pulses and capillary refill
- Weight
- Orthostatic vital signs:
  - Measure BP and pulse with client supine; leave cuff in place and allow to remain flat for 3 to 5 minutes.
  - Have client sit up; immediately measure BP and pulse.
  - After another 3 to 5 minutes, have client stand; measure BP and pulse.
  - A BP drop of 10 to 15 mm Hg and increase in pulse of 10 BPM indicates orthostatic or postural hypotension (an indicator of hypovolemia).
- Mental status, level of consciousness
- Color and moisture of skin and mucous membranes; skin temperature
- Observe jugular veins.
- Assess skin turgor: Gently pinch up a fold of skin on the forearm or over the sternum. Turgor is good if the skin returns immediately to previous shape; poor when it remains tented.
- Auscultate breath and bowel sounds.

FLUID	TONICITY	USES
0.9% NaCl (Normal saline)	Isotonic	Restore intravascular volume Replace extracellular fluid Replace sodium losses
0.45% NaCl (½ normal saline)	Hypotonic	Replace water losses Maintain sodium and chloride levels
3% NaCl	Hypertonic	Correct sodium depletion
5% dextrose in water (D_5W)	Isotonic	Replace water losses Correct hypernatremia (excess sodium)
10% dextrose in water ($D_{10}W$)	Hypertonic	Replace water losses Provide calories (340 kcal/L)
20% dextrose in water ($D_{20}W$)	Hypertonic	Promote diuresis Provide calories (680 kcal/L)
50% dextrose in water ($D_{50}W$)	Hypertonic	Treat severe hypoglycemia Provide calories (1,700 kcal/L)
5% dextrose in 0.45% NaCl (D_5½ NS)	Isotonic	Maintenance fluid Replace water losses Maintain sodium and chloride levels
Ringer's solution (balanced electrolyte solution)	Isotonic	Replace fluids Maintain intravascular volume
Lactated Ringer's solution (electrolyte solution with buffer)	Isotonic	Replace fluid losses Prevent acidosis

TABLE 5-3   COMMONLY ADMINISTERED INTRAVENOUS FLUIDS

DIAGNOSING, PLANNING, AND IMPLEMENTING

DEFICIENT FLUID VOLUME

- Monitor intake and output (I&O). Report a urine output of less than 30 mL per hour to the charge nurse or primary care provider. *Urine output of less than 30 mL per hour indicates poor kidney perfusion and a risk for renal failure.*
- Measure urine specific gravity. *Urine specific gravity is normally 1.010 to 1.035. A reading higher than 1.025 may indicate fluid volume deficit.*
- Assess vital signs, CVP, and peripheral pulses every 4 hours. *Hypotension, tachycardia, and weak peripheral pulses indicate hypovolemia. CVP is used to evaluate fluid replacement.*
- Weigh daily with standard conditions (same time of day, approximately the same clothing, balanced scale). *Rapid weight changes often reflect changes in fluid balance.*
- If a fluid challenge is ordered, assess vital signs, urine output, breath sounds, and mental status prior to fluid administration, and every 10 to 15 minutes during the challenge. *A large amount of fluid may be given very rapidly in a fluid challenge. Clients with impaired cardiac or renal status may develop signs of a fluid overload during the challenge.*
- Provide oral fluids as ordered. Identify the client's beverage preferences; monitor fluid intake. *Oral fluids are used to replace lost fluids and relieve thirst.*

- Administer intravenous fluids as ordered. *Clients with severe fluid volume deficit or who are unable to tolerate oral fluids may require intravenous fluid replacement to restore blood volume.*
- Assess laboratory values: electrolytes, serum osmolality, and hematocrit. *Electrolyte levels, serum osmolality, and hematocrit may fall with rehydration. Continue to assess these values to ensure they remain within normal limits.*

RISK FOR INJURY

- Institute safety precautions, including keeping the bed in low position, using side rails, and raising the client slowly from supine to sitting or sitting to standing position. *The client with orthostatic hypotension is at risk for dizziness, fainting, or falling with rapid position changes.*
- Teach client to get up slowly, sitting on the side of the bed for several minutes before standing. *These measures reduce orthostatic hypotension and the client's risk for injury.*

EVALUATING

Collect data related to fluid volume status (such as stable vital signs and weight) and safety to evaluate the effectiveness of nursing measures for the client with a fluid volume deficit.

Discharge Considerations

Assess the client's resources for home care and for preventing future problems with fluid losses (Box 5-4). Provide verbal and written instructions including:

■ Recommended fluid intake.
■ Avoid overexposure to heat and exercise (adjust activity level and fluid intake in hot weather).
■ If vomiting, take small frequent amounts of ice chips or clear liquids (weak tea, flat cola, or ginger ale).
■ Be aware that coffee, tea, alcohol, and large amounts of sugar increase urine output and can cause fluid loss.
■ Replace fluids lost through diarrhea with fruit juices or bouillon rather than large amounts of tap water.
■ Monitor weight, reporting changes of more than 3 to 5 pounds in a week to primary care provider.

Teach older adults and their caregivers to prevent fluid volume deficit. Suggest offering preferred fluids on a regular basis throughout the day and using alternative sources of liquid (such as gelatin, broth, or ice cream). Discuss the importance of providing additional water to clients who are receiving enteral nutrition via tube feedings.

BOX 5-4
ASSESSING FOR DISCHARGE

FLUID VOLUME IMBALANCE
Client

• Self-care: Ability to perform activities of daily living (ADLs), access fluids
• Knowledge:
  • Risks for fluid deficit (e.g., vomiting, diarrhea, strenuous exercise during hot weather, diuretic therapy, chronic diseases like diabetes mellitus); preventive measures; early manifestations
  • Risks for fluid excess (e.g., heart, kidney, or liver failure; medications); preventive measures; early manifestations; low-sodium diet, fluid restriction
• Home environment: Appropriate heating and cooling; access to clean water and other fluids; cooking facilities

Family

• Availability and knowledge of caregivers to assist with ADLs, monitor fluid intake, assist with fluid or dietary restrictions as ordered

Community

• Resources for aged, debilitated, or homebound clients
• Access to health care resources

BOX 5-5
FOODS HIGH IN SODIUM

HIGH IN ADDED SODIUM

• *Processed meat and fish*—Bacon, sausage, smoked fish, luncheon meat and other cold cuts
• *Selected dairy products*—Buttermilk, cottage cheese, cheeses, ice cream
• *Processed grains*—Graham crackers, most dry cereals
• *Canned goods*—Meats, vegetables, soups
• *Snack foods*—Salted popcorn, nuts, potato chips/pretzels, gelatin desserts
• *Condiments and food additives*—Barbecue sauce, saccharin, catsup, pickles, chili sauce, soy sauce, meat tenderizers, salted margarine, Worcestershire sauce, salad dressings

NATURALLY HIGH IN SODIUM

• Brains, kidney, oysters, shrimp, clams, crab, lobster
• Dried fruit
• Spinach, carrots

Fluid Volume Excess

Fluid volume excess usually results from sodium and water retention. It is rarely a problem in healthy adults. However, older adults, people with chronic or debilitating illnesses, and clients receiving intravenous therapy are at risk.

BOX 5-6
NURSING CARE CHECKLIST

FLUID RESTRICTION GUIDELINES

☑ Subtract requisite fluids (e.g., ordered IV fluids, fluid in which IV medications are mixed) from total daily allowance
☑ Divide remaining fluid allowance:
  • Day shift: ½ of total
  • Evening shift: ¼ to ⅓ of total
  • Nights: Remainder
☑ Explain the fluid restriction to the client and family members
☑ Work with client to determine preferred fluids and intake pattern
☑ Offer fluids in small glasses (allows perception of a full glass)
☑ Offer ice chips (which, when melted, are approximately half of the frozen volume)
☑ Provide frequent mouth care and opportunities to rinse mouth
☑ Provide sugarless chewing gum (if allowed) to reduce thirst

PATHOPHYSIOLOGY

Fluid volume excess is caused by excess sodium in the body that leads to water retention. Sodium and water are retained in approximately the same proportion as is present in ECF. The excess fluid tends to remain within the extracellular space, leading to the primary manifestations of **hypervolemia** (excess intravascular fluid) and interstitial **edema** (excess fluid in body tissues). Manifestations of fluid volume excess are listed in Table 5-2.

COLLABORATIVE CARE

Because sodium retention is a primary cause of fluid volume excess, a sodium-restricted diet often is prescribed. People require about 500 mg of sodium per day, but Americans typically consume about 4 to 5 grams daily, mostly from salt, processed foods, and foods themselves. A mild sodium restriction can be achieved by reducing the amount of salt in recipes by half, by not using the salt shaker at the table, and by avoiding foods that contain high levels of sodium either naturally or because of processing (Box 5-5). In moderate and severely sodium-restricted diets, salt and all foods containing significant amounts of sodium are avoided altogether.

Fluid intake also may be restricted in clients who have fluid volume excess. The amount of fluid allowed per day is prescribed by the care provider. All fluid intake must be calculated, including fluid in meals and fluid used to administer medications orally or intravenously. Box 5-6 provides guidelines for clients on a fluid restriction.

Diuretics, which promote sodium and water excretion, may be prescribed. Three classes of diuretics are commonly used: loop diuretics, thiazide diuretics, and potassium-sparing diuretics (Table 5-4 ◆).

TABLE 5-4 NURSING IMPLICATIONS FOR PHARMACOLOGY: CLIENTS WITH FLUID VOLUME EXCESS

DRUG GROUP/DRUGS	ACTION/USES	NURSING IMPLICATIONS *(FOR ALL DRUG GROUPS)*	CLIENT TEACHING *(FOR ALL DRUG GROUPS)*

Loop diuretics
  Furosemide (Lasix)
  Ethacrynic acid
    (Edecrin)
  Bumetanide (Bumex)
	Loop diuretics inhibit sodium and water reabsorption in the loop of Henle and increase potassium loss in the distal tubule. As a result, loop diuretics promote sodium, chloride, potassium, and water excretion.	Obtain baseline weight and vital signs.
		Monitor intake and output, weight, VS, skin turgor, and edema.
		Report manifestations of volume depletion: dizziness, orthostatic hypotension, tachycardia, muscle cramping.
		Loop and thiazide diuretics cause potassium wasting.
		Monitor serum electrolytes (especially potassium) and blood glucose. Notify physician of abnormal values.
		Notify the physician if the client is receiving a loop diuretic with another ototoxic drug such as an aminoglycoside antibiotic.
			The drug will increase the amount and frequency of urination.
			Take the drugs in the morning and afternoon to avoid having to get up at night to urinate.
			Change position slowly to avoid dizziness.
			Report the following to your primary health care provider: flulike symptoms, weakness, dehydration, thirst, dizziness; trouble breathing; or swelling of face, hands, or feet.
			Weigh yourself at the same time every day, and report sudden gains or losses.
			Try to avoid using the salt shaker when eating.
			If the drug increases potassium loss, eat foods high in potassium, such as orange juice and bananas.
			Unless restricted, drink 6 to 8 glasses of water daily.

Thiazide diuretics
  Bendroflumethiazide
    (Naturetin)
  Polythiazide (Renese)
  Chlorothiazide
    (Diuril)
  Chlorthalidone
    (Hygroton)
  Hydrochlorothiazide
    (HydroDIURIL)
  Metolazone (Diulo)
	Thiazide diuretics promote the excretion of sodium, chloride, potassium, and water by decreasing their reabsorption in the distal tubule.		

Potassium-sparing diuretics
  Spironolactone
    (Aldactone)
  Amiloride HCl
    (Midamor)
	Potassium-sparing diuretics promote excretion of sodium and water by inhibiting sodium–potassium exchange in the distal tubule.		

NURSING CARE

ASSESSING

Preventing fluid volume excess and early identification of its manifestations are important nursing responsibilities. Assessment data to collect for clients at risk for or with fluid volume excess are listed in Box 5-7.

DIAGNOSING, PLANNING, AND IMPLEMENTING

EXCESS FLUID VOLUME

Monitoring clients with fluid volume excess is important, and is particularly critical in older clients because of age-related changes in cardiac and renal function.

■ Monitor daily weights and intake and output. Report weight or fluid gain to the charge nurse or physician. *Daily weights are one of the most important gauges of fluid balance. Two kilograms (approximately 1 lb.) of weight gain is equivalent to 2 liters of fluid gain.*

■ Monitor edema, particularly in the lower extremities and the sacral and periorbital areas. *Localized edema tends to occur in dependent tissues such as the lower extremities of ambulatory clients and the sacrum in bedridden clients. Periorbital edema indicates generalized edema.*

■ If fluid restriction is prescribed, carefully monitor fluid intake. Instruct the client and significant others about the restriction and how to accurately measure fluid intake. *All sources of fluid intake, including ice chips, should be strictly monitored to avoid excess fluid.*

■ Provide oral hygiene as needed. *Oral hygiene contributes to client comfort and keeps mucous membranes intact; it also helps relieve thirst if fluids are restricted.*

■ Encourage the client to rest frequently in bed or a recliner with the feet elevated. *Bed rest promotes excretion of excess fluid by promoting its reabsorption into blood vessels and excretion by the kidneys.*

■ Place in semi-Fowler's or Fowler's position if dyspnea is present. *Semi-Fowler's position improves lung expansion and promotes fluid excretion.*

RISK FOR IMPAIRED SKIN INTEGRITY

Edema, which results from excess fluid in the interstitial spaces, decreases the delivery of nutrients to tissues and increases their susceptibility to injury.

■ Reposition at least every 2 hours. *Frequent change of position minimizes tissue pressure.*

■ Assess vulnerable pressure areas—particularly tissues over bony prominences—with each position change, and provide skin care. *Edematous tissue over bony prominences is more prone to tissue breakdown.*

■ Minimize tissue pressure by providing egg crate mattresses, foot cradles, and other devices. *An egg crate mattress distributes pressure over a wider area of the body surface and reduces pressure over bony prominences. A foot cradle minimizes the pressure that bedding can exert on the feet and lower extremities.*

EVALUATING

To evaluate the effectiveness of nursing care for clients with fluid volume excess, collect assessment data, evaluating for changes in vital signs, weight, ease of breathing, and relief of edema. Assess skin integrity and the need for additional measures to protect skin and underlying tissues from injury.

Discharge Considerations

Assess the client's and family's readiness and ability to provide home care after an episode of fluid volume excess (see Box 5-4). Focus on prevention in teaching. Emphasize the importance of taking medications as prescribed and avoiding foods that are high in sodium. Instructions for a low-sodium diet are found in Box 5-8. Provide verbal and written instructions, including:

■ Amount and type of fluids allowed, with a specific plan if fluids are restricted.

■ Ways to reduce sodium intake when buying and preparing foods.

■ To reduce dependent edema, change positions often, elevate feet and legs when sitting, avoid crossing legs, and

---

BOX 5-7
ASSESSING FOR FLUID VOLUME EXCESS

SUBJECTIVE DATA

- Complaints of cough, shortness of breath, difficulty sleeping or breathing when lying down
- Recent changes in fluid intake, output, or weight
- Risk factors such as renal failure, heart failure, cirrhosis of the liver, or an endocrine disorder; medications such as corticosteroid drugs (e.g., prednisone), nonsteroidal anti-inflammatory drugs (NSAIDs)

OBJECTIVE DATA

- Vital signs, peripheral pulses, and weight
- Mental status, level of consciousness
- Presence of peripheral or facial edema; color and moisture of skin and mucous membranes
- Observe for distended jugular or distal veins
- Auscultate breath sounds for crackles, wheezes; heart sounds for S_3 (heard immediately after S_2) and/or S_4 (heard immediately before S_1)

BOX 5–8
TEACHING FOR DISCHARGE

TEACHING CLIENTS ABOUT A LOW-SODIUM DIET

- The body needs less than 1 teaspoon (about 500 mg) of salt per day. About one third of sodium intake comes from adding salt during cooking and at the table; one fourth to one third comes from processed foods; and the rest comes from food and fluids naturally high in sodium.
- In place of salt or salt substitutes, use herbs, spices, lemon juice, vinegar, and wine as flavoring when cooking. The taste for salt will eventually diminish.
- Use salt substitutes sparingly; they often taste bitter instead of salty in large amounts.
- Low-sodium salt substitutes may contain half the sodium of regular salt.
- Read labels. Salt, monosodium glutamate, baking soda, and baking powder contain significant amounts of sodium. Processed foods list the sodium content. Some nonprescription drugs (such as laxatives and antacids) contain high amounts of sodium.

wear support hose and clothing that does not impair circulation.

- To reduce the risk of damage to edematous tissue, shop in the afternoon for shoes that do not require "breaking in," and avoid walking barefoot.
- Use more than one pillow or a recliner chair for sleeping if orthopnea is a problem.
- Weigh daily and report sudden increases of more than 2 lb to your doctor.

Nursing Process Case Study
▪ CLIENT WITH EXCESS FLUID VOLUME

Dorothy Rainwater is a 45-year-old former high school principal who is hospitalized with acute renal failure. She is expected to recover from this acute illness, but she currently has very little urine output.

Assessment Mike Penning, Ms. Rainwater's evening shift nurse, notes that her output for the previous 24 hours is 250 mL; this low output has been constant for the past 8 days. She has gained 1 lb (0.45 kg) in the past 24 hours. Ms. Rainwater is on a fluid restriction of 500 mL plus the amount of her output for the previous day.

Mr. Penning collects the following assessment data: T 98.6 F, BP 160/92, P 102, with obvious neck vein distention, R 28, with crackles and wheezes; head of bed elevated 30

degrees; periorbital and sacral edema noted, 3+ pitting edema in feet bilaterally; skin pale and shiny. Alert and oriented; responds appropriately to questions; states she is thirsty, slightly nauseated, and extremely tired.

Diagnosis The current nursing diagnoses for Ms. Rainwater are as follows:

- *Excess Fluid Volume* related to acute renal failure
- *Risk for Impaired Skin Integrity* related to edema
- *Risk for Impaired Gas Exchange* related to pulmonary congestion
- *Activity Intolerance* related to fluid volume excess, fatigue, and weakness

Expected Outcomes The expected outcomes specify that Ms. Rainwater will

- Regain fluid balance, as evidenced by weight loss, decreasing edema, and normal vital signs.
- Experience decreased dyspnea.
- Maintain intact skin and mucous membranes.
- Increase activity levels as prescribed.

Planning and Implementation The following nursing interventions are planned and implemented:

- Weigh q 12 hr at 0600 and 1800.
- Monitor vital signs and breath sounds q 4 hr.
- Intake and output q 4 hr.
- Restrict fluids as follows: 375 mL 0700 to 1500; 275 mL 1500 to 2300; 100 mL 2300 to 0700. Prefers water or apple juice.
- Turn every 2 hours, following schedule posted at the head of bed. Inspect skin, and provide skin care when turned; avoid vigorous massage.
- Provide oral care every 2 to 4 hours; allow to brush own teeth (caution not to swallow water). Use moistened applicators as desired.
- Keep head of bed at 30 to 40 degrees; prefers two small soft pillows under her head.
- Up at bedside in recliner for 20 minutes bid. Monitor carefully for fatigue and weakness as activity level increases.

Evaluation At the end of the shift, Mr. Penning notes that Ms. Rainwater gained no weight, and her urinary output during his shift is 300 mL. Her vital signs remain unchanged, but her crackles and wheezes have decreased, and she states that she can breathe more easily. Her skin and mucous membranes are intact. She enjoyed sitting in the chair at her bedside and did not experience any shortness of breath.

Critical Thinking in the Nursing Process

1. Why are Ms. Rainwater's respiratory rate, blood pressure, and pulse elevated?
2. Explain how elevating the head of the bed 30 degrees makes breathing easier.
3. Outline a plan for teaching Ms. Rainwater about diuretics.

4. Suppose Ms. Rainwater says, "I would really like to have all my fluids at once instead of spreading them out." What would be your reply, and why?

Sodium Imbalance

Sodium, the most plentiful electrolyte in ECF, has a normal serum range of 135 to 145 mEq/L. Sodium regulates ECF volume and distribution, and contributes to neuromuscular activity and acid–base balance. Because of the close relationship between sodium and water balance, disorders of fluid volume and sodium often occur together. Sodium imbalances affect the osmolality of ECF. When sodium levels are low (*hyponatremia*), water is drawn into the cells of the body, causing them to swell. In contrast, high sodium levels in ECF (*hypernatremia*) draw water out of body cells, causing them to shrink (see Figure 5-4).

Although the body requires only about 500 mg of sodium per day, many people consume more than 10 times that amount. Sodium excretion is controlled by the kidneys. The kidneys work together with the renin–angiotensin–aldosterone system and atrial natriuretic factor to retain or excrete sodium. They usually maintain ECF sodium concentration within its usual range despite variations in daily intake.

HYPONATREMIA

Hyponatremia (serum sodium < 135 mEq/L) usually results from loss of sodium from the body. It may also be caused by water gains that dilute ECF. Hyponatremia affects the function of voluntary and involuntary muscles (such as the gastrointestinal tract). Brain cells swell, leading to neurologic manifestations such as headache and possible brain damage. The causes, manifestations, and laboratory values of hyponatremia are shown in Table 5-5 ◆.

Collaborative Care

Serum electrolyte and *osmolality* levels are drawn. A *24-hour urine specimen* may be ordered to evaluate sodium excretion and help identify the cause of hyponatremia. Procedure 5-1 lists steps to take when collecting a 24-hour urine specimen.

If hyponatremia is mild, increased intake of foods high in sodium may restore normal sodium balance (see Box 5-5). Oral fluids often are restricted. If the client is unable to eat or drink, or if hyponatremia is severe, sodium-containing intravenous fluids may be administered. Normal saline (0.9% NaCl) may be given, or a 3% or 5% NaCl solution may be used cautiously to replace sodium and draw fluid out of the intracellular fluid compartment. A loop diuretic such as furosemide (see Table 5-4) may be administered along with sodium replacements to remove excess water.

HYPERNATREMIA

Hypernatremia (serum sodium concentration > 145 mEq/L) almost never occurs in people with an intact thirst mechanism and access to water. Hypernatremia results either from a gain of sodium in excess of water or from a loss of water in excess of sodium. Because excess sodium causes ECF to become hyper-

TABLE 5-5	**SODIUM IMBALANCES**		
		HYPONATREMIA	**HYPERNATREMIA**
CAUSES		Excess sodium loss through kidneys, skin, or GI tract (vomiting, diarrhea, gastric suctioning or irrigation, enemas with water) Excess sodium excretion due to diuretic medications, kidney or endocrine disorders Water gains related to kidney disease, heart failure, or cirrhosis of the liver Syndrome of inappropriate secretion of antidiuretic hormone (SIADH) Excessive hypotonic IV fluids	Altered thirst or inability to respond to thirst Hyperventilation Profuse sweating Diarrhea Diabetes insipidus Oral electrolyte solutions or hyperosmolar tube-feeding formulas Excess IV fluids such as normal saline, 3% or 5% sodium chloride, or sodium bicarbonate
MANIFESTATIONS		Anorexia, nausea, vomiting, abdominal cramping, and diarrhea Headache Mental status changes Hyperreflexia, muscle twitching, and tremors Convulsions and coma	Thirst Restlessness, weakness Altered mental status, decreasing level of consciousness, seizures Muscle irritability Dry, sticky mucous membranes Postural hypotension Hot, dry skin, fever, and decreased sweating
Lab values (normal 135–145 mEq/L)		Serum sodium < 135 mEq/L *Other lab values* Serum osmolality < 280 mOsm/kg	Serum sodium > 145 mEq/L *Other lab values* Serum osmolality > 295 mOsm/kg

| PROCEDURE 5-1 | Collecting a 24-Hour Urine Specimen |

■ BEFORE THE PROCEDURE

- Obtain a specimen container with preservative (if indicated). Label with the client's identifying information, the test to be performed, the time started, and the time of completion.
- Obtain a clean commode, bedpan, or urine collection device and place in the client's room.
- Post notices—on the client's chart, in the Kardex, on the door, over the client's bed, and over the toilet—alerting all personnel that all urine is to be saved.
- When the collection is to begin, have the client completely empty the bladder and discard this urine.

■ DURING THE PROCEDURE

- Save all urine produced during the 24-hour period in the container, refrigerating it or keeping it on ice as indicated.

- Instruct the client to urinate (and save the urine) before defecating and to avoid discarding any tissue in the urine container.
- When the collection period ends, have the client empty the bladder completely and save this specimen as part of the total. Take the full specimen with requisition to the lab for analysis.

■ SAMPLE DOCUMENTATION

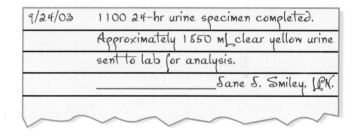

9/24/03   1100 24-hr urine specimen completed.
Approximately 1850 mL clear yellow urine
sent to lab for analysis.
                                        Jane S. Smiley, LPN.

---

osmolar, water moves out of cells, leading to cellular dehydration. Dehydration of brain cells causes neurologic manifestations such as confusion and a decreasing level of consciousness. Cellular dehydration also causes dry, sticky mucous membranes. Causes of excess water loss or excess sodium intake, as well as manifestations and laboratory values of hypernatremia, are summarized in Table 5-5.

Collaborative Care

Hypernatremia is treated by adding water (oral or hypotonic intravenous solutions such as D_5W or 0.45% NaCl) to correct any water deficit. Diuretics may also be given to increase sodium excretion, and a low-sodium diet may be prescribed. Hypernatremia is corrected slowly (over a 48-hour period) to avoid a rebound cerebral edema as water shifts back into the dehydrated brain cells.

 NURSING CARE

ASSESSING

Nurses need to identify and monitor clients at risk for sodium imbalances. Hyponatremia is often associated therapeutic measures such as IV fluid administration, gastrointestinal suction, or tap-water enemas. Diuretics such as furosemide and thiazide diuretics cause increased sodium excretion and contribute to a risk for hyponatremia.

DIAGNOSING, PLANNING, AND IMPLEMENTING

RISK FOR IMBALANCED FLUID VOLUME

- Monitor intake and output, and weigh daily. *Fluid excess or deficit may occur in clients with sodium disorders.*
- Maintain oral and intravenous fluid intake as prescribed. Monitor serum sodium levels and osmolality. Report rapid changes in serum sodium and osmolality. *Body water and sodium are replaced gradually to prevent cerebral edema or fluid volume excess.*
- In clients who are receiving normal saline or IV solutions with a higher sodium concentration, monitor for signs of hypervolemia (increased blood pressure and CVP, tachypnea, tachycardia, gallop rhythm, shortness of breath, crackles). *Hypertonic saline solutions may cause fluid retention and lead to heart failure, particularly in the elderly or people with preexisting heart problems.*
- Explain ordered fluid restrictions, how much fluid is allowed over 24 hours, and how to measure fluid volumes. *Fluid intake may be restricted in clients with a sodium imbalance; teaching increases understanding and compliance.*

RISK FOR INJURY

- Assess muscle strength and tone by asking client to squeeze your fingers, to hold the arms flexed while you pull downward, and to push both feet against your hands. *Muscle weakness resulting from sodium imbalance increases the risk for falling.*

- Assess for mental status changes, such as lethargy, altered or decreased level of consciousness, confusion, and seizures. Monitor behavior, mental status, and orientation. *Baseline data and ongoing assessments are critical because changes in serum sodium and serum osmolality may affect neurologic status and safety.*

- Maintain a quiet environment, and institute seizure precautions as indicated: keep the bed in its lowest position, side rails up and padded, and airway at the bedside. *A quiet environment reduces neurologic stimulation. Seizures often occur unexpectedly. Safety precautions reduce risk of injury from seizure.*

EVALUATING

To evaluate the effectiveness of nursing interventions for clients with sodium imbalances, collect data related fluid balance, serum sodium level, and freedom from injury.

Discharge Considerations

Athletes, people who do heavy labor in a hot environment, and older adults without access to air conditioning during hot weather are at risk for developing hyponatremia if they replace fluid losses with water. Teaching to prevent hyponatremia includes the following:

- Manifestations of mild hyponatremia, including nausea, cramps in the abdomen, and muscle weakness
- The importance of drinking liquids containing sodium and other electrolytes (such as GatorAid and other sports drinks) at frequent intervals when perspiring heavily, when environmental temperatures are high, or if experiencing prolonged watery diarrhea
- The importance of regular checkups to monitor electrolytes if taking a potent diuretic or on a low-sodium diet

People with impaired thirst or a condition that interferes with normal sodium balance require teaching to prevent hypernatremia. Emphasize the importance of adequate water intake and discuss ways to ensure that water needs are met. Teach clients and caregivers about a low-sodium diet if prescribed (see Box 5-8). When helping the client plan a low-sodium diet, include cultural foods and identify nondietary sources of sodium, such as softened water or over-the-counter medications.

Potassium Imbalance

Potassium (K^+), the primary intracellular cation, is vital for cell metabolism and for cardiac and neuromuscular function. The normal serum (ECF) potassium level is 3.5 to 5.0 mEq/L, while the potassium concentration of intracellular fluid is 140 to 150 mEq/L. The sodium–potassium pump sustains this significant difference in concentrations between ICF and ECF.

To maintain normal potassium levels in the body, potassium must be replaced every day. Virtually all foods contain potassium, although some foods and fluids are richer sources than others. The kidneys eliminate potassium very efficiently; even when potassium intake is stopped, the kidneys continue to excrete potassium. The hormone aldosterone contributes to potassium regulation by the kidneys. When aldosterone is present, more potassium is excreted; when it is absent, potassium is retained.

Potassium shifts into and out of the cells constantly. For example, it shifts into or out of the cells in response to changes in hydrogen ion concentration (pH, discussed later in this chapter), as the body strives to maintain a stable acid–base balance. This movement can significantly affect the serum potassium level.

HYPOKALEMIA

Hypokalemia (abnormally low serum potassium, < 3.5 mEq/L) usually results from excess potassium loss. However, many hospitalized clients are at risk for hypokalemia because of inadequate intake. Clients who are NPO for extended periods, as well as clients with anorexia nervosa (see Chapter 18) are at risk for inadequate intake of potassium.

Excess potassium may be lost through the kidneys or the gastrointestinal (GI) tract (Table 5-6 ◆). Drugs such as diuretics, corticosteroids, and some antibiotics are a major cause of excess potassium loss from the kidneys. GI losses may be caused by severe vomiting, diarrhea, or excessive ileostomy drainage.

A temporary shift of potassium into the intracellular space may occur because of alkalosis, rapid tissue repair (e.g., following a burn or trauma), or high blood insulin levels.

Hypokalemia affects the transmission of nerve impulses and the normal contractility of smooth, skeletal, and cardiac muscle. All clients with serum potassium values of 3.5 mEq/L or less should be closely monitored. Manifestations of hypokalemia generally are not seen until the serum K+ level falls below 3.0 mEq/L. Serious and potentially life-threatening cardiac dysrhythmias are a major concern, particularly in clients who are receiving digitalis to treat heart failure (see Chapter 22). The manifestations of hypokalemia are summarized in Table 5-6.

Collaborative Care

Serum potassium levels are drawn. *Arterial blood gases (ABGs)* may be ordered to determine acid–base status, because hydrogen ion balance (pH) and serum potassium levels are linked. An *electrocardiogram (ECG)* is done to evaluate cardiac rhythm and assess for characteristic changes associated with hypokalemia.

Potassium replacement therapy (by mouth or intravenously) is implemented both to prevent and to treat

TABLE 5-6

POTASSIUM IMBALANCES

	HYPOKALEMIA	HYPERKALEMIA
CAUSES	Excess GI losses: vomiting, diarrhea, ileostomy drainage Renal losses: diuretics, corticosteroids; hyperaldosteronism Inadequate intake (NPO, anorexia nervosa) K^+ shift into cells (alkalosis, tissue repair)	Renal failure Potassium-sparing diuretics Adrenal insufficiency Excess potassium intake (e.g., excess potassium replacement) Administering aged blood K^+ shift out of cells (acidosis, tissue damage)
MANIFESTATIONS	Dysrhythmias and ECG changes Nausea and vomiting Anorexia Decreased bowel sounds or ileus Muscle weakness or leg cramps	Tall, peaked T waves, dysrhythmias, heart block, cardiac arrest Nausea, abdominal cramping, diarrhea Muscle weakness, paresthesias, flaccid paralysis
Lab values (normal 3.5–5.0 mEq/l)	Serum potassium < 3.5 mEq/L	Serum potassium > 5.0 mEq/L

hypokalemia. Commonly prescribed potassium supplements, their actions, and nursing implications are described in Table 5-7 ◆. Several days of therapy may be required to correct hypokalemia.

Increased intake of foods high in potassium may be recommended for clients at risk for hypokalemia, either to prevent its occurrence or to supplement pharmacologic therapy. Box 5-9 lists foods and fluids that are high in potassium.

TABLE 5-7

NURSING IMPLICATIONS FOR PHARMACOLOGY: CLIENTS WITH HYPOKALEMIA

DRUG GROUP/DRUGS	ACTION/USES	NURSING IMPLICATIONS	CLIENT TEACHING

POTASSIUM SOURCES
  Potassium acetate (Tri-K)
  Potassium bicarbonate (K+ Care ET)
  Potassium citrate (K-Lyte)
  Potassium chloride (K-lease, Micro-K10, Apo-K)
  Potassium gluconate (Kaon Elixir, Royonate)
	Potassium is used to prevent and treat hypokalemia. It is rapidly absorbed from the gastro-intestinal tract. Potassium chloride is the agent of choice, because low chloride levels often accompany low potassium.	When giving oral potassium:
		a. Dilute or dissolve effervescent, soluable, or liquid potassium in fruit or vegetable juice or cold water.
		b. Chill to increase palatability.
		When giving parenteral potassium:
		a. Administer slowly.
		b. Do not administer undiluted.
		c. Assess injection site frequently for pain and inflammation.
		d. Use an infusion control device.
		Monitor intake and output.
		Monitor serum potassium levels; do not administer if serum K^+ is > 5.0 mEq/L.
			Take as prescribed; do not skip a dose or double your prescribed dose unless instructed to do so by your physician.
			Take potassium supplements with meals to reduce gastric irritation.
			Do not chew enteric-coated tablets or allow them to dissolve in the mouth; this may affect the potency and action of the medications.
			Do not use salt substitutes when taking potassium (most salt substitutes are potassium based).
			Do not take potassium supplements if you are also taking a potassium-sparing diuretic.

HYPERKALEMIA

Hyperkalemia (abnormally high serum potassium, > 5 mEq/L), results from inadequate potassium excretion, excessive potassium intake, or a shift of potassium from the ICF to the ECF. The major cause of hyperkalemia is impaired renal excretion (see Table 5-6). Excess potassium intake often occurs when people use potassium-based salt substitutes while taking potassium-sparing diuretics. Administration of aged blood can also lead to hyperkalemia, because the potassium concentration of blood increases during storage. Burns and crushing injuries release potassium from cells into ECF. In acidosis, hydrogen ion moves into the cells and potassium shifts out into ECF as the body attempts to maintain a normal pH.

Hyperkalemia alters neuromuscular function. Its most harmful effects are on cardiac function, with a risk for dysrhythmias, heart block, and cardiac arrest. The strength of cardiac contractions decreases as the potassium level rises. It also affects skeletal and smooth muscle, causing weakness and GI symptoms.

CLINICAL alert

Remember: Both *hypo*kalemia and *hyper*kalemia affect cardiac function and can result in serious, even fatal dysrhythmias.

Collaborative Care

Managing hyperkalemia focuses on returning the serum potassium level to normal by treating the underlying cause and avoiding additional potassium intake. *Serum electrolytes* are monitored, because low calcium and sodium levels may increase the effects of hyperkalemia. *ABGs* are measured to determine whether acidosis is present. *ECG monitoring* of heart rate and rhythm is performed to evaluate the effects of hyperkalemia on cardiac function.

Mild hyperkalemia may be reversed by treating the cause (e.g., correcting acidosis) or by discontinuing drugs that caused it. Loop diuretics such as furosemide (Lasix) promote renal excretion of potassium. A cation exchange resin, sodium polystyrene sulfonate (Kayexalate), may be given orally or rectally (by enema) to remove excess potassium by exchanging sodium for potassium in the intestinal tract. In the client with renal failure, hemodialysis and peritoneal dialysis are used to manage hyperkalemia (see Chapter 21).

For moderate to severe hyperkalemia, intravenous insulin and glucose may be given to drive potassium into the cells. Intravenous sodium bicarbonate has a similar effect. Calcium gluconate may also be given block the effects of hyperkalemia on the heart.

NURSING CARE

ASSESSING

Nursing care focuses on early identification and reporting of abnormal serum potassium levels and monitoring cardiac status. Ask about potassium-wasting diuretics (such as loop and thiazide diuretics; see Table 5-4) and other drugs associated with potassium loss (e.g., corticosteroids). Question the client about compliance with prescribed potassium supplements and dietary intake of foods and fluids.

DIAGNOSING, PLANNING, AND IMPLEMENTING

RISK FOR INJURY

- Carefully monitor serum potassium levels in clients at risk for imbalances, and notify the charge nurse or physician of abnormal levels (< 3.5 mEq/L or > 5 mEq/L). *Early identification of a potassium imbalance allows prompt treatment and reduces the risk for injury from very high or very low potassium levels.*
- Monitor for manifestations of potassium imbalance, such as muscle weakness, nausea and anorexia, abdominal cramping, or decreased bowel sounds. *Weakness and GI manifestations of potassium imbalance increase the risk for injury from falls or aspiration of vomitus.*
- Closely monitor clients receiving sodium bicarbonate or sodium polystyrene sulfonate (Kayexalate) for fluid volume excess. *Increased sodium levels can cause water retention.*
- Closely monitor the ECG of clients receiving calcium gluconate, particularly if the client also is on digitalis. *Digitalis toxicity may develop when calcium gluconate and digitalis are given concurrently.*

DECREASED CARDIAC OUTPUT

- Monitor vital signs, including apical pulse. Chart and report any irregularities. *Disruptions of heart rhythm are more easily detected by listening to the apical pulse than by palpating peripheral pulses.*
- Place on a cardiac monitor and observe for changes in heart rhythm or pattern (e.g., prolonged PR interval, ST segment and T wave changes, and the presence of U waves). (See Chapter 22 for more explanation of ECG waveforms.)

Notify the physician of changes. *A monitor allows early identification and intervention for life-threatening dysrhythmias.*

- Monitor clients taking digitalis for signs of digitalis toxicity (see Chapter 22). *Hypokalemia increases the risk for digitalis toxicity.*

- Monitor intravenous potassium infusions closely. Dilute intravenous potassium as recommended, and administer using an electronic infusion device. *A rate above 40 mEq of potassium per hour is not safe.*

CLINICAL alert

Do not administer undiluted potassium directly into the vein. Potassium usually is mixed to a concentration of 20 to 40 mEq/L of solution and should not exceed 60 mEq/L. The rate of infusion should not exceed 20 to 40 mEq of potassium per hour. Evaluate the serum potassium level during therapy. In clients requiring rapid potassium replacement, monitor the ECG. Too rapid administration of intravenous potassium may cause cardiac dysrhythmias and death.

- Promote comfort by slowing the intravenous infusion rate or applying an ice pack to the IV site if necessary. *Potassium may cause local irritation to the vein wall.*

EVALUATING

Collect data related to the client's serum potassium level, safety, and cardiovascular status to evaluate the effectiveness of nursing interventions for clients with potassium imbalances.

Discharge Considerations

Discharge planning for clients with potassium imbalances focuses on teaching about prescribed medications (potassium supplements or diuretics), diet, and the importance of regular follow-up assessments. Include the family, a significant other, or a caregiver in teaching as indicated. Provide both written and verbal instructions. Provide a list of salt substitutes and foods high in potassium, with instructions for their use (see Box 5-9). Instruct clients taking supplemental forms of potassium and potassium-sparing diuretics to avoid salt substitutes that contain potassium. Instruct clients with chronic renal failure to avoid foods high in potassium. Discuss measures to make potassium supplements more palatable: Dilute liquid potassium supplements with water or juices, or mix with sherbet or gelatin. Emphasize the importance of regular laboratory tests as ordered by the physician. Teach the client taking digitalis to count the pulse before taking the medication. Report a rate of less than 60 to the primary health care provider.

Nursing Process Case Study
■ CLIENT WITH HYPOKALEMIA

Rose Ortiz is a 72-year-old woman who is being treated for mild heart failure with digoxin (Lanoxin) 0.125 mg, hydrochlorothiazide (Oretic) 75 mg orally (PO) daily, and a mildly sodium-restricted diet (2 g daily). For the last several weeks, Ms. Ortiz has been feeling weak and sometimes faint, light-headed, and dizzy. Her physician ordered serum electrolytes drawn, which showed a potassium level of 2.4 mEq/L. Potassium chloride solution (Kaochlor, 20 mEq/15 mL) PO twice daily is prescribed, and the clinic nurse does a nursing assessment prior to teaching Ms. Ortiz about her care.

Assessment Ms. Ortiz has adhered to her sodium-restricted diet and has been taking her prescribed medications. She occasionally takes an additional "water pill" when her ankles swell. She says she is reluctant to take the potassium the doctor has ordered because her neighbor says it causes "heartburn." Physical assessment findings include T 98.4, P 70, R 20, and BP 138/84.

Diagnosis The following nursing diagnosis is identified for Ms Ortiz:

- *Risk for Ineffective Health Maintenance* related to lack of knowledge of side effects of diuretic therapy and of foods high in potassium

Expected Outcomes The expected outcomes specify that Ms. Ortiz will:

- Have a potassium level within normal limits (3.5 to 5.0 mEq/L).
- Verbalize understanding of the side effects of diuretic therapy.
- State measures to avoid gastrointestinal irritation when taking oral potassium.
- Identify potassium-rich foods.

Planning and Implementation The following nursing interventions are planned and implemented:

- Discuss the side effects of diuretic therapy, and explain how taking additional diuretics may have contributed to her hypokalemia.
- Explain the need for the prescribed potassium and its role in reversing her muscle weakness.
- Instruct to take the potassium supplement after breakfast and supper, diluted in 4 oz of juice or water, and sipped slowly over a 5- to 10-minute period. Instruct her to call if gastric irritation occurs.
- Discuss dietary sources of potassium, and provide a list of potassium-rich foods (see Box 5-9).

Evaluation On a follow-up visit 1 week later, Ms. Ortiz says that her symptoms have been resolved. She is taking her prescribed drugs as directed. She also reports that she has increased her intake of potassium-rich foods. Her potassium level is within normal limits.

 Critical Thinking in the Nursing Process

1. What did Ms. Ortiz do that contributed to her hypokalemia?
2. What additional teaching at the time that digitalis and hydrochlorothiazide were prescribed might have prevented Ms. Ortiz from developing hypokalemia? How could the nurse reinforce this teaching?

Calcium Imbalance

Calcium is one of the most abundant ions in the body. Most of it is in the bones and teeth; a small amount is in the ECF. The normal adult total serum calcium concentration is 8.5 to 10.0 mg/dL. About half of extracellular calcium is ionized; the rest is bound to protein, phosphate, or other ions.

Ionized calcium is essential to a number of body processes. It affects neuromuscular irritability, nerve impulse transmission, muscle contraction and relaxation, blood clotting, and hormone secretion. It is vital in maintaining heart rhythm and contraction.

Three hormones interact to regulate serum calcium levels: parathyroid hormone (PTH), calcitriol (a metabolite of vitamin D), and calcitonin. When serum calcium levels fall, the parathyroid glands secrete PTH. PTH mobilizes calcium from the bones, increases calcium absorption in the intestines, and promotes calcium reabsorption by the kidneys (Figure 5-10 ◆). Calcitriol assists these processes.

Calcitonin is secreted by the thyroid gland in response to high serum calcium levels. Calcitonin has the opposite effect of PTH: It inhibits the movement of calcium out of bone, reduces intestinal absorption of calcium, and promotes urinary calcium excretion.

HYPOCALCEMIA

Hypocalcemia is a serum calcium of less than 8.5 mg/dL. People at risk for hypocalcemia include those who have had their parathyroid glands removed, older adults (especially women), and alcoholics. Older adults often consume less milk and milk products (good sources of calcium) and may have less exposure to the sun (a source of vitamin D). They may be less active, which promotes calcium loss from bones. They are more likely to be taking drugs that interfere with calcium absorption or promote calcium excretion (e.g., furosemide). Older women are at particular risk after menopause because of estrogen deficiency. Alcohol consumption reduces intestinal absorption of calcium and interferes with other processes that help maintain serum calcium levels.

Hypocalcemia can result from decreased total body calcium stores or low levels of calcium in ECF with normal amounts of calcium stored in bone. Many disorders can cause hypocalcemia (Table 5-8 ◆). *Hypoparathyroidism,* usually due

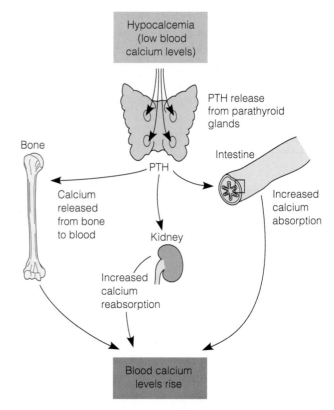

Figure 5-10. ◆ Low serum calcium levels stimulate parathyroid hormone release, increasing serum calcium levels by triggering its release from bone, absorption in the intestine, and reabsorption in the kidneys.

to surgical removal of the parathyroid glands, is the most common cause. Hypoparathyroidism also may result from total thyroidectomy or radical neck surgery. Hypocalcemia is common in clients with acute pancreatitis (see Chapter 19). It often accompanies hypomagnesemia, common in malnourished alcoholics.

The manifestations of hypocalcemia are caused by insufficient ionized calcium in ECF. Calcium has a sedative effect on neuromuscular transmission. When calcium levels are low, neuromuscular excitability increases. **Tetany** (a group of symptoms caused by this increased excitability) is the most characteristic and serious consequence of hypocalcemia. Manifestations of tetany are *paresthesias* (numbness and tingling around the mouth and in the hands and feet) and muscle spasms. Chvostek's sign (facial muscle spasm when the facial nerve is tapped in front of the ear) and Trousseau's sign (carpal spasm that occurs when blood flow to the lower arm is restricted) also may be present. Other manifestations are listed in Table 5-8.

Collaborative Care

The *total serum calcium* will be less than 8.5 mg/d, and ionized calcium (the active form) generally is about 50% of that. *Serum magnesium* is measured because hypocalcemia is often associated with hypomagnesemia. *Serum phosphate* is measured because there is a relationship between phosphorus and calcium levels (i.e., the serum level of one often rises as the other falls, and vice versa). *Parathyroid hormone (PTH)* is measured to

TABLE 5-8   CALCIUM IMBALANCES

	HYPOCALCEMIA	HYPERCALCEMIA
CAUSES	Parathyroidectomy or neck surgery Acute pancreatitis Inadequate dietary intake Lack of sun exposure (vitamin D) Lack of weight-bearing exercise Drugs: loop diuretics, calcitonin, furosemide Hypomagnesemia (alcohol abuse, some chemotherapy)	Hyperparathyroidism Some cancers (lung, breast, multiple myeloma) Prolonged immobilization Paget's disease Excess milk or antacid intake Renal failure
MANIFESTATIONS	Neuromuscular ▪ Tetany: paresthesias, muscle spasms, laryngospasm, seizures ▪ Positive Chvostek's sign ▪ Positive Trousseau's sign ▪ Anxiety, confusion, psychoses Cardiovascular ▪ ↓ Cardiac output ▪ ↓ BP ▪ Dysrhythmias Gastrointestinal ▪ Abdominal cramping ▪ Diarrhea	Neuromuscular ▪ Muscle weakness ▪ ↓ Deep tendon reflexes Behavioral ▪ Confusion, impaired memory, bizarre behavior ▪ Psychoses Gastrointestinal ▪ Constipation ▪ Anorexia, nausea, vomiting Cardiovascular ▪ Dysrhythmias ▪ ↑ BP ▪ Renal ▪ ↑ Urine output
Lab values (normal 8.5–10.0 mg/dL)	Serum calcium < 8.5 mg/dL	Serum calcium > 10 mg/dL

identify hypoparathyroidism as a possible underlying cause. The *ECG* shows changes in the waveforms and dysrhythmias, such as bradycardia (slow heart rate) or ventricular tachycardia (a very rapid ventricular rate).

Oral calcium preparations, increased dietary intake of calcium, and oral vitamin D are used to increase calcium levels in clients with chronic hypocalcemia. Vitamin D may be given as well to increase GI absorption of calcium.

In acute hypocalcemia, intravenous calcium (calcium chloride, calcium gluconate, or calcium gluceptate) is given to prevent or treat tetany. Calcium may be given by slow IV push or by infusion. It is given with caution to clients taking digitalis, because it increases the risk of digitalis toxicity. (See Table 5-9 ◆.)

HYPERCALCEMIA

Hypercalcemia (serum calcium > 10.0 mg/dL) usually results from increased calcium release *(resorption)* from the bones. Increased calcium intake and decreased renal excretion of calcium are other causes.

Increased resorption of calcium from the bones may result from *hyperparathyroidism* and excess PTH secretion, prolonged immobilization, or certain malignancies (such as lung and breast cancers and multiple myeloma). Excess PTH also impairs renal excretion of calcium, as does kidney failure. Other causes of hypercalcemia are listed in Table 5-8.

The effects of hypercalcemia largely depend on the degree of serum calcium elevation and the length of time over which it develops. The primary effects are neuromuscular. Calcium has a sedative effect on neuromuscular transmission, which affects skeletal, smooth, and cardiac muscles. Excess calcium in cerebrospinal fluid affects behavior, and excess calcium in the urine can lead to kidney stones. Review Table 5-8 for the manifestations of hypercalcemia by body systems.

CLINICAL alert

Remember, calcium has a sedative effect on neuromuscular transmission. Therefore:

Hypocalcemia → *Increased* neuromuscular excitability, muscle twitching, spasms, and possible tetany

Hypercalcemia → *Decreased* neuromuscular excitability, muscle weakness, and fatigue

Hypercalcemia can lead to complications such as peptic ulcer disease and pancreatitis. Extremely high serum calcium levels may cause complete heart block and cardiac arrest.

Collaborative Care

Hypercalcemia is diagnosed by measuring *serum calcium levels*. *Serum PTH* is measured to identify possible hyperparathyroidism. Levels are increased in hyperparathyroidism but may

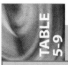

TABLE 5-9 NURSING IMPLICATIONS FOR PHARMACOLOGY: CLIENTS WITH HYPOCALCEMIA			
DRUG GROUP/DRUGS	**ACTION/USES**	**NURSING IMPLICATIONS**	**CLIENT TEACHING** *(FOR ALL DRUG GROUPS)*

Oral calcium
    Calcium carbonate
    (BioCal, Calsam,
    Caltrate, OsCal, Tums)
    Calcium gluconate
    Calcium lactate
	Oral calcium
	    preparations are
	    used to increase
	    calcium levels in the
	    body.
		Administer oral calcium
		    1–1.5 hours after meals.
		Calcium absorption is
		    improved by concurrent
		    administration
		    of vitamin D.
			A daily intake of 1,000–1,500
			    mg of calcium is
			    recommended for adults.
			Older adults should take in
			    1,500 mg/day.
			Milk and milk products are a
			    good source of calcium.
			If you have a tendency to form
			    kidney stones, talk to your
			    doctor before taking calcium
			    supplements.
			Smoking and alcohol
			    consumption interfere with
			    calcium absorption.
			Regular physical exercise that
			    involves weight bearing
			    (walking, bicycling, weight
			    training) helps maintain
			    calcium stores in the bone
			    and can help prevent
			    osteoporosis.

Intravenous calcium
    Calcium gluconate
    Calcium chloride
	Intravenous calcium is
	    used to treat acute
	    hypocalcemia. It also
	    may be ordered
	    postoperatively
	    for clients who
	    have had neck
	    surgery such as
	    parathyroidectomy,
	    thyroidectomy, or
	    radical neck surgery.
		Administer into a central
		    line or large peripheral
		    vein.
		Dilute calcium solutions
		    with normal saline or
		    administer by infusion
		    to reduce irritation of
		    the vein.
		Monitor IV site closely; stop
		    the infusion if infiltration
		    occurs.
		Closely monitor ECG and
		    serum calcium levels.	

be low in other cases of hypercalcemia. An *ECG* is done to identify changes in impulse transmission and rhythm related to hypercalcemia.

In acute hypercalcemia, intravenous normal saline solution (0.9% NaCl) is given to restore fluid volume and dilute plasma calcium. Diuretics such as furosemide (Lasix) or ethacrynic acid (Edecrin) may be given to promote calcium excretion by the kidneys.

When hypercalcemia is due to excess bone resorption, *biphosphonates* may be used. This group of drugs, including etidronate (Didronel) and pamidronate (Aredia), inhibit bone resorption and can reduce serum calcium levels with few side effects. Phosphates may be prescribed to inhibit bone resorption and reduce intestinal absorption of calcium. Other drugs used to treat hypercalcemia include calcitonin or intravenous plicamycin (Mithracin) to inhibit bone resorption, and glucocorticoids to decrease GI absorption of calcium and increase its excretion.

NURSING CARE

ASSESSING

Clients who have or are at risk for calcium imbalance are assessed for the following:

- Heart rate and rhythm
- Respiratory rate and effort; laryngeal *stridor* (a high-pitched, harsh sound heard during inspiration)
- Mental status and neuromuscular function
- Manifestations of tetany (tingling around mouth and fingers, muscle twitching or cramps, hyperactive reflexes)
- Serum calcium, magnesium, phosphate, and albumin levels

DIAGNOSING, PLANNING, AND IMPLEMENTING

RISK FOR INJURY

- Institute safety precautions for clients who have mental changes resulting from hypercalcemia. *Changes in mental status may impair the client's judgment and ability to maintain his or her own safety.*
- Frequently monitor airway and respiratory status. Report any changes, such as respiratory stridor or increased respiratory rate and effort. *These may indicate laryngeal spasm, a respiratory emergency that requires immediate intervention to maintain adequate ventilation of the lungs.*
- Monitor cardiovascular status, including heart rate and rhythm and blood pressure. *Calcium imbalances can affect heart contractility, leading to decreased cardiac output, dysrhythmias, and hypotension.*
- Place clients receiving intravenous calcium replacement on a cardiac monitor. *Clients receiving intravenous calcium may develop dysrhythmias.*
- Provide a quiet environment. Institute seizure precautions: Raise padded side rails and keep an airway at the bedside. *A quiet environment reduces central nervous system stimuli. The client with tetany is at risk for developing seizures.*

- If excess bone resorption has occurred, use caution when turning, transferring, or ambulating the client. *Bone may fracture more easily if excess calcium has been lost.*
- Ambulate clients as soon as allowed and encourage weight-bearing activity. *These measures help move calcium into bone, lowering serum calcium levels and reducing the risk of fracture.*
- Promote fluid intake to keep the client well hydrated and maintain dilute urine. Encourage fluids such as prune or cranberry juice. *The client is at risk for developing calcium renal stones. These juices help maintain acid urine.*
- Keep emergency resuscitation equipment available. *Cardiac arrest may occur with extremely high serum calcium levels.*

EVALUATING

In addition to monitoring serum calcium levels, collect assessment data such as mental status, muscle strength, deep tendon reflexes, and cardiovascular status to evaluate the effectiveness of interventions for clients with calcium imbalances.

Discharge Considerations

Assess risk factors for future episodes of calcium imbalance, such as poor dietary intake, cigarette smoking, alcohol consumption, lack of exposure to sunlight, and lack of weight-bearing exercise. Evaluate the client's knowledge and understanding of measures to prevent calcium imbalances. Discuss dietary sources of calcium and vitamin D; provide a list of foods that are high in calcium (Box 5-10).

Encourage taking prescribed oral calcium and vitamin D replacements as directed; caution to avoid excess doses of vitamin D supplements. Advise the client to increase fluid intake to 2,000 to 3,000 mL over 24 hours. Instruct clients who are at high risk for renal stone formation to increase the intake of fluid and acid-ash foods (meats, fish, poultry, eggs, cranberries, plums, prunes). Discuss the relationship between weight-bearing activities and maintaining bone calcium. Help the client identify activities that fit with his or her lifestyle. Finally, instruct to increase dietary fiber and fluid to maintain normal bowel function and avoid constipation.

BOX 5-10
FOODS HIGH IN CALCIUM

- Milk and milk products
- Canned salmon and sardines
- Rhubarb
- Broccoli, collard greens, spinach
- Soy flour, tofu

Magnesium Imbalance

About two thirds of the magnesium in the body is in bones; one third is within the cells; 1% is in ECF. The normal serum magnesium concentration is 1.3 to 2.1 mEq/L or 1.6 to 2.6 mg/dL. Magnesium is critical to intracellular metabolism. Extracellular magnesium affects neuromuscular irritability and contractility. Excess ECF magnesium depresses skeletal muscle contraction and central nervous system activity. A deficit causes increased irritability of the nervous system, cardiac dysrhythmias, and peripheral vasodilation.

Magnesium enters the body in the foods we eat. It is abundant in green vegetables, grains, nuts, meats, and seafood. The kidneys regulate extracellular magnesium levels by conserving or excreting it as needed.

HYPOMAGNESEMIA

Hypomagnesemia (serum magnesium < 1.3 mEq/L or 1.6 mg/dL) is usually due to a total body deficit of magnesium. In fact, body stores of magnesium may be depleted even when the serum magnesium level is within normal limits.

Chronic alcoholism is one of the most common causes of hypomagnesemia. (See Table 5-10 ♦.)

Hypomagnesemia has direct effects on body processes; it also affects potassium and calcium metabolism. Manifestations of hypomagnesemia usually do not occur until the serum level drops below 1 mEq/L. Neuromuscular excitability is increased in hypomagnesemia. Electrical conduction in the heart is affected, as is central nervous system function. The manifestations of hypomagnesemia are also listed in Table 5-10.

HYPERMAGNESEMIA

Hypermagnesemia (serum magnesium level > 2.1 mEq/L or 2.6 mg/dL) is often caused by renal insufficiency or failure. It also may develop in clients who take excess amounts of magnesium-containing antacids or laxatives, and when magnesium solutions are given to treat complications of pregnancy.

Elevated serum magnesium levels interfere with neuromuscular transmission and depress the central nervous system. Hypermagnesemia also affects the cardiovascular system and respiratory function. With mild hypermagnesemia, nausea and vomiting, hypotension, facial flushing, sweating, and a feeling of warmth occur. Table 5-10 summarizes the manifestations of hypermagnesemia.

Collaborative Care

Prevention is important for both hypomagnesemia and hypermagnesemia. Identifying clients at risk and treatments that increase the risk of altered serum magnesium levels can prevent adverse effects.

In clients who are able to eat, a mild deficiency may be corrected by increasing the intake of magnesium-rich foods (Box 5-11), or by using oral magnesium supplements (for example, magnesium-containing antacids). The use of these supplements is limited by their tendency to cause diarrhea.

TABLE 5-10   MAGNESIUM IMBALANCES

	HYPOMAGNESEMIA	HYPERMAGNESEMIA
CAUSES	Chronic alcoholism GI losses (intestinal suction, vomiting and diarrhea, ileostomy) Impaired intestinal absorption Increased renal excretion: drugs (loop diuretics, aminoglycoside antibiotics), kidney disease	Renal insufficiency or failure Excess intake of antacids, laxatives Excess magnesium administration
MANIFESTATIONS	*(Generally seen with serum levels < 1 mEq/L)* Neuromuscular ■ Muscle weakness, tremors ■ Tetany ■ Positive Chvostek's and Trousseau's signs Gastrointestinal ■ Dysphagia Cardiovascular ■ Dysrhythmias ■ Peripheral vasodilatation ■ ECG changes CNS ■ Seizures ■ Mental status changes	Neuromuscular ■ Muscle weakness ■ ↓ Deep tendon reflexes Gastrointestinal ■ Nausea and vomiting Cardiovascular ■ Vasodilation (facial flushing, sweating, feeling of warmth) ■ ↓ BP ■ Bradycardia ■ Cardiac arrest CNS ■ Lethargy, drowsiness ■ Respiratory depression, paralysis ■ Coma
Lab values (normal 1.6–2.6 mg/dL or 1.3–2.1 mEq/L)	Serum magnesium < 1.6 mg/dL (1.3 mEq/L)	Serum magnesium > 2.6 mg/dL (2.1 mEq/L)

Magnesium also can be given intravenously or by deep intramuscular injection. Serum magnesium levels and deep tendon reflexes are monitored frequently during treatment. Depressed deep tendon reflexes indicate high serum magnesium levels and a need to stop treatment.

Hypermagnesemia is treated by withholding all medications and solutions that contain magnesium. In clients with renal failure, excess magnesium is removed by hemodialysis or peritoneal dialysis (see Chapter 21). With extremely high magnesium levels, intravenous calcium is given to counteract the cardiac effects of magnesium. Some clients may require mechanical ventilation to maintain respirations.

NURSING CARE

Nursing interventions for clients with magnesium imbalances focus on carefully monitoring individuals at risk, assessing signs and symptoms, implementing safety measures, teaching the client and family, and administering prescribed medications.

Assess clients at risk for magnesium imbalances for:

■ Serum magnesium levels and other electrolytes, particularly potassium, calcium, and phosphate.
■ Manifestations of neuromuscular excitability, such as muscle twitching, tremors, grimaces, paresthesias, leg cramps, and hyperactive reflexes.
■ Changes in GI function, such as nausea, vomiting, anorexia, diarrhea, and abdominal distention.
■ Changes in cardiovascular function, such as hypotension, dysrhythmias, and changes in cardiac conduction. In clients receiving digitalis, monitor for digitalis toxicity.

Closely monitor serum magnesium levels and deep tendon reflexes in clients receiving intravenous magnesium solutions. Refer to the section on calcium imbalances for measures to reduce the risk of injury related to increased neuromuscular excitability.

**BOX 5-11
FOODS HIGH IN MAGNESIUM**

• Green, leafy vegetables
• Legumes
• Whole grains
• Bananas, oranges, grapefruit
• Dairy products
• Meat
• Seafood

Discharge Considerations

Teach clients about foods that are high in magnesium (see Box 5-11) and provide information about magnesium supplements. Teach clients who have high magnesium levels to avoid magnesium-containing medications, including antacids, mineral supplements, cathartics, and enemas. Provide a list of magnesium-containing medications. Refer clients for whom alcohol abuse is a problem to a treatment program. Discuss support systems for alcoholics such as Alcoholics Anonymous, Al-Anon, and/or Al-a-Teen.

Phosphorus Imbalance

The normal serum phosphorus level in adults is 2.5 to 4.5 mg/dL. Phosphorus is found in all body tissues, but most of it is combined with calcium in bones and teeth. Phosphorus is the primary anion in ICF. Within cells, phosphorus is important for energy (ATP) production, metabolism, and red blood cell function. Although a very small portion of phosphorus (1%) is in ECF, it is essential for normal neuromuscular activity. Phosphate, the ionized form of phosphorus, is responsible for its physiologic effects. Phosphate is abundant in many foods, including meat, fish, poultry, eggs, milk products, and legumes. The kidneys regulate serum phosphorus levels, excreting excess phosphorus or retaining it if phosphate intake is low. An inverse relationship exists between phosphorus and calcium levels: When one increases, the other decreases. Thus, regulatory mechanisms that maintain calcium levels in the body also affect phosphorus levels.

Hypophosphatemia (serum phosphorus < 2.5 mg/dL) may indicate a phosphorus deficit, or it may occur when phosphate shifts out of ECF into the cells. Decreased absorption of phosphate from the GI tract or increased excretion of phosphate by the kidneys can lead to a deficit of phosphorus. Iatrogenic (treatment-related) causes of hypophosphatemia are common (Table 5-11 ◆). Alcoholism can cause severe hypophosphatemia.

The manifestations of hypophosphatemia (see Table 5-11) are caused by a lack of intracellular phosphate. Cellular

TABLE 5-11

PHOSPHORUS IMBALANCES

	HYPOPHOSPHATEMIA	HYPERPHOSPHATEMIA
CAUSES	<ul><li>Decreased GI absorption or increased renal excretion</li><li>Shift from ECF into cells</li><li>Alcoholism</li></ul> Iatrogenic causes <ul><li>IV glucose administration</li><li>Total parenteral nutrition without phosphorus</li><li>Aluminum- or magnesium-based antacids</li><li>Insulin administration</li><li>Diuretic therapy</li></ul>	Acute or chronic renal failure Impaired excretion Increased phosphate intake or absorption Shift into ECF from: <ul><li>Chemotherapy</li><li>Muscle tissue trauma</li><li>Sepsis</li><li>Severe hypothermia</li><li>Heat stroke</li></ul>
MANIFESTATIONS	Neurologic <ul><li>Irritability, confusion</li><li>Paresthesias</li><li>Ataxia, lack of coordination</li><li>Seizures, coma</li></ul> Hematologic <ul><li>Tissue hypoxia</li><li>Hemolytic anemia</li><li>↓ WBC function, ↑ risk of infection</li></ul> Muscle <ul><li>Muscle pain, weakness</li><li>Respiratory failure</li></ul> Cardiac <ul><li>Chest pain</li><li>↓ Cardiac output</li><li>Dysrhythmias</li></ul>	Circumoral and peripheral paresthesias Muscle spasms Tetany Soft tissue calcification
Lab values (normal 2.5–4.5 mg/dL)	Serum phosphorus < 2.5 mg/dL	Serum phosphate > 4.5 mg/dL

energy resources for vital processes are depleted. The ability of red blood cells to transport oxygen is affected, resulting in tissue hypoxia.

Hyperphosphatemia (serum phosphate > 4.5 mg/dL) usually results from acute or chronic renal failure and impaired phosphorus excretion. It may be caused by increased phosphate intake or absorption. Phosphate is released into ECF when cells are damaged or destroyed (see Table 5-11).

When serum phosphate levels are high, the excess phosphate combines with calcium. The primary manifestations of hyperphosphatemia (Table 5-11) relate to the resulting hypocalcemia rather than to high phosphate levels themselves.

Management of phosphate imbalances focuses on preventing an imbalance in clients at risk and treating any underlying disorder causing phosphate imbalance.

For mild hypophosphatemia improved nutrition may be enough. Unless contraindicated, milk may be recommended because it supplies phosphate, calcium, and potassium. Oral phosphorus supplements may be prescribed, but common adverse effects (nausea and diarrhea) may limit their effectiveness. For severe hypophosphatemia, intravenous phosphate solutions may be ordered.

For hyperphosphatemia, agents such as aluminum hydroxide (Amphogel) that bind with phosphate may be used to lower serum phosphate levels. Dialysis may be used to remove excess phosphate. In clients with adequate renal function, intravenous normal saline may promote phosphate excretion. In severe hyperphosphatemia, glucose and insulin may be given to drive phosphate into the cells, lowering the serum phosphate level.

Identifying clients at risk for phosphate imbalances is an important nursing responsibility. Monitor serum phosphorus levels closely in malnourished clients, alcoholics, clients with renal failure, and clients being treated for diabetic ketoacidosis. Assess for and report manifestations of phosphate imbalance (paresthesias, muscle weakness and pain, or changes in mental status). Protect clients with severe hypophosphatemia from infection. Administer intravenous phosphate solutions carefully, observing for signs of hyperphosphatemia or other electrolyte imbalances (particularly potassium and calcium).

Teach at-risk clients and their families how to prevent and recognize manifestations of phosphate imbalance. Discuss the effects of phosphorus-binding antacids and phosphate-containing laxatives and enemas. Provide information about appropriate alternatives to these products and directions for their use. Teach clients that a well-balanced diet provides adequate phosphate. Milk and milk products, meats, and legumes (such as dried beans) are particularly rich in phosphate. Stress the importance of good nutrition, particularly with clients for whom alcohol is a problem. Provide information about alcohol treatment programs such as Alcoholics Anonymous. Instruct clients to mix powdered oral phosphorus supplements with very cold water or juice to make them more palatable.

Acid–Base Disorders

For optimal cell function, the concentration of hydrogen ions (H^+) in body fluids must remain relatively constant. Hydrogen ions determine the relative acidity of body fluids. Acids release hydrogen ions in solution; bases (or alkalis) accept hydrogen ions in solution. The hydrogen ion concentration of a solution is measured as its **pH,** from 0 to 14, with 7 being neutral. The relationship between hydrogen ion concentration and pH is inverse; that is, as hydrogen ion concentration increases, the pH falls, and the solution becomes more acidic. As hydrogen ion concentration falls, the pH rises, and the solution becomes more alkaline or basic. The normal pH of body fluids is slightly basic, ranging from 7.35 to 7.45.

Acid–Base Regulation

Acids are continually produced by metabolic processes in the body. These acids may be either volatile or nonvolatile acids. *Volatile acids* can be eliminated from the body as a gas.

Carbonic acid (H_2CO_3) is the only volatile acid produced in the body. It dissociates into carbon dioxide (CO_2) and water (H_2O). The carbon dioxide is eliminated from the body through the lungs. All other acids produced in the body (e.g., lactic acid, hydrochloric acid, phosphoric acid, and sulfuric acid) are *nonvolatile acids.* These must be metabolized or excreted from the body in fluid. Most acids and bases in the body are weak (close to a pH of 7).

Three systems work together in the body to maintain a normal pH despite continuous acid production: buffers, the respiratory system, and the renal system.

BUFFER SYSTEMS

Buffers prevent major changes in pH by attaching to or releasing hydrogen ion. When body fluid becomes excessively acid, buffers bind with hydrogen ions to minimize the change in pH. If body fluids become too basic or alkaline, buffers release hydrogen ion, restoring the pH. Although buffers act within a fraction of a second, their capacity to maintain pH is limited. The major buffer systems of the body are the bicarbonate–carbonic acid buffer system, phosphate buffer system, and protein buffers.

Bicarbonate is a weak base; when an acid is added to the system, it combines with bicarbonate, and the pH changes only slightly. Carbonic acid is a weak acid produced when carbon dioxide dissolves in water. If a base is added to the system, it combines with carbonic acid, and the pH remains within the normal range. The normal serum bicarbonate level is 24 mEq/L, and that of carbonic acid is 1.2 mEq/L. Thus, the ratio of bicarbonate to carbonic acid is 20:1. As long as this ratio is maintained, the pH remains within the 7.35 to 7.45 range (Figure 5-11 ◆). When a strong acid is added to ECF, bicarbonate is depleted, changing the 20:1 ratio. The pH then drops below 7.35. If a strong base is added, carbonic acid is depleted, the 20:1 ratio is altered, and the pH rises above 7.45.

Inorganic phosphates and plasma proteins serve a lesser role as buffers in ECF, although they are important intracellular buffers. Within red blood cells, hemoglobin also acts as a buffer.

RESPIRATORY SYSTEM

The respiratory system (including the respiratory center of the brain) regulates carbonic acid in the body by eliminating or retaining carbon dioxide. Carbon dioxide is a potential acid; when combined with water, it forms carbonic acid. Acute increases in either carbon dioxide or hydrogen ions in the blood stimulate the respiratory center in the brain to increase the rate and depth of respirations. This eliminates carbon dioxide from the body; carbonic acid levels fall, bringing the pH to a more normal range. This compensation for increased hydrogen ion concentration occurs within minutes. It becomes less effective over time, however. Clients with chronic lung disease may have consistently high carbon dioxide levels in their blood.

Alkalosis, by contrast, depresses the respiratory center. The rate and depth of respirations decrease, and carbon diox-

ide is retained. The retained carbon dioxide then combines with water to restore carbonic acid levels and bring the pH back within the normal range.

RENAL SYSTEM

The renal system responds more slowly to changes in pH (hours to days). It is responsible for the long-term regulation of acid–base balance in the body. The kidneys regulate bicarbonate levels in ECF and can either excrete or retain hydrogen ion as needed. When excess hydrogen ions are present and the pH falls, the kidneys excrete hydrogen ions and retain bicarbonate. When bicarbonate levels are high, the kidneys retain hydrogen ion and excrete bicarbonate to restore acid–base balance.

Types of Acid–Base Imbalances

Acid–base imbalances fall into two major categories: *acidosis* and *alkalosis.* **Acidosis** occurs when the hydrogen ion concentration increases above normal and the pH falls below 7.35. **Alkalosis** occurs when the hydrogen ion concentration decreases below normal and the pH rises above 7.45. Acid–base imbalances are further classified as *metabolic* or *respiratory* disorders. In *metabolic disorders,* the primary change is in bicarbonate concentration. In metabolic acidosis, the amount of bicarbonate is decreased in relation to the amount of acid in the body (Figure 5-12A ◆). *Metabolic alkalosis,* by contrast, occurs when there is an excess of bicarbonate (Figure 5-12B). In *respiratory disorders,* the primary change is in the concentration of carbonic acid. *Respiratory acidosis* occurs when carbon dioxide is retained, increasing the amount of carbonic acid in the body (Figure 5-13A ◆). When too much carbon dioxide is "blown off," carbonic acid levels fall, and *respiratory alkalosis* develops (Figure 5-13B).

Acid–base disorders are further defined as primary (simple) and mixed. *Primary (simple) disorders* usually are due to one cause. For example, respiratory failure often causes respiratory acidosis; renal failure usually causes metabolic acidosis. With

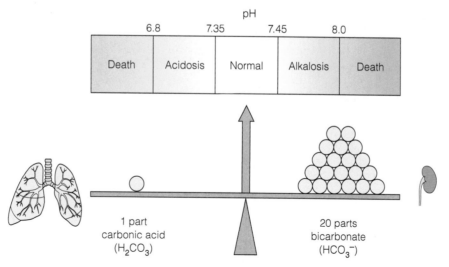

Figure 5-11. ◆ As long as the ratio of bicarbonate to carbonic acid is 20:1, the pH remains within the normal range of 7.35 to 7.45.

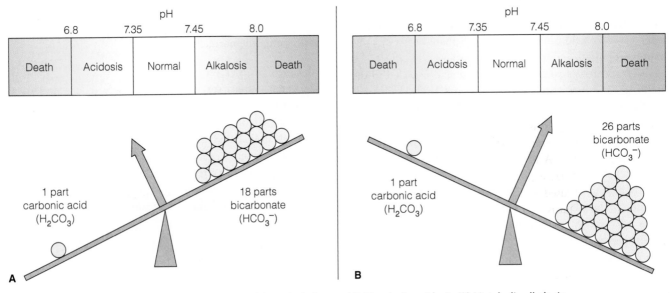

Figure 5-12. ◆ Metabolic acid–base imbalances. (A) Metabolic acidosis. (B) Metabolic alkalosis.

primary disorders, the amount of change in pH may be minimized by *compensatory* responses by the acid–base regulatory system. The kidneys compensate for simple respiratory imbalances by altering bicarbonate production and hydrogen ion excretion; the lungs compensate for simple metabolic imbalances by changing the rate and depth of respirations. *Mixed disorders* occur when both metabolic and respiratory imbalances are present. For example, a client in cardiac arrest develops a mixed respiratory and metabolic acidosis due to respiratory arrest and hypoxia of body tissues that affects normal cell metabolism.

ASSESSMENT OF ACID–BASE BALANCE
Acid–base balance is evaluated by measuring *arterial blood gases (ABGs)*. The elements measured are the $PaCO_2$, the PaO_2, bicarbonate, and pH. Arterial blood is used because it reflects acid–base balance throughout the entire body and allows evaluation of oxygenation.

CLINICAL alert

In contrast to veins, arteries are high-pressure vessels. ABGs are drawn by a registered nurse, respiratory therapist, or laboratory technician who has had specialized training. After the sample has been drawn, apply firm pressure to the puncture site for at least 5 minutes to prevent bleeding into the surrounding tissues.

The $PaCO_2$ measures the amount of dissolved carbon dioxide in the blood. The $PaCO_2$ is regulated by the lungs. The

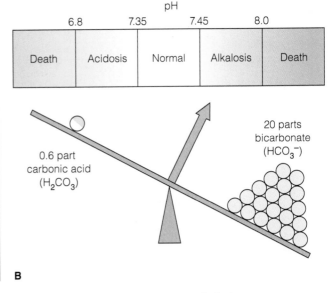

Figure 5-13. ◆ Respiratory acid–base imbalances. (A) Respiratory acidosis. (B) Respiratory alkalosis.

normal value is 35 to 45 mm Hg. A $PaCO_2$ of less than 35 mm Hg is known as *hypocapnia;* a $PaCO_2$ greater than 45 mm Hg is *hypercapnia.*

The PaO_2 measures the amount of oxygen dissolved in the plasma. Only about 3% of oxygen in the blood is in solution; most oxygen is carried by hemoglobin. However, it is the dissolved oxygen that is available to the cells for metabolism. As dissolved oxygen diffuses out of plasma into the tissues, more is released from hemoglobin. The normal value for PaO_2 is 80 to 100 mm Hg. A PaO_2 less than 80 mm Hg indicates **hypoxemia.** The PaO_2 is valuable for evaluating respiratory function but is not used as a primary measurement in determining acid–base status.

CLINICAL alert

The abbreviations $PaCO_2$ and PaO_2 often are used interchangeably with PCO_2 and PO_2. The "P" stands for partial pressure: the pressure exerted by the gas dissolved in the blood. The "a" indicates that the sample is arterial blood. Because these measurements rarely are done on venous blood, the "a" often is deleted from the abbreviation.

The serum bicarbonate (HCO_3^-) reflects the renal regulation of acid–base balance. It often is referred to as the *metabolic component* of arterial blood gases. The normal HCO_3^- is 22 to 26 mEq/L.

The *base excess (BE)* also may be reported on ABGs. It reflects the degree of acid–base imbalance; it represents the amount of acid or base that must be added to a blood sample to achieve a pH of 7.4. The normal base excess is −3.0 to +3.0.

ABGs are analyzed to identify acid–base disorders and their probable cause, determine the extent of the imbalance, and monitor treatment. When analyzing ABG results, it is important to use a systematic approach (see Box 5-12). First, evaluate each individual measurement, then look at the interrelationships to determine the client's acid–base status.

Metabolic Acidosis

Metabolic acidosis may be caused by excess acid or inadequate bicarbonate in the body. It is characterized by a low pH (< 7.35) and a low bicarbonate (< 22 mEq/L). When metabolic acidosis develops, the respiratory system attempts to return the pH to normal by increasing the rate and depth of respirations. Carbon dioxide elimination increases, and the $PaCO_2$ falls (< 35 mm Hg).

PATHOPHYSIOLOGY

Metabolic acidosis rarely is a primary disorder; it usually develops during the course of another disease (Table 5-12 ◆). Insufficient oxygen to support cell metabolism leads to the production of lactic acid. When inadequate glucose is available for cell metabolism (due to starvation or a lack of insulin), the body breaks down fatty tissue to meet its metabolic needs.

BOX 5-12
NURSING CARE CHECKLIST

INTERPRETING ARTERIAL BLOOD GASES

1. Look at the pH.
   - ☐ pH < 7.35 = acidosis
   - ☐ pH > 7.45 = alkalosis

2. Look at the $PaCO_2$.
   - ☐ $PaCO_2$ < 35 mm Hg = hypocapnia; more carbon dioxide is being exhaled than normal.
   - ☐ $PaCO_2$ > 45 mm Hg = hypercapnia; carbon dioxide is being retained.

3. Evaluate the pH–$PaCO_2$ relationship for a possible respiratory problem.
   - ☐ If the pH is < 7.35 (acidosis) and the $PaCO_2$ is > 45 mm Hg (hypercapnia), retained carbon dioxide is causing *respiratory acidosis.*
   - ☐ If the pH is > 7.45 (alkalosis) and the $PaCO_2$ is < 35 mm Hg (hypocapnia), low carbon dioxide levels are causing *respiratory alkalosis.*

4. Look at the bicarbonate.
   - ☐ If the HCO_3^- is < 22 mEq/L, bicarbonate levels are lower than normal.
   - ☐ If the HCO_3^- is > 26 mEq/L, bicarbonate levels are higher than normal.

5. Evaluate the pH, HCO_3^-, and base excess (BE) for a possible metabolic problem.
   - ☐ If the pH is < 7.35 (acidosis), the HCO_3^- is < 22 mEq/L, and the BE is < −3 mEq/L, low bicarbonate levels are causing *metabolic acidosis.*
   - ☐ If the pH is > 7.45 (alkalosis), the HCO_3^- is > 26 mEq/L, and the BE is > +3 mEq/L, high bicarbonate levels are causing *metabolic alkalosis.*

6. Look for compensation.
   - *Renal compensation:*
     - ☐ In respiratory acidosis (pH < 7.35, $PaCO_2$ > 45 mm Hg), the kidneys retain HCO_3^- to buffer the excess acid, so the HCO_3^- is > 26 mEq/L.
     - ☐ In respiratory alkalosis (pH > 7.45, $PaCO_2$ < 35 mm Hg), the kidneys excrete HCO_3^- to minimize the alkalosis, so the HCO_3^- is < 22 mEq/L.
   - *Respiratory compensation:*
     - ☐ In metabolic acidosis (pH < 7.35, HCO_3^- < 22 mEq/L), the rate and depth of respirations increase, increasing carbon dioxide elimination, so the $PaCO_2$ is < 35 mm Hg.
     - ☐ In metabolic alkalosis (pH > 7.45, HCO_3^- > 26 mEq/L), respirations slow, and carbon dioxide is retained, so the $PaCO_2$ is > 45 mm Hg.

In this process, fatty acids are released. Renal failure, which impairs the body's ability to excrete excess hydrogen ion and form bicarbonate, is a common cause of metabolic acidosis.

TABLE 5-12 CAUSES AND MANIFESTATIONS OF PRIMARY ACID–BASE IMBALANCES

IMBALANCE	LAB VALUES	COMMON CAUSES	MANIFESTATIONS
Metabolic acidosis	pH < 7.35 HCO_3^- < 22 mEq/L Compensation: $Paco_2$ < 35 mm Hg Serum K^+ usually > 5 mEq/L	Increased acid production ■ Lactic acidosis ■ Ketoacidosis (diabetes, starvation, or alcoholism) ■ Salicylate toxicity Decreased acid excretion ■ Renal failure Increased bicarbonate loss ■ Diarrhea, ileostomy drainage, intestinal fistula Increased chloride ■ Sodium chloride IV solutions ■ Renal tubular acidosis	CNS ■ Headache ■ Confusion ■ Decreased level of consciousness GI ■ Anorexia ■ Nausea and vomiting Cardiovascular ■ Vasodilation; warm, flushed skin ■ Decreased cardiac output Respiratory (compensatory) ■ Increased rate and depth (hyperventilation)
Metabolic alkalosis	pH > 7.45 HCO_3^- > 26 mEq/L Compensation: $Paco_2$ > 45 mm Hg Serum potassium often < 3.5 mEq/L	Increased acid loss or excretion ■ Vomiting, gastric suction ■ Hypokalemia Increased bicarbonate ■ Alkali ingestion (bicarbonate of soda) ■ Excess bicarbonate administration	■ Dizziness ■ Paresthesias (around mouth and fingers and toes) ■ Carpopedal spasm (+ Trousseau's sign) ■ Hyperactive DTRs (deep tendon reflexes) ■ Depressed respirations (compensatory)
Respiratory acidosis	pH < 7.35 $Paco_2$ > 45 mm Hg Compensation: HCO_3^- > 26 mEq/L	Acute respiratory acidosis ■ Acute respiratory conditions ■ Narcotic overdose ■ Chest trauma ■ Respiratory arrest Chronic respiratory acidosis ■ Chronic respiratory conditions ■ Multiple sclerosis, other neuromuscular diseases ■ Stroke	Acute respiratory acidosis ■ Feeling of fullness in head ■ Mental cloudiness, decreasing level of consciousness ■ Dizziness, muscle twitching, seizures ■ Warm, flushed skin ■ Cardiac dysrhythmias Chronic respiratory acidosis ■ Dull headache ■ Weakness
Respiratory alkalosis	pH > 7.45 $Paco_2$ < 35 mm Hg Compensation: HCO_3^- < 22 mEq/L	■ Anxiety-induced hyperventilation ■ Fever ■ Early salicylate intoxication ■ Hyperventilation with mechanical ventilator	↓ Cerebral blood flow ■ Lightheadedness ■ Inability to concentrate ↓ Calcium ionization ■ Paresthesias around mouth and distal extremities Hyperventilation syndrome ■ Palpitations, shortness of breath, chest tightness ■ Tremulousness, sweating, dry mouth ■ Feeling of panic ■ Loss of consciousness, seizures

Bicarbonate-rich fluid from the small intestine can be lost through intestinal suction, severe diarrhea, ileostomy drainage, or fistulas. Administering excess chloride solutions (e.g., NaCl or ammonium chloride) can lead to metabolic acidosis as well.

In all acid–base imbalances, the manifestations may be subtle. Metabolic acidosis primary affects the central nervous system, GI tract, and cardiovascular function. See Table 5-12 for the manifestations of metabolic acidosis.

COLLABORATIVE CARE

The focus of treatment for acute metabolic acidosis is the underlying cause. (See Chapter 17 for treatment of diabetic ketoacidosis and Chapter 21 for treatment of renal failure.)

In addition to ABGs, *serum electrolytes* are measured. The serum potassium is usually greater than 5 mEq/L as potassium ions shift out of cells in exchange for hydrogen ions. Serum potassium levels are measured throughout treatment for metabolic acidosis because hypokalemia can develop as the acidosis is corrected. An *ECG* is done to evaluate the effects of metabolic acidosis on cardiac function.

Bicarbonate may be given to correct the acid–base imbalance. Overtreatment is avoided, as it may lead to metabolic alkalosis, hypokalemia, dysrhythmias, and possible tetany. Other basic solutions that may be given to correct metabolic acidosis include lactate, acetate, or citrate solutions.

NURSING CARE

ASSESSING

Collect subjective assessment data, including symptoms of anorexia, nausea, abdominal discomfort, fatigue, or lethargy. Ask about precipitating factors such as diarrhea, aspirin ingestion, chronic diseases such as diabetes or renal failure, and current medications.

Obtain objective data including mental status and level of consciousness; vital signs including respiratory rate and depth; apical and peripheral pulses; skin color and temperature; and urine output.

DIAGNOSING, PLANNING, AND IMPLEMENTING

DECREASED CARDIAC OUTPUT

Metabolic acidosis decreases the strength of heart contractions, slows the heart rate, and increases the risk of dysrhythmias.

■ Monitor vital signs, peripheral pulses, and capillary refill. *Hypotension, diminished pulse strength, and slowed capillary refill may indicate decreased cardiac output.*
■ Monitor ECG pattern for dysrhythmias. Notify the physician of changes. *Dysrhythmias further decrease cardiac output, which may worsen acidosis.*
■ Monitor laboratory values, including arterial blood gases, serum electrolytes, serum creatinine, and blood urea nitrogen (BUN). *Frequent monitoring of laboratory values helps evaluate treatment effectiveness and identify potential problems.*

RISK FOR EXCESS FLUID VOLUME

Administering bicarbonate to correct acidosis increases the risk for hypernatremia and fluid volume excess.

■ Obtain daily weights. *Daily weights are an accurate indicator of fluid balance.*
■ Monitor intake and output. Obtain hourly urine outputs as indicated, reporting an output of less than 30 mL/hr. *Heart failure and inadequate renal perfusion may lead to decreased urine output.*

■ Monitor respiratory status and CVP. *Increasing dyspnea, adventitious lung sounds, and high CVP readings indicate excess fluid volume. Report to the care provider.*
■ Assess for edema in dependent tissues and periorbital areas. *Dependent or generalized edema may indicate excess fluid volume.*

RISK FOR INJURY

■ Monitor mental status, level of consciousness, and muscle strength. *As the pH falls, mental function declines, causing confusion and a decreasing level of consciousness. This increases the risk for injury.*
■ Institute safety precautions as necessary—keep the bed in its lowest position, side rails up. *These measures help protect the client from injury resulting from confusion or disorientation.*
■ Keep clocks, calendars, and familiar objects at the bedside. Orient to time, place, and circumstances as needed. Allow significant others to remain with the client as much as possible. *An unfamiliar environment and altered thought processes can further increase the risk for injury. Significant others provide a sense of security and reduce anxiety.*

Nursing care also includes measures to treat the underlying disorder, such as diabetic ketoacidosis. Refer to the chapters on diabetes (Chapter 17) and renal failure (Chapter 21) for specific interventions.

EVALUATING

In order to evaluate the effectiveness of nursing care, monitor the client's cardiac output, safety, and fluid balance.

Discharge Considerations

Discharge planning focuses on the underlying cause of the metabolic acidosis. Teach the client who has developed ketoacidosis as a result of diabetes mellitus, starvation, or alcoholism about diet and medications. Refer for treatment of alcoholism and to a support group such as AA. Discuss the importance of day-to-day management of renal failure (e.g., diet and dialysis) to prevent future problems with metabolic acidosis. With clients who developed acidosis as a result of diarrhea or ileostomy drainage, provide information about strategies to prevent or treat diarrhea, and when to call their primary care provider.

Metabolic Alkalosis

Metabolic alkalosis may be caused by loss of acid or excess bicarbonate in the body. It is characterized by a high pH (> 7.45) and a high bicarbonate (> 26 mEq/L). When metabolic alkalosis develops, the respiratory system attempts to return the pH to normal by slowing the respiratory rate. Carbon dioxide is retained, and the $PaCO_2$ increases (> 45 mm Hg).

PATHOPHYSIOLOGY

Vomiting or gastric suction often leads to loss of hydrogen ions from the body. Gastric secretions are highly acidic (pH 1–3). Hypokalemia also reduces hydrogen ion concentration, as the kidneys excrete hydrogen ion in exchange for potassium. In addition, when potassium shifts out of the cells to maintain potassium levels in ECF, hydrogen ion shifts into the cells.

Excess bicarbonate usually results from ingestion of antacids that contain bicarbonate (such as soda bicarbonate or Alka-Seltzer) or overzealous administration of bicarbonate to treat metabolic acidosis. Review Table 5-12 for common causes of metabolic alkalosis.

Alkalosis affects calcium ionization in ECF. Because of this, the manifestations of both metabolic and respiratory alkalosis are similar to those of hypocalcemia. As the respiratory system compensates for metabolic alkalosis, respirations are depressed (see Table 5-12).

COLLABORATIVE CARE

Treatment of metabolic alkalosis focuses on diagnosing and correcting the underlying cause. Serum electrolytes are monitored; hypokalemia (< 3.5 mEq/L) and hypochloremia (< 95 mEq/L) are often present. The potassium level is closely monitored during treatment, because correcting the alkalosis may affect serum potassium.

Treatment includes restoring normal fluid volume and administering sodium chloride solutions. Chloride is necessary for the kidney to excrete excess bicarbonate. Potassium may be ordered to restore potassium levels.

NURSING CARE

ASSESSING

Obtain the following assessment data related to metabolic alkalosis:

■ Current symptoms, such as numbness and tingling, muscle spasms, or dizziness; any precipitating factors such as bicarbonate ingestion or vomiting, current medications.
■ Objective data: Vital signs including apical pulse, rate and depth of respirations; muscle strength; and deep tendon reflexes.

DIAGNOSING, PLANNING, AND IMPLEMENTING

RISK FOR IMPAIRED GAS EXCHANGE

Respiratory compensation for metabolic alkalosis depresses the respiratory rate and depth. The client is at risk for impaired gas exchange, especially if chronic lung disease also is present.

■ Monitor respiratory rate, depth, and effort. Monitor oxygen saturation continuously; report an oxygen saturation level

of less than 95% (or as ordered). *Depressed respirations can lead to hypoxemia and impaired tissue oxgenation. An oxygen saturation of less than 90% indicates significant problems.*
■ Monitor mental status and level of consciousness (LOC). Report decreasing LOC or behavior changes such as restlessness, agitation, or confusion. *Changes in mental status or behavior may be early signs of hypoxia.*
■ Place in semi-Fowler's or Fowler's position as tolerated. *Elevating the head of the bed improves ventilation and gas exchange.*
■ Schedule nursing care activities to allow rest periods. *The hypoxemic client has limited energy reserves, requiring frequent rest and limited activities.*
■ Administer oxygen as ordered or necessary to maintain oxygen saturation levels. *Supplemental oxygen can help maintain blood and tissue oxygenation despite depressed respirations.*

DEFICIENT FLUID VOLUME

Clients with metabolic alkalosis often have an accompanying fluid volume deficit.

■ Assess intake and output; monitor hourly if indicated. *Urine output less than 30 mL per hour indicates inadequate renal perfusion and an increased risk for acute renal failure and inadequate tissue perfusion.*
■ Monitor vital signs, CVP, and peripheral pulses at least every 4 hours. *Hypotension, tachycardia, low CVP, and weak, easily obliterated peripheral pulses indicate hypovolemia.*
■ Weigh daily. *Rapid weight changes accurately reflect fluid balance.*
■ Administer intravenous fluids as ordered using an infusion pump. Monitor for dyspnea, tachypnea, tachycardia, increased CVP, jugular vein distention, and edema. *Rapid fluid replacement may lead to hypervolemia.*
■ Monitor serum electrolytes, osmolality, and ABG values. *Rehydration and administration of potassium chloride will affect both acid–base and fluid and electrolyte balance. Careful monitoring is important to identify changes.*

EVALUATING

Collect data related to the client's respiratory status, tissue oxygenation, and fluid balance to evaluate the effectiveness of nursing interventions for clients with metabolic alkalosis.

Discharge Considerations

Planning and teaching for home care of the client who has experienced metabolic alkalosis focuses on the underlying cause of the imbalance. Teach clients how to prevent and manage problems such as acute gastroenteritis that can lead to excessive vomiting (see Chapter 18). Discuss the importance of adequate potassium in the diet, foods high in potassium (see Box 5-9), and potassium supplements with clients for whom hypokalemia contributed to metabolic alkalosis. Teach clients to avoid using bicarbonate-based antacids, and suggest alternatives.

Respiratory Acidosis

Respiratory acidosis is caused by an excess of dissolved carbon dioxide, or carbonic acid. It is characterized by a pH of less than 7.35 and a $PaCO_2$ greater than 44 mm Hg. Respiratory acidosis may be either acute or chronic in nature. In chronic respiratory acidosis, the bicarbonate is higher than 26 mEq/L as the kidneys compensate by retaining bicarbonate.

PATHOPHYSIOLOGY

Both acute and chronic respiratory acidosis are caused by alveolar hypoventilation leading to carbon dioxide retention. Hypoxemia (low oxygen in the arterial blood) frequently accompanies respiratory acidosis.

Acute respiratory acidosis occurs due to an acute failure of ventilation. Chest trauma, aspiration of a foreign body, acute pneumonia, and overdoses of narcotic or sedative medications can lead to acute respiratory acidosis. In acute respiratory acidosis, the $PaCO_2$ rises rapidly and the pH falls markedly. The serum bicarbonate initially is unchanged because the compensatory response of the kidneys occurs over hours to days.

Chronic respiratory acidosis is associated with chronic respiratory or neuromuscular conditions such as chronic obstructive pulmonary disease (COPD), asthma, cystic fibrosis, or multiple sclerosis. These conditions affect alveolar ventilation because of airway obstruction, structural changes in the lung, or limited chest wall expansion. Most clients with chronic respiratory acidosis have chronic obstructive pulmonary disease with chronic bronchitis and emphysema (see Table 5-12). In chronic respiratory acidosis, the $PaCO_2$ increases over time and remains elevated. The kidneys retain bicarbonate, increasing bicarbonate levels, and the pH often remains close to the normal range.

The manifestations of acute and chronic respiratory acidosis differ. An acute rise in $PaCO_2$ causes manifestations of hypercapnia (elevated serum carbon dioxide levels). Carbon dioxide dilates cerebral blood vessels, causing a feeling of fullness in the head and mental cloudiness. Rapid and dramatic changes in ABGs can lead to unconsciousness and cardiac arrest.

Clients with chronic respiratory acidosis may have few symptoms because carbon dioxide levels rise gradually, allowing compensatory changes to occur. See Table 5-12 for other manifestations of acute and chronic respiratory acidosis.

CLINICAL alert

In clients with chronically high blood levels of carbon dioxide, hypoxemia becomes the primary stimulus to breathe. Administering oxygen at a high flow rate may suppress respirations and lead to acute respiratory failure.

COLLABORATIVE CARE

Clients with acute respiratory failure usually require treatment in the emergency department or intensive care unit to restore adequate ventilation and gas exchange. Hypoxemia often accompanies acute respiratory acidosis, so oxygen is administered as well. Supplemental oxygen is used with caution for clients with chronic respiratory acidosis.

Bronchodilator drugs may be given to open the airways. Antibiotics may be ordered to treat respiratory infections. If excess narcotics or anesthetic has caused acute respiratory acidosis, drugs to reverse their effects may be given. Pulmonary hygiene measures, such as breathing treatments or percussion and drainage, may be used to clear airways and support ventilation. Adequate hydration is important to promote removal of respiratory secretions. Intubation and mechanical ventilation may be necessary for some clients in respiratory acidosis. (See Chapter 26 for more information about mechanical ventilation and its nursing implications.)

NURSING CARE

ASSESSING

Assessment data related to respiratory acidosis includes the following:

- *Subjective data:* Current symptoms such as headache, difficulty thinking, blurred vision; any precipitating factors such as drug use or infection; chronic diseases such as cystic fibrosis or COPD; current medications.
- *Objective data:* Mental status and LOC; vital signs; skin color and temperature; rate and depth of respirations, lung sounds.

DIAGNOSING, PLANNING, AND IMPLEMENTING

IMPAIRED GAS EXCHANGE

- Frequently assess respiratory status (rate, depth, effort, and oxygen saturation levels) and LOC. *Decreasing respiratory rate, effort, oxygen saturation level, and LOC may indicate worsening of the client's condition.*
- Promptly report ABG results to the physician and respiratory therapy. *Rapid changes in carbon dioxide or oxygen levels may indicate a need to modify the treatment plan.*
- Place in semi-Fowler's to Fowler's position as tolerated. *Elevating the head of the bed promotes lung expansion and gas exchange.*
- Administer oxygen as ordered. Carefully monitor response. Reduce the oxygen flow rate or percentage and immediately report decreased level of consciousness. *Supplemental oxygen can suppress the respiratory drive in clients with chronic respiratory acidosis.*

INEFFECTIVE AIRWAY CLEARANCE

- Frequently auscultate breath sounds. *Increasing adventitious sounds or decreasing breath sounds (faint or absent) may indicate worsening airway clearance due to obstruction or fatigue.*
- Encourage the client with chronic respiratory acidosis to use pursed-lip breathing. *Pursed-lip breathing helps maintain open airways throughout exhalation, promoting carbon dioxide elimination.*
- Frequently reposition and encourage client to get out of bed as tolerated. *Movement and ambulation promote airway clearance and lung expansion.*
- Encourage fluid intake of up to 3,000 mL per day as tolerated or allowed. *Fluids help liquefy secretions and hydrate respiratory mucous membranes, promoting airway clearance.*
- Administer medications such as inhaled bronchodilators as ordered. *Inhaled bronchodilators help relieve bronchial spasm, dilating airways.*
- Provide percussion, vibration, and postural drainage as ordered. *Pulmonary hygiene measures such as these help loosen respiratory secretions so they can be coughed out of airways.*

EVALUATING

Collect data such as ABG results, oxygen saturation levels, skin color, lung sounds, activity tolerance, and ease of respirations to evaluate the effectiveness of nursing interventions for the client with respiratory acidosis.

Discharge Considerations

Planning and teaching for discharge focus on the problem that caused the client to develop respiratory acidosis. Clients with acute respiratory acidosis resulting from acute pneumonia or chest trauma may need only teaching to prevent future problems. If acute respiratory acidosis was secondary to a narcotic overdose, determine if the drug was prescribed or an illicit street drug. Provide teaching to the client who requires narcotic medication on a continuing basis. Refer the client using illicit drugs to a substance abuse counselor, treatment center, or Narcotics Anonymous as appropriate.

For clients with chronic lung disease, discuss ways to avoid future episodes of acute respiratory failure. Encourage the client to be immunized against pneumococcal pneumonia and influenza. Discuss ways to avoid acute respiratory infections and measures to take when respiratory status is further compromised.

Respiratory Alkalosis

Respiratory alkalosis is always caused by hyperventilation leading to a carbon dioxide deficit. It is characterized by a pH greater than 7.45 and a $PaCO_2$ of less than 35 mm Hg.

PATHOPHYSIOLOGY

In acute respiratory alkalosis, the pH rises rapidly as the $PaCO_2$ falls. The bicarbonate level remains within normal limits because the kidneys require time to increase bicarbonate elimination. Anxiety-induced hyperventilation is the most common cause of acute respiratory alkalosis. Other causes are listed in Table 5-12. Low carbon dioxide levels cause cerebral blood vessels to constrict, reducing blood flow. The manifestations of respiratory alkalosis relate to this cerebral vasoconstriction and decreased calcium ionization (which also occurs in metabolic alkalosis). Table 5-12 lists the manifestations of respiratory alkalosis.

COLLABORATIVE CARE

Anxiety-induced respiratory alkalosis is treated by instructing the client to breathe slowly into a paper bag or rebreather mask. This allows the client to rebreathe exhaled carbon dioxide, which increases $PaCO_2$ levels and reduces the pH. A sedative or antianxiety agent may be given. In other cases, such as salicylate intoxication or excessive ventilation by a mechanical ventilator, treatment is aimed at the underlying cause of the hyperventilation.

NURSING CARE

INEFFECTIVE BREATHING PATTERN

- Assess respiratory rate, depth, and ease. Monitor vital signs (including temperature) and skin color. *Assessment data can help identify the underlying cause, such as a fever or hypoxia.*
- Obtain subjective assessment data such as circumstances leading up to the current situation, current health and recent illnesses or medication use, as well as current manifestations. *Subjective data provide cues to the cause and circumstances of hyperventilation.*
- Reassure the client that he or she is not having a heart attack and that symptoms will resolve when breathing returns to normal. *Manifestations of hyperventilation and respiratory alkalosis such as dyspnea, chest tightness or pain, and palpitations can mimic those of a heart attack.*
- Instruct client to maintain eye contact and breathe with you to slow the respiratory rate. *These measures help make the client aware of respirations and provide a sense of support and control* (Ackley & Ladwig, 2002).
- Have the client breathe into a paper bag. *This allows the client to rebreathe exhaled carbon dioxide, increasing the $PaCO_2$ and decreasing the pH.*
- Protect from injury. *If hyperventilation continues, the client may lose consciousness, causing respirations and acid–base balance to return to normal.*
- Refer clients with repeated episodes of hyperventilation or a chronic anxiety disorder for counseling. *Counseling can help the client develop strategies for dealing with anxiety.*

Discharge Considerations

Planning and teaching for home care are directed toward the underlying cause of hyperventilation. If anxiety precipitated the episode, discuss anxiety-management strategies. Refer the client and family to a counselor if appropriate. Teach how to identify a hyperventilation reaction and breathe into a paper bag to manage it at home.

Nursing Interventions Classification

The following nursing interventions (McCloskey & Bulechek, 2000) may be appropriate for clients with fluid, electrolyte, and acid–base disorders:

- Acid–Base Management
- Anxiety Reduction
- Electrolyte Management
- Fluid Management
- Intravenous (IV) Therapy
- Medication Administration
- Nutritional Counseling
- Oxygen Therapy
- Seizure Precautions
- Teaching: Prescribed Diet
- Teaching: Prescribed Medication

(*Note:* The bibliography listings for this and all chapters have been compiled at the back of the book.)

Chapter Review

 key terms by topic

Use the CD-ROM disk enclosed with your textbook to hear the pronunciation of key terms in the chapter.

Fluid and electrolyte balance
homeostasis, electrolytes, intracellular fluid (ICF), extracellular fluid (ECF)

Body fluid movement
osmosis, diffusion, filtration, active transport

Fluid volume excess
hypervolemia, edema

Potassium imbalance
hypokalemia, hyperkalemia

Calcium imbalance
tetany

Acid–base disorders
pH, buffers, acidosis, alkalosis, metabolic acidosis/alkalosis, respiratory acidosis/alkalosis, hypoxemia

key points

- The volume and composition of body fluid is normally maintained by a balance of fluid and electrolyte intake; elimination of water, electrolytes, and acids by the kidneys; and hormonal influences. Change in any of these factors can lead to a fluid, electrolyte, or acid–base imbalance that affects health.

- Fluid, electrolyte, and acid–base imbalances can affect all body systems, especially the cardiovascular system, the central nervous system, and the transmission of nerve impulses.

- Fluid and sodium imbalances commonly are related; both affect serum osmolality.

- Both hypokalemia and hyperkalemia affect cardiac conduction and function. Carefully monitor cardiac rhythm and status in clients with very low or very high potassium levels.

- Calcium imbalances primarily affect neuromuscular transmission: Too little calcium causes increased neuromuscular irritability; too much calcium depresses neuromuscular transmission. Magnesium imbalances have a similar effect.

- Acid–base imbalances may be caused by either metabolic or respiratory problems.

- Buffers, lungs, and kidneys work together to maintain acid–base balance in the body. Buffers respond to changes almost immediately; the lungs respond within minutes; the kidneys, however, require hours to days to restore normal acid–base balance.

- The lungs compensate for metabolic acid–base imbalances by excreting or retaining carbon dioxide. This is accomplished by increasing or decreasing the rate and depth of respirations.

- The kidneys compensate for respiratory acid–base imbalances by producing and retaining or excreting bicarbonate, and by retaining or excreting hydrogen ions.

- Careful monitoring of respiratory and cardiovascular status, mental status, neuromuscular function, and laboratory values is an important nursing responsibility for all clients with fluid, electrolyte, or acid–base imbalances.

 Medialink

Additional interactive resources for this chapter can be found on the Companion Website at www.prenhall.com/burke. Click on Chapter 5 and "Begin" to select the activities for this chapter.

For NCLEX review questions and an audio glossary, access the accompanying CD-ROM in this book.

for further study

For more on water reabsorption and urine concentration, see Chapters 16 and 21.

For more information on diabetic ketoacidosis, see Chapter 17.

For more about ECG waveforms and cardiac disorders, see Chapter 22.

For more information on clients with renal failure, see Chapter 21.

For more on clients with acute pancreatitis, see Chapter 19.

For more about mechanical ventilation, see Chapter 26.

Critical Thinking Care Map

Caring for a Client with Acute Respiratory Acidosis
NCLEX-PN Focus Area: Physiological Adaptation

Case Study: Marlene Hitz, age 76, is eating lunch with her friends when she suddenly begins to choke and is unable to breathe. After several minutes of trying, an attendant at the senior center successfully dislodges some meat caught in Ms. Hitz's throat using the Heimlich maneuver. Ms. Hitz is taken by ambulance to the emergency department for follow-up.

Nursing Diagnosis: Impaired Gas Exchange

COLLECT DATA

Subjective

_____
_____
_____
_____
_____
_____

Objective

_____
_____
_____
_____
_____
_____

Would you report this data? Yes/No

If yes, to: _____

Nursing Care

_____
_____
_____
_____
_____
_____
_____
_____

How would you document this? _____
_____
_____

Data Collected
(use those that apply)

- T 98.2° F, P 102, R 36 and shallow, BP 146/92
- Skin warm and dry
- Alert but not oriented to time or place
- Responds slowly to questions
- Restless
- Oxygen at 4 L/min per nasal cannula
- D5 ½ NS running intravenously at 50 mL/hr
- Chest x-ray normal
- ABGs: pH 7.38 (normal 7.35 to 7.45), $Paco_2$ 48 mm Hg (normal 35 to 45 mm Hg), Pao_2 92 mm Hg (normal 80 to 100 mm Hg), HCO_3 24 mEq/dL (normal 22 to 26 mEq/L)

Nursing Interventions
(use those that apply)

- Monitor ABGs, to be redrawn in 2 hours.
- Monitor respiratory status and vital signs every 15 minutes for the first hour, then hourly.
- Assess mental status, LOC, and color of skin, nail beds, and oral mucous membranes hourly.
- Maintain a calm, quiet environment.
- Reorient to setting and explain all activities.
- Keep side rails in place, and place call bell within reach.

NCLEX-PN Exam Preparation

TEST-TAKING TIP

Memorizing electrolyte imbalances is a difficult task. Learn the basic electrolytes and their functions in the body. Imbalances occur when the blood level of the electrolyte is either too high or too low. If you are familiar with one state, the other state generally manifests in the opposite direction.

1. Which of these clients would most likely develop dehydration after surgery?
   a. 24-year-old male diagnosed with an inguinal hernia
   b. 60-year-old female with ovarian cancer
   c. 29-year-old morbidly obese female
   d. 19-year-old male with Crohn's disease

2. A client has been diagnosed with a deficiency in the antidiuretic hormone. Which condition should the nurse anticipate?
   a. increase in serum osmolality
   b. dilute urine
   c. decreased thirst
   d. normal blood pressure

3. The nurse assists in the assessment of a client who has just arrived in the emergency room. The physical assessment reveals dry, sticky mucous membranes; hypovolemia; and tachycardia. The primary nursing diagnosis should be:
   a. Deficient Fluid Volume
   b. Impaired Skin Integrity
   c. Risk for Injury
   d. Decreased Cardiac Output

4. A client was admitted to the medical floor with muscle spasms and a positive Chvostek's sign. During the client history, the nurse discovers that the client had a thyroidectomy 6 weeks ago. Based on this finding, the nurse anticipates that the physician will order a lab test for:
   a. sodium
   b. calcium
   c. iron
   d. potassium

5. The nurse anticipates that the low magnesium level in the client with chronic alcoholism will most likely manifest as
   a. negative Trousseau's sign:
   b. bradycardia
   c. vasodilation
   d. tetany

6. A client is hyperventilating due to anxiety. Which of the following lab values indicates an altered acid–base balance?
   a. pH > 7.45
   b. $Paco_2$ > 35 mm Hg
   c. HCO_3 > 22
   d. Pao_2 95

7. The nurse knows that a client's low bicarbonate level may be caused by:
   a. gastrointestinal suction
   b. constipation
   c. use of baking soda for indigestion
   d. alcohol abuse

8. A client with hypercalcemia was admitted to the medical floor. Which of the following findings from the assessment would be the most likely cause of hypercalcemia?
   a. lack of vitamin D
   b. prescribed loop diuretic
   c. excessive use of the antacid tums
   d. menopause

9. The nurse administered the prescribed dose of Lasix. To evaluate the effectiveness of the drug, the nurse should assess:
   a. weight
   b. apical pulse
   c. breath sounds
   d. PO intake

10. The nurse is admitting an 84-year-old client with dehydration. Which of the following would be an expected assessment finding?
    a. peripheral edema
    b. bounding pulses
    c. poor skin turgor
    d. elevated blood pressure

chapter

6

Caring for Clients in Pain

"Listen to your client. Ask questions to clarify and validate what you hear and observe."

Carol Strysick, RN, BSN • Practical Nursing Instructor • Moraine Park Technical College • Beaver Damn, Wisconsin

LEARNING outcomes

After completing this chapter, you will be able to:
- Define pain.
- Describe the steps of pain conduction: transduction, transmission, perception, and modulation.
- Identify the characteristics of acute and chronic pain.
- Differentiate the characteristics among the four types of acute pain.
- Identify factors that may affect a client's response to pain.
- Explain the nurse's role in administering pharmacologic measures to reduce or relieve pain.
- Describe nonpharmacologic interventions clients may use in reducing or relieving pain.
- Describe pain rating scales and their use in assessing pain.
- Identify several myths and misconceptions about pain and pain management.
- Use the nursing process in care of clients experiencing pain.

MediaLink

www.prenhall.com/burke

Use the above address to access the free, interactive Companion Website created for this textbook. Get hints, instant feedback, and textbook references to chapter-related multiple choice questions. Link to other interesting sites.

Pain—the "Fifth Vital Sign"

There are many accepted definitions of pain. The International Association for Study of Pain describes **pain** as an unpleasant sensory and emotional experience associated with actual or potential tissue damage. This definition is misleading, because pain may not always result from actual or potential tissue damage. For instance, psychogenic pain and some forms of headache pain are not caused by tissue damage.

McCaffery and Beebe (1989, p. 7) define pain as "whatever the person experiencing it says it is, and existing whenever the person says it does." This definition recognizes that the client is the only person who can accurately describe his or her own pain. If the client says he or she has pain, the client is in pain. All pain should be considered real. It is a well-known fact that pain can negatively affect the whole body. This definition considers the person as its main focus and should guide nursing assessment and care.

Pain is a subjective response to physical and psychological stressors. All people feel pain at some point during their lives. Although pain is unwelcome, it often serves as a warning of potentially health-threatening conditions. Each pain event is a unique, personal experience. It can be affected by biologic, psychological, cognitive, social, cultural, and spiritual factors. Pain is the most common reason for seeking health care.

Because it is subjective, pain presents a real challenge to nurses. Usually nurses assess clear objective manifestations of a disorder, like skin color or decreased pulse. In assessing pain, however, the nurse must rely on the client's description and nonverbal cues to indicate the type, location, duration, and intensity of pain.

Unfortunately, pain management can be inadequate in all types of health care settings. Several factors influence how pain is perceived and managed. Often, physicians and nurses do not understand the newer concepts about pain management. The public and health care professionals fear addiction. The nurse's own bias can positively or negatively affect how a client's pain is managed. Because pain is subjective, the nurse may judge whether the client is actually experiencing pain. This is not the nurse's role. Nurses have an obligation to react positively to the client's report of pain and a responsibility to minimize or eliminate pain.

In 1997, the American Pain Society proposed making pain assessment a fifth vital sign. Because vital signs are routinely monitored, it was felt that by including pain, more client problems would be addressed. Slowly, health care facilities and nursing organizations are adopting and implementing this proposal.

National and state regulating agencies are recognizing the importance of assessing and treating pain. Standards for pain management have been developed by the Agency for Health Care Policy and Research, and the Joint Commission for the Accreditation of Healthcare Organizations (JCAHO). Nurses working in JCAHO-accredited facilities are expected to comply with these standards. These standards focus on the client's right to appropriate pain assessment and intervention and the health care professional's responsibility to treat pain.

PHYSIOLOGY OF PAIN

The ability of the body to produce pain depends on **nociceptors.** Nociceptors are nerve endings in the skin, viscera, blood vessels, muscle, and joints that are activated when *noxious* (unpleasant) stimuli are applied. Various noxious stimuli start the pain process (Table 6-1 ◆). Once tissue damage occurs from the noxious stimuli, inflammation begins. Inflammation causes the release of bradykinin and prostaglandins, which also activate the nociceptors. So pain impulses are initiated both by direct tissue damage and by the release of internal chemicals. The intensity and duration of the stimuli determine the sensation. Long-lasting, intense stimulation produces greater pain than does brief, mild stimulation.

Pain Conduction

The conduction of pain impulses involves four steps: transduction, transmission, perception, and modulation (Figure 6-1 ◆).

TRANSDUCTION. Transduction is the change of a noxious stimulus into an electrical action potential that sends impulses throughout the central nervous system. Pain is transmitted through large afferent A-delta and small C nerve fibers to the spinal cord. A-delta fibers are *myelinated* (covered with an insulating sheath). They transmit impulses rapidly and produce the sharp, well-defined pain sensations usually associated with acute pain. A-beta fibers also carry impulses for touch from the skin. C fibers are not myelinated; they transmit pain impulses more slowly. C-fiber pain is diffuse, usually chronic, and described as dull, burning, or aching.

Both A-delta and C fibers are involved in most injuries. For example, if a person bangs an elbow, A-delta fibers transmit this pain stimulus within 0.1 second. The person feels this pain as a sharp, localized, smarting sensation. One or more seconds after the blow, the person experiences a duller, aching, diffuse sensation of pain impulses carried by the C fibers.

TABLE 6-1 PAIN STIMULI	
CAUSATIVE FACTOR	**EXAMPLE**
Inflammation	Sore throat
Impaired blood flow	Angina
Invasive tumor	Colon cancer
Obstruction	Kidney stone
Spasm	Colon cramping
Stretching or straining	Sprained ankle
Fractures	Fractured hip

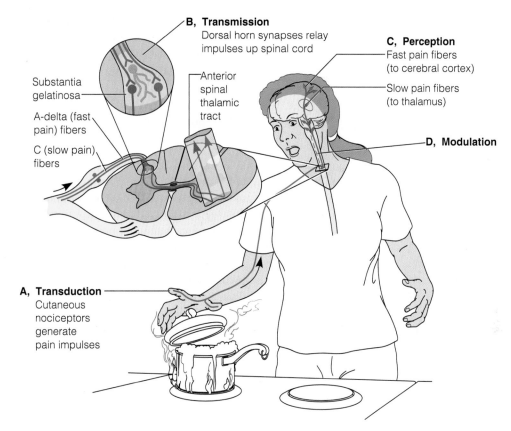

Figure 6-1. ◆ Pain conduction. (A) **Transduction:** Cutaneous nociceptors send impulses to spinal cord. (B) **Transmission:** Impulses synapse in the substantia gelatinosa. (C) **Perception:** Pain impulses processed in the thalamus and cerebral cortex. (D) **Modulation:** Along efferent fibers from cerebral cortex to substantia gelatinosa, pain may be inhibited or modulated.

TRANSMISSION. Transmission, the second step, involves sending the impulses from the afferent neurons to the dorsal horn in the spinal cord, where they *synapse* (transmit an impulse) in the substantia gelatinosa. Substance-P helps send the impulse across the synapse. From here the impulses travel to the spinothalamic tracts and ascend to the thalamus and cerebral cortex.

PERCEPTION. Perception is the processing of pain impulses in the thalamus and cerebral cortex. During this step, pain impulses are perceived and interpreted. The client experiences pain when the sensation reaches a conscious level.

Pain reactions are affected by an individual's pain threshold and pain tolerance. **Pain threshold** is the point at which each person recognizes pain. This was thought to be fairly consistent among individuals, but newer research suggests that pain intensity and duration vary among people. If a client reports more pain than is expected, the nurse should investigate further.

Pain tolerance is the amount and duration of pain a person can stand before seeking relief. Again, pain tolerance varies. Sometimes mild pain can be tolerated longer than severe, intense pain. Each person's tolerance is not to be judged as acceptable or unacceptable by health care providers. Instead, it should be accepted as a basis for pain management.

MODULATION. Modulation is the last step of pain conduction, in which the body attempts to decrease the perception of pain. Descending pathways of efferent fibers run from the cerebral cortex to the substantia gelatinosa in the dorsal horn. Along these fibers, pain may be inhibited or modulated. The body's naturally occurring **endorphins** (endogenous morphines) are released in response to afferent noxious stimuli or from efferent impulses. Endorphins bind with opiate receptors on the neurons and inhibit the release of substance-P. This process stops the pain impulse transmission (Figure 6-2 ◆).

Gate-Control Theory of Pain

In 1965, Melzack and Wall developed the *gate-control theory* of pain. This theory states that when pain impulses travel from the skin to the substantia gelatinosa in the dorsal horn of the spinal cord, the substantia gelatinosa can either open or close the "gate" to transmit pain impulses to the brain.

Whether the gate is opened or closed in the substantia gelatinosa depends on the amount of stimulation the large and small nerve fibers receive. If more small-diameter C fibers are stimulated, the gate is open, and pain impulses travel uninhibited to the brain. In contrast, if more large-diameter A-delta fibers are stimulated, the gate is closed and pain is inhibited (Figure 6-3 ◆).

Stimulation of the A-beta or touch fibers closes the gate and "turns away" pain impulses. Massaging a stubbed toe acti-

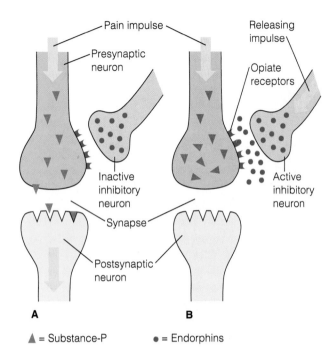

▲ = Substance-P   ● = Endorphins

Figure 6-2. ◆ (A) Substance-P transmits pain impulse across synapse between presynaptic neuron and postsynaptic neuron. (B) During modulation, endorphins are released from inhibitory neuron, which prevents the release of substance-P, and pain impulse is inhibited.

vates A-beta fibers, so it reduces intensity and duration of the pain.

Pain impulses may be inhibited in the brain stem. It is believed that cells in the midbrain can be activated by distrac-

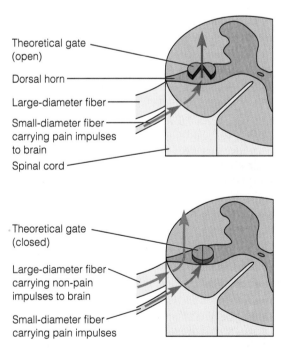

Figure 6-3. ◆ Diagram of gate-control theory. When small-diameter C fibers are stimulated, the gate is open and pain is transmitted. When large-diameter A-delta fibers are stimulated, the gate is closed and pain transmission is stopped.

tion, imagery, or relaxation techniques. These pain-reducing techniques signal receptors in the medulla. The medulla receptors stimulate nerve fibers in the spinal cord to block the transmission of pain fibers. This brain stem regulation may explain why a client who experiences severe pain may not feel it under certain circumstances. For example, an athlete often fails to notice an injury until the competition is over.

TYPES OF PAIN
Acute Pain

Acute pain is usually temporary, has a sudden onset, and is localized. It normally lasts for less than 6 months and has an identified cause. Acute pain is caused by tissue injury from trauma, surgery, or inflammation. Examples of acute pain include sprains, toothache, needle sticks, and muscle spasms. Acute pain may warn of actual or potential injury to tissues. Pain can initiate the fight-or-flight response. Physical responses to pain include tachycardia, rapid and shallow respirations, increased blood pressure, dilated pupils, sweating, and pallor. The person with acute pain may be anxious and fearful. The four major types of acute pain are:

1. *Cutaneous or superficial pain* arises from the skin or superficial tissues. This type of pain is described as sharp, cutting, burning, and well localized. When blood vessels are involved, individuals may describe the pain as throbbing.
2. *Somatic pain* results from injury to muscles, bones, ligaments, tendons, and joints. It is characterized as dull and diffuse.
3. *Visceral pain* comes from the body organs lined with viscera. Visceral pain is dull and poorly localized and is associated with nausea and vomiting, hypotension, and restlessness. It often radiates or is referred.
4. *Referred pain* starts in one site but is perceived in another area, distant from the site of the stimuli (Figure 6-4 ◆).

Chronic Pain

Chronic pain is prolonged pain, usually lasting longer than 6 months. There may not be an identifiable cause, and often it is unresponsive to conventional medical treatment. Chronic pain is more complex than acute pain. Clients with chronic pain are often depressed, withdrawn, immobile, irritable, or controlling. They may experience social withdrawal, fatigue, and reduced activity level. The autonomic nervous system is unaffected because the body adapts to the constant presence of pain.

Chronic pain may be nonmalignant pain or malignant pain. *Chronic nonmalignant pain* is "pain that has lasted 6 months or longer, is on-going, is not due to life-threatening causes, has not responded to currently available treatments, and may continue for the remainder of the patient's life" (McCaffery and Pasero, 1999, p. 471). Examples of this category include low back pain, arthritis, chronic abdominal pain (Crohn's disease), migraine headache, peripheral neuropathy, and neuralgia.

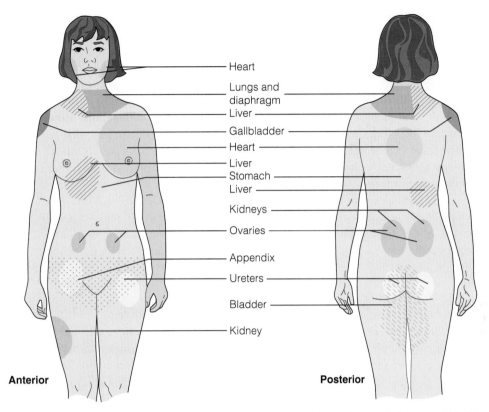

Anterior   **Posterior**

Figure 6-4. ◆ Referred pain begins in one site but is felt in another area. For example, pain from an inflamed gallbladder may be felt in the shoulder, or angina from ischemia of the heart muscle may be felt in the left arm or jaw.

Chronic malignant pain or *cancer pain* is due to cancer. Cancer pain can result from factors associated with disease progression (tumor pressing on nerves or other structures, stretching of viscera, or metastasis to the bones). It may be associated with chemotherapy and radiation therapy. Cancer pain requires multiple pharmacologic and nonpharmacologic

approaches, discussed below. (A comparison of the characteristics of acute and chronic pain is found in Table 6-2 ◆.)

Neuropathic Pain

Neuropathic pain is pain caused by damage to the central nervous system or peripheral nerves. Brain tumors, stroke, or

TABLE 6-2   COMPARISON OF ACUTE AND CHRONIC PAIN

ACUTE PAIN	CHRONIC PAIN
Pain lasts less than 6 months.	Pain lasts more than 6 months.
Results from specific tissue injury (e.g., surgery, trauma).	Chronic malignant from cancer; chronic nonmalignant (e.g., low back pain, headache).
Pain is localized.	Pain areas are hard to identify.
Resolves when specific injury heals.	May have no foreseeable end except for death.
Autonomic Responses	*Autonomic Responses*
Blood pressure, pulse, and respiration are increased.	Vital signs are normal.
Pupils are dilated.	Pupils are normal.
Skin is diaphoretic, pale, cool.	Skin is dry, warm, normal color.
Psychological Responses	*Psychological Responses*
Anxious, facial grimacing, guarding, crying.	Sense of depression, hopelessness, frustration.
	Decreased sleep and appetite.

trauma can result in central nerve injury, causing burning or tingling pain sensations in the affected area. **Allodynia** (pain that results from a stimulus that usually would not cause pain) is a unique feature of neuropathic pain. The other common type of neuropathic pain is peripheral neuropathy, a complication of diabetes. (See Chapter 17 for further discussion of peripheral neuropathy.)

Phantom limb pain occurs following surgical or traumatic amputation of a limb. The client experiences pain in the missing body part even though there is complete awareness that the limb is gone. This pain may include itching, tingling, or pressure sensations, or it may be more severe, including burning or stabbing sensations. It may be due to stimulation of the severed nerves at the site of the amputation. Treatment is complex and often unsuccessful.

Psychogenic Pain

Psychogenic pain is pain that results from emotional rather than physical causes. Typically, the client has had a long history of severe pain complaints that are real. If psychogenic pain persists, it may lead to physiologic changes, such as muscle tension, which may produce further pain. This condition may result from interpersonal conflicts or a desire to avoid a stressful or traumatic situation. Depression is often present.

FACTORS AFFECTING CLIENT RESPONSE TO PAIN

Just as individual pain thresholds differ, so do responses to pain. A person's response is shaped by age, sociocultural factors, emotional state, past experiences with pain, the meaning of pain, and the client's knowledge base. Pain tolerance may be decreased by repeated episodes of pain, fatigue, anger, anxiety, and sleep deprivation. On the other hand, it may be increased by medications, alcohol, warmth, distraction, and spiritual practices.

Age

In the past it was assumed that as people age, pain perception decreases. There is no scientific evidence to prove that age reduces pain perception or sensitivity to pain. What is true is that older adults have at least one chronic disease condition associated with pain. Chronic diseases that are more common in the elderly include arthritis, low back pain, and diabetic neuropathy. Elders tend to underreport pain. They may believe that pain is a part of growing older or that it is unacceptable to show pain. They might fear drug addiction. They may ignore pain or self-medicate with over-the-counter medications. If they do report pain, health care providers often discount it. All of these factors increases the older adult's risk of injury or serious illness.

Sociocultural Factors

Family and culture strongly influence a person's response to pain. From childhood, people learn from their families what behavior is expected when they experience pain. Expected behaviors range from being stoic to feeling comfortable requesting pain medication. Pain behaviors are the way a client expresses his or her pain. They should not be used to judge the amount of pain an individual client has. Despite many misconceptions, men and women respond similarly to pain. Cultural standards play a powerful role in how much pain an individual should tolerate, what types of pain to report and to whom, and what kind of treatment to seek. In some cultures, one family member or the entire extended family may expect to be involved in pain management decisions.

The nurse's sociocultural values and beliefs also influence pain treatment. If these values and beliefs differ from the client's, the nurse may have difficulty accepting the client's pain behaviors. It is important for the nurse to understand how ethnicity and culture affect pain expression and management, and to respect cultural differences.

Emotional Status

Pain perception can be affected by the client's emotional status. Different emotional factors affect how a person handles pain. Clients experiencing acute pain usually have some degree of anxiety. The anxious client can develop tense muscles that can add to the pain. This is why relaxation and guided imagery are helpful in relieving or decreasing pain. The presence or absence of support people can influence how a client perceives pain.

Past Experiences with Pain

Previous experiences with pain influence how the person reacts to a current pain episode. If the person's childhood experiences with pain were positive, then the adult usually will have a healthy attitude toward pain. If, however, the person's experiences were unfavorable, then future responses to pain will be negative.

Nurses play an important role in how clients view their pain. When the nurse is helpful and caring, the client is less anxious about future pain. However, when the client has unrelieved pain or a nonsupportive nurse, the client fears how future pain will be managed. The client's anxiety, in turn, increases pain.

Meaning of Pain

The meaning associated with the pain affects the pain experience. For example, the pain of labor to deliver a baby is experienced differently from the pain following removal of a major organ for cancer. Individuals usually associate pain with the potential for disability, loss of role, and death. For this reason, it is important for clients to understand the *etiology* (source) and *prognosis* (predicted outcome) of their pain.

The client who perceives advantages from the sick role may be motivated to maintain pain. These advantages, called *secondary gain,* may include support from others and avoidance of disagreeable work or stressful social obligations. Such clients may require assistance not only to treat the pain but also to learn new ways for handling personal stresses.

Knowledge Deficit

Misunderstanding the source, outcome, and meaning of pain can negatively affect the pain experience. If the client understands pain, it is easier for the nurse to teach the client about pain and pain management strategies. It is important for the nurse to assess the client's readiness to learn, use teaching methods appropriate for the client and family, and evaluate the level of learning. Teaching content should include the pain process and the plan of care. The nurse should encourage clients to describe what pain relief measures work best for them. Also, clients should learn how to let family know about their pain and how they can help promote effective pain management.

COLLABORATIVE CARE

Effective pain relief involves collaboration among a variety of health care professionals. Pain clinics are independent centers, run by a team of health care professionals who use a variety of approaches to manage chronic pain. These therapies may include medications, herbs, biofeedback, hypnosis, acupuncture, and massage. Hospice provides care and support for terminally ill clients and their families.

Pharmacology

Medication is the most common approach to pain management. These drugs include nonopioids, opioids, and adjuvant analgesics. The nurse is responsible for assessing the side effects of the medications, evaluating the medication's effectiveness, and providing client teaching. The nurse's role in pain relief also includes being a client advocate as well as a direct caregiver.

Types of Medications

Analgesics are pharmacologic agents used to relieve or reduce pain. The pharmacologic agents most commonly ordered to provide *analgesia* (pain relief) are the nonopioids, opioids, and adjuvant analgesics.

NONOPIOIDS. Nonopioids are drugs used for pain that are not derived from opium. They include acetaminophen (Tylenol) and nonsteroidal anti-inflammatory drugs (NSAIDs). Acetaminophen reduces pain and fever but does not have an anti-inflammatory effect. It does not produce adverse effects on the kidney, gastric lining, or platelets.

NSAIDs act on the peripheral nervous system. They reduce pain by interfering with prostaglandin synthesis. Examples are aspirin, ibuprofen, and ketorolac. NSAIDs are the treatment of choice for mild pain and continue to be effective when combined with narcotics for moderate to severe pain. However, they have an *analgesic ceiling.* This means that increasing the dose beyond a certain number will not increase its pain relief effect. NSAIDs can cause gastric ulcers and increase bleeding. (Nursing implications and client teaching guidelines for acetaminophen and NSAIDs are found in Table 6-3 ◆.)

OPIOIDS. Opioids are derivatives of the opium plant. They produce analgesia by binding to opioid receptors in the central nervous system, especially the brain and spinal cord. Opioids are subdivided into two groups: opioid agonists (e.g., morphine, meperidine, and codeine) and opioid agonist-antagonists (e.g., buprenorphine and nalbuphine). Both opioid categories are given for moderate to severe pain. Nursing responsibilities and client teaching recommendations for opioids are found in Table 6-3.

ADJUVANT ANALGESICS. Adjuvant analgesics are drugs with other specific uses that can provide analgesia in clients with chronic nonmalignant and cancer pain. They include anticonvulsants, antidepressants, systemic anesthetics, corticosteroids, and psychostimulants. Anticonvulsants include such drugs as carbamazepine (Tegretol), clonazepam (Klonopin), and phenytoin (Dilantin). Antidepressants include amitriptyline (Elavil) and doxepin (Sinequan). An example of a systemic anesthetic is bupivacaine (Marcaine). Corticosteroids include dexamethasone (Decadron), and methylprednisolone (Solu-Medrol). The psychostimulant methylphenidate (Ritalin) is also useful.

Anticonvulsants are used for diabetic neuropathy and neuralgia. *Antidepressants* promote normal sleeping patterns in clients with chronic pain. They are useful in treating neuropathic pain. *Systemic anesthetics* can be injected into nerves for a nerve block or given via the intraspinal route for cancer pain. Metastatic bone cancer pain may be relieved by using *corticosteroids. Psychostimulants* decrease sedation from opioids without decreasing pain relief in persons with cancer.

Routes of Administration

The route of administration affects the amount of medication needed to relieve pain. For example, oral doses of some narcotics may need to be five times greater than parenteral doses to achieve the same amount of pain relief. Of course, different narcotics have different recommended dosages. Consulting an equianalgesic dosage chart helps to ensure that dosages of different narcotics given by different routes will have the same analgesic effect (Table 6-4 ◆).

ORAL. The oral (PO) route is usually the simplest to administer for the client and the nurse, although special nursing care may be required when the client has difficulty swallowing or is confused. The nurse must know whether medications are given with food or can be chewed. In addition, the nurse is responsible for making sure that the medication is actually swallowed.

RECTAL. The rectal route is useful for clients who cannot swallow. Morphine, hydromorphone, and oxymorphone are available in this form. To be effective, any rectal medication must be placed above the rectal sphincter. The rectal route is effective and simple, but the client may not accept it.

TRANSDERMAL. The transdermal ("patch") form of medication is simple and painless and delivers a continuous level of

TABLE 6-3 NURSING IMPLICATIONS FOR PHARMACOLOGY: CLIENTS RECEIVING ACETAMINOPHEN, NSAIDS, OPIOIDS

CLASS/DRUGS	PURPOSE	NURSING RESPONSIBILITIES	CLIENT TEACHING
Acetaminophen (Tylenol)	It is given to decrease pain and fever but not inflammation.	Give with a full glass of water.	Take with a full glass of water.
NSAIDs ▪ Aspirin ▪ Ibuprofen (Motrin) ▪ Piroxicam (Feldene) ▪ Ketorolac (Toradol) ▪ Naproxen (Naprosyn)	NSAIDs are given for mild to moderate pain; antipyretic and anti-inflammatory effects.	Give with meals or a full glass of water. Do not give aspirin with other NSAIDs. Monitor for signs of GI bleeding. If given for fever, monitor client's temperature.	Take with meals or a full glass of water. Do not take more than the recommended amount. Do not take aspirin or alcohol with other NSAIDS. Monitor for GI bleeding (e.g., black stools).
Opioid Agonists ▪ Codeine ▪ Fentanyl ▪ Hydrocodone ▪ Hydromorphone (Dilaudid) ▪ Meperidine (Demerol) ▪ Morphine sulfate ▪ Oxymorphone (Numorphan) ▪ Propoxyphene (Darvocet) **Opioid Agonist–Antagonists** ▪ Buprenorphine (Buprenex) ▪ Nalbuphine (Nubain)	Opioids are used to manage moderate to severe pain. They bind to opiate receptors in the brain to alter the perception of pain. They are addictive, causing psychological and physical dependence.	Record the appropriate information in the narcotic inventory sheet. Follow institution policy for wasting any narcotic. Monitor for side effects of sedation, respiratory depression, urinary retention, constipation, nausea, and vomiting. Keep naloxone available to treat respiratory depression.	Opioids used to treat severe pain are unlikely to cause addiction. Do not drink alcohol. Do not take over-the-counter drugs without MD approval. Increase fluids and fiber to prevent constipation. The drugs often cause dizziness, drowsiness, and impaired thinking; use caution when driving or making decisions. Do not increase dosage or take extra doses without discussing with MD.

medication (Figure 6-5 ◆). Transdermal medications are expensive but easy to store and apply. The only opioid available for the transdermal route is fentanyl (Duragesic). The fentanyl patch is used to treat moderate to severe cancer pain. If breakthrough pain occurs, short-acting medications are added.

SUBLINGUAL. Sublingual medications are placed beneath the tongue. The only drug currently available in this form is buprenophrine (Buprenex).

NASAL. The intranasal route has limited use for pain control. The only available analgesic in the United States for the nasal route is butorphanol (Stadol).

INTRAMUSCULAR. Although the intramuscular (IM) route is still used for pain management, it has limited usefulness. It has several problems, including uneven absorption from the muscle and pain during administration.

INTRAVENOUS. The intravenous (IV) route provides the most rapid onset, usually ranging from 1 to 15 minutes. Medication can be given by drip, bolus, or **patient-controlled analgesia (PCA),** a pump with a handheld button that allows clients to manage their own pain (Figure 6-6 ◆). The medication dose and interval between doses are programmed into the PCA pump so that the client does not receive an overdose. The PCA pump allows clients to feel somewhat in control of their pain relief. The commonly ordered drugs include morphine, hydromorphone, fentanyl, and meperidine.

SUBCUTANEOUS. The subcutaneous continuous infusion (SCCI) route is used as an alternative for chronic cancer pain management. A subcutaneous needle, placed in the upper arm or thigh, is connected to a continuous infusion of medication. This route is painful and usually is disliked by clients.

INTRASPINAL. The intraspinal route delivers drugs directly into the spinal column and then to the brain. This method is

TABLE 6-4   EQUIANALGESIC DOSAGE CHART

ANALGESIC	DOSAGE (MG)	DURATION (HOURS)	NURSING CONSIDERATIONS
Opioid Agonists Morphine sulfate	10 IM 30 PO	4–5 IM 4–5 PO	**MS 10 mg IM is the analgesic dose to which all other IM and PO doses in this table are considered equianalgesic.**
Codeine	130 IM 200 PO	4 IM 4 PO	Often given together with aspirin or acetaminophen for mild to moderate pain.
Hydrocodone	30 PO	4–6	Combined with acetaminophen (Vicodin) for mild to moderate pain.
Hydromorphone (Dilaudid)	1.5 IM 7.5 PO	4–5 IM 4 PO	More potent than morphine for severe pain; monitor client closely during first doses.
Meperidine (Demerol)	75 IM 300 PO	2–4 IM 2–4 PO	Produces a metabolite, normeperidine, causing CNS irritability and tremors. Occurs with chronic or high-dose therapy. PO dose of 300 mg not recommended.
Oxycodone	20 PO	3–4	Combined with acetaminophen (Tylox, Percocet) for mild to moderate pain.
Oxymorphone (Numorphan)	1 IM	3–6	Used for moderate to severe pain.
Propoxyphene (Darvon)	500 PO	4–6	Give only recommended dose of 65–130 mg PO for short-term mild pain. **Never** give 500 mg due to risk of toxicity.
Opioid Agonist-Antagonists Buprenorphine (Buprenex)	0.4 IM	6	Used for moderate to severe pain.
Butorphanol (Stadol)	2 IM	3–4	Given preop and postop for moderate to severe pain.
Nalbuphine (Nubain)	10 IM	3–6	Given preop and postop for moderate to severe pain.
Pentazocine (Talwin)	60 IM 180 PO	2–3 IM 3 PO	May be used for moderate to severe pain but has limited use due to short half-life.

Source: Data compiled from Deglin, J. H., & Vallerand, A. H. (2001). *Davis's drug guide for nurses* (7th ed). Philadelphia: Davis; LeMone, P., & Burke, K. M. (2000). *Medical-surgical nursing.* Upper Saddle River, NJ: Prentice Hall Health; and McCaffery, M., & Pasero, C. (1999). *Pain: Clinical manual.* St. Louis, MO: Mosby.

invasive and requires experienced nursing care. Box 6-1 provides nursing implications for clients receiving intraspinal analgesia.

NERVE BLOCKS. In a nerve block, local anesthetics are injected into or near a nerve to reduce unrelenting pain. Sometimes this procedure is used to locate the source of pain before permanent blocking is done. Permanent nerve blocking is done with a neurolytic agent that destroys the nerve. Neurolytic blocks are reserved for terminally ill clients because of the risks of weakness, paralysis, and bowel and bladder dysfunction. Temporary nerve blocks may give the client enough relief to feel hopeful that pain relief is possible.

Surgery

As a pain-relief measure, surgery is performed only after all other methods have failed. Clients need to understand thor-

oughly the implications of surgery for pain relief. The common surgical procedures (Figure 6-7 ◆) are as follows:

CORDOTOMY. A *cordotomy* is an incision into the anterolateral tracts of the spinal cord to interrupt the transmission of pain. It is difficult to isolate the nerves responsible for upper body pain, so this surgery is most often performed for pain in the abdominal region and legs, including severe pain from terminal cancer.

NEURECTOMY. A *neurectomy* is the removal of a nerve. It is sometimes used for pain relief. A peripheral neurectomy is the severing of a nerve at any point distal to the spinal cord.

SYMPATHECTOMY. Because sympathetic nerves produce and transmit the pain sensation, a *sympathectomy* may reduce pain by destroying the involved sympathetic nerve with an injec-

Figure 6-5. ◆ Transdermal patch. To apply the patch, clip any hair from the upper body, clean the site with clear water, and dry it. Apply immediately after opening the package by placing it in the palm and pressing firmly onto the prepared site for 30 seconds. Be sure that contact is complete around the edges. A patch lasts for 72 hours, and the next patch is applied on a different site.

tion or incision. Usually, nerves in the lumbar or cervical region are considered for this procedure.

RHIZOTOMY. Rhizotomy is severing of the dorsal spinal roots to relieve the pain of cancer of the head, neck, or lungs. This is done by surgically cutting the nerve fibers, injecting a chemical such as alcohol or phenol into the subarachnoid space, or using a radio frequency current to selectively destroy pain fibers.

Figure 6-6. ◆ PCA unit allows the client to self-manage severe pain. It can be mounted on an intravenous pole.

Complementary Therapy

Nonpharmacologic interventions are often used together with analgesics. They may be used for all types of pain, but their success is highly individual. Nonpharmacologic methods include relaxation, distraction, cutaneous stimulation, transcutaneous electrical nerve stimulation, acupuncture, biofeedback, and hypnotism.

RELAXATION. Relaxation involves learning to relax the body and mind. The primary goal of relaxation is to decrease muscle tension and anxiety. Some examples of relaxation activities are as follows:

- *Diaphragmatic breathing.* The client assumes a comfortable position in a quiet room and keeps the eyelids closed. The client inhales and exhales slowly, using the diaphragm to help extend the breath. (The technique for diaphragmatic breathing is described and illustrated in Chapter 7.)
- *Progressive muscle relaxation.* The client is taught to tighten one group of muscles slowly and then relax them completely. The client should repeat the sequence for all parts of the body. Audiotapes may guide the client through this process.
- *Guided imagery.* To distract clients from their pain and produce relaxation, clients use their imagination to create a scene that is pleasurable and relaxing. The nurse assists the client through the steps of imagery. Clients should understand that several sessions may be necessary before they experience some pain relief.
- *Meditation.* The client empties the mind of all sensory data and may concentrate on a single object, word, or idea. This activity can produce a deeply relaxed state. A variety of exercises can induce the meditative state, and all are relatively easy to learn. Many books and tapes on meditation are available commercially.

DISTRACTION. Distraction focuses the client's attention away from the pain and onto something that the client finds more pleasant. It is often used in labor and is best used when the pain is mild to moderate. Examples of distracting activities are listening to music, tapping out a musical rhythm with the fingers or foot, and humor. Humor is known to be highly effective in pain relief. Laughing for 20 minutes or more produces an increase in endorphins that may continue pain relief even after the client stops laughing.

CUTANEOUS STIMULATION. Cutaneous stimulation seems to be an effective pain reliever because it closes the "gate" in the substantia gelatinosa. Cutaneous stimulation may be accomplished by massage and the application of heat and cold (Table 6-5 ◆).

TRANSCUTANEOUS ELECTRICAL NERVE STIMULATION (TENS). A **transcutaneous electrical nerve stimulation (TENS)** unit is a low-voltage transmitter connected by wires to electrodes that are placed on the client (Figure 6-8 ◆). The client

BOX 6-1
NURSING CARE OF THE CLIENT RECEIVING INTRASPINAL ANALGESIA

Intraspinal analgesia is used to manage chronic, cancer, and severe postoperative pain. The intraspinal route may be either intrathecal (into the subarachnoid space) or epidural (into the epidural space). Opioids such as morphine and fentanyl and local anesthetics like bupivacaine (Marcaine) are given. Opioids act on the opiate receptors in the central nervous system; anesthetics block conduction of pain impulses. This method provides complete pain relief but produces side effects. The opioids cause pruritus (itching), urinary retention, nausea, sedation, and respiratory depression. Local anesthetics can cause motor and sensory deficits.

PROCEDURE

The physician places a catheter into the epidural space, attaches a tube to an infusion pump, and starts the medication infusion. A portable or implantable pump may deliver a narcotic infusion that lasts for a few days.

NURSING CARE

- Monitor pulse, blood pressure, respirations, and pulse oximetry every 15 minutes for the first 2 to 3 hours and then every hour for the first 24 hours.
- Have naloxone, a narcotic antagonist, at bedside to reverse respiratory depression.
- Monitor for effectiveness of pain relief.
- Monitor intake and output.
- Monitor for motor and sensory deficits.

Placement of catheter in the epidural space.

experiences a vibrating sensation at the electrodes, which decreases pain. Clients can adjust the voltage to achieve maximum pain relief. The advantages of TENS units are avoidance of drug side effects and client control. Disadvantages are its cost (it is not reimbursed by insurance) and the need for training.

A TENS unit is most commonly used to relieve chronic benign pain and acute postoperative pain. The nurse or physical therapist explains the manufacturer's directions, where to place the electrodes, and the importance of placing the electrodes on clean, unbroken skin. The client is taught how to assess the skin daily for signs of irritation.

ACUPUNCTURE. Acupuncture is an ancient Chinese system of pain relief that involves inserting needles into specific points on the body. It is believed that acupuncture enhances energy flow (Qi) along pathways called meridians, which restores the body's healing mechanisms. Only care

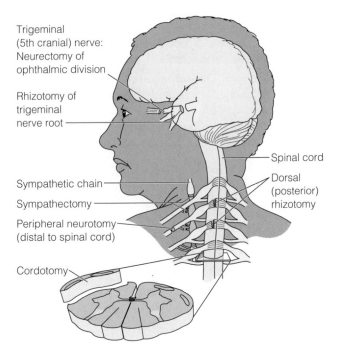

Trigeminal
(5th cranial) nerve:
Neurectomy of
ophthalmic division

Rhizotomy of
trigeminal
nerve root

Spinal cord

Dorsal
(posterior)
rhizotomy

Sympathetic chain

Sympathectomy

Peripheral neurotomy
(distal to spinal cord)

Cordotomy

Figure 6-7. ◆ Surgical procedures are used to treat severe pain that does not respond to other types of management. They include cordotomy, neurectomy, sympathectomy, and rhizotomy.

Figure 6-8. ◆ TENS unit. Electrodes that deliver low-voltage electrical stimuli are placed directly on the client over painful areas.

providers with special training can use this method. Acupuncture and acupressure are fairly well accepted therapies for pain.

BIOFEEDBACK. Biofeedback uses electronic instruments to measure brain waves, muscle contraction, and skin temperature, and then "feeds" this information back to the client. Electrodes are placed on the client's skin and an amplification unit transforms data into visual cues, such as colored lights. The client learns to recognize stress-related responses and to replace them with relaxation responses. The goal is for the client to initiate those actions that cause relaxation independently.

HYPNOTISM. Hypnosis is a trance-like state in which the mind becomes extremely suggestible. For this technique to work, the client must be fully relaxed and believe in the concept. It usually requires a skilled practitioner, but some clients can hypnotize themselves. Hypnosis has been successful in modifying pain.

NURSING CARE

Nursing care of the client in pain presents more of a challenge than other illnesses or injuries. Whether pain is acute or chronic, the goal of nursing care is to assist the client to achieve optimal control of the pain. To accomplish pain con-

	METHODS OF CUTANEOUS STIMULATION		
METHOD	**TECHNIQUE**	**USES**	**NURSING IMPLICATIONS**
Massage	The nurse performs massage to back, shoulders, or feet.	May be soothing and relaxing to decrease pain.	Ask the client about accepting a massage.
Heat	Nurse applies a hot-water bottle, heating pad, or hot moist towels to client's body. A hot shower or bath may also be effective.	May reduce muscle spasms and pain. Works best for localized pain.	Protect the client from burns. Heat should be applied for about 20–30 minutes.
Cold	Nurse applies waterproof bags filled with ice, gel packs, or cool damp towels to the client's body.	May reduce muscle spasm and arthritic joint pain. Usually more effective than heat for pain relief.	Monitor for excessive redness or blisters. Cold should be applied for about 20–30 minutes.

TABLE 6-5

trol, the nurse uses a combination of medications and non-pharmacologic pain-relief strategies.

ASSESSING

The first step in relieving the client's pain is to conduct an accurate, unbiased, and thorough assessment of the client's pain. A comprehensive pain assessment ensures adequate and appropriate interventions. The nurse should assess the client's perceptions, physiologic responses, and behavioral responses.

CLIENT PERCEPTIONS

Because pain is subjective, the client's perceptions provide the most reliable indicator about the type and degree of pain. The McGill Pain Questionnaire is one tool for assessing the client's pain (Figure 6-9 ◆). A thorough pain assessment will ensure a complete database for pain management (Box 6-2).

Pain intensity is assessed by using a pain rating scale (several scales are illustrated in Figure 6-10 ◆). For clients who do not understand English or numerals, a scale using colors may be helpful. Another resource is the "Wong–Baker Faces Pain Rating Scale," which ranges from a happy face to one with a huge frown.

The nurse must thoroughly explain the purpose of the pain rating scale. When a word descriptor scale is used, verify that the client can read and understand the language being used. If a numerical scale is used, be sure the client can count to 10. It is often helpful to use the client's own words when describing the pain. The client should understand that reporting pain is important for recovery, not just for achieving temporary comfort.

PHYSIOLOGIC RESPONSES

Physiologic changes result from stimulation of the sympathetic nervous system. Objective manifestations include muscle tension; tachycardia; rapid, shallow respirations; increased blood pressure; dilated pupils; sweating; and pallor. They usually occur in the presence of acute pain. However, absence of physiologic signs does not mean absence of pain. In clients

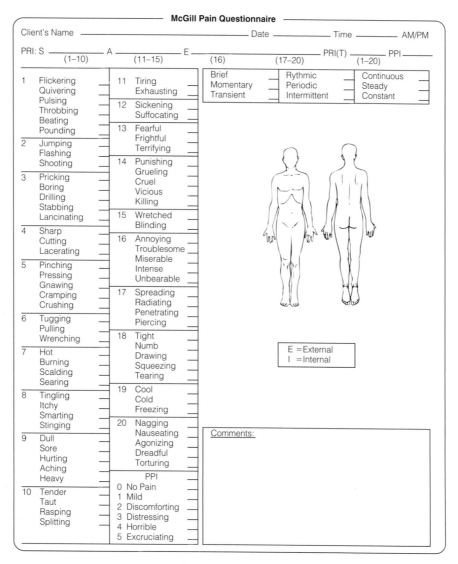

Figure 6-9. ◆ The McGill Pain Questionnaire.

BOX 6-2
ASSESSING FOR PAIN

SUBJECTIVE DATA

Location

- Where does it hurt?
- Does the pain radiate?
- Is the pain superficial or deep?

Onset, Pattern, Duration, Quality

- When did the pain start?
- Did it begin gradually or suddenly?
- Is it constant or intermittent?
- Does it occur in cycles (e.g., same time each day)?
- How often does it appear?
- How long does the pain last?
- Is the pain throbbing, dull, aching, sharp, stabbing, prickling, burning?

Precipitating, Aggravating, and Relieving Factors

- What seems to trigger the pain?
- What seems to make the pain worse (e.g., movement, position changes, coughing, straining, or eating)?
- What seems to make the pain better (e.g., rest, sleep, food, pain medications, standing, or sitting)?

Intensity

- How strong is your pain? (Have client rate the pain using a rating scale.)

Other Problems

- Does the pain cause nausea, vomiting, anorexia, or insomnia?
- Does pain interfere with activities at home, work, or social interactions?
- Are there other diseases or conditions (e.g., arthritis)?

Methods of Pain Relief

- What has helped control pain in the past?
- What has not worked to relieve the pain?

OBJECTIVE DATA

- Vital signs: blood pressure, pulse, respirations
- Assess skin moisture and color; pupils for dilation.
- Observe appearance for signs of: grimacing, clenching jaws or fist, guarding, drawing up into fetal position, lying rigidly, restlessness.
- Observe behavioral responses: moaning, sighing, crying, becomes quiet, withdraws from others, appears frightened, has sad facial expression.
- Gently palpate painful area; identify possible trigger points.

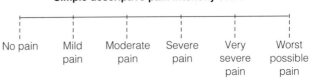

Figure 6-10. ◆ Examples of commonly used pain scales. Other examples include pictures of faces (from happy and relaxed to sad and frowning), or colors from bright red (terrible pain) to light blue (no pain).

with prolonged pain, the body adapts to the pain stimulus and there may not be physiologic changes. The client with chronic pain may have an unexpressive, tired facial appearance.

BEHAVIORAL RESPONSES

Behavioral responses to pain may or may not match the client's report of pain. The nurse must accept the client's pain rating regardless of the client's behaviors. For example, one client may rate pain at an 8 on a 0 to 10 scale while laughing or walking down the hall; another may deny pain completely while tachycardic, hypertensive, and grimacing. Discrepancies between the client's report of pain and behavioral responses may result from cultural factors, coping skills, fear, denial, or the use of relaxation or distraction techniques.

Clients often deny pain for a variety of reasons. They may fear injections. Fears of developing addiction or physical dependence may exist. Sometimes clients believe they will be labeled as an addict if they ask for analgesics. **Addiction** is a condition of seeking drugs habitually (other than for a medical purpose) and of not being able to give them up without adverse effects. **Physical dependence** occurs when the body adapts to chemical substances over an extended period of time; abrupt cessation of the substance causes withdrawal symptoms (see Chapter 11).

Sometimes there is a misinterpretation of terms. The client may think that aching, soreness, or discomfort does not qualify as pain. Also, clients may think that health care providers know when they are experiencing pain. Some clients may deny pain as an attempt to deny that anything is wrong with them. Other clients believe that "as needed" medications are given only if their pain rating is high.

The nurse should not assume that a sleeping client is without pain. Pain is physically exhausting. Unrelieved pain leaves clients fatigued. Sometimes clients sleep out of fatigue rather than because they are pain free.

DIAGNOSING, PLANNING, AND IMPLEMENTING

Numerous misconceptions about pain and its management exist among clients and health care professionals. Before appropriate nursing care can be delivered, the nurse must explore these misconceptions and understand the facts. Box 6-3 lists a few common misconceptions and their corrections.

Managing pain in the older adult requires special considerations. Box 6-4 lists guidelines and rationale for managing pain in the elderly.

ACUTE PAIN

- Believe the client is experiencing pain. *By believing the client, the nurse reduces anxiety, which may lessen pain.*
- Discuss with the client his or her desired level of pain relief and any fears about proposed interventions. *Understanding the client's goals and fears will help the nurse determine suitable pain relief methods.*
- Individualize the choice of medication, route, dose, and interval between doses. *Because each client absorbs, metabolizes, and excretes medications differently, the nurse carefully selects an analgesic based on the client's needs. When frequent injections are needed, the intravenous route should be considered.*
- Adjust the analgesic regimen by using a flow sheet (Figure 6-11 ◆). The dose can be adjusted within prescribed limits according to the client's response. Adjustments should be considered:
  - When the client feels most of his or her pain an hour after administration (dose too low)
  - When dose causes significant side effects such as respiratory depression (dose too high)
  - When most of the pain returns before the next scheduled dose (interval too long)
    The pain flow sheet records the effectiveness of each pain intervention. It is the nurse's role to inform the physician if the prescribed medication, route, dose, and interval does not meet the client's needs.
- Use a preventive approach. Administer pain analgesics at regular, scheduled intervals around the clock (ATC) when the client's pain is expected for at least 12 of the next 24 hours. PRN (as-needed) administration is appropriate for unpredictable pain. It should be administered before pain becomes severe and before painful procedures such as a dressing change or physical activities. *Preventive approaches allow clients to know that their pain needs will be met. They help reduce anxiety about the return of pain and may result in decreased doses, fewer side effects, and less time in pain. Physical activity may increase, so problems caused by immobility can be avoided.*

BOX 6-3
MISCONCEPTIONS ABOUT PAIN MANAGEMENT

Misconception	Correction
People who frequently ask for opioid pain medications are addicted.	Research shows that addiction from opioids is rare. If the client is asking for pain medication, pain relief is probably inadequate.
It is best to wait until a client has pain before giving medication.	Anticipating pain and offering pain relief ahead of time can significantly lessen the pain.
Postoperative pain is best treated with intramuscular injections.	The most commonly ordered postoperative pain medication is meperidine (Demerol) IM. This is a poor choice because it is short-acting, can irritate tissues, and produces normeperidine, a central nervous system (CNS) stimulant.
It is dangerous to give an opioid and a nonsteroidal anti-inflammatory drug (NSAID) at the same time.	These medications do not need to be given at different times. The opioid acts on the CNS; the NSAID acts on the peripheral nervous system. By combining them, the client receives better pain management.
Opioid medication is too risky to be used in chronic pain.	Other methods should be tried first; if they prove ineffective, opioids should be added.

Sources: Data compiled from Agency for Health Care Policy and Research. (1992). *Acute pain management: Operative or medical procedures and trauma.* Rockville, MD: U.S. Department of Health and Human Services; McCaffery, M., & Pasero, C. (1999). *Pain: Clinical manual.* St. Louis, MO: Mosby; and LeMone, P., & Burke, K. M. (2000). *Medical–surgical nursing.* Upper Saddle River, NJ: Prentice Hall Health.

- Use a balanced analgesia approach by administering medications from all three classes (nonopioids, opioids, and adjuvants) when ordered. *Nonopioids act on the peripheral nervous system; opioids act on the central nervous system. A combination of these medications can improve pain relief and lower the incidence of side effects.*
- Demonstrate use of self-administered PCA. *PCA allows clients more control over their pain relief.*

population
FOCUS

Pain Management Guidelines for the Older Adult

Guideline	Rationale
• Reduce initial opioid dose by 25%, then carefully titrate dose based on client response.	• Drug absorption, distribution, metabolism, and excretion decrease with age; therefore, monitor dosages carefully.
• Avoid administering benzodiazepines such as diazepam (Valium) or lorazepam (Ativan).	• They cause delirium, increasing the risk for injury.
• Use all NSAIDs with caution and monitor for side effects.	• The elderly are four times more likely to develop peptic ulcers.
• Closely monitor long-term use of acetaminophen.	• Acetaminophen can accumulate and cause liver toxicity.
• Choose NSAIDs like ibuprofen (Motrin) and naproxen (Naprosyn).	• They have shorter half-lives, so they will not accumulate and cause toxicity.
• Avoid using meperidine and propoxyphene (Darvon).	• They produce toxic metabolites with long half-lives, leading to more adverse effects.
• Choose morphine or hydromorphone for moderate to severe pain.	• They have short half-lives and less chance for toxicity.
• Monitor closely for sedation and respiratory depression with opioid use.	• Decreased renal and liver clearance rates increase potential opioid side effects.
• Avoid the IM route.	• It is painful, absorption is unreliable, and there is less muscle mass in the elderly.
• Assess frequently for signs of constipation.	• Elderly are prone to constipation before adding opioids, which also cause constipation.

- Teach the client to request pain medication before the pain becomes severe. *This strategy prevents the client from experiencing highs and lows of pain relief.*
- Use an equianalgesic dosage chart when changing doses or medications. *If the client is receiving inadequate pain relief or is being switched from a parenteral to an oral route, an* **equianalgesic dose** *chart helps the client maintain adequate pain relief.*
- Monitor effectiveness of pain relief measures at least every 2 hours and ATC. *Planned assessments prevent inconsistent pain relief for the client.*

CHRONIC PAIN

Chronic nonmalignant pain can occur throughout the body. This type of pain may accompany chronic diseases or occur as the result of an injury (e.g., low back pain). Because chronic pain is prolonged, different interventions are used by the nurse.

- Discuss client's expectations about pain relief and management. *The nurse and the client need to understand whether the pain can be resolved or significantly lessened.*
- Teach the client and family about the nature of chronic pain and various pain relief methods. *Inclusion of the family enables them to support the client better.*
- Administer nonopioids, adjuvant, and opioid pain medications as ordered and needed. *The type of chronic pain determines the combination of analgesics needed by the client.*
- When opioid analgesics are ordered, use the oral route. *Chronic pain is usually long term, so the parenteral route is unacceptable.*
- Encourage the client to use noninvasive methods of pain management, such as relaxation, distraction, and cutaneous stimulation. *These techniques are useful in managing chronic pain.*
- Promote rest and proper nutrition. *Chronic pain is physically exhausting.*
- Consult with health care team about referral to multidisciplinary pain management facility. *Clients with unresolved pain problems may need more advanced pain management techniques or referral to a pain clinic.*

- Use nonpharmacologic measures (e.g., relaxation, distraction, heat, or cold) as appropriate. *Nondrug measures by the nurse or client's family can provide pain relief with minimal risk to the client. They should not be substituted for medications but rather combined with them.*
- Provide comfort measures, such as changing positions, back massage, oral care, skin care, and changing bed linens. *Basic comfort measures promote physical and emotional well-being.*
- Avoid actions that increase pain, for example, jarring the bed, moving the client too quickly out of bed. *By avoiding actions that increase pain, the nurse shows a caring attitude.*

CANCER PAIN

Clients with cancer usually do not develop pain until the later stages of the disease. Their pain may be acute or chronic. Cancer-related pain requires many different approaches. (Chapter 8 discusses care of the client with cancer.)

- Discuss goals of care with the client. *These goals may include the amount of pain the client will tolerate in order to participate in activities of daily living. The nurse needs to understand these goals and help the client meet them.*
- Encourage client and family to express concerns about opioid use. *Fears of addiction may prevent the client from obtaining adequate pain relief.*

PAIN FLOWSHEET

Client: Mrs. J **Age:** 55 **Physician:** Dr. Masson **Date:** 4/12/03
Diagnosis: 4/12/03 Abdominal hysterectomy
Pain rating scale: 0 to 10 (0 = no pain, 10 = worst pain)
Analgasic ordered: Morphine 6-12 mg. IM q 4 hours

Date and Time	Pain rating	Analgesic	Vital signs R, P, BP	Level of arousal	Other: Nausea and vomiting, bowel function	Initials
4/12/03 14:00	10	MS 10 mg. IM	24, 90, 138/88	Awake, "I have sharp pain in my stomach. It really hurts to move."	Denies nausea and vomiting. No bowel tones since returning from surgery at 13:00.	KC
14:30	8		22			KC
15:00	4		20	"The pain is much less than before."		KC
16:30	4		18	"Pain is about the same."		EB
17:45	7		20	"The pain is coming back."	No nausea or vomiting.	EB
18:10	8	MS 10 mg. IM	20, 88, 130/82	"The pain isn't quite as bad as before, but it still hurts a lot."		EB
18:30	8		20	"Pain is a little less."		EB

Figure 6-11. ◆ A flowsheet for nursing documentation of pain management.

- Administer a combination of nonopioid, adjuvant, and opioid analgesics according to the World Health Organization analgesic ladder (Figure 6-12 ◆). *The three steps of the analgesic ladder are used progressively until the cancer pain is relieved or at least reduced to an acceptable level.*

- Give analgesics ATC. *Clients with cancer pain usually have persistent pain. Consistent administration should prevent peaks and valleys of pain relief.*

- Have analgesics available for breakthrough pain. *As cancer progresses, clients will experience breakthrough pain. They need fast-acting analgesics to control it.*

- Give analgesics orally. *Oral route is safe and easy to administer. When clients cannot take their medications orally, the transdermal, rectal, intravenous, and intraspinal routes should be used. The IM route is avoided because it is painful.*

- Teach the patient about opioid **tolerance**—the loss of effectiveness with chronic use. For the client to receive the same amount of pain relief, increased doses are required. *Clients need to understand why they need increased doses.*

- Aggressively treat adverse effects of analgesics (see following nursing diagnosis). *Sedation, respiratory depression, nausea, and constipation are the common adverse effects of opioids.*

- Add noninvasive pain management strategies. *Noninvasive strategies are helpful in managing cancer pain.*

- Refer to support groups and pastoral counseling. *Clients and families need emotional and spiritual resources.*

RISK FOR INJURY: SIDE EFFECTS OF OPIOID ANALGESICS

The four main side effects of opioid therapy are sedation, respiratory depression, constipation, and nausea. Usually, side effects develop at the beginning of narcotic therapy. Only sedation and respiratory depression may subside with long-term use.

- *Sedation* often occurs at the start of opioid therapy or when the dose is increased. This results from opioids acting on the central nervous system. Assess the client's sedation level every 1 to 2 hours for the first 8 to 12 hours. *Sedation precedes respiratory depression. Monitor the client frequently during initial opioid therapy or increased dosage changes.*

- If pain relief is adequate and sedation is clinically significant, consult with physician about reducing the dose. *The goal is to decrease sedation, yet maintain pain relief.*

Freedom from pain

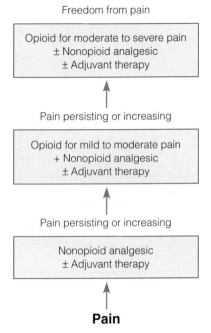

Opioid for moderate to severe pain
± Nonpioid analgesic
± Adjuvant therapy

Pain persisting or increasing

Opioid for mild to moderate pain
+ Nonpioid analgesic
± Adjuvant therapy

Pain persisting or increasing

Nonopioid analgesic
± Adjuvant therapy

Pain

Figure 6-12. ◆ The WHO three-step analgesic ladder.

- Add a mild stimulant such as caffeine during the day. *Mild stimulants may offset the opioid sedative effects.*
- All opioid analgesics are capable of causing *respiratory depression.* Most of the time the altered respiratory function is not life threatening or clinically significant. Monitor sedation and respiratory rate and depth q 1 to 2 hours during the first 24 hours the client receives opioids. *Clients are at risk for respiratory depression when they start on opioids.*

CLINICAL alert

Respiratory depression is clinically significant when there is a decrease in rate and depth of respirations from the client's baseline.

- Encourage deep breathing and use of incentive spirometry. *These measures help counteract respiratory depression.*
- If the client is unresponsive to physical stimulation, has shallow respirations, and respiratory rate of less than 8 breaths per minute with pinpoint pupils, naloxone (Narcan) may be required. *Naloxone, an opioid antagonist, reverses the effects of opioids.*
- *Constipation* is the most common side effect of opioids. They decrease gastric emptying and peristalsis, which increases the client's risk for developing constipation. Auscultate abdomen for presence of bowel tones. *Reduced bowel tones mean decreased peristalsis.*
- Encourage at least eight glasses of water per day. *Increased fluid intake promotes moist, soft stool.*

- Encourage a diet high in bulk and fiber such as beans, carrots, bran cereals and breads, and prunes. *This type of diet improves stool consistency and promotes passage through the colon.*
- Promote activity and exercise as tolerated. *Increased movement stimulates peristalsis.*
- Give a stool softener or stimulant during the opioid therapy. *An aggressive bowel regimen is needed to prevent and treat opioid-induced constipation.*
- Monitor client's bowel pattern carefully. *Monitoring is essential to prevent further complications of constipation.*
- *Nausea* may occur during the beginning of opioid therapy but usually decreases with longer use. It is caused by stimulation of a trigger zone in the brain and slowed gastric motility. Give an antiemetic such as ondansetron (Zofran) or prochlorperazine (Compazine). *These medications decrease nausea.*
- Provide frequent oral care. *Oral care helps to decrease bad tastes in the mouth.*
- Provide a clean-smelling environment. *Reducing unpleasant odors decreases the potential for nausea.*
- Have patient try to eat dry toast or crackers. *Dry foods tend to decrease nausea.*
- If nausea continues from opioid use, add a nonopioid or adjuvant medication before reducing opioid dose. *To maintain client's pain relief yet decrease nausea, add other pain medications.*
- For chronic nausea with advanced cancer, give metoclopramide (Reglan). *This medication increases gastric motility.*

EVALUATING

Evaluation focuses on determining the effectiveness of pain management strategies. The nurse collects data on the client's report of pain relief, physical responses, and emotional behaviors.

 Discharge Considerations

Clients can learn to manage most types of pain at home. The nurse should explain about expected pain, when it will happen, what it feels like, and what to do to help oneself during the event. Education should decrease anxiety about the unknown and provide the client with a means of controlling the pain. Box 6-5 lists the assessment data to consider when planning discharge.

All instructions should be in writing so that the client can take them home. The following teaching points should be included for the client and family:

- Specific drugs, including the frequency, potential side effects, possible drug interactions, and any special precautions such as taking with food or avoiding alcohol

- How to administer the drugs (if given by any route other than oral)
- The importance of taking pain medications before the pain becomes severe
- How to manage adverse effects of opioids (e.g., constipation)
- How to keep a diary or log about pain, including what makes it better or worse
- An explanation about addiction and drug tolerance
- The importance of scheduling periods of rest and sleep
- Contact person with phone number if pain becomes worse
- Reminder to store narcotics away from small children or grandchildren

The client and family may need additional information about pain clinics or support groups in the community. Also, they may need help with finding resources for finances, care, and hospice.

Nursing Process Case Study
■ CLIENT WITH PAIN

Susan Akers, 37 years old, is being seen at an outpatient clinic for a 3-year history of neck and shoulder pain. She believes the pain is caused by lifting heavy objects at work, but she says now household chores make it worse. She misses work about three times a month from her pain. About twice a month the pain becomes so intense that she needs Demerol injections at the local emergency department. She takes Darvocet-N 100 and Valium usually two to three times a day without complete relief.

Assessment Ms. Akers rates her pain during an acute episode as a 7 on a 0 to 10 scale. When she raises her arms above shoulder level, it causes sharp pain.

Diagnosis The main nursing diagnosis for Ms. Akers is: Chronic pain related to muscle inflammation.

Expected Outcomes The expected outcomes for the plan of care are that Ms. Akers will

- After 5 days on regularly scheduled analgesics report a decrease in pain from 7 to 3–4 on a 0–10 scale.
- Modify activities at work and at home, especially when pain is intense.

Planning and Implementation The following interventions are implemented for Ms. Akers:

- Consult with a physician for new opioid and nonopioid analgesic prescription.
- Teach Ms. Akers about her medications, as well as the side effects and how to treat them.
- Teach Ms. Akers relaxation and distraction techniques.
- Discuss with Ms. Akers and her children ways for dividing the household tasks between everyone.

BOX 6-5
ASSESSING FOR DISCHARGE

PAIN
Client

- Self-care: Ability to perform activities of daily living (ADLs) independently; to use a pain rating scale; to self-administer prescribed medications; to perform nonpharmacologic therapies (e.g., distraction, relaxation, heat and cold).
- Knowledge: Prescription medications; nonpharmacologic therapies; high-fiber diet and adequate fluid intake; indications for seeking medical care.
- Home environment: Appropriate heating and cooling; electricity; telephone; access to clean water for drinking and handwashing.

Family

- Members of household: Supportive and caring.
- Caregivers: Availability and willingness to provide care and assist with household chores; ability to administer prescribed medications and nonpharmacologic therapies; availability of transportation services.
- Financial resources: Income; availability of sick leave; resources for medications, equipment such as TENS, and medical care required.

Community

- Access to health care resources, especially a pharmacy.
- Availability of neighbors, community support groups, church groups.
- Availability of respite care for caregivers.

Evaluation A week later Ms. Akers reports that the pain medications have decreased her pain to a 2–3 on a 0–10 scale. She says she has been reassigned to a position that requires no lifting and that her children are helping with the household tasks.

💡 Critical Thinking in the Nursing Process

1. Ms. Akers asks you how often she should take her pain medications. You tell her to (a) take them on a regular basis or (b) wait until she experiences pain. Which action would you choose, and why?
2. If Ms. Akers experienced acute pain, what assessment findings would the nurse expect to see?
3. What suggestions should the nurse give to Ms. Akers for treating constipation?

Nursing Interventions Classification

Some of the following nursing interventions may be considered for the client in pain (McCloskey & Bulechek, 2000):

- Active Listening
- Environmental Management: Comfort
- Heat/Cold Application
- Transcutaneous Electrical Nerve Stimulation (TENS)

(*Note:* The bibliography listings for this and all chapters have been compiled at the back of the book.)

Chapter Review

key terms by topic

Use the CD-ROM disk enclosed with your textbook to hear the pronunciation of the key terms in the chapter.

Client in pain
pain

Physiology of pain
nociceptors, pain threshold, pain tolerance, endorphins

Types of pain
acute pain, referred pain, chronic pain, allodynia, neuropathic pain, psychogenic pain

Types of medication
analgesics, nonopioids, opioids, patient-controlled analgesia (PCA), transcutaneous electrical nerve stimulation (TENS) unit

Nursing care
addiction, physical dependence, equianalgesic dose, tolerance, drug tolerance

key points

- Pain affects an individual both physically and emotionally.
- Pain is transmitted through the four steps of transduction, transmission, perception, and modulation.
- Acute pain is usually a short-term event while chronic pain is prolonged.
- Pain management includes medications such as nonopioids, opioids, and adjuvant analgesics and nonpharmacologic therapies including relaxation, distraction, massage, and TENS.
- Nonopioids are used to manage mild to moderate pain; opioids are given for moderate to severe pain; and adjuvant analgesics are used in chronic pain.
- Clients receiving opioids must be monitored for side effects of sedation, respiratory, nausea, and constipation.
- The nurse assumes an important role in assessing the client's pain and working collaboratively with the physician to implement appropriate pain reducing methods.
- All pain relief measures must incorporate an individualized and preventive approach.

 ## Medialink

Additional interactive resources for this chapter can be found on the Companion Website at www.prenhall.com/burke. Click on Chapter 6 and "Begin" to select the activities for this chapter.

For NCLEX review questions and an audio glossary, access the accompanying CD-ROM in this book.

for further study

For further discussion of peripheral neuropathy, see Chapter 17.

The technique for diaphragmatic breathing is described and illustrated in Chapter 7.

For in-depth discussion about care of the client with cancer, see Chapter 8.

Critical Thinking Care Map

Caring for a Client with Pain
NCLEX Focus Area: Physiological Adaptation

Case Study: Mrs. Bruski, 98 years old, has returned to her room following a colon resection. Four hours later the nurse enters Mrs. Bruski's room and finds her lying on her side with her eyes closed. When the nurse asks about her pain, she says, "It hurts right here," as she points to her lower abdomen. She describes the pain as dull and rates it at a 7 on a 0–10 scale. She complains of feeling thirsty and cold. She says, "I just wish I could sleep. I feel so tired."

Nursing Diagnosis: Acute Pain

COLLECT DATA

Subjective

_____

_____

_____

_____

_____

Objective

_____

_____

_____

_____

_____

Would you report this data? Yes/No

If yes, to: _____

Nursing Care

_____

_____

_____

_____

_____

_____

_____

_____

How would you document this? _____

_____

_____

Data Collected
(use those that apply)

- Says she feels cold
- Pulse 100
- Dull pain in lower abdomen
- Temperature 99° F
- "It hurts right here."
- Blood pressure 150/92
- Rates pain at a 7
- Lying on her side with eyes closed
- Complains of being thirsty
- "I'm tired. I wish I could sleep."

Nursing Interventions
(use those that apply)

- Teach Mrs. Bruski to use the incentive spirometer.
- Give acetaminophen (Tylenol) 650 mg PO q 4 hours PRN.
- Offer a back massage at HS.
- Give morphine sulfate 8 mg IM q 4 hours PRN.
- Listen attentively to Mrs. Bruski.
- Teach Mrs. Bruski a relaxation technique.

NCLEX-PN Exam Preparation

1. Client reports a history of constant low back pain for the past 7 months. In planning care for client, the nurse recognizes this type of pain as:
   a. acute pain
   b. chronic pain
   c. superficial pain
   d. neuropathic pain

2. A client complains of pain in her abdomen radiating to the left shoulder. The nurse explains this type of pain is:
   a. visceral
   b. somatic
   c. referred
   d. cutaneous

3. Client has pain related to a brain tumor that required multiple pharmacologic approaches. This pain is classified as:
   a. acute pain
   b. neuropathic pain
   c. referred pain
   d. chronic malignant pain

4. Client has a below the knee amputation of her right leg. She reports pain in her right foot and requests pain medication. The appropriate nursing intervention is to:
   a. report the symptoms to the charge nurse
   b. remind the client that her foot has been amputated
   c. administer pain medication
   d. offer a back rub

5. Client has a history of gastric ulcer. The nurse recognizes this client should avoid which of the following analgesics?
   a. Motrin (ibuprofen)
   b. Tylenol (acetaminophen)
   c. Demerol (meperidine)
   d. Codeine (codeine sulfate)

6. Client complains of pain in his surgical incision. To assess the severity of his pain, which of the following would be MOST effective?
   a. observe his facial expressions
   b. assess his vital signs
   c. ask if the pain is mild, moderate, or severe
   d. ask the client to describe the pain using a scale of 0–10

7. Client, age 75, complains of arthritis pain in her left hip. Which of the following analgesics will provide the least risk of accumulation and toxicity for this client?
   a. Demerol (meperidine)
   b. Motrin (ibuprofen)
   c. Tylenol (acetaminophen)
   d. Darvon (propoxyphene)

8. Client receives morphine sulfate 10 mg intravenously for severe abdominal pain. Thirty minutes later client is unresponsive to physical stimulation. His breathing is shallow. His vital signs are: T 98, P 100, R 8, BP 90/60. Which of the following medications would the nurse expect to be administered?
   a. Ativan (lorazepam)
   b. Valium (diazepam)
   c. Narcan (naloxone)
   d. Toradol (ketorolac)

9. A client is prescribed Naprosyn (naproxen) 500 mg for treatment of osteoarthritis. Teaching for home care should include:
   a. discontinuing the medication when the pain is relieved
   b. limiting alcohol intake to three servings/day
   c. taking with meals to decrease gastric irritation
   d. combining with aspirin to enhance analgesic effect

10. Client, age 67, is receiving Codeine 60 mg PO every 3 to 4 hours PRN for pain. A priority nursing implication is to:
    a. assess bowel sounds every 4 hours
    b. limit fluids to 1,000 mL/day
    c. assess respiratory rate every 4 hours
    d. monitor for evidence of gastrointestinal bleeding

Answers for Review Questions, as well as discussion of Case Study Critical Thinking questions, appear in Appendix V.

Cultural Care STRATEGIES

Responding to Pain as a Cross-Cultural Variable

Mr. Chu, a 48-year old Chinese client, refused pain medication following surgery. When asked by the nurse about whether he needed pain medication, he said his discomfort was bearable and he could survive without any medication. Later, the nurse noticed he was restless and perspiring. Again, the nurse offered pain medication. Again, he refused, saying her responsibilities were far more important than his discomfort and he did not want to impose. The nurse knew that many Chinese are taught self-restraint and that some Chinese view the needs of the group as more important than individual needs. She also knew that some Chinese individuals have been taught it is polite to say no the first time an offer is extended. The nurse said, "Mr. Chu, it will help you recover sooner if you are able to relax. I have time to get it for you and would like to do that. If I bring you some medication, will you take it?" Mr. Chu smiled, look relieved, and said, "Yes, you are very kind."

Pain is a universal experience of human existence, but it is not a concrete entity. McCaffery and Thorpe (1988) stated: "Pain is whatever the experiencing person says it is, existing whenever the experiencing person says it does." Today, this phrase is often quoted when holistic pain management is discussed.

Holistic pain management involves consideration of the physical, emotional, social, and spiritual components of pain. It also includes consideration of the client in the context of family, culture, past experiences, and the meaning of the event being experienced (Davidhizar, Shearer, & Giger, 1997). Culture shapes beliefs and behaviors related to pain and influences the way pain is expressed.

Affective Response to Pain

Cultural responses to pain have been divided into two categories: stoic and emotive. Stoic clients are those who tend to "grin and bear it." Emotive people are more likely to verbalize their feelings of pain. A child raised in a Jewish home may react to a physical injury stoically, saying, "It does not hurt much," while a child raised in a Hispanic home may react to the same injury very demonstratively.

Communication of Pain

Words used to describe symptoms differ among cultures. A nurse may understand what is said by a client from the same cultural background, but have less understanding of a client from another culture who uses different terms, is less fluent in English, or speaks another language.

Nonverbal communication also differs among cultures. A client may feel that he or she is communicating the level of pain nonverbally and does not need to describe it. However, the nurse may not recognize culturally unique communications of pain (Giger & Davidhizar, 1999).

Biological Variations and Cultural Reaction to Pain

People within cultural groups may differ biologically in their reaction to pain and to pain medication. For example, when white clients and Chinese clients were compared for reactions to morphine, white clients reported less pain but greater incidence of drug-induced gastrointestinal effects (Levy, 1993).

Nursing Implications

- **Assess individuals in pain from a holistic and cultural perspective.** A "meaning-centered" approach must be used when assessing the client in pain. This approach includes an assessment not only of what the client is saying verbally and nonverbally, but also of personal meanings that pain may have for that person.
- **Avoid reacting judgmentally to the client who is demonstrative about pain.** When a client's reaction to pain appears excessive, the nurse should appreciate that the behavior may be customary in the client's culture and that any other behavior would be considered abnormal. The nurse should react with sensitivity and provide emotional support.
- **Provide appropriate care to promote health in a client who may have a stoic reaction to pain.** When the client is stoic, the nurse may need to be more directive in controlling pain. The nurse should assess for physiological symptoms of pain and tell the client why intervention will help recovery.
- **Recognize differences in responses to pain among health team members.** If team members are stoic themselves, they may be less responsive to complaints of pain by clients.

Self-Reflection Questions

1. What is your attitude toward pain—your own and others'?
2. How do you think your family has shaped your attitude toward pain?
3. How do you react when you are around people who have different reactions to pain than yours?

chapter

7

Caring for Clients Having Surgery

CARING tip

"Make sure you receive sufficient orientation. Ask for help until you feel comfortable in your position."

Margaret Walker, BSN, MA, RN • Associate Dean, Academic Affairs • SUNY Brockport/Rochester Educational Opportunity Center • Rochester, New York

LEARNING outcomes

After completing this chapter, you will be able to:

- Describe the classifications of surgical procedures.
- Identify laboratory and diagnostic tests used in the perioperative period.
- Describe nursing implications for medications prescribed for the surgical client.
- Discuss appropriate nursing care for the client in the preoperative, intraoperative, and postoperative phases of surgery.
- Identify variations in perioperative care for the older adult.
- Describe principles of pain management for postoperative pain control.
- Compare and contrast outpatient and inpatient surgery.
- Use the nursing process to provide care for the client undergoing surgery.

MediaLink

www.prenhall.com/burke

Use the above address to access the free, interactive Companion Website created for this textbook. Get hints, instant feedback, and textbook references to chapter-related multiple choice questions. Link to other interesting sites.

Surgery is an invasive medical procedure performed to diagnose, treat, or cure illness, injury, or deformity. Although surgery is a medical treatment, the nurse assumes an active role in caring for the client before, during, and after surgery. The licensed vocational/practical nurse (LVN/LPN) collaborates with members of the health care team to prevent complications and promote optimal recovery of the surgical client.

Perioperative nursing care incorporates the three phases of the surgical experience: preoperative, intraoperative, and postoperative. The **preoperative phase** begins when the decision for surgery is made and ends when the client is transferred to the operating room. The **intraoperative phase** begins with the client's entry into the operating room and ends with admittance to the postanesthesia care unit (PACU, or recovery room). The **postoperative phase** begins with the client's admittance to the postanesthesia recovery area and ends with the client's complete recovery from the surgical intervention.

Surgical procedures can be classified according to purpose, risk factor, and urgency (Table 7-1 ◆). Based on this information, nursing care can be individualized to meet client needs well.

Although health care professionals collaborate to identify and meet the client's needs, the perioperative nurse has the primary responsibility and accountability for nursing care of the client undergoing surgery.

The client may have either inpatient surgery or outpatient surgery. **Inpatient surgery** is surgery requiring admission to a hospital before and after the procedure. **Outpatient surgery** is defined as a surgical procedure performed on a nonhospitalized client under local or general anesthesia. (Most of this chapter discusses care of the client having inpatient surgery. Special outpatient considerations are discussed at the end of the chapter.) Inpatient surgery may be a planned event or an unanticipated emergency situation. Although the length of stay for surgical clients has declined during the past two decades, many major procedures still require inpatient stays of 4 days or more following surgery.

The complexity of the inpatient surgical experience requires exceptional collaborative and independent nursing care. Most clients have a strong emotional response to the prospect of surgery, and this may lead to physical and psychological responses. The situation is complicated further when the surgery occurs as an emergency, and the client has limited time to prepare. The role of the perioperative nurse is to assist the client to achieve and maintain the best possible state of health before, during, and after surgery.

Preoperative Phase

The *preoperative phase* begins when the decision for surgery is made and ends when the client is transferred to the operating room. Nursing care during this phase focuses on assessment of the client's readiness for surgery and establishing a plan of care

TABLE 7-1 CLASSIFICATION OF SURGICAL PROCEDURES

	CLASSIFICATION	FUNCTION	EXAMPLE
Purpose	Diagnostic	Determine or confirm a diagnosis	Breast biopsy
	Ablative	Remove diseased organ or extremity	Appendectomy, amputation
	Constructive	Build tissue/organs that are absent (congenital anomalies)	Repair of cleft palate
	Reconstructive	Rebuild tissue/organ that has been damaged	Skin graft after a burn, total joint replacement
	Palliative	Alleviate symptoms of a disease (not curative)	Bowel resection in client with terminal cancer
	Transplant	Replace organs/tissue to restore function	Heart, lung, liver, kidney transplant
Risk Factor	Minor	Minimal physical assault with minimal risk	Removal of skin lesions, dilation and curettage (D&C), cataract extraction
	Major	Extensive physical assault and/or serious risk	Transplant, total joint replacement, cholecystectomy, colostomy, nephrectomy
Urgency	Elective	Suggested though no foreseen ill effects if postponed	Cosmetic surgery, cataract surgery, bunionectomy
	Urgent	Necessary to be performed within 1 to 2 days	Heart bypass surgery, amputation resulting from gangrene, fractured hip
	Emergency	Performed immediately	Obstetric emergencies, bowel obstruction, ruptured aneurysm, life-threatening trauma

to prevent complications during and after the surgical procedure.

COLLABORATIVE CARE
Laboratory and Diagnostic Tests

Laboratory and diagnostic tests are performed prior to surgery to provide baseline data and to detect problems that may place the client at risk during and after surgery. Laboratory studies and diagnostic procedures are performed in a preadmission clinic within a week prior to elective surgery, and immediately prior to surgery in emergency situations. The surgeon and anesthesiologist use this information when choosing the type of anesthetic. The surgeon and nursing staff use laboratory and diagnostic data in the preparation and recovery phases.

The most common preoperative laboratory and diagnostic tests performed are *complete blood count* (CBC), *electrolytes* (Na+, K+, Cl−), *coagulation studies* (prothrombin time [PT], partial thromboplastin time [PTT]), *urinalysis, chest x-ray,* and *electrocardiogram* (ECG/EKG) (Table 7-2 ◆). Additional laboratory tests are performed as needed. For example, if the client

TABLE 7-2	LABORATORY TESTS FOR PERIOPERATIVE ASSESSMENT			
TEST	**NORMAL VALUE**	**SIGNIFICANCE OF INCREASED VALUES**	**SIGNIFICANCE OF DECREASED VALUES**	**NURSING IMPLICATIONS**
Hemoglobin (Hgb)	12–16 g Females 14–18 g Males	Dehydration, excessive plasma loss	Fluid overload, excessive blood loss, anemia	Monitor intake and output, vital signs, assess for bleeding.
Hematocrit (Hct)	37–47% Females 40–54% Males	Polycythemia		
White blood cell count (WBC)	5–10 mm³	Infection/ inflammatory process	Immune deficiencies	Monitor for signs of inflammation and infection.
Platelet count	200,000–300,000	Malignancies	Clotting deficiency disorders, chemotherapy	Assess for signs of bleeding at incision site and drainage tubes. Assess for hematoma.
Potassium (K+)	3.5–5.0 mEq/L	Renal failure, dehydration	Renal damage, dehydration	Monitor cardiac status; monitor intake and output.
Chloride (Cl−)	98–106 mEq/L	Dehydration, renal dysfunction	Side effects of diuretics, vomiting, NG suctioning	Monitor lab values; monitor intake and output.
Sodium (Na+)	135–145 mEq/L	Kidney dysfunction, normal saline containing IV fluids	Side effects of diuretics, vomiting, NG suctioning	Monitor lab values; monitor intake and output.
Prothrombin time (protime, or PT) and partial thromboplastin time (PTT)	10–13 sec 22–32 sec	Defect in mechanism for blood clotting, anticoagulant therapy, side effects of other drugs affecting clotting time	May lead to thrombus formation in the veins	Monitor lab values. Assess for bleeding from incision, urine, and hematoma formation.
Urinalysis	Glucose negative Protein negative WBC negative RBC negative Bacteria negative Ketones negative	Varied	Varied	Used to detect abnormal substances in the urine.

has a history of diabetes mellitus, blood glucose levels are monitored before, during, and after surgery.

The chest x-ray examination provides baseline information about the size, shape, and condition of the heart and lungs. Pulmonary complications, such as chronic lung disease or pneumonia, may require postponement of surgery for further evaluation or treatment. If findings are abnormal and surgery cannot be postponed, the x-ray information can be used to determine the safest form of anesthesia.

The electrocardiogram (ECG/EKG) is ordered routinely on clients who are undergoing general anesthesia, are over age 40, or have a history of cardiovascular disease. The ECG is used to evaluate the cardiac status of the client as well as either new or preexisting cardiac conditions. The client's surgery may be postponed or canceled if a life-threatening cardiac condition is discovered.

CLINICAL alert

monitor
Monitor laboratory test values and results of diagnostic tests for the preoperative patient.
report
Report abnormal values to the charge nurse or physician.

Pharmacology

The surgical client may be given preoperative medications 45 to 60 minutes before the scheduled surgery. Preoperative drugs may be ordered to sedate the client, reduce client anxiety, enhance the actions of anesthetics, induce amnesia to minimize unpleasant surgical memories, increase comfort during preoperative procedures, reduce gastric acidity and volume, increase gastric emptying, decrease nausea and vomiting, and reduce the incidence of aspiration by drying oral and respiratory secretions. (Table 7-3 ◆ outlines commonly prescribed preoperative medications.) The nurse is responsible for administering these drugs prior to surgery. Preoperative medications should be administered *at the time ordered by the physician,* so that the desired effects can be obtained. Any delay must be reported to operating room personnel immediately.

Physical and Psychological Preparation

The nurse must begin by assessing the needs of the client and the factors that may increase risks associated with surgery. The nurse collects data on admission and performs a physical examination. From this information the nurse prioritizes baseline data and collaborates with the registered nurse to identify physical needs, teaching needs, and psychological support for the client and family. Interventions planned by the nurse (Table 7-4 ◆) are determined by the type of surgical procedure and its associated risks.

For example, if a client is admitted for surgery on the right knee, it is of concern to the nurse that this client has diabetes, smokes two packs of cigarettes per day, has numbness in the right foot, and takes insulin. This information must be incorporated into a care plan, using appropriate nursing diag-

TABLE 7-3

PREOPERATIVE MEDICATIONS AND NURSING IMPLICATIONS

GENERIC NAME	TRADE NAME	DOSE AND ROUTE	ACTION	NURSING IMPLICATIONS
Benzodiazepines				
■ Midazolam	Versed	3–5 mg IM	Decreases anxiety and produces sedation	Monitor for respiratory depression, hypotension, drowsiness, and lack of coordination.
■ Diazepam	Valium	5–20 mg PO	Induces amnesia	
■ Lorazepam	Ativan	1–4 mg IM or IV	May induce substantial amnesia	
Opioid Analgesics				
■ Morphine	Morphine	5–15 mg IM, IV	Decreases anxiety, provides analgesia, allows decreased anesthetics	Monitor for respiratory depression, nausea, vomiting, orthostatic hypotension, and pruritus.
■ Meperidine	Demerol	50–150 mg IM, IV		
H_2 Receptor Antagonists				
■ Cimetidine	Tagamet	300 mg IV, IM, PO	Reduces gastric acid volume and concentration	Monitor for confusion and dizziness in older adults.
■ Famotidine	Pepcid	20 mg IV		
■ Ranitidine	Zantac	50 mg IV, IM, PO		

TABLE 7-3 PREOPERATIVE MEDICATIONS AND NURSING IMPLICATIONS (CONTINUED)

GENERIC NAME	TRADE NAME	DOSE AND ROUTE	ACTION	NURSING IMPLICATIONS
Antiemetics ▪ Metroclopramide ▪ Droperidol	Reglan Inapsine	10 mg IV 2.5–10 mg IM	Enhances gastric emptying Tranquilizer	Monitor for sedation and extrapyramidal reaction (involuntary movement, muscle tone changes, and abnormal posture).
Anticholinergic ▪ Atropine sulfate ▪ Glycopyrrolate	Atropine sulfate Robinul	0.4–0.6 mg IM, IV 0.1–0.3 mg IM, IV	Reduces oral and respiratory secretions to decrease risk of aspiration; decreases vomiting and laryngospasm	Monitor for confusion, restlessness, and tachycardia. Prepare client to expect a dry mouth.

TABLE 7-4 NURSING IMPLICATIONS FOR SURGICAL RISK FACTORS

FACTOR	ASSOCIATED RISK	NURSING IMPLICATIONS
Advanced age	Older adults have age-related changes that affect physiologic, cognitive, and psychosocial responses to the stress of surgery; decrease tolerance of general anesthesia and postoperative medications, and delay wound healing.	Thorough assessment of response to anesthesia and medications. Monitor level of consciousness and orientation. Monitor renal status.
Obesity	The obese client is at increased risk for delayed wound healing, wound dehiscence, infection, pneumonia, atelectasis, thrombophlebitis, dysrhythmias, and heart failure.	Promote weight reduction if time permits. Monitor closely for wound, pulmonary, and cardiovascular complications postoperatively. Encourage coughing, turning, and diaphragmatic breathing exercises and early ambulation.
Malnutrition	Reserves may not be sufficient to allow the body to respond satisfactorily to the physical assault of surgery; organ failure and shock may result. Increased metabolic demands may result in poor wound healing and infection.	With the physician and dietitian, promote weight gain by providing a well-balanced diet high in calories, protein, and vitamin C. Daily weights.
Dehydration/ electrolyte imbalance	Depending on the degree of dehydration and/or type of electrolyte imbalance, cardiac dysrhythmia or heart failure may occur. Liver and renal failure may also result.	Administer intravenous fluids as ordered. Monitor intake and output. Monitor for signs of electrolyte imbalance.
Cardiovascular disorders	Increases risk of hemorrhage and shock, hypotension, thrombophlebitis, pulmonary embolism, stroke, and fluid volume overload.	Monitor vital signs, especially pulse rate, regularity, and rhythm, and general condition of the client. Assess skin color. Assess for chest pain, lung congestion, and peripheral edema. Provide early postoperative ambulation.

(continues)

TABLE 7-4   NURSING IMPLICATIONS FOR SURGICAL RISK FACTORS (CONTINUED)

FACTOR	ASSOCIATED RISK	NURSING IMPLICATIONS
Respiratory disorders	Respiratory complications such as bronchitis, atelectasis, and pneumonia are some of the most common postoperative complications. Respiratory depression from general anesthesia and acid–base imbalance may also occur.	Closely monitor respirations, pulse, and breath sounds. Encourage coughing, turning, deep-breathing exercises, and early ambulation.
Diabetes mellitus	Increases risk for cardiovascular disease, delayed wound healing, and wound infection; life threatening hypoglycemia or ketoacidosis.	Monitor blood glucose levels. Assess for signs of hypoglycemia and hyperglycemia.
Renal and liver dysfunction	Poor tolerance of general anesthesia, fluid and electrolyte imbalance, decreased metabolism and excretion of drugs.	Monitor fluid status. Monitor response to drugs. Monitor intake and output.
Alcoholism	Client may be malnourished; may require more general anesthesia; at risk for hemorrhage and delayed wound healing.	Monitor for signs of delirium tremens. Monitor diet. Assess for evidence of bleeding.
Smoking	Increased risk for respiratory complications such as pneumonia, atelectasis, and bronchitis because of increased mucus secretions and a decreased ability to expel them.	Encourage the client to quit smoking. Monitor for respiratory complications. Encourage coughing and breathing exercises. Promote early ambulation.
Medications	Anesthesia interaction with some medications can cause respiratory difficulties, hypotension, and circulatory collapse. Other medications can produce side effects that may increase surgical risk.	Inform the anesthesiologist of all prescribed or over-the-counter medications.
Anticoagulants	May cause intraoperative and postoperative hemorrhage.	Monitor for bleeding. Assess PT/PTT values.
Diuretics	May lead to fluid and electrolyte imbalances, producing altered cardiovascular response and respiratory depression.	Monitor intake and output and electrolytes. Assess cardiovascular and respiratory status.
Antihypertensives	Increase the hypotensive effects of anesthesia.	Closely monitor blood pressure.
Antidepressants	Increase the hypotensive effects of anesthesia.	Closely monitor blood pressure.
Antibiotics	May cause apnea and respiratory paralysis.	Monitor respirations.

noses and interventions to meet all of the client's needs and assist the client toward full postoperative recovery.

Surgery is a significant and stressful event in the life of the client and family. Whether it is major or minor surgery, it creates anxiety. The level of anxiety the client and family experiences is unique and depends on the significance of the procedure to the individuals. For example, a client scheduled to have a biopsy to rule out cancer may be more anxious than a client undergoing gallbladder removal.

The nurse's ability to listen actively to both verbal and nonverbal messages is essential to establishing a trusting relationship with the client and family. Therapeutic communication can help the client and family identify fears and concerns. The nurse can then plan nursing interventions and supportive care to reduce the client's anxiety level and assist the client to cope successfully with the stressors encountered during the perioperative period.

Physical preparation of the client for surgery may include the following:

■ *Skin preparation* involves shave prep of the surgical area and scrubbing the area with an antiseptic solution. The purpose of skin preparation is to reduce the number of bacteria on the skin in the surgical area. New growth of bacteria occurs soon after completion of skin prep. Therefore, these procedures are usually performed in the operating room immediately prior to the procedure. Care must be taken with shave preps, because any nicks in the skin can result in introduction of bacteria. The areas to be prepped are determined by the type and location of surgery to be performed.

■ *Insertion of an indwelling (Foley) catheter* reduces the risk of injury to the bladder during abdominal surgery. It also provides a means to assess urinary output accurately during extensive surgery.

- *Bowel preparation* may be necessary to prevent introduction of bacteria into the peritoneum during surgery on the bowel. This may include administration of enemas or medications (e.g., GoLytely) to evacuate the bowel prior to surgery. Bowel prep may be initiated by the client prior to admission to the hospital or by the nurse for inpatients. The nurse should explain the procedures thoroughly to the patient and document evaluation of patient understanding.
- *Witholding of food and fluids* may be part of preparation for surgery. Patients may be instructed to withhold food and fluids 8 to 10 hours prior to surgery. This reduces the risk of aspiration of stomach contents during surgery, especially if the patient receives general anesthesia. The nurse should explain the importance of following these instructions and the risks if instructions are not followed. Clients with a history of chronic medical problems such as diabetes mellitus, hypertension, or heart disease may be allowed to take their medications prior to surgery. The nurse must verify this with the physician and instruct the client to take the medications with a minimal amount of water.

Informed Consent

Informed consent (operative permit) is a legal document required for certain diagnostic procedures or therapeutic measures, including surgery. This legal document serves to protect the client, nurse, physician, and health care facility. Informed consent includes the following information:

- The need for the procedure in relation to the diagnoses
- A description and purpose of the proposed procedure
- Possible benefits and potential risks
- Likelihood of a successful outcome
- Alternative treatments or procedures available
- Anticipated risks should the procedure not be performed
- Physician's advice as to what is needed
- Right to refuse treatment or withdraw consent

The surgeon who performs the procedure is responsible for obtaining the client's informed consent. The surgeon should discuss the above information with the client and family in language they can understand. Ideally, the nurse should be present during this time. Later, the nurse can discuss what was presented. If the client's questions or concerns were not answered, or if the nurse questions the client's understanding, the nurse should contact the surgeon. The surgeon is responsible for supplying further information before the client signs the informed consent form. After a thorough discussion of the informed consent, the nurse witnesses the client's signature on the form (Figure 7-1 ◆). The nurse also signs the form, indicating that the correct person signed the form and that the client was alert and aware of what was being signed.

The LPN/LVN should refer to hospital policy to determine appropriate criteria and procedure for signing the surgical consent. These policies identify who can sign the consent, circumstances in which the consent may be signed by someone other than the client, and the procedure to follow if the signature cannot be obtained. Most states require clients age 18 and over to sign their own consent, and a parent or legal guardian to sign for clients under age 18. Married minors may sign their own consent for surgery, regardless of age. **Emancipated minors** (individuals under age 18 who are responsible for their own welfare and live independently from their parents) also sign their own consent. Mentally challenged adults, as well as adults determined by the courts to be incompetent to make their own medical decisions, must have a legal guardian sign for them. In life-threatening situations when surgery is required but the client is unable to sign the consent, every effort is made to contact *next of kin* for consent. (The definition of next of kin is specified in most facility policies related to informed consent.) If next of kin cannot be located and continued delay of surgical intervention would be life threatening, a court order may be obtained, or the surgeon may assume responsibility for proceeding without consent. The nurse must thoroughly document the steps taken to obtain consent and the circumstances dictating the need for surgery.

The decision to have surgery is a major event in any person's life, especially in the older client who faces additional risks. Therefore, the nurse should allow adequate time for the client to process information, ask questions, and make decisions with the assistance of professionals and family members. The input of adult children and other family members is almost always represented in the older adult's decision to proceed with surgery. The nurse works closely with both the client and family members to provide teaching and emotional support.

CLINICAL alert

Follow facility policy related to signing of informed consent. Spouses, children, and significant others cannot sign the informed consent instead of the capable, adult surgical client.

NURSING CARE

The LPN/LVN plans care with the registered nurse to meet the needs of the client. Refer to the facility's position description to determine the role of the practical/vocational nurse in applying the nursing process.

ASSESSING

Thorough assessment by the nurse is critical for the preoperative client. Data collected during this phase can identify physiologic and psychological alterations that require nursing and/or medical intervention. The nurse should collect data related to medical and social history, assessment of all body systems, and psychosocial status.

M.R. # _____

Saint Francis Medical Center

Informed Consent to Operation, Administration of Anesthetics, and the Rendering of Other Medical Services

1.   I do hereby authorize and direct _____ M.D./D.O./D.D.S., my physician, and/or such associates or assistants of his choice, to perform the following operation or procedure:

_____

_____

upon _____ (client's name). I understand that the above named physician and his associates or assistants are employed by me and will be occupied solely with performing such operation or procedure.

2.   The nature of the operation or procedure has been explained to me and no warranty or guarantee has been made as to result or cure. I have been advised that additional surgical and/or medical procedures or treatment may be deemed necessary during the course of the operation or procedure consented hereto, and I fully consent to such additional procedures and treatment which, in the opinion of my physician, are deemed necessary or desirable for the well-being of the client. The possible risks and complications of the operation or procedure have been explained to me. The physician has explained to me the above medical terminology and I satisfactorily understand the type of operation/procedure.

3.   I hereby authorize and direct the above named physician and/or his associates or assistants or those working under his direction to provide for _____ (client's name) such additional services as he or they may deem reasonable and necessary, including, but not limited to, the administration and maintenance of anesthesia, blood or blood derivatives, and the performance of services involving pathology and radiology and I hereby consent thereto. The possible risks and complications of blood transfusions and the administration of anesthetics have also been explained to me.

4.   I understand also that the persons in attendance at such operation or procedure for the purpose of administering anesthesia, and the radiologists in attendance at such operation or procedure for the purpose of performing radiological (x-ray) service are not the agents, servants, or employees of St. Francis Medical Center nor of any physician, but are independent health care providers who are employed by me in the same way that my surgeon and physician are employed by me.

5.   I hereby authorize the Medical Center pathologist or personnel to use their discretion in the disposal of any severed tissue or member.

6.   I hereby grant permission for St. Francis Medical Center to obtain clinical photographs for educational purposes or for my patient record as deemed necessary by my physician.

7.   **The exception to this consent:** (If none, write "none.") _____

_____ and I assume full responsibility for these exceptions.

_____   _____
       CLIENT'S SIGNATURE   **DATE**

If the client is a minor or incompetent or is unable to sign, the following must be completed:

I hereby certify that I am the (relationship) _____ of the above named client who is unable to sign because _____ and I am fully authorized to give the consent herein granted.

_____   _____
           SIGNATURE   DATE

_____   _____
   WITNESSED BY/DATE   **WITNESSED BY/DATE**

If signed in the physician's office, the following MUST be completed by the Medical Center.

_____   _____
  REVIEWED BY (CLIENT NAME)/DATE   WITNESSED BY/DATE

Figure 7-1. ◆ Informed consent to operation, administration of anesthetics, and the rendering of other medical services.

DIAGNOSING, PLANNING, AND IMPLEMENTING

The nurse identifies problems, plans care, and develops nursing interventions to meet client needs and prevent complications during the perioperative period.

DEFICIENT KNOWLEDGE

- Assess client's current level of knowledge. *This allows the nurse to prioritize teaching, provide new information, and reinforce prior knowledge about surgical procedure and postoperative course of treatment.*
- Assist the client to obtain information about expectations during the intraoperative and postoperative phase. Refer the client to the physician for detailed information about the surgical procedure. *The surgeon provides information so the client can make an informed decision about care.*
- Teach postoperative breathing exercises, turning, coughing, deep breathing, and leg exercises. *This knowledge helps prevent postoperative complications.*
- Collaborate with physician concerning postoperative pain control. Communicate this information to the client. *This assures the client that pain will be managed.*

ANXIETY

- Assess specific source(s) of anxiety. *Common fears include loss of control, pain, death, disfigurement, disability, and disturbing diagnosis and prognosis. The unfamiliar environment increases anxiety. Assessment provides the basis for planning specific nursing interventions.*
- Answer all questions thoroughly and honestly. Refer to appropriate resource as needed. *Honesty establishes trust and helps relieve anxiety.*
- Allow expression of fears. Use active listening. *Listening helps the client identify fears and clarify concerns.*
- Refer to clergy or spiritual support of client's choice. *Spiritual support provides comfort to most clients.*

DISTURBED SLEEP PATTERN

- Assess usual sleep pattern. *This identifies alterations in pattern. Anxiety prior to surgery often results in sleep disturbance.*
- Provide environment with minimal stimuli prior to surgery. *A relaxing environment encourages sleep.*
- Collaborate with physician to obtain sleep medication. *Adequate rest reduces the risk of complications and contributes to more effective induction of anesthesia.*

EVALUATING

The nurse evaluates the client's success in meeting expected outcomes.

- Client demonstrates preoperative exercises according to teaching plan.
- Client verbalizes understanding of surgical procedure.
- Client states that he or she understands anticipated pain management techniques.
- Client states that anxiety is decreased.
- Client sleeps 8 hours without interruption the night before surgery.

Preoperative Teaching

Client teaching is an essential nursing responsibility in the preoperative period. Client education combined with emotional support has positive physical and psychological effects. In an analysis of 102 case studies, surgical clients receiving client education and/or supportive interventions had less pain and anxiety, experienced fewer complications, were discharged sooner, were more satisfied with their care, and returned to normal activities sooner than clients who did not receive this type of care. These positive outcomes may be attributed in part to the perceived sense of control the client gains through the nurse's teaching.

Nurses develop and implement the preoperative teaching plan. Client teaching should begin as soon as the client is aware of the upcoming surgery. Most teaching is carried out prior to surgery, because postsurgical pain and the effects of anesthesia greatly diminish the client's ability to learn.

The amount of information desired varies from client to client. The nurse must assess the client's need for and readiness to accept information. The teaching is determined partly by the particular surgical procedure being performed. Client teaching that helps to reduce postsurgical risk for most patients is included in Box 7-1.

Besides teaching measures to decrease the risk of complications, the nurse provides other preoperative information to prepare the client and family for surgery:

- List of laboratory and diagnostic tests to be performed, including reason for the tests and preparations
- Time family should arrive if surgery is scheduled in early morning
- Preparations for the day of surgery: nothing by mouth (NPO) after midnight prior to a morning surgery, skin preparation, indwelling catheter or bladder elimination, start of intravenous infusion, preoperative medication, handling of valuables (e.g., rings, watch, money)
- Sedative/hypnotic medication to be taken the night before surgery to promote rest and sleep
- Informed consent
- Expected timetable for surgery and the recovery room
- Procedure for transfer to the surgery department
- Location of the surgical waiting room
- Procedure for transfer to recovery room
- Anticipated postoperative routine and devices or equipment (drains, tubes, equipment for intravenous infusions, oxygen or humidifying mask, dressings, splints, casts)
- Plans for postoperative pain control

A nursing care checklist for the day of surgery is provided in Box 7-2.

BOX 7-1
PREOPERATIVE CLIENT TEACHING

DIAPHRAGMATIC BREATHING EXERCISE

Diaphragmatic (abdominal) breathing exercises help to prevent pulmonary complications. Risk factors for atelectasis or pneumonia include general anesthesia, abdominal or thoracic surgery, history of smoking, chronic lung disease, obesity, and advanced age.

1. Explain to the client that the diaphragm is a muscle that makes up the floor of the abdominal cavity and assists in breathing. When the client breathes in deeply, the diaphragm expands down and out, promoting lung expansion, ventilation, and blood oxygenation. When the client exhales, the diaphragm contracts inward and upward and helps to expel air.
2. Position the client in a high or semi-Fowler's position (see figure), with hands placed lightly on the abdomen.

Diaphragmatic breathing exercise.

Splinting abdomen while coughing.

3. Ask the client to place hands lightly on the abdomen.
4. Instruct the client to breathe in deeply through the nose, allowing the chest and abdomen to expand.
5. Have the client hold the breath for a count of 5.
6. Tell the client to exhale completely through pursed (puckered) lips, allowing the chest and abdomen to deflate.
7. Have the client repeat the exercise five times consecutively. Encourage the client to perform diaphragmatic breathing exercises every 1 to 2 waking hours if possible.

COUGHING EXERCISE

Coughing exercises are also taught to clients at risk for pulmonary complications. The purpose of coughing is to loosen, mobilize, and remove pulmonary secretions. *Splinting* (holding something firm over) the incision decreases the discomfort associated with coughing.

1. Assist the client in following steps 1 through 4 for diaphragmatic breathing.
2. Ask the client to splint the incision with interlocked hands or a pillow (see figure).
3. Tell the client to take three deep breaths and then cough forcefully.
4. Have the client repeat the exercise five times consecutively every 2 hours while awake, taking short rest periods between coughs, if necessary.

LEG, ANKLE, AND FOOT EXERCISES

Leg exercises are taught to clients at risk for developing thrombophlebitis (inflammation of a vein, associated with formation of blood clots). Risk factors for developing thrombophlebitis include decreased mobility preoperatively or postoperatively; a history of difficulties with peripheral circulation; and cardiovascular, pelvic, or lower extremity surgeries.

As the leg muscles contract and relax, blood is pumped back to the heart, promoting cardiac output and reducing venous stasis. Besides promoting venous blood return from the extremities, leg exercises also maintain muscle tone and range of motion, which facilitates early ambulation.

Teach the client to perform the following exercises while lying in bed (see drawings):

1. Muscle pumping exercise: Contract and relax calf and thigh muscles at least 10 times in a row.
2. Leg exercises:
    a. Bend the knee and raise it toward the chest.
    b. Straighten out leg and hold for a few seconds before lowering the leg back to the bed.
    c. Repeat exercise five times with one leg, then do them with the other leg.

Leg exercises.   Ankle and foot exercises.

3. Ankle and foot exercises:
    a. Rotate both ankles by making complete circles, first to the right and then to the left. Repeat five times and then relax.
    b. With feet together, point toes toward the head and then to the foot of the bed. Repeat this pumping action 10 times, and then relax.

Encourage the client to perform leg, ankle, and foot exercises every 1 to 2 hours while awake, depending on the client's needs and ambulatory status, the physician's preference, and institutional protocol.

TURNING IN BED

Clients at risk for circulatory, respiratory, or gastrointestinal dysfunction following surgery are taught to turn in bed. This normally simple task may be very difficult after surgery, particularly abdominal surgery. The client may need to splint the incision with the hand and a small pillow or blanket. Analgesics can be given to ease postoperative discomfort involved with turning. Encourage the client to turn every 2 hours while awake.

1. Tell the client to grasp the side rail toward the direction to be turned, to rest the opposite foot on the mattress, and to bend the knee.
2. Instruct the client to roll over in one smooth motion by pulling on the side rail while pushing off with the bent knee.
3. Pillows may need to be positioned behind the client's back to help the client maintain a side-lying position. The older client may also need padding over pressure points between the knees and ankles to prevent decubitus ulcer formation.

Nursing Process Case Study
■ PREOPERATIVE CARE FOR CLIENT HAVING INPATIENT SURGERY

Martha Overbeck is a 74-year-old widow of German descent who lives alone in a senior citizens' housing complex. She is active in the housing complex's activities, as well as in the Lutheran church. She is in good health and is independent; however, she has become progressively less active as a result of arthritic pain and stiffness. Mrs. Overbeck has degenerative joint changes that have particularly affected her right hip. On the recommendation of her physician and following a discussion with her friends, Mrs. Overbeck has been admitted to the hospital for an elective right total hip replacement. Her surgery has been scheduled for 8:00 A.M. the following day.

Mrs. Eva Jackson, a close friend and neighbor, accompanies Mrs. Overbeck to the hospital. Mrs. Overbeck explains that her friend will help in her home and assist her with the wound care and prescribed exercises.

BOX 7-2
NURSING CARE CHECKLIST

DAY OF SURGERY

☑ Assist with bathing, grooming, and changing into operating room gown.

☑ Ensure that the client takes nothing by mouth (NPO).

☑ Provide additional teaching, and reinforce prior teaching.

☑ Ensure that identification, blood, and allergy bands are correct, legible, and secure.

☑ Remove nail polish and makeup to facilitate circulatory assessment during and after surgery.

☑ Remove hair pins and jewelry. A wedding ring may be worn if it is removed from the finger, covered with gauze, and then taped to the finger.

☑ Complete skin or bowel preparation as ordered.

☑ Insert an indwelling catheter, intravenous line, or nasogastric tube as ordered.

☑ Remove dentures, artificial eye, and contact lenses, and store them in a safe place.

☑ Leave a hearing aid in place if the client cannot hear without it, and notify the operating room nurse.

☑ Verify that the informed consent has been signed prior to administering preoperative medications.

☑ Verify that the client's height and weight are recorded in the chart (for dosage of anesthesia).

☑ Verify that all ordered laboratory and diagnostic test reports are in the chart.

☑ Have the client empty the bladder immediately before the preoperative medication is administered (unless an indwelling catheter is in place).

☑ Administer preoperative medication as scheduled (see Table 7-3).

☑ Ensure the safety of the client once the medication has been given by placing the client on bed rest with the side rails up and by placing the call light within reach.

☑ Obtain and record vital signs.

☑ Provide ongoing supportive care to the client and the client's family.

☑ Complete the preoperative surgical checklist. Document all preoperative care in the appropriate location, such as the preoperative surgical checklist, the medication record, and the nurses' notes.

☑ Verify the client's identity with the surgical personnel, and verify that all client information is documented appropriately.

☑ Assist the surgical personnel in transferring the client from the bed to the gurney.

☑ Prepare the client's room for postoperative care, including making the surgical bed and ensuring that anticipated supplies and equipment are in the room.

Assessment Gloria Nobis, LVN, completes the admission assessment for Mrs. Overbeck. Mrs. Overbeck appears to be an alert, oriented, healthy 74-year-old client. She is 30 pounds over her ideal weight. Mrs. Overbeck states she has pain and some stiffness in her weight-bearing joints, particularly her right hip. Enteric-coated aspirin 650 mg four times daily is the only medication she has been taking. Preadmission laboratory tests are normal except for a slightly elevated clotting time (which suggests an increased risk for bleeding). The x-ray film of her right hip reveals degenerative joint changes indicative of osteoarthritis.

Mrs. Overbeck confides that although she has faith that her surgery will be successful, she feels uneasy. She cannot identify exactly why she is apprehensive. She states she has had a number of restless nights since her decision to have surgery. She has never had major surgery and is not familiar with the hospital routine.

Diagnosis The following nursing diagnoses are identified for Mrs. Overbeck and are included in her preoperative plan of care:

■ *Anxiety* related to unfamiliar environment (hospital) and upcoming surgery

■ *Deficient Knowledge* related to lack of information about the perioperative surgical experience

■ *Disturbed Sleep Pattern* related to environmental changes (hospitalization) and anxiety response

Expected Outcomes The expected outcomes established in the plan of care specify that Mrs. Overbeck will

■ Describe an increase in psychological and physiologic comfort

■ Verbalize an understanding of perioperative events to occur

■ Demonstrate turning, coughing, deep-breathing exercise, and leg exercises

■ Report sleeping soundly from 10:00 P.M. to 7:00 A.M.

Planning and Implementation Ms. Nobis plans and implements the following interventions to assist Mrs. Overbeck in the preoperative surgical phase:

■ Establish a therapeutic relationship with Mrs. Overbeck and her friend.

■ Provide reassurance and comfort by acknowledging concerns and conveying understanding.

■ Familiarize Mrs. Overbeck with hospital routines.

■ Initiate perioperative teaching to include:
  ■ Preparation for surgery
  ■ A visit from the operating room nurse and anesthesiologist
  ■ Coughing, turning, and deep-breathing exercises
  ■ Leg exercises
  ■ Written materials describing total hip replacements

■ Help Mrs. Overbeck identify factors that interfere with her ability to sleep.

■ Decrease noise, lighting, and disturbances between 10:00 P.M. and 7:00 A.M.

- Encourage the use of prescribed hypnotic/sedative medications to assist in sleep prior to surgery.

Evaluation By the end of the shift, Ms. Nobis assesses that Mrs. Overbeck's anxiety has diminished. Mrs. Overbeck confirms that she feels more comfortable about the upcoming surgery. She is able to describe the preoperative preparations that will occur the following morning, events that are most likely to occur in surgery and the recovery room, and routine postoperative nursing care following her total hip replacement. She states that she will take the hypnotic/sedative prescribed to help her sleep. She asks Ms. Nobis to convey to the evening and night nurses that she would like to have her door closed and lights off except for the one in the bathroom.

Critical Thinking in the Nursing Process

1. What teaching would you implement with Mrs. Overbeck and her friend to prepare them for the first 72 hours of postoperative recovery?
2. What consultations may be appropriate for you to make to other health care providers to assist Mrs. Overbeck before and after surgery?
3. Develop a care plan for Mrs. Overbeck for the nursing diagnosis *Knowledge Deficit* related to lack of information about preoperative care.

Intraoperative Phase

The **intraoperative phase** begins when the client is admitted to the operating room and ends when the client is admitted to the PACU. Nursing care during this phase focuses on maintenance of physiologic function and client safety.

COLLABORATIVE CARE
Pharmacology

The anesthesiologist visits the surgical client in the preoperative phase to discuss anesthesia. Factors that influence the type of anesthesia used include type of surgery to be performed, client's medical and surgical history, client's age and medical status, and client preference. **Anesthesia** is the use of chemical substances to produce loss of sensation, reflex loss, or muscle relaxation during a surgical procedure, with or without the loss of consciousness. *General anesthesia* produces all of the above effects including unconsciousness. *Regional anesthesia* results in loss of sensation, reflex loss, and muscle relaxation in a particular area but does not cause the client to lose consciousness. *Local anesthesia* provides loss of sensation around the area to be treated. An anesthesiologist (physician) or certified registered nurse anesthetist (CRNA) administers the anesthetics during the intraoperative phase of surgery.

GENERAL ANESTHESIA. General anesthesia is administered by inhalation or the intravenous route. It produces central nervous system depression resulting in loss of consciousness and amnesia. The client perceives no pain, skeletal muscles relax, and reflexes diminish. Advantages to general anesthesia include rapid excretion of the anesthetic agent and prompt reversal of its effects when desired. Additionally, general anesthesia can be used with all age groups and any type of surgical procedure.

Disadvantages of general anesthesia include risks associated with circulatory and respiratory depression. Clients with serious respiratory or circulatory diseases, such as emphysema or congestive heart failure, are at greater risk for these complications.

The phases of general anesthesia are divided into three distinct categories:

1. The *induction phase* begins when the client receives the anesthetic agent and ends when the client is ready for the surgical procedure to begin. During this phase, airway patency is achieved with endotracheal intubation. The client is positioned and the skin is prepared during this phase.
2. The *maintenance phase* begins with surgical incision and continues until the procedure nears completion. The anesthesiologist maintains the proper depth of anesthesia while constantly monitoring such parameters as heart rate, blood pressure, respiratory rate, temperature, and oxygen and carbon dioxide levels.
3. The *emergence phase* begins as the client "emerges" from the anesthetic agents and continues until the client is ready to leave the operating room. The endotracheal tube is removed (*extubated*) once the client has reestablished voluntary breathing. Airway patency is critical during this period, because extubation may cause bronchospasm or laryngospasm.

REGIONAL ANESTHESIA. In regional anesthesia, medication is instilled around the peripheral nerves to block transmission of nerve impulses in a particular area. Regional anesthesia produces analgesia, relaxation, and reduced reflexes. The client is awake and conscious during the surgical procedure but does not perceive pain. Regional anesthesia has several subclassifications:

- *Surface or topical.* Anesthesia is applied to the skin or mucous membranes to block nerve impulses at that site. Wounds of the skin or burns are anesthetized using a cocaine solution, lidocaine (Xylocaine), or benzocaine.
- *Local nerve infiltration.* Lidocaine or tetracaine is injected around a local nerve to depress nerve sensation over a limited area of the body. This technique may be used when a skin or muscle biopsy is obtained or when a small wound is sutured.
- *Nerve blocks.* An anesthetic agent is injected at the nerve trunk to produce a lack of sensation over a specific body area, like the hand.
- *Epidural blocks.* Local anesthetic agents are injected into the epidural space, outside the dura mater of the spinal cord.

This may be used for surgeries of the abdomen and lower extremities.

■ *Spinal anesthesia.* A local anesthetic is injected into the subarachnoid space. Surgeries of the lower abdomen, perineum, and lower extremities are likely to use this type of regional anesthesia. Leakage of cerebrospinal fluid (CSF) from the needle insertion site may cause reduced CSF pressure and postoperative headaches. Bed rest, maintaining hydration, and applying pressure to the infusion site combat this common side effect.

CONSCIOUS SEDATION. **Conscious sedation** is a type of anesthesia that provides analgesia and amnesia but allows the client to remain conscious. An increasing number of surgical and diagnostic procedures are performed using conscious sedation. A combination of intravenous medications with opioids and sedatives produce the pharmacologic effects. Opioids include morphine sulfate, meperidine hydrochloride (Demerol), and fentanyl (Sublimaze). Sedatives include diazepam (Valium) and midazolam (Versed). During conscious sedation, the client can independently maintain an open airway and respond to verbal and physical stimulation.

Common adverse side effects include venous thrombosis, phlebitis, local irritation, confusion, drowsiness, hypotension, and apnea. Naloxone hydrochloride (Narcan) and flumazenil (Romazicon) are used as needed as reversal agents to enhance the safety of conscious sedation. The client must be monitored before, during, and after the procedure when using conscious sedation.

The Surgical Team

All surgical team members have a vital role in the success of the procedure. The surgeon and anesthesiologist maintain primary roles, but nurses are responsible for maintaining the safety of the client and the environment, and for providing physiologic monitoring and psychological support.

The surgeon, surgical assistant(s), anesthesiologist and certified registered nurse anesthetist, circulating nurse, scrub nurse, and certified surgical technologist (CST) constitute the surgical team. Because the intraoperative environment is so complex, members must function as a coordinated unit.

The *surgeon* is the physician performing the procedure and the head of the surgical team. All medical actions and judgments are the surgeon's responsibility.

The *surgical assistant* works closely with the surgeon in performing the operation. The number of assistants varies according to the complexity of the procedure. The assistant may be another physician, a nurse, a physician's assistant, or other trained personnel. The LPN/LVN may assume this role with specialized training. The assistant performs such duties as exposing the operative site, retracting nearby tissue, sponging or suctioning the wound, ligating bleeding vessels, and suturing or assisting with suturing of the surgical wound.

The *anesthesiologist* or the certified registered nurse anesthetist (CRNA) allows the surgeon to focus on the technical aspects of the procedure by assuming responsibility for the client's general well-being. The anesthesiologist or CRNA evaluates the client preoperatively, administers the anesthesia and other required medications, transfuses blood or blood products, infuses intravenous fluids, continuously monitors the client's physiologic status, alerts the surgeon to developing problems and treats them as they arise, and supervises the client's recovery in the PACU.

The *circulating nurse* is a registered nurse who coordinates and manages a wide range of activities before, during, and after the surgical procedure. The circulating nurse oversees the physical aspects of the operating room and its equipment. The circulating nurse assists with transferring and positioning the client, preparing the client's skin, ensuring that no break in aseptic technique occurs, and counting all sponges and instruments. The circulating nurse helps all other team members and is responsible for thorough documentation of intraoperative nursing activities, medications, blood administration, placement of drains and catheters, and length of the procedure. The circulating nurse is at all times an advocate for the safety and well-being of the client.

The role of the *scrub nurse* (Figure 7-2 ◆) primarily involves technical skills, manual dexterity, and in-depth knowledge of the anatomic and mechanical aspects of a particular surgery. LPNs/LVNs often assume the role of scrub nurse. Nurses acquire the necessary skills through facility training programs or formal surgical technology programs. The scrub nurse handles sutures, instruments, and other equipment immediately adjacent to the sterile field. (The "scrub nurse" does not need to be a nurse; a certified surgical technologist [CST] may also assume this role.)

SURGICAL ATTIRE. Strict dress codes are necessary in the surgical department to provide infection control within the operating suites, to reduce cross-contamination between the surgery department and other hospital units or departments,

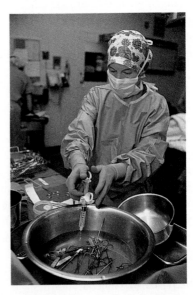

Figure 7-2. ◆ A scrub nurse in the operating room.

and to promote the health and safety of both client and personnel. All personnel in the surgical department must wear proper surgical attire, which minimizes bacterial shedding and reduces wound contamination.

The area in the surgical department is divided into three zones:

1. Unrestricted zones that permit access by those in hospital uniforms or street clothes, and may allow limited access for communicating with operating room personnel.
2. Semirestricted zones that require scrub attire, including a scrub suit, shoe covers, and a cap or hood (Figure 7-3A ◆). Hallways, work areas, and storage areas are considered semirestricted.
3. Restricted zones that are located within operating rooms. Personnel there must wear masks, sterile gowns, and gloves in addition to appropriate scrub attire (see Figure 7-3B). The entire surgical attire is changed between procedures or whenever it becomes soiled or wet.

THE SURGICAL SCRUB. The surgical scrub is performed to render hands and arms as clean as possible in preparation for a procedure. All personnel who participate directly in the procedure must perform a surgical scrub with a brush and antimicrobial soap. Skin cannot be rendered sterile, but it can be considered "surgically clean" following the scrub. The purposes of the surgical scrub are to

- Remove dirt, skin oils, and transient microorganisms from hands and forearms.
- Increase client safety by reducing microorganisms on surgical personnel.

Figure 7-3. ◆ (A) Surgical attire. (B) Sterile surgical attire.

- Leave an antimicrobial residue on the skin to inhibit growth of microbes for several hours.

Following the 5- to 10-minute surgical scrub, hands and arms are dried with sterile towels.

PREPARING THE CLIENT. The client's skin is cleansed in the surgical department to decrease microorganisms on the skin and reduce the possibility of wound infection. The surgeon also may order the skin shaved in and around the proposed incision area (Figure 7-4 ◆). Generally, the area shaved is wider than the planned incision because of the possibility of unexpected extension of the incision. Disposable, sterile supplies are used, in accordance with aseptic techniques. Hospital policy and surgeon preference should be followed.

Preparing the client for surgery also includes positioning the client on the operating table (Table 7-5 ◆). Positioning allows for exposure of the operative site and access for administration of anesthesia. Proper positioning is crucial to prevent injury to the client. Pressure, rubbing, or shearing forces can damage the tissue over bony prominences. If positioning causes normal joint range of motion to be exceeded, injury to muscles and joints can occur. Improper positioning also can lead to sensory and motor dysfunction and nerve damage. Pressure on peripheral blood vessels can decrease venous return to the heart and negatively affect the client's blood pressure. Oxygenation of the blood can be decreased if the client is not properly positioned to promote lung expansion.

The anesthetized client cannot respond to discomfort. It is the surgical team's responsibility to position the client not only for the best surgical advantage but also for client safety and comfort. The circulating nurse follows hospital policy, the surgeon's preference, and the client's history to ensure optimal positioning, and continuously assesses the client. Box 7-3 lists special considerations for the older adult undergoing surgery.

NURSING CARE

Maintenance of the client's physiologic and psychological safety is the priority during the intraoperative period. The nurse shares this responsibility with all members of the surgical team.

CLINICAL alert

Carefully identify the client on admission to the operating room. Ensure that the surgical consent accurately describes the scheduled procedure.

ASSESSING

The nurse is responsible for assessing the client for medical/surgical or social history that may increase the risk of complications during the intraoperative phase. Pertinent history would include cardiovascular or respiratory disorders, arthritis, and altered sensory perception.

Figure 7-4. ◆ Surgical areas to be shaved. (A) Head surgery. (B) Abdominal surgery. (C) Thoracoabdominal surgery. (D) Gynecologic surgery. (E) Genitourinary surgery. (F) Forearm, elbow, or hand surgery. (G) Hip surgery. (H) Lower leg or foot surgery.

DIAGNOSING, PLANNING, AND IMPLEMENTING

The nursing care plan for the intraoperative client is established by the registered nurse in collaboration with other members of the surgical team.

RISK FOR PERIOPERATIVE POSITIONING INJURY

■ Assess client for potential risk factors, including history of arthritis or other musculoskeletal disorders and lack of

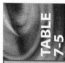

TABLE 7-5   COMMON SURGICAL POSITIONS

POSITION AND USE	POSSIBLE ADVERSE EFFECTS AND NURSING INTERVENTIONS
(a) The *dorsal recumbent or supine position* is used for many abdominal surgeries (e.g., colostomy and herniorrhaphy) as well as for some thoracic surgeries (e.g., open heart surgery) and some surgeries on the extremities.	This position may cause excessive pressure on posterior bony prominences, such as the back of the head, scapulae, sacrum, and heels. Pad these areas with soft materials. To avoid compression of blood vessels and sluggish circulation, ensure that the knees are not flexed. Use trochanter rolls or other padding to avoid internal or external rotation of the hips and shoulders.
(b) The *semi-sitting position* is used for surgeries on the thyroid and neck areas.	This position can lead to postural hypotension and venous pooling in the legs. It may promote skin breakdown on the buttocks. Sciatic nerve injury is possible. Assess for hypotension. Ensure that knees are not sharply flexed. Use soft padding to prevent nerve compression.
(c) The *prone position* is used for spinal fusion and removal of hemorrhoids.	This position causes pressure on the face, knees, thighs, anterior ankles, and toes. Pad bony prominences, and support the feet under the ankles. To promote optimum respiratory function, raise the client's chest and abdomen and support with padding. Corneal abrasion could occur if the eyes are not closed or are insufficiently padded.
(d) The *lateral chest position* is used for some thoracic surgeries as well as hip replacements.	This may cause excessive pressure on the bony prominences on the side on which the client is positioned. Ensure adequate padding and support, especially on the downside arm. The weight of the upper leg may cause peroneal nerve injury on the downside leg. Both legs must therefore be padded.
(e) The *lithotomy position* is used for gynecologic, perineal, or rectal surgeries.	This position causes an 18% decrease (from a standing position) in vital capacity of the lungs. Monitor respirations, and assess for hypoxia and dyspnea. The lithotomy position can lead to joint damage, peroneal nerve damage, and damage to peripheral blood vessels. To avoid injury, ensure adequate padding, and manipulate both legs into the stirrups simultaneously.
(f) The *jackknife position* is used for proctologic surgeries, such as removal of hemorrhoids, and for some spinal surgeries.	This position causes a 12% decrease (from a standing position) in vital capacity of the lungs. Monitor respirations, and assess for hypoxia and dyspnea. In this position, the greatest pressure is felt at the bends in the table. Therefore, the client is supported with pads at the groin and knees, as well as at the ankles. Padding of the chest and knees helps prevent skin breakdown. Padding and proper positioning help prevent pressure on the ear, the neck, and the nerves of the upper arm.

population
FOCUS

Older Adult Undergoing Surgery

Because of *cardiovascular and tissue changes* that result from aging, surgeries lasting longer than 2 hours place the older adult at increased risk for complications. The older adult is more prone to hypotension, hypothermia, and hypoxemia resulting from anesthesia and the cool temperature in the operating room.

Other complications experienced by the older adult result from *positioning*. Intraoperative positioning of arthritic joints can result in postoperative joint pain that is unrelated to the operative site. The older client is at increased risk for developing skin breakdown because of decreased subcutaneous fat tissue and reduced peripheral circulation. Elderly clients who remain in the same position for an extended period of time have increased risk of this complication.

Some older adults have *hearing or visual impairment*. Sensory impairments, coupled with an unfamiliar environment, can make the operating room a frightening, disorienting place. By effectively communicating with the client, the nurse can provide support and reassurance to minimize these factors.

optimal tissue integrity due to aging or nutritional status. *Information provides a basis for planning.*

■ Report data to the physician if condition requires adjustment to planned position. *This ensures patient safety yet provides the means to accomplish surgical procedure.*

■ Use safety belts to secure client to stretcher and operating room table. *Belts reduce risk of falls when client's awareness is decreased.*

■ Provide padding to bony prominences on patient at risk for tissue breakdown due to prolonged pressure. *Padding prevents excessive pressure on body parts.*

RISK FOR INFECTION

■ Assess sterility status of all instruments and supplies used in the operating room. *Decreases risk of introduction of pathogens during the surgical procedure.*

■ Report results of lab studies that may indicate systemic infection. *Client may require prophylactic antibiotics.*

■ Follow instructions related to surgical shaves and skin prep. *Preparation reduces bacteria at surgical site.*

■ Inform any member of the surgical team if breaks or potential breaks in technique are observed (e.g., tears in sterile gloves, contamination of equipment or surgical instruments). *The circulating nurse is responsible for assuring strict aseptic technique is followed in the operating room.*

RISK FOR IMBALANCED BODY TEMPERATURE

Surgical clients are at risk for injury due to the cool environment of the operating room. Hyperthermia may occur from the effects of anesthesia or from medications used during the intraoperative phase.

■ Assess client's temperature prior to induction of anesthesia. *This provides baseline data.*

■ Assess environmental temperature and patient response. *Temperature can be modified to maintain client's body temperature.*

■ Note changes in client's temperature, and intervene as soon as possible (e.g., provide cooling or warming blanket). *Prompt response reduces risk for injury.*

RISK FOR ASPIRATION

■ Assess NPO status. *Data provide a basis for decision making about postponing or canceling surgery. A nasogastric tube may be inserted.*

■ Report noncompliance with NPO status to the surgeon or anesthesiologist. *Surgery may have to be delayed or canceled.*

■ Insert nasogastric tube if ordered. *Clients requiring emergency surgery may have eaten. Anesthetic agents may also contribute to aspiration risk. Removal of stomach contents reduces risk of aspiration.*

EVALUATING

The nurse evaluates whether or not expected outcomes are met. Validation includes:

■ Client is free from injury during the intraoperative period.
■ Client's body temperature remains within normal limits during the intraoperative period.
■ No evidence of breaks in aseptic technique during the intraoperative period.

Postoperative Phase

COLLABORATIVE CARE
Pharmacology

Pharmacologic management of acute postoperative pain is of primary concern to the client, surgeon, and nurse. Established, severe pain is more difficult to treat than pain that is at its onset. Initially, postoperative analgesics should be administered at regular intervals to maintain a therapeutic blood level. As-needed (PRN) administration allows for a lowering of this therapeutic level; delays in medication administration further increase pain intensity. (Chapter 6 discusses care of the client in pain.)

Nonsteroidal anti-inflammatory drugs (NSAIDs) (e.g., ibuprofen, Toradol) should be administered to treat mild to moderate postoperative pain. They should be given soon after surgery (orally, parenterally, or rectally) along with opioids unless contraindicated. NSAIDs may not control pain completely, but they allow for lower dosages of opioid analgesics and, therefore, fewer side effects. NSAIDs can be given safely to older clients, but the nurse should observe closely for side effects, especially gastric, hepatic, and renal toxicity.

Opioid analgesics, such as morphine and meperidine (Demerol), are the foundation for managing moderate to severe postoperative pain. Opioid dosage requirements vary greatly from one client to another, so the dosage must be individually tailored.

Contrary to the belief of many health care providers, physical dependence and tolerance to opioid analgesics are uncommon in short-term postoperative use. Also, when opioid analgesics are used to treat acute pain, they rarely lead to psychological dependence and addiction.

Older clients tend to experience a higher peak effect and longer duration of pain control with opioids.

Common Postoperative Complications

A number of factors place the client at risk for postoperative complications. Nursing care before, during, and after surgery is aimed at preventing and/or minimizing the effects of these complications.

CARDIOVASCULAR COMPLICATIONS

Shock. **Shock** is a life-threatening postoperative complication that results from an insufficient blood flow to vital organs. *Hypovolemic shock,* the most common type in the postoperative client, results from a decrease in circulating fluid volume from loss of blood, severe vomiting, or prolonged diarrhea. The greater the loss of fluid volume, the more severe the symptoms. (See section on shock in Chapter 10.)

Hemorrhage. **Hemorrhage** is excessive loss of blood. A concealed hemorrhage occurs internally from a blood vessel that is no longer sutured or cauterized, or from a drainage tube that has eroded a blood vessel. An obvious hemorrhage occurs externally from a dislodged or ill-formed clot at the wound. Hemorrhage also may result from abnormalities in the blood's ability to clot, either because of illness or as a side effect of medications.

A venous hemorrhage oozes out quickly and is dark red. An arterial hemorrhage spurts bright red blood with each heartbeat. Either type of hemorrhage will cause hypovolemic shock if enough blood is lost from the circulation.

Assessment findings depend on the amount and rate of blood loss. Restlessness and anxiety are observed in the early stage of hemorrhage. Frank bleeding will be present if the hemorrhage is external. Manifestations of hypovolemic shock also will be noted (see Box 10-3).

Deep Venous Thrombosis (DVT). *DVT* is the formation of a *thrombus* (blood clot) that occurs in association with inflammation in deep veins. This complication occurs most often in the lower extremities of the postoperative client. It may result from a combination of factors, including trauma during surgery, pressure applied under the knees, and sluggish blood flow during and after surgery. Clients particularly at risk for developing DVT include those who:

- Have undergone orthopedic surgery to lower extremities; urologic, gynecologic, or obstetric surgeries; or neurosurgery
- Have varicose veins
- Have a history of thrombophlebitis or pulmonary emboli

- Are over age 40
- Are obese
- Have an infection
- Have a malignancy

Common assessment findings of DVT reveal pain or cramping in the involved calf or thigh. Redness and edema of the entire extremity may occur along with a slightly elevated temperature. A positive *Homans' sign* (pain in the calf on dorsiflexion of the affected foot; see Box 23-14) may be noted.

Pulmonary Embolism. A *pulmonary embolism* is a blood clot or other substance that lodges in a pulmonary artery. For the postoperative client with DVT, the threat that a portion of the thrombus may dislodge and travel to the lung, heart, or brain is a constant concern. Early detection of this potentially life-threatening complication depends on the nurse's careful, continuing assessment of the postoperative client.

Signs and symptoms of a pulmonary embolism include mild to moderate dyspnea, chest pain, diaphoresis, anxiety, restlessness, rapid respirations and pulse, dysrhythmias, cough, and cyanosis. Sudden death can occur if a major pulmonary artery becomes completely blocked.

RESPIRATORY COMPLICATIONS.
Common postoperative respiratory complications include pneumonia and atelectasis.

Pneumonia. *Pneumonia* (inflammation of lung tissue) is caused either by an infection or by the presence of a foreign substance in the lung, which leads to an infection. Factors involved in the development of pneumonia include aspiration, infection, retained pulmonary secretions, failure to cough deeply, impaired cough reflex, and decreased mobility.

Common assessment findings (see also Box 26-4) of the client with pneumonia include:

- High fever
- Rapid pulse and respirations
- Chills (may be present initially)
- Productive cough (depending on the type of pneumonia)
- Dyspnea
- Chest pain
- Crackles and wheezes

Treating the pulmonary infection, supporting the client's respiratory efforts, promoting lung expansion, and preventing the organisms' spread are the goals in caring for the client with pneumonia.

Atelectasis. Atelectasis is an incomplete expansion or collapse of lung tissue. It results in inadequate ventilation and buildup of pulmonary secretions. Assessment findings commonly observed include dyspnea, diminished breath sounds over the affected area, anxiety, restlessness, crackles, and cyanosis. Promoting lung expansion and systemic oxygenation of tissues is a goal in the care of the client with atelectasis (see also Chapter 26).

COMPLICATIONS IN ELIMINATION. Common postoperative complications associated with elimination include urinary retention and altered bowel elimination. Urinary retention may occur postoperatively as a result of the recumbent position, effects of anesthesia and narcotics, inactivity, altered fluid balance, anxiety, or surgical manipulation in the pelvic area.

Bowel elimination frequently is altered after abdominal or pelvic surgery and sometimes after other surgeries as well. Return to normal gastrointestinal function may be delayed by general anesthesia, narcotic analgesia, decreased mobility, or altered fluid and food intake during the perioperative period.

WOUND COMPLICATIONS

Normal Wound Healing. Wounds heal by primary, secondary, or tertiary intention (Figure 7-5 ◆):

1. Healing by **primary intention** takes place when the wound is uncomplicated and clean and has sustained little tissue loss. The edges of the incision are well *approximated* (have come together well) with sutures or staples.

Primary intention

Clean incision

Early suture

"Hairline" scar

Secondary intention

Gaping wound with blood clot

Granulation tissue fills in wound

Large scar

Tertiary intention

Contaminated wound

Granulation tissue

Closure with wide scar

Figure 7-5. ◆ Wound healing by primary, secondary, and tertiary intention.

This type of incision heals quickly with very little scarring.

2. **Secondary intention** refers to the healing that occurs when the wound is large, gaping, and irregular. Tissue loss prevents wound edges from approximating, so granulation takes place to fill in the wound. This type of wound takes longer to heal, is more prone to infection, and develops more scar tissue.

3. Healing by **tertiary intention** occurs when substantial time passes before a wound is sutured. Infection is more likely. Wound edges are not approximated, so tissue is replaced by granulation. Closure of the wound may result in a wide scar.

Healing time varies according to many factors, such as age, nutritional status, general health, and the type and location of the wound.

Wound Drainage. Wound drainage *(exudate)* results from the inflammatory process that occurs in the first two stages of wound healing. The drainage is from the rich blood supply that surrounds the wound tissue and is composed of escaped fluid and cells. The drainage is described as serous, sanguineous, or purulent.

- *Serous drainage* contains mostly the clear portion of the blood. The drainage appears clear or slightly yellow and is thin in consistency.
- *Sanguineous drainage* contains a combination of serum and red blood cells and has a thick, reddish appearance. This is the most common drainage from a noncomplicated surgical wound.
- *Purulent drainage* is composed of white blood cells, tissue debris, and bacteria. Purulent drainage is the result of infection and tends to be of a thicker consistency, with various colors specific to the type of organism. It also may have an unpleasant odor.

Other common assessment findings of an infected wound include redness, warmth, and edema around the edges of the incision. The client may have a fever, chills, and increased respiratory and pulse rates.

Nursing care of the postoperative client with a surgical wound focuses on preventing and monitoring for wound complications. The nurse assumes a leading role in supporting the wound-healing process, providing emotional support to the client, and teaching wound care to the client. Box 7-4 describes and illustrates wound drainage devices that decrease pressure in the wound area by removing excess fluid.

Dehiscence. **Dehiscence** is a separation in the layers of the incisional wound (Figure 7-6A ◆). When dehiscence occurs, the wound should be covered immediately with a sterile dressing moistened with normal saline. Treatment depends on the extent of wound disruption. If the dehiscence is extensive, the incision must be resutured in surgery.

BOX 7-4
WOUND DRAINAGE DEVICES

A Penrose (A) **drain,** used for passive wound drainage, promotes healing from the inside to the outside (see figure). The use of the drain decreases the chance of abscess formation. The safety pin in the Penrose drain prevents the exposed end from slipping down into the wound.

Wound care focuses on cleaning around the drain with a prescribed solution, such as sterile normal saline, and replacing the precut gauze dressing as necessary to keep the surrounding skin dry and to encourage further drainage. An absorbent dressing is placed over the drain and gauze (not shown).

Wound **suction** devices promote drainage of fluid from the incision site, decreasing pressure on healing tissues and reducing abscess formation. Shown are the Jackson Pratt (B) and Hemovac (C) wound suction devices (see figures).

The frequency with which the nurse empties the device depends on the time elapsed since surgery, type of surgery, amount of drainage, and hospital policy. For example, immediately after surgery the nurse may empty the device every 15 to 60 minutes. As drainage decreases, the device is emptied every 2 to 4 hours (per hospital policy). Amount, color, consistency, and odor of drainage are documented.

Usually, the nurse removes the drain on the second to fourth day after surgery (depending on hospital policy). Removal causes minor client discomfort. The drain site is cleaned, and a sterile dressing is applied.

Evisceration. Evisceration is the protrusion of body organs from a wound dehiscence (see Figure 7-6B). Like dehiscence, this serious complication may result from delayed wound healing, may occur immediately following surgery, or may occur after forceful straining (coughing, sneezing, or vomiting). Emergency surgery is performed to repair evisceration.

The nurse or physician removes sutures or staples after the wound has healed sufficiently (usually 5 to 10 days after surgery). Removal is performed using medical aseptic technique. Strips of tape (or Steri-Strips) may be applied to provide additional support to the incision, as directed by institutional policy or by the physician.

Special Considerations for Older Adults. The older adult is at increased risk for postoperative complications because of physiologic, cognitive, and psychosocial changes associated with the aging process. The nurse must be aware of these normal changes and must modify nursing care accordingly to provide safe, supportive care.

CLINICAL alert

Monitor the elderly client for response to medication and treatment. Common symptoms include acute confusion, restlessness, changes in level of consciousness, and withdrawal from the environment.

NURSING CARE

ASSESSING

Postoperative care begins when the client is transferred from the operating room to the PACU. The nurse monitors the client's respiratory and cardiovascular status, vital signs, surgical site, and level of consciousness to determine the response to

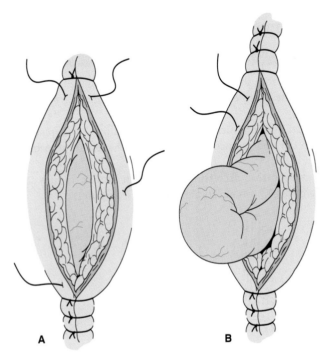

Figure 7-6. ◆ Wound complications. (A) Dehiscence.
(B) Evisceration.

the surgical procedure and anesthesia. In addition, the PACU nurse assesses the client's pain level. Careful administration of analgesics provides comfort yet does not compound the potential side effects from the anesthesia.

After the client is stabilized and awakens, the client is transferred to his or her room. Prior to the client's arrival, the PACU nurse communicates specific information about the client's condition and postoperative orders to the unit nurse. This prepares the nurse for any additional problems or needed equipment.

The hospital policy or physician's orders dictate the frequency of follow-up assessments. After major surgery, the nurse generally assesses the client every 15 minutes during the first hour and, if the client is stable, every 30 minutes for the next 2 hours, and then every hour during the subsequent 4 hours. Then assessments are carried out every 4 hours, unless the client's condition changes or protocol for the particular surgical procedure says otherwise.

After carrying out the initial assessment and ensuring the client's safety by lowering the bed, raising the side rails, and placing the call light within reach, the nurse notes the physician's postoperative orders. These orders guide the nurse in the specific care of the postoperative client. They specify activity level, diet, medications for pain and nausea, antibiotics, continuation of preoperative medications, frequency of vital sign assessments, administration of intravenous fluids, and laboratory tests such as hemoglobin and potassium level. In most institutions, orders written prior to surgery must be reordered following surgery because the client's condition is assumed to have changed.

DIAGNOSING, PLANNING, AND IMPLEMENTING

Nursing care planning during the postoperative phase should focus on prevention of postoperative complications.

ACUTE PAIN

Pain is expected after surgery. Managing acute postoperative pain is an important nursing role before, during, and after surgery. It involves cooperation of the client, physician, and nurse. Preoperatively, the client should be made aware of how much pain to anticipate and what methods are available to control pain (see Chapter 6). After discussing options with the client, health care providers must respect the client's personal preferences.

■ Assess level of pain at least every 4 hours. Have patient describe pain on a scale of 0 to 10 (where 0 is no pain and 10 is the worst pain). *Controlling postoperative pain not only promotes comfort but also facilitates coughing, turning, deep-breathing exercises, and early ambulation. Rating the pain provides a more objective description and helps the nurse to choose pain medication appropriate to severity of the pain.*

■ Identify location and source of pain. *Assessment data are used to plan interventions.*

■ Administer pain medication as prescribed. *Medication provides comfort and allows the client to rest.*

■ Initiate nonpharmacologic approaches to pain management such as relaxation, distraction, and imagery techniques. *These techniques complement pain medication.*

■ Evaluate effectiveness of pain medication within 30 to 45 minutes. *Effectiveness may indicate a need for change of dosage or medication.*

■ Document administration of pain medication. Communicate to all members of the health care team. *Documentation and communication ensure continuity of care.*

RISK FOR INJURY (HEMORRHAGE)

■ Apply one or more sterile gauze pads and a snug pressure dressing to the area. If external bleeding is severe, apply mechanical pressure with gloved hands. *Pressure assists the coagulation process. Increased pressure may be necessary to achieve coagulation.*

■ Notify physician of events. *Medical intervention is needed to correct the complication.*

■ Monitor vital signs frequently. *Data are used to assess physiologic response to the event.*

■ Establish or maintain intravenous access. *Rapid infusion of fluids may be necessary to maintain or replace fluid volume.*

■ Prepare client and family for emergency surgery. *Surgery may be necessary to locate and repair the source of bleeding.*

INEFFECTIVE TISSUE PERFUSION

Deep vein thrombosis usually occurs in the postoperative patient due to venous stasis as a result of immobility. Nursing care focuses on prevention of this life-threatening complication.

- Assess the Homans' sign at least every 4 hours. Evaluate positive response and report findings to the physician. *This provides early detection of signs of DVT.*
- Encourage postoperative leg exercises at least every 2 hours. Encourage early ambulation. *Exercise prevents venous stasis, and enhances venous return.*
- Administer anticoagulants as prescribed. *Anticoagulants prevent platelet aggregation and decrease the risk of clot formation.*
- Monitor laboratory values for clotting times. *This information is used to determine dosage of anticoagulant medications.*
- Apply thigh-high antiemboli stockings or prescribed devices. *Stockings stimulate venous return.*

IMPAIRED GAS EXCHANGE (PULMONARY EMBOLUS)

- Immediately notify the charge nurse and physician. *Stabilizing respiratory and cardiovascular functioning while preventing the formation of additional emboli is of utmost importance. Additional nursing care and medical care assistance are needed.*
- Frequently assess and record general condition and vital signs. *This monitors physiologic response and determines whether there is a need for additional intervention.*
- Maintain the client on bed rest, and keep the head of the bed elevated. *This position facilitates breathing and prevents extension of the condition.*
- Provide oxygen as ordered and monitor pulse oximetry. *This supports respiratory status and detects a deteriorating condition early.*
- Administer prescribed intravenous fluids. *Circulating volume must be maintained.*
- Administer prescribed anticoagulants. *This prevents development of additional clots.*

INEFFECTIVE BREATHING PATTERN (PNEUMONIA OR ATELECTASIS)

- Position client with the head of the bed elevated. *This facilitates lung expansion.*
- Encourage the client to turn, cough, and perform deep-breathing exercises at least every 2 hours. *This mobilizes secretions and supports airway clearance.*
- Assist with and encourage incentive spirometry, intermittent positive pressure breathing (IPPB), and nebulizer treatments as ordered. *These expand alveoli and facilitate airway clearance.*
- Ambulate client as condition permits and as prescribed. *Ambulation reduces the risk of complications related to immobility.*
- Administer oxygen as ordered. *This improves gas exchange and oxygenates the tissues.*
- Assess vital signs, breath sounds, and general condition. *Chronically ill or malnourished clients, clients with a history of chronic lung disease, and the elderly are at increased risk for these complications. Data allow treatment to be evaluated.*
- Maintain fluid intake to at least 2,000 mL/day if condition permits. *Fluid liquefies secretion for easier clearance.*

RISK FOR INFECTION (SURGICAL INCISION)

- Maintain medical asepsis (use good handwashing technique). Observe aseptic technique during dressing changes and handling of tubes and drains. *Asepsis reduces risk of introducing microorganisms into surgical wounds.*
- Assess vital signs, especially temperature. *Elevated temperature may indicate development of infection.*
- Evaluate the characteristics of wound discharge (color, odor, and amount). *They indicate presence or absence of wound infection.*
- Assess the condition of the incision (approximation of the edges, sutures, staples, or drains). *Integrity of the incision site reduces risk factors.*
- Maintain the client's hydration and nutritional status. *Nutrition facilitates healing.*

RISK FOR URINARY RETENTION

- Assess for bladder distention if the client has not voided within 7 to 8 hours after surgery or if the client is urinating small amounts frequently. *Early detection of urinary retention provides information for intervention.*
- Increase daily oral fluid intake to 2,500 to 3,000 mL if the client's condition permits. *This facilitates renal function.*
- Insert a straight or indwelling catheter if ordered. *Emptying the bladder provides comfort.*
- Assist patient to void by:
  - Assisting and providing privacy when the client uses a bedpan.
  - Helping the client to use the bedside commode or to walk to the bathroom.
  - Assisting male clients to stand to void.

These promote normal urinary elimination.

RISK FOR CONSTIPATION

- Auscultate bowel sounds every 4 hours while the client is awake. Assess the abdomen for distention. Determine whether the client is passing flatus. Monitor for passage of stool, including amount and consistency. *A distended abdomen with absent or high-pitched bowel sounds may indicate paralytic ileus. These measures evaluate presence or absence of peristalsis.*
- Encourage early ambulation within prescribed limits. *Mobility stimulates peristalsis.*
- Facilitate a daily fluid intake of 2,500 to 3,000 mL (unless contraindicated). *Fluids provide moisture and facilitate passage of stool.*

■ Provide privacy when the client is using the bedpan, bedside commode, or bathroom. *Privacy provides relaxation and facilitates bowel elimination.*

EVALUATING

Careful evaluation of the postoperative client's progress is essential to prevent development of complications and prompt intervention should they occur. Expected outcomes include:

■ Client is free of wound or systemic infection.
■ Homans' sign is negative.
■ Oxygen saturation remains at least 90%.
■ Client voids at least 1,000 mL in 24 hours.
■ Breath sounds remain clear.
■ Client performs incentive spirometry exercises at least every 4 hours.
■ Client voids within 7 hours of returning to the nursing unit.
■ Bowel sounds are active in all four quadrants within 24 hours of abdominal surgery.

Discharge Considerations

Because the postoperative phase does not end until the client has recovered completely from the surgical intervention, the nurse's role is vital as the client nears discharge. To prepare the client to recuperate at home, the nurse provides information and supports the client to meet self-care demands. Written guidelines, directions, and information should accompany all aspects of teaching, especially when teaching involves a large amount of unfamiliar detail. The nurse must be organized in order to educate the client and family during the brief hospital stay. The most common teaching needs are as follows:

■ *Wound care.* Teaching is more effective if the nurse first demonstrates and explains the procedure, then asks the client and family to participate in the care. The nurse should ask the client or caregiver to demonstrate the procedure in return. Ideally, teaching is carried out over several days, evaluated, and reinforced.
■ *Signs and symptoms of a wound infection.* Teach the client what is normal and what should be reported to the physician.
■ *Method and frequency of taking one's temperature.*
■ *Limitations or restrictions on activities* (lifting, driving, bathing, sexual activity, return to work or school, and other physical activities).
■ *Control of pain.* If analgesics are prescribed, instruct the client in the dosage, frequency, purpose, common side effects, and symptoms to report to the physician. Reinforce the use of relaxation, distraction, imagery, or other pain-control techniques that the client has found useful in controlling postoperative pain.

Outpatient Surgery

Outpatient, ambulatory, or same-day surgery is performed on a nonhospitalized client under local or general anesthesia. The surgical procedure is short, usually lasting 15 to 90 minutes. Following the surgical procedure, the client may be discharged immediately or remain for a short period of postoperative recovery and observation. Surgeries such as cataract removal with or without lens implant, hernia repair, tubal ligation, vasectomy, dilation and curettage (D&C), and biopsy are routinely performed on an outpatient basis.

The number of outpatient surgeries has grown rapidly in the past decade as part of the effort to contain the high costs of surgery. Increasingly complex surgeries on clients with complicated medical problems are now commonly performed on an outpatient basis. There are advantages and disadvantages to outpatient surgery. This increase in number of procedures and acuity level of the clients presents a challenge to the perioperative nurse.

Many similarities exist in nursing care of the inpatient and outpatient surgical client. Physical care is provided in much the same manner in the preoperative, intraoperative, and postoperative phases of surgery.

The major differences lie in the degree of teaching and emotional support that must be provided. In addition to the physiologic insult of surgery, the outpatient surgical client must cope with the additional stress produced by the need to learn a great deal of information in a short span of time. The nurse teaches the client and family in both the preoperative and postoperative periods, to enable the client to perform self-care following discharge. More extensive teaching and emotional support are required as clients with complicated health problems undergo complex surgical procedures as outpatients. (Figure 7-7 ◆ shows a standard outpatient care plan form.)

Following outpatient surgery, the client is discharged after meeting the institution's criteria. Discharge criteria may include:

■ Vital signs are stable.
■ Client is able to stand and begin to walk without dizziness or nausea.
■ Pain is controlled or alleviated.
■ Client is able to urinate.
■ Client is oriented (returned to preoperative mental status).
■ Client and family/caregiver demonstrate understanding of postoperative instructions.

Nursing Interventions Classification

Some of the following nursing interventions (McCloskey & Bulechek, 2000) may also be useful in planning and implementing care for the client undergoing surgery:

OUTPATIENT CARE PLAN

Outpatient Surgery Center
Directions: Each unit, please check "Yes" or "No" and initial
appropriate space in column on right.

Client's Name _____ Date _____

NURSING DIAGNOSES	CLIENT OUTCOME STANDARDS	Goal Met		OPTI	PREOP	OR	PACU	OBS
I. A. Anxiety related to knowledge deficit regarding surgical procedure. B. Fear related to risk of death, alteration of body image, or change in lifestyle. C. Impaired verbal communication related to anxiety. D. Impaired verbal communication related to preoperative medication/sedation. E. Impaired verbal communication related to language barrier. F. Ineffective individual or family coping related to perceived threat of surgery or surgical outcome. G. Noncompliance related to sensory alteration, fear, anxiety. H. Sensory–perceptual alteration related to inadequate tissue perfusion, or preexisting deficits.	**I.** The client demonstrates knowledge of the physiologic and psychological responses to surgical intervention. Comments _____ _____ _____ _____ _____ _____	Yes						
		No						
II. A. Potential for infection related to: Type of operative procedure Wound classification Tissues transected Length of procedure Preexisting disease process Obesity Length of preoperative hospitalization Implants Presence/insertion of invasive/indwelling lines	**II.** The client is free from infection. Comments _____ _____ _____ _____	Yes						
		No						
III. A. Potential for impaired skin integrity related to: Positioning Preexisting disease process Pooling of prep solutions under client Improper placement of electrical dispersive pad Impaired circulation Poor tissue perfusion Allergic reactions to chemical agents	**III.** The client's skin integrity is maintained. Comments _____ _____ _____	Yes						
		No						
IV. A. Potential for injury related to: Electrical hazards Positioning Retained foreign objects External constriction of peripheral circulation Chemical agents (ETO or Glutaraldehyde residuals, irritants, allergans) B. Impaired gas exchange related to: Positioning Inadequate airway Obesity C. Impaired physical mobility related to positioning.	**IV.** The client is free from injury related to positioning; extraneous objects; or chemical, physical, and electrical hazards. Comments _____ _____ _____ _____	Yes						
		No						
V. A. Potential for fluid and electrolyte imbalance related to: Type of surgical procedure Excessive blood loss Shock, trauma	**V.** The client's fluid and electrolyte balance is maintained. Comments _____ _____ _____	Yes						
		No						
VI. A. Potential for altered or ineffective participation in rehabilitation related to: Ineffective coping mechanisms Anxiety due to surgical outcomes Lack of resources for self-care after discharge	**VI.** The client participates in the rehabilitation process. Comments _____ _____ _____	Yes						
		No						

Figure 7-7. ◆ Outpatient care plan form.

- Coping Enhancement
- Decision-Making Support
- Embolus Precautions
- Intravenous (IV) Therapy
- Discharge Planning

- Lab Data Interpretation
- Medication Administration
- Learning Facilitation

(*Note:* The bibliography listings for this and all chapters have been compiled at the back of the book.)

Chapter Review

key terms by topic

Use the CD-ROM disk enclosed with your textbook to hear the pronunciation of the key terms in the chapter.

Surgery
preoperative phase, intraoperative phase, postoperative phase, inpatient surgery, outpatient surgery

Intraoperative phase
anesthesia

key points

■ Perioperative nursing includes care of the client through three phases: preoperative, intraoperative, postoperative.

■ Care of the surgical client should focus on psychological as well as physiologic risk factors.

■ Thorough nursing assessment is key to identifying potential risk factors that may lead to perioperative complications.

■ Nursing interventions are developed to prevent development of perioperative complications.

■ Control of postoperative pain is a major concern of the surgical client.

■ Patient education is a critical tool to prepare the client for the perioperative experience. Inclusion of family members and caregivers is essential for success of the nursing plan of care.

■ Major postoperative complications include respiratory and cardiovascular disorders, infection, hemorrhage, and elimination disorders.

■ Collaboration of all members of the health care team is essential to achieve an optimal outcome for the surgical client.

Medialink

Additional interactive resources for this chapter can be found on the Companion Website at www.prenhall.com/burke. Click on Chapter 7 and "Begin" to select the activities for this chapter.

For NCLEX review questions and an audio glossary, access the accompanying CD-ROM in this book.

for further study

For more information about assessing and managing pain in clients, see Chapter 6.

For illustration of assessment of Homans' sign, see Box 23-14.

For further study about nursing care of constipation, see Chapter 20; and for urinary retention, see Chapter 21.

For more about promoting lung expansion and systemic oxygenation, see Chapter 26.

Critical Thinking Care Map

Caring for a Client After Surgery
NCLEX-PN Focus Area: Safety and Infection Control

Case Study: Mrs. Wilson, age 80, is 3 days post total hip replacement of her right hip. Daniel Moore, LPN, is assigned to her care. Mr. Moore performs a complete head-to-toe assessment and determines that Mrs. Wilson is alert and oriented. Her skin is warm and moist. Mrs. Wilson states she has slight discomfort with incisional pain of 3 on a 0- to 10-point scale. She complains of feeling warm and has chills. Vital signs are: T 101° F, P 100, R 24, BP 134/82. She is on a soft diet and states she is "drinking lots of fluids." An intravenous solution of dextrose and water is infusing at 100 mL/h per infusion pump. No redness or edema is noted at the infusion site. Mrs. Wilson is receiving ciprofloxacin hydrochloride (Cipro) PO every 8 hours. She has a gauze dressing to the right hip incision. The dressing is intact with a 3-cm area of light brown drainage. Mr. Moore removes the dressing and notes the incision to be red and edematous with a 2-cm opening. Steri-Strips are in place, and a Jackson Pratt drain is in place. Mr. Moore empties 25 mL of dark red drainage from the device. Mrs. Wilson has a Foley catheter in place with 250 mL of clear, light amber urine in the bag.

When assessing Mrs. Wilson's lower extremities, Mr. Moore finds her feet pink and warm with rapid capillary refill. Dorsalis pedis and posterior tibial pulses are strong and equal bilaterally. Mr. Moore notes slight pitting edema in the right foot and ankle. Sensation and ability to move both extremities are noted. Review of lab work reveals Hgb 11.3 g, Hct 38.4%, WBC 13,000 mm^3.

Nursing Diagnosis: Risk for Infection

COLLECT DATA

Subjective	Objective
_____	_____
_____	_____
_____	_____
_____	_____
_____	_____
_____	_____

Would you report this data? Yes/No

If yes, to: _____

Nursing Care

_____
_____
_____
_____
_____
_____

How would you document this? _____
_____
_____

Data Collected
(use those that apply)

- Alert and oriented
- Incisional pain
- T 101° F, P 100
- Jackson Pratt drain in place
- WBC 13,000 mm^3
- IV infusing at 100 mL/h
- Pedal pulses strong
- Light brown drainage on dressing
- Foley has 250 mL clear, light amber urine
- Incision red, edematous, 2-cm opening
- Complains of feeling warm and has chills
- Cipro 250 mg q 8 h
- States she is "drinking lots of fluids"

Nursing Interventions
(use those that apply)

- Empty Jackson Pratt drain q 4 h.
- Monitor vital signs, especially temperature and pulse, q 4 h. Report temperature above 100° F to charge nurse.
- Assess pedal pulses q 8 h.
- Provide extra blankets for warmth.
- Change dressing, using aseptic technique, twice per day.
- Assess wound status with each dressing change.
- Tylenol 325 mg PO q 4 h for temperature above 100° F.
- Cleanse wound with normal saline qd, per physician's order.
- Monitor urinary output.
- Maintain fluid intake at least 2,000 mL/day.
- Administer pain medications as needed.
- Administer antibiotics as ordered.
- Collect sample of wound drainage, send to lab for culture and sensitivity.

NCLEX-PN Exam Preparation

1. A client is scheduled for a thyroidectomy. Which of the following would be an appropriate preoperative nursing diagnosis?
   a. Infection, Risk for (surgical wound)
   b. Aspiration, Risk for
   c. Knowledge Deficit (surgical procedure)
   d. Urinary Elimination, Altered (urinary retention)

2. A man is admitted to the ambulatory surgery unit in preparation for a hernia repair. Which of the following lab results noted by the nurse may require medical intervention?
   a. hemoglobin 13.4, hematocrit 44
   b. potassium 2.8
   c. platelets 280,000
   d. blood urea nitrogen (BUN) 10

3. A client asks the nurse to explain possible complications she might experience as a result of her total abdominal hysterectomy. The MOST appropriate response by the nurse would be:
   a. "I will contact your physician to discuss this with you."
   b. "Let's not worry about complications. You will be just fine."
   c. "Why are you worried about complications?"
   d. "There are many potential complications. Let's discuss them."

4. A client is 5 hours postoperative. He has an IV infusing at 125 mL/hr. He has not voided and complains of pain in his lower abdomen. The nurse's FIRST action should be to:
   a. assist Mr. Harris to stand to void
   b. assess the bladder for distention
   c. take his vital signs
   d. administer pain medication

5. A client has been taught coughing exercises prior to surgery. Which one of the following actions indicates need for further teaching?
   a. He splints his incision with a pillow.
   b. He takes a deep breath through his nose prior to coughing.
   c. He positions himself supine and flat in bed.
   d. He coughs forcefully after the deep breath.

6. The client's surgical incision is healing by primary intention. Which assessment finding should the nurse expect?
   a. The wound is large, gaping, and irregular.
   b. Wound exudate is present.
   c. Wound edges are approximated.
   d. Granulation tissue is evident.

7. A teenage girl, age 16, and her husband, age 23, present to the outpatient center to complete her preoperative procedures. The appropriate procedure for completion of the surgical consent would be to:
   a. have the husband sign the consent for the wife
   b. have the girl sign the consent
   c. have the husband co-sign the consent
   d. contact the girl's parents to sign the consent

8. The nurse assesses the postoperative client on return to the nursing unit. The following data are collected:
   1:15 P.M.: T 99° F, P 92, R 20, BP 120/80, alert, oriented
   1:30 P.M.: T 98° F, P 100, R 24, BP 116/68, sleeping
   1:45 P.M.: T 98° F, P 116, R 28, BP 100/54, restless
   2:00 P.M.: T 97° F, P 130, R 32, BP 90/50, restless, drowsy

   The appropriate INITIAL nursing action would be to:
   a. assess the surgical dressing
   b. notify the physician
   c. position the client flat with the feet elevated 8 to 12 inches
   d. increase the IV infusion rate

9. A client had a right total hip replacement 3 days ago. The LPN/LVN assesses a positive Homans' sign in the left leg. The MOST important action by the nurse at this time would be to:
   a. document the findings
   b. notify the physician
   c. place the client on complete bed rest
   d. assess the extremity for signs of thrombus formation

10. A client asks if she should take her medications for hypertension and diabetes the morning of surgery. The MOST appropriate response by the nurse would be:
    a. "No, the anesthesiologist will monitor your blood pressure and blood glucose."
    b. "NPO means nothing by mouth."
    c. "Yes, take them with no more than a glass of water."
    d. "I will clarify this with your physician."

chapter **8**

Caring for Clients with Cancer

LEARNING outcomes

After completing this chapter, you will be able to:

- Define cancer and differentiate benign from malignant neoplasms.
- Discuss the pathophysiology of cancer and factors associated with carcinogenesis.
- Describe the effects of cancer on the body.
- Describe the laboratory and diagnostic tests used to diagnose cancer.
- Discuss the use of surgery, radiation therapy, chemotherapy, and biotherapy in the treatment of cancer.
- Provide teaching for the client and family experiencing cancer.
- Use the nursing process as a framework for providing individualized care for the client with cancer.

Cancer is a family of complex diseases with manifestations that vary according to the body system affected and the type of tumor cells involved. People of any age, gender, ethnicity, or geographic region can be affected by this disease. Despite research that has shed more light on this dreaded disease, cancer fatality is still 41%. The fear caused by even a possible diagnosis of cancer is considerable. Cancer, "the big C," brings forth feelings of dread and helplessness.

This chapter looks at cancer disease and treatment. It discusses nursing care that is appropriate for most clients with cancer. Discussions of cancers that affect specific body systems (e.g., laryngeal cancer, lung cancer) are found in corresponding chapters in the text.

Cancer, the Nurse, and the Health Care Team

Cancer is a disease that results when normal cells mutate into abnormal, deviant cells and continue to reproduce within the body. Because cancer can affect any body tissue and has many different manifestations, care of the client with cancer can be a complex process.

Nursing focuses on cancer not as one disease, but as many diseases. The nurse recognizes that cancer is a disruptive process that affects the whole person and that person's significant others. Nursing interventions reflect the fact that cancer is a chronic condition with acute episodes, that the client is often treated in the home, and that the client is treated with a combination of therapeutic modalities. Equally important, the nurse recognizes that caring for the client with cancer involves prevention, detection, rehabilitation, long-term follow-up, and terminal care.

Oncology is the study of cancer; *oncologists* are physicians who specialize in caring for clients with cancer. Oncologists may be medical doctors, surgeons, radiologists, immunologists, or researchers. Often, the client with cancer has the benefit of a team of physicians, nurses, and other health care professionals who collaborate to provide the most effective treatment.

Cancer Incidence and Trends

Only heart disease has a higher mortality rate than cancer. Despite continuing research, the rates of death from some forms of cancer are rising. Statistics from the American Cancer Society (ACS) show that in the United States, approximately 25% of all deaths in the year 2001 were attributable to cancer. It was estimated that 1.26 million new cases of cancer would occur that year, with a projected death rate of 553,400 (ACS, 2001).

Lung cancer continues to be the leading cause of cancer deaths. In 2001, the most commonly diagnosed cancers were prostate (198,100 new cases), breast (193,700 new cases), lung (169,500 new cases), and colorectal cancer (135,400 new cases). The incidence rates for prostate, breast, and colon cancer have begun to level off or decline. One of the most rapidly increasing cancers is melanoma (51,400 new cases), which has increased an average of 3% per year since 1981. The mortality rates for different cancers vary according to their incidence. Information about the most recent cancer cases and mortality rates are available on the World Wide Web at *www.cancer.org*.

Race and economic factors affect survival rates. The 5-year survival rate for all cancers together is 60%, but African Americans are 33% more likely to die of cancer than whites (ACS, 2001).

The number of new cancer cases and cancer deaths is declining in the United States, and the 5-year survival rate for individual cancers continues to improve. Still, the gains are not equal for men and women nor for European Americans versus African Americans. For example, although breast cancer occurs more commonly in white women than in black women, the survival rate is 86% for white women but only 71% for African Americans. Similar disparities can be seen in survival rates for colorectal, prostate, and endometrial cancers.

Cancer is a disease associated with aging; 80% of cancer diagnoses occur after age 55. This fact is very significant for health care as our elderly population increases.

PATHOPHYSIOLOGY

The cell is the basic structural unit of all life. Mature normal cells are uniform in size and have nuclei characteristic of the tissue to which the cells belong. Within the nucleus of normal cells, chromosomes containing deoxyribonucleic acid (DNA) molecules carry the genetic information that controls the synthesis of proteins. The genetic information coded in the DNA of every gene is translated into the protein structures that determine the type, maturity, and function of a cell. Any change or disruption in a gene can result in an inaccurate "blueprint" that can produce an abnormal cell, which may then become cancerous.

Benign and Malignant Neoplasms

A **neoplasm** is a mass of abnormal cells that grows independently of its surrounding structures and has no physiologic purpose. It is often called a *tumor* (from the Latin word for "swelling"). Neoplasms grow at a rate uncoordinated with the needs of the body, do not benefit the host, and in some cases are actively harmful. Neoplasms typically are classified as benign or malignant, based on their potential to damage the body and on their growth characteristics.

Benign neoplasms are localized growths with well-defined borders; they are frequently encapsulated. Benign neoplasms tend to respond to the body's controls. They grow slowly and often remain stable in size. Because they are usually encapsulated, they often are easily removed and tend not to recur. However, they can be destructive if they crowd surrounding tissue and obstruct the function of organs. For example, a benign meningioma (from the meninges of the brain and spinal cord) can cause severely increased intracranial pressure and progressively impair the person's cerebral function. Unless the meningioma is successfully removed, rising intracranial pressure will eventually lead to coma and death.

In contrast, *malignant neoplasms* grow aggressively and do not respond to the body's controls. They have an irregular shape and cut through surrounding tissues, causing bleeding, inflammation, and *necrosis* (tissue death) as they grow. When health care professionals use the term *cancer,* they are referring to a malignant neoplasm. Malignant neoplasms can recur after surgical removal of the primary and secondary tumors and after other treatments. (Table 8-1 ◆ lists the comparison of benign and malignant neoplasms.)

Malignant tumors compress, and cancer cells easily separate from the neoplasm, allowing them to move into surrounding body fluids and tissues. Malignant cells may break away from the primary tumor, traveling through the blood or lymph to invade other tissues of the body. The ability of cancer cells to invade adjacent tissues and travel to distant organs is considered their most dangerous characteristic. Both the secondary tumor they form and the process by which malignant neoplasms spread are called **metastasis.**

Metastasis can travel as an embolism in the blood or lymph or shed cells into body cavities. A blood or lymph-borne metastasis allows a new tumor to be established in a distant organ (Figure 8-1 ◆). The malignant cells enter the circulation, survive in the blood, exit the circulation, and implant in a new tissue. About 60% of metastatic lesions occur in this manner. Also, malignant cells from a colon cancer may be seeded into the peritoneal cavity, establishing a new tumor in the mesenteric epithelium.

For metastasis to occur, the cancerous cells must avoid detection by the immune system. Thus, impairment or alteration of the immune system is a major factor in the establishment of metastatic lesions. The most common sites of metastasis are the lymph nodes, liver, lungs, bones, and brain (Table 8-2 ◆).

It is estimated that 50% of all cancers have already metastasized by the time the tumor is identified. This may

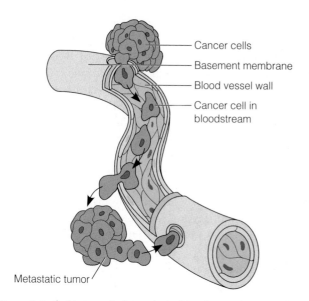

Figure 8-1. ◆ Metastasis through the bloodstream. Cancer cells disrupt the basement membrane in the blood vessel and gain access into the circulation. Once in the blood, only about 1 cell in 1,000 escapes immune detection, but that can be enough. Undetected cells move out of the blood, entering new tissue. Once in the new site, the malignant cells multiply and establish a metastatic tumor.

account for the current 41% death rate and supports the need for client education to speed early diagnosis. The time it takes for metastasis to occur is extremely variable and often difficult to predict. Some cancers, such as basal cell carcinomas, do not metastasize. The aggressiveness and location of the tumor, as well as the state of the immune system, determine whether and how rapidly metastasis takes place.

ETIOLOGY

Factors that cause cancer are both external (chemicals, radiation, and viruses) and internal (hormones, immune conditions, and inherited mutations). Causal factors may act together or in

TABLE 8-1	COMPARISON OF BENIGN AND MALIGNANT NEOPLASMS	
BENIGN	**MALIGNANT**	
Local	Invasive	
Cohesive	Noncohesive	
Well-defined borders	Does not stop at tissue border	
Pushes other tissues out of the way	Invades and destroys surrounding tissues	
Slow growth	Rapid growth	
Encapsulated	Metastasizes to distant sites	
Easily removed	Not always easy to remove	
Does not recur	Can recur	

TABLE 8-2	VARIOUS CANCERS AND SITES OF METASTASES	
PRIMARY TUMOR	**COMMON METASTATIC SITES**	
Bronchogenic (lung)	Spinal cord, brain, liver, bone	
Breast	Regional lymph nodes, vertebrae, brain, liver	
Colon	Liver, lung, brain, ovary	
Prostate	Bladder, bone (especially vertebrae), liver	
Malignant melanoma	Lung, liver, spleen, regional lymph nodes	

sequence to initiate or promote carcinogenesis. Ten or more years often pass between exposures or mutations and detectable cancer. Intensive research has led to increasingly credible and interrelated theories. In addition, research has identified numerous **carcinogens** (cancer-causing agents) that may contribute to the development of the disease.

Theories of Carcinogenesis

One theory suggests that carcinogens cause mutations in cellular DNA. The period of time between the damage to the DNA and the manifestation of a tumor may be as long as 10 to 20 years, a fact that may explain why many cancers tend to occur in older adults. Also, some researchers believe it takes several generations of mutant cells to result in enough damage to produce a cancer.

Most cancer researchers believe that all cells in the body have **oncogenes** (genes capable of triggering cancerous characteristics), which normally are repressed. Invading viruses or other carcinogens may "switch on" a cell's oncogenes, accelerating the cell's rate of multiplication and enabling it to invade other tissues. According to another theory, oncogenes are held in check after birth by the body's *T lymphocytes* (a class of white blood cells).

The expression of oncogenes may be allowed by a decrease in the body's immunity (e.g., during times of stress) or in response to certain carcinogens. For example, clients with acquired immune deficiency syndrome (AIDS), who have a decreased number of helper T lymphocytes, have a much higher than normal incidence of certain cancers.

Some researchers suspect that cancerous cells form continuously within the body. The healthy immune system recognizes these cells as "foreign" and destroys them. A tumor takes hold and grows only when it escapes immune surveillance (e.g., people who are immunocompromised).

KNOWN CARCINOGENS. Viruses, drugs, hormones, and chemical and physical agents are known to cause cancer or have strong links to certain kinds of cancers. Certain *viruses* can cause cancer by modifying the genes of the cells they invade. Human immunodeficiency virus (HIV) infects helper T lymphocytes and monocytes, and impairs the person's protection against cancers like lymphoma and Kaposi's sarcoma. Hepatitis B virus is believed to cause primary liver cancer. Papillomaviruses, which cause benign warts, are associated with malignant melanoma and cervical, penile, and laryngeal cancers. Vaccines to prevent virus-induced cancers are under investigation. The preliminary results of the use of vaccines to treat malignancies, such as melanoma, are encouraging.

Certain *drugs* and *hormones* are also related to the development of cancer. Chemotherapeutic drugs and recreational drugs, (e.g., heroin) cause immune suppression. Hormones, such as estrogen, have been linked to cervical, endometrial, and breast cancers.

Many *chemicals* have been identified as carcinogens. Many of them are occupational hazards encountered in the workplace. Examples of environmental carcinogens include poly-cyclic hydrocarbons, found in soot; arsenic, found in pesticides; wood and leather dust; polymer esters, used in plastics and paints; carbon tetrachloride; and asbestos. Some foods also contain carcinogens that are added during preparation or preservation. Examples include the sugar substitute sodium saccharine and nitrosamines and nitrosindoles, which are found in pickled, salted foods. In some cases, food contaminants produce carcinogenic chemicals.

Excessive *exposure to radiation* causes increased rates of cancer. Both solar radiation from ultraviolet rays and ionizing radiation from industrial or medical sources are carcinogenic. Radon, a naturally formed radioactive gas found in the basements of many homes, is also a known carcinogen. People who have lived in areas where nuclear weapons testing has been carried out or whose ground water has been polluted by nuclear wastes are also at increased risk for developing cancers.

Although everyone comes into contact with a vast number of substances that are considered carcinogenic, not everyone develops cancer. Other factors, such as genetic predisposition, impairment of the immune response, and repeated exposure to the carcinogen, are all necessary for a cancer to develop.

RISK FACTORS. Risk factors make an individual or a population vulnerable to a specific disease or other unhealthy outcome. Some risk factors are controllable; others are not. Knowledge and assessment of risk factors are especially important in counseling clients and families about measures to prevent cancer.

Noncontrollable Risk Factors. Noncontrollable risk factors include: heredity, age, gender, and poverty. Inherited genetic defects have been identified in some types of cancer (breast, colorectal, lung, and prostate). Although heredity plays a lesser role in a person's susceptibility to cancer than other factors, people with familial predisposition should be counseled about health promotional behaviors. For example, if there is a family history of lung cancer, a client should be counseled to avoid smoking and to avoid areas where smoking is allowed.

Age is a risk factor; about 80% of all cancers occur in people over age 55. One possible factor involved in this increased risk is that at least five cycles of genetic mutations seem to be necessary to cause permanent damage to afflicted cells. Evidence indicates that the immune response is altered with aging, and cells are damaged over time. Also, long-term exposure to carcinogenic agents is usually necessary for cancer to take hold. Hormonal changes that occur with aging can be associated with cancer. Postmenopausal women receiving exogenous estrogen have an increased risk for breast and uterine cancers. Older men are at risk for prostate cancer, possibly due to breakdown of testosterone into carcinogenic forms. See Box 8-1 for a discussion about cancer and older adults.

Gender is a risk factor for certain types of cancer. For example, thyroid cancer occurs more commonly among females; bladder cancer is seen more often among males.

population FOCUS

BOX 8-1

Older Adults with Cancer

Nurses need to be aware of how cancer and cancer treatments affect older adults. Cancer is the second leading cause of death in people over age 65. The incidence of cancer increases with age, probably as a result of the accumulated exposure to carcinogens and to age-related declines in the action of the immune system. Hormonal changes (estrogen, testosterone) may also predispose older adults to cancer. The most commonly seen cancers in older women are colorectal, breast, lung, pancreatic, and ovarian. In older men, lung, colorectal, prostate, pancreatic, and gastric cancers occur most frequently.

The importance of screening and early detection of cancer does not diminish with age. Unfortunately, some health care providers may believe that cancer screening is not as important as it is for the younger client. Older adults may not participate in screening programs or seek treatment for cancer due to fear, depression, cognitive impairments, poor access to health care, or financial constraints. Some older adults (and health care providers) mistake cancer symptoms for normal age-related changes and do not seek appropriate health care. When they do seek treatment, chronic conditions may mask the usual symptoms associated with cancer.

Older adults are at greater risk for side effects associated with cancer treatment (especially chemotherapy) because of age-related physiologic changes and chronic conditions associated with aging. Older adults have increased incidence of cardiotoxicity and toxicity of the central nervous system, plus fatigue, problems related to immobility and functional decline, and risk for infection. The nurse must be aware of potential problems and monitor the client closely. The nurse needs to consider how the aging process will alter the response to the disease and treatment plan.

Teach the older client and family about the warning signs of cancer. Stress the importance of seeking health care if any of the warning signs develop. Encourage clients to schedule an annual physical examination. Teach women how to perform a breast self-exam and instruct them to perform the exam every month. Teach men to perform a prostate self-examination; encourage them to do this exam every month. Also, tell men to schedule a prostate-specific antigen (PSA) screening for prostate cancer.

Cancer statistics show that *poverty* is a risk factor for cancer. Inadequate access to health care, especially preventive screening and counseling, may be a major factor. Some factors that usually come under the category of controllable risks, such as diet and stress, are frequently not controllable in this population.

Controllable Risk Factors. Controllable risk factors include: emotion, diet, weight, occupation, infection, drug and alcohol use, and sun exposure. Continuous unmanaged *stress* can keep certain hormones (e.g., epinephrine and cortisol) at high levels; this can result in systematic "fatigue" and weaker immunologic surveillance. Emotional and physical isolation, unexpressed anger, depression, and hopelessness tend to shut down the energizing chemicals in the body and depress immune responses.

Some *foods* such as nitrosamines and nitrosindoles are considered carcinogenic. Excessive frying or broiling of foods increases the cancer risk considerably. Other substances that are believed to increase cancer risk include sodium saccharine, red food dyes, and coffee. *Obesity* has been linked to hormone-dependent cancers. Obese people often have excessive amounts of the hormones that feed malignancies of the breast, bowel, ovary, endometrium, and prostate.

Occupational risk may be considered either controllable or uncontrollable because choice of occupation is often limited by education and ability. Although federal standards exist to protect workers from hazardous substances, many feel they lack the power to prevent violations. Outdoor workers (farmers, construction workers) are exposed to solar radiation. Health care workers (x-ray technicians, biomedical researchers) are exposed to ionizing radiation and carcinogenic substances. People who work in old buildings may be exposed to asbestos in the walls.

Avoiding specific *infections* decreases the risk of cancer. For example, genital herpes and papillomavirus-induced genital warts (linked to cancer) can often be avoided by following safe-sex practices (e.g., use of condoms). Lung cancer is highly preventable because of the relationship of *smoking* and lung cancer. The larger the dose and the longer the use, the higher the risk for developing cancer. The carcinogenic substances in tobacco are weak; therefore, stopping smoking can reverse the damage. Research has shown a significantly lower lung cancer death risk for former smokers compared to current smokers. Smokers who quit before age 50 decrease their death risk by 50% in the next 15 years (ACS, 2001). Tobacco is also related to oropharyngeal, esophageal, laryngeal, gastric, pancreatic, and bladder cancers. It is well documented that long-term exposure to secondhand smoke increases the risk for lung or bladder cancers in nonsmokers.

Alcohol promotes cancer by modifying the metabolism of carcinogens in the liver and esophagus, increasing their effectiveness. People who both smoke and drink a considerable amount of alcohol daily have an increased risk for oral, esophageal, and laryngeal cancers. *Recreational drugs* suppress the immune system, and drug use often promotes an unhealthy lifestyle that increases general cancer risk. Furthermore, marijuana has been demonstrated to cause chromosomal damage.

As the protective ozone layer thins, more of the sun's damaging *ultraviolet radiation* reaches the earth. Since the early 1970s, the incidence rate of melanoma has increased an average of 4% per year. Incidence rates are more than 10 times higher in whites than in blacks. Sun-related skin cancers are now considered to be a problem for all people, regardless of skin color, but people of Northern European extraction with very fair skin, blue or green eyes, and light-colored hair are

BOX 8-2
AMERICAN CANCER
SOCIETY CAUTION MODEL

The American Cancer Society has established the following seven common symptoms that could lead to a diagnosis of cancer.

1. A change in bowel or bladder function.
2. Sores that do not heal.
3. Unusual bleeding or discharge.
4. Thickening or lump in breast or other parts of the body.
5. Indigestion or difficulty swallowing.
6. Recent change in a wart or mole.
7. A nagging cough or hoarseness.

Source: American Cancer Society.

BOX 8-3
AMERICAN CANCER SOCIETY
RECOMMENDATIONS
FOR CANCER CHECKUPS

BREAST

- Routine monthly breast self-examination starting at age 20
- Breast examination by a health care professional every 3 years from age 20 to 39 and yearly thereafter
- Screening mammography every year from age 40

COLON AND RECTUM

- Fecal occult blood test every year beginning at age 50
- Flexible sigmoidoscopy every 5 years with digital rectal exam
- Colonoscopy every 10 years. Double-contrast barium enema every 5 years

CERVIX/UTERUS

- Yearly pelvic examination and Papanicolaou (Pap) test for sexually active girls and any women over 18; less often for women with three consecutive negative results
- At age 35, women with risk for hereditary non-polyposis colon cancer should be offered endometrial biopsy annually to screen for endometrial cancer

PROSTATE

- Digital rectal exam yearly beginning at age 50
- Prostate-specific antigen (PSA) test yearly beginning at age 50

Source: American Cancer Society.

most vulnerable. Elderly people with decreased pigment are also more at risk, even those with darker skin.

EARLY DETECTION

Early detection and treatment are the factors that influence the prognosis of people with cancer most. Many people do not seek early diagnosis and treatment because of denial, fear and anxiety, stigma, or the absence of specific early signs. Screening procedures (mammograms, occult blood stool tests, etc.) may be lifesaving.

The ACS promotes early detection through the CAUTION model (Box 8-2), which lists signs and symptoms that are characteristic of cancer. For people without symptoms, the ACS recommends a cancer checkup every 3 years from age 20 to 39, yearly for those over 40, and more frequently if a person is at special risk due to heredity, environment, occupation, or lifesrvle.

The routine cancer check should include counseling to improve health behaviors, physical examination, and instructions for self-examination when possible. Box 8-3 lists tests recommended for a cancer checkup. Nurses have a special role in public education. They should encourage all clients to schedule regular cancer checkups.

Physiologic and Psychological Effects of Cancer

Much of the nursing care for clients with cancer is related to the generalized effects of cancer on the body and the side effects of the treatments. Although pathophysiologic effects vary with the type and location of the cancer, certain effects are usually observed.

Acute pain is often the primary symptom associated with diagnosis. Acute pain may also be related to cancer treatment (surgery, radiation, chemotherapy).

Chronic pain may be related to cancer treatment or be a consequence of progression of the disease. It may be preexisting pain related to other disorders. Chronic pain may be related to a history of drug abuse. The cancer-related pain in the dying client is also chronic pain (Foley, 1985).

Disruption of function may be due to obstruction or pressure (e.g., urine retention from prostatic tumors obstructing bladder neck or urethra). Resulting anoxia and necrosis cause loss of function of the involved organ or tissue.

Hematologic alterations impair normal blood cell function. In leukemia the immature leukocytes cannot perform protective functions, so immunity is compromised. Also, excessive numbers of immature leukocytes in the bone marrow cause a drop in erythrocyte and thrombocyte (platelet) production; this results in secondary anemia and clotting disorders.

Infection is a common effect. Tumors may connect two incompatible organs, such as the bowel and bladder. They may become necrotic, and septicemia may result. Tumors that grow near the surface of the body may erode through to the surface, providing a site for the entry of microorganisms. Any malignant involvement of immune-system organs or tissues can seriously impair the immune response.

Hemorrhage may be caused by tumor erosion through blood vessels. Hemorrhage can be serious enough to cause life-threatening hypovolemic shock.

The **anorexia–cachexia syndrome** describes the effect of cancer cells on the client's metabolism. Metabolism increases in response to increased cancer cell reproduction, but the cancer cells divert nutrition to their own use. In addition, they inhibit food intake. The tumor secretes substances that alter taste and smell and produce early satiety. Pain, infection, and depression also contribute to anorexia. Cancer cells support their growth processes by breaking down *(catabolizing)* body tissue and muscle proteins (Figure 8-2 ◆). Unexplained rapid weight loss is often the first symptom that brings the client to a health care provider.

Creation of ectopic sites of hormone production is a characteristic of some cancers (e.g., breast, ovarian, and renal cancers may set up sites that produce parathyroid hormones, causing severe hypercalcemia).

Pain is ranked as one of the most serious concerns of clients, families, and oncology health care professionals. Cancer pain may be acute, with a well-defined pattern of onset, and related to the diagnosis or treatment. It may be chronic, lasting more than 6 months and frequently lacking the objective manifestations of acute pain. Chronic pain may alter personality, functional abilities, and lifestyle; it may disrupt compliance with treatment and quality of life.

Cancer pain may be due to direct tumor involvement (about 70% of pain experienced by people with cancer). It may be affected by preexisting pain or a history of drug abuse. For the dying client, pain may be intensified by issues regarding hopelessness and death.

PHYSICAL STRESS

The immune system mounts an all-out assault on the foreign invader. The immune system can destroy a microscopic neoplasm. However, a neoplasm of 1 cm is large enough to over-

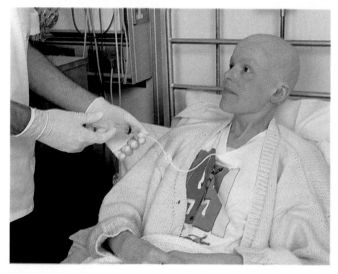

Figure 8-2. ◆ Cachexic person with cancer. Cancer robs its host of nutrients and increases body catabolism of fat and muscle to meet its demands.

whelm most immune systems. The body fights until it is exhausted. This is why many clients with cancer present with fatigue, weight loss, anemia, dehydration, and altered blood chemistries.

PSYCHOLOGICAL STRESS

People exhibit a variety of psychological and emotional responses to a diagnosis of cancer. Some see it as a death sentence; they experience overwhelming grief and often give up. Others feel guilt and consider cancer a punishment for past behaviors. Common emotions are anger, powerlessness, fear, isolation, and concern about body image and sexual dysfunction.

COLLABORATIVE CARE

Collaborative care begins with a variety of specialized tests. The ACS identifies four major goals of medical treatment: (1) to eliminate the tumor or malignant cells, (2) to prevent metastasis, (3) to reduce cellular growth and tumor burden, and (4) to promote functional abilities and provide pain relief to those whose disease does not respond to treatment.

Laboratory and Diagnostic Tests

TUMOR IDENTIFICATION. To provide some standardization in diagnosis and treatment protocols, an identification system has been developed. It consists of *tumor classification* (naming its origin), *tumor grading* (describing its aggressiveness), and *tumor staging* (describing its spread within or beyond the tissue of origin):

1. *Classification.* Tumors are classified and named by the tissue or cell of origin; adjectives are added to further specify the location. Other names for tumors incorporate the name of the discoverer of that particular cancer, such as Burkitt's lymphoma or Hodgkin's disease. *Hematopoietic* (blood cell) malignancies are usually named by the type of immature blood cell that predominates. An example is myelocytic leukemia, named for the immature form of the granulocyte.
2. *Grading.* Grading of tumors evaluates the amount of differentiation of the cell and estimates the rate of growth. Cells that are the most differentiated are the least malignant and earn a grade of 1. Grade 4 is reserved for the least differentiated and most aggressively malignant cells. Grading criteria may vary with different locations and types of tumors.
3. *Staging.* Staging refers to the relative size of the tumor and extent of the disease. Tumors are most often staged by the TNM classification system (Table 8-3 ◆). T stands for the relative tumor size, N indicates the presence and extent of lymph node involvement, and M denotes distant metastases. Table 8-3 shows the basic outline of the TNM system. Although the TNM system is generalized for all solid tumors, it is frequently adapted for specific types of cancers.

Other systems use specific coding to differentiate types and locations of tumors. These provide a shorthand for staging

TABLE 8-3 TNM STAGING CLASSIFICATION SYSTEM		
STAGE		**MANIFESTATIONS**
Tumor	T_0	No evidence of primary tumor
	T_{IS}	Tumor in situ
	T_1, T_2, T_3, T_4	Ascending degrees of tumor size and involvement
Nodes	N_0	No abnormal regional nodes
	N_{1a}, N_{2a}	Regional nodes—no metastasis
	N_{1b}, N_{2b}, N_{3b}	Regional lymph nodes— metastasis suspected
	N_x	Regional nodes cannot be assessed clinically
Metastasis	M_0	No evidence of distant metastasis
	M_1, M_2, M_3	Ascending degrees of metastatic involvement of the host including distant nodes

and grading tumors and provide guidelines for treatment. For example, oncologists may use either an A-B-C-D staging system (which includes grading numbers) or a modified TNM system for evaluating prostate cancer.

Several procedures are used to diagnose cancer. X-ray imaging, computed tomography, ultrasonography, and magnetic resonance imaging can locate abnormal tissues or tumors. However, only microscopic histologic examination of the tissue reveals the type of cancer. Tissue samples are acquired through biopsy, shedded cells, or collections of secretions. Lymph nodes are also biopsied to determine whether metastasis has begun. Simple blood screening procedures, such as the prostatic-specific antigen (PSA), can aid in the diagnosis. Increased enzymes or hormones may also aid in the diagnosis of cancer. Tumor markers are used both for early diagnosis and for devising immunologic treatments.

Cytologic Examination. For malignant tissues to be identified by name, grade, and stage, they must first be subjected to histologic and cytologic examination. Biopsy specimens are collected by exfoliation (a Papanicolaou smear or bronchial washings), aspiration of fluid (like pleural or cerebrospinal fluid), or needle aspiration (solid tumors of breast, lung, or prostate). Body secretions, such as sputum or urine, are also examined.

Tumor Markers. A tumor marker is a biochemical indicator of the presence of a malignancy. High levels of certain proteins are suspicious and require follow-up diagnostic studies. For example, PSA is used to screen for prostate cancer in men over 40. The primary use of tumor markers, however, is to determine the client's response to therapy and to detect residual disease.

X-Ray Imaging. Considered the least expensive and least invasive diagnostic procedure for screening, x-ray studies are useful to reassure the client (if findings are negative) or to encourage follow-up studies (if findings are suspicious). X-ray imaging cannot distinquish well between cysts and tumors; also, it does not usually detect tumors smaller than 1 cm in size, which is late in their development.

Computed Tomography. Computed tomography (CT) scans reveal subtle differences in tissue densities and are much more accurate. Although more expensive than x-ray, CT scans are useful in screening for renal cell, most gastrointestinal tumors, and lymph node involvement.

Magnetic Resonance Imaging. Magnetic resonance imaging (MRI) produces images from radio frequency signals emitted by the body. It is expensive, but it is the tool of choice for head and neck tumors. Some clients become claustrophobic during the MRI because it requires being placed inside the diagnostic imaging machine, an experience that has been likened to being encased in a small tube. In addition, some machines make loud thumping sounds that can be frightening if the client is not informed beforehand that this is normal.

Ultrasonography. Ultrasonography measures the sound waves as they bounce off body structures. It is useful in detecting early prostate cancers, or masses in the denser breast tissue of young women.

Radioisotope Scans. Radioisotope scans involve the use of a special scanner and ingestion or injection of specific radioactive isotopes. For clients with newly diagnosed cancer, it is often used to check for possible metastases and to help determine treatment. Antiemetics for nausea and antianxiety medication for difficulty lying still during the scan may be prescribed. Client preparation may include allowing nothing by mouth or clear fluids only after midnight.

Angiography. Angiography is expensive and invasive; it is performed when the tumor's location cannot be identified precisely by other methods or the tumor must be visualized before surgery. Fluoroscopy or serial x-ray films trace the movement of radiopaque dye injected into a major blood vessel. Dye flow blockage indicates the tumor's location. Dye may also identify blood vessels that supply the tumor, allowing the surgeon to know where to ligate vessels safely. Preparation for the test includes: ensuring that the client takes only fluids the day of the test; performing skin preparation at the insertion site; administering sedative drugs prior to the procedure; and informing the client that injection of the dye may cause a hot, flushing sensation or nausea and vomiting. Angiography is usually done on an outpatient basis, but the client is monitored for several hours for complications such as bleeding at the catheter insertion site.

Monoclonal Antibodies. These antibodies can detect specific cancer antigens. They have been important in the diagnosis of several solid tumors, lymphomas, and leukemias.

Direct Visualization. Direct visualization procedures are invasive but do not require radiography. They allow the visual identification of the organs within the limits of a flexible fiberoptic scope and usually permit biopsy of suspicious lesions or masses. *Sigmoidoscopy* (viewing the sigmoid colon), *cystoscopy* (viewing the urethra and bladder), and *endoscopy* (viewing the upper gastrointestinal tract) all require some client preparation (e.g., food restriction, bowel cleaning), cause some discomfort, and may require sedation or even anesthesia. Some may be performed in the physician's office.

Exploratory surgery with biopsy is a more radical method of direct visualization of suspected malignancies. The client undergoes the usual preoperative preparation for the type of surgery anticipated (see Chapter 7). When the tumor is exposed, a sample of tissue (biopsy) is sent to the pathology laboratory for a rapid "frozen-section" histologic examination. If the initial report is negative, the benign mass is usually removed to prevent further symptoms. If the report is positive for cancer, the tumor, often adjacent lymph nodes, and any other suspicious tissue are resected. These are sent to the pathology laboratory for further analysis. The client then receives the usual postoperative care.

OTHER LABORATORY TESTS. Certain laboratory tests of blood, urine, and other body fluids—when used in conjunction with other diagnostic studies—can be useful in screening for pathologic conditions or validating the cancer diagnosis. These include the enzymes alanine aminotransferase (ALT) and lactic dehydrogenase (LDH) for liver metastases; and the tumor markers PSA for prostate cancer and CEA for colon cancer.

Psychological Support During Diagnosis

Preparing for and awaiting the results of diagnostic tests can create extreme anxiety. In addition to coping with the possibility of a life-threatening disease, or at least a life-altering one, clients often also face the prospect of uncomfortable, even painful, diagnostic procedures. They have important decisions to make that hang on the outcome of those tests. Many unspoken questions may exist:

■ Do I have cancer?
■ If so, what kind, and how serious?
■ Has it spread?
■ Will I survive?
■ What kind of treatment is needed?
■ How will this affect my lifestyle?
■ How will this affect family members and friends?

The nurse can provide valuable help during this very difficult stage by keeping clients actively involved in managing their life and disease. Sitting down with clients as soon as they enter the health care system, asking what they know already about what is going to happen, and soliciting questions is a good way to start. Initiating the interaction with objective questions and encouraging clients to share what

knowledge and experience they have, allows the client to maintain control. From there, the nurse can obtain the information needed.

It is essential that clients thoroughly understand the preparation required for their tests, especially if they will be preparing at home. They also need to be informed of any unusual effects that may occur with the test, such as nausea from radioactive dye. If possible, a phone call the evening before to verify the client's understanding of the procedure and answer questions can be very supportive.

As clients begin to feel more comfortable with the nurse, they may express concerns, fears, and other emotions. The nurse should avoid giving advice and false reassurance, but rather just listen and be supportive, sharing appropriate information when needed. For clients who are not ready to discuss concerns or for those who appear angry, being nonjudgmental and providing nonverbal support may facilitate more open communication. An atmosphere of calmness, warmth, caring, and respect can ease the tension and often unspoken terror of this initial period.

Support of and communication with the client's significant others is extremely important. Often, they try to be strong for the client but have many fears and emotional concerns they do not feel comfortable expressing. The nurse needs to be available to the family without the client present, to allow them to talk without the need to edit for the client's benefit. This can help them manage their own difficulties in coping with their loved one's potential cancer diagnosis.

Cancer Treatment

The goals of cancer treatment are aimed at cure, control, or palliation of symptoms. These goals may overlap. Cancer may be treated through surgery, radiotherapy, chemotherapy, and biotherapy.

SURGERY. Surgery is used for diagnosis and staging of more than 90% of all cancers and for primary treatment of more than 60%. Whenever possible, the tumor is removed entirely. This sometimes requires creation of new structures for body function. For example, if the sigmoid colon and rectum are removed, the remaining healthy segment of the bowel is brought out through a *stoma* (a created opening) in the abdominal wall, providing a permanent *colostomy* for bowel elimination. Surgery can also destroy nerves and alter normal functioning; for example, prostate surgery may result in incontinence and impotence.

Not all cancer surgery is so radical. Surgery may remove a nonessential portion of organ or tissue. It may remove an organ whose function can be replaced chemically, like the thyroid. It may remove one of a pair of organs, and the unaffected organ can take over (e.g., the lung).

If the tumor is *nonresectable* (cannot be removed) or has metastasized, surgery may be only a palliative measure, to allow the involved organs to function as long as possible, to relieve pain, or to reduce the bulk of the tumor so that other modalities can be more effective. Surgery is often used along with other treatments to effect a more secure cure. For example, radiation may be used to shrink a brain tumor prior to surgery for removal. Surgery may be done after radical mastectomy to reconstruct the breast. Reconstructive surgery corrects the defect caused by the original surgery.

RADIATION THERAPY. Radiation therapy is still the treatment of choice for some tumors. Radiation causes lethal injury to DNA. It is used to kill the tumor, to reduce its size, to decrease pain, or to relieve obstruction, and when beginning metastasis is suspected. *External radiation* places the source of radiation at a distance from the client and delivers a relatively uniform dose. *Brachytherapy* is internal; the radioactive material *(implant)* is placed directly into the tumor site, delivering a high dose to the tumor and a lower dose to the normal tissues around it. It requires special safety measures (Box 8-4). A combination of these two therapies is often used.

Radiation sources are placed into the affected tissue or body cavity and are sealed in tubes, containers, wires, seeds, capsules, or needles. An implant may be temporary or permanent. Internal radiation may also be ingested or injected as a solution into the bloodstream or a body cavity or be introduced into the tumor through a catheter. The radioactive substance may transmit rays outside the body or be excreted in body fluids.

Implanted or ingested radiation can be dangerous for those living with, caring for, or treating the client. Box 8-5 discusses nursing care for the client receiving radiation therapy.

Radiation may cause skin changes (blanching, erythema, sloughing), ulcerations of mucous membranes, vulnerability to infection, gastrointestinal effects (nausea, vomiting, diarrhea, bleeding), interstitial exudate in the lungs, (called *radiation pneumonia*), and sometimes fistulas or necrosis of adjacent tissues.

CHEMOTHERAPY. Chemotherapy disrupts the cell cycle in various phases by interrupting cell metabolism and replication. It reduces the malignant cell's ability to synthesize needed enzymes and chemicals. It may work during specific phases of the cell cycle or through the entire cell cycle

Chemotherapy can effect a cure in some cancers (leukemias, lymphomas, some solid tumors). It may be used to decrease tumor size, as an adjunct to surgery or radiation, or to prevent or treat suspected metastases. Chemotherapy is also being used in conjunction with *biologic response modifiers* (BRMs) in some types of advanced cancers. BRMs modify the antitumor response of the body. All chemotherapy has side effects or toxic effects; the type and severity depend on the drugs used.

Most chemotherapy involves combinations of drugs given over varying periods of time. Treatment is given in cycles with rest periods in between. Treatment is continued until the disease goes into remission or the particular protocol is abandoned and a new one is tried.

Several courses of chemotherapy are necessary because the chemotherapy kills a fixed percentage of cells each time. Each course lessens the tumor burden. The goal is to reduce the number of cells until the body's immune system can finish the job. For this reason, oncologists usually give the maximum amount of chemotherapy the client can tolerate.

Classes of Chemotherapeutic Drugs. The major classes of chemotherapeutic agents are: alkylating agents, antimetabolites, cytotoxic antibiotics, plant derivatives, and hormones (Tortorice, 2000). (Table 8-4 ◆ gives the classifications of chemotherapeutic drugs, common examples, target malignancies, adverse effects and side effects, and nursing implications.)

PREPARATION AND ADMINISTRATION. Chemotherapeutic drugs can be administered orally, intramuscularly, intravenously, or by direct injection into intraperitoneal or intrapleural body cavities. They are prepared and administered under specific safety guidelines established by the federal government or the Oncology Nursing Society. Many clients now receive vascular access devices (VADs), especially when they must have several cycles of treatment over weeks or months. VADs are also useful for parenteral nutrition, for pain management (see Chapter 6), or for frequent blood drawing to monitor blood counts. Different types of VADs include: peripherally inserted central catheters; catheters into a major vein, such as

---

BOX 8-4
SAFETY PRINCIPLES FOR CAREGIVERS OF CLIENTS RECEIVING INTERNAL RADIATION

- Maintain the greatest possible distance from the source of radiation.
- Spend the minimum amount of time close to the radiation source.
- Shield yourself from the radiation with lead gloves and aprons whenever possible.
- If you are pregnant, do not come into contact with any radiation sources.
- If you work routinely near radiation, wear a monitoring device to measure whole-body exposure.
- Avoid direct exposure to radioisotope containers (do not touch the container).
- Keep clients with implanted radioisotopes in a private room with private bath and as far away from other hospitalized persons as possible.
- Use special care to dispose of body fluids of clients with unsealed implanted radioisotopes. Use specially marked containers for disposal.
- Handle bed linen and clothing with care and according to agency protocol.
- Use long-handled forceps to place any dislodged implants into a lead container.
- Consult with the radiation therapy department if there are questions or problems in caring for these clients.

BOX 8-5
NURSING CARE CHECKLIST

CLIENTS RECEIVING RADIATION THERAPY

Nursing Responsibilities for Both External and Internal Radiation Therapy

☑ Carefully assess and manage any complications, usually in collaboration with the radiation oncologist.

☑ Assist in documenting the results of the therapy; for example, clients receiving radiation for metastases to the spine will show improved neurologic functioning as tumor size diminishes.

☑ Provide emotional support, relief of discomfort, and opportunities to talk about fears and concerns. For some clients, radiation therapy is a last chance for cure or even just for relief of physical discomfort.

External Radiation

Prior to the start of treatments, the treatment area will be specifically located by the radiation oncologist and marked with colored semipermanent ink. Treatment is usually given 5 days per week for 15 to 30 minutes per day over 2 to 7 weeks.

Nursing Responsibilities

☑ Monitor for adverse effects: skin changes, such as blanching, erythema, desquamation, sloughing, or hemorrhage; ulcerations of mucous membranes; nausea and vomiting, diarrhea, or gastrointestinal bleeding.

☑ Assess lungs for abnormal sounds. Observe for any dyspnea or changes in respiratory pattern.

☑ Identify and record any medications that the client will be taking during the radiation treatment.

☑ Monitor white blood cell counts and platelet counts for significant decreases.

Client and Family Teaching

☑ Wash skin that is marked as the radiation site only with plain water, no soap; do not apply deodorant, lotions, medications, perfume, or powder to the site during the treatment period. Take care not to wash off the treatment marks.

☑ Do not rub, scratch, or scrub treated skin areas. If it is necessary to shave the treated area, use only an electric razor.

☑ Apply neither heat nor cold to the treatment site.

☑ Inspect the skin for damage or changes, and report these to the radiologist or physician.

☑ Wear loose, soft clothing over the treated area.

☑ Protect skin from sun exposure during and for at least 1 year after radiation therapy. Cover skin with protective clothing during treatment; after treatment, use sun-blocking agents with a sun protection factor (SPF) of at least 15.

☑ External radiation poses no risk to other people for radiation exposure, even with intimate physical contact.

☑ Be sure to get plenty of rest and eat a balanced diet.

Internal Radiation

Nursing Responsibilities

☑ Place the client in a private room.

☑ Limit visits to 10 to 30 minutes; have visitors sit at least 6 feet from the client.

☑ Monitor for side effects such as burning sensations, excessive perspiration, chills and fever, nausea and vomiting, or diarrhea.

☑ Assess for fistulas or necrosis of adjacent tissues.

Client and Family Teaching

☑ While a temporary implant is in place, stay in bed and rest quietly to avoid dislodging the implant.

☑ For outpatient treatments, avoid close contact with others during treatment.

☑ If the radiologist indicates the need for such measures, dispose of excretory materials in special containers or in a toilet not used by others.

☑ Carry out daily activities as able; get extra rest if feeling fatigued.

☑ Eat a balanced diet; frequent, small meals often are better tolerated.

☑ Contact the nurse or physician for any concerns or questions after discharge.

---

a Hickman or Groshong; and surgically implanted ports, such as Mediport.

During chemotherapy, a number of psychological issues that can cause emotional distress may arise. The need to plan activities around chemotherapy treatments and the side effects can impair the client's ability to work, manage a household, function sexually, or participate in social and recreational activities. Weight loss and alopecia may prompt feelings of powerlessness and depression. The nurse can assist by carefully evaluating symptoms, providing specific interventions as

TABLE 8-4   NURSING IMPLICATIONS FOR PHARMACOLOGY: CLIENTS RECEIVING CHEMOTHERAPEUTIC DRUGS

DRUG CLASSIFICATIONS/ DRUGS	TARGET MALIGNANCIES	ADVERSE EFFECTS OR SIDE EFFECTS	NURSING IMPLICATIONS
Alkylating Agents Mechlorethamine (Mustargen)	Hodgkin's disease Lymphosarcoma Lung cancer Chronic leukemia	Nausea and vomiting Leukopenia Thrombocytopenia Hyperuricemia	Maintain good hydration. Alkalinize urine. Administer antiemetics prior to chemotherapy. Monitor WBC, uric acid. Assess for infection.
Busulfan (Myleran)	Chronic myelogenous leukemia	Leukopenia Thrombocytopenia Renal failure Pulmonary fibrosis	Monitor WBCs, BUN. Maintain adequate fluid intake. Assess for infection. Assess lungs for fibrotic (coarse, loud) rales.
Cyclophosphamide (Cytoxan)	Lymphomas Multiple myeloma Leukemias Adenocarcinoma of lung and breast	Hemorrhagic cystitis Renal failure Alopecia Stomatitis Liver dysfunction	Encourage daily fluid intake of 2 to 3 L during treatment. Monitor WBCs, BUN, liver enzymes. Teach ways to manage hair loss.
Antimetabolites Methotrexate	Acute lymphoblastic leukemia Osteosarcoma Gestational trophoblastic carcinoma	Oral and gastrointestinal ulcerations Anorexia and nausea Leukopenia Thrombocytopenia Pancytopenia	Monitor CBC, WBC with differential, BUN, uric acid, creatinine. Assess oral mucous membranes; treat ulcers PRN. Assess for infection, bleeding.
5-Fluorouracil (5-FU)	Colon carcinoma Rectal carcinoma Breast carcinoma Gastric carcinoma Pancreatic cancer	Stomatitis Alopecia Nausea and vomiting Gastritis Enteritis Diarrhea Anemia Leukopenia Thrombocytopenia	Monitor CBC with differential, BUN, uric acid. Administer antiemetics PRN. Assess for bleeding; check stool occult blood. Evaluate hydration and nutrition status. Teach oral care for stomatitis. Assess for infection. Teach care for hair loss.
Antitumor Antibiotics Doxorubicin (Adriamycin)	Acute lymphoblastic leukemia (ALL) Acute myeloblastic leukemia Neuroblastoma Wilms' tumor Breast, ovarian, thyroid, lung cancer	Stomatitis Alopecia Nausea and vomiting Gastritis Enteritis Diarrhea Anemia Leukopenia Thrombocytopenia Cardiac toxicity	Monitor ECG; assess for arrythmias, gallops, and congestive heart failure (CHF). Monitor CBC with differential, BUN, uric acid. Administer antiemetics PRN. Assess for bleeding; check stool for occult blood. Evaluate hydration and nutrition status. Teach oral care for stomatitis. Assess for infection. Teach care for hair loss.

TABLE 8-4   NURSING IMPLICATIONS FOR PHARMACOLOGY: CHEMOTHERAPEUTIC DRUGS (CONTINUED)

DRUG CLASSIFICATIONS/ DRUGS	TARGET MALIGNANCIES	ADVERSE EFFECTS OR SIDE EFFECTS	NURSING IMPLICATIONS
Bleomycin (Blenoxane)	Squamous cell carcinoma Lymphosarcoma Reticulum cell sarcoma Testicular carcinoma Hodgkin's disease	Mucocutaneous ulcerations Alopecia Nausea and vomiting Chills and fever Pneumonitis and pulmonary fibrosis	Check for fever 3 to 6 hours after administration. Have chest x-ray films taken every 2 to 3 weeks. Assess respiratory status, and check for coarse rales. Evaluate hydration and nutrition status. Teach oral care for stomatitis. Assess for infection. Teach care for hair loss.
Plant Alkaloids Vincristine (Oncovin)	Combination therapy for acute leukemia, Hodgkin's and non-Hodgkin's lymphomas, rhabdomyosarcoma, neuroblastoma, Wilm's tumor	Areflexia Muscle weakness Peripheral neuritis Constipation Paralytic ileus Mild bone marrow depression	Assess neuromuscular function. Monitor CBC with differential. Evaluate gastrointestinal function. Manage constipation.
Vinblastin (Velban)	Combination therapy for Hodgkin's disease, lymphocytic and histocytic lymphoma, Kaposi's sarcoma, advanced testicular carcinoma, unresponsive breast cancer	Areflexia Alopecia Nausea and vomiting Bone marrow depression	Assess neuromuscular function. Monitor CBC with differential. Administer antiemetics PRN. Teach ways to manage hair loss.
Etoposide, also called VP-16 (VePesid)	Nonresponsive testicular tumors Small-cell lung cancer	Alopecia Hypotension with rapid infusion	Hydrate adequately before administration. Administer for 60 minutes. Monitor vital signs every 15 minutes during administration and every 2 to 4 hours thereafter. Teach ways to manage hair loss.
Prednisone	Combination therapy for many tumors Leukemia Lymphoma	Fluid retention Hypertension Steroid diabetes Emotional lability Silent bleeding ulcers Increased risk for infection	Monitor vital signs. Administer diuretics PRN. Check blood glucose regularly. Evaluate mental status. Administer oral medications with food. Administer hydrogen ion antagonist drugs (antacids) as ordered. Monitor WBC with differential. Check for signs of systemic infection.

(continues)

TABLE 8-4 NURSING IMPLICATIONS FOR PHARMACOLOGY: CHEMOTHERAPEUTIC DRUGS (CONTINUED)

DRUG CLASSIFICATIONS/ DRUGS	TARGET MALIGNANCIES	ADVERSE EFFECTS OR SIDE EFFECTS	NURSING IMPLICATIONS
Diethylstilbestrol (DES)	Advanced breast and prostrate cancers	Fluid retention Feminization Uterine bleeding	Monitor vital signs. Administer diuretics PRN as ordered. Explain reason for feminization to men, bleeding to women. Monitor for excessive bleeding.
Tamoxifen (Nolvadex)	Breast cancer	Hot flashes Nausea and vomiting	Teach ways to manage hot flashes. Explain reason for hot flashes. Administer antiemetics as ordered.
Paclitaxel (Taxol)	Ovarian cancer, breast cancer, non–small-cell lung cancer, head and neck cancer	Hypersensitivity reactions including: dyspnea, urticaria, flushing, and hypotension Cardiotoxicity Peripheral neuropathy Alopecia Mucositis Nausea and vomiting	Administer prophylactic antiallergic medications. Monitor for arrythmias, chest pain, palpitations, and changes in hemodynamic status. Assess neuromuscular function. Teach care for hair loss. Teach oral care for stomatitis. Administer anitemetics PRN.
Miscellaneous Drugs Cisplatin (CDDP) (Platinol)	Combination and single therapy for metastatic testicular and ovarian cancers, advanced bladder cancer, head and neck tumors, non–small-cell lung carcinoma, osteogenic sarcoma, neuroblastoma	Bone marrow depression: leukopenia and thrombocytopenia Renal tubular damage Deafness	Monitor WBC with differential and platelets, BUN, creatinine, uric acid. Watch for bleeding. Monitor for signs of infection. Evaluate hearing; check for tinnitus. Ensure that client is well hydrated before drug is administered. Encourage 2 to 3 L of fluid intake daily.

indicated, and allowing clients opportunities to express their fears, concerns, and feelings. The nurse can also encourage clients to participate in their care and maintain control over their life as much as possible (McDaniel & Rhodes, 1998). Specific interventions will be discussed later in the chapter under the appropriate nursing diagnoses. Table 8-4 includes nursing implications for specific adverse effects of common chemotherapy drugs.

BIOTHERAPY. Biotherapy is immunotherapy used to treat solid tumors, hematologic malignancies, bone marrow transplants, and as supportive therapy for myelosuppresive chemotherapy. Biotherapy includes injection of monoclonal antibodies, cytokines, hematopoietic growth factors, and natural killer cells (Battiato & Wheeler, 2000).

As promising as biotherapy is, it is accompanied by serious side effects and toxic effects. Interleukin-2 can cause acute alterations in renal, cardiac, liver, gastrointestinal, and mental functioning. Alpha-interferon causes mental slowing, confusion, and lethargy. When used in combination with 5-fluorouracil or interleukin-2, it may cause severe flulike symptoms, with chills and fever of 103° F to 106° F (39.4° C to 41.1° C), nausea, vomiting, diarrhea, anorexia, severe fatigue, and stomatitis. The toxic effects are probably exaggerations of the normal systemic effects that these substances cause when fighting infection. Nursing care of clients receiving immunotherapy is discussed in Box 8-6.

BONE MARROW TRANSPLANTATION. Bone marrow transplantation (BMT) is an accepted treatment to stimulate nonfunctioning marrow or to replace marrow. BMT is given as an intravenous infusion of cells obtained from a donor or the patient himself. BMT was originally used for leukemias or aplastic anemia. The therapy has been expanded to include treatment of solid tumors, such as breast and ovarian cancer.

BOX 8-6
NURSING CARE CHECKLIST

CLIENT RECEIVING IMMUNOTHERAPY

Immunotherapy can consist of various substances used alone (interleukin-2) or combination biotherapy (e.g., alpha-interferon with 5-fluorouracil). The nurse's role is to enhance the client's quality of life.

Nursing Responsibilities

☑ Monitor for side effects: Alpha-interferon may cause mental slowing, confusion, and lethargy. Combination therapy of 5-fluorouracil or interleukin-2 and alpha-interferon may cause severe flulike symptoms, with chills and fever of 103° F to 106° F (39.4° C to 41.1° C), nausea, vomiting, diarrhea, anorexia, severe fatigue, and stomatitis. Erythropoietin may cause acute hypertension.

☑ Monitor enzymes and other appropriate biochemical indicators for acute alterations in renal, cardiac, liver, or gastrointestinal functioning (potential side effects of interleukin-2).

☑ Evaluate response to therapy by conducting a thorough evaluation of client's symptoms.

☑ Assess client's coping behaviors and teach new strategies as needed.

☑ Manage fatigue and depression.

☑ Encourage self-care and participation in decision making.

☑ Provide close supervision for clients with altered mental functioning, either by caretakers or frequent nursing visits to the client's home.

☑ If client is unable to manage alone, teach medication administration and care of equipment to caregivers.

Client and Family Teaching

☑ Minimize symptoms by managing fever and flulike symptoms: increase fluid intake, take analgesic and antipyretic medications, and maintain bed rest until symptoms abate.

☑ Seek help for serious problems not managed by usual means, such as dehydration from diarrhea.

☑ Use correct technique for providing subcutaneous injections.

☑ Identify how to work and care for ambulatory pumps when medication is administered through an inter-catheter or vascular access device.

NURSING CARE

Nurses should educate all clients about preventive measures and lifestyle changes to reduce the risk of cancer. At the same time, they must reassure clients with cancer that they are not responsible for having acquired cancer. Once a cancer diagnosis is established, nurses have the responsibility of assisting and supporting clients during their recovery and rehabilitation. In cases of terminal cancer, nurses provide comfort and facilitate positive growth for the client and significant others.

ASSESSING

During a focused interview, the nurse collects significant data about the client, including the following:

■ History of the client's disease, including the signs and symptoms that led the client to seek health care
■ Other current diseases, such as diabetes
■ Current physical or psychological problems resulting from the cancer, such as pain or depression
■ Understanding of the treatment plan
■ Expectations of the treatment plan
■ Functional limitations and effect on current lifestyle of illness or treatment
■ Support systems or caretakers the client can rely on
■ Coping strategies and how well they are working

Specific interview questions for assessing a client with cancer are listed in Box 8-7. If the client is not expected to survive, it is important to ask about end-of-life decisions.

As soon as the client is admitted to the health care service or agency, a complete physical assessment should be conducted to establish a baseline against which to evaluate later changes. It is especially important to document the nutritional status of the client using anthropomorphic measurements (i.e., frame size, height, weight, body fat, and muscle mass), and to evaluate laboratory results and note any specific signs and symptoms. Signs and symptoms include wasted appearance, considerable weight loss over a relatively short period of time, anthropometric measurements below 85% of standard for fat and muscle tissue, decreases in serum proteins, and negative responses to antigen testing. (Table 8-5 ◆ compares the signs and symptoms of good nutrition with those of malnutrition.)

It is also important to assess the client's hydration status, especially if the client is not taking oral food and fluids well or is having bouts of vomiting. Specific assessments include intake and output, skin turgor, venous filling, tongue furrows and moisture, eyeball softness, lung sounds, and laboratory values. Manifestations of cancer, or of side effects of treatment, can be found in Box 8-8.

DIAGNOSING, PLANNING, AND IMPLEMENTING

Nursing goals focus on supporting the client and managing specific physical and emotional problems. They also focus on promoting rehabilitation for survivors and helping others maintain their dignity in the dying process. Nursing care includes the whole family from the onset of diagnosis through

BOX 8-7
MEETING INDIVIDUALIZED
NEEDS: CLIENTS WITH CANCER

INTERVIEW QUESTIONS FOR A CLIENT WITH CANCER

The following are appropriate questions to ask during the initial interview and at subsequent visits:

- "What brought you in to see the doctor?" Some clients may need more specific questions ("Did pain or any specific problem cause you to seek health care?").
- "Do you have any other medical conditions or problems that are troubling you at this time?"
- "What physical problems are you having at this time? Do you have pain? Have you lost weight? Are you discouraged because of your illness?" For each positive response, ask follow-up questions to define the exact nature of the problem.
- "What options has your physician suggested for treating your cancer?" (The answer may indicate a need for the nurse to collaborate with the physician to clarify information.)
- "What do you expect to happen as a result of this treatment?"
- "What effect is the disease or treatment having on your ability to carry out your usual daily activities?" (The response may indicate the need to collaborate with other professionals.)
- "Who is available to help you at home? To run errands? To provide transportation? To listen or just be a comfortable companion? Is there someone you would like to make health care decisions for you if there is a time when you cannot make them for yourself?"
- "How do you manage your stress or your feelings of discomfort? Do these measures work well for you?"
- If the client is not expected to survive the cancer: "Have you made a will? Have you thought about your last wishes for a funeral and burial? Have you discussed them with others?"

need medical intervention with appropriate medications. Those with moderate or even severe anxiety can probably be managed through listening, counseling, and teaching new skills.

- Convey warmth and empathy, and listen nonjudgmentally. *A client who feels safe will more easily express feelings and thoughts, and may be more willing to try new behaviors as suggested.*
- Encourage the client to acknowledge and express feelings, no matter how inappropriate they may seem. *Expressing feelings helps the client diminish anxiety and direct energy toward healing. Acknowledging feelings helps the client lay the groundwork for new coping behaviors.*
- Review the client's past coping strategies and introduce new strategies as appropriate. Explain why inappropriate strategies (repressing anger, turning to alcohol) are not helpful. *The client will be more willing to build on strategies that worked in the past. The client will be more able to reject inappropriate strategies if shown why they did not work in past crises.*
- Identify community resources, such as crisis hotlines and support groups. *The client may not have support systems, or the support system may be having their own difficulties dealing with the cancer diagnosis. Programs such as "I Can Cope," sponsored by the ACS, provide education, counseling, and support in a group setting with other cancer patients.*
- Provide specific information for the client about the disease, treatment, and what may be expected, especially for those clients with obvious misinformation. Avoid advice and false reassurance. *Knowing what to expect gives the client a sense of control and the ability to make decisions. Knowing that every effort will be made to help the client manage symptoms can do a great deal to relieve anxiety.*
- Provide a safe, calm, and quiet environment for the client in panic. Stay with the client, and administer antianxiety medications as ordered. *Staying with the client and displaying calmness and confidence can protect the client from injury and prevent further panic. If the panic does not subside, report to the physician for medication management.*
- Use crisis intervention theory to promote growth in the client and significant others, regardless of the outcome of the disease. A referral to mental health professional may be helpful. *With help, people can transform a major crisis from an experience of defeat and despair to one of personal and spiritual growth.*

treatment and the ultimate outcome. Only the most common diagnoses are discussed here.

ANXIETY

Clients, especially those with poor coping skills, may exhibit overt signs of anxiety, such as trembling, irritability, increased blood pressure, pallor, or poor eye contact. The client may report insomnia and feelings of tension, or express concerns about perceived changes caused by the disease and fear of future events.

- Carefully assess the client's level of anxiety versus the real threats of the client's current situation. *A client in panic may*

DEFICIENT KNOWLEDGE

- Before surgery, give the client the opportunity to ask questions and to discuss concerns and fears. *In some cases, the client may want to discuss alternative treatment options that are available.*
- Explain the specific surgical procedure and any anticipated alterations to the client's body. *Some surgeries will require major lifestyle adjustments, such as a colostomy.*
- Prior to surgery, set up a conference for the client with the oncologist and surgeon. *This will provide an opportunity to clarify the planned surgery and follow-up treatment.*

TABLE 8-5   SIGNS OF NUTRITIONAL STATUS

SYSTEM	GOOD NUTRITION	POOR NUTRITION
General	Alert, energetic, good endurance, psychologically stable Weight within range for height, age, body size	Withdrawn, apathetic, easily fatigued, irritable Over- or underweight
Integumentary	Skin glowing, good turgor, smooth, free of lesions Hair shiny, lustrous, minimal loss	Skin dull, pasty, scaly-dry, bruises, multiple lesions Hair brittle, dull, falls out easily
Head, eyes, ears, nose, and throat	Eyes bright, clear, no fatigue circles Oral mucous membranes pink-red and moist Gums pink, firm Tongue pink, moderately smooth, no swelling	Eyes dull, conjunctiva pale, discoloration under eyes Oral mucous membranes pale Gums red, spongy, and bleed easily Tongue bright to dark red, swollen
Abdomen	Abdomen flat, firm	Abdomen flaccid or distended (ascites)
Musculoskeletal	Firm, well-developed muscles Good posture No skeletal changes	Flaccid muscles, wasted appearance Stooped posture Skeletal malformations
Neurologic	Good attention span, good concentration, astute thought processes Good reflexes	Inattentive, easily distracted, impaired thought processes Paresthesias, reflexes diminished or hyperactive

■ Teach clients and family members to observe for: redness, swelling, pain, or exudate at the insertion site; and swelling of the neck or skin near the VAD. Teach them to flush catheters and provide site care on a regular basis. *The*

risk of infection, catheter obstruction, and extravasation are the main problems associated with VADs.

■ Assess and monitor client for signs and symptoms of toxic side effects of chemotherapy. *This will alert the nurse to the onset of toxicity. Indicators of organ toxicities, such as nephrotoxicity or cardiac toxicity, must be reported immediately to the physician.*

■ Teach clients undergoing chemotherapy to dispose of used equipment and excretions safely. *Excretion of chemotherapy is primarily through the urine.*

BOX 8-8
MANIFESTATIONS OF CANCER OR CANCER TREATMENT

- Hair loss
- Depression
- Fever
- Bleeding gums
- Oropharyngeal ulcerations
- Stomatitis
- Anorexia
- Nausea and vomiting
- Diarrhea
- Emaciation
- General weakness
- Flaccid muscles
- Stooped posture
- Pallor
- Excessive bruising
- Radiation burns
- Visible tumor (abdomen)
- Odor of decay
- Hypotension

DISTURBED BODY IMAGE

■ Discuss with the client the meaning of the loss or change. *Doing so helps the nurse discover the best approach for each client and involves the client more actively in interventions. A seemingly trivial loss may have a big impact on the client's life. Likewise, a major loss may not be as important as the nurse imagines. The nurse must evaluate each situation in terms of the reactions of the specific client.*

■ Observe and evaluate the client's interaction with significant others. *People may unintentionally reinforce negative feelings about body image. Also, the client may perceive rejection where none exists.*

■ If the client won't acknowledge the body change, allow the client to engage in denial, but do not participate in it. (If a client won't look at the wound, the nurse may say, "I am going to change the dressing to your breast incision now.") *Denial is a protective mechanism and should not be challenged, but it also should not be promoted. A matter-of-fact and sympathetic attitude will help the client's accept the change.*

■ Encourage the client and significant others to express their feelings about the situation and to identify new coping strategies. Give matter-of-fact responses to questions and concerns, and enlist family and friends in reaffirming the client's worth. *A supportive, safe environment promotes acceptance and encourages new coping strategies. It also reaffirms that the client's worth is not lessened by any physical changes.*

■ Teach the client or significant others to participate in care of the afflicted body area. Support and validate their efforts. *Active involvement in providing care empowers the client and significant others. It promotes closeness and reduces the risk of rejection. Positive reinforcement encourages these behaviors to continue.*

■ Teach the client specific strategies for minimizing physical changes, (skin care during radiation therapy, dressing to enhance appearance and disguise change in a body part). *Early intervention can limit negative side effects and promote the client's recovery. Involvement gives the client some control in a difficult situation.*

■ Teach clients ways to reduce the *alopecia* (hair loss) from chemotherapy or radiation therapy and to enhance their appearance until hair grows back:

  ■ Discuss the pattern and timing of hair loss. *This allows the client to cope with changes and incorporate them into daily activities.*

  ■ Encourage the client to wear cheerful head coverings, coordinated with client's usual clothing. *Attractive head coverings protect the head while allowing the client to feel well dressed.*

  ■ Teach the client that hair will grow back after chemotherapy, but that its color and texture may be different. Refer the client to a good wig shop before the client experiences hair loss. *Hair color and texture can be matched to minimize obvious changes in appearance. The client who knows what to expect may experience less anxiety and distress.*

  ■ Refer the client to support programs such as "Look Good . . . Feel Better," which is sponsored by the ACS and the Cosmetic, Toiletry, and Fragrance Association Foundation. *A support group can diminish feelings of isolation and provide practical tips for managing problems. For a list of community resources available to clients with cancer, refer to a local phone book.*

ANTICIPATORY GRIEVING

■ Use active listening, silence, and nonverbal support to provide an open environment to discuss feelings realistically and to express anger or other negative feelings. *This helps the client and family members get in touch with their feelings and confront the possibility of the loss or death. Although 59% of people with cancer recover fully, facing death and making preparations can be a healthy response that allows the client and family to work through the dying process and achieve growth, or to cope with changes in body image and lifestyle (see Chapter 9).*

■ Answer questions about illness and prognosis honestly, always encouraging hope. *This allows them to assess their situation realistically and make plans. It also helps combat feelings of hopelessness and depression.*

■ Encourage the dying client to make funeral and burial plans ahead of time and to be sure the will is in order. Make sure the necessary phone numbers can be easily located. *This gives the client a sense of control and frees family members of these concerns when the client is most in need of their support.*

■ Encourage the client to continue taking part in activities he or she enjoys, including keeping a job as long as possible. *The client keeps a sense of continuity of life even in the face of severe losses.*

RISK FOR INFECTION

■ Monitor the client's vital signs. *Fever and sympathetic nervous system responses, such as increased pulse and respiration, are usual early signs of impending infection. However, severely immunosuppressed patients may have infection without fever.*

■ Monitor white blood cell counts frequently, especially for the client receiving chemotherapy that causes bone marrow suppression. *This allows the nurse to notify the physician at the first sign of diminishing white blood cell counts, so that corrective action can be taken.*

■ Teach the client and significant others to avoid crowds, small children, and people with infections when the client's white blood cell count is at *nadir* (lowest point) and to practice careful personal hygiene. *During periods of leukopenia, the client may lose immunity to home flora. Careful attention to hygiene reduces the risk. Even minor infections can be very dangerous for the immunosuppressed client.*

■ Protect skin and mucous membranes from injury. Teach good hygiene, use of moisturizing lotion to prevent dryness and cracking, frequent position changes for the bedfast client, and immediate attention to skin breaks or lesions. *Intact skin is the first line of defense against infection.*

■ Encourage the client to consume a diet high in protein, minerals, and vitamins, especially vitamin C. *Improved nutrition decreases the risk of infection. Vitamin C has been shown to help prevent certain infections.*

RISK FOR INJURY

■ Assess the client frequently for signs and symptoms indicating problems with obstruction (e.g., the brain, lungs, or liver). *Early detection allows the nurse to seek medical help for the client before the problem evolves into a crisis.*

■ Teach the client and family to differentiate minor from serious problems. Box 8-9 provides guidelines to identify problems that must be reported to the nurse or physician or that require a call to 911. *Having guidelines for when to call the doctor provides an anxiety-reducing safety net for the client and family and promotes early detection of complications.*

■ Monitor laboratory values that may indicate the presence of ectopic functioning. Report abnormal findings to physicians immediately. *If the cancer creates ectopic sites of hormones, elevated hormone levels can injure the client in a variety of ways (hypercalcemia, fluid retention, pulmonary edema).*

TEACHING FOR DISCHARGE

WHEN TO CALL FOR HELP

Instruct the client or family member to call the nurse or physician if any of the following signs or symptoms occur:

- Oral temperature greater than 101.5° F (38.6° C)
- Severe headache; significant increase in pain at usual site, especially if the pain is not relieved by the medication regimen; or severe pain at a new site
- Difficulty breathing
- New bleeding from any site, such as rectal or vaginal bleeding
- Confusion, irritability, or restlessness
- Withdrawal, greatly decreased activity level, or frequent crying
- Verbalizations of deep sadness or a desire to end life
- Changes in body functioning, such as the inability to void or severe diarrhea or constipation
- Changes in eating patterns, such as refusal to eat, extreme hunger, or a significant increase in nausea and vomiting
- Appearance of edema in the extremities or significant increase in edema already present

Instruct the client or family member to call 911 if the client:

- Is having much difficulty breathing or if the lips or face has a bluish tinge
- Becomes unconscious or has a convulsion
- Exhibits unmanageable behavior, such as being physically abusive, hurting self, or engaging in uncontrollable activity

IMBALANCED NUTRITION: LESS THAN BODY REQUIREMENTS

- Assess the client's current eating patterns, including likes and dislikes, and identify factors that impair food intake. *This permits an individualized plan based on the client's needs and preferences.*
- Evaluate degree of malnutrition:
  - Check laboratory values for total serum protein, serum albumin and globins, total lymphocyte count, serum transferrin, hemoglobin, and hematocrit. *These values are most likely to decrease with malnutrition.*
  - Evaluate immunologic response by antigen skin testing using common antigens such as *Candida,* purified protein derivative (PPD), mumps, and tetanus. *A positive response (> 5 mm of induration and redness at the site of the intradermal injection) indicates immunocompetence. Nonreaction indicates depressed immune function. Immune response suppression can be related to malnutrition.*

- Calculate nitrogen balance and creatinine-height index. Calculate skeletal muscle mass, and compare findings to normal ranges. *Urinary creatinine is an index of lean body mass and decreases in malnutrition. Lean muscle mass is catabolized for energy in clients with cancer.*
- Teach the client the principles of maintaining good nutrition by using the Food Pyramid (see Figure 18-4) and adapting the diet to the client's medical restrictions and current preferences. *Clients comply better with food plans that are tailored to their needs.*
- Manage problems that interfere with eating:
  - Encourage the client with food aversions to eat whatever is appealing. *It is better for the client to eat something even if it is not nutritionally balanced.*
  - Eat small, frequent meals. *These are more easily digested and absorbed and usually better tolerated by the client with anorexia.*
  - Encourage the client to try icy cold foods (such as ice cream) or more highly seasoned dishes if food has no taste. *Chemotherapy and radiation therapy may harm tastebuds. Strong seasonings and coldness make food more enjoyable to the client.*
  - Encourage cold, bland semisoft and liquid foods for the client with painful oropharyngeal ulcers. Have the client use an anesthetic mouthwash prior to eating. *These foods are less irritating to sensitive mucous membranes. Deadening the pain can make chewing and swallowing easier.*
  - Administer antiemetic medications. Encourage the client to eat low-fat meals with dry foods such as crackers and toast; to avoid liquids with meals; and to sit upright for an hour after meals. Remove emesis basins and encourage oral hygiene before eating. *Dry, low-fat foods are more readily tolerated by the nauseated client. Removing odors and supplies associated with nausea and vomiting can reduce nausea.*
- Teach the client and family to supplement meals with nutritional supplements (Ensure, Isocal) and to take multivitamin and mineral tablets with meals. Suggest increasing calories by adding ice cream or frozen yogurt to the liquid supplement or commercial protein–carbohydrate powders to milk or fruit juice. *Food intake of most cancer clients is usually less than what is needed to maintain or gain weight. These supplements can add calories in a manner often tolerated by the client.*
- Teach client and family to keep a food diary to document client's daily intake. *When clients see how little is being consumed, they may eat more. A food diary also helps the nurse keep a calorie count and alerts the physician if more drastic nutritional measures, such as parenteral nutrition, need to be instituted.*

IMPAIRED TISSUE INTEGRITY

- Carefully assess and evaluate the type of tissue impairment present. Identify possible causes. Manifestations may include small ulcers on the edges of the tongue and throughout the mouth and throat (due to chemotherapy); herpes simplex type I lesions; fungal infections, like thrush (*Candida* infections), seen as a white, yellow, or tan coating with dry, red, fissured tissue underneath; red, swollen, gums that bleed with minimal or no trauma; or *xerostomia* (excessive dryness of the oral mucous membranes) due to chemotherapy or radiation. *This allows the nurse to implement appropriate corrective measures.*

■ Implement and teach measures for preventing oropharyngeal infection:

■ Observe for systemic signs of infection. Be suspicious of any fever that has no apparent cause. *This aids early identification of an infection before it spreads.*

■ Have client clean teeth gently and use a mouthwash after waking in the morning, after any oral intake, and before bedtime. The client should soak dentures nightly in hydrogen peroxide and floss gently with waxed floss after meals and bedtime (this measure is contraindicated for people with leukemia or thrombocytopenia). *Disrupted mucous membranes allow the normal oral bacterial flora into the systemic circulation; this can result in sepsis in the immunocompromised person. Reducing the oral flora by frequent hygiene decreases the risk of infection.*

■ Culture any oral lesions, and report the problem to physician. *Herpes lesions may not follow a typical pattern in immunosuppressed clients. Identifying the cause of the infection, whether viral, fungal, or bacterial, allows the physician to prescribe the appropriate treatment.*

■ Implement and teach measures for reducing trauma to delicate tissues:

■ Counteract xerostomia with lubricating and moisturing agents, such as Gatoraid, sugarless gum, and Blistex. Avoid putting sharp instruments or utensils in the mouth. Teach that dental work should be done by dental oncologists. Brush teeth with a very soft toothbrush, and obtain a new toothbrush monthly. If gums are bleeding, clean teeth with toothpaste and a soft cloth over finger. Chlorhexidine mouthwash (Peridex) may be used. *These measures protect gums from trauma and decrease risk of hemorrhage.*

■ Administer specific medications as ordered to control infection or pain: Acyclovir (viral infections), systemic antibiotics (bacterial infections), Nystatin or clotrimazole solution or lozenges (fungal infections), or viscous Xylocaine or various combination mouthwashes before meals and as needed. *These agents reduce pain and inflammation. Knowing the contents of each mouthwash can prevent hypersensitivity reactions (e.g., to lidocaine).*

CHRONIC PAIN

■ Provide relief that allows clients to function as they wish and, for terminally ill clients, to die relatively free of pain. Pain may be associated with direct tumor involvement (e.g., metastatases, nerve compression), with treatment; or with an unrelated cause (like diabetic neuropathy). *Providing pain relief allows the client to maintain control and function at an optimal level.*

■ Begin pain management with combinations of nonnarcotic drugs (such as aspirin or ibuprofen) and adjuvants (such as corticosteroids or antidepressants). Progress to stronger

drugs as needed, from mild narcotics such as oxycodone (Percodan) or propoxyphene (Darvon) to strong narcotics such as morphine or hydromorphone (Dilaudid). *A combination of medications may be required to manage the client's pain.*

■ Continue to try combinations and escalate dosages until maximal pain relief is achieved, balanced with client's need to function. *When narcotic doses are increased gradually, there is no limit to the amount the client can receive, as long as adverse reactions can be managed.*

■ Administer medication on a regular time schedule (e.g., every 4 hours) with additional medication to cover breakthrough pain. *A regular schedule of medication will provide the patient with greater pain relief.*

EVALUATING

Evaluating the effectiveness of nursing care for the client with cancer will require ongoing assessment throughout the nursing process. Measures that are ineffective, such as pain management, will need to be changed and the effectiveness evaluated over time. The family or significant others can also provide data about the effectiveness of the plan of care.

Discharge Teaching

PREVENTION

The ACS makes specific recommendations for prevention, in addition to the screening measures discussed earlier in this chapter. Based on these recommendations, nurses should provide the following teaching:

■ Avoid tobacco, secondhand smoke, and excessive alcohol use.
■ Avoid obesity and eat a low-fat, high-fiber diet.
■ Consume ample amounts of antioxidant foods, such as those containing beta carotene (a vitamin A precursor), vitamins E and C, and omega-3 oils.
■ Avoid foods with carcinogenic additives, dyes, or chemicals used in processing (salt-cured, smoked, and nitrate-cured foods).
■ Take certain medications and hormones, such as estrogen or tamoxifen, only under close medical supervision.
■ Limit exposure to radiation, including sun exposure.
■ Use extreme caution if employed in an industry that uses carcinogenic chemicals or airborne particles (smoke). Seek new employment if you are at risk for related cancers.
■ Protect yourself from viral diseases known to cause cancer.
■ Improve immunity by maintaining a healthy lifestyle and managing stress.

In addition, encourage people to report to the public health department any known leaking of chemicals or radioactive materials into the water or air. Also report any noted increase in the incidence of cancer, especially of one specific type, in the community.

REHABILITATION

Rehabilitation from cancer not only involves regaining strength, recovering from surgery or chemotherapy, and learning to live with an altered body part or appliance, but also entails recovering from associated psychological and emotional turmoil.

Rehabilitation centers provide physical therapy, occupational therapy, speech therapy, job retraining, and an opportunity to rest before resuming life responsibilities. In addition, many clients convalesce at home and receive in-home support in the form of nursing supervision, direct care, and teaching. Hygiene and home maintenance can be provided by a certified home health aide. Physical and occupational therapists provide muscle strengthening and mobility training (especially with prostheses), and home safety teaching.

Psychological rehabilitation of cancer survivors addresses quality-of-life issues. Employment may be a problem, health insurance may be canceled, and life insurance may be difficult to get following a diagnosis of cancer. Relationships may have suffered from the strain the illness placed on significant others and the essential self-focusing required for recovery. However, both the client and significant others may have undergone personal and spiritual growth that ushers in a new and enriching period of their lives.

Self-help groups are emerging in many communities to support others through their cancer experience. Clients and families need to be informed about the many resources that are available through community agencies as well as the survivor support groups.

HOME CARE

Teach the client and significant others or caregivers how to manage the client at home. Discuss problems that may result from the type of cancer and the treatment received. Provide information on how to manage these problems and when to call the physician. Teach wound care to the client with an open wound or draining lesion, and provide a referral to a home health nurse to monitor progress. Explain special diets clearly, or refer the client to a dietitian before discharge. Carefully review home care instructions with the client and family, making sure they understand medications to be taken, any other treatments, and when to see the doctor for follow-up care. Provide or order equipment and supplies needed for home care, especially any special bed or equipment for mobility and safety in the home. For the client who needs complex care, such as parenteral nutrition, provide a referral to a home health nurse before discharge. Because the hospital stay is often short, make follow-up phone calls for several days after the client arrives home, and provide the client and family with a number to call for concerns and questions.

HOSPICE CARE

The increased availability of hospice programs has made it easier for cancer clients with terminal disease to elect to die at home. When a client and family choose hospice care, they are usually deciding against additional hospitalizations, except those required to manage reversible problems. Hospice clients also refuse resuscitation measures (see Chapter 9). The multidisciplinary hospice team usually consists of the following members:

- A nurse case manager, who works directly with the client and family, and coordinates the activities of the other disciplines. The nurse is usually on call 24 hours a day and makes home visits frequently. The nurse is often with the family when the client dies.
- A physician, who may make periodic home visits and collaborates with the nurse case manager about medications and treatments.
- An anesthesiologist or pharmacist, who manages pain control and watches for drug interactions.
- An infusion therapist, who provides equipment, supplies, solutions, and expertise for intravenous medications or nutrition administered to the client. This person is usually on call 24 hours a day to trouble-shoot equipment problems.
- A social worker, who helps with resources for the client and family, with grief work, and with general support and counseling as needed.
- A physical therapist, who teaches how to manage the immobilized client.
- A home health aide, who provides physical care to the client and assists the family with household chores.
- Volunteers, who provide companionship for the client and give respite to the family for short periods of time.

Many hospice services are connected with an inpatient respite care unit, where the client can receive 24-hour care for up to several weeks. This source provides the necessary care to the client if a family member becomes ill or needs to be relieved temporarily of the tremendous burden of caring for a dying loved one.

Nursing Process Case Study
■ CLIENT WITH CANCER

James Casey is a 72-year-old man who has been under medical care for chronic obstructive pulmonary disease, post-myocardial infarction, and Type 1 diabetes mellitus for over 15 years. He lost his wife due to lung cancer 5 years ago and still "misses her terribly." He reports smoking two packs of cigarettes a day for 52 years, one to two six-packs of beer a week, one "bourbon and water" a night, and "a lot of sugar-free junk food." He quit smoking 2 years ago, when he could no longer walk a block without considerable shortness of breath, and just quit drinking alcohol a few weeks ago at his physician's insistence. About a year ago, he had a basal-cell carcinoma removed from his right ear. Six months ago, he underwent two 6-week courses of chemotherapy for bladder cancer. The latest report indicates that the cancer has returned and no further chemotherapy would be useful. Surgery was considered but his other medical problems would compromise his chances of survival, so Mr. Casey decided to forgo further treatment and to be managed at home through hospice care. His daughter, Mary Walsh, and her family have moved in with him to provide care and support during his final months. The daughter says she is glad to be able to spend this time with her father. She has been informed of the physical and emotional stress this will entail.

Data Collection The hospice nurse, Ms. Jackson, completes a health history and physical examination during her first two home visits. She gathers this information over 2 days to conserve his strength and allow more time for him and his daughter to talk about their concerns.

During the assessment, Ms. Jackson notes that Mr. Casey is pale and thin, with a wasted appearance and a worried facial expression. His blood pressure is 90/50; apical pulse is 102 and regular; respiratory rate 24; breath sounds are clear but diminished in the bases; oral temperature is 96.8° F.

Last week a tunneled Groshong catheter as a VAD was placed in the right anterior chest. There is no drainage, redness, or swelling at the site.

Mr. Casey states that he spends most of his time either in bed or sitting up in a chair in his room. He says he has no energy and is unable to walk to the bathroom alone or take care of his own personal hygiene. He complains of severe back pain no longer adequately relieved by alternating Percodan and Vicodin every 2 to 4 hours. The nurse rates Mr. Casey's functional level as: capable of only limited self-care, confined to bed or chair 50% or more of waking hours. He tells the nurse that his daughter "is working day and night to help me and is looking awfully tired."

Ms. Walsh reports that Mr. Casey is eating very poorly: He has a small bowl of oatmeal for breakfast, soup and crackers for lunch, and only fruit juice for dinner. Mr. Casey says that he has no appetite and eats just to please his daughter. He does drink at least three to four glasses of water a day plus juice. His finger-stick blood sugars remain within normal range. His current weight is 120 pounds, down from 180 pounds a year ago. He has lost about 30 pounds over the last 2 months.

Laboratory values from his visit with the doctor show the following:

Total protein: 4.1 (Normal range: 6.0 to 8.0 g/dL)
Albumin: 2.2 (Normal range: 3.5 to 5.0 g/dL)
Hemoglobin: 10.2 (Normal range: 13.5 to 18.0 g/dL)
Hematocrit: 30.5 (Normal range: 40.0 to 54.0%)
Blood urea nitrogen (BUN): 30 (Normal range: 5 to 25 mg/dL slightly higher in older people)
Creatinine: 2.2 (Normal range: 0.5 to 1.5 mg/dL)

Diagnosis The nursing diagnoses for Mr. Casey (and significant others) include the following:

■ Imbalanced Nutrition: Less Than Body Requirements related to anorexia and fatigue
■ Risk for Caregiver Role Strain related to severity of her father's illness and lack of help from other family members
■ Chronic Pain related to progression of disease process
■ Impaired Physical Mobility related to pain, fatigue, and beginning neuromuscular impairment
■ Risk for Impaired Skin Integrity related to impaired physical mobility and malnourished state

Expected Outcomes The expected outcomes established in the plan of care specify that

■ Mr. Casey will increase his oral intake and show improvement in his serum protein values.
■ His daughter will be able to maintain her supportive caretaking activities as long as Mr. Casey needs them.
■ Mr. Casey will have minimal pain for the rest of his life.
■ Mr. Casey will be able to continue his current activity level.
■ Mr. Casey will have intact skin.

Planning and Implementation The following interventions are planned and implemented during Mr. Casey's care:

■ Ask Mr. Casey what his favorite foods are, and ask his daughter to offer him a small portion of one of these foods each day.
■ Encourage Mr. Casey to drink up to four cans of Ensure Plus with Fiber a day, sipping them throughout the day.
■ Talk with the physician about trying a medication to stimulate the appetite.
■ Have a home health aide assist with personal care and some household tasks.
■ Talk with Ms. Walsh about her adult children providing some assistance. Offer to talk with them if she is uncomfortable doing so.
■ Request a volunteer to spend up to 4 hours a day, twice a week with Mr. Casey so that Ms. Walsh can attend to outside activities and chores.
■ Talk with the physician, and work out a pain-control program fusing the VAD and a patient-controlled analgesia (PCA) infusion pump with a continuous morphine infusion.
■ Call the infusion therapist to set up the equipment and supplies (including the medication) for the morphine infusion.
■ Teach Mr. Casey and his daughter how to use the pump and about the side effects of the morphine infusion, including those requiring assistance.
■ Leave detailed instructions regarding medication storage and care of the pump, along with the telephone number of the infusion therapist.
■ Instruct Ms. Walsh to allow ample rest periods between each activity Mr. Casey must carry out, such as taking a shower or using the commode.

- Order a hospital bed, a special foam pad for Mr. Casey's bed and chair and a bedside commode from the medical supply house.
- Instruct Ms. Walsh and the home health aide in proper skin care, and to report any beginning lesions immediately to the nurse.

Evaluation Mr. Casey increased his oral intake a little and drank one or two cans of Ensure a day. His weight remained at about 120 pounds until his death 2 weeks later. Ms. Walsh was very grateful for the extra help from the home health aide and the volunteer, but could not bring herself to ask her son and daughter for help and did not want the nurse to do so. She did become more rested and reported that "we had some wonderful 3:00 A.M. talks when he couldn't sleep."

Mr. Casey was started on 20 mg of morphine per hour with boluses of 10 mg four times a day. This medication relieved his pain quite well; after 2 days he was alert enough most of the time to carry on a normal conversation and able to walk to the bathroom with help until 2 days before he died.

The hospital bed simplified Mr. Casey's care and made it much easier for him to rest comfortably and change position. His skin remained intact and in good condition. Mr. Casey died peacefully in his sleep, about 2 weeks after care was started.

Critical Thinking in the Nursing Process

1. What other tests could have been done to evaluate Mr. Casey's nutritional status?
2. Mr. Casey had severe back pain. What were the possible pathophysiologic reasons for his pain?
3. If Mr. Casey's daughter, Ms. Walsh, had a nursing diagnosis of Ineffective Individual Coping, what would you include in a teaching plan to help her learn new coping strategies?

Nursing Interventions for Oncologic Emergencies

In caring for clients with cancer, nurses may encounter a number of emergency situations in which their role may be crucial to the client's survival. Most of these emergencies require astute observation, accurate judgment, and rapid action once the problem has been identified (Hogan & Rosenthal, 1998). In all cases, notifying the physician or emergency team immediately is the first step. A brief description of some of the more common oncologic emergencies with nursing interventions follows.

PERICARDIAL EFFUSION AND NEOPLASTIC CARDIAC TAMPONADE

Malignant *pericardial effusion* may occur secondary to lung or esophageal cancers or due to metastases. It can compress the heart, restrict heart movement, and result in a cardiac tamponade. The signs of cardiac tamponade are those of circulatory collapse or cardiogenic shock: hypotension, tachycardia, tachypnea, dyspnea, cyanosis, increased central venous pressure, anxiety, restlessness, and impaired consciousness. Interventions include the following:

- Start oxygen and alert respiratory therapy for other respiratory support as needed.
- Monitor vital signs and initiate hemodynamic monitoring.
- Bring crash cart to bedside.
- Set up for and assist physician with a pericardial tap (pericardiocentesis).
- Reassure the client.

SUPERIOR VENA CAVA SYNDROME

The superior vena cava can be compressed by mediastinal tumors or adjacent thoracic tumors. The most common cause is lung cancer. Signs and symptoms may develop slowly. Facial and arm edema are early signs. As the problem progresses, pleural effusion and tracheal edema cause respiratory distress, dyspnea, cyanosis, and, eventually, altered consciousness and neurologic deficits. Nursing measures include the following:

- Provide respiratory support with oxygen, and prepare for tracheostomy.
- Monitor vital signs.
- Administer corticosteroids (e.g., dexamethasone) to reduce edema.
- If the disorder is due to a clot, administer antifibrinolytic or anticoagulant drugs, as ordered.
- Provide a safe environment, including seizure precautions.

After the emergency is managed, the client often receives radiation or chemotherapy to reduce the tumor size.

SEPSIS AND SEPTIC SHOCK

Tumor necrosis coupled with an immunosuppressed and/or malnourished state can result in sepsis. Bacteria gain entrance to the blood, grow rapidly, and produce septicemia. The sepsis, which is usually gram-negative, progresses to systemic shock and eventually results in multisystem failure (see Chapter 10). Signs and symptoms appear in two phases. The first phase is characterized by vasodilation with vascular dehydration; high fever; peripheral edema; hypotension; tachycardia; tachypnea or Kussmaul's respirations; hot, flushed skin with creeping mottling beginning in the lower extremities; and anxiety or restlessness. Without treatment, the shock progresses to the second phase and more classic signs of shock: hypotension; rapid, thready pulse; respiratory distress; cyanosis; subnormal temperature; cold, clammy skin; decreased urinary output; and altered mentation. Identifying the problem while the client is still in the first phase is crucial to the client's survival. Interventions include the following:

- Monitor infusion of colloidal solutions (plasma volume expanders, such as albumin) and balanced salt solutions as ordered.

■ Monitor hemodynamic functioning to evaluate the effects of rehydration and to detect early signs of overload.

■ Provide oxygen and other respiratory support as needed.

■ Assist with obtaining cultures of the source of infection and blood cultures.

■ Administer prescribed broad-spectrum antibiotics until the specific organism is identified.

■ Provide a safe environment for the client with altered mentation; provide support and reassurance for the anxious client.

SPINAL CORD COMPRESSION

Spinal cord compression is most commonly associated with pressure from expanding tumors of the breast, lung, or prostate; lymphoma; or metastatic disease. It has the potential for irreversible paraplegia. Early symptoms include progressive back and leg pain, numbness, paresthesias, and coldness. Later, bowel and bladder dysfunction occur and, finally, neurologic dysfunction progressing to weakness and paralysis. Treatment often consists of radiation or surgical decompression, but early detection is essential. Nursing responsibilities include the following:

■ Perform neurologic checks every shift for clients with advanced cancers of the breast, lung, prostate, or lymphoma.

■ Thoroughly assess all complaints of back pain or sensory changes.

■ Notify physician if spinal cord compression is suspected, and prepare for magnetic resonance imaging (MRI).

■ Administer cortisteroids (e.g., dexamethasone) to reduce cord edema and protect function.

OBSTRUCTIVE UROPATHY

Clients with intra-abdominal, retroperitoneal, or pelvic malignancies (prostate, cervical, or bladder cancers), may experience obstruction of the bladder neck or the ureters. Bladder neck obstruction usually manifests as urinary retention, flank pain, hematuria, or persistent urinary tract infections; ureteral obstruction is often not evident until the client is in renal failure. Interventions include the following:

■ Investigate complaints of flank pain or urinary retention.

■ Monitor serum BUN, creatinine, and potassium for elevated levels.

■ Send a specimen of any foul-smelling urine for culture.

■ Report hematuria to the physician immediately.

■ Catheterize the client with acute retention as ordered.

HYPERCALCEMIA

Hypercalcemia is associated with cancers of the breast, lung, esophagus, thyroid, head, and neck and with multiple myeloma. Bone metastases may also cause hypercalcemia. (Hypercalcemia is discussed in detail in Chapter 5.) Clients

often present with nonspecific symptoms (fatigue, anorexia, polyuria, constipation). Neurologic symptoms include muscle weakness, lethargy, and diminished reflexes. Without treatment, hypercalcemia progresses to alterations in mental status, psychotic behavior, cardiac dysrythmias, seizures, coma, and death. Nursing interventions include the following:

■ Monitor serum calcium, phosphate, alkaline phosphatase, electrolytes, BUN, and creatinine levels.

■ Monitor pulse.

■ Administer intravenous solutions of normal saline to increase urinary calcium excretion.

■ Administer corticosteroids and calcitonin.

■ Maintain the client on bed rest until calcium levels decrease.

HYPERURICEMIA

Hyperuricemia usually is a complication of rapid necrosis of tumor cells after vigorous chemotherapy for lymphomas and leukemias. Uric acid crystals are deposited in the urinary tract, causing renal failure and uremia. Symptoms of hyperuricemia include nausea, vomiting, lethargy, and oliguria. Nursing actions focus on prevention and include the following:

■ Increase intravenous hydration to ensure urinary output of approximately 3 L a day for 48 hours prior to chemotherapy.

■ Administer allopurinol (antigout drug) per recommended dosage and schedule for 48 hours prior to chemotherapy.

■ Administer daily sodium bicarbonate to alkalinize the urine and thereby prevent uric acid crystallization.

■ Monitor serum uric acid levels and urine pH.

■ If signs of uremia occur, insert a Foley catheter and monitor urinary output as well as serum BUN, creatinine, and potassium levels.

Nursing Interventions Classification

The following interventions (McCloskey & Bulechek, 2000) may also be appropriate for the client with cancer:

■ Caregiver Support
■ Coping Enhancement
■ Nausea Management
■ Fluid Management
■ Home Maintenance Assistance
■ Hope Instillation
■ Self-Care Assistance

(*Note:* The bibliography listings for this and all chapters have been compiled at the back of the book.)

Chapter Review

 ## key terms by topic

Use the CD-ROM disk enclosed with your textbook to hear the pronunciation of the key terms in the chapter.

Cancer
cancer, oncology, neoplasm, metastasis, carcinogens

Theories of carcinogenesis
oncogenes

Physiologic effects of cancer
anorexia–cachexia syndrome

key points

- Cancer can affect people of any age, gender, ethnicity, or geographic region.
- Many cancer risk factors are controllable; prevention is key.
- Clients with cancer need a great deal of emotional support because fear and anxiety are common responses to a diagnosis of cancer.
- Cancer treatment is aimed at cure, control, or palliation of symptoms.
- Cancer may be treated through surgery, radiotherapy, chemotherapy, and biotherapy.
- Early detection and treatment influence the prognosis of people with cancer most.
- All people should have regular cancer checkups.
- Cancer pain is the most feared symptom.

 ## Medialink

Additional interactive resources for this chapter can be found on the Companion Website at http://www.prenhall.com/burke. Click on Chapter 8 and "Begin" to select the activities for this chapter.

For NCLEX review questions and an audio glossary, access the accompanying CD-ROM in this book.

for further study

For more information on preoperative preparation, see Chapter 7.

For more information about caring for clients in pain, see Chapter 6.

For more on the death and dying issues and hospice care, see Chapter 9.

For more information on infection, see Chapter 12.

For more about electrolyte imbalances, see Chapter 5.

For more information about endocrine disorders, see Chapter 16.

For more about nutrition and the Food Guide Pyramid, see Figure 18-4.

For more information on shock and multisystem failure, see Chapter 10.

For more information on hypercalcemia, see Chapter 5.

Critical Thinking Care Map

Caring for a Client Undergoing Chemotherapy for Cancer
NCLEX-PN Focus Area: Physiological Integrity: Reduction of Risk Potential

Case Study: Maria Hernandez, a 78-year-old Hispanic woman, was diagnosed with colon cancer and had a colon resection 6 months ago. When she comes in for chemotherapy, she reports that she has been progressively anorexic and nauseated since beginning chemotherapy of 5-fluorouracil (5-FU). She states "I just can't eat. My mouth is so sore and it hurts to swallow. I've lost so much weight."

Nursing Diagnosis: Imbalanced Nutrition: Less Than Body Requirements

COLLECT DATA

Subjective

Objective

Would you report this data? Yes/No

If yes, to: _____

Data Collected (use those that apply)

- Height: 5', 4"
- Weight: 102 lbs.
- Pale skin with poor turgor
- Blood pressure: 134/76
- Apical pulse: 88, regular
- Lungs clear to auscultation
- Pale skin with poor turgor
- Hemoglobin: 13.4
- White blood count: 6,500
- Oral mucous membranes red and swollen
- Bowel sounds present in all four quadrants
- Hair dry and brittle
- Concentrated urine

Nursing Care

How would you document this? _____

Nursing Interventions (use those that apply)

- Administer pain medications.
- Administer antiemetics.
- Assist Mrs. Hernandez with ambulation.
- Assess hemoglobin and hematocrit.
- Encourage fluid intake.
- Monitor vital signs every 4 hours.
- Suggest referral for counseling.
- Suggest eating soft bland foods at room temperature.
- Offer high-protein drinks.
- Instruct on using soft toothbrush or toothette for oral hygiene.
- Administer pain medications.

NCLEX-PN Exam Preparation

TEST-TAKING TIP

Assisting clients to meet their psychological needs in relation to cancer is important. However, when answering NCLEX questions that require implementation, meeting physiologic needs is of greater priority.

1. A client has a history of lung cancer. Cells from the lung tumor have traveled to his liver. This process is called:
   a. carcinogenesis
   b. metastasis
   c. encapsulation
   d. mutation

2. A client is diagnosed with colon cancer. She asks the nurse if her diet of high-fat, low-fiber, and fried foods may have contributed to this condition. The nurse's response is based on the knowledge that:
   a. food has no link to development of colon cancer
   b. The client's diet is linked to lung cancer, not colon cancer
   c. research has established that a high-fat, low-fiber diet contributes to development of colon cancer
   d. baked, high fiber foods contribute to development of colon cancer

3. A client diagnosed with lung cancer reports he is having difficulty sleeping and often feels tense. The most appropriate initial nursing intervention would be to:
   a. offer an antianxiety drug such as Ativan (lorazepam)
   b. encourage the client to express his or her feelings concerning the diagnosis of cancer
   c. document the client's status in the medical record
   d. collaborate with the physician to obtain an order for sleep medication

4. Following surgery to remove a colon tumor, a client refuses to care for his colostomy. Appropriate nursing intervention would be to:
   a. teach a family member to perform colostomy care
   b. inform the client that he must learn to change the colostomy bag
   c. tell the client to turn his head away while colostomy care is performed
   d. refer the client for psychological counseling

5. A client anticipates alopecia as a result of chemotherapy. The nurse can BEST assist her to cope with this result by:
   a. encouraging her to choose a wig or other head cover before losing her hair
   b. discussing the advantages of being bald
   c. scheduling a consultation with a hairdresser when she loses her hair
   d. purchase a wig for the client

6. A client reports a 15-pound weight loss due to anorexia during a course of chemotherapy. The serum albumin level is 2.0. The MOST effective nursing action would be to:
   a. report the lab finding to the physician
   b. request double portion meals for the client
   c. assess food likes and dislikes and encourage small frequent meals
   d. encourage hot foods such as soup and broth to provide calories

7. A client is receiving internal radiation to the cervix. The nurse discovers the implant in the client's bed. The appropriate action would be to:
   a. remove the client from the room
   b. use long-handled forceps to place the implant in a lead container
   c. discard the implant in the trash receptacle
   d. flush the implant in the toilet

8. A client is receiving external radiation for treatment of lung cancer. Client teaching for care of the skin in the marked area includes:
   a. apply antibacterial ointment daily
   b. cleanse the skin with mild soap and water
   c. avoid rubbing or scratching treated skin areas
   d. avoid contact with others to eliminate radiation risk

9. A client complains of nausea and vomiting following her daily chemotherapy treatment. The MOST appropriate nursing intervention would be to:
   a. provide antiemetic medication 30 to 40 minutes prior to each treatment
   b. place the patient NPO until after each treatment
   c. schedule chemotherapy for bedtime
   d. provide clear liquids until chemotherapy is finished

10. A client experiences bone marrow depression as a result of chemotherapy. Which of the following would the nurse expect to find?
    a. nausea and vomiting
    b. alopecia
    c. temperature 102° F
    d. platelet count 200,000

Cultural Care STRATEGIES

Responding to Beliefs Related to Death, Dying, and Grief from a Cultural Perspective

Mr. Fazil, 68, a Muslim from Afghanistan, is dying of pancreatic cancer. His brother remains constantly at the bedside where he recites verses from the Koran. When staff offer to sit with Mr. Fazil so the brother can go to the cafeteria, he refuses, saying his voice reciting the Koran must be the last words Mr. Fazil hears before he dies. The nurse offers to bring him some food and he accepts this offer, provided he is able to perform handwashing rites before eating. The brother requests that a private room be provided for other family members including the women of the family where they can meet and grieve together. The brother also requests that he be given all the information concerning Mr. Fazil's status so that he can give this information to the other family members. The women in the family are not permitted in Mr. Fazil's room.

One of the most challenging aspects of providing care for dying people and their families is rendering care that is relevant to cultural, racial, ethnic, and religious needs. (Dowd, Poole, Davidhizar, & Giger, 1998). There is no universally applicable view of grief. Rather, grief practices and responses to death and dying vary depending on cultural orientation. It is important to determine how the nurse can assist in bereavement and the dying process in a culturally competent manner.

Mourning practices and methods of communicating grief vary across and within cultural groups. For example, for some Chinese individuals, wailing is an essential part of proper mourning. Among African-Americans, it has been said that wailing shows how much the family cared about the individual (Perry, 1993). Buddhists use chanting during the dying process. Chanting is thought to facilitate a calm and peaceful atmosphere for the caregivers, thus indirectly helping the dying person. Crying is the most common expression of grief among cultures. Crying serves to bind individuals who mourn together. In some cultures, grief is expressed through singing and dancing.

Mourning customs related to social organization are important. Individuals may wish to mourn in private, with family members, or with a community group. In some families, such as many Asian families, having the extended family present and involved in decision making is important. This can be problematic when the head of the family group is still resident in Asia (Dowd et al., 1998). Talamanes, Lawler, and Espino (1995) note that involving Hispanic family members in decision making is important. Issues related to gender role must also be considered. For example, Hispanic, Amish, and Asian-American families may have male-dominated decision making. In some cultures grief expression

may be related to the social position, age, and sex of the deceased. In a country with high infant mortality, the death of an infant may not be considered as "important" as it is in Western culture. In Chinese society, husbands require "greater mourning" than wives. Rosenblatt et al. (1976) suggested that this might be a cross-cultural constant, since the average time of mourning by widows was found to be 304 days, and by widowers 215 days.

Many cultures are rich in rituals surrounding death. For instance, some Hindus perceive death as a passage from one existence to another. Thus, preparation of the body for cremation involves bathing the remains in a milk and yogurt solution, which symbolically cleanses the soul of the deceased. When a married Indian women dies, she traditionally is placed in a white wedding sari; a man is dressed in a plain off-white East Indian suit. Religious prayers and chanting are continuous before and after death to promote safe passage of the soul. Russian family members—after washing, dressing, and placing the body in the coffin—may keep vigil over the coffin for hours prior to the wake and funeral. They may place a black wreath on the door of the deceased person's home. If the individual is Catholic or Russian Orthodox, a priest uses holy oil to anoint the deceased person while making the sign of the cross and saying specific prayers. At the funeral, each member of the Russian Orthodox family may symbolically place a few grains of soil into the coffin.

Nursing Implications

- **Assess individuals for personal beliefs related to death and dying.** Nurses should appreciate that clients' practices related to grief, dying, and death may be significantly different from their own and may be related to cultural practices.
- **Assist the client and family to grieve and practice death rituals to meet individual needs.** By respecting personal beliefs, the nurse can facilitate grieving in a culturally appropriate manner.

Self-Reflection Questions

1. What beliefs related to grief, death, and dying do you have?
2. Are you flexible in allowing people from different cultures to practice their own traditions in relation to bereavement, the dying process, and death rituals?
3. What can you do to increase your knowledge of bereavement and death practices?

Loss, Grief, and End-of-Life Care

LEARNING outcomes

After completing this chapter, you will be able to:

- Define loss, grief, and death.
- Describe the stages of loss, with commonly experienced emotional responses.
- Discuss factors that influence responses to loss and reflect on one's own responses to loss and death.
- Discuss legal and ethical issues of dying, including advance directives, living wills, do-not-resuscitate orders, and euthanasia.
- Describe physiologic changes in the dying client and signs of death.
- Use the nursing process to collect data and provide interventions for the client who is experiencing loss and is at the end of life.

MediaLink

 www.prenhall.com/burke

Use the above address to access the free, interactive Companion Website created for this textbook. Get hints, instant feedback, and textbook references to chapter-related multiple choice questions. Link to other interesting sites.

Loss, Grief, and Death

Loss occurs when a valued object, person, body part, or situation that was formerly present is lost or changed and can no longer be seen, felt, heard, known, or experienced. A loss may be temporary or permanent, complete or partial, subjective, physical, or symbolic. Losses that occur in any phase of the life cycle may produce grief responses as intensely painful as those observed in the death experience. Only the person who experiences it can determine the meaning of the loss.

The order of importance varies, but people most commonly fear the loss of the following:

- Health
- Social status
- Possessions
- Lifestyle
- Sexual functioning
- Body part
- Death
- Marital relationship (i.e., through divorce)
- Reproductive functioning
- Stable relationships

The stress of loss may initiate physical or emotional changes in a person or family. To deal with the resulting changes, people must resolve their feelings about the loss, through a process called *grief work.*

Grief is the emotional response to loss and its accompanying changes. *Grieving* may be thought of as the internal process the person uses to work through the response to loss. *Mourning* describes the actions or expressions of the bereaved (symbols, clothing, and ceremonies) that make up the outward signs of grief.

Death is defined in a variety of ways. A commonly used definition of death is an irreversible cessation of circulatory and respiratory functions or irreversible cessation of all functions of the entire brain, including the brain stem. Generally, the following characteristics must be present (in some cases for at least 24 hours) for death to be declared: a lack of responsiveness, a lack of movement or breathing, a lack of reflexes, and a flat encephalogram.

Although death is an inevitable part of life, it is often an immensely difficult loss both for the person who is dying and for his or her loved ones. Death may be accidental (such as from trauma or a drug overdose). It may be the end of a long and painful struggle with a terminal illness such as cancer, AIDS, or heart disease. It may also be purposeful, if a person commits suicide.

EXPERIENCING AND RESOLVING LOSS

Medical–surgical nurses practicing in all types of settings care for clients who are in various stages of the grieving process. Grief is highly individual. The grief process may range from discomforting to debilitating; it may last a day or a lifetime, depending on what the loss means to the person experiencing it.

Kübler-Ross's (1969, 1978) research on death and dying provides one framework for understanding the stages of coping with an impending or actual loss. Kübler-Ross was careful to state that not all people dealing with a loss go through these stages or go through them in the sequence described. She identified stages of death and dying, but repeatedly stressed the danger of labeling a "stage" prematurely. She emphasized that her goal was to describe observations of how people come to terms with loss. She observed that some or all of the following stages may occur during the grieving process and may reappear as the person experiences the loss.

Denial

A person may react with shock and disbelief after receiving word of an actual or potential loss. People may make such statements as, "This can't be happening to me" or "This can't be true." This initial stage of denial serves as a buffer. During denial, the person or family mobilizes defenses to cope with the situation.

Anger

In the anger stage, the person resists the loss. The anger, described as "acting out," is often directed toward family and health care providers.

Bargaining

The bargaining stage serves as an attempt to delay the reality of the loss. The person makes a secret bargain with God, expressing a willingness to do anything to postpone the loss or change the prognosis. This is the individual's plea for an extension of life or the chance to "make everything right" with a dying family member or friend.

Depression

When the person realizes the full impact of the actual or perceived loss, the person enters a stage of depression and prepares for the impending loss by working through the struggle of separation. While grieving over "what cannot be," the person may either talk freely about the loss or withdraw from others.

Acceptance

Some people who are dying reach a stage of acceptance in which they may appear to have no emotions. The struggle is past, and the emotional pain is gone. If the person has experienced the loss of a loved one or other valued object, he or she begins to come to terms with the loss and resumes activities with an air of hopefulness for the future.

Differences in a person's understanding of and reaction to loss are affected by the person's developmental stage. In general, as people age and experience life transitions, they are more able to understand and accept the losses associated with those transitions (Table 9-1 ◆).

FAMILY AND OTHER SUPPORT SYSTEMS

Grieving is painful and lonely. Reactions to loss are affected by how much social support people feel they have. Lack of a sup-

TABLE 9-1	DEVELOPMENT OF THE CONCEPT OF DEATH	
AGE	**BELIEFS/ATTITUDES ABOUT DEATH**	
3	Fears separation; lacks comprehension of permanent separation.	
3–5	Believes death is like sleeping and is reversible. Expresses curiosity about what happens to the body.	
6–10	Understands finality of death. Views own death as avoidable. Associates death with violence. Believes wishes can be responsible for death.	
11–12	Reflects views of death expressed by parents. Expresses interest in afterlife as an understanding of mortality develops. Recognizes death as irreversible and inevitable.	
13–21	Usually has a religious and philosophic view of death but seldom thinks about it. Views own death as distant or a challenge, acting out defiance through reckless behavior. Previously held developmental awareness of death may still be present.	
22–45	Does not think about death unless confronted with it. Emotionally distances self from death. Attitude toward death influenced by religious and cultural beliefs.	
46–65	Experiences the death of parents or friends. Accepts own mortality. Experiences waves of death anxiety. Puts life in order to prepare for death and decrease anxiety.	
66 and older	Fears lingering, incapacitating illness. Views death as inevitable but from a philosophical viewpoint, that is, as freedom from pain and illness or as a spiritual reunion with decreased friends and loved ones.	

port system has been identified as one factor that may delay grief work (Carpenito, 2000). Even if the client is reacting to the loss in an expected manner, feelings of isolation and withdrawal behaviors are often observed. Clients need encouragement to reestablish contact with significant others in their lives to allow them to share their grief. If the client is not making progress in grief work, the nurse may need to explain to the client the benefit of sharing their grief with significant others. Some losses may lead to social isolation, placing clients at high risk for dysfunctional grief reactions. For example, survivors of people with AIDS often report feeling excluded by the deceased person's family and by health care providers. Factors that can interfere with successful grieving include:

- Perceived inability to share the loss
- Lack of social recognition of the loss
- Ambivalent relationships prior to the loss
- Traumatic circumstances of the loss

A well-functioning family usually rallies after the initial shock and disbelief and the family members provide support for each other during all phases of the grieving process. After a loss, the well-functioning family is able to shift roles, levels of responsibility, and ways of communicating.

The nurse needs to be alert for the negative as well as positive effects the family may have on the grieving client. For example, the dying client may ask someone the family perceives as an outsider to be near, and the family may respond with anger to this "intrusion." Similarly, certain family members may have hurt feelings or be angry if the client is unresponsive to them. Well-meaning family members also may try to shield the client from the pain of grieving. Because no two people grieve alike, the nurse must assess the individual family members' reactions to the loss. The family and the client rarely experience anger, denial, and acceptance in unison. While one member is in denial, another may be angry because "not enough is being done."

SPIRITUALITY

Spirituality is at the core of human existence, integrating and transcending the physical, emotional, intellectual, and social dimensions (Reed, 1996). The principles, values, personal philosophy, and meaning of life may be called into question when the client responds to an actual or perceived loss. Because of a fear of intruding on personal beliefs and practices, the nurse often feels at a loss in implementing interventions that would help the client respond to a loss and meet spiritual needs.

Developing a trusting relationship with the client and family helps the nurse overcome discomfort in dealing with the spiritual aspects of care, even when the client and nurse have different views. For example, the nurse should be accepting and nonjudgmental if the client initially expresses a belief that the loss is punishment for some past misdeed or failure "to do right." Even spiritually healthy clients need time to challenge their beliefs and values before moving on to the next stage of grieving.

As the client becomes aware of the full impact of the loss, spiritual beliefs and rituals often provide comfort and help the client to find meaning in the loss. The nurse provides spiritual support by listening as the client analyzes beliefs and values, begins to put the loss in perspective, and expresses interest in getting on with life.

NURSES' SELF-ASSESSMENT

To give effective nursing care, nurses need to take time to analyze their own feelings and values related to loss and the expression of grief. The nurse's conscious or unconscious reactions to the client's responses to the loss will influence the outcome of interventions. When assessing the physical symptoms of grief, for example, the nurse may believe the client's behavior is exaggerated and out of proportion to the loss suffered. However, even a brief moment of self-reflection will help the nurse approach the interaction more objectively.

End-of-Life Considerations

Nurses care for dying clients in intensive care units, emergency rooms, hospital units, long-term care facilities, and the home. Regardless of the setting, the client's wishes about death should be respected. *The Dying Person's Bill of Rights* states that each person has "the right to be cared for by caring, sensitive, knowledgeable people who will attempt to understand my needs and will be able to gain some satisfaction in helping me face my death" (Barbus, 1975, p. 99).

LEGAL AND ETHICAL ISSUES

Issues such as those involved in advance directives and living wills, euthanasia, and quality of life are especially important to nurses in upholding the specific care requests of their clients.

Advance Directives and Living Wills

Advance directives are legal documents that allow a person to plan for health care and/or financial affairs in the event of incapacity. A **durable power of attorney for health care** (or *health care proxy*) is a legal document written by a competent (mentally healthy) adult that gives another competent adult the right to make health care decisions on his or her behalf if he or she cannot. The legal authority is limited to decisions about health care. A **living will** is a legal document that formally expresses a person's wishes regarding life-sustaining treatment in the event of terminal illness or permanent unconsciousness (Figure 9-1 ◆). It is not a type of durable power of attorney and usually does not designate a substitute decision maker. It is the responsibility of the nurse as client advocate to request and record the client's preference for care and include it in the plan of care. The nurse's documentation helps communicate these preferences to the other members of the health care team.

All facilities that receive Medicare and Medicaid funds are required to provide all clients with written information and counseling about advance directives and the institution's policies governing them. The specific terms of this requirement are found in the *Patient Self-Determination Act (PSDA)*. A copy of the signed advance directive must be kept in the client's medical record, but clients do not have to sign it in order to be treated. Nurses are the ones in close contact with clients, so they are often left with unresolved feelings about the moral, ethical, and legal aspects of their actions. Although advance directives do not ease the pain of seeing clients die, they do help nurses provide clients with the care the clients have chosen.

Do-Not-Resuscitate Orders

A **do-not-resuscitate** (DNR, or "no-code" order) is written by the physician for the client who is near death. This order is usually based on the wishes of the client and family that no cardiopulmonary resuscitation be performed for respiratory or cardiac arrest. A **comfort measures only** order indicates that no further life-sustaining interventions are necessary and that the goal of care is a comfortable, dignified death. Confusing or conflicting DNR orders create dilemmas, because nurses are involved in resuscitation and either begin CPR or ensure that unwanted attempts do not occur. The ANA has made specific recommendations related to a DNR order (Box 9-1). The ANA further recommends that guidelines and policies be developed to help resolve conflicts between clients and their families, between clients and health care professionals, and among health care professionals.

Euthanasia

Euthanasia (from the Greek for painless, easy, gentle, or good death) is now commonly used to signify a killing that is prompted by some humanitarian motive. There are many arguments for and against euthanasia, and nurses have often found themselves at the center of the debate. As a result, nurses have pushed for the development of appropriate guidelines and procedures for DNR orders. When no such orders exist, the nurse faces a dilemma. Certainly, there are situations in which the nurse's role is clear. For example, it is considered malpractice to participate in "slow codes" (in which the nurse does not hurry to alert the emergency team when a terminally ill client without a DNR order stops breathing).

The natural death laws seek to preserve the notion of voluntary versus involuntary euthanasia. In *voluntary euthanasia,* the competent adult client and a physician, nurse, or adult friend or relative make the decision to terminate life. *Involuntary euthanasia* ("mercy killing") is performed without the client's consent. Because care settings offer many complex and technologic interventions, it is not likely that the ethical aspects of euthanasia will soon be resolved. However, advance directives do give clients a much more active role in decisions about their own care.

HOSPICE

Hospice is a model of care (rather than a place of care) for clients and their families when faced with a limited life expectancy. Hospice care is initiated for clients as they near

---

Directive

I, _____ recognize that the best health care is based on a partnership of trust and communication with my physician. My physician and I will make health care decisions together as long as I am of sound mind and able to make my wishes known. If there comes a time that I am unable to make medical decisions about myself because of illness or injury, I direct that the following treatment preferences be honored:

If, in the judgment of my physician, I am suffering with a terminal condition from which I am expected to die within six months, even with available life-sustaining treatment provided in accordance with prevailing standards of medical care:

_____ I request that all treatment other than those needed to keep me comfortable be discontinued or withheld and my physician allow me to die as gently as possible; OR

_____ I request that I be kept alive in this terminal condition using available life-sustaining treatment. (This Selection Does Not Apply To Hospice Care)

If, in the judgment of my physician, I am suffering with an irreversible condition so that I cannot care for myself or make decisions for myself and am expected to die without life-sustaining treatment provided in accordance with prevailing standards of care:

_____ I request that all treatment other than those needed to keep me comfortable be discontinued or withheld and my physician allow me to die as gently as possible; OR

_____ I request that I be kept alive in this irreversible condition using available life-sustaining treatment. (This Selection Does Not Apply To Hospice Care)

Additional request:
_____
_____

After signing this directive, if my representative or I elect hospice care, I understand and agree that only those treatments needed to keep me comfortable would be provided and I would not be given available life-sustaining treatment.

If I do not have a Medical Power of Attorney, and I am unable to make my wishes known, I designate the following person(s) to make treatment decisions with my physician compatible with my personal values:

1. _____
    (name of person)

2. _____
    (name of second person)

SIGNED _____ DATE _____
    (your name)   (date)

City, County, State of Residence

_____ , _____ , _____
  (city)   (county)   (state)

WITNESS #1: _____

WITNESS #2: _____

Excerpted. *Texas Directive to Physicians and Family or Surrogates.* Courtesy of Partnership for Caring, Inc., 1620 Eye Street, NW, Suite 202, Washington, DC 20006 800-989-9455

Figure 9-1. ◆ Sample living will.

the end of life; it emphasizes quality rather than quantity of life. The client and the family are included in the plan of care. Emotional, spiritual, and practical support is provided based on the wishes of the client and the needs of the family.

Hospice regards dying as a normal part of life; it provides support for a dignified and peaceful death. It is *palliative* (takes care of the comfort needs of the whole person) rather than curative.

BOX 9-1
THE ANA POSITION ON NURSING CARE AND DO-NOT-RESUSCITATE DECISIONS

- The choices and values of the competent patient should always be given highest priority, even when these wishes conflict with those of health care providers and families.
- In the case of the incompetent or never competent patient, any existing advance directives or the decisions of surrogate decision makers acting in the patient's best interest should be determinative.
- The DNR decision should always be a subject of explicit discussion among the patient, the family, . . . any designated surrogate decision maker acting in the patient's best interest and the health care team and include consideration of the efficacy and desirability of cardiopulmonary resuscitation (CPR), a balancing of benefits and burdens to patients, and therapeutic goals.
- DNR orders must be clearly documented, reviewed, and updated periodically to reflect changes in the patient's condition.
- Nurses have a responsibility to educate patients and their families about various forms of advance directives such as living wills, durable power of attorney, and the like.
- If it is the nurse's personal belief that her moral integrity is compromised by her professional responsibility to carry out a particular DNR order, she should transfer the responsibility for the patient's care to another nurse.

Source: Task Force on the Nurse's Role in End of Life Decisions. (1992). New position statement. Adopted by the ANA Board of Directors.

End-of-Life Care

End-of-life nursing care that ensures a peaceful death was mandated by the International Council of Nurses' (1997) and further supported by the American Association of Colleges of Nursing [AACN] (1999). The principles of hospice care are basic to end-of-life care: that people live until the moment they die, that care until death may be offered by a variety of health care professionals, and that such care is coordinated, sensitive to diversity, offered around the clock, and incorporates the physical, psychological, social, and spiritual concerns of the patient and the patient's family. Listed below are selected competencies necessary for nurses to provide high-quality end-of-life care as defined by the AACN (1999).

- Promote the provision of comfort care to the dying as an active, desirable, and important skill, and an integral component of nursing care.

- Communicate effectively and compassionately with the patient, family, and health care team members about end-of-life issues.
- Recognize one's own attitudes, feelings, values, and expectations about death and the individual, cultural, and spiritual diversity existing in those beliefs and customs.
- Demonstrate respect for the patient's views and wishes during end-of-life care.
- Use scientifically based standardized tools to assess symptoms (e.g., pain, dyspnea [breathlessness], constipation, anxiety, fatigue, nausea/vomiting, and altered cognition) experienced by patients at the end of life.
- Use data from symptom assessment to plan and intervene in symptom management using state-of-the-art traditional and complementary approaches.
- Assist the patient, family, colleagues, and oneself to cope with suffering, grief, loss, and bereavement in end-of-life care.

PHYSIOLOGIC CHANGES IN THE DYING CLIENT

Death may occur rapidly or slowly. Physiologic changes are a part of the dying process. As death nears, these changes result in any or all of the manifestations listed in Box 9-2.

- *Weakness and fatigue.* Weakness and fatigue cause discomfort, especially in joints, and contribute to an increased risk for pressure ulcers (see Chapter 17).
- *Anorexia and decreased food intake.* Although anorexia and a decrease in food intake are normal in the dying client, the family often views this as "giving up." Anorexia may be a protective mechanism; the breakdown of body fats results in ketosis, which leads to a sense of well-being and helps decrease pain. Parenteral or enteral feedings do not improve symptoms or prolong life and may actually cause discomfort. As weakness and difficulty in swallowing progress, the gag reflex is decreased and clients are at increased risk for aspiration if oral foods are given.
- *Fluid and electrolyte imbalances.* Decreased oral fluid intake is normal at the end of life and does not cause distress.

BOX 9-2
MANIFESTATIONS OF IMPENDING DEATH

- Difficulty talking or swallowing
- Nausea, flatus, abdominal distention
- Urinary and/or bowel incontinence, constipation
- Decreased sensation, taste, and smell
- Weak, slow, and/or irregular pulse
- Decreasing blood pressure
- Decreased, irregular, or Cheyne–Stokes respirations
- Changes in level of consciousness
- Restlessness, agitation
- Coolness, mottling, and cyanosis of the extremities

Parenteral fluids are sometimes given to decrease delirium, but they may cause increased edema, breathlessness, cough, and respiratory secretions. If the client has edema or *ascites* (a collection of fluid in the abdominal cavity), excess body water is present, so dehydration is not a problem.

■ *Hypotension and renal failure.* As cardiac output decreases, so does intravascular blood volume. As a result, renal perfusion decreases and the kidneys cease to function. Urinary output is scanty. The client will have tachycardia, hypotension, cool extremities, and cyanosis with skin mottling.

■ *Neurologic dysfunction.* Neurologic dysfunction results from any or all of the following: decreased cerebral perfusion, hypoxemia, metabolic acidosis, sepsis, an accumulation of toxins from liver and renal failure, the effects of medications, and disease-related factors. These changes may result in decreased level of consciousness or agitated delirium. Clients with terminal delirium may be confused, restless, or agitated. Moaning, groaning, and grimacing often accompany the agitation and are often misinterpreted as pain. Level of consciousness often decreases to the point where the client cannot be aroused. Although decreased consciousness and agitation are both normal states at the end of life, they are very distressing to the client's family. A client near death often has altered cerebral function, so the nurse must stand near the bedside and speak clearly.

CLINICAL alert

Hearing is thought to be the last sense a dying client loses; the nurse should never whisper or engage in conversation with the family as if the client were not there.

■ *Respiratory changes.* Respiratory changes are normal at this time. The client may have dyspnea, *apnea* (periods of not breathing), or Cheyne–Stokes respirations (see Chapter 26), and may use accessory muscles to breathe. Fluids accumulated in the lungs and oropharynx may lead to what is sometimes called "the death rattle." Oxygen may not relieve these manifestations.

■ *Bowel and bladder incontinence.* Loss of sphincter control may lead to incontinence of feces, urine, or both.

■ *Pain.* Pain is a common problem for clients at the end of life, and is what people often say they fear the most. It is of utmost importance to keep the client comfortable through general comfort measures and by administering ordered medications for pain and anxiety.

CLINICAL alert

At the end of life, there is no maximum allowable dose for opioids such as morphine sulfate; the dose should be increased to whatever is necessary to relieve pain (Rabow & Brody, 1999). (See Chapter 6 for further information about pain medications.)

SUPPORT FOR THE CLIENT AND FAMILY

As the client's condition deteriorates, the nurse's knowledge of the client and family guides the care provided. It may be necessary to provide opportunities for clients to express personal preferences about where they want to die and about funeral and burial arrangements. If the family feels that this is morbid, the nurse explains that it helps clients to keep a sense of control as they approach death.

The client needs the opportunity to say goodbye to others. The nurse encourages and supports the client and family as they terminate relationships as a necessary part of the grief process. The nurse acknowledges that termination is painful and, if the client or family desires, stays with them during this time. Family members are often afraid to be present at the moment of death, yet dying alone is the greatest fear expressed by clients.

DEATH

The manifestations listed in Box 9-3 are seen after death occurs and are the basis for pronouncing death. They appear gradually and not in any special order. Pronouncement of death is legally required by a physician or other health care provider to confirm death. The time of death, with any related data, is documented in the client's chart.

The nurse may also fear being present at the moment of the client's death. In fact, Kübler-Ross (1969) noted that the nurse's fear of death frequently interferes with the ability to provide support for the dying client and family. Thoughts such as, "Please, God, don't let him die on my shift" are common, and they express the nurse's emotional turmoil in dealing with the task. Nurses who have worked through their own feelings about death and dying are more at ease in assisting the dying client toward a peaceful death.

After the death, the family is encouraged to acknowledge the pain of loss. The nurse's presence and support as the bereaved express their sorrow, anger, or guilt can help them resolve their grief. It is important for the bereaved not to suppress the pain of grieving with drugs. By accepting variations in the expression of grief, the nurse supports the family's grief reactions and helps prevent dysfunctional grieving. Dysfunctional grieving is an extended and unsuccessful resolution of grief.

BOX 9-3
MANIFESTATIONS OF DEATH

- Absence of respirations, pulse, and heartbeat
- Fixed and dilated pupils; eyes may stay open
- Release of stool and urine
- Waxen color (pallor) as blood settles to dependent areas
- Drop in body temperature
- Lack of reflexes
- Flat encephalogram

Resolution of grief begins with acceptance of the loss. The nurse can encourage this acceptance by maintaining open, honest dialogue and by providing the family with the opportunity to view, touch, hold, and kiss the person's body (Carpenito, 2000). As family members realize the finality of the death, they are often comforted by the presence of the nurse who cared for the client during the final days.

Postmortem Care

Normally, the nurse documents the time of death (required for the death certificate and all official records), notifies the physician, and assists the family (if needed) in choice of a funeral home. If the client dies at home, death must be pronounced before the body is removed. In some states and in some situations, nurses can pronounce death. For specifics, consult state practice acts, laws, and agency policy. All jewelry, except a wedding ring, is removed and given to the family. The body is kept in place until the family is ready and gives permission. If an autopsy is required or requested, the body must be left undisturbed (e.g., do not remove any tubes) for transportation to the medical examiner.

CLINICAL alert

The bodies of deceased clients with known infections that require body and body fluid precautions or isolation (such as tuberculosis or AIDS) should be tagged accordingly. Soiled items should be disposed of appropriately, and nondisposable items should be cleaned.

Documentation of the death is completed by sending a completed death certificate to the funeral home (for a death in the home), or by completing the required paperwork and sending the body to the morgue or funeral home (for a death in the hospital or long-term care setting).

Nurses' Grief

The nurse who has developed a close relationship with the client who has died may experience strong feelings of grief. Crying with families (at one time considered unprofessional) is now recognized as simply an expression of empathy and caring. Sharing grief with the family after the death of a loved one helps both the nurse and family to cope with their feelings about the loss. Taking time to grieve after the death of a client provides a release that can help prevent "blunting" of feelings, a problem often experienced by nurses who care for terminally ill clients.

Nurses working with critically or terminally ill clients should be aware that witnessing a client's death and the family's grief may reactivate feelings about some unresolved grief in their own lives. In these cases, nurses may need to reflect on their responses to their own losses. Also, nurses who work with dying clients need support from peers and other professionals to work through the often overwhelming feelings that result from dealing with death, grief, and loss (Figure 9-2 ◆).

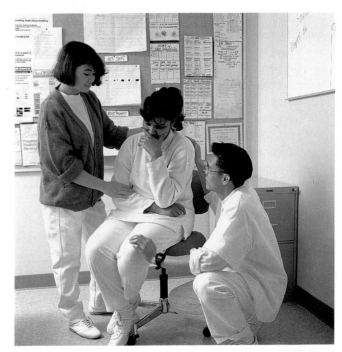

Figure 9-2. ◆ Nurses who work with dying clients need support from their colleagues to work through their often overwhelming feelings of grief.

Rituals of Mourning

The rituals of mourning are an important part of the work of mourning and grieving a loss. Culture is the primary factor that dictates the rituals of mourning (Table 9-2 ◆). The funeral ceremony serves the needs of the bereaved as they gather together to share their loss. Through the ceremony, people symbolically express triumph over death and deny the fear of death. Through rituals, the survivors publicly adapt to the loss. This adaptation does not decrease the suffering they will continue to feel, but it does move them toward reinvesting emotionally in the future.

COLLABORATIVE CARE

Interventions for loss and grief may be planned and implemented by any or all members of the health care team. Nurses and social workers may provide interventions to help clients or families adapt to a loss. They may also make referrals to mental health professionals (grief counselors, social services), support groups, chaplains, or legal or financial assistance agencies.

NURSING CARE

Nursing care of clients and family members who are experiencing loss, grief, or death must be holistic; that is, it must consider physical, emotional, cultural, and spiritual needs. The nursing process is used to organize a plan of care to provide comfort and facilitate grief resolution. Comfort measures for the client nearing death are outlined in Box 9-4.

TABLE 9-2   CULTURAL ASPECTS OF DYING AND DEATH

CULTURE/ETHNICITY	NURSING INTERVENTIONS
Native American	Some tribes prefer not to openly discuss terminal prognosis and DNR decisions, as negative thoughts may make inevitable loss occur sooner. Suggest a family meeting to discuss care and end-of-life issues. If the family feels comfortable, all members of the family and close friends may remain 24 hours a day (eating, joking, singing). Mourning is done in private, away from the dying person. After death, the family may hug, touch, sing, and stay close to the deceased.
Black/African American	Suggest that the family have a family meeting or talk with their minister or family elder. Client may decide to have older family member disclose a poor prognosis. Care for the dying family member is often done at home until death is imminent.
Chinese American	Ensure the head of the family is present when terminal illness is discussed. The client may not want to discuss approaching death. Special amulets or cloths may be brought from home. Family members may prefer to bathe the body after death.
Iranian	Information about a terminal illness should be presented by a trusted member of the health care team to the family, and never to the client when he or she is alone. Most Iranians believe in *tagdir* (will of God) in life and death as a predestined journey. When death occurs, notify the head of the family first. DNR decisions are often made by the family. The family may want to bathe the body.
Mexican American	Based on the belief that worry may make health worse, the family may want to protect the client from seriousness of illness. The information is often handled by an older daughter or son. Extended family members are obligated to pay respects to the sick and dying, although pregnant women do not care for dying persons or attend funerals. May prefer that the client die at home. Prayers, amulets, and rosary beads are used, and the priest should be notified. Death is seen as an important spiritual event. The family may bathe the body and spend time with the body.
Vietnamese	Consult head of family before telling client about a terminal illness. Entire family will make DNR decision, often with assistance from the priest or monk. Often prefer to die at home. Family should have extra time with the body, and may cry loudly and uncontrollably. Spiritual/religious rites are often conducted in the room.

Source: Adapted from Lipson, J. G., Dibble, S. L., & Minarik, P. A. (Eds.). (1996). *Culture & nursing care: A pocket guide.* San Francisco: UCSF Nursing Press.

ASSESSING

Before collecting data to plan and implement care for the client experiencing a loss, the nurse must consider the individual response. Approaches for collecting data depend on the age of the client and the circumstances under which the nurse encounters the client. The nurse observes for changes in sensory processes and asks questions about the client's sleeping and eating patterns, activities of daily living, general health status, and pain.

Clients may experience one or more physical reactions as they become aware of a loss. Gastrointestinal symptoms occur frequently (indigestion, nausea or vomiting, anorexia, weight gain or loss, constipation, or diarrhea). The shock and disbelief that accompany a loss may cause shortness of breath, a choking sensation, hyperventilation, or loss of strength. Some clients also report insomnia, preoccupation with sleep, fatigue, and decreased or increased activity level (Carpenito, 2000).

Crying and sadness are normal during grieving. Crying may make the client feel exhausted and may interfere with carrying out daily activities. However, a person who is unable to cry may have difficulty completing the mourning process.

The nurse must assess the client's concerns about pain, especially if the client has cancer or another painful illness. Knowledge of pain theories and pain assessment can help the nurse assess the need for pain medication (see Chapter 6).

It is important for the nurse to explore the client's spiritual beliefs and practices, because they greatly influence people's reaction to loss. The spiritually healthy client has inner resources that help him or her work through the grief process. Faith, prayer, trust in God or a superior being, perception of a purpose in life, or belief in immortality are examples of the inner resources that may sustain the client during an actual or perceived loss (Reed, 1996).

Clients often perceive a loss as punishment from God for wrongdoing or for failing to remain faithful to their religious practices. Clients may suddenly turn to religion to seek comfort or to cope with feelings of despair, helplessness, hopelessness, or guilt. They may utter anguished statements such as "Why, God?" or "Please help me, God." The nurse assesses and reports the client's verbalization of such feelings.

It is more important for the nurse to focus on the meaning of the loss to the client than to place the client in a stage

BOX 9-4
PROVIDING PHYSICAL COMFORT FOR THE CLIENT NEARING DEATH

☑ Maintain clean skin and bed linens.

☑ Use a draw sheet to turn the client as often as possible and is comfortable for the client.

☑ Position the client to promote comfort and protect bony areas with padding. Reposition the client and raise the head of the bed if fluids accumulate in the upper airways and back of the throat.

☑ Use bed pads or insert a Foley catheter (if ordered) for urinary incontinence.

☑ Use gentle massage to improve circulation and shift edema.

☑ Provide small, frequent sips of fluids, ice chips, or Popsicles.

☑ Provide oral care, using a soft moist brush or glycerin swab.

☑ Clean secretions from the eyes and nose.

☑ Administer ordered pain medications as needed to maintain comfort.

☑ Administer oxygen as prescribed to relieve dyspnea.

or phase of grief. The caring and sensitivity of the nurse's questions will influence the amount of information the client will be willing to reveal. Asking such questions as, "Why do you feel this way?" or "What does this loss mean to you?" is less helpful than making a statement such as, "This must be difficult for you." This last sentence conveys the nurse's genuine interest in hearing how the client feels about the loss.

The nurse may not be able to collect much information during a brief initial contact. However, as trust is built, the client may reveal the meaning of the relationship and the circumstances surrounding the loss. By establishing trust during the first stages of the nurse–client relationship, the nurse will be better able to assess the impact of the loss. If the relationship was a significant one, the nurse will observe intense grief. The client may state, "I know I can't go on without him/her." The client may even feel anger at the person for having left, whether through death, divorce, or separation. The losses associated with changes in body image or work role may produce similar feelings.

DIAGNOSING, PLANNING, AND IMPLEMENTING

ANTICIPATORY GRIEVING

Anticipatory grieving is a combination of intellectual and emotional responses and behaviors by which people adjust their self-concept in the face of a potential loss. Their response may be normal or problematic. Anticipatory grieving may be

a response to one's own future death; to potential loss of body parts or functions; to potential loss of a significant person, animal, or possession; or to potential loss of a social role.

- Assess for factors that are causing or contributing to the grief. Ask about support systems, how many losses have occurred, relationship with the lost person, significance of the body part, and previous experiences with loss and grief. *Grief and mourning occur when a person experiences any type of loss.*

- Use open-ended questions to encourage the person to share concerns and the possible effect on the family unit. *Grief resolution cannot occur until the client acknowledges the loss.*

- Promote a trusting nurse–client relationship by:
  - Allowing enough time for communications
  - Speaking clearly, simply, and to the point
  - Listening
  - Being honest in responses to questions, and not giving unrealistic hope
  - Offering support
  - Demonstrating respect for the person's age, culture, religion, race, and values

  An effective nurse–client relationship begins with acceptance of the client's feelings, attitudes, and values related to the loss. If the client is ready to talk, then the nurse's listening and presence are the most appropriate interventions (Figure 9-3 ◆).

- Ask about the client's strengths and weakness in coping with the anticipated loss. *Current responses are influenced by past experiences with loss, illness, and death. Socioeconomic and cultural background, as well as cultural and spiritual beliefs and values, affect a person's ability to adapt to loss.*

- Teach the client and family the stages of grief. *This helps them to be aware of their emotions in each stage, and reassures them that their reactions are normal.*

- Provide time for decision making. *In periods of stress, people may need extra time to make informed decisions.*

- Provide information about appropriate resources, including support from family, friends, and support groups, community resources, and legal/financial aides. *Support from others decreases feelings of loneliness and isolation and facilitates grief work.*

DEATH ANXIETY

Death anxiety is worry or fear related to death or dying. It may be present in clients who have an acute life-threatening illness, who have a terminal illness, who have experienced the death of a family member or friend, or who have experienced multiple deaths in the same family.

- Explore the client's knowledge of the situation. For example, ask, "What has your doctor told you about your condition?" *This informs you about the client's knowledge base about the condition and about his or her ability to make informed decisions.*

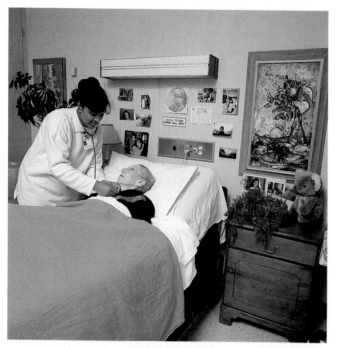

Figure 9-3. ◆ The nurse establishes a trusting nurse–client relationship through therapeutic communications and by demonstrating respect for the person's age, culture, religion, race, and values.

■ Ask the client to identify specific fears about death. *This provides data about any unrealistic expectations or misperceptions.*

■ Determine the client's perceptions of strengths and weakness in coping with death. *Identifying past strengths can help the client cope with loss, illness, and death.*

■ Ask the client to identify needed help. *This determines whether available resources are adequate.*

■ Encourage independence and control in decisions about treatment and care. *This promotes self-esteem, decreases feelings of powerlessness, and allows the client to retain dignity in dying.*

■ Facilitate client's access to culturally appropriate spiritual rituals and practices. *This provides spiritual comfort.*

■ Explain advance directives and assist with them if necessary. *Advance directives help ensure that the client's wishes for end-of-life care are carried out.*

■ Encourage life review and reminiscence. *Life review is self-affirming.*

■ Encourage activities such as listening to music, aromatherapy, massage, or relaxation exercises. *These activities decrease anxiety.*

■ Suggest keeping a journal or leaving a written legacy. *A written document provides continuing support to others after death.*

EVALUATING

Evaluate the effectiveness of nursing care for loss and grief by collecting data from statements by the client that support

grief resolution, such as "I am beginning to accept the fact that my father is gone." The plan of care for the dying client is effective if the client has had a comfortable and dignified death.

Discharge Considerations and Teaching

Nurses teach clients and families to carry out the physical skills that are necessary to the client's care. They also provide information on identifying signs of deterioration and obtaining additional sources of support (from hospice, home health care agencies, and public health departments). Encourage families to identify friends and other family members who can help out either routinely or occasionally. At discharge, provide the client or family with information for contacting the appropriate support groups. Box 9-5 provides general guidelines for teaching clients and families about grief.

Nursing Process Case Study
■ CLIENT EXPERIENCING LOSS

Pearl Rogers is a 79-year-old African American woman who is admitted to the Methodist Home Nursing Center. Mrs. Rogers lived with her husband of 58 years until his death 9 months ago. She had one son, who died in an auto accident 2 years ago, and she has one daughter who lives nearby. After her husband's death, Mrs. Rogers lived with her daughter until her admission to the Nursing Center. Mrs. Rogers has become increasingly agitated and helpless, complaining constantly of pain. Her daughter states that Mrs. Rogers is chronically constipated, has difficulty sleeping, and has stopped taking part in all social activities, including weekly church services. She cries frequently. Extensive medical testing prior to her admission to the Nursing Center revealed Mrs. Rogers has arthritis but no other pathologic disorder.

Assessment When Mrs. Rogers arrives at the Nursing Center, she is admitted by Sandy Sutphin, LPN. Mrs. Rogers tells Ms. Sutphin, "I'm a sick woman, and no one will listen to me! I can't walk, I'm so weak. My head hurts, and I'm always sick at my stomach. I haven't had a bowel movement in a week, and I never sleep more than 3 hours a night." Ms. Sutphin completes data collection and works with her manager to develop a plan of care for Mrs. Rogers.

Diagnosis The following nursing diagnoses are made for Mrs. Rogers:

■ *Dysfunctional Grieving* related to stress of husband's death
■ *Sleep Pattern Disturbance* related to grieving
■ *Constipation* related to inactivity

BOX 9-5
TEACHING FOR DISCHARGE

TEACHING FOR CLIENTS EXPERIENCING A LOSS

- Encourage both children and adults to discuss expected or impending loss and to express feelings.
- Teach problem-solving skills.
  - Define what the possible changes and problems are related to the predicted loss.
  - Develop potential strategies for dealing with problems.
  - List pros and cons of each strategy.
  - Decide which strategies might be most useful to try first to solve potential problems associated with loss.
- Identify persons who are at risk for potential dysfunctional grieving: those who present a brave, stoic front; clients with a history of multiple losses; socially isolated individuals; people who feel their social network is not supportive; and clients with a history of dealing ineffectively with loss.
- Teach individuals and families how to support a person who is dealing with an impending loss:
  - Explain what to expect with a loss: sadness, fear, rejection, anger, guilt, and loneliness.
  - Teach signs of grief resolution:
    - No longer living in the past, becoming future oriented
    - Breaking ties with the lost object or person (Acute stage often shows signs of resolving in 6 to 12 months.)
    - The possibility of having painful "waves" of grief years after the loss, especially on the anniversary of the loss and in response to "triggers" such as pictures, events, songs, or memories
- Identify community agencies that may be helpful to people responding to loss.

Expected Outcomes The expected outcomes established in the plan of care are that Mrs. Rogers will:

- Discuss her losses, use constructive coping mechanisms, and discuss positive and negative aspects of the loss
- Fall asleep within 20 to 30 minutes after retiring and remain asleep for 7 to 8 hours
- Have a bowel movement at least every other day

Planning and Implementation The following interventions are planned and implemented during care of Mrs. Rogers:

- Promote trust: Show empathy and caring, demonstrate respect for her culture and values, offer support and reassurance, be honest, engage in active listening.

- During one-to-one interactions, encourage Mrs. Rogers to recognize normal grieving behavior. Assist her in labeling her feelings: anger, fear, loneliness, guilt, and isolation.
- Explore previous losses and the ways in which the client has coped.
- Encourage Mrs. Rogers to express her feelings of anger. Do not become defensive, and explain to her family that anger helps her feel as though she has some control over her environment, even though she has no control over her loss.
- Encourage Mrs. Rogers to participate in her spiritual practices.
- Provide afternoon activities for Mrs. Rogers as indicated by the occupational therapist.
- Provide evening care: warm sponge bath; clean, warm bed; night-light; soft music for relaxation; closed door.
- Provide measures that assist in bowel function: Encourage exercise as tolerated, including walks and rocking in a rocking chair. Offer foods that stimulate bowel movements (such as fruits, vegetables, and high-fiber cereals). Increase fluid intake. Provide privacy: Close the door, ensuring that the emergency call bell is within reach, and do not interrupt. Assure Mrs. Rogers that a nurse will be there to help her clean herself if she needs one, and have toilet paper, soap, warm water, and a cloth available to promote her dignity.
- Administer a mild laxative and/or stool softener to Mrs. Rogers, if ordered and necessary, but discontinue as soon as possible.

Evaluation After 4 weeks at the Nursing Center, Mrs. Rogers states, "I don't feel any better, but I know I have to accept my situation." Although Mrs. Rogers states that she doesn't feel better, she now walks the length of the hall several times a day, is sleeping better, and has regular bowel movements. Mrs. Rogers is also less withdrawn, has greatly reduced the time she spends crying, and has openly discussed her feelings related to her husband's death, including her anger at the loss of her son and her husband less than 2 years apart. She has attended chapel services on Sunday for the past 2 weeks. She plays bridge with the other residents 2 or 3 afternoons a week.

Critical Thinking in the Nursing Process

1. How might the nursing staff involve Mrs. Rogers's daughter in developing and implementing her mother's plan of care?
2. Suppose Mrs. Rogers said that she did not want any help, that she just wanted to be left alone to die. How would you respond?
3. What factors in Mrs. Rogers's current life would support the nursing diagnosis of *Social Isolation?*

Nursing Interventions Classification

Some of the following nursing interventions from the Nursing Interventions Classification Project (McCloskey & Bulechek, 2000) may also be useful in planning and implementing care for clients experiencing loss, grief, and end-of-life care:

- Dying Care
- Grief Work Facilitation
- Simple Guided Imagery
- Spiritual Support
- Values Clarification

(*Note:* The bibliography listings for this and all chapters have been compiled at the back of the book.)

Chapter Review

key terms by topic

Use the CD-ROM disk enclosed with your textbook to hear the pronunciation of key terms in the chapter.

Loss, grief, and death
loss, grief, death

End-of-life considerations
advance directives, durable power of attorney for health care, living will, do-not-resuscitate orders, comfort only measures, euthanasia, hospice

key points

- When a valued object, person, body part, or situation is lost or changed, the experience of loss occurs. Grief is the emotional response to loss. Grieving responses are individualized to each person, but commonly include the stages of denial, anger, bargaining, depression, and acceptance.

- Death is an immensely difficult loss for both the person who is dying and for his or her loved ones. Grief work is often facilitated by family, friends, and spiritual practices.

- The dying person may control his or her own care through advance directives, living wills, and a durable power of attorney for health care. The client and family may request that the physician write a do-not-resuscitate (DNR) order.

- As death nears, specific physiologic changes take place. These changes result in manifestations that indicate impending death. Death is pronounced when respiratory and circulatory functions stop or when all brain function ceases.

- Nursing care for clients who experience loss, grief, or death is implemented to meet the physical, emotional, and spiritual needs of the client and family. Nurses must also be aware of their own responses to these experiences to provide care more effectively.

Medialink

Additional interactive resources for this chapter can be found on the Companion Website at www.prenhall.com/burke. Click on Chapter 9 and "Begin" to select the activities for this chapter.

For NCLEX review questions and an audio glossary, access the accompanying CD-ROM in this book.

for further study

For further information about fear of pain, see Chapter 6.

For further information about pressure ulcers, see Chapter 13.

For further information about respiratory changes, see Chapter 26.

Critical Thinking Care Map

Caring for a Client Experiencing a Loss
NCLEX-PN Focus Area: Psychosocial Adaptation

Case Study: Tom Moore was involved in a serious automobile accident on his way to work and was pronounced dead on arrival at the emergency room. Tom and his wife, Sara, were married for more than 30 years. During that time, Sara did not work outside the home and Tom took care of all the finances. One year after Tom's death, Sara has her annual physical check-up.

Nursing Diagnosis: Dysfunctional Grieving

COLLECT DATA

Subjective

Objective

_____   _____
_____   _____
_____   _____
_____   _____
_____   _____
_____   _____

Would you report this data? Yes/No

If yes, to: _____

Nursing Care

_____
_____
_____
_____
_____
_____
_____

How would you document this? _____
_____
_____

**Data collected
(use those that apply)**

• Weight loss of 25 lbs.
• B/P 110/70
• States "I can't stand being alone."
• States "I am still angry at Tom for dying."
• Difficulty sleeping
• States "My knees sometimes feel like sandpaper inside."
• Unable to continue normal routines
• Has joined a grief support group at her church

**Nursing Interventions
(use those that apply)**

• Discuss time needed to resolve a loss.
• Explain grief reactions.
• Ignore statements and conduct basic physical assessment.
• Encourage expression of feelings.
• State "I can't talk about that right now—I'm too busy."
• State "This must have been very difficult for you."
• State "I know it's hard, but you will be okay."

NCLEX-PN Exam Preparation

TEST-TAKING TIP

Select answers in which the nurse promotes the client's ability to cope with stress or illness.

1. The grief process may range from discomforting to debilitating, and it may last a day or a lifetime, depending on:
   a. whether the loss is temporary or permanent
   b. what the loss means to the person experiencing it
   c. what religion the person experiencing the loss is
   d. the educational level of the person experiencing the loss

2. A client has been diagnosed with terminal cancer and is reacting with hostility and abruptness to her family and the hospital staff. She tells them to leave her alone. The client is most likely in the stage of:
   a. denial
   b. anger
   c. bargaining
   d. acceptance

3. Factors that affect an individual's reaction to loss include:
   a. age and availability of a support system
   b. socioeconomic status and age
   c. self-esteem and family support available
   d. mental stability and employment status

4. A do-not-resuscitate order is written for the client who is near death by:
   a. the client
   b. the family
   c. the nurse
   d. the physician

5. Regardless of the setting, the client's wishes about death should:
   a. be kept private
   b. be respected
   c. conform to the cultural norm
   d. be the same as his or her family's wishes

6. A model of care initiated for clients as they near the end of life, emphasizing quality rather than quantity of life, is known as:
   a. hospice
   b. euthanasia
   c. advance directive
   d. the patient's bill of rights

7. To provide high-quality end-of-life care, it is necessary for the nurse to:
   a. control his or her own emotions about death
   b. maintain a sense of detachment
   c. agree with the client's values and beliefs
   d. provide comfort and symptom-management interventions

8. Respiratory changes to be expected near death include:
   a. tachypnea and coughing episodes
   b. periods of apnea and Cheyne–Stokes respiration
   c. loss of sphincter control and anorexia
   d. rapid respirations and edema

9. Grief before a loss actually occurs is called:
   a. dysfunctional
   b. functional
   c. adaptive
   d. anticipatory

10. The best response for the nurse to help grieving family members express their grief would be:
    a. "I know just how you feel."
    b. "Things will get better over time."
    c. "Tell me how you are feeling."
    d. "Let me know if there is anything I can do to help."

Caring for Clients Experiencing Shock, Trauma, or Critical Illness

chapter 10

CARING tip

66 Remember the patient is an individual who has put a lot of trust in you to help calm his or her fears about getting better. 99

Josephine Henry, LPN • St. Albans Primary Extended Care • St. Albans, New York • Graduate, Vocational Education Extension Board • Long Island, New York

LEARNING outcomes

After completing this chapter, you will be able to:
- Identify the three stages of shock.
- Identify the common causes for each type of shock: hypovolemic, anaphylactic, cardiogenic, septic, and neurogenic.
- Describe the pathophysiology and manifestations of the five types of shock.
- Explain the nursing care of the client in shock.
- State the nursing implications for administering fluid replacement solutions.
- Identify common traumatic injuries.
- Describe emergency management of clients with traumatic injuries.
- Use the nursing process to collect data, establish outcomes, provide individualized care, and evaluate responses for the client experiencing shock or trauma.
- Describe the effects of a critical care unit on the client and family.
- Discuss the legal and ethical considerations of organ donation.

MediaLink

 www.prenhall.com/burke

Use the above address to access the free, interactive Companion Website created for this textbook. Get hints, instant feedback, and textbook references to chapter-related multiple choice questions. Link to other interesting sites.

The Client in Shock

Shock is a life-threatening condition that is characterized by inadequate blood flow to the tissues and cells. Shock is identified according to its underlying cause. Types of shock include the following:

- **Hypovolemic shock** (low-volume shock)—caused by lack of circulating blood volume
- **Anaphylactic shock**—caused by immunologic reactions that trigger abnormal dilation of blood vessels
- **Cardiogenic shock**—caused by failure of the heart's pumping action
- **Septic shock**—caused by toxins produced from an overwhelming infection
- **Neurogenic shock**—caused by changes in sympathetic tone of blood vessels

All types of shock progress through the same stages and exert similar effects on body systems.

PATHOPHYSIOLOGY

All cells require a consistent supply of oxygen and removal of metabolic wastes. This process *(homeostasis)* is maintained by the cardiovascular system. Homeostasis requires three basic factors: an adequate blood flow, a correctly functioning heart (pump), and normal blood vessel diameter. When one of these functions is altered, normal cell function is disrupted. The body's mechanisms compensate to prevent damage to the vital organs of the heart and brain. When shock is prolonged or severe, **hypoxemia** (inadequate cell oxygenation) occurs. The cells become *hypoxic* and die. If shock is not halted, organ failure and death may result.

Stages of Shock

There are three stages of shock: compensated, progressive, and irreversible. Box 10-1 lists the fairly distinct manifestations of each stage. Early treatment focuses on preventing the client from reaching the irreversible stage.

COMPENSATED STAGE. The *compensated stage* of shock occurs when decreased blood volume significantly reduces the heart's cardiac output. As a result, blood pressure drops and normal tissue perfusion cannot be maintained. At this point, the body initiates several mechanisms to maintain blood pressure and preserve the vital organs:

1. Baroreceptors (in the aortic arch) sense the drop in blood pressure and stimulate the sympathetic nervous system (SNS). The SNS releases epinephrine and norepinephrine. These "fight-or-flight" hormones constrict arterial blood vessels and increase the heart's rate and ability to contract. Arterial constriction causes the body to *shunt* (push) blood from the kidneys, skin, and gastrointestinal tract to the heart and brain. All these effects increase venous return to the heart, increase cardiac output, and increase oxygen supply to the body's tissues.

2. Reduced blood flow to the kidneys activates the **renin–angiotensin system** (a blood pressure regulation system activated when there is reduced blood flow to the kidneys; see also Chapters 5 and 21). Renin stimulates the production of angiotensin II, a potent vasoconstrictor that raises blood pressure. Angiotensin II signals the adrenal cortex to release aldosterone. Aldosterone causes the kidneys to reabsorb water and sodium. When circulating blood volume increases, so does the blood pressure.

3. Low blood volume stimulates the posterior pituitary gland to release antidiuretic hormone (ADH) or vasopressin. ADH increases water reabsorption and helps to increase blood pressure.

If effective treatment is provided at the compensated stage, the client should not experience any permanent damage. When the underlying cause cannot be reversed, shock advances to the progressive stage.

PROGRESSIVE STAGE. When the compensatory mechanisms fail, the progressive stage of shock occurs. Without adequate tissue perfusion, the body's organ functions deteriorate. Unless this stage of shock is treated rapidly, the client's prognosis is poor.

The progressive stage produces numerous effects on the body's organs (Figure 10-1 ◆):

1. *Cardiovascular:* A decrease in cardiac output reduces blood flow to the coronary arteries. The myocardium receives less oxygen. The imbalance between oxygen supply and demand results in muscle ischemia, arrhythmias, and a myocardial infarction.

2. *Respiratory:* Decreased pulmonary blood flow alters the exchange of oxygen and carbon dioxide between the alveoli and capillaries. Oxygen levels decrease, carbon dioxide levels increase, and respiratory acidosis occurs (see Chapter 5). When this condition is prolonged, a complication develops that is called adult respiratory distress syndrome (ARDS, or "shock lung"). ARDS is discussed under Complications.

3. *Gastrointestinal (GI) and liver:* When blood is shunted from the GI tract and liver to the heart and brain, the GI organs become ischemic and the gastric mucosa ulcerates. Stress ulcers can develop (see Chapter 18). With increased gastric permeability, intestinal bacteria can enter the abdominal cavity and progress into the circulation. Impaired gastric and intestinal motility may cause paralytic ileus.

   Shock alters the metabolism of drugs, fats, and protein by the liver. Because the liver cannot process bilirubin, the client may become jaundiced. The liver's Kupffer cells (phagocytes that destroy bacteria) cannot function, so bacteria can multiply, and an overwhelming bacterial infection can occur.

4. *Neurologic:* Decreased blood flow to the brain alters mental status and orientation. The client's level of conscious-

BOX 10-1
MANIFESTATIONS FOUND IN EACH STAGE OF SHOCK

Clinical Manifestation	Compensated Stage	Progressive Stage	Irreversible Stage
Level of consciousness	Oriented, can follow simple commands; restless	Confused; listless; decreased response to painful stimuli	Lethargy to coma; no reflex response
Speech	Clear	Slurred	Incoherent to absent
Blood pressure	Normal to slightly decreased	< 90 mm Hg	Falling to unobtainable
Pulse rate	> 100 beats/min	> 150 beats/min, irregular	Slow and irregular
Peripheral pulses	Thready	Weak, thready	Absent
Respirations	> 20 per min	> 30 per min, shallow, possible crackles	Slow with Cheyne–Stokes respiration
Skin	Pale, cool, moist	Cold, clammy; possible cyanosis	Cold, cyanotic, mottled
Urinary output	< 30 mL per hour	< 20 mL per hour	Anuria
Bowel sounds	Decreased	Absent	Absent

ness deteriorates and may progress to coma. Cerebral edema and irreversible brain cell damage may occur.

5. *Renal:* Blood shunting to the heart and brain reduces flow through the kidneys. Urine output decreases, and the client may develop oliguria. Prolonged renal hypoperfusion leads to acute tubular necrosis and acute renal failure.

6. *Skin and temperature:* In most types of shock, blood vessels in the skin are vasoconstricted. Skin color changes develop. Caucasian clients appear pale. Persons with darker skin (such as those of African, Hispanic, or Mediterranean descent) have pale lips, oral mucous membranes, nail beds, and conjunctiva. With activation of the sweat glands, the skin is cool and moist and may become cold. As metabolism decreases, so does the body's temperature.

IRREVERSIBLE STAGE. If shock progresses to the irreversible stage, tissue and cellular death becomes so widespread that no treatment can reverse the damage. **Multiple organ dysfunction syndrome (MODS)** is an irreversible complication of shock in which the body's systems fail and the client eventually dies.

Types of Shock
HYPOVOLEMIC SHOCK. Hypovolemic shock is the most common type, and is caused by a decrease in intravascular volume. Normally, about two thirds of the body's fluids are found in the intracellular compartment and the remaining third is in the extracellular compartment. The extracellular compartment is divided into intravascular and interstitial fluids. To remain in balance, each compartment must maintain the correct amount of fluid (see Chapter 5).

Box 10-2 lists the most frequent causes of hypovolemic shock. Hypovolemic shock can occur alone or develop along with other types of shock (Figure 10-2 ◆).

Manifestations of hypovolemic shock vary depending on the client's age, general health, severity of injury or illness, length of time before treatment is provided, and the rate of loss. Hypovolemic shock from hemorrhage is classified according to the volume of blood lost (Box 10-3). Hypovolemic shock caused by dehydration or internal fluid shifts may have more subtle manifestations than hypovolemic shock caused by hemorrhage.

ANAPHYLACTIC SHOCK. Anaphylactic shock, or anaphylaxis, is caused by a severe allergic reaction. Almost any *antigen* (foreign substance) can trigger an anaphylactic response. Antigens can enter the body by injection, ingestion, or through the skin or respiratory tract. Some common causes of anaphylactic shock are:

- Foods, such as legumes (nuts, seeds), shellfish, egg whites, milk, chocolate, tomatoes, and strawberries
- Stings and bites of insects
- Snake venom
- Substances used to diagnose and treat disease, such as antibiotics, vaccines, local anesthetics, iodine dyes, blood, and narcotics
- Other substances like latex, pollen, and molds or food additives

When a person is first exposed to an antigen, the body produces antibodies against it. The initial antigen–antibody response usually produces no harmful effects, but it sensitizes the person to the antigen. With each future exposure, the antigen reacts with the antibodies and anaphylaxis may occur.

CLINICAL alert

Anaphylactic reactions are more severe when the antigen enters the body by the intravenous route or when a second exposure occurs.

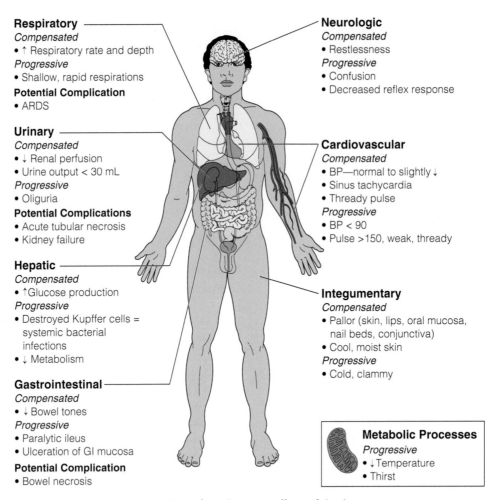

Respiratory
Compensated
- ↑ Respiratory rate and depth
Progressive
- Shallow, rapid respirations
Potential Complication
- ARDS

Urinary
Compensated
- ↓ Renal perfusion
- Urine output < 30 mL
Progressive
- Oliguria
Potential Complications
- Acute tubular necrosis
- Kidney failure

Hepatic
Compensated
- ↑Glucose production
Progressive
- Destroyed Kupffer cells = systemic bacterial infections
- ↓ Metabolism

Gastrointestinal
Compensated
- ↓ Bowel tones
Progressive
- Paralytic ileus
- Ulceration of GI mucosa
Potential Complication
- Bowel necrosis

Neurologic
Compensated
- Restlessness
Progressive
- Confusion
- Decreased reflex response

Cardiovascular
Compensated
- BP—normal to slightly ↓
- Sinus tachycardia
- Thready pulse
Progressive
- BP < 90
- Pulse >150, weak, thready

Integumentary
Compensated
- Pallor (skin, lips, oral mucosa, nail beds, conjunctiva)
- Cool, moist skin
Progressive
- Cold, clammy

Metabolic Processes
Progressive
- ↓Temperature
- Thirst

Figure 10-1. ◆ Multisystem effects of shock.

An antigen–antibody reaction stimulates mast cells to release histamine and other chemical mediators into the circulation. These substances cause widespread vasodilation and make capillaries more permeable. The shift of fluids results in hypotension and **relative hypovolemia** (fluid shift from the vasculature into the interstitial space, so that blood pools in the tissues). Blood volume is reduced, tissue perfusion is impaired, and cell metabolism is altered. Other effects include inflammation, bronchoconstriction, and cutaneous reactions. Manifestations of anaphylactic shock may begin within 20 minutes of contact with an antigen. Anaphylactic shock is a life-threatening emergency that requires immediate intervention to prevent death within a matter of minutes. People with known allergies should wear a Medic-Alert bracelet. Health care providers should carefully assess and document allergies or previous drug reactions. A summary of the manifestations found in anaphylactic shock is listed in Box 10-4.

CARDIOGENIC SHOCK. Cardiogenic shock occurs when the heart fails to act as an effective pump, so cardiac output and adequate tissue perfusion cannot be maintained. Myocardial infarction is the most common cause of cardiogenic shock. The amount of myocardial damage determines the severity and progression of shock. (Other cardiac disorders that can cause cardiogenic shock are discussed more thoroughly in Chapter 22.)

In cardiogenic shock, the ventricles fail to pump blood into the circulatory system. This leads to a decreased **stroke volume** (the amount of blood ejected from the heart each

---

BOX 10-2
CAUSES OF HYPOVOLEMIC SHOCK

- Hemorrhage (loss of blood volume): Trauma, major fractures of pelvis or femur, surgery, hemophilia, GI bleeding, hemothorax
- Internal Fluid Shifts (third-spacing): Cirrhosis with ascites, pleural effusion, pancreatitis, intestinal obstruction
- Burns (loss of plasma proteins through the skin)
- Dehydration (body fluid loss): Profuse diaphoresis; massive diuresis from diuretics or diabetes insipidus; GI loss from persistent and severe vomiting, diarrhea, or continuous nasogastric suctioning; prolonged inadequate fluid intake

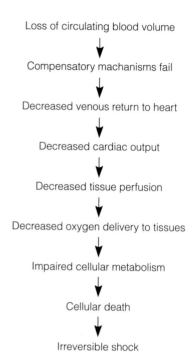

Loss of circulating blood volume

↓

Compensatory machanisms fail

↓

Decreased venous return to heart

↓

Decreased cardiac output

↓

Decreased tissue perfusion

↓

Decreased oxygen delivery to tissues

↓

Impaired cellular metabolism

↓

Cellular death

↓

Irreversible shock

Figure 10-2. ◆ The pathophysiology of hypovolemic shock.

> **BOX 10-4**
> **MANIFESTATIONS OF ANAPHYLACTIC SHOCK**
>
> • **Cutaneous:** Generalized itching, flushing, sensation of warmth, urticaria (hives), angioedema (edema of eyelids, lips, and tongue)
> • **Neurologic:** Restlessness, apprehension, anxiety, decreased level of consciousness
> • **Respiratory:** Difficulty breathing, wheezing, laryngospasm, stridor, rales
> • **Cardiovascular:** Hypotension, tachycardia
> • **Gastrointestinal:** Nausea, vomiting, diarrhea

---

minute). Excess blood is left in the ventricle with each beat. This blood backs up into the lungs, leading to pulmonary edema. When cardiac output drops, the client becomes hypotensive. A compensatory rise in heart rate increases myocardial oxygen consumption and decreases coronary perfusion. This burdens an already overworked myocardium, so eventually it fails. Common manifestations of cardiogenic shock are listed in Box 10-5.

SEPTIC SHOCK. Septic shock is shock that results from an overwhelming bacterial infection (i.e., *Pseudomonas, Escherichia*

coli, Klebsiella). Sometimes gram-positive infections (e.g., *Staphylococcus* and *Streptococcus*) may be the underlying cause. Common sources of pathogens include the hospital environment and health care workers. Various predisposing risk factors increase the chance for developing septic shock (Box 10-6).

Septic shock begins with **septicemia** (the presence of pathogens and their toxins in the blood). The invading bacteria multiply faster than the body can kill them. As bacteria are destroyed, endotoxins are released into the bloodstream. The endotoxins damage tissues and starve the cells of oxygen and nutrients. The damaged cells release histamine and other chemicals to dilate peripheral blood vessels and increase capillary permeability. As in anaphylactic shock, fluids shift from intravascular space to interstitial space, resulting in relative hypovolemia. *Microemboli* (tiny blood clots) form in the capillaries, causing further cell damage and death. Septic shock has an early phase and a late phase; manifestations are summarized

---

> **BOX 10-3**
> **MANIFESTATIONS OF HYPOVOLEMIC SHOCK CAUSED BY HEMORRHAGE**
>
> | | Class I | Class II | Class III | Class IV |
> |---|---|---|---|---|
> | *Blood Loss (mL)* | Up to 750 | 750–1,500 | 1,500–2,000 | > 2,000 |
> | *% Blood Volume* | Up to 15% | 15–30% | 30–40% | > 40% |
> | *Pulse Rate* | < 100 | > 100 | > 120 | > 140 |
> | *Blood Pressure* | Normal | Normal | Decreased | Severe hypotension |
> | *Capillary Refill* | Normal | Delayed | Delayed | Delayed |
> | *Skin Circulation* | Pale pink, slightly cool | Slightly pale, cool | Pale, cold, moist | Cyanotic, cold, clammy |
> | *Respiratory Rate* | 14–20 | 20–30 | 30–40 | > 40 |
> | *Urine Output* | ≥ 30 | 20–30 | 5–15 | Negligible |
> | *Mental Status* | Slightly anxious | Mildly anxious | Anxious, confused | Confused, lethargic |
>
> *Source:* Adapted from American College of Surgeons Committee on Trauma. (1993). *The advanced trauma life support student manual* (p. 18). Chicago: American College of Surgeons.

BOX 10-5
MANIFESTATIONS OF CARDIOGENIC SHOCK

- Systolic pressure < 90 mm Hg
- Rapid, weak, thready pulse
- Distended neck veins
- Rapid, labored respirations; crackles
- Pale, cold, moist skin
- Restlessness, agitation, or disorientation
- Oliguria to anuria

BOX 10-7
MANIFESTATIONS OF SEPTIC SHOCK

EARLY (WARM) SEPTIC SHOCK

- Normal to decreased blood pressure
- Tachycardia
- Rapid respirations
- Warm, flushed, dry skin
- Alert, anxious
- Normal urine output
- Elevated body temperature

LATE (COLD) SEPTIC SHOCK

- Profound hypotension
- Rapid, thready pulse; arrhythmias
- Rapid, shallow respirations with crackles
- Cold, cyanotic extremities
- Confused to lethargic to comatose
- Oliguria to anuria
- Decreased body temperature

in Box 10-7. Death may result from respiratory, cardiac, or renal failure.

Toxic shock syndrome (TSS) is caused by a toxin-producing form of *Staphylococcus aureus.* It usually affects menstruating women between 15 and 19 who use tampons. Toxins from the bacteria enter the bloodstream and circulate throughout the body, causing the septic shock process to begin. The client may have a high fever, vomiting, and diarrhea. The client's condition worsens and can be fatal without treatment.

NEUROGENIC SHOCK. Neurogenic shock is shock that occurs when there is interruption in the sympathetic nervous system. The problem can result from damage to the vasomotor center in the medulla or from loss of impulse transmission (seen in a spinal cord injury above the T6 level). Other causes include head injury, spinal anesthesia, opiate drug overdose, and hypoglycemia.

Without sympathetic nervous system impulses, the blood vessels dilate, leading to massive peripheral vasodilation. Blood pools in the venous and capillary beds, leading to inadequate tissue perfusion. Thermoregulation is impaired because the cutaneous blood vessels lose vasomotor tone. Without appropriate treatment, organ failure and death can occur. Manifestations of neurogenic shock are listed in Box 10-8.

Complications of Shock

The two most common complications of shock are **adult respiratory distress syndrome (ARDS)** and **disseminated intravascular coagulation (DIC).** Both disorders usually develop once the client has entered the progressive stage of shock.

ARDS is characterized by acute respiratory failure due to damage to the alveoli. When alveolar capillaries become more permeable, fluid and proteins leak into the alveoli, causing a type of pulmonary edema. The client with ARDS may require mechanical ventilation.

DIC is an acute condition characterized by abnormal platelet *aggregation* (clumping of red blood cells) and excessive clotting in the body's capillaries. There is simultaneous bleeding and clotting throughout the body. The clumping reduces capillary blood flow to the skin and causes *mottling* (discoloration). Because most of the clotting factors are consumed by aggregation, generalized bleeding begins. Initially, the client

BOX 10-6
PREDISPOSING RISK FACTORS FOR SEPTIC SHOCK

- Extremes of age (< 1 year, > 65 years)
- Chronic debilitating diseases or conditions:
  - Cancer, AIDS, or malnutrition
  - Burns or decubitus ulcers
  - Diabetes mellitus
- Surgery or invasive diagnostic procedures
- Invasive lines or tubes (IV or central venous lines, urinary catheters, tracheostomy or endotracheal tube)
- Drug therapy (chemotherapy, antibiotic therapy, corticosteroids)

BOX 10-8
MANIFESTATIONS OF NEUROGENIC SHOCK

- Hypotension
- Bradycardia
- Warm, dry skin
- Anxiety, restlessness
- Decreased urine output
- Lowered body temperature

bleeds from puncture sites and incisions. Treatment is aimed at replacing the platelets and clotting factors while protecting the client from injury.

COLLABORATIVE CARE

Successful management of shock requires early recognition and treatment. The nurse is expected to identify early manifestations of shock. Once a diagnosis of shock is made, medical management focuses on treating the underlying cause, increasing oxygenation, and improving tissue perfusion. The common interventions include oxygen therapy, fluid and blood replacement, and pharmacologic therapy.

No single laboratory and diagnostic test can determine shock. However, the following laboratory tests may be ordered to help identify the type of shock and to assess the client's physical status:

- Blood hemoglobin and hematocrit, to identify decreases associated with hypovolemic shock resulting from hemorrhage.
- Arterial blood gases (ABGs), to measure oxygen and carbon dioxide levels and pH. As shock progresses, metabolic acidosis develops from anaerobic metabolism.
- Serum sodium and serum potassium levels; the first decreases and the second increases in the progressive stage.
- Blood glucose levels; these increase in early shock but decrease as shock worsens.
- Blood urea nitrogen (BUN) and serum creatinine levels, to measure renal function. Decreased renal perfusion reduces renal function, so the BUN and creatinine levels increase.
- Blood cultures, to identify the causative organism in septic shock.
- White blood cell count (WBC), this is elevated in the client with septic shock.
- Serum cardiac isoenzymes (creatine kinase CK-MB) and troponin (a myocardial muscle protein); these are elevated following a myocardial infarction and in cardiogenic shock.
- X-ray studies, computerized tomography (CT) scans, magnetic resonance imaging (MRI), and peritoneal lavage may determine the extent of injury or locate sites of internal hemorrhage.

Oxygen Therapy

To reverse shock, adequate oxygenation and tissue perfusion must be restored. The first step is to ensure that the client has a patent airway. If necessary, a nasal or oral airway may be inserted. When excess secretions obstruct the airway, the nurse must be prepared to suction the client.

All clients in shock should receive oxygen therapy. This may be given by a nonrebreather mask at 12 to 15 L/min to maintain the PaO_2 greater than 90 mm Hg. If the client develops respiratory distress, the nurse should anticipate endotracheal intubation and mechanical ventilation. (Care of the client requiring ventilatory assistance is discussed in Chapter 26.)

Hypovolemic Shock

Hypovolemic shock resulting from trauma or hemorrhage requires immediate emergency care. This care begins as soon as medical rescuers arrive on the accident scene and continues through transport to the emergency department (ED). At the emergency scene, intravenous fluids are started and pneumatic antishock garments may be applied. Because shock can progress so rapidly, treatment needs to begin within the first hour following an injury if at all possible (the "golden hour" of trauma care). Failure to begin emergency treatment within the first hour increases the client's risk for death. Box 10-9 summarizes the prehospital emergency care for a client in hypovolemic shock.

PNEUMATIC ANTISHOCK GARMENT. The **pneumatic antishock garment (PASG)**, also called military antishock trousers (MAST), is applied following a traumatic injury (Figure 10-3 ◆). The device is used to raise blood pressure and can be used to stabilize pelvic and femoral fractures. Only specially trained personnel can apply or remove PASGs.

> ## BOX 10-9
> ## PREHOSPITAL EMERGENCY CARE OF THE CLIENT EXPERIENCING HEMORRHAGE
>
> 1. Scan the area for potential hazards (e.g., fire).
> 2. Call for help.
> 3. Ensure adequate airway; assist with ventilation as needed.
> 4. Assess for cause of hemorrhage.
> 5. Control external bleeding by applying direct pressure to the local site. If an extremity is involved, elevate it to stop venous bleeding. When bleeding continues, apply pressure to an arterial pressure point.
> 6. Apply a tourniquet *only as a last resort.*
> 7. Assess for manifestations of shock, which may include:
>   a. Decreased blood pressure
>   b. Rapid, thready pulse
>   c. Rapid, shallow respirations
>   d. Cool, pale, moist skin
>   e. Thirst
>   f. Restlessness
>   g. Changes in level of consciousness
> 8. Keep the client's trunk and head flat and legs slightly elevated. (Use this position *only* when no head injury exists.)
> 9. Cover the client to maintain warmth.
> 10. Do not give the client anything by mouth.
> 11. Use touch and verbal communication to reduce apprehension and anxiety.

1 Wrap left leg compartment around client's left leg.

2 Fasten velcro strips.

Tubing from abdominal air chamber to foot pump

4 Wrap and fasten abdominal compartment.

3 Wrap and fasten right leg compartment around right leg.

Tubing from right and left leg air chambers

Figure 10-3. ◆ Pneumatic antishock garments provide rapid, emergency treatment of shock.

FLUID REPLACEMENT. The main goal for clients with hypovolemic shock is to restore intravascular volume. Intravenous fluids are used alone or in combination with colloids, blood, or blood products. The type and amount of fluid chosen depends on the type of fluid lost. Usually, fluid replacements are given in a 3:1 ratio (300 mL fluid for every 100 mL of fluid loss).

Crystalloid solutions contain electrolytes dissolved in water. The most commonly ordered intravenous solutions are normal saline (0.9%) and lactated Ringer's. Both isotonic solutions increase volume in the intravascular and the interstitial spaces.

These solutions are given during the emergency phase while the client's blood is being typed and cross-matched.

CLINICAL alert

Large infusions of crystalloid solutions can lead to pulmonary edema. The client must be monitored closely for signs of respiratory distress.

Colloid solutions contain proteins that increase osmotic pressure. (Osmotic pressure holds fluid within the vessels so that the plasma volume expands.) Colloid solutions include albumin, plasma protein fraction, dextran, and hetastarch. (Nursing implications for administering colloids are discussed in Table 10-1 ◆.)

Blood and blood products used in treating hemorrhage are obtained from a donor and given as a *transfusion* (an infusion of blood or blood components) to the client (Table 10-2 ◆). State and institution policies vary about whether LPNs can administer transfusions. Nurses are responsible for knowing their state's scope of practice.

Each person has one of four blood types: A, B, AB, and O. Blood group antigens A and B form the basis for ABO blood categorization. The presence or absence of these inherited antigens determines one's blood type (type A has A antigen, type B has B antigen, and type AB has both). Persons with neither antigen have blood type O.

A protein on the red blood cell membrane determines the Rh of a person's blood. Rh positive blood has the protein, Rh negative blood does not (Table 10-3 ◆).

Before a client can receive a blood transfusion, a blood **type and cross-match** (test to determine donor and recipient ABO types and Rh groups) must be done. Blood is also tested for hepatitis A, hepatitis B, and human immunodeficiency virus (HIV).

TABLE 10-1	NURSING IMPLICATIONS FOR PHARMACOLOGY: CLIENTS RECEIVING COLLOID SOLUTIONS		
DRUG GROUP/DRUGS	**ACTION**	**NURSING IMPLICATIONS**	**CLIENT TEACHING**
Colloid solutions (plasma expanders) ▪ Albumin 5% or 25% (Albuminar, Buminate) ▪ Plasma protein fraction (Plasmanate) ▪ Dextran 40 or 70 (Gentran 40 or 70) ▪ Hetastarch (Hespan)	▪ Colloid solutions expand blood volume and are used to treat hypovolemic shock. ▪ Albumin and plasma protein fraction come from healthy human donors. ▪ Dextran and hetastarch are made synthetically.	▪ Before infusion, take client's vital signs and assess lung and heart sounds. ▪ Take vital signs according to institutional policy (usually every 15–60 minutes). ▪ Monitor for manifestations of congestive heart failure or pulmonary edema (dyspnea, cyanosis, cough, crackles, wheezes). If these appear, notify the physician immediately.	▪ The solutions are helping to maintain blood volume. ▪ Vital signs are takenfrequently to ensure the client's safety.

TABLE 10-2   BLOOD AND BLOOD PRODUCTS

TYPE	COMPOSITION	USE
Whole blood	Contains RBCs, plasma, and clotting factors	Replaces blood volume and increases oxygen-carrying capacity in hemorrhage and shock
Packed red cells	Contains some platelets; very little plasma	Increases oxygen-carrying capacity of blood
Platelets	Contains only platelets	Controls bleeding in clients with platelet deficiencies
Fresh frozen plasma	Contains all clotting factors except platelets	Expands blood volume; can be administered to any blood group or type, because it contains no RBCs; takes 30–60 minutes to thaw
Cryoprecipitate	Contains factor VIII, factor XIII, and fibrinogen	Treats clients with clotting factor deficiencies

Note: Each hospital has its own policy about blood transfusions. The nurse must learn and follow those policies.

Despite rigorous type and cross-matching procedures, blood transfusion reactions may still occur. The most common is a febrile reaction, which typically begins during the first 15 minutes of the transfusion. In *febrile reaction,* the client's antibodies react to the donor's white blood cells, causing fever and chills. (General guidelines for monitoring blood transfusions are found in Table 10-4 ◆.)

When hemorrhage causes hypovolemic shock, the client may receive whole blood or red blood cells (RBCs). The goal is to increase the client's hematocrit and hemoglobin levels to near-normal values. Trauma victims may receive a type O blood transfusion while the type and cross-match is done.

Some emergency departments and trauma centers use autotransfusion for the client with multiple injuries and/or severe shock. **Autotransfusion** is the collection, filtration, and retransfusion of a client's own blood. Blood from the chest cavity is the typical source for an autotransfusion.

Anaphylactic Shock

When an anaphylactic reaction develops, the client needs immediate intervention. First priorities are a patent airway and supplemental oxygen, followed by drug therapy.

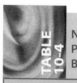

TABLE 10-3   BLOOD GROUP AND RH TYPES AND COMPATIBILITIES

BLOOD GROUP	COMPATIBLE DONOR BLOOD GROUPS
O	O
A	A, O
B	B, O
AB	A, B, AB, O
Rh	*Compatible Donor*
Rh positive	Rh Pos, Rh Neg
Rh negative	Rh neg

Note: Group O is often called the universal donor, and group AB is called the universal recipient. Do not infuse if types are not compatible according to the chart!

TABLE 10-4   NURSING IMPLICATIONS FOR PHARMACOLOGY: CLIENTS RECEIVING BLOOD TRANSFUSIONS

NURSING IMPLICATIONS	CLIENT TEACHING
▪ Take and record baseline vital signs. ▪ Stay with the client during the first 15 minutes of the transfusion. ▪ Monitor for manifestations of a transfusion reaction. ▪ Take and record vital signs according to institutional policy. ▪ If a transfusion reaction occurs, take the following actions: 　a. Stop the transfusion immediately, and notify the nurse. Start normal saline slowly. 　b. Take vital signs and assess for manifestations. 　c. Follow institutional policy for saving the blood bag, returning it to the laboratory, and collecting urine and venous blood samples. 　d. Continue to monitor the client and provide prescribed interventions to treat the reaction according to physician orders.	Immediately report any warm feelings, chills, itching, feelings of weakness or fainting, or difficulty breathing.

Epinephrine is the drug of choice to restore arterial blood pressure and promote bronchodilation. Antihistamines like diphenhydramine (Benadryl) reverse the effects of histamine. Corticosteroids are given to prevent a delayed reaction to the antigen. If respiratory distress continues, aminophylline is ordered. Once the client's condition is stable, the client must be monitored for reappearance of signs and symptoms of anaphylaxis. The effects of the causative antigen may last for hours.

Cardiogenic Shock

Cardiogenic shock usually results from an acute myocardial infarction. Oxygen is given to prevent further heart muscle damage. Drug therapy and mechanical devices are prescribed to raise blood pressure and improve cardiac output. These clients are acutely ill and are best managed in a critical care unit. Several intravenous medications are used to treat cardiogenic shock. **Adrenergic drugs** mimic the fight-or-flight response of the sympathetic nervous system. This drug group includes vasopressor drugs and positive inotropic drugs. **Vasopressor drugs** (alpha-adrenergic) produce vasoconstriction, which raises the client's blood pressure. Vasopressors include dopamine (Intropin) and norepinephrine (Levophed). **Positive inotropic drugs** (beta-adrenergic) increase the force of myocardial contraction so that cardiac output increases. Dobutamine (Dobutrex) and amrinone (Inocor) are positive inotropic drugs. Nitroglycerin (Tridol) and nitroprusside (Nipride) may also be ordered to improve the pumping action of the heart. Diuretics and digoxin (Lanoxin) may be given if the client shows signs of heart failure. Antiarrhythmic drugs regulate the client's heart rhythm.

In addition to medications, two mechanical devices can also help improve blood circulation: the intra-aortic balloon pump (IABP) and the ventricular assist device (VAD). (See Chapter 22 for further discussion.)

Septic Shock

One of the first steps in managing septic shock is to identify the causative organism. Using aseptic technique, specimens of blood, urine, wounds, and sputum are collected and sent for culture and sensitivity. Intravenous fluids are given to counteract the massive vasodilation caused by the release of bacterial endotoxins. Intravenous antibiotics (such as aminoglycosides and third-generation cephalosporins) are started immediately. Once the organism is positively identified, antibiotic therapy may be changed. If clients become unstable, they should be transferred to the critical care unit.

Neurogenic Shock

Treatment of neurogenic shock varies according to its cause. Intravenous fluids are ordered to reverse the peripheral vasodilation, so blood pressure and tissue perfusion are restored. If neurogenic shock is caused by severe pain, appropriate analgesics should be given. Clients receiving spinal anesthesia should have the head of the bed raised to prevent the anesthetic from moving up the spinal cord. (Management of clients with spinal cord injury is presented in Chapter 30.)

NURSING CARE

The nurse assumes an important role in preventing shock as well as potential complications.

ASSESSING

Assessment data collected by the nurse can determine the severity of the shock condition. The manifestations for each type of shock can be found in the previous discussion. Each client's condition will determine how frequently assessments are conducted.

DIAGNOSING, PLANNING, AND IMPLEMENTING

Nursing care for the client in shock focuses on monitoring overall tissue perfusion and on meeting the psychosocial needs of the client and family. Two major nursing diagnoses appropriate for the client with hypovolemic shock are: Ineffective Tissue Perfusion and Anxiety.

INEFFECTIVE TISSUE PERFUSION: CARDIOPULMONARY, PERIPHERAL, CEREBRAL, RENAL

■ Monitor skin color, temperature, turgor, and moisture. *Decreased tissue perfusion is shown by pale, cool, moist skin. When hemoglobin levels drop, cyanosis may occur.*

■ Monitor cardiopulmonary function every 15 to 30 minutes by assessing blood pressure, heart rate and rhythm, rate and depth of respirations, lung sounds, and peripheral pulses (include presence, equality, rate, rhythm, and quality). If unable to palpate pulses, use a Doppler ultrasound device. If a line is inserted, measure central venous pressure (CVP). *Vital signs help identify the stage of shock. As shock progresses, BP drops; the pulse becomes rapid, weak, and thready. Decreased lung perfusion causes crackles, wheezes, and dyspnea. Capillary refill is prolonged. Peripheral pulses (dorsalis pedis and posterior tibial) are weak or nonpalpable. CVP measures fluid status; low findings indicate decreased blood volume (normal = 5 to 15 cm).*

■ Monitor oxygen saturation by attaching a pulse oximeter to the client. *Oxygen saturation should be maintained between 94% and 100% with oxygen therapy.*

■ Assess for restlessness, confusion, mental status changes, and decreased level of consciousness. *These indicate decreased cerebral perfusion.*

■ Monitor intake and urinary output per Foley catheter hourly, using a urimeter. Measure daily weight and fluid loss such as emesis and gastric and chest tube drainage. Estimate fluid loss from profuse perspiration and wound drainage. *This evaluates fluid status and renal blood flow. Urinary output less than 30 mL per hour indicates reduced renal perfusion.*

■ Monitor bowel sounds, abdominal distention, and abdominal pain. *Decreased gastrointestinal blood flow reduces bowel motility and peristalsis; paralytic ileus may result.*

■ Assess for sudden sharp chest pain, dyspnea, cyanosis, anxiety, and restlessness. *Hemoconcentration and increased platelet aggregation may result in pulmonary emboli.*

■ Assess for irregular heart rate and chest pain. *These indicate decreased coronary artery perfusion and increased risk for myocardial infarction.*

■ Monitor body temperature. *An elevated body temperature increases oxygen requirements.*

■ Maintain client on bed rest, and provide a calm, quiet environment. Place the client in a modified Trendelenburg position as tolerated (Figure 10-4 ◆). *Bed rest decreases the workload of the heart. The modified Trendelenburg position increases venous return to the heart. Do not use this position for clients in cardiogenic shock.*

ANXIETY

Clients with hypovolemic shock may have experienced a traumatic injury that has required major surgery and a transfer to a critical care unit. Throughout these events, the client and family are frightened, anxious, and often emotionally isolated. While the nurse's first priority must be to provide emergency care, the psychosocial needs of the client and family also must be met.

■ Acknowledge the client's anxiety and fear. *This helps validate the client's feelings.*

■ Remain with and explain procedures to the client. Listen carefully to client. Speak slowly and calmly, using short sentences. Use touch to provide support. *These measures provide reassurance to the client and help reduce anxiety.*

■ Provide comfort measures (e.g., calm, quiet environment, back rub). *Comfort measures can reduce the client's anxiety.*

■ Provide time, space, and privacy for family members. *Allowing the family access to the client reduces anxiety and gives both the client and the family some feeling of control.*

Figure 10-4. ◆ Modified Trendelenburg position. Position the client with the lower extremities elevated approximately 20 degrees (knees straight), trunk horizontal, and the head elevated about 10 degrees.

■ Provide anticipatory guidance to prepare for recovery or death. *If the prognosis is poor, this helps the family begin the grieving process.*

■ Keep the client's family informed. *They need information on which to make their decisions.*

EVALUATING

Evaluate the effectiveness of care by noting whether the client's vital signs are stabilized. Also, the nurse notes the client's tissue perfusion: alert and oriented; warm, dry skin, urine output > 30 mL/hr, and palpable pedal pulses.

Discharge Considerations

Shock must be fully resolved before a client can be discharged. Although the client has survived the shock episode, recovery from the original medical problem may be delayed. Teach the family that a lengthy recovery often leads to depression and that the client will need a supportive and nurturing environment. Teach clients who have experienced an anaphylactic reaction how to prevent a future reaction. Box 10-10 highlights key points to teach these clients before discharge.

Nursing Process Case Study
■ CLIENT WITH SEPTIC SHOCK

Huang Mei Lan is a 43-year-old single woman who had surgery four days ago for recurrent breast cancer. She is under-

---

BOX 10-10
TEACHING FOR DISCHARGE

TEACHING CLIENTS HOW TO PREVENT ANAPHYLAXIS

- Avoid known allergens.
- Notify health care professionals of allergies.
- If allergic to insect stings, avoid wearing bright colors, perfumes, and scented hair sprays when outdoors.
- If allergic to foods, read package labels. When eating out, ask how meals are prepared and what ingredients are used.
- Wear a Medic-Alert bracelet or necklace.
- Advise client to carry an emergency kit for anaphylaxis.
- Review manifestations of anaphylaxis.
- Seek medical attention immediately when symptoms occur.

weight, weak, and depressed. Despite her multiple problems, she never complains or asks for pain medication. A central line and a urinary catheter are in place. On her fourth postoperative day, Mrs. Canote, her primary nurse, finds Ms. Huang huddled in the middle of the bed, shivering violently.

Assessment T 104° F, P 110, R 30, and BP 96/66. Her skin is hot, dry, and flushed with poor turgor. She is alert and oriented, but is restless and appears anxious. She is nauseated and has diarrhea. Her WBC count is elevated. Blood, sputum, urine, and wound cultures are collected. She is diagnosed as having septic shock. Intravenous solutions of lactated Ringer's and of a broad-spectrum antibiotic are begun until the organism and its portal of entry are identified. Ms. Huang's condition worsens. Her blood pressure continues to drop, her skin becomes cool and cyanotic, and she has periods of disorientation. She is transferred to the critical care unit. As she is being prepared for the transfer she begins to cry and asks, "Am I going to die?"

Diagnosis The following nursing diagnoses are established for Ms. Huang:

- Deficient Fluid Volume related to vomiting, diarrhea, high fever, and hypotension
- Impaired Gas Exchange related to rapid respirations
- Ineffective Tissue Perfusion related to hypotension and massive vasodilation
- Anxiety related to feelings that illness is worsening and is potentially life threatening

Expected Outcomes The expected outcomes for the plan of care are that Ms. Huang will:

- Maintain adequate circulating blood volume.
- Regain and maintain blood gas parameters within normal limits.
- Regain and maintain stable hemodynamic levels.
- State her feelings of fear and anxiety.

Planning and Implementation The following nursing interventions are implemented for Ms. Huang. Assessments are done frequently to monitor her condition.

- Monitor mental status and level of consciousness.
- Monitor arterial blood pressure; rate, rhythm, and quality of pulses; central venous pressure; pulmonary artery pressure; and cardiac output.
- Assess color and character of skin.
- Monitor results of arterial blood gases, blood counts, clotting times, and platelet counts.
- Monitor respiratory rate, rhythm, and breath sounds.
- Monitor temperature every 2 hours.
- Monitor urinary output hourly, reporting any output of less than 30 mL per hour.
- Explain procedures and provide oral and skin care, turning, and positioning.

Evaluation Despite intensive nursing and medical care, Ms. Huang's condition remains critical. The interventions are continued.

 Critical Thinking in the Nursing Process

1. What stage of shock was Ms. Huang experiencing when Ms. Canote first entered her room? Provide supporting evidence.
2. Why was the lactated Ringer's solution started on Ms. Huang?
3. Why would the nursing diagnosis Altered Skin Integrity be appropriate for Ms. Huang?

The Client Experiencing Trauma

Persons who need urgent medical care enter the medical system through the emergency department (ED). Severely injured clients may require transport to a regional trauma center. Treatment in the ED is provided by nurses and doctors with special training in emergency care. Emergency nurses take care of clients of all ages with a wide range of medical problems. This type of nursing requires a broad knowledge base, solid observation skills, and the ability to provide care in an unpredictable environment.

The goals of emergency care are to stabilize the critically ill, prevent deterioration of a client's condition, and promote optimal function. In order to accomplish these goals, clients must be prioritized when they enter the ED. **Triage** systems identify who will receive medical attention first. The most common triage categories are emergent, urgent, and nonurgent. During disasters like earthquakes or tornados, a tag triage system is used. Clients are tagged as "red" *(emergent),* "yellow" *(urgent),* "green" *(nonurgent),* and "black" *(dead or expected to die).*

CAUSES AND TYPES OF TRAUMA

Trauma is defined as an injury caused by physical force (motor vehicle crashes, falls, drowning, gunshots, burns, stabbing, or other physical assaults). Trauma is the number one cause of death for persons under the age of 35 and is the fifth leading cause of death in the United States for all age groups. At highest risk are males between the ages of 15 and 24 years; geriatric clients are also at risk (Box 10-11). Traumatic injuries can result in temporary physical impairment, permanent disability, or death.

Traumatic injury occurs suddenly, leaving the client and family with little time to prepare for its consequences. Nurses serve as a vital communication link between the injured client and the family. They help the client and family cope with the client's current injury, as well as understand the potential long-term effects of this injury.

Minor or Major Trauma

Whether intentional or accidental, trauma causes injury to one or more body parts. *Minor trauma* involves a single body part or system and is usually treated in the ED. A fractured collarbone, a small second-degree burn, and a cut requiring

population
FOCUS

Geriatric Risks for Trauma

The elderly are hospitalized for trauma twice as often as the general population. Falls commonly cause trauma in those over age 65. The fall may be caused by acute or chronic medical conditions, environmental factors, or simply the aging process. Persons over age 75 also experience a high fatality rate following a motor vehicle crash. Elderly pedestrians are at a higher risk for being struck by a motor vehicle, because they don't move as quickly when crossing the street or cannot see traffic lights well.

Figure 10-5. ◆ Intubation with insertion of an endotracheal tube (ETT). When a client is experiencing respiratory distress, oxygen can be given into the external opening of the tube.

stitches are all considered minor trauma. *Major* or *multiple trauma* involves serious single-system injury (such as traumatic amputation of a leg) or multiple-system injuries. Multiple trauma victims require immediate emergency care.

Blunt or Penetrating Trauma

Trauma also may be classified as blunt or penetrating. *Blunt trauma* does not cause a break in the skin. It can result in greater internal damage than appears on the surface. Common blunt forces are motor vehicle crashes, falls, assaults, and contact sports. *Penetrating trauma* results from foreign objects that pierce the body. The most common sources are knives, bullets, shotgun blast, or impaled, sharp objects. The penetrating object often damages the intestines, liver, spleen, and vascular system. Again, the external appearance of the wound does not determine the extent of internal damage.

EFFECTS OF TRAUMATIC INJURY

Traumatic injuries have serious consequences that must be identified and treated rapidly. Some common effects of traumatic injury are the following:

- *Airway obstruction* can be caused by blood, teeth, the tongue, or vomitus in a client's airway. Once the cervical spine is immobilized, oxygen is given. If equipment is available, the airway is suctioned. Clients with severe airway obstruction may require intubation with an endotracheal tube (Figure 10-5 ◆).

- *Pneumothorax* results from air in the pleural space causing partial or complete lung collapse. Blunt and penetrating injuries to the chest may be the cause. A *tension pneumothorax* develops when air continually enters the chest cavity but cannot exit. In the ED, a chest tube is inserted to reinflate the lung.

- *Hemorrhage* in the trauma client may be external or internal (see the classes of hemorrhage in Box 10-3 and prehospital care in Box 10-9). When an artery is severed, the bleeding must be controlled immediately (Figure 10-6 ◆). Internal hemorrhage may lead to blood pooling in several body cavities. For example, chest trauma may cause bleeding into the pleural space. A pelvic fracture may lead to bleeding in the

retroperitoneal region. The nurse must identify the cause, location, and extent of blood loss.

- *Hypovolemic shock* may be caused by hemorrhage from blunt or penetrating injuries, long-bone or pelvic fractures, major

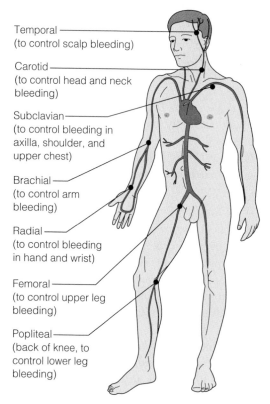

Figure 10-6. ◆ The major pressure points used to control bleeding.

vessel injuries, traumatic amputation, or plasma loss from burns or crush injuries (see above discussion).

■ Among *neurologic injuries,* traumatic brain injuries (TBIs) are one of the most common; spinal cord injuries occur less frequently. Both injuries can have a permanent, devastating outcome. Most head and spinal cord injuries result from motor vehicle crashes; other causes include falls, sports injuries, and assault.

■ *Gastrointestinal and genitourinary injuries* to the abdominal organs can be caused by blunt and penetrating injuries. Liver and spleen injuries are the main sources of life-threatening hemorrhage. Peritonitis can occur when damaged intestines leak bile and stool into the peritoneum. Motor vehicle crashes cause most of the renal injuries.

CLINICAL alert

Never remove a penetrating object. Removal may cause internal injuries or possible nerve damage.

■ *Musculoskeletal injuries* are frequently seen in the ED. Injury includes damage to bone, soft tissue, nerves, or blood vessels. Common manifestations of musculoskeletal injuries are swelling, bone protrusion, obvious deformity, abnormal motion, pain, and a pulseless extremity.

■ *Integumentary injuries* are not usually as serious, except for burns (see Chapter 15). The nurse must assess both the skin and the underlying structures for any sign of injury. Injuries to the integument are often contaminated with dirt, debris, or foreign objects that increase the client's risk for infection. The four main skin injuries are contusions, abrasions, puncture wounds, and lacerations (Figure 10-7 ◆).

■ *Psychosocial effects on the family* are a consequence of trauma. Death or serious injury may change family dynamics. The suddenness and seriousness of the event predispose families to psychological crisis. Families may exhibit shock, fear, numbness, anxiety, guilt, hostility, or anger.

COLLABORATIVE CARE

The trauma client requires collaborative care at the accident scene before arriving in the ED (see Box 10-9). This type of care may be provided by emergency medical technicians (EMTs), paramedics, flight nurses, or physicians. Flight nurses are educated in trauma care and air transport techniques. They can perform advanced techniques such as intubation or chest tube insertion.

At the accident scene, life-threatening problems must be identified and treated immediately. Before other treatments are started, the client may require basic life support and advanced cardiac life support. The client's cervical spine is immobilized at once by placing the client on a spine board and applying a cervical collar (Figure 10-8 ◆). If the client's

Figure 10-7. ◆ (A) Contusions (bruises) do not cause a break in the skin. (B) Abrasions (scrapes) occur when a partial layer of skin is removed. (C) Puncture wounds occur when the integument is penetrated by a sharp or blunt object. (D) Lacerations are irregular tears in the skin.

airway is patent, high-flow oxygen is started. Direct pressure may be applied to control active external bleeding. One or two intravenous lines with IV fluids are started.

As soon as the client's condition is stabilized, the client is transported rapidly to the ED or trauma center. Ground ambulances and air ambulances (e.g., specially staffed and equipped helicopters) are used. Once the trauma client arrives at the ED, team members provide medical and nursing care. These team members may include an ED physician, ED

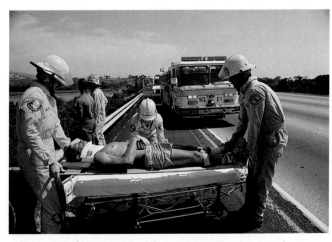

Figure 10-8. ◆ Application of a cervical collar at an accident scene immobilizes the cervical spine and prevents further injury to the spinal cord.

nurses, trauma surgeon, anesthesiologist, laboratory technicians, radiologist, and respiratory therapist.

Laboratory and Diagnostic Tests

The type of laboratory and diagnostic tests obtained depend on the client's injuries. Besides the tests used to rule out shock, the following tests may be ordered:

■ Blood alcohol levels measure the amount of alcohol in a client's blood (20% to 50% of people who are injured may be intoxicated).

■ Drug screen test determines the presence of cocaine, heroin, or amphetamines.

■ Pregnancy test for any woman of childbearing age rules out the potential for pregnancy and fetal injury.

■ Diagnostic peritoneal lavage identifies the presence of blood in the peritoneal cavity, which may indicate abdominal injury.

■ Computerized tomography (CT) scan locates injuries to the brain, skull, spinal cord, chest, and abdomen.

■ Magnetic resonance imaging (MRI) identifies brain and spinal cord injuries.

Emergency Surgery

Surgery is indicated when the client remains in shock despite resuscitation and there is no obvious sign of blood loss. Nurses prepare the client for emergency surgery by undressing the client and removing jewelry, dentures, or other loose objects. Place an identification bracelet on the client. Report the extent of the injury, allergies and past medical history (if obtainable), and completed nursing interventions to the operating room nurse.

It is important for the emergency or trauma nurse to speak with the family as soon as possible and keep them informed about what is happening to their family member. Unfortunately, family members or significant others may not have time to see their loved one before transfer to the operating room.

Forensic Considerations

Sometimes injuries involve criminal activity that requires legal investigation. The nurse's role is to identify, store, and properly transfer potential evidence for medical–legal investigations. All evidence must be marked and sealed in tamper-proof containers.

The nurse must not cut through any clothing containing potential evidence such as blood stains or bullet holes. Each clothing item is placed in an individual breathable container, such as a paper bag, and labeled appropriately. Bullets or knives are labeled with the identifying source and given to the proper authorities. Entrance and exit wounds must be recorded in the chart.

The client's hands may yield important evidence, such as powder burns on the skin or tissue or hair samples beneath the fingernails. Paper bags should be placed over the client's hands if the presence of evidence is suspected. Photographs may be needed of wounds and clothing.

NURSING CARE

Nursing care of the client who has suffered a serious injury starts with a primary assessment and includes collaborative interventions to manage any life-threatening injuries.

ASSESSING

In the emergency department, the nurse ensures that the cervical spine is immobilized and then performs a five-step assessment: **A**irway, **B**reathing, **C**irculation, **D**isability, and **E**xposure. The ABCs are assessed and managed first. Then the nurse assesses for the degree of disability related to neurological functioning. A baseline neurologic assessment should include the client's level of consciousness and pupillary function. In the exposure step, the nurse removes the client's clothes and examines all body surfaces for obvious injuries. The nurse also obtains a brief history, client allergies, and past medical history.

A Foley catheter is inserted to monitor urinary output. If there is a risk for aspiration, a nasogastric tube is placed. The client is attached to a cardiac monitor. At least two lines are used to give IV fluids, blood components, inotropic drugs, and vasopressors as needed, to treat hypovolemic shock. The emergency nurse monitors the client closely for shivering or chills. Warm blankets and warmed IV solutions are used to prevent hypothermia. If the client has penetrating wounds, a tetanus prophylaxis such as tetanus toxoid or human toxin–antitoxin may be given.

DIAGNOSING, PLANNING, AND IMPLEMENTING

The post-trauma client has many nursing care problems. Two of the most common are: actual or potential problems with infection, and mobility.

RISK FOR INFECTION

Traumatic injuries often occur in a dirty environment. Projectiles entering the body carry dirt and debris into the wound. Open fractures provide an entry point for bacteria and dirt. Even after surgery, wounds can remain contaminated.

■ Use strict aseptic technique when inserting catheters, suctioning, or changing dressings. *Trauma clients are at a greater risk for infection.*

■ Monitor wounds for odor, redness, heat, swelling, purulent drainage, increased pain under casts, and increased drainage over the wound area. Be sure dressings do not restrict circulation. Avoid tape; instead, use mesh or stretch gauze to hold dressings in place. Prevent cross-contamination between wounds. *Because the skin is the first line of defense against infection, the nurse must monitor for signs of infection and prevent any new breaks in the skin.*

- Take vital signs and temperature every 2 to 4 hours. *An elevated body temperature and pulse are indicators of an infection.*
- Provide adequate fluids and nutrition. *Adequate fluids, calories, and protein are essential to wound healing.*
- Monitor for manifestations of sepsis. *Clients with traumatic injuries are at a high risk for developing sepsis.*

IMPAIRED PHYSICAL MOBILITY

- Provide active or passive exercises to affected and unaffected extremities at least once every 8 hours. Do not perform exercises if active bleeding or edema is present. *Exercise improves muscle tone, maintains joint mobility, improves circulation, and prevents contractures. Immobility due to trauma increases the risk for complications of the skin, cardiovascular, gastrointestinal, respiratory, musculoskeletal, and renal systems.*
- Assist the client to turn, cough, and deep breathe at least every 2 hours. *Changing positions, coughing, and deep breathing reduce the risk of skin and respiratory complications.*
- When the client cannot be moved and positioned easily, consult with the physician for using a specialty bed like the kinetic continuous rotation bed (Figure 10-9 ◆). *Continuous motion helps prevent pneumonia, venous stasis, urinary stasis, and bone loss.*
- Monitor the lower extremities every 8 hours for deep vein thrombosis (DVT): heat, swelling, and pain. Measure the circumference of the thigh and calf each day. Remove antiemboli stockings for one hour during each shift and assess the skin for changes. *When injury occurs to the vein and blood flow becomes sluggish, a thrombus (clot) forms. DVT is a major risk for pulmonary embolism.*

EVALUATING

Evaluate the effectiveness of nursing care by collecting data related to the absence of infection and complications from immobility. As the client recovers, evaluate the client's progress toward maximum wellness.

Discharge Considerations

The nurse's main responsibility is to prepare the client and family for discharge and promote maximum wellness. Before discharge, determine potential home modifications. (For example, if the client's bedroom is on an upper floor, first floor sleeping arrangements may be necessary until healing has occurred.) Review when and how to take the medications and their potential side effects. Provide information as needed about special diets. Discuss the client's rehabilitation plan and identify transportation concerns. Emphasize the need for follow-up appointments with the physician. Discuss with the family emotional changes that the client may experience

Figure 10-9. ◆ A kinetic continuous rotation bed reduces complications of immobility for a client with multiple injuries.

(e.g., insomnia, nightmares, and reliving the incident). If the family has lost a loved one, provide a referral for grief counseling.

PREVENTIVE HEALTH TEACHING

Injury is a major health problem in the United States. The nurse is in a unique position to provide preventive education, after assessing for individual risk factors (weakness, poor vision, and risky behaviors). Safety education should be taught in emergency departments, doctors' offices, clinics, schools, and health fairs. Because many injuries occur at home, individuals should also know how to make their homes safer. Box 10-12 lists common safety tips.

Nursing Process Case Study
■ CLIENT WITH MULTIPLE INJURIES

Jane Souza, a 25-year-old married woman with two children, is involved in a head-on collision. Ms. Souza, who is not wearing a seat belt, is thrown forward against the steering wheel.

Her lower legs are trapped under the dashboard. Ms. Souza is transported to the local trauma center. She is conscious, is receiving high-flow oxygen by mask, and has one intravenous line in place.

Assessment   Airway is patent, with high-flow oxygen in place. Breathing rate is 36; breath sounds on the right side are decreased (multiple bruises and abrasions on right side of chest); she complains of difficulty breathing. Circulation indi-

cates palpable systolic blood pressure of 80, pulse rate of 120, and palpable pedal pulses. No active external bleeding noted. Skin is pale, cool to the touch, and diaphoretic. Pupils are equal and react to light. Ms. Souza has limited extremity movement because of a broken right arm and an open fracture of the left ankle.

Because of Ms. Souza's respiratory distress, she is intubated and connected to a ventilator with 100% oxygen. Another intravenous line is inserted and O-negative blood is given. Her blood pressure continues to decrease, and she is immediately taken to surgery.

Diagnosis   The emergency nursing staff make the following nursing diagnoses for Ms. Souza:

- Ineffective Breathing Pattern related to respiratory rate of 36, multiple bruises on the right side of her chest, decreased breath sounds on the right, and respiratory difficulty.
- Deficient Fluid Volume related to acute internal blood loss.

Expected Outcomes   The expected outcomes established in the plan of care specify that Ms. Souza will:

- Maintain adequate oxygenation
- Maintain adequate circulating blood volume

Planning and Implementation   The following nursing interventions are implemented for Ms. Souza by the emergency nurses:

- Monitor Ms. Souza's airway and assist the physician with the intubation.
- Explain all procedures to Ms. Souza.
- Monitor any changes in Ms. Souza's blood pressure and pulse.
- Prepare Ms. Souza for transfer to the operating room for emergency surgery.
- Keep Ms. Souza's family informed about her condition.

Evaluation   In the operating room, it is determined that Ms. Souza has a ruptured spleen and a serious pelvic fracture. Ms. Souza's treatment continues in the operating room.

 Critical Thinking in the Nursing Process

1. Explain why O-negative blood was used in the emergency department.
2. Why did the emergency nursing staff think Ms. Souza had internal bleeding?
3. Suggest two nursing interventions to assist Ms. Souza's family in coping with this traumatic event.

ENVIRONMENTAL INJURIES

A variety of medical emergencies can result from excessive exposure to heat or cold. This section presents prehospital and basic ED intervention for clients with environmental emergencies.

Hyperthermia (elevated core body temperature) occurs when the body is exposed to excessive heat. Normally, the body regulates its temperature through sweating and peripheral vasodilation. When the temperature and humidity exceed the body's regulatory mechanisms, heat exhaustion and heat stroke develop. *Heat exhaustion* results from increased sweating and electrolyte loss, which causes hypovolemia. It is characterized by profuse sweating, weakness, nausea, and cool skin. Individuals with heat exhaustion should be placed in a cool area and given oral fluids. Loosen clothing and apply cool, wet towels. Victims who are very young or elderly, or who do not improve within 30 minutes, should be taken to the nearest hospital.

Heat stroke involves a rapid rise in temperature, often above 106° F, because the body cannot cool itself. It is not common but is a medical emergency. Manifestations include altered mental status, loss of coordination, hypotension, tachycardia, and seizures. Heat stroke victims must be cooled immediately. This is done by removing the client's clothes and placing cold packs to the groin, axillae, and back of the neck. The client can be misted with cool water but never immersed in icy water (shivering produces more heat). As soon as possible, the client is transported to an emergency department. If the temperature has not dropped to 102° F, a cooling blanket is used. Shivering is treated with chlorpromazine (Thorazine). The client is monitored closely for seizures.

Hypothermia (core body temperature is below 95° F) results from exposure to cold temperatures. Infants are at higher risk because they have less body fat. Older adults also have an increased risk. Mild hypothermia is characterized by shivering and slowed mental functioning. As the victim's temperature drops, muscle coordination is lost and cardiorespiratory and neurological function slows; eventually death results.

In cases of mild hypothermia, move the client to a warm place, remove wet clothing, and cover with warm blankets. Clients with moderate to severe hypothermia should be transported immediately to a nearby hospital. On arrival in the ED, the client is warmed slowly with blankets, radiant heat lamps, or an external warming blanket. Warmed intravenous solutions may be given, along with warmed peritoneal lavage. Respiratory therapy includes warmed, humidified oxygen. The client is monitored closely for signs of cardiac arrest.

POISONINGS

A *poison* is any chemical substance that damages body structures. Poisons enter the body through ingestion, inhalation, and skin contamination. Common ingested poisons include corrosives such as lye, toilet bowl cleaners, and bleach; plants; and drugs like aspirin, antidepressants, and benzodiazepines. Most inhalation injuries occur in the home from carbon monoxide, natural gas, chlorine, and some pesticides. Skin contamination occurs from pesticides and industrial chemicals.

When poisoning is suspected, call the local poison control center immediately. They can provide guidelines for

---

BOX 10-13
TEACHING FOR DISCHARGE

GUIDELINES TO PREVENT POISONING

- Use dangerous chemicals only in well-ventilated areas.
- Wear protective clothing such as gloves and goggles.
- Do not mix common household cleaning products.
- Keep all products in their original containers with the label attached.
- Use poison symbols to identify dangerous substances.
- Keep all poisons and medicines locked away.
- Identify poisonous plants and keep them away from children.
- Never call medicine "candy."
- Use childproof safety caps.
- Always take medications in a well-lit room to prevent an error.
- Post the local Poison Control Center telephone number by the phone.

---

appropriate treatment. Some poisonings can be managed at home, but most require treatment in the ED. When the client arrives in the ED, the first priority is to assess the client's airway, breathing, and circulation, and then to identify the poison. The medical staff will recommend the appropriate antidote or an elimination method.

Ingested poisons may be treated by giving activated charcoal orally or through a gastric lavage; this binds to the poison for expulsion in the stool. Syrup of ipecac induces vomiting but its use has decreased over the past decade. It is contraindicated for corrosive poison, which must be diluted with milk or water. Other elimination methods include gastric lavage, cathartics, whole-bowel irrigation, and hemodialysis. Clients who have inhaled poisonous substances need supplemental oxygen. Contaminated skin must be drenched immediately with running water and all clothes must be removed. Anyone assisting the client should wear protective clothing to prevent secondary exposure.

Poisonings can be prevented. Box 10-13 summarizes prevention tips.

The Client Experiencing a Critical Illness

Clients with shock or traumatic injuries are best treated in a critical care unit or *intensive care unit (ICU)*. These highly specialized units are designed to provide care to clients in the critical phase of an illness. ICU nurses and physicians have advanced knowledge in the latest medical and technological methods. The critical care nurse constantly monitors the acutely ill client for life-threatening situations and initiates nursing actions as needed. Because of the critical condition of these clients, the ICU nurse may care for only one or two clients.

PSYCHOSOCIAL EFFECTS

The critical care environment is overwhelming to clients. They are under artificial lighting and are attached to strange machines that make sounds. The environment and the constant nursing care often lead to sensory overload and sleep deprivation. Unfamiliar voices and the lack of personal touch from family members result in sensory deprivation and increase the client's stress level.

The nurse can reduce sensory overload by monitoring noise levels and limiting conversation directly to the client. Adding a calendar and clock to the client's room, or playing a favorite radio station or tape, may reorient the client. The client's psychological well-being can be increased by encouraging the family to touch the client. Uninterrupted rest periods are beneficial, but rest must be balanced with the client's need for family and with the need for hourly monitoring.

ICU psychosis (acute confusion after 2 to 3 days in the ICU) develops rapidly and is generally reversible. Older adults are more prone to this condition. Common features include altered attention span, memory loss, confusion, and visual and auditory hallucinations. Sedatives or psychotropic drugs may be given, but often they can make the condition worse. ICU psychosis usually decreases once the client's sensory-perceptual problems and sleep deprivation are resolved, but it is distressing to the client and family.

Although a critical illness affects the client most, it also affects family roles and functions. The family fears death of a loved one. They are anxious about all of the equipment surrounding the client and the potential for pain. They worry about finances and permanent changes in family roles. The nurse can assist the family by giving them a short status report every time they visit. If possible, involve the family in the client's daily care. Each family member should be assessed for signs of exhaustion. When necessary, the nurse should consult a social worker and chaplain to help obtain resources for the family. When the family's needs can be met, they are able to provide greater support to the client.

ORGAN DONATION

Under the Uniform Anatomical Gift Act, consent for organ donation may be given not only by the donor but also by a spouse, adult child, parent, adult sibling, or guardian. Most states require health care providers to ask family members about organ donation. Nurses should know their hospital's organ and tissue donation policies. The following organs and tissues can be donated: kidneys, heart, lungs, pancreas, intestines, liver, cornea, bones, bone marrow, and skin.

BOX 10-14 BRAIN DEATH CRITERIA

- Cause of coma accounts for loss of brain function
- Irreversible condition
- Unresponsive coma (absence of motor and reflex movements)
- No spontaneous respirations; $PaCO_2$ greater than 60 mm Hg
- Absent brain stem functions (no pupillary, corneal, and gag reflexes)
- Isoelectric (flat) electroencephalogram (EEG)
- Persistence of these signs for 30 minutes to 1 hour

Before donation is considered, the family is notified of the client's grave prognosis. They should be given the option of donating the client's organs but should realize that organ donation is an option, not an obligation. The family should be encouraged to ask questions and express their feelings in making this difficult decision. A grief counselor or clergy can provide emotional support to the family. Even if the client carries an organ donor card, many institutions will not remove any organs without a signature from a family member or other authorized person.

Before organs can be removed, the client must be declared brain dead. **Brain death criteria** are clinical signs used to determine whether a comatose client is brain dead (Box 10-14). Once brain death has been confirmed, the family must also agree with the diagnosis and be allowed time to prepare for the client's death as well as they can.

When the decision has been made to proceed with organ donation, the Organ Procurement Organization is notified (1-800-24-DONOR). Nurses should know the agency in their region that is responsible for organ procurement.

Nursing Interventions Classification

Some of the following Nursing Interventions from the Nursing Interventions Classification Project (McCloskey & Bulechek, 2000) may also be useful in planning and implementing care for clients experiencing shock, trauma, or critical illness:

- Oxygen Therapy
- Vital Sign Monitoring
- Fluid/Electrolyte Management
- Pain Management
- Family Support

(*Note:* The bibliography listings for this and all chapters have been compiled at the back of the book.)

Chapter Review

 ## key terms by topics

Use the CD-ROM disk enclosed with your textbook to hear the pronunciation of key terms in the chapter.

Client in shock
shock, hypoxemia, renin–angiotensin system, multiple organ dysfunction syndrome (MODS)

Types of shock
hypovolemic shock, anaphylactic shock, relative hypovolemia, cardiogenic shock, stroke volume, septic shock, septicemia, neurogenic shock

Complications of shock
adult respiratory distress syndrome (ARDS), disseminated intravascular coagulation (DIC)

Collaborative care
pneumatic antishock garment, type and cross-match, autotransfusion, adrenergic drugs, vasopressor drugs, positive inotropic drugs

Client experiencing trauma
triage, heat stroke

Client experiencing a critical illness
ICU psychosis, brain death criteria

key points

- Shock is characterized by inadequate blood flow and oxygen to cells and tissues.
- Without immediate recognition and treatment, shock progresses through the compensated, progressive, irreversible stages and can result in death.
- Nursing management of hypovolemic shock includes providing oxygen therapy; intravenous fluids, blood or blood products, cardiac support, and client support.
- Trauma is the leading cause of death in young people. It can be prevented by following common safety guidelines such as wearing a seat belt or helmet when riding a bicycle.
- Clients experiencing a traumatic accident, are assessed in the emergency department for Airway, Breathing, Circulation, Disability, and Exposure.
- The critical care unit is overwhelming to clients and families. The nurse plays an important role in reducing the psychosocial effects while caring for the acutely ill client.

 ## Medialink

Additional interactive resources, including animations and video, for this chapter can be found on the companion website at http://www.prenhall.com/burke. Click on Chapter 10 and "Begin" to select the activities for this chapter.

For NCLEX review questions and an audio glossary, access the accompanying CD-ROM in this book.

for further study

For further information about regulatory systems and their effects on the kidneys, see also Chapters 5 and 21.

For further information about changes with respiratory acidosis, see Respiratory Acidosis section in Chapter 5.

For more information about how stress ulcers develop, see Ulcer section in Chapter 18.

For further information about fluid compartments, see Chapter 5.

For more information about cardiac disorders that can cause cardiogenic shock, see Chapter 22.

For more information about care of the client requiring ventilatory assistance, see Chapter 26.

For more information about the intra-aortic balloon pump (IABP) and the ventricular assist device (VAD), see Chapter 22.

For more information about management of clients with spinal cord injury, see Chapter 30.

Critical Thinking Care Map

Care for a Client at an Accident Scene
NCLEX-PN Focus Area: Physiological Integrity

Case Study: You are driving down a rural road and see a car swerve back and forth across the road. It hits a patch of ice and strikes a utility pole. There is no one else in sight and you stop. You find a young man alone in the car who says his name is Paul Thompson. He is not wearing a seat belt.

Nursing Diagnosis: Risk for Ineffective Tissue Perfusion

COLLECT DATA

Subjective

_____
_____
_____
_____
_____
_____

Objective

_____
_____
_____
_____
_____
_____

Would you report this data? Yes/No

If yes, to: _____

Data Collected
(use those that apply)

- Scalp is bleeding
- Allergic to penicillin
- Skin slightly pale and dry
- Is awake
- Complains of being thirsty
- Left leg is twisted at an odd angle
- Shallow, slow respirations
- Does not drink alcohol
- Rapid radial pulse rate
- Says his dad will be really mad that he wrecked the car
- Denies any difficulty breathing
- Complains of left leg pain
- Wears glasses

Nursing Care

_____
_____
_____
_____
_____
_____
_____
_____

How would you document this? _____
_____
_____

Nursing Interventions
(use those that apply)

- Splint Paul's left leg.
- Ask how the accident happened.
- Give him a few sips of water.
- Cover scalp wound with a clean cloth.
- Cover client with a blanket.
- Keep head and neck in neutral position.
- Assist him out of the car.
- Call for help.
- Lay him on the ground and elevate his feet and legs.
- Look for hazards in the area.

NCLEX-PN Exam Preparation

1. Your client has an order to receive 2 units of packed red blood cells (PRBCs) for postoperative induced anemia. During the transfusion of the first unit, your client tells you that he is having chills. Which of the following nursing interventions should be your first priority?
   a. Retake the client's vital signs.
   b. Notify your charge nurse.
   c. Slow the infusion rate of the blood.
   d. Stop the infusion.

2. A client was admitted to your medical floor during the early morning hours after sustaining numerous facial and chest lacerations as a result of a motor vehicle accident. One of her diagnoses is hypovolemia due to blood loss. At 10:00 A.M. you observe that the client's Foley catheter bag has approximately 75 cc of dark, tea-colored urine. Which of the following actions would be the most appropriate at this time?
   a. Ask the client if she feels unusually light-headed.
   b. Check the client's medical records for CBC results.
   c. Assess the client's pain level.
   d. Check the Foley catheter tubing for kinks.

3. Your client has been admitted to the intensive care unit following surgery for an abdominal aneurysm. Her vital signs are stable and her dressing is dry and intact. Your client is restless and repeatedly states that she might die. Which of the following nursing diagnoses would be the most appropriate to add to her care plan?
   a. Infection, Risk for
   b. Anxiety
   c. Deficient Knowledge
   d. Confusion, Acute

4. You are working in a community hospital ED and have been assigned to care for a 50-year-old man with a diagnosis of a first-degree burn to the left forearm. Your client is complaining that he has been waiting to be seen for 3 hours. Your best response would be:
   a. "I know, this place has a history of long waiting times."
   b. "There are other clients here that are a lot worse than you and they are not fussing."
   c. "I understand your concerns. I will check to see how much longer it will be."
   d. just ignore the client and he will stop complaining

5. A client broke her pelvis when she was thrown from the horse she was riding. Her son found her several hours after the accident had occurred. When she arrived at the ED she was confused and her skin was cold and clammy. No bowel sounds were present. Her apical pulse was 180 with thready and weak radial pulses. In which stage of shock might the client's condition be categorized?
   a. noncompensated
   b. compensated
   c. progressive
   d. irreversible

6. A 65-year-old man on your unit is diagnosed with advanced cirrhosis of the liver. Vital signs: P 130, R 32, BP 110/60, T 100.4° F. The physician states that the client is in shock. Which of the following would most accurately describe this type of shock?
   a. anaphylactic
   b. hypovolemic
   c. septic
   d. cardiogenic

7. Which of the following statements by a client being treated for a severe reaction to a bee sting indicates that additional teaching might be needed?
   a. "I'm going to order a Medic-Alert bracelet right away."
   b. "My pharmacist can tell me which anti–bee sting medication will be best for me."
   c. "I'll just stay away from bees and not worry about them."
   d. "I'm going to tell my family what to do if I get stung again."

8. When assessing a female client who has ARDS, which findings would indicate acute respiratory distress?
   a. blood hemoglobin within the normal range
   b. severely decreased arterial oxygen blood gas level
   c. decreased white blood cell count
   d. increased serum sodium

9. When managing cardiogenic shock and heart failure, the nurse expects to administer several medications including a diuretic such as Lasix. Which of the following conditions indicates that the diuretic is effective?
   a. The client's blood pressure increases.
   b. There is a significant increase in urine output.
   c. The client's level of consciousness improves dramatically.
   d. The client's irregular heartbeat has stabilized.

10. Your elderly client has recovered from a traumatic injury to the right hip from a fall in the bathroom at his apartment. He will be going home with a walker for ambulation. Which of the following should be your most important priority for assessment and discussion prior to the discharge?
    a. transportation to his home
    b. the client's ability to ambulate with his walker
    c. social services consult for Meals-on-Wheels
    d. home safety tips

Answers for Review Questions, as well as discussion of Case Study Critical Thinking questions, appear in Appendix V.

chapter **11**

Caring for the Client with Substance Abuse or Dependency

LEARNING outcomes

After completing this chapter, you will be able to:

- Define substance abuse, substance dependency, tolerance, and withdrawal.
- Identify commonly abused drugs.
- Be aware of potential adverse interactions between commonly abused substances and medications used in surgery or trauma care.
- Assess the client with substance abuse problems.
- Provide appropriate nursing interventions for a client in withdrawal.

MediaLink

  www.prenhall.com/burke

Use the above address to access the free, interactive Companion Website created for this textbook. Get hints, instant feedback, and textbook references to chapter-related multiple choice questions. Link to other interesting sites.

Problem of Substance Abuse

Throughout human history, people have used substances to alter their perceptions; elevate mood; relieve pain, fear, anxiety, or boredom; and to aid in religious ceremonies. Alcohol, the most commonly used psychoactive substance, can be used responsibly and enjoyably. Only when substance use interferes with an individual's ability to function at work or at home, when it causes legal problems, or when it puts the individual in danger is there a substance-related disorder.

Substance abuse is one of the most important health problems in the United States in the twenty-first century. As many as 20% of the adult population of the United States may meet the diagnostic criteria for an alcohol- or substance-related disorder (American Psychiatric Association [APA], 2000). Add to this number the family members, employers and co-workers, people injured or killed by substance abusers, and babies born to women who abuse alcohol and other substances, and you can see how many people are affected. The annual cost to society is in the hundreds of billions of dollars.

The exact number of people with substance abuse and dependency (also called *addiction*) is not known. The reason for this lack of information is that **denial** (refusal to acknowledge the existence of a real situation or feelings) is a common coping mechanism for people with these disorders and for health professionals who work with them.

People with substance-related disorders do not tend to seek treatment. Health professionals often do not ask the questions that could determine who is affected by substance use. Sometimes health professionals are not aware of how they can help. This chapter helps to identify clients with substance-related disorders and how nurses can intervene to help them.

The Diagnostic and Statistical Manual of Mental Disorders, 4th edition, Text Revision *(DSM-IV-TR)* (APA, 2000) is the standard for the diagnosis and terminology of mental disorders, including substance-related disorders. The definitions from the *DSM-IV-TR* are relevant to all substances of abuse and dependence.

TYPES OF SUBSTANCE ABUSE
Substance Abuse

The *DSM-IV-TR* defines **substance abuse** as a maladaptive pattern of substance use leading to significant impairment or distress manifested by one or more of the following:

1. Inability to fulfill major role obligations at work, school, and home (poor work performance, expulsions from school, neglect of children)
2. Recurrent substance use in physically hazardous situations (driving a car, operating a machine)
3. Recurrent legal or interpersonal problems
4. Continued use despite persistent social and interpersonal problems caused by use of the substance, such as fights or arguments with spouse about intoxication (APA, 2000)

Substance Dependency

Substance dependency is a maladaptive pattern of substance use leading to significant impairment or distress, manifested by three or more of the following:

1. Tolerance to the substance
2. Withdrawal syndrome
3. Substance either taken in higher amounts or for longer periods than intended
4. Unsuccessful or persistent desire to cut down or control use
5. A great deal of time spent in obtaining, using, and recovering from effects of the substance
6. Reduction of important social, occupational, or recreational activities due to substance use
7. Continued substance use despite knowledge of a persistent physical or psychological problem that is likely caused by the substance (APA, 2000)

Compulsive Substance Use

Compulsive substance use is repetitive substance use behavior for the purpose of reducing distress. Compulsive use is often unwanted and time consuming (APA, 2000).

Commonly Abused Substances

Substances that rapidly alter the mental state, by either stimulating or depressing the central nervous system (CNS), are the most commonly abused. The *DSM-IV-TR* lists 11 substances of abuse:

1. Alcohol
2. Opioids
3. Sedatives, hypnotics, and anxiolytics
4. Cocaine
5. Amphetamines and similar drugs
6. Hallucinogens
7. Phencyclidine (PCP) and similar drugs
8. Inhalants
9. Cannabis
10. Caffeine
11. Nicotine

(Tables 11-1 ◆ and 11-2 ◆ provide summaries of the effects of these substances.)

ALCOHOL

Ethyl alcohol (ethanol, beverage alcohol) is the most commonly abused substance. It is a CNS depressant that is quickly absorbed into the blood after drinking. Initial symptoms of alcohol **intoxication** (a reversible set of physical, psychological, and behavioral symptoms caused by use of the substance) are relaxation, loss of inhibition, **euphoria** (an exaggerated feeling of well-being), and decreased mental concentration. With increased use, symptoms progress to slurred speech, **ataxia** (staggering gait), **labile** (changeable) mood, aggressive behavior, incoherent speech, vomiting, coma, respiratory

TABLE 11-1

COMPARISON OF COMMONLY ABUSED CNS DEPRESSANTS AND STIMULANTS

DRUG	EFFECTS OF USE	OVERDOSE SYMPTOMS	WITHDRAWAL SYMPTOMS AND THEIR ONSET (AFTER LAST DOSE)

CNS DEPRESSANTS
Alcohol, Beer,
    Wine, Liquor
	Euphoria, loss of
	    inhibition, ataxia, lack
	    of coordination,
	    reduced cognition,
	    impaired judgment,
	    nausea
		Respiratory depression,
		    mental confusion,
		    unconsciousness,
		    death
			6-8 hours
			CNS irritability, anxiety,
			    increased vital signs (T, P, R,
			    BP), tremors, ataxia,
			    diaphoresis, slurred speech,
			    GI disturbance, disorientation,
			    hallucinations, seizures death

Opioids
    (narcotics)
Morphine,
    Methadone,
    Hydromorphone,
    Heroin
	Analgesia, cough
	    suppression,
	    constipation,
	    constricted pupils,
	    same as alcohol
		Same as alcohol	12–72 hours
			Watering eyes
			Same as alcohol, less likely to
			    cause death

Sedatives,
    Hypnotics,
Anxiolytics
Barbiturates,
    Benzodiazepines
	Sedation, same as alcohol
	Anxiolytics cause less
	    sedationin low doses
		Same as alcohol	Onset depends on type of
			    sedative (short or long acting)
			Same as alcohol

CNS STIMULANTS
Cocaine
	Sudden rush of euphoria,
	    elation, energy,
	    talkativeness, anorexia,
	    weight loss, elevated
	    vital signs, grandiosity
		Chest pain, slurred speech,
		    mental confusion,
		    vomiting, hallucinations,
		    myocardial infarction,
		    severe elevation of BP and
		    P, shock, death
			Acute depression, craving drug,
			    fatigue, irritability, suicidal
			    thoughts, loss of pleasure
			    (anhedonia), not life
			    threatening

Amphetamines	Same as cocaine	Same as cocaine	As with cocaine, withdrawal
			    severity depends on
			    amount of drug use

depression, and death. See Box 11-1 for blood alcohol concentrations.

Tolerance and Withdrawal

With continued use, the user develops tolerance. **Tolerance** is defined by either of the following:

1. A need for increased amounts of the substance to achieve the same effect
2. Diminished effect with continued use of the same amount of the substance (APA, 2000)

If an individual drinks large amounts of alcohol regularly, the CNS experiences depression. Through an effective mechanism for maintaining homeostasis for survival, the CNS increases its own stimulation. The client experiences increased blood pressure, pulse, respiratory rate, temperature, and psychomotor stimulation. The individual then requires more alcohol to achieve intoxication of the stimulated CNS. The process of increasing tolerance develops over years of alcohol

dependency, until the individual must drink almost constantly to avoid the distressing symptoms of CNS stimulation.

Withdrawal occurs when a person discontinues or reduces heavy and prolonged use of a substance. Withdrawal may include the following events:

1. A substance-specific withdrawal syndrome develops (see Table 11-1).
2. The same or related substance is taken to relieve or avoid withdrawal symptoms.
3. Significant distress or impairment in social or occupational functioning occurs (APA, 2000).

When the alcohol-dependent individual stops drinking, the CNS is still stimulated. The homeostatic mechanism that balanced the depressant effects of the alcohol takes time to return to normal, and the individual suffers withdrawal symptoms. The alcohol withdrawal syndrome includes elevated vital signs, anxiety, tremors, diaphoresis, slurred speech, GI disturbances (vomiting, cramping, diarrhea), ataxia, nystag-

TABLE 11-2 EFFECTS, OVERDOSE SYMPTOMS, AND WITHDRAWAL SYMPTOMS OF HALLUCINOGENS, INHALANTS, CANNABIS, CAFFEINE, AND NICOTINE

SUBSTANCE	EFFECTS OF USE	OVERDOSE SYMPTOMS	WITHDRAWAL SYMPTOMS
HALLUCINOGENS LSD, Mescaline, MDMA (Ecstasy)	Hallucinations and distorted perceptions, distortions of time and space, illusions, emotional lability, tremor, nausea and vomiting	Panic (may be drug reaction, not OD), seizures (rare)	No withdrawal, may experience flashbacks for several months after last dose
Phencyclidine (PCP)	Bizarre perceptions, disorientation, hallucinations, agitation, grandiosity, withdrawn or agitated or both, paranoid, dilated pupils, dry red skin	Seizures, coma, death	No withdrawal
INHALANTS AND CANNABIS *Inhalants* Hydrocarbons: Glue, gasoline, aerosol spray, solvents	Euphoria, impaired judgment, nystagmus, ataxia, slurred speech, perceptual changes, sense of invulnerability	Stupor, coma, cardiac depression & dysrhythmia, respiratory arrest, renal complications	Similar to alcohol
Nitrites: Amyl nitrite, nitrous oxide	Postpone or enhance intercourse	Panic, hypotension Both: Brain damage	
Cannabis Marijuana Hashish	Mild euphoria, pleasure, confidence, grandiosity, relaxation, red eyes, dry mouth, increased appetite	None	No physical withdrawal May have craving
CAFFEINE AND NICOTINE Caffeine	Increased alertness	None	Headache, fatigue
Nicotine	Pleasure, alertness, increased BP, P, decreased blood flow to heart muscle	None	Anxiety, depressed mood, anger, craving, increased appetite

mus, disorientation, and, at its most severe, hallucinations, seizures, and death.

Alcohol withdrawal delirium (delirium tremens or DTs) is diagnosed when withdrawal is associated with severe cognitive symptoms such as confusion, delusions, and terrifying hallucinations. This delirium happens to people with a long (5- to 15-year) history of alcoholism. It is a medical emergency.

Note that the symptoms of alcohol withdrawal are generally the opposite of those of alcohol intoxication. The individual takes the CNS depressant substance; the CNS stimulates itself to maintain homeostasis. When the substance is withdrawn, the CNS is still stimulated, and the individual has CNS stimulation symptoms until the CNS eventually regains homeostasis without alcohol, and the symptoms subside. Alcohol withdrawal syndrome usually lasts about 4 days (see Table 11-1).

The alcohol-dependent individual (alcoholic) may experience many episodes of withdrawal symptoms that he or she treats with alcohol. The statement, "I feel bad (nervous, tired, angry, lonely, etc.); I need a drink," may be evidence of withdrawal symptoms. Nurses should be aware that substance withdrawal symptoms are often behind a patient's desire to leave the hospital against medical advice.

Pattern of Use

The pattern of use of alcohol varies from one individual to another. Some people start drinking alcohol in childhood or adolescence, some in old age. Some drink daily, starting with "one or two drinks with dinner" and progressing to greater amounts and frequency. Some drink heavily on weekends or may abstain for long periods and then have a drinking binge.

Jellinek described four phases of drinking behavior in alcoholics (1960). Models of disease processes cannot predict

---

BOX 11-1
MANIFESTATIONS OF ALCOHOL INTOXICATION BY BLOOD ALCOHOL CONCENTRATION

Blood Alcohol Concentration	Manifestations
0.05–0.10 (0.08–0.10 is legal level of intoxication in most states)	Relaxation, euphoria, decreased inhibitions, impaired judgment, changeable mood, decreased mental concentration, decreased fine motor coordination
0.15–0.25 g/dL	Slurred speech, decreased motor function, ataxia, mood outbursts, aggressive behavior
0.3 g/dL	Incoherent speech, mental confusion, stupor, vomiting, labored breathing
0.4 g/dL	Unconsciousness, coma
0.5 g/dL	Respiratory depression, death

the behavior of individuals, but this one gives an interesting perspective on substance abuse and dependency as a progressive disease. The following are Jellinek's phases.

THE PREALCOHOLIC PHASE. Drinking alcohol begins with a social motivation. Alcohol is used to relieve the everyday stress of life. People deny that alcohol is a problem, despite evidence otherwise, and despite tolerance.

THE EARLY ALCOHOLIC PHASE. This phase begins with memory blackouts. The alcohol is no longer a source of pleasure or relief, but a drug that is required by the individual. Commonly people in this phase begin to drink alone, or drink secretly. They experience withdrawal symptoms. They wake up in the morning and need a drink to control tremors (an "eye-opener"). Denial is still the defense mechanism.

THE CRUCIAL PHASE: THE TRUE ALCOHOLIC. In this phase, the individual completely loses control over the ability to choose whether or not to drink. Experiences include isolation from others, anger, aggression, loss of interest in any activity that previously brought pleasure, and malnutrition. The individual is willing to give up everything to maintain the addiction. It is common for people in this phase to have lost their jobs, families, friends, and self-respect.

THE CHRONIC PHASE. This phase is characterized by emotional and physical disintegration. The individual may experience psychosis and impairment in reality testing. Every body system is affected by life-threatening complications. Abstention from alcohol results in the torture of full-blown, life-threatening withdrawal. Thoughts of suicide are common.

Long-Term Physical Effects

Chronic use of alcohol takes a toll on the body. All body systems are affected over a period of years. The gastrointestinal (GI) system is one of the first to show the effects of chronic alcoholism. Alcohol causes *gastritis* by inflaming the stomach lining. The protective mucous lining of the stomach is damaged by alcohol, allowing hydrochloric acid to erode the stomach wall. If the vascular structure in the stomach wall is involved, bleeding can occur. Ulcers may form in the stomach. Symptoms include gastric distress, nausea, vomiting, black stools, and abdominal distention. *Esophagitis,* inflammation of the esophagus, is caused by the irritant effect of alcohol on the esophagus and by frequent vomiting. The primary symptom is esophageal pain.

Pancreatitis, either acute or chronic, may also be caused by chronic alcohol use. Chronic pancreatitis leads to pancreatic insufficiency, which causes malnutrition, weight loss, and diabetes mellitus. Acute pancreatitis happens one or two days after a binge of drinking alcohol. The symptoms include severe, constant epigastric pain, nausea, vomiting, and abdominal distention.

Alcoholic hepatitis affects an already damaged liver, usually after a prolonged binge of excessive alcohol consumption. The patient has right upper quadrant abdominal pain, jaundice, an enlarged liver and spleen, vomiting, weakness, profound fatigue, and possibly ascites. *Cirrhosis* of the liver is the worst alcohol-related liver disorder. It is the end stage of chronic alcoholic liver disease. Liver cells are severely damaged and destroyed. They are replaced by scar tissue, which makes this disease irreversible. Cirrhosis causes portal hypertension, ascites, *esophageal varices* (varicose veins in the esophagus that can rupture and hemorrhage), and hepatic encephalopathy. *Hepatic encephalopathy* is caused by accumulation of ammonia (due to the damaged liver's inability to metabolize protein). It results in impaired mental function and progresses to death.

The cardiovascular system is also affected by chronic alcohol use. *Cardiomyopathy* (muscle abnormality and weakening causing enlargement of the heart), heart failure, and cardiac dysrhythmias may occur. The risk of *hemorrhagic stroke* is increased. Other cardiovascular manifestations include *hypertension* (especially diastolic elevation), *tachycardia,* and *edema.*

Chronic use of alcohol produces changes in the neurologic system as well. *Blackouts* are an early sign of alcoholism. The affected individual remains conscious and appears to be functioning normally, but is completely unable to remember anything that occurs while intoxicated. After many years of alcohol abuse, a person may develop Korsakoff's syndrome and Wernicke's syndrome, which affect the entire neurologic system. These syndromes usually occur together, and are often called *Wernicke–Korsakoff's syndrome.*

Korsakoff's syndrome is a group of symptoms caused by a deficiency in the B vitamins, including thiamine, riboflavin, and folic acid. Amnesia, disorientation to time and place, confabulation (falsification of memory to fill in the gaps), and severe peripheral neuropathy characterize it. Symptoms of the neuropathy include tingling; muscle weakness; sore, burning muscles; abnormal sensation; and pain with movement. The extremities are affected, especially the legs. Because of their extreme pain, care must be taken when moving these patients.

Wernicke's syndrome (alcoholic encephalopathy) is characterized by ataxia, paralysis of eye muscles, nystagmus, and mental confusion. It is the result of severe vitamin B_1 deficiency from lack of adequate nutritional intake. Early in the disorder, it may respond well to large doses of parenteral thiamine. If not treated early, it progresses to an irreversible, fatal condition that requires custodial care.

The reproductive system is affected as well. Men may become *impotent.* Women may stop menstruating and become infertile. Further, the unborn child of a pregnant woman may be seriously affected. Box 11-2 describes effects of fetal alcohol syndrome.

When the musculoskeletal system is affected, *osteoporosis* can develop. Also, acute or chronic **myopathy** may occur, characterized by muscle cramps of sudden onset and later development of pain, tenderness, and edema of the skeletal muscles, especially of the legs. In chronic myopathy, there is wasting and weakness of the skeletal muscles.

OTHER CNS DEPRESSANTS

Other depressants of the central nervous system are similar to alcohol in their effects on the CNS, intoxication symptoms, tolerance effects, and withdrawal symptoms (see Table 11-1).

The Opiates

Opiates are naturally occurring substances derived from opium (e.g., morphine), semisynthetics (e.g., heroin), and drugs that resemble them (e.g., methadone, meperidine, or codeine). Opiates are narcotic drugs prescribed to relieve pain or diarrhea, or to reduce cough. These drugs have alleviated immeasurable human pain, but when abused they have caused immense suffering as well.

Opiate drugs (see Table 11-1) can cause physical dependence (tolerance and withdrawal). Intoxication symptoms are similar to those of alcohol. Common symptoms include drowsiness, analgesia, euphoria, mood changes, nausea, and pupillary constriction.

The opiate drugs decrease GI peristalsis, so they can be used therapeutically to treat severe diarrhea. When opiates are abused, *constipation* can be severe, including fecal impaction. The *nausea and vomiting* that are commonly caused by opiates are due to stimulation of the medulla of the brain.

In therapeutic doses, opiates have little effect on the heart. Morphine is often used to treat cardiac patients for pain or to divert blood flow to the peripheral circulation, decreasing the work of the heart. In high doses, they cause *hypotension* by affecting the heart or reducing vascular resistance.

Opioids also affect *sexual functioning.* People who use opioids regularly in high doses have decreased libido and may have lack of orgasm. Men can have ejaculation abnormalities and impotence. Women often have menstrual irregularities and infertility.

Nurses especially need to know about the respiratory effects of opioids. These drugs, which are used therapeutically to suppress cough, depress the respiratory center in the medulla of the brain. *Respiratory depression* is not likely to happen in therapeutic doses unless the patient is *narcotic naïve* (has not been exposed to opiates recently). With high doses, though, respiratory depression may be life threatening. Chronic respiratory depression predisposes the patient to pneumonia and other respiratory infections.

Opiate overdose is a medical emergency. Symptoms can include pinpoint pupils, depressed (slow, shallow) respiration, seizures, and coma. Death can result from respiratory arrest and hypoxia. The treatment for opiate overdose is to administer a narcotic antagonist drug, such as naloxone hydrochloride (Narcan). This drug competes for opiate receptors and blocks or reverses the action of narcotic analgesics (opiates).

BOX 11-2
MANIFESTATIONS OF FETAL ALCOHOL SYNDROME

- Low birth weight
- Microcephaly (small head circumference, small brain)
- Facial anomalies
  - Flat midface
  - Flat nasal bridge
  - Small eyes
  - Short palpebral fissures (narrow eye openings)
  - Short nose
  - Flat philtrum (indistinct infranasal depression)
  - Thin upper lip
- Neurodevelopmental disorders
  - Developmental delay
  - Learning disabilities
  - Poor coordination
  - Distractibility/impulsivity

CLINICAL alert

The nurse must be aware that naloxone has a shorter duration of action than narcotics. Additional doses may need to be given if the initial dose of naloxone is no longer effective and the client still has active narcotics in the blood.

PATTERNS OF USE. While alcohol is legal and readily available, the opiates are either available only by prescription (narcotic analgesics) or are illegal under all circumstances (heroin). Opiate dependence is typically associated with a history of crimes committed to obtain drugs or the money to buy them. Health care professionals who are opiate dependent may steal medications from patients or their employers, write prescriptions for themselves, or manipulate physicians to write prescriptions for them.

Opioid dependence may begin at any age, but problems are most commonly observed in the late teens or early 20s (APA, 2000). Dependence develops over a period of many years, with periods of **abstinence** (complete lack of drug use). **Relapse** (returning to drug use after abstinence) is very common. Men are more commonly affected than women. Opiate-dependent individuals also experience other risks, such as developing hepatitis B or C, HIV infection, or other blood-borne diseases from needle use. Mortality in opiate-dependent people may be 2% per year. Death often results from overdose, accidents, or injuries (APA, 2000).

Sedatives, Hypnotics, and Anxiolytics

Sedatives, hypnotics, and anxiolytics include the benzodiazepines, the barbiturates, and similar drugs. Prescription sleeping medications and almost all of the anxiolytic (antianxiety) drugs are included. Like alcohol and the opiates, these substances depress the CNS.

OVERDOSE. It is important for nurses to know that CNS depressant drugs have additive effects when taken together. For example, when people use alcohol and a sedative drug at the same time, the CNS depressant effect is beyond what either substance would cause alone. Although the amount of sedative may be usual and the amount of alcohol may be what the person usually drinks, the two together could cause fatal respiratory depression. It is not uncommon for people to die as a result of this additive effect.

CLINICAL alert

Nurses who work in emergency or trauma care must assess every client for substance use to prevent additive CNS depression. A client may be treated with prescribed narcotics, sedatives, or anesthetics while still under the influence of alcohol or other CNS depressant drugs.

Prescribed Demerol for pain + heroin or alcohol = respiratory depression.

It is also common for the substance-dependent individual to have a drug of choice, but to use a variety of other substances, including alcohol. This combination of abused substances is called **polysubstance abuse** (see Table 11-1). Benzodiazepines alone in overdose are rarely fatal, but barbiturates in overdose are often fatal, due to cardiac or respiratory arrest.

A relatively new, quick-acting sedative drug is flunitrazepam (Rohypnol). It is called the "date rape drug," because it can rapidly incapacitate a rape victim. One or two tablets dissolved in alcohol can render a person unconscious within minutes. The affected individual then has amnesia for several hours.

CNS STIMULANTS
Cocaine and Amphetamines

The clinical usefulness of this group of drugs is limited to the treatment of attention deficit–hyperactivity disorder. Cocaine especially is a popular drug of abuse because of the immediate euphoria it induces. Intoxication with stimulants includes euphoria, hyperactivity, talkativeness, grandiosity, hyperactivity, anger, aggression, impaired judgment, and possibly hallucinations. Physical effects include elevated blood pressure, nausea, chest pain, dilated pupils, confusion, and cardiac dysrhythmias.

WITHDRAWAL. Just as the brain creates homeostasis by elevating its stimulation in response to regular use of depressants, it can also depress its function to balance regular use of a stimulant. When the stimulant-dependent individual abstains suddenly from stimulants, the withdrawal syndrome includes CNS depression. The individual feels lethargic and depressed (see Table 11-1). Withdrawal from stimulants is uncomfortable but not life threatening. The affected individual may experience depressive symptoms for several days.

Hallucinogens

Hallucinogens distort the user's perception of reality. The most common hallucinogens are lysergic acid diethylamine (LSD), mescaline, and phencyclidine (PCP). The CNS effects are unpredictable and may be influenced by the expectations of the user. (Table 11-2 summarizes effects of use, symptoms of overdose, and manifestations of withdrawal.) Some individuals have frightening psychotic experiences. Hallucinations can lead to violent behavior.

There is no withdrawal syndrome associated with hallucinogens. However, flashbacks can occur for months after the last dose is used. In the flashback experience, the individual has similar symptoms to those associated with use of the drug.

Synthetic or "designer" drugs are becoming increasingly popular. MDMA or Ecstasy is derived from amphetamine and methamphetamine, so it acts as both a stimulant and a hallucinogen.

Inhalants

A variety of volatile substances have become popular inhalants since "glue sniffing" in the 1950s. (Table 11-2 summarizes effects of use of inhalants, the symptoms of overdose, and manifestations of withdrawal.) Methods of use include directly spraying the substance into the mouth and inhaling, bagging (pouring substance into a plastic bag and inhaling), and huffing (soaking a cloth with the substance, putting cloth in mouth and inhaling). The user of inhalants may be identified by the strong odors of the inhaled substances or the presence of the substance (such as spray paint) on the face and hair (Sullivan, 1995).

Because inhalants are readily available legally, they are often the drug of choice for younger users (10 to 15 years old). They act on the CNS, causing intoxication and euphoria at lower doses. Death may result from toxicity, aspiration of gastric contents, suffocation, or erratic/risk-taking behavior.

Cannabis

Delta-9-tetrahydrocannabinol (THC) is thought to be the chemical responsible for the psychoactive effects of marijuana and hashish. Cannabis effects include euphoria, a sense of serenity, and perceptual changes in vision, hearing, taste, touch, or smell. (See Table 11-2 for a summary of effects of use, symptoms of overdose, and manifestations of withdrawal.)

Cannabis is the most widely used illegal substance in the United States. It has been therapeutically used to treat the anorexia, nausea, and vomiting associated with AIDS and cancer. Some people have proposed that it be approved for use as a treatment for glaucoma, because it lowers intraocular pressure. This approval is very unlikely because other effective drugs to treat glaucoma are available. The constant cannabis intoxication that would be required for treatment is not necessary.

Caffeine and Nicotine

It may be surprising to find caffeine and nicotine on the list of substances of abuse. Still, these substances fit the model of dependence defined in the *DSM-IV-TR*. Both substances cause tolerance and withdrawal (see Table 11-2).

Caffeine is the most commonly used stimulant drug. The physiologic effects of caffeine explain why it is so popular as a performance enhancer. It prolongs the time the user can continue to work, improves mental alertness, and elevates mood. However, it also increases anxiety and can cause insomnia, irritability, diuresis, and tachycardia. Effects and the development of tolerance are dependent on the amount used. Withdrawal symptoms include headache, fatigue, irritability, and nervousness.

Nicotine dependence is the most common substance dependence in the United States (American Society of Addiction Medicine, 1997). Smoking is especially common in the population of people who use alcohol and other substances. Symptoms of use include increased performance, decreased appetite, reduced anxiety, and increased alertness initially, followed by relaxation.

The consequences of nicotine use are also due to other substances present in tobacco. The incidence of cancer of the lungs, oral cavity, esophagus, pancreas, and prostate is increased significantly in tobacco users. The risk of cardiovascular disease, including stroke, myocardial infarction, and peripheral arterial disease, is increased by tobacco use as well. Accidents related to fire are also a concern (smoking in bed while drinking alcohol can be deadly). Withdrawal symptoms include irritability, restlessness, drowsiness, anxiety, craving, and a transient increase in appetite.

One implication for nurses is that hospitalized clients are likely to experience caffeine or nicotine withdrawal. The headache clients have after surgery may be better treated with a cup of coffee than medication. Some clients may consider checking themselves out of the hospital against medical advice so they can smoke cigarettes. These situations require the nurse's problem-solving skills.

Another implication of the likelihood of caffeine and nicotine withdrawal is that nurses should teach the consequences of substance use to all clients. Nurses need to realize that physiologic dependence on nicotine is a major factor in the difficulty people have when they try to quit smoking. The following five "Rs" (Gordon, Williams, & Lapin, 2001) may be of use with smokers who are currently unwilling to quit:

- Provide motivational information that is personally **relevant** to the client.
- Discuss the **risks** associated with smoking and the **rewards** of quitting, such as improvements in functioning and self-efficacy.
- Ask the client about **roadblocks** or barriers to quitting.
- **Repeat** motivational strategies at every clinic visit because most smokers need to make repeated quit attempts to be successful.

COLLABORATIVE CARE

Medical treatment of the client in the acute phase of alcohol withdrawal focuses on physiologic safety issues: symptom management, seizure prevention, stabilizing vital signs, and minimizing the effects of CNS stimulation. Management of the client in the rehabilitation phase is supportive. Physicians take a cooperative role with nurses, therapists, social workers, and others on the health care team.

Pharmacology

Medical management includes prescription of medications and therefore must include consideration of drug interactions and cross-tolerance. Clients who use drugs or alcohol regularly are at risk for withdrawal, and those who have used drugs or alcohol recently are at risk for additive effects with prescribed drugs.

Nurses and physicians in emergency departments need to know that any client who is under the influence of drugs or alcohol on arrival is at risk for an overdose of CNS depressants. Clients who are taking narcotics (morphine, Demerol, codeine, methadone, Dilaudid, other prescribed narcotic analgesics), other CNS depressants (alcohol, barbiturates, sedatives, prescription sleep aids), or illegal drugs that depress the CNS (heroin, "downers") are at high risk of additive CNS depression. Commonly prescribed medications that cause additive CNS depression are the narcotic analgesics, sedatives, benzodiazepines, sleep agents, and anesthetic agents.

A person who is dependent on heroin or alcohol will be tolerant not only to these, but to other CNS depressants as well. This phenomenon is called **cross-tolerance.** Cross-tolerance is important to the anesthesiologist, who may find that the client needs more than the usual anesthetic to put him or her to sleep. It is also important to physicians and nurses, because the client may need a higher-than-usual analgesic dose to relieve pain.

Treatment Phases

There are several theories about chemical dependency and its causes. Current treatment methods are based on the concept that substance dependency is a chronic, progressive medical illness that is characterized by remissions and relapses, and that is eventually fatal if untreated. The etiology of substance abuse is a combination of genetic factors and cultural influences (nature and nurture). People who are dependent on substances have learned to use them to cope with their problems. These clients must have new skills to replace the functions substances play in their lives. A promise of abstinence alone is not a long-term solution. The ultimate goals of substance dependency treatment are: (a) abstinence from substance use and (b) development of effective coping mechanisms to replace the need for substances as solutions to problems.

ACUTE PHASE. Substance dependency treatment has two major phases: acute and rehabilitation. In the *acute phase,* the person may be in a hospital or another inpatient or outpatient setting. The client often enters treatment while intoxicated. **Detoxification,** or removal of the substance from the body, begins the acute phase. The withdrawal syndrome also occurs acutely. Medical and nursing support are often needed during withdrawal.

Medications are used in the acute phase of treatment to provide safe withdrawal. For clients whose primary substance of abuse is alcohol, vitamin B_1 is given to prevent Wernicke–Korsakoff's syndrome.

Alcohol withdrawal is usually managed with a benzodiazepine anxiolytic agent, which is given in a decreasing dose over several days to treat and prevent withdrawal. Some health care workers have the attitude that if clients are allowed to suffer agonizing withdrawal, they will "learn a lesson" about why they should stop using drugs. On the contrary, withdrawal causes preoccupation and craving for the substance. There is no ethical justification for allowing clients to suffer needlessly. Alcohol and barbiturate withdrawals can be life threatening.

REHABILITATION PHASE. The second phase of substance dependency treatment is **rehabilitation.** This phase continues indefinitely. When clients have detoxified and are abstaining from substance use, rehabilitation begins.

Medications used in the rehabilitation phase of treatment are for the purpose of preventing relapse. Disulfiram (Antabuse) may be prescribed to deter clients from drinking alcohol. It causes a severe, uncomfortable reaction when the client drinks (flushing, throbbing headache, nausea, and vomiting).

Methadone, a synthetic opiate, is used as a replacement for heroin. A regular dose is prescribed, and the client basically trades one dependency for another. The goal is to prevent the risks of intravenous drug use (methadone is given orally) and the socially inappropriate behaviors associated with obtaining heroin (prostitution, burglary, robbery, etc.).

Naltrexone (ReVia) is an opioid antagonist used to treat opiate overdose. It blocks the effects of any opioids used by the client. It has been found to reduce the cravings for alcohol in abstinent clients (Freed & York, 1997).

Clonidine (Catapres) is an antihypertensive drug. It is given to clients with opiate dependence to prevent some of the symptoms of withdrawal. Nurses should take the client's blood pressure before each dose, and hold the drug if the person is hypotensive.

The tasks of rehabilitation are to:

- Maintain sobriety (abstinence)
- Develop new coping skills
- Make a plan for relapse prevention
- Live life with all its responsibilities, joys, and frustrations

Relapse is common. The best response to relapse is for the person to learn from the experience and to begin again on rehabilitation.

Many people with substance abuse and dependency respond well to treatment. The most popular treatment program is Alcoholics Anonymous (AA). This is a self-help group for alcoholics that is based on 12 steps, thus the name "12-step program." Box 11-3 lists the Twelve Steps of Alcoholics Anonymous. AA itself is for alcoholics only. Other 12-step programs are based on their principles. In all these anonymous groups, people with similar problems share experience, strength, and hope. The groups offer a sense of community and unconditional support.

There are thousands of AA groups. Refer clients to their local telephone book or directory assistance for the closest meeting. There are also AA meetings for special-interest groups, such as nonsmokers, women, lesbians, teachers, people who want to focus on religious aspects of recovery, and so on. Other 12-step programs include Overeaters Anonymous, Narcotics Anonymous, and Cocaine Anonymous.

Al-Anon is a group for family members, especially spouses, of alcoholics. Al-ateen is a similar group for teenage children of alcoholics. Substance dependency is certainly a family illness; these groups have helped many family members.

Dual Diagnosis

The term **dual diagnosis** refers to clients who have both a substance use disorder and a serious mental illness. El-Mallakh (1998) reports that up to 51% of people with severe mental illnesses also have substance use disorders. These individuals have two separate chronic illnesses, and they have a higher level of functional impairment than the general population of people with substance dependency. Many people self-medicate their psychiatric symptoms with alcohol or drugs. Both the mental disorder and the substance use must be treated together.

Substance Dependency Among Nurses

It may seem unlikely for nurses to have problems with substance use, because they should know better. In fact, many

We

1. Admitted that we were powerless over alcohol, that our lives had become unmanageable.
2. Came to believe that a Power greater than ourselves could restore us to sanity.
3. Made a decision to turn our wills and lives over to the care of God as we understood Him.
4. Made a searching and fearless moral inventory of ourselves.
5. Admitted to God, to ourselves, and to another human being the exact nature of our wrongs.
6. Were entirely ready to have God remove all these defects of character.
7. Humbly asked Him to remove our shortcomings.
8. Made a list of all persons we had harmed, and became willing to make amends to them all.
9. Made direct amends to such people whenever possible, except when to do so would injure them or others.
10. Continued to take personal inventory and when we were wrong promptly admitted it.
11. Sought through prayer and meditation to improve our conscious contact with God as we understood Him, praying only for knowledge of His will for us and the power to carry that out.
12. Having had a spiritual awakening as a result of these steps, we tried to carry this message to alcoholics and to practice these principles in all our affairs.

Source: Alcoholics Anonymous World Services, 1952. The Twelve Steps are reprinted with permission of Alcoholics Anonymous World Services, Inc. (A.A.W.S.). Permission to reprint the Twelve Steps does not mean that A.A.W.S. has reviewed or approved the contents of this publication, or that A.A.W.S. necessarily agrees with the views expressed herein. A.A. is a program of recovery from alcoholism *only*—use of the Twelve Steps in connection with programs and activities which are patterned after A.A., but which address other problems, or in any other non-A.A. context, does not imply otherwise.

nurses do use substances. Some reasons our profession is at especially high risk for substance use disorders are that:

■ Nurses see medications as a solution to problems.
■ Nurses have access to drugs at work, and to physicians who prescribe them.
■ Nurses often believe that they should work even when they are tired or sick, so they may use drugs to increase their ability to continue working.

■ Nurses experience pressure, emotional pain, anger, and frustration, which are symptoms that respond to drugs in the short term.
■ Nurses think that if they know about drugs and drug abuse, addiction will not happen to them.

If nurses had adequate understanding of addiction and its early signs, we could identify it earlier in our co-workers and ourselves. Signs of **impaired nursing** include changes in the nurse's *behavior* (mood changes, irritability, forgetfulness, isolation from co-workers, inappropriate behavior). *Work performance* may be affected (multiple medication errors, missed deadlines, sloppy charting, inattention to detail, absenteeism, poor judgment, volunteering to give other nurses narcotics, excessive wasting of narcotics, client complaints that pain medications are not effective, tampering with drug packaging, going to bathroom after administering narcotics). The nurse may also have *signs of drug use or withdrawal* (alcohol on breath, heavy use of breath mints and perfume, red eyes, ataxia, restlessness, anxiety, slurred speech, hyperactivity, family problems that interfere with work, tremors, runny nose).

Substance dependency is a chronic physiologic illness that requires treatment. Affected nurses deserve to be diagnosed and treated before they hurt their clients or themselves. If you suspect that a peer is impaired, notify a manager or hospital supervisor. The nurse is unlikely to be able to manage the problem alone. Check to see if your state board of nursing has a nurse-monitoring or treatment program that can help affected nurses recover and return to the profession.

In the acute situation, your duty as a nurse is to protect your clients from an impaired nurse. In the big picture of caring for colleagues in your profession, your duty is to help your peers get treatment. The intervention to reach each of these outcomes is the same: Tell a supervisor (not just the unit charge nurse for the day), so clients will be safe and the nurse will be treated. This is no time to engage in denial.

NURSING CARE

ASSESSING

It is important to assess the substance use history of every client. The nurse can notify the physician of recent use or regular use so appropriate measures can be taken to adjust doses. Nursing assessment questions are listed in Box 11-4. Note that the substance use assessment does not ask, "Do you drink?" Because alcohol and drug use is associated with strong negative attitudes by society and with guilt by users, the client is most likely to believe that the right answer is "no." People use denial to cope with their substance abuse problems, and they often lie about or underestimate their use. The nurse must present a nonjudgmental attitude and be accepting of clients as people, whether they use drugs or not.

BOX 11-4
ASSESSING FOR SUBSTANCE USE

- How many cigarettes a day do you smoke?
- How often do you drink alcohol?
- About how much do you drink?
- What kind of drugs do you use that are not pre-scribed?
- What is your method of use (oral, smoking, inhaling, injecting)?
- What purpose do these substances serve for you (relaxation, fun, to help you get through the day)?
- Have you had any problems because of drinking or drug use (social, job, or legal)?
- When was the last time you used alcohol or any drug, what was it, and how much?

Note: This is a screening assessment. A more thorough assessment would be indicated in a substance abuse treatment setting.

Notice the assessment question that asks the client what purpose the substance serves. This promotes the nurse's ability to help the client find other choices for coping or entertainment.

A general screening tool for whether a client has problems with alcohol is the CAGE questionnaire (Ewing, 1984). Further inquiry is necessary if the client answers "yes" to one of the following questions:

- Have you ever felt you ought to *C*ut down on your drinking?
- Have people *A*nnoyed you by criticizing your drinking?
- Have you ever felt bad or *G*uilty about your drinking?
- Have you ever had a drink first thing in the morning to steady your nerves or get rid of a hangover (*E*ye-opener)?

DIAGNOSING, PLANNING, AND IMPLEMENTING

INEFFECTIVE PROTECTION

- Take vital signs frequently. If they are elevated (temperature, pulse, respiration, and blood pressure may be involved), medicate with ordered benzodiazepines according to physician's orders. *Benzodiazepines either treat or prevent symptoms of alcohol withdrawal by balancing the CNS stimulation with a depressant effect until the client's CNS can return to homeostasis without alcohol.*
- Assess for other withdrawal symptoms (anxiety, agitation, sweating, nausea, vomiting, tremors, and ataxia). *Treat with PRN benzodiazepines as above. If withdrawal is so severe that the client has hallucinations or seizures, call the physician immediately. These may be symptoms of life-threatening withdrawal.*
- If the client is nauseated, do not push fluids. Offer small amounts of fluids frequently. Offer high-calorie feedings. Assess for dehydration. *Clients in withdrawal are at risk for fluid and electrolyte disturbances. They are also at risk for inade-*

quate nutrition. It is easier for the nauseated client to take foods and fluids in small amounts than in big meals.

- Assist the client with activities of daily living (ADLs). *Clients experiencing withdrawal are likely to be weak and possibly too tired to perform ADLs independently.*
- Maintain a low-stimulation environment for the client. *Clients in withdrawal are experiencing CNS stimulation. They will be more comfortable and less likely to have a seizure if they are in a quiet room with dim lights.*
- Encourage expression of feelings about drinking or about what the client is experiencing. *People with alcohol dependency often have difficulty understanding their own feelings. Expressing them can begin the process of behavior change.*

DEFICIENT KNOWLEDGE

- Assess what clients know and what they need to learn. Teach them about the process of drug abuse and dependency, and how people use drugs for coping, recreation, and company. Review the *consequences to the client* of substance use. *Because so many people deny the severity of the problem, nurses must be honest about what the consequences are (job loss, divorce, family estrangement, disease of every body system, etc.) When people know what the problem is physiologically and realistically, they can begin to do something about it.*

INEFFECTIVE INDIVIDUAL COPING

- Help plan for new healthy coping strategies to replace substance use. *The client may need to meet new people to make new friends if all his old friends only get together to drink or use drugs. People need alternatives to substance use when they become too Hungry, Angry, Lonely, or Tired. (HALT is an acronym for feelings that lead to relapse into drug use.)*
- Help make a list of fun, recreational activities. *Clients may not even know what to do for fun. Be sure the list is realistic and includes the client's preferences (taking a walk, calling a friend on the phone, listening to music, hiking, bike riding, outdoor work, reading, community service, spiritual activities, dancing, carpentry, painting, and appreciating nature are some ideas).*
- Help clients identify their resources for various needs and stressful situations (e.g., a ride to the grocery store or the doctor's office, help caring for the cat if the client is in the hospital). His (her) sponsor from Alcoholics Anonymous may be the one to call if he (she) feels like drinking again, or if he (she) wants to talk about how hard life is. *A practical list like this may be the thing the client turns to instead of drinking when he or she has a problem and cannot think of what to do.*

Other nursing diagnoses that commonly apply to people with substance use disorders are:

- Interrupted Family Processes
- Chronic Low Self-Esteem
- Powerlessness
- Fear
- Denial, Ineffective

- Imbalanced Nutrition, Less Than Body Requirements
- Risk for Injury
- Disturbed Sleep Pattern
- Social Isolation
- Spiritual Distress
- Disturbed Sensory Perceptions
- Risk for Violence

EVALUATING

To evaluate whether nursing interventions for clients with substance use disorders are effective, look at the outcomes. Desired outcomes include:

- Client will have a plan for healthy alternatives to substance use for coping.
- Clients will identify resources for obtaining help when they need it (family, friends, Alcoholics Anonymous, social service agencies).
- Client will identify risk factors for relapse and plan for relapse prevention.
- Client will identify and verbalize feelings.
- Client will assume responsibility for own behavior.
- Client will use peer support to maintain sobriety.

 Discharge Considerations

When people with substance use disorders are discharged from the hospital, there must be follow-up of their substance use issues. Clients may benefit from a written list of telephone numbers for counseling resources, drug abuse treatment, or Alcoholics Anonymous. When a person is not expected to abstain from substance use, the physician must consider this when prescribing medications for use at home. If a client is going to be discharged with sedatives or other medications that could interact with drugs of abuse, discuss the potential risks with the physician.

Nurses should remind clients that they are in control of their own behavior. Clients should be given resources for outpatient support. A promise "never to use again" will not make the person successful. People with substance dependency should always be referred to Social Service for assistance with discharge planning. Also see the list of resources for clients and families.

RESOURCES FOR NURSES, CLIENTS, AND FAMILIES

Alcoholics Anonymous World Services
475 Riverside
New York, NY 10115
www.aa.org
www.recovery.org/aa

Al-Anon Family Group Headquarters
1600 Corporate Landing Parkway
Virginia Beach, VA
1-888-4ALANON
www.Al-Anon-Alateen.org

International Nurses Anonymous
1020 Sunset Drive
Lawrence, KS 66044
(913) 842-3893
www.suresite.com

National Clearinghouse for Alcohol and Drug Information (NCADI)
Prevline: Prevention Online
This is the Website for the Center for Substance Abuse Prevention, Substance Abuse and Mental Health Services Administration, and Center for Substance Abuse Treatment.
www.health.org/

National Institute on Drug Abuse (NIDA)
American Self Help Clearing House
www.nida.nih.gov

Nursing Process Case Study
■ CLIENT WITH INEFFECTIVE INDIVIDUAL COPING

A 30-year-old woman was hospitalized for hematemesis (vomiting blood) and abdominal pain 3 days ago. The medical diagnosis is acute gastritis due to chronic alcohol use. Her husband is a truck driver and is away from home most of the time.

Assessment The nurse did a substance use assessment and found that the woman uses alcohol most days. She drinks a bottle of wine at night after her children go to bed. She sometimes has a few drinks in the morning after they go to school. She drinks because the only time she feels good is when she is drinking. Her parents were both alcoholics. She has no hobbies and states that her only reason for living is her children. The client states, "I don't even know what I like to do. The only time I feel good is when I'm drunk." Vital signs are T 99.2° F, P 90, R 18, BP 118/80.

Diagnosis The nursing diagnosis is Ineffective Individual Coping, related to inadequate role modeling and ineffective skills.

Expected Outcomes The client will:
- Relate her feelings about alcohol dependency.
- List three resources for help when she needs it.
- Plan for four possible alternatives to drinking alcohol when she is under stress.
- Contact Alcoholics Anonymous while in the hospital, and plan to attend a meeting on the day she is discharged.
- List at least three things that she enjoys doing.

Planning and Implementation The nurse will implement the following interventions:

- Spend time each shift talking with the client.
- Help the client make a list of people who can help her in various everyday situations (caring for the children, driving her to an AA meeting, being available to talk on the phone if she is lonely).
- Help the client make a list of alternatives to drinking. These items will be thing that the client agrees that she would actually do. They may include going for a walk, writing a letter, working outdoors, taking the children to the park or the library, playing a game, listening to music, dancing, exercise, journaling, volunteering, and so on.
- Show the client how to find the telephone number of the local Alcoholics Anonymous group in the phone book, and encourage the client to contact them.
- Assist the client to make a list of thing she would enjoy doing. The nurse may make suggestions, but the client should choose the enjoyable things. These also become alternatives to drinking.

Evaluation The client was discharged after 6 days in the hospital. She started attending Alcoholics Anonymous, but quit because she did not feel comfortable in the group meetings. Her sponsor convinced her to try an AA group for women only, which she likes and continues to attend. She and her husband are in couples counseling. He is scheduling his work so he can be at home more often. She has not had any alcohol since she left the hospital 4 weeks ago.

 Critical Thinking in the Nursing Process

1. What are the situations that would put this client at greatest risk for relapse into drinking again?
2. What role did alcohol play in this woman's life?
3. If the client called the hospital unit and told the nurse that she feels like drinking and doesn't know what to do, what should the nurse say?

Nursing Interventions Classification

The following nursing interventions (McCloskey & Bulechek, 2000) may also be useful in caring for a person with substance abuse problems:

- Family Support
- Fluid/Electrolyte Management
- Seizure Precautions
- Nutritional Management
- Spiritual Support
- Values Clarification

(*Note:* The bibliography listings for this and all chapters have been compiled at the back of the book.)

Chapter Review

key terms by topic

Use the CD-ROM disk enclosed with your textbook to hear the pronunciation of the key terms in the chapter.

Problems of substance abuse
denial, substance abuse, substance dependency, addiction

Commonly abused substances
intoxication, euphoria, ataxia, labile, tolerance, withdrawal

Long-term physical effects
Korsakoff's syndrome, Wernicke's syndrome, myopathy

Patterns of use
abstinence, relapse, polysubstance abuse

Treatment
cross-tolerance, detoxification, rehabilitation, dual diagnosis, impaired nurse

key points

- Substance abuse is a maladaptive pattern of substance use despite adverse outcomes. Substance dependency involves continuing to use the substance despite significant substance-related problems, including tolerance, withdrawal, and compulsive use.

- The *DSM-IV-TR* lists 11 substances of abuse: alcohol; opioids; sedatives, hypnotics, and anxiolytics; cocaine; amphetamines and similar drugs; hallucinogens; phencyclidine (PCP) and similar drugs; inhalants; cannabis; caffeine; and nicotine.

- The CNS depressant effects of prescribed drugs in the hospital, combined with effects of drugs or alcohol the client used before admission, may cause severe respiratory depression.

- People who are tolerant to alcohol or narcotics need more analgesics than usual to obtain pain relief.

- Nurses should assess the substance use history of each client on admission.

- When dual diagnosis exists (a person has both a mental disorder and a substance use disorder), both disorders must be treated together.

- Understanding the personal consequences of drug and alcohol use is necessary for client rehabilitation.

- When substance abuse and dependency occur among nurses and other health care professionals, the first responsibility of the nurse is client safety and the second is to seek help for your colleague.

- The goal of substance use treatment is abstinence from substance use and development of skills to replace drug use for coping, enjoyment, or companionship.

- Clients with substance dependency need referral to Social Services for assistance and follow-up after discharge.

- Many people respond well to treatment for substance-related disorders: keep hope alive.

Medialink

Additional interactive resources for this chapter can be found on the Companion Website at www.prenhall.com/burke. Click on Chapter 11 and "Begin" to select the activities for this chapter.

For NCLEX review questions and an audio glossary, access the accompanying CD-ROM in this book.

for further study

For more information about gastritis, see Chapter 18.
For discussion of pancreatitis, see Chapter 19.
For further study about cardiac disorders, see Chapter 22.
For more about musculoskeletal disorders, see Chapter 28.

Critical Thinking Care Map

Care for a Client with Substance Dependency
NCLEX-PN Focus Area: Psychosocial Integrity: Coping and Adaptation

Case Study: A 24-year-old male client is admitted to the medical-surgical unit with multiple trauma suffered in an automobile accident that happened while he was drinking. He has been on the unit for 4 days. His vital signs are stable now, although he has experienced alcohol withdrawal syndrome over the past several days. The substance use history reveals that he drinks beer every day, usually "about two six-packs or so." The client states, "I don't have a drinking problem. I can quit whenever I want!"

Nursing Diagnosis: Ineffective Denial

COLLECT DATA

Subjective	Objective
_____	_____
_____	_____
_____	_____
_____	_____
_____	_____
_____	_____

Would you report this data? Yes/No

If yes, to: _____

Nursing Care

_____
_____
_____
_____
_____
_____
_____
_____

How would you document this? _____
_____
_____

Data Collected
(use those that apply)

- States "I don't have a drinking problem. I can quit whenever I want!"
- Vital signs stable
- Blood alcohol content on admission 0.24 mg/dL
- Weight 165 lbs.
- Skin warm, dry
- Requests pain medication (ordered q4h PRN) about q1h
- States "I feel nervous."
- Has insomnia (sleeps < 4 hours per night)
- Had seizures as a child
- Poor appetite: Eats less than 50% of meals
- States "If you don't let me out of here tomorrow, I'm leaving anyway."

Nursing Interventions
(use those that apply)

- Assess client's knowledge about alcoholism.
- Teach client about the disease of substance dependency.
- Weigh the client daily.
- Provide effective pain management.
- Minimize the amount of narcotics given to this client because he is an addict.
- Offer frequent feedings of high-protein foods.
- Confront the client with the reality of the consequences of alcoholism.
- Encourage the client to express his feelings about drinking and alcoholism.
- Ask the client why he wants to leave the hospital. If he doesn't say so, ask if he wants to drink alcohol.
- Ask the physician for an order for a sleeping medication for the client to take now and when he goes home.

NCLEX-PN Exam Preparation

1. A client discovers he needs more than his usual pint of liquor to achieve the same effect. This phenomenon is called:
   a. tolerance
   b. intoxication
   c. addiction
   d. abuse

2. A woman client is admitted with a diagnosis of alcohol withdrawal. The nurse expects to find which of the following on assessment:
   a. B/P 110/70, P 72, R 20
   b. cooperative behavior
   c. anxiety, tremors
   d. warm, dry skin

3. A male client is admitted with alcoholic encephalopathy (Wernicke's syndrome). The nurse prepares to administer which of the following medications?
   a. Demerol (meperidine)
   b. Valium (diazepam)
   c. Thiamine (vitamin B_1)
   d. Dilantin (phenytoin)

4. The physical assessment of a client admitted to the emergency department reveals pinpoint pupils, depressed respirations, and confusion. The physician diagnoses morphine overdose. Treatment includes:
   a. Thiamine (vitamin B_1)
   b. Narcan (naloxone HCl)
   c. Librium (chlordiazepoxide)
   d. $D_{50}W$

5. A client is prescribed Xanax (alprazolam) for treatment of anxiety. Which of the following MUST the LPN/LVN include in the teaching plan?
   a. Take the drug every 4 hours.
   b. Avoid alcohol while taking the drug.
   c. The drug can cause drowsiness.
   d. Avoid driving until effects are known.

6. An LVN suspects her co-worker is diverting narcotics on the nursing unit. What action by the nurse would be MOST effective?
   a. Confront the nurse with her suspicions.
   b. Notify the physician.
   c. Notify the charge nurse.
   d. Notify the nursing supervisor.

7. The nurse establishes a nursing diagnosis of Knowledge Deficit for a client with a history of substance abuse. The LPN/LVN reinforces a teaching plan to include:
   a. signs and symptoms of withdrawal
   b. consequences to client of continued substance abuse
   c. safe levels of drug use
   d. antidotes to opiates

8. A 28-year-old woman presented to the emergency department for treatment of cocaine addiction. The nurse expects her to exhibit which of the following behaviors during withdrawal from cocaine?
   a. anxiety
   b. hypertension
   c. depression
   d. seizures

9. The LPN/LVN confronts a client about her suspicion that the client is using alcohol while in the hospital. Based on the most common coping mechanism in substance abuse, the client's most likely response would be:
   a. "This is not your concern."
   b. "You can't tell anyone about this."
   c. "I will drink at any time I choose."
   d. "I have not had a drink since admission."

10. A 22-year-old presents to the emergency department after attending an event at a local night club. The nurse suspects he is exhibiting signs of MDMA (Ecstasy) use. The BEST indicator of the use of this drug is:
    a. hallucinations
    b. watery eyes
    c. pinpoint pupils
    d. depression

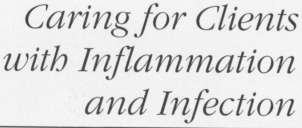

chapter

12

Caring for Clients with Inflammation and Infection

CARING tip

❝The ten worst offenders in the spread of infection are your ten fingers.❞

Vivian Bingman, RN, MEd • Director, Practical Nursing Program • Mid-Del Technology Center • Midwest City, Oklahoma

LEARNING outcomes

After completing this chapter, you will be able to:

- Explain the steps of the inflammatory process.
- State the five cardinal manifestations of acute inflammation.
- Identify the purpose of the laboratory tests used to diagnose inflammation and infection.
- Describe the chain of infection.
- Identify common nosocomial infections.
- Explain age-related changes in older adults that increase their risk for infection.
- Identify the common antimicrobial medications, nursing implications, and client teaching guidelines.
- Describe the guidelines for standard–hand transmission-based precautions.
- Use the nursing process to collect data, establish outcomes, provide individualized care, and evaluate responses for clients with inflammation and infections.

MediaLink

 www.prenhall.com/burke

Use the above address to access the free, interactive Companion Website created for this textbook. Get hints, instant feedback, and textbook references to chapter-related multiple choice questions. Link to other interesting sites.

Inflammation

Inflammation is a "nonspecific" response to an injury, meaning the same sequence of events occurs regardless of the cause. Inflammation brings fluid, dissolved substances, and blood cells into the interstitial tissues where an injury has occurred. Its purpose is to destroy the harmful agent, limit spread to other tissues, and begin the healing process. Inflammation develops as soon as one or more harmful invaders injure the body's cells.

PATHOPHYSIOLOGY

Normally, the skin and mucous membranes act as the body's first line of defense, preventing an invasion by external organisms. Mucous membranes lining the inner surfaces of the body trap microorganisms and other foreign substances. These are removed by other protective mechanisms such as ciliary movement in the respiratory tract or the washing action of tears and urine. Many body fluids contain bactericidal substances that provide barrier protection. These include acid in the gastric fluid and lysosomes in tears, nasal secretions, and saliva.

External or internal agents can destroy the body's defense mechanisms and trigger the inflammatory process. Inflammation can be caused by the following factors:

- Mechanical injuries, such as cuts or surgical incisions
- Physical damage, such as burns
- Chemical injury from toxins or poisons
- Microorganisms, such as bacteria, viruses, or fungi
- Extremes of heat or cold
- Immunologic responses, such as hypersensitivity reactions
- Ischemic damage or trauma, such as a stroke or myocardial infarction

The inflammatory response involves three steps:

1. *Vascular response.* Initially, the blood vessels around the injured area constrict briefly. Then they dilate as chemical mediators, such as histamine, bradykinin, and prostaglandins, are released. Blood flow to the injured area increases, causing redness and warmth. It also raises local hydrostatic pressure, so capillaries leak fluid into surrounding tissues. The result is edema at the injury site and dilution of the organisms or toxins in the area. The chemical mediators and edema are responsible for pain and impaired function.
2. *Cellular response.* As blood flow increases to the injured tissues, white blood cells (WBCs) move into the area. *Neutrophils,* the first white blood cells to respond, usually arrive within 90 minutes. They move from inside the capillary to the injured tissue by a process known as **diapedesis** (Figure 12-1 ◆).

   Neutrophils and **macrophages** (large white blood cells that develop from monocytes) ingest harmful bacteria and dead tissue cells in a process called **phagocytosis** (see Figure 12-2 ◆). Once neutrophils have ingested their full capacity of bacteria, they die. The accumulation of

B Emigration

Figure 12-1. ◆ (A) Leukocytes in the circulation. (B) Diapedesis, the process of leukocytes moving from inside the capillary to injured tissue.

dead neutrophils, dead bacteria, and tissue debris forms *pus.* Bacteria such as staphylococci, streptococci, and neisseriae often cause purulent drainage.

3. *Healing and tissue repair.* After neutrophils die, macrophages clean up the site for healing. In minor injuries, the inflammatory process and healing restore normal structure and function. If the injury is more

Figure 12-2. ◆ Phagocytosis—the bacterium is bound to and engulfed by the phagocyte.

extensive, new cells are produced to replace the functional tissue. Most cells can regenerate or reproduce (except for nerve, skeletal muscle, and cardiac muscle cells). When regeneration is impossible, collagen scar tissue replaces the destroyed tissue through a process known as repair. Scar tissue, which is composed of a different cell type from the original cell, fills in the empty space left by the injury. It often has less strength than the original tissue, and so is more vulnerable to future injury. (See Chapter 7 for more on the healing process.) Box 12-1 discusses age-related changes related to inflammation in the older adult.

Acute Inflammation

Inflammation may be either acute or chronic. *Acute inflammation* is a short-term reaction of the body to any tissue damage. It is immediate and usually lasts less than 1 to 2 weeks. Once the harmful agent is removed, the inflammation subsides. Healing and tissue repair occur, and the body returns to normal or near-normal function. Acute inflammation produces local and systemic manifestations.

LOCAL MANIFESTATIONS. Local manifestations develop at and around the site of injury. The degree of functional loss depends on the location and extent of the injury. Increased tissue damage results in more swelling, pain, and functional impairment. The amount of prostaglandin release determines whether pain is immediate or delayed.

Sometimes the inflammatory process does not end immediately with healing and tissue repair. **Cellulitis** develops if inflammation spreads to the surrounding connective tissues. In other circumstances, pus develops and accumulates in pockets called **abscesses**. Abscesses are the body's way of walling off the infection. Abscesses may need to be artificially drained with a procedure called **incision and drainage** (I&D). Inflammation may also cause the formation of a **fistula** (an abnormal tubelike passage from one body cavity to another cavity). More extensive treatment is necessary to manage a fistula.

Clients with diabetes mellitus are at an increased risk for poor wound healing and cellulitis. High blood glucose levels seem to alter phagocytic function and to damage the capillaries. Both these changes impair wound healing. Once a wound heals, it loses some of its original strength, so the diabetic client has a higher incidence of leg and foot ulcers.

SYSTEMIC MANIFESTATIONS. One systemic response to inflammation is enlargement of the lymph nodes (**lymphadenitis**). This process occurs when bacteria, phagocytes, and destroyed lymph tissue accumulate in the affected lymph node. Enlarged lymph nodes are palpable in the groin, axillae, and neck (Figure 12-3 ◆). Loss of appetite and fatigue develop as the body tries to conserve energy during the inflammatory process. **Leukocytosis** (increased WBC production) supports inflammation and phagocytosis.

Another systemic manifestation is fever. Fever inhibits the growth of many microorganisms and may increase tissue repair. Macrophages release chemicals called **endogenous pyrogens** that act on the temperature control center in the hypothalamus to elevate the temperature set-point. As the temperature rises, the client complains of being cold and shivers because the blood vessels constrict to conserve heat. Once the new set-point is reached, the body attempts to cool itself by vasodilation and sweating. Fever should end when the microorganism is destroyed or antibiotics or antipyretics are given. Clients who are immunosuppressed may not experience a fever.

CLINICAL alert

In 25% of the elderly, fever is low grade or absent. Older clients may have a serious infection with a 98.6° F temperature. The best indicator of a serious infection is delirium or a change in mental function.

Local and systemic manifestations of inflammation are summarized in Box 12-2.

Chronic Inflammation

Chronic inflammation is slower in onset and lasts weeks to months or years. It may develop when the acute inflammatory process has been ineffective in removing the offending agent. For example, in tuberculosis, the mycobacteria resist phagocytosis. *Mycobacterium tuberculosis* can survive for many years and emerge only when the client's immune system is compromised. Chronic inflammation may also develop from constant irritation by chemicals or physical irritants such as talc, asbestos, or silica.

COLLABORATIVE CARE

Management of the client with an inflammation focuses on promoting healing. Care is generally supportive, allowing the client's own physiologic processes to remove foreign matter and damaged cells. The client is encouraged to rest and drink more fluids. A well-balanced diet with vitamin supplements

BOX 12-1

population
FOCUS

Inflammatory Changes in the Older Adult

In the older adult, the skin becomes thinner, drier, and more fragile, increasing the potential for injury. The combination of decreased blood flow from atherosclerosis and fewer macrophages results in slower wound healing. The phagocytic activity of the neutrophils lessens with age and impairs local resistance to infection. Older adults also take more medications that interfere with inflammation and healing. The cardinal signs of inflammation—redness, heat, and swelling—tend to be diminished or absent in older adults.

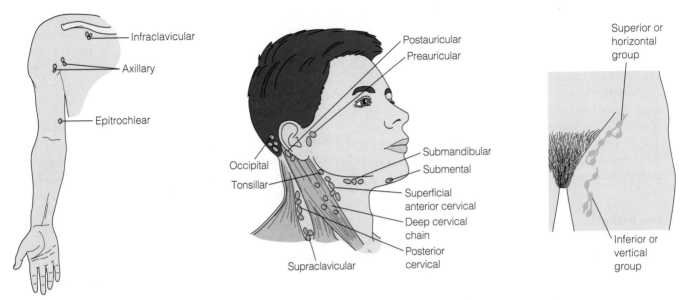

Figure 12-3. ◆ Lymph nodes that may be assessed by palpation.

also promotes healing. The client may receive anti-inflammatory medications and antibiotics.

Laboratory and Diagnostic Tests

Laboratory and diagnostic tests can identify the source and extent of inflammation. The following laboratory tests may be ordered:

- *WBC count with differential* provides information about five leukocytes: neutrophils, eosinophils, basophils, monocytes, and lymphocytes. It measures the percentage of the total WBC made up by each type of leukocyte and provides clues about the type of inflammation (Table 12-1 ◆). With inflammation, **leukocytosis** (a WBC count of > 10,000/

mm^3) typically occurs. **Leukopenia** (a WBC count of < 4,500/mm^3) may indicate a viral infection.

- *Erythrocyte sedimentation rate* (ESR or sed rate) is a nonspecific test that can detect generalized inflammation.
- *C-reactive protein* (CRP) test can identify the presence of active inflammation and tissue necrosis but cannot specify the site. It may show inflammation quicker that the ESR.
- *Cultures* of the blood and other body fluids are also ordered to determine whether infection is the cause of inflammation.

Pharmacology

The medications prescribed to relieve the effects of inflammation include antibiotics, acetaminophen, anti-inflammatory agents, and corticosteroids.

Antibiotics are used to treat infection and prevent infection from interfering with the healing process. If an infection is present, a culture and sensitivity test is done to determine the most effective antibiotic. Anti-infective therapy is discussed in greater depth later in the chapter under infectious diseases.

Acetaminophen (Tylenol) does not have an anti-inflammatory effect. It is used by clients to reduce the pain associated with inflammation. Acetaminophen does have an antipyretic effect. It decreases fever by acting directly on the hypothalamic heat-regulating center.

Although inflammation is a beneficial process to prepare injured tissue for healing, it can have harmful effects. When inflammation presents a danger to the client, anti-inflammatory medications are prescribed. Anti-inflammatory medications fall into three broad groups: salicylates; other nonsteroidal anti-inflammatory drugs (NSAIDs), and corticosteroids.

Aspirin (acetylsalicylic acid, or ASA) and NSAIDs have a similar action. They produce anti-inflammatory, antipyretic,

---

BOX 12-2
MANIFESTATIONS
OF INFLAMMATION

LOCAL MANIFESTATIONS

- Redness
- Warmth
- Edema
- Pain
- Loss of function

SYSTEMIC MANIFESTATIONS

- Fever
- Tachycardia
- Increased respiratory rate
- Loss of appetite
- Fatigue
- Enlarged lymph nodes
- WBC count > 10,000/mm^3

TABLE 12-1 WHITE BLOOD CELL COUNT AND DIFFERENTIAL

CELL TYPE AND NORMAL VALUE	INCREASED	DECREASED
Total WBCs: 4,500–10,000 per mm³	*Leukocytosis:* Acute infection, tissue necrosis, trauma, stress	*Leukopenia:* Anemia, viral infections, autoimmune diseases
Neutrophils: 50–70%	*Neutrophilia:* Acute infection, inflammatory diseases, acute pancreatitis	*Neutropenia:* Viral diseases, leukemia, anemia
Eosinophils: 1–3%	*Eosinophilia:* Allergies, parasitic diseases, cancer, phlebitis	*Eosinopenia:* Stress, Cushing's syndrome
Basophils: 0.4–1%	*Basophilia:* Inflammation, leukemia reactions	*Basopenia:* Acute stress, hypersensitivity
Monocytes: 4–6% diseases, leukemia	*Monocytosis:* Viral diseases, parasitic marrow depression	*Monocytopenia:* Lymphocytic leukemia, bone
Lymphocytes: 25–35%	*Lymphocytosis:* Lymphocytic leukemia, viral infections, chronic bacterial infection	*Lymphocytopenia:* Cancer, leukemia, Cushing's syndrome, multiple sclerosis, renal failure

Source: Data compiled from Kee, J. L. (2001). *Handbook of laboratory and diagnostic tests* (4th ed.) Upper Saddle River, NJ: Prentice Hall.

and analgesic effects. Clients receive varying degrees of relief with aspirin and different NSAIDs. Sometimes several different drugs are tried before the client reports any relief. All of these medications can produce gastrointestinal (GI) irritation and the possibility of bleeding. Indomethacin is the most toxic NSAID; it should be limited to short-term therapy (see Table 12-2 ◆).

CLINICAL alert

Aspirin should not be given to children with chickenpox or influenza, because it can cause Reye's syndrome.

Corticosteroid therapy is prescribed for acute hypersensitivity reactions, such as poison oak, or for inflammation unrelieved by aspirin or NSAIDs. They are also used to manage chronic inflammatory diseases such as arthritis, but they do not cure disease. Steroid medications cause adverse reactions. They suppress the immune and inflammatory responses as well as delay healing; therefore, they should be used cautiously. Remember the following principles when administering corticosteroids:

- Use the smallest effective dose.
- An alternate-day dose schedule may decrease suppression of adrenal gland activity.
- Never stop steroid therapy abruptly. Taper the dose gradually so that adrenal gland function can return to normal.
- Harmful side effects increase with higher doses and prolonged therapy.

The nursing implications of caring for a client receiving corticosteroid medications are presented in Chapter 16 (see Table 16-4).

Wound Care

Minor wounds may require no more then gentle cleansing with soap and water. If wounds are more extensive, wound care may involve irrigations and debridement of necrotic tissue. To prevent additional wound damage, the nurse cleanses the site with sterile normal saline or commercially prepared nontoxic wound cleansers such as Comfeel (Coloplast Corporation) or ClinisWound (Sage Laboratories). Hydrogen peroxide, povidone–iodine (Betadine), and sodium hypochlorite (Dakin's solution) have a drying effect on the tissue. They can also inhibit the healing process. They should be used as a last resort. Because granulation tissue in a healing wound is fragile and bleeds easily, wound care must be performed gently. (See wound care in Chapter 7.)

Nutrition

Inflammation and wound healing require adequate nutrition, blood supply, and oxygenation. *Malnutrition* makes the phagocytes ineffective so that there is a delayed inflammatory response. The macrophages cannot prepare the wound site for healing. If an infection develops, it interferes with effective wound healing. *Inadequate circulation* cannot deliver sufficient oxygen and nutrients or remove waste products. Without normal circulation the injury site cannot heal properly.

The client with an inflammation or wound requires a well-balanced diet to promote healing. When clients develop protein deficiency, their risk for poor wound healing and infection increases. Inflammation produces **catabolism,** a condition in which body tissues are broken down. During healing, the desired result is tissue building (**anabolism**). Diets low in calories and essential nutrients lead to catabolism and impaired healing.

Encourage the client to eat a diet high in carbohydrates, protein, and vitamins. Carbohydrates are important to meet

TABLE 12-2 NURSING IMPLICATIONS FOR PHARMACOLOGY: CLIENTS RECEIVING ANTI-INFLAMMATORY DRUGS

DRUG GROUP/DRUGS	PURPOSE	NURSING RESPONSIBILITIES	CLIENT TEACHING
Salicylates ▪ Aspirin (acetylsalicylic acid)	Aspirin is a nonsteroidal anti-inflammatory drug (NSAID) with analgesic, antipyretic, and antiplatelet effects.	Do not give to clients with peptic ulcers, with gastritis, or taking anti-coagulants. Give with food or milk to prevent gastric irritation. Notify the physician for signs of black or bloody stools, coffee-ground emesis, or tinnitus.	Take with food or milk to avoid gastric irritation. Report any dark stools, unusual bleeding, bruising, blurred vision, or ringing in the ears. Do not use with other drugs containing aspirin. Discard tablets with vinegar-like odor.
Nonsteroidal Anti-Inflammatory Drugs (NSAIDs) ▪ Fenoprofen calcium (Nalfon) ▪ Ibuprofen (Motrin, Advil) ▪ Indomethacin (Indocin) ▪ Ketorolac (Toradol) ▪ Naproxen (Anaprox, Naprosyn) ▪ Piroxicam (Feldene) ▪ Ketoprofen (Orudis)	NSAIDs are used to reduce pain and inflammation.	Give cautiously to patients with bleeding disorders, peptic ulcers or gastritis, and renal disease. Give with food or milk to decrease gastric irritation. Monitor for heartburn, gastrointestinal bleeding, a change in urination or bloody urine.	Take with food or milk as ordered. Report changes in vision or hearing; a change in urination or bloody urine; coffee-ground emesis or blood in the stool. Avoid the use of alcohol while taking NSAIDs.

energy demands and to support leukocyte function. Protein is necessary for tissue healing and the production of antibodies and WBCs. Some vitamins and minerals are also important. Vitamin A fosters capillary formation and tissue growth. B-complex vitamins promote wound healing. Vitamin C is necessary for collagen synthesis. Vitamin K is essential for blood clotting. Minerals, especially zinc, are important for tissue growth, skin integrity, and immune function.

NURSING CARE

The nursing care needs of the client with an inflammatory process are related to the manifestations of inflammation and altered tissue integrity. Priority nursing diagnoses include Pain, Impaired Tissue Integrity, and Risk for Infection.

ASSESSING

The nurse must collect assessment data to help determine the extent to which the inflammatory process is interfering with the client's life. Data can also identify risk factors for compli-

cations and can determine the type of medical intervention (Box 12-3).

DIAGNOSING, PLANNING, AND IMPLEMENTING

ACUTE PAIN

Along with redness, warmth, swelling, and impaired function, pain is one of the cardinal manifestations of inflammation. Depending on the cause, affected area, and degree of inflammation, pain may be acute and immobilizing or chronic.

- Give anti-inflammatory medications as prescribed. *These medications can lessen the pain resulting from inflammation.*
- Give mild analgesic medications as prescribed. *Although most analgesics do not reduce inflammation, they may decrease pain perception.*
- Remind the client that rest is important for acutely inflamed tissue. *Strenuous activity or exercising an inflamed body part may increase discomfort and cause tissue damage.*
- Apply cold or heat therapy as ordered. Remove ice pack or heating pad after 10 minutes and check the client's skin. (For cold, note bluish color or a feeling of numbness; for

■ Encourage the client to eat a well-balanced diet with adequate carbohydrates, protein, vitamins, and minerals. If the client is NPO or unable to eat an adequate diet, suggest parenteral nutrition, between-meal supplements, or multivitamin supplements. *A well-balanced diet promotes immune function and healing.*

RISK FOR INFECTION

The inflammatory response is meant to protect the client against microorganisms. However, when intact skin is broken (as in a healing wound), the risk for infection increases.

■ Monitor the client's temperature, pulse, and respirations at least every 4 hours. *Increased vital signs usually indicate inflammation. A temperature of 101°F (38.3°C) or above indicates infection.*

■ Culture purulent or odorous wound drainage. *Wound culture is used to determine the infectious organism and appropriate antibiotic therapy.*

■ Provide fluid intake of 2,500 mL per day unless otherwise contraindicated. *Adequate hydration helps maintain blood flow and nutrient supply to the tissues. Fluids may be limited for the client with congestive heart failure.*

■ Use proper handwashing techniques (including at least 15 seconds of friction). *Handwashing is the fundamental tool for preventing the spread of infection to a susceptible person.*

■ Wear sterile gloves when providing wound care. *Sterile gloves prevent further wound contamination and the spread of infection to other clients.*

EVALUATING

To evaluate the effectiveness of care for a client with acute inflammation, collect data about the presence of redness, heat, swelling, loss of function, and swelling. For the client with systemic inflammation, note vital signs, appetite, energy level, and lymph nodes.

Discharge Considerations

Client and family teaching should focus on understanding the inflammatory process, its cause, and its management. Teaching is also important to prevent actions that could lead to infection. Box 12-4 lists assessment data to consider when planning home care.

Provide the client with the following verbal and written instructions:

■ Increase fluid intake to 2,500 mL (approximately 2½ quarts) per day, unless contraindicated.

■ Eat a well-balanced diet that is high in carbohydrates, protein, vitamins, and minerals.

■ Use good handwashing techniques (wash for at least 15 seconds with friction) when caring for wounds and after using the bathroom.

BOX 12-3
ASSESSING CLIENTS
WITH INFLAMMATION

SUBJECTIVE DATA

• Present health status:
  • General health and nutritional status
  • Describe any injuries
  • Describe any redness, warmth, swelling, or pain
  • Is drainage associated with current injury or previous procedure? Is drainage clear or purulent?
  • Changes in appetite or energy level
• Past medical history:
  • Any frequent infections?
  • Use of anti-inflammatory medications, corticosteroids, or antibiotics

OBJECTIVE DATA

• Vital signs: Blood pressure, pulse, respirations, temperature
• Height and weight
• Observe client for fatigue and listlessness
• Assess ability to move injured area and amount of pain
• Assess circulation to affected area
• Inspect skin and surrounding area of injury for redness and warmth, purulent drainage, odor, and poor healing
• Measure size (depth and width) of wounds
• Palpate the skin for the presence of edema
• Palpate for enlarged lymph nodes

---

heat, observe for redness.) *For an acute injury, cold reduces swelling and relieves pain. After the initial stage, heat increases blood flow to the affected tissue promotes absorption of edema. It is important to monitor the client's skin for untoward effects and to prevent injury to the skin.*

■ Elevate the inflamed area if possible. *Elevation promotes venous return and reduces swelling.*

IMPAIRED TISSUE INTEGRITY

Both an injury and the inflammatory response to it can lead to impaired skin integrity. The nurse must prevent any additional skin problems.

■ Provide protective devices, such as an eye patch, over the injured area. *Protective devices aid in comfort and healing.*

■ Clean inflamed tissue gently; use water or normal saline only. *Soap and harsh cleansing agents can cause drying and further tissue damage.*

■ Encourage the client to balance rest with active and passive exercises. *Rest decreases metabolic demands and promotes cell growth. Activity promotes circulation.*

BOX 12-4
ASSESSING FOR DISCHARGE

INFLAMMATION
Client

- Self-care: Ability to perform ADLs independently; to plan rest periods and prepare nutritional meals; to self-administer prescribed medications; to perform wound care
- Knowledge: Disease process; prescription and over-the-counter medications; well-balanced diet; indications for seeking medical care
- Home environment: Appropriate heating and cooling; access to clean water for drinking and handwashing; safe environment to minimize risk of injury

Family

- Members of household: Individuals with infections
- Caregivers: Availability and willingness to provide care as needed; assist with meals and home maintenance
- Financial resources: Income; availability of sick leave; resources for drugs and medical care needed

Community

- Access to health care resources

- Elevate the inflamed area to reduce swelling and pain.
- Apply heat or cold for no longer than 20 minutes at a time to reduce the risk of tissue damage from burns or frostbite.
- Take all medications as prescribed. Review the use, expected effects, and side effects of anti-inflammatory medications. Notify the physician if adverse effects occur.
- Rest acutely inflamed tissue. Do not engage in strenuous activity until the inflammation has subsided.

Infection

Microorganisms invade humans in order to grow and reproduce. Contact between humans and microorganisms is often beneficial to both. For example, the normal flora of the skin, mucous membranes, and gastrointestinal tract play an important part in the body's defense system. However, all microorganisms are capable of producing **infection** (growth and invasion of microorganisms that leads to disease), especially when an individual is in poor health.

Infectious diseases have existed throughout history. Modern medicine, antibiotic therapy, immunizations, and public health measures that protect food and water supplies have significantly reduced the prevalence of infectious diseases in many parts of the world. Smallpox, once a deadly disease, has been eliminated. However, malaria, typhoid, and tuberculosis are still common in many developing nations. In spite of vac-

cines and anti-infective drugs, new strains of bacteria for sexually transmitted diseases (STDs), tuberculosis, and antibiotic-resistant strains of *Staphylococcus* have emerged. Tuberculosis is on the rise in the United States because organisms are resistant to antitubercular medications. New diseases such as human immunodeficiency virus (HIV), legionnaires' disease, Lyme disease, and *Hantavirus* are challenging modern medicine to find new treatments. Even diseases that once were unrelated to microorganisms now have an infectious disease connection; for example, *Helicobacter pylori* seems to be the underlying cause of chronic gastritis. Bioterrorism adds another dimension, as diseases like anthrax are used for hostile political ends.

To a certain extent, modern medicine has contributed to the development of microorganisms. For example, invasive procedures that use metal and plastic prosthetic devices provide potential sites for infection. **Immunosuppression** (inability of the immune system to provide adequate immunity) is part of the medical consequence for organ recipients. Clients who receive immunosuppressive therapy following organ transplant or chemotherapy are, therefore, more susceptible to infection.

PATHOPHYSIOLOGY
Chain of Infection

For an individual to develop an infection, the chain of infection must be in place. Key elements of the chain include: (1) a microorganism, (2) a reservoir, (3) a portal of exit from the reservoir, (4) a mode of transmission from the reservoir to the host, and (5) an entry point into a susceptible host (Figure 12-4 ◆). Each element is presented in more detail in the following discussion.

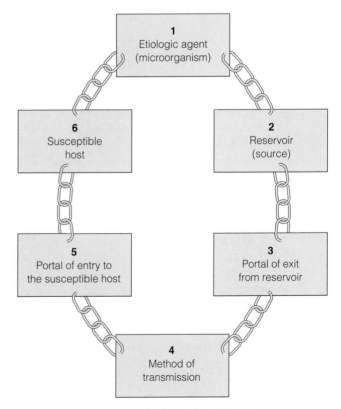

Figure 12-4. ◆ The chain of infection.

MICROORGANISMS. **Pathogens** are microorganisms that are capable of causing disease. Common pathogens include bacteria, mycoplasma, rickettsia, chlamydia, viruses, fungi, protozoa, helminths, and arthropods (Box 12-5). Each organism causes a different reaction in the host.

For microorganisms to result in disease, several factors are required, including virulence and invasiveness. **Virulence** is the power of a microorganism to cause infection. It is affected by the number of organisms, the host's health, and whether toxins are produced. For example, measles has a low virulence, but rabies has a high virulence. An organism's ability to invade and multiply in a host determines its **invasiveness.** Microorganisms that produce enzymes or toxins are bet-ter able to resist the host's defenses and can easily invade the body. For example, *Staphylococcus aureus* releases an enzyme that increases its resistance to certain antibiotics.

Bacteria may release **exotoxins** (from *Staphylococcus, Streptococcus,* or tetanus bacteria) or **endotoxins** (from gram-negative bacteria). Also, diseases such as botulism and cholera release deadly bacterial exotoxins. Gram-negative organisms that produce endotoxins can cause septic shock. (Common infections and their causative organisms are noted in Table 12-3 ♦.)

RESERVOIR AND PORTAL OF EXIT. The reservoir is where the pathogen lives and multiplies. Humans, animals, insects, and

---

BOX 12-5
PATHOGENIC ORGANISMS

BACTERIA

Bacteria are single-celled organisms. They have different shapes: round *(cocci),* rod-shaped *(bacilli),* or spiral *(spirochete).* Bacteria can adapt to different environments: *aerobes* require oxygen for survival; *anaerobes* survive without oxygen. In the laboratory, they are classified by staining properties: *gram-positive* bacteria stain purple and *gram-negative* bacteria stain red. Common bacterial infections include *Streptococcus pneumoniae, Staphylococcus aureus,* and *Escherichia coli.*

MYCOPLASMA

Although similar to bacteria, mycoplasma are smaller. They are more resistant to antibiotics such as penicillins and cephalosporins.

RICKETTSIAE AND CHLAMYDIA

Rickettsiae and chlamydia have some features similar to bacteria and viruses. Rickettsiae infect the cells of arthropods (e.g., fleas, ticks, and lice) without causing disease. When they are transmitted from these vectors to humans, they cause diseases like typhus. Chlamydia are transmitted by direct contact and can cause sexually transmitted diseases.

VIRUSES

Viruses are the smallest pathogens. They are incapable of reproducing outside of a living cell. They use the host's metabolic and reproductive materials to multiply. Viruses consist of a protein shell around a DNA or RNA core. Some viruses are short-lived, such as rhinovirus (the common cold). Latent viruses remain dormant in the host until they are reactivated, for example, herpes zoster (shingles) and fever blisters (cold sores). Human immunodeficiency virus (HIV) is classed as a retrovirus. Oncogenic viruses may be able to transform normal cells into cancer cells.

FUNGI

Fungi are prevalent throughout the world, but few are capable of causing disease in humans. They grow in two forms: yeasts and molds. Fungal infections can be mild, affecting the skin and subcutaneous tissue. Some fungi, such as *Pneumocystis carinii,* can cause life-threatening opportunistic infections in the immunocompromised host.

PROTOZOANS, HELMINTHS, AND ARTHROPODS

Protozoa, helminths, and arthropods are considered parasites. Protozoa are single-celled organisms transmitted from host to host, indirectly through contaminated water, or by an arthropod vector. Helminths are wormlike parasites (e.g., roundworms, tapeworms, and flukes). They are transmitted via eggs or larvae that usually are excreted by humans in urine or feces. They enter other humans through food contaminated by urine or feces or through broken skin. Arthropod parasites, such as scabies (mites), lice, and fleas, typically infest external body surfaces, causing localized tissue damage and inflammation. Transmission is by direct contact with the arthropod or its eggs.

Sources: Data adapted from Bullock, B. A., & Heet, R. L. (2000). *Focus on pathophysiology.* Philadelphia: Lippincott; and Porth, C. M. (1998). *Pathophysiology: Concepts of altered health states* (5th ed.). Philadelphia: Lippincott.

TABLE 12-3	**COMMON INFECTIOUS DISEASES AND THE CAUSATIVE ORGANISM**

DISEASE	CAUSATIVE ORGANISM
Chickenpox	Varicella zoster
Gonorrhea	*Neisseria gonorrhoeae*
Foodborne hepatitis	Hepatitis A virus
Bloodborne hepatitis	Hepatitis B, C, or D
Herpes simplex	Human herpesvirus 1 and 2
Impetigo	*Staphylococcus aureus*
Influenza	Influenza virus A, B, or C
Lyme disease	*Borrelia burgdorferi*
Meningitis	*Haemophilus influenzae*
Meningococcal meningitis	*Neisseria meningitidis*
Pneumococcal pneumoniae	*Streptococcus pneumoniae*
Rabies	Rabies virus
Respiratory synctial disease	Respiratory synctial virus
Ringworm	*Microsporum* species
Rubella	Rubella virus
Streptococcal pharyngitis	*Streptococcus pyogenes*, Group A
Syphilis	*Treponema pallidum*
Tetanus	*Clostridium tetani*
Tuberculosis	*Mycobacterium tuberculosis*

nonliving or inanimate objects such as equipment, needles, and utensils act as reservoirs. Infectious diseases are usually transmitted from human sources who have the clinical disease. People who have the disease but do not show any clinical manifestations are called **carriers.** For an infection to escape its reservoir, it must have a portal of exit. Pathogens exit humans through respiratory secretions, gastrointestinal and genitourinary body fluids, skin or mucous membrane lesions, or the blood.

MODE OF TRANSMISSION. Pathogens move from their reservoir to a susceptible host by several routes: direct or indirect contact, droplet or airborne transmission, or a vector. *Direct contact* includes person-to-person spread or contact with infected body fluids or contaminated food or water. *Indirect contact* occurs when the infectious agent is carried on inanimate objects, such as dirty eating utensils.

Droplet transmission involves large, moist droplets released during sneezing, talking, and coughing. Contaminated droplets can be sprayed to another person within a 2- to 3-foot radius. In *airborne transmission,* small respiratory particles are carried by air currents and then inhaled by the host. For example, tuberculosis is spread by airborne transmission. *Vectors* are insects and animals (such as flies, mosquitoes, or rodents) that act as intermediate hosts between the source and host.

Pathogenic organisms must be able to survive their transport from the reservoir to a host. Over time, they have developed mechanisms to resist drying and unfavorable temperatures (e.g., tetanus bacteria produce spores).

PORTAL OF ENTRY. An organism needs a portal of entry to gain access into the host. Portals of entry include eyes; mouth; respiratory, gastrointestinal, and genitourinary tracts; broken skin; and blood.

HOST. The susceptible host is the final link in the chain of infection. The concepts of normal flora, colonization, infection, and disease are important to how bacteria can affect a host. Normal flora (resident bacteria) work in harmony with the host and provide a benefit such as the normal flora in the intestinal tract. **Colonization** occurs when pathogenic microorganisms live in the host but do not cause injury or initiate the inflammatory response. For example, *Staphylococcus aureus* may colonize on the skin. Infection indicates that pathogenic bacteria have triggered the inflammatory process, such as when *S. aureus* enters a surgical wound, causing redness, heat, and pain. *Infectious disease* is the illness that results from an infection.

Whether an infection develops depends on microbe virulence and host resistance. The following factors help the host resist infection:

- Physical barriers, such as the skin and mucous membranes
- Hostile environment created by acid stomach secretions, urine, and vaginal secretions
- Antimicrobial factors in saliva, tears, and prostatic fluid
- Coughing, sneezing, and the cilia in the respiratory tract
- Neutrophils and macrophages

When host resistance is compromised, the host becomes *susceptible* to infection. Invasive procedures (urinary catheters, chest tubes, IV lines) penetrate the body's physical barriers. The very young and very old may have underdeveloped or failing immune systems. Clients who are malnourished, have AIDS, or have cancer and are being treated with chemotherapy or radiation therapy have increased susceptibility. Susceptibility is lowered when a person receives an immunization or has previously developed the disease.

Stages of the Infectious Process

Infectious disease usually follows a predictable course through five stages as it develops in the host:

1. The *initial stage* is the incubation period. The pathogen actively reproduces but does not cause symptoms. Some diseases have short incubation periods (like food poison-

ing due to *Salmonella*). On the other hand, HIV infection has an incubation period of months to years.

2. In the *prodromal stage,* symptoms begin to appear, although they are often vague and nonspecific. The client will report general malaise, fever, muscle aches and pains, headache, and fatigue.

3. During the *acute stage,* the pathogen continues reproducing and disperses rapidly. Manifestations become obvious and reflect the specific organism and site. Usually, the client develops a fever, chills, tachycardia, and tachypnea. Infections of an internal organ cause an inflammatory response. The client may have tenderness over the site or show signs of altered function, such as hematuria in kidney infections. If the infectious process continues over an extended period, clients show signs of increased catabolism and malnutrition. They lose weight and their muscles become weak. Sometimes products of the immune process, formed in other sites than the primary infection, cause an inflammatory reaction. For example, a sore throat caused by a streptococcal infection may result in glomerulonephritis.

4. In the *convalescent stage,* the infection is contained and the pathogen is continually destroyed. At this point, affected tissues are repaired and symptoms disappear.

5. During the last stage, *resolution,* the infection is totally eliminated from the body without residual manifestations. Clients with chronic infections never reach the convalescent and resolution stages.

Complications

Complications may be associated with the type of infecting organism and its virulence. They also may be related to the physical condition of the host. As discussed above, if the host is immunosuppressed, the body's normal defenses are missing. Immunosuppression causes not only poor wound healing but also slower disease resolution.

Microorganisms such as bacteria, fungi, and viruses can enter the bloodstream causing *bacteremia, fungemia,* or *viremia.* If gram-negative organisms release their toxins into the bloodstream, the client develops *septicemia* (infection in the blood). Septicemia in an immunosuppressed host can lead to septic shock. Septic shock is a systemic inflammatory response to infection resulting in inadequate blood flow to the internal organs; unless treated aggressively, it can lead to widespread cell and tissue injury, organ failure, and death. (See in-depth discussion in Chapter 10.)

NOSOCOMIAL INFECTIONS. Nosocomial infections are infections acquired in a health care setting, such as a hospital or long-term care facility. Over 2 million clients a year develop a nosocomial infection while hospitalized. Hospital-acquired infections increase the client's hospital stay and are costly in terms of diagnosis and treatment. The frequency of nosocomial infections varies according to the type of clients, the severity of illness, and the number of health care workers within each facility.

Numerous factors can affect whether the hospitalized client develops a nosocomial infection (Box 12-6). In addition, clients in the hospital are exposed to numerous health care personnel who may transmit microorganisms between clients. Often, visitors carry infectious diseases that they unknowingly transmit to ill clients. Even such items as thermometers, blood pressure cuffs, and wheelchairs also can carry nosocomial organisms. Some of the pathogens that typically cause nosocomial infections include: *Escherichia coli, Stapylococcus aureus,* Group A streptococci, and *Enterococcus.* Urinary tract infections are the number-one infection, usually due to urinary catheterization and urologic procedures. Postoperative infections may result from wound contamination during surgery. For example, *E. coli,* normally found in the colon, is accidentally transferred to another site via contaminated instruments. Other common infection sites are the respiratory tract and the bloodstream.

The nurse assumes a key role in recognizing clients who are at risk for nosocomial infections. It is the nurse's responsibility to use consistently the principles of medical and surgical asepsis and assist other health care personnel to follow these principles when caring for clients. When necessary, limit visitors to prevent overcrowding in the client's room.

Another factor contributing to the rise in nosocomial infections is long-term or inappropriate use of antibiotics. Every time an antibiotic is given, a few hardy bacteria survive. When these bacteria reproduce, they pass along their antibiotic resistance. If a client does not complete the course of antibiotic therapy, an entire generation of resistant bacteria can survive to reproduce. Then, when a new infection occurs, the client may need a stronger antibiotic. This process, if repeated frequently

BOX 12-6
RISK FACTORS FOR NOSOCOMIAL INFECTIONS

- Chronic diseases (e.g., renal disease, lung disease, cancer, AIDS, diabetes, peripheral vascular disease, pressure ulcers, dermatitis)
- Morbid obesity
- Long-term use of corticosteroids, chemotherapy, radiation therapy
- History of frequent antibiotic use
- Major surgery such as cardiothoracic or intra-abdominal surgeries, or organ transplant
- Invasive procedures (e.g., urinary catheter, peripheral and central IV lines, respiratory care procedures, percutaneous endoscopic gastrostomy (PEG) feeding tube, dialysis)
- Prosthetic devices: Vascular grafts, heart valves, orthopedic joints
- Infections in other sites
- Burns
- Length of hospital stay
- Very young and very old age

enough, can establish a pattern of *multidrug resistance*. The most common multidrug-resistant microorganisms include: methicillin-resistant *Staphylococcus aureus* (MRSA) and vancomycin-resistant *Enterococcus* (VRE). MRSA, VRE, and *Clostridium difficile*–associated diarrhea (CDAD, another nosocomial infection) are discussed in the following section.

Methicillin-Resistant *Staphylococcus aureus* (MRSA).

Staphylococci normally live in the mucous membranes of the respiratory tract and on the skin. MRSA is a type of staphylococcal infection that survives the antibiotic methicillin. The general population and health care workers can be silent carriers, because the colonized bacteria grow in the anterior part of the nose.

In health care facilities, MRSA is transmitted on the hands of health care workers. After exposure, it can live on a person's hands for more than 3 hours. Clients with MRSA infections are isolated using contact precautions (see Table 12-7 for further guidelines). When providing direct care, gowns and gloves must be worn. Serious MRSA infections are treated with intravenous vancomycin. However, vancomycin may be losing its effectiveness. Since 1997, four cases of *vancomycin intermediate Staphylococcus aureus (VISA)* have occurred in the United States. They were successfully treated with other antibiotics, but the medical community fears that new, totally antibiotic-resistant microorganisms will emerge.

Vancomycin-Resistant *Enterococcus* (VRE).

Enterococci are primarily found in the GI and female genital tracts as part of the normal flora. VRE, the second most common nosocomial infection, developed in the past 10 years from overuse of different antibiotics. VRE is spread by direct contact from client to client or health care worker to client. The bacteria can live on equipment or environmental surfaces like overbed tables. Clients and health care workers can carry the colonized bacteria into a health care facility.

Once VRE is confirmed, the client is isolated using contact precautions (see Table 12-7). These include wearing gloves and gowns when providing direct care and dedicating essential equipment (a thermometer, blood pressure cuff, and stethoscope) to the affected client.

Clostridium difficile–Associated Diarrhea (CDAD).

Clostridrium difficile is an anaerobic gram-positive bacillus that produces two endotoxins causing damage to the mucosal lining of the bowel. Because the organism forms spores, it can live for months on environmental sources. Antibiotic therapy reduces the bowel's normal flora, allowing the growth of *C. difficile*.

Manifestations may range from mild diarrhea to the life-threatening condition of pseudomembranous colitis. The client is placed in a private room with contact precautions (see Table 12-7). Again, gowns and gloves are worn when providing direct client care. Because CDAD is easily transmitted, equipment such as thermometer, stethoscope, and blood pressure cuff must be left in the client's room. Mild diarrhea is treated with fluid and electrolyte replacement and discontinuation of any antibiotic therapy. Clients with severe cases

receive metronidazole (Flagyl) as well as fluids, electrolytes, and nutritional support.

COMMUNITY-ACQUIRED INFECTIONS. Community-acquired infections are usually referred to as *communicable diseases,* because they can be transmitted to other people. Smallpox, diphtheria, polio, mumps, measles, rubella, pertussis, and tetanus are long-standing communicable diseases. Other community-acquired infections include influenza, community-acquired pneumonia, hepatitis A, and tuberculosis. Smallpox is the only communicable disease to have been completely eradicated. In the United States, most of these communicable diseases are under control through immunization programs. (See Chapter 13 for more information on immunizations.)

Communicable diseases are monitored from an international to a local level. The World Health Organization (WHO) focuses on controlling disease throughout the world. In Atlanta, Georgia, the Centers for Disease Control and Prevention (CDC) (a federal government agency) is responsible for monitoring, controlling, and preventing infectious diseases. It routinely publishes guidelines and recommendations to use in caring for clients with infections. State and local health departments work cooperatively with the CDC to manage diseases in their area. Physicians and health care facilities are expected to report any communicable disease to their local health department.

Emerging Infectious Diseases.

Emerging infectious diseases are defined as diseases that have increased in the past 20 years or threaten to increase in the near future. Several factors contribute to this threat: worldwide food supply and distribution, international travel, increased crowding in cities, resistant microorganisms, and poor sanitation.

Public health officials remain concerned about multidrug-resistant tuberculosis (TB) and HIV. In addition, diarrheal diseases seem to be increasing throughout the world and the United States. Infectious diarrhea results from organisms such as *E. coli, Salmonella, Shigella, Campylobacter,* and *Giardia,* which are transmitted by contaminated food or water.

WHO and CDC are responsible for protecting the public from infectious diseases. The role of nursing is education and prevention of the spread of infectious diseases. Through the efforts of the health care community, the battle against these new infections may be won.

INFECTIOUS PROCESS IN OLDER ADULTS. Infections are a leading cause of disease and death in older adults. Those older than 75 years of age have a higher rate of infections. The geriatric client is especially prone to several infectious diseases. Part of their increased risk is related to physiologic changes of aging. (Common infections in older adults, as well as associated factors, are outlined in Table 12-4 ◆.)

In addition to physiologic changes, the following factors can increase the risk for infectious disease:

- Decreased activity level related to musculoskeletal, neurologic, or balance problems

TABLE 12-4   SPECIAL POPULATION: COMMON INFECTIOUS DISEASES IN OLDER ADULTS, AGE-RELATED CHANGES, AND NURSING IMPLICATIONS

DISEASE WITH CONTRIBUTING FACTORS	AGE-RELATED CHANGES	NURSING IMPLICATIONS
Urinary Tract Infections Leading cause of bacteremia and sepsis. Often due to poor hygiene, improper cleansing after bowel elimination, and the presence of a urinary catheter.	Loss of bladder tone, reduced bladder contractility, and decreased mucosal barrier lead to UTIs. Also, incomplete bladder emptying causes residual urine that provides a breeding ground for bacteria.	Monitor for manifestations of burning and urgency. Teach clients to clean properly after bowel elimination. Increase fluids to increase urinary output unless contraindicated by cardiac status. Provide cranberry juice to reduce UTI. Give antibiotics as ordered.
Pneumonia and Influenza Older adults are prone to community-acquired and nosocomial pneumonia. Influenza A and pneumococcal pneumonia can be deadly to those with chronic cardiac and respiratory diseases.	Decreased ciliary action, poor chest expansion, shallow breathing, and reduced cough inhibit removal of inhaled organisms. Impaired swallow reflex from CVA increases risk of aspiration pneumonia.	Monitor for manifestations of increased respiratory rate, listlessness, anorexia, and confusion. (Cough and pleuritic chest pain are often absent.) Recommend annual influenza vaccine and pneumococcal vaccine every 7 years. Give antibiotics as ordered.
Tuberculosis Increased incidence especially in long-term care facilities. Usually recurs from a previous infection.	Altered immune function with decreased phagocytosis reduces ability to ward off TB infection. See other respiratory changes above.	Monitor for weight loss, anorexia, and weakness. (Classic signs of night sweats and fever are absent.) Give anti-TB drugs and monitor closely for side effects.
Skin Infections Due to *S. aureus* and *Streptococcus* A and B; and fungal infections causing candidiasis.	Thinning of skin, loss of elasticity, and decreased sensation increase the skin's vulnerability and invasion of organisms.	Wash hands for 15 seconds with friction to reduce disease transmission. Give antibiotics or antifungals as ordered.
Herpes Zoster or Shingles Reactivation of a latent varicella (chickenpox) virus.	Altered immune system function reduces ability to prevent virus reactivation.	Give analgesics, steroids, antivirals, and topical ointments to alleviate symptoms.
Decubitus Ulcers Increased risk due to chronic diseases, reduced mobility, dehydration, and poor nutrition.	Thinning of skin, loss of elasticity, and decreased sensation reduce skin integrity.	Maintain skin integrity by: turning, removing wet linens and clothing, using pressure mattresses, and gently massaging reddened skin areas. Perform wound care as indicated.

- Poor nutrition and an increased risk of dehydration
- Chronic diseases, such as diabetes mellitus, cardiac disease, and renal disease
- Chronic medication use
- Lack of recent influenza and pneumococcal vaccinations
- Altered mental status and dementias
- Hospitalization or residence in a long-term care facility

Although the older adult is at increased risk for infection, he or she may not exhibit the classic manifestations of infection. Fever may be mild or absent. (It is not unusual for a client's normal temperature to range from 96 to 98° F.) The white blood cell count may be only slightly elevated. Confusion is a frequent atypical sign of infection in older adults, along with restlessness, fatigue, and mild behavioral changes. Even older adults with sepsis may only appear slightly disoriented and tachypneic.

If an infection is suspected, the physician will order chest x-ray, urinalysis and culture, and complete blood count. The nurse must complete a baseline assessment and be alert for subtle changes in the client's mental status or behavior. Other important data to collect includes: fluid and diet intake, urinary output, respiratory and cardiovascular assessment, and activity level. Early diagnosis and prompt treatment will improve outcomes for the older adult. Nursing implications for common infectious diseases are provided in Table 12-4.

COLLABORATIVE CARE

Most infectious diseases need little or no medical care. However, medical treatment can be lifesaving in an overwhelming infection or an immunocompromised host.

The client's history and manifestations can limit the number of possible infectious agents. Asking about recent activities may provide the necessary clues. For instance, family members who all came down with vomiting and diarrhea within 12 hours after a picnic probably do not have the flu.

Once the infecting agent and disease are identified, the type of therapy is selected for each client. Viral infections may need only supportive care, such as providing rest and fluids. Skin infections may respond to a topical agent. Severe systemic infections may require long-term intravenous antibiotic therapy.

Laboratory and Diagnostic Tests

Laboratory studies assess the client's response to infection, identify the infecting organism, and monitor progress of the medical intervention. The following laboratory tests may be ordered:

- *WBC count* provides clues about the infecting organism and the body's immune response to it (see Table 12-1).

The normal WBC count ranges from 4,500 to 10,000 per mm^3.

- *WBC differential* is also ordered. During acute infections, more mature neutrophils are produced. If the infection is severe, the body may require more neutrophils than are made. The bone marrow responds by releasing immature neutrophils called *bands*. This condition is termed *a shift to the left* (Figure 12-5 ◆). Eventually the band cells mature and assist in fighting the infection.

- *Cultures of the wound, blood, or other infected body fluids* may be obtained. Using sterile technique, a specimen is collected and immediately taken to the laboratory. There, it is placed in or on a special culture medium. The culture is placed in an incubator to encourage growth of the organism outside the body. Most cultures take 24 to 36 hours to grow. Then the culture is examined under the microscope to identify the offending microorganism.

- *Sensitivity studies* determine which antibiotics are most effective against the identified pathogen. Often, several antibiotics are listed. The health care professional selects the appropriate drug based on host and pathogen factors. (See Pharmacology section below for additional information.)

- *Antibiotic peak and trough levels* monitor therapeutic blood levels of a prescribed medication, especially aminoglycosides. It is important to maintain drug levels within a **therapeutic range** (the amount of drug that will effectively destroy pathogens while producing few toxic effects). By measuring blood levels at the predicted *peak* (1 hour after IM injection and 30 minutes after IV infusion) and *trough* (lowest level, usually just before the next scheduled dose), the physician can determine whether the client is maintaining a level within the therapeutic range.

Diagnostic studies may confirm an infectious diagnosis in a specific organ. Two of the common tests are:

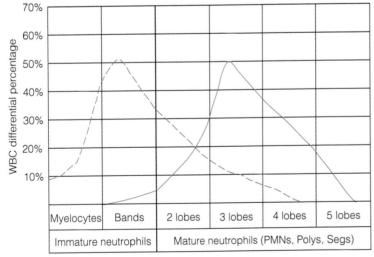

Type of WBC	Normal differential	Shift to left
Myelocytes	0%	Present
Band neutrophils (Bands)	3 to 5%	Increased
Mature neutrophils (Segs, Polys, PMNs)	50 to 65%	May be stable, increased, or decreased

Figure 12-5. ◆ Neutrophils by stage of maturity and normal distribution in the blood versus shift to left caused by severe infection.

■ *Lumbar puncture,* done to obtain cerebrospinal fluid (CSF) for examination and culture if meningitis or encephalitis is suspected

■ *Ultrasound examination,* used to detect abscesses or evaluate organ function. An echocardiogram assesses cardiac function and is ordered when pericarditis, or endocarditis is suspected. Renal ultrasonography may reveal defects in the urinary tract that would predispose the client to infection.

Pharmacology

Management of infectious diseases focuses on administering *antimicrobials* (drugs capable of killing or incapacitating pathogens). Antimicrobial therapy includes antibiotic, antifungal, antiviral, or antiparasitic drugs. Antibiotics are classified according to the way they interfere with bacterial growth. **Bacteriostatic** agents inhibit the growth of microorganisms. Tetracyclines, macrolides, and sulfonamides are bacteriostatic preparations. **Bactericidal** agents kill the microorganism and include penicillin, cephalosporin, and aminoglycoside antibiotics. In addition, antibiotics have either a narrow spectrum or broad spectrum of action. **Narrow-spectrum antibiotics** act against a limited number of pathogens, while **broad-spectrum antibiotics** inhibit a wide variety of microbes.

Antimicrobials can be applied topically or administered by oral, intramuscular, intravenous, interperitoneal, or intrathecal routes. Oral and intravenous routes are most commonly used.

A culture and sensitivity test should be done before antimicrobial therapy is started. If antibiotics are started before the culture is collected, they could interfere with organism growth on the culture medium. When clients are scheduled for surgery or invasive procedures that could cause an infection, they are started on **prophylactic** (preventive) anti-infective therapy.

Selection of an appropriate antimicrobial is based on its effectiveness, low toxicity, ease of administration, and cost effectiveness. The health care professional must also consider several factors about the client, such as:

■ History of allergic reactions
■ Client's age and childbearing status
■ Client's present health status; presence of malnutrition, cancer, or AIDS
■ Renal and hepatic function
■ Site and extent of the infection
■ History of chronic diseases and other drug therapy

Many microorganisms can develop resistance to one or more antimicrobial agents. This means that the pathogen lives and grows in the presence of the antimicrobial. Resistance occurs because the pathogen develops a new form or **mutation,** allowing the organism to survive. Overuse of antibiotics and insufficient medication doses are the most frequent causes.

Several factors contribute to antimicrobial resistance. Clients may expect to receive antibiotics every time they are ill, no matter whether the organism is bacterial or viral. When antibiotics are given for viral infections, bacteria learn to thrive in an antibiotic environment. Also, the use of broad-spectrum rather than narrow-spectrum drugs can lead to multidrug-resistant strains of bacteria.

Finally, the way the client takes an antibiotic can contribute to drug resistance. When a client fails to take all of the prescribed doses, the pathogen is inadequately destroyed, and new microbe mutations can occur. The nurse must teach clients the importance of completing their drug prescriptions.

As with all drug therapy, antimicrobials can cause adverse reactions. Allergic responses, toxicity to the liver, kidneys, ears and bone marrow, and superinfections may develop. A **superinfection** is a new infection that appears because the antibiotic has eliminated normal bacterial flora. For example, yeast infections called candidiasis (or *thrush*) will appear in the mouth or vaginal area.

ANTIBIOTIC DRUGS. Medications used to treat bacterial infections are generally known as **antibiotics.** They were first developed over 50 years ago. New antibiotics are constantly being developed to overcome the multidrug-resistant bacteria. Antibiotics fall into different classes of drugs with related chemical structure and activity. Some are effective only against gram-positive bacteria; others are effective only against gram-negative organisms. Newer broad-spectrum antibiotics have activity against a wide variety of bacteria, including both gram-positive and gram-negative forms. (Antibiotic drugs, action, nursing implications, and client teaching for each class are summarized in Table 12-5 ◆.)

ANTIFUNGAL AGENTS. Fungal infections can be superficial or systemic. Topical antifungal preparations are used to treat superficial infections such as candidiasis, tineas, and ringworm. One of the most frequently ordered drugs is nystatin (Mycostatin) for treating candidiasis. Vaginal preparations are available to treat vaginal yeast infections.

Amphotericin B (Fungizone) is a systemic antifungal agent for parenteral administration. It is used to treat severe, life-threatening fungal infections including histoplasmosis, coccidioidomycosis, and candidiasis. Fluconazole (Diflucan) is preferred over amphotericin B because it is less toxic and is available in oral and parenteral forms. (Nursing responsibilities are listed in Table 12-6 ◆.)

ANTIVIRAL DRUGS. Viral infections can be as mild as the common cold, chronic like herpes infections, or life threatening like acquired immunodeficiency syndrome (AIDS). Antiviral therapy is relatively new and quite limited because new viruses can reproduce before a drug is developed. The drugs in this class are expensive and fairly toxic to the client. Common antiviral agents are summarized in the Table 12-6.

ANTIPARASITIC AGENTS. Drugs used to treat parasitic infections are as varied as the organisms that cause them. Generally, these drugs are expensive and often toxic. Quinine

TABLE 12-5 NURSING IMPLICATIONS FOR PHARMACOLOGY: CLIENTS RECEIVING ANTIBIOTIC THERAPY

CLASS/DRUGS	PURPOSE	NURSING RESPONSIBILITIES	CLIENT TEACHING
Penicillins *Natural* ▪ Penicillin G ▪ Penicillin V *Penicillinase-Resistant* ▪ Cloxacillin (Tegopen) ▪ Dicloxacillin (Dynapen) ▪ Nafcillin (Unipen) ▪ Oxacillin (Prostaphlin) *Ampicillins* ▪ Amoxicillin (Amoxil) ▪ Ampicillin (Polycillin) *Extended-Spectrum* ▪ Carbenicillin (Geocillin) ▪ Mezlocillin (Mezlin) ▪ Piperacillin (Pipracil) ▪ Ticarcillin (Ticar) *Penicillin/* *Beta-Lactamase* *Inhibitors* ▪ Amoxicillin and clavulanate (Augmentin)	Penicillins are bactericidal and effective against streptococci, staphylococci, meningococci, and gonococci organisms. They are safe, effective, and have a low toxicity. Penicillin is ordered in units or milligrams. They are available in PO, IM, and IV forms.	Check for allergies before giving the first dose. Do not give to anyone with an allergy to penicillin or cephalosporins. Assess the client for an allergic response: rashes, hives, and itching. Notify the MD immediately. Monitor for anaphylaxis. In an outpatient setting, ask client to wait 30 minutes after an IM injection. Monitor for white patches in mouth or a vaginal discharge due to candidiasis. An antifungal drug may be needed while the antibiotic is continued.	Take as ordered to prevent developing resistant organisms. Shake suspensions well before pouring them. Take with a full glass of water 1 hour before or 2 hours after meals. If any signs of an allergic reaction occur, stop the drug and contact the physician. Notify the physician if white patches are noted on the oral mucosa or if vaginitis develops. Eat yogurt or buttermilk to prevent fungal infection but do not take these products within 1 hour of taking the drug.
Cephalosporins *First Generation* ▪ Cefadroxil (Duricef) ▪ Cefazolin (Ancef) ▪ Cephalexin (Keflex) *Second Generation* ▪ Cefaclor (Ceclor) ▪ Cefoxitin (Mefoxin) ▪ Cefuroxime (Zinacef) *Third Generation* ▪ Cefoperazone (Cefobid) ▪ Cefotaxime (Claforan) ▪ Ceftazidime (Fortaz) ▪ Ceftizoxime (Cefizox) ▪ Ceftriaxone (Rocephin) *Fourth Generation* ▪ Cefepime (Maxipime)	Cephalosporins are related structurally to the penicillins so there may be a cross-sensitivity between them. First generation act against gram-positive organisms; second and third generation are more effective against gram-negative orgnaisms; fourth generation act against gram-positive and -negative organisms. They are used preoperatively and to treat skin, soft tissue, respiratory and urinary tract.	Check for allergic response to cephalosporins or penicillins. Give with food or milk to reduce GI upset. Give IM injections into large muscle site. Monitor IV site for phlebitis or local pain at IM site. Monitor for decreased output and elevated blood urea nitrogen (BUN) in older clients. Monitor for diarrhea; if blood or mucus appears, notify MD immediately.	Take all of the prescribed drug as ordered. Take with food or milk to reduce GI upset. Eat yogurt or drink buttermilk to prevent oral or vaginal infections. Notify MD if skin rashes, hives, vomiting, severe diarrhea, anal or vaginal itching, or mouth sores develop.

CLASS/DRUGS	PURPOSE	NURSING RESPONSIBILITIES	CLIENT TEACHING
Aminoglycosides ▪ Amikacin (Amikin) ▪ Netilmicin (Netromycin) ▪ Gentamicin (Garamycin) ▪ Streptomycin (Stepolin) ▪ Kanamycin (Kantrex) ▪ Tobramycin (Nebcin)	Aminoglycosides are used against gram-negative organisms; *Pseudomonas, E. coli, Klebsiella.* They are combined with other antibiotics to provide a greater effect.	Monitor for ototoxicity (ringing in the ears) and nephrotoxocity (decreased urine output, elevated BUN and serum creatinine). Monitor peak and trough levels. Increase fluid intake to 2,000–3,000 mL/day. Give IV drugs one hour apart from other IV antibiotics. Give IM deep into a large muscle.	If adverse effects occur, stop the drug and notify the MD. Monitor daily weights. A sudden weight gain may indicate adverse effects on the kidney.
Fluoroquinolones ▪ Ciprofloxacin (Cipro) ▪ Gatifloxacin (Tequin) ▪ Levofloxacin (Levaquin)	Fluoroquinolones act against gram-positive and gram-negative organisms to treat respiratory, GI, and genitourinary (GU) infections. They are given in PO and IV forms.	Increase fluid intake to 2,000–3,000 mL/day. Monitor for decreased urine output.	Check label before taking with food. Drink 6–8 glasses of water per day. Avoid exposure to sunlight; notify MD if skin rashes or redness occur.
Tetracyclines ▪ Tetracycline (Achromycin) ▪ Demeclocycline (Declomycin) ▪ Doxycycline (Vibramycin)	Tetracyclines are active against gram-positive and gram-negative bacteria to treat chlamydia, severe acne, and when the client is allergic to other antibiotics. Tetracyclines should not be used during pregnancy or in children under 5 to prevent tooth discoloration.	Do not give with milk/milk products or antacids. Monitor for signs of epigastric burning, nausea, vomiting, and diarrhea. Monitor for thrush, vaginal or anal itching. Report signs to the physician.	Do not take with milk/milk products or antacids. Take dose with a full glass of water. Avoid sun exposure and wear protective clothing to reduce risk of sunburn. Avoid exposing drug to light, extreme heat, and humidity.
Sulfonamides ▪ Sulfamethiazole (Thiosulfil Forte) ▪ Sulfamethoxazole (Gantanol) ▪ Trimethoprim-sulfamethoxazole (Bactrim, Septra) ▪ Sulfisoxazole (Gantrisin) ▪ Mafenide (Sulfamylon)	Oral sulfonamides treat UTIs by bacteriostatic action. Trimethoprim-sulfamethoxazole is used for *Pneumocystis carinii* pneumonia (PCP). Sulfamylon is applied topically for burns.	Give with a full glass of water. Increase fluid intake to 2,000–3,000 mL/day. Monitor for skin rash, itching, easy bruising, or bleeding gums and notify MD. For burns, apply thin layer of sulfamylon with sterile gloves.	Take drug with full glass of water. Drink 2–3 quarts of fluids per day. Protect skin from sun exposure with clothing and sunscreen to reduce sunburn. Notify physician if skin rash, itching, hives, easy bruising, or bleeding gums develop.

(continues)

TABLE 12-5   NURSING IMPLICATIONS FOR PHARMACOLOGY: CLIENTS RECEIVING ANTIBIOTIC THERAPY (CONTINUED)

CLASS/DRUGS	PURPOSE	NURSING RESPONSIBILITIES	CLIENT TEACHING
Macrolides ■ Erythromycin (E-Mycin, Ilosone) ■ Azithromycin (Zithromax) ■ Clarithromycin (Biaxin)	Macrolides are used for gram-positive and gram-negative organisms causing skin/soft tissue and respiratory infections; for clients allergic to penicillin. Zithromax and Biaxin act longer and have less GI side effects.	Give with a full glass of water. Check whether to give with or without food. Monitor for nausea, vomiting, diarrhea, dark urine, jaundice. Use cautiously in pregnancy and those with liver disease.	Take with a full glass of water. Check label for taking with or without food. Notify physician if GI upset is severe or if dark urine or yellowish-tinge of eyes appear.
Miscellaneous Drugs ■ Metronidazole (Flagyl) ■ Vancomycin (Vancocin)	It is effective for protozoa causing amebiasis, giardiasis, and trichomoniasis. It is given prophylactically for anaerobic gram-negative bacteria before and after colon surgery. It is used for severe gram-positive infections such as MRSA.	Give with meals to decrease GI upset. Inform client that drug causes a metallic taste and urine turns dark. Increase fluid intake to 2,000–3,000 mL/day. Notify MD if dizziness, headache, tingling of extremities, or seizures occur. Give IV dose over 1–2. hours and monitor closely for Red Man syndrome— severe rash, flushing, and hypotension. Monitor for ototoxicity and nephrotoxicity.	Take with meals to decrease GI upset. Drink 2–3 quarts of water daily. Avoid alcohol during therapy to prevent flushing, nausea, vomiting, and headache. Notify physician if dizziness, headache, tingling of extremities, or seizures occur. Take oral doses as prescribed. Report dizziness, tinnitus, or hearing loss immediately.

was one of the first antiparasitic drugs developed to treat malaria. Quinine is very toxic, but newer forms such as chloroquine (Aralen), primaquine, and hydroxychloroquine (Plaquenil) are widely used as antimalarial drugs. Metronidazole (Flagyl) is used to treat protozoan infections and is discussed in Table 12-4.

Infection Prevention and Control Techniques

Prevention is the most important control measure for nosocomial infections and begins with health care workers. Health care personnel wear clean clothing and follow good hygiene practices. Most infectious organisms are spread by direct contact with health care workers. *Effective handwashing (at least 15 seconds, with friction) is the single most important measure in infection control.* They also should keep immunizations current and should not care for clients when ill with an infectious disease or open skin lesions. The nurse also assumes an important role in determining when invasive procedures such as urinary

catheterization are needed. Catheterization increases the incidence of urinary tract infection (UTI), so the nurse must decide whether another choice for managing incontinence might be workable.

Controlling the spread of infectious diseases in the hospital or long-term care setting is essential. Each health care facility follows infection control guidelines developed by the CDC. Each institution also develops its own specific policies for handling biologic waste disposal, housekeeping and sterilization procedures, and employee health standards. Other policies outline the frequency for changing urinary drainage bags or intravenous bags and tubing. For instance, intravenous bags are changed every 24 hours and tubing every 24 to 72 hours.

The Occupational Safety and Health Administration (OSHA) is responsible for reducing the risk of exposure to infectious diseases. It publishes mandatory guidelines about routine training to prevent bloodborne pathogens and TB.

TABLE 12-6 NURSING IMPLICATIONS FOR PHARMACOLOGY: CLIENTS RECEIVING ANTIFUNGAL AND ANTIVIRAL DRUGS

CLASS/DRUGS	PURPOSE	NURSING RESPONSIBILITIES	CLIENT TEACHING
Antifungal Drugs ■ Amphotericin B (Fungizone) ■ Clotrimazole (Lotrimin) ■ Fluconazole (Diflucan) ■ Ketoconazole (Nizoral) ■ Miconazole (Monistat) ■ Nystatin (Mycostatin)	Antifungals treat oral and vaginal candidiasis, ringworm, histoplasmosis, and cryptococcosis. May be applied topically or given PO and IV.	Follow standard precautions when cleaning skin lesions and applying topical medications. Have client swish Nystatin suspension in mouth for 2–3 minutes before swallowing. Premedicate with Tylenol and/or Demerol to prevent rigors with amphotericin B.	For topical agents, wash and dry the area before applying the medication. Swish Nystatin suspension in mouth for 2–3 minutes before swallowing. Follow instructions for using vaginal preparations. Notify physician of unusual fatigue, decreased appetite, vomiting, dark urine, jaundice, or diarrhea.
Antiviral Drugs ■ Amantadine (Symmetrel) ■ Acyclovir (Zovirax) ■ Ganciclovir (Cytovene) ■ Ribavirin (Virazole) ■ Vidarabine (Vir-A) ■ Zidovudine (AZT, Retrovir)	Antivirals treat influenza A, herpesvirus, and opportunistic viral infections in AIDS. Specific antiretroviral drugs reduce viral loads in HIV. May be given PO, IV, or topical.	Apply topical agents with gloves. For IV acyclovir: increase fluid intake to 2,000–3,000 mL/day and monitor for fatigue, headache, and seizures. Monitor for signs of bone marrow suppression. See Chapter 13 for discussion of antiretroviral drugs.	Take drugs as prescribed. Cleanse area and apply topical ointment with gloves. Keep acyclovir in tight, light-resistant container. Report unusual fatigue, headache, and seizures. Discuss sexual abstinence during active herpes infection.

Institutions that do not follow OSHA standards face penalties and fines.

ISOLATION PRECAUTIONS. The CDC developed and implemented two tiers of isolation precautions to be used in health care facilities. These two tiers are: standard precautions and transmission-based precautions. To determine the need for isolation precautions, the nurse must consider the microorganism, the mode of transmission, and susceptibility of hospital staff and other clients. For example, clients with active tuberculosis are highly contagious and must be placed in airborne precautions.

STANDARD PRECAUTIONS. Standard precautions are guidelines to protect the health care worker as well as prevent transmission to other clients. These guidelines are used with all clients, whether they are known to have an infectious disease or not. All health care workers who have direct contact with clients or with their body fluids or have indirect contact, such as by emptying trash, changing linens, or cleaning the room must use standard precautions. Standard precautions apply to (a) blood; (b) all body fluids, secretions and excretions except sweat, regardless of whether they contain visible blood; (c) nonintact skin; and (d) mucous membranes.

Barrier protection prevents exposure of skin and mucous membranes to blood and body fluids. Barrier protection involves using gloves, gowns, masks, or goggles as appropriate. Standard precautions are outlined in Box 12-7.

TRANSMISSION-BASED PRECAUTIONS. Some infectious diseases require added techniques in addition to standard precautions. The three types of **transmission-based precautions** are: airborne precautions, droplet precautions, and contact precautions. Transmission-based precautions may be combined for diseases that have multiple routes of transmission. (Specific guidelines for transmission-based precautions are outlined in Table 12-7 ◆.)

NURSING CARE

Nursing management of clients with an infection or infectious disease focuses on prevention, health promotion, and health maintenance. Prevention includes assessing the client's risk for infection, immune function, and the need for immunizations. Health promotion and maintenance activities include: monitoring vital signs; administering prescribed antibiotics; using aseptic technique and infection control measures; and promot-

BOX 12-7
STANDARD PRECAUTION GUIDELINES

- Wash hands immediately after touching blood, body fluids, secretions and excretions, mucous membranes, nonintact skin, and contaminated items; between client contact; and after removing gloves.
- Wear clean, nonsterile gloves when touching blood, body fluids, secretions and excretions, mucous membranes, nonintact skin, and contaminated items.
- Change gloves between tasks on the same client.
- Wear mask, eye protection, face shield, gown, or plastic apron to avoid being splashed or sprayed with blood, body fluids, secretions, and excretions.
- Remove soiled protective clothing as soon as client care is completed.
- Do not recap or break needles; dispose of needles and other sharp objects in puncture-proof containers. Use one-handed "scoop" technique or a special needle-recapping device.
- Clean spills immediately with 1:10 bleach solution or facility-recommended germicide.
- Handle used client equipment and linen carefully to prevent self- and clothing contamination, and transfer of organisms to other clients. Place in leakproof bags and follow institution's policies regarding double-bagging.
- Place the client, who may contaminate the environment, in a private room with a private bathroom.

Source: Adapted from Taylor, C., Lillis, C., & LeMone, P. (2001). *Fundamentals of nursing* (4th ed.). Philadelphia: Lippincott; and Smith, S., Duell, D., & Martin, B. (2000). *Clinical nursing skills* (5th ed.). Upper Saddle River, NJ: Prentice Hall Health.

ing rest, activity, and nutritional intake. Priority nursing diagnoses are Risk for Infection, Altered Nutrition, and Altered Body Temperature.

ASSESSING

Before implementing nursing care, the nurse must collect assessment data. These data can help determine the extent to which an infection or infectious disease is interfering with the client's life, can identify risk factors for complications, and can be used by the physician to determine the type of medical intervention needed (Box 12-8). The nurse must also assess for risks of nosocomial infection from invasive procedures and therapies.

DIAGNOSING, PLANNING, AND IMPLEMENTING

Individuals with an acute infection or infectious disease may require hospitalization until the crisis is resolved. Those with

chronic infections or side effects from the infectious disease process may need care in long-term care facilities or at home.

RISK FOR INFECTION

Clients may enter health care facilities with inadequate physical defenses, malnutrition, or chronic diseases. In addition, they may be exposed to drug-resistant microorganisms. It is vital that nurses in health care facilities follow all of the standards for infection prevention and control.

- Admit clients with known or suspected infections to a private room. *This minimizes risk to other clients.*
- Wash hands thoroughly on entering and leaving the client's room. *Handwashing removes microorganisms from the skin and prevents transmission of infection to or from the client.*
- Use standard precautions for all clients. *Standard precautions significantly reduce the risk of disease transmission during client care.*
- Use transmission-based precautions when appropriate. *Transmission-based precautions reduce the spread of disease by airborne, droplet, or direct and indirect methods.*
- Explain to the client and family the reasons for isolation precautions. *Clients with isolation precautions may feel neglected or dirty. Explaining the reasons and procedures can enhance understanding and acceptance.*
- Place a mask on the client or cover all infectious lesions or wounds completely when transporting the client to other parts of the facility for diagnostic or treatment procedures. *These measures minimize air contamination and the risk to visitors and personnel.*
- Collect a culture and sensitivity (C&S) specimen as ordered. *C&S can identify infectious organisms and determine the most effective antibiotics.*
- Administer prescribed antimicrobial agents. *Antimicrobial agents are given to destroy invading microorganism.*
- Notify all personnel who have contact with the client about the diagnosis. *Personnel must take appropriate precautions, particularly for clients with diseases requiring category-specific isolation.*
- Make sure that visitors wear appropriate protective garments before they enter the client's room. *Protective wear reduces visitors' risk of infection.*
- Follow facility guidelines for disposal of contaminated tissues, dressings, or other material, and for removal of soiled linens and equipment from the client's room. *These measures prevent the transmission of pathogenic organisms.*

IMBALANCED NUTRITION

Fever, especially prolonged high fever, increases the body's metabolism. Inadequate nutrition may prolong the infectious process.

- Encourage a high-calorie, high-protein diet. *Increased calories and protein are needed to meet increased metabolic demands.*
- Provide liquid or soft, easily digested foods. *Difficult-to-digest foods increase heat production. If the client has a sore throat, liquids and soft food are easier to swallow.*

TABLE 12-7   **TRANSMISSION-BASED PRECAUTIONS**

CATEGORY	INFECTIOUS DISEASES	PURPOSE	PRECAUTIONS
Airborne precautions	Pulmonary tuberculosis, varicella (chickenpox), measles	Reduce transmission of airborne droplets or dust particles containing the infectious agent.	Private room with private bathroom. Use negative pressure (pulls air from hall inward when someone enters the room); otherwise, keep door closed. Particulate air filter for TB cases. Place mask on client if transport needed.
Droplet precautions	Meningitis, pneumonia, influenza, mumps, pertussis, diphtheria, adenovirus	Reduce transmission of large droplets generated during coughing, sneezing, talking, or procedures such as suctioning. Can infect others if droplets land on conjunctivae, nasal mucosa, or mouth.	Private room with bathroom facilities. Wear mask when working within 3 feet of client. Place mask on client if transport is required.
Contact precautions	Acute diarrhea including VRE, CDAD; MRSA; herpes and varicella; respiratory syncytial virus (RSV); skin, wound, or urinary tract infection with multidrug-resistant organisms; *Staphylococcus aureus* infections; hepatitis A in incontinent clients	Reduce transmission by direct skin-to-skin contact or indirect contact with a contaminated object. Direct contact may occur between clients or during direct care activities such as bathing or turning clients.	Private room with bathroom facilities. Don gloves when entering room and remove before leaving room. Change gloves after contact with infective material. Wear gown and gloves when giving direct care or touching contaminated surfaces. Leave blood pressure cuff, stethoscope, and thermometer in room. Wash hands immediately after removing gloves.

- Encourage client to choose appealing foods. *Clients with a systemic infection often lose their appetite. If they can choose foods they like, it may stimulate their appetite.*
- Minimize offensive odors from draining wounds. *Decreasing odors may increase the client's appetite.*

INEFFECTIVE THERMOREGULATION

Clients with an infectious disease usually develop a fever. Although fever serves a useful purpose, abnormally high fevers can put the client at risk for other complications.

- Monitor temperature, pulse, and respirations at regular intervals. *This helps to determine the fever pattern and effects on other body systems.*
- Increase oral fluid intake to 2,500 mL/day, as appropriate, for the client's cardiopulmonary status. *Fever can cause dehydration; increased fluid intake reduces this risk. Fluids are given*

cautiously to clients with cardiopulmonary disease to prevent fluid overload.
- Administer IV fluid and electrolytes as ordered. *If fluid loss is severe, client will need IV electrolyte solutions.*
- Record intake and output at least every 8 hours. *Decreased urine output may indicate dehydration.*
- Give prescribed antipyretics as ordered for an elevated temperature. *Antipyretics lower the body's temperature; however, they decrease WBC activity, especially phagocytosis. Some microorganisms can be destroyed when the body reaches a certain temperature.*
- Provide tepid baths, place ice packs in the groin and axilla, or cover with a hypothermia blanket only if temperature is greater than 104° F. *These methods can reduce fever too rapidly, causing more shivering and increased temperature. Be sure to wrap ice bags in a towel to prevent tissue damage.*
- Maintain bed rest. *Bed rest conserves energy and reduces metabolic demands.*

BOX 12-8
ASSESSING CLIENTS WITH INFECTION

SUBJECTIVE DATA

- Present health status:
  - General health and nutritional status
  - Fever: How long has the fever existed? Has client had chills?
  - Describe cough and/or sputum
  - Sore throat, congestion, runny or stuffy nose
  - Anorexia, nausea, vomiting, abdominal pain, diarrhea
  - Weakness, malaise, muscle aches, joint pains, headache
  - Pain on urination, odor, urgency, frequency, flank pain
  - Vaginal discharge—color, odor, itching
  - Describe any rash
  - Presence of animal or insect bite
- Past medical history:
  - Any infections or exposure to infectious person
  - Treatment for tuberculosis or sexually transmitted disease
  - Has the client been tested for HIV?
  - Use of antipyretics, antimicrobials
  - Immunization history
  - Any travel overseas?

OBJECTIVE DATA

- Vital signs: Blood pressure, pulse, respirations, temperature
- Height and weight
- Observe client for fatigue, shortness of breath, and altered mental status
- Assess for dehydration: increased thirst, dry mucous membranes, decreased skin turgor
- Auscultate chest for crackles and wheezes
- Inspect sputum, stool, genitourinary excretions for amount, color, consistency, and odor
- Inspect throat for redness
- Palpate the skin for the presence of any rash
- Palpate for enlarged lymph nodes

- When the client becomes diaphoretic, bathe and replace wet gowns and linen. *Personal hygiene promotes client comfort.*
- Monitor the client for decreased level of consciousness and seizures. *High fevers can cause dehydration, leading to an altered mental status and seizures.*

EVALUATING

Evaluate effectiveness of nursing care by collecting the following data: temperature remains normal for 24 hours, no signs of dehydration, clear breath sounds, and cultures negative for pathogens. Also, evaluate whether the client takes precautions to prevent spread of an infection and is completing any ordered antibiotics.

Discharge Considerations

Client and family teaching focuses on promoting client recovery, preventing spread of infection to others, and preventing potential complications. Box 12-9 outlines assessment data to consider for discharge planning.

Include the following verbal and written instructions:

- Wash hands after touching infected wounds or lesions, coughing, sneezing, blowing the nose, using the bathroom, before preparing food or eating, or before wound care.
- Take all prescribed antibiotics until the prescription is completed even after symptoms are relieved. Notify your health care provider if any of the following occurs:
  - No improvement in symptoms within 24 to 48 hours after antibiotic therapy is started, or recurring symptoms after antibiotic therapy is completed.

BOX 12-9
ASSESSING FOR DISCHARGE

INFECTION
Client

- Self-care: Ability to perform ADLs independently; to plan rest periods and prepare nutritional meals; to self-administer prescribed medications; to monitor temperature
- Knowledge: Disease process; prescription and over-the-counter medications; well-balanced diet; need for current immunizations; indications for seeking medical care
- Home environment: Appropriate heating and cooling; access to clean water for drinking and handwashing; safe environment to minimize risk of injury

Family

- Members of household: Individuals with infections
- Caregivers: Availability and willingness to provide care as needed; ability to apply infection control precautions; assist with meals and home maintenance; ability to administer long-term antimicrobial therapy; restrict visitors with infections
- Financial resources: Income; availability of sick leave; resources for drugs and medical care needed

Community

- Access to health care resources

- Itching, rash, difficulty breathing; signs of superinfection such as vaginitis, oral candidiasis, or diarrhea; persistent high fever, change in alertness, or activity.
- Adverse reactions, such as gastrointestinal distress, that interferes with completion of the prescription.

- Do not share medication with family members or others.
- Wear Medic-Alert bracelet noting medication allergies.
- Increase fluid intake to at least 2.5 quarts per day and eat a well-balanced diet.
- Prevent the spread of infection to others by:
  - Avoiding crowds and contact with infectious persons
  - Using disposable tissues when coughing or sneezing
  - Practicing safe food handling practices
  - Not sharing personal hygiene items
  - Using safe sex practices
  - Keeping the home clean; disinfecting with 1:10 bleach solution for blood spills
- Keep immunizations current. If they are not up to date, discuss where immunizations can be obtained.

Nursing Process Case Study
■ CLIENT WITH MRSA INFECTION

Mr. Frank Kendall, 87 years old, is transferred from a nearby long-term care facility to the medical unit of the community hospital. Mr. Kendall has been in the long-term care facility for 6 months following a cerebrovascular accident (CVA). Two months ago he was in the hospital for urosepsis. He has been widowed for 9 months. One daughter lives 1,000 miles away and has visited him only once in the past 6 months.

The nurse from the long-term care facility reports that he is too weak to get out of bed by himself. He has a poor appetite and seems frail. About 1 month ago he developed a large decubitus ulcer on the sacral area that is not healing.

Assessment   On admission, vital signs are: BP 150/84, P 92, R 24, T 100° F (37.7° C), weight 165 lbs., and height 5′10″. He is listless, with decreased right arm and leg movement, thin extremities, and poor skin turgor. He answers the nurse's questions without looking at her. The decubitus ulcer on the sacral area measures 7 cm long, 4 cm wide, 1.5 cm deep, with yellowish-green drainage. The wound edges are red and tender. He grimaces as the nurse assesses the wound. An intravenous line is inserted and 5% dextrose/0.45 normal saline is started at 75 mL/hour. After 24 hours a preliminary culture report shows MRSA in the decubitus ulcer. The nurse implements contact precautions for Mr. Kendall.

Diagnosis   The following nursing diagnoses are developed for Mr. Kendall:

- Imbalanced Nutrition: Less Than Body Requirements related to poor appetite

- Impaired Skin Integrity related to large decubitus ulcer
- Acute Pain related to decubitus ulcer
- Hopelessness related to recent widowhood and CVA

Expected Outcomes   The expected outcomes established in the plan of care specify that:

- Mr. Kendall will increase dietary intake.
- Wound will show signs of healing.
- Wound cultures will no longer show a MRSA infection.
- Mr. Kendall will report that pain is decreased.
- He will communicate feelings about his situation.

Planning and Implementation   Ms. Thompson, RN, implements the following interventions:

- Monitor daily weight, intake and output, and hydration status.
- Assess for risk of aspiration during eating and drinking.
- Identify foods Mr. Kendall likes and dislikes.
- Provide small, frequent, high-protein meals.
- Consult with a dietitian regarding supplemental foods such as Ensure.
- Monitor serum albumin levels.
- Assess skin every 8 hours; keep clean and dry.
- Turn at least every 2 hours; minimize time Mr. Kendall lies on his back; and prevent shearing.
- Consult with physician for an air/water mattress or specialized bed (e.g., Clinitron Bed).
- Follow contact precautions; meticulously wash hands before and after care.
- Premedicate before dressing changes or wound care.
- Use aseptic technique to provide wound care to decubitus ulcer.
- Administer antibiotics as ordered.
- Determine level of pain using a 0 to 10 pain scale.
- Administer pain medications PRN.
- Encourage Mr. Kendall to discuss his feelings and concerns.
- Arrange for social services to talk to his daughter.

Evaluation   After a month in the hospital Mr. Kendall's wound culture is negative for MRSA. The wound is showing signs of healing. His daughter has visited him twice. He smiles occasionally and interacts with the staff more positively. Mr. Kendall's appetite has improved and he no longer needs supplemental feedings. He reports that his pain is tolerable. He understands that he has to return to the long-term care facility until his wound heals completely. His daughter plans to move him to her home sometime in the near future.

Critical Thinking in the Nursing Process

1. What type of isolation garments should the nurse wear while providing care to Mr. Kendall?
2. How did Mr. Kendall contract MRSA?
3. List three strategies to prevent the transmission of MRSA to other clients.

Nursing Interventions Classification

The following nursing interventions (McCloskey & Bulechek, 2000) may be considered for the client with inflammation and infection:

- Fluid Monitoring
- Wound Care
- Wound Irrigation
- Health Education

(*Note:* The bibliography listings for this and all chapters have been compiled at the back of the book.)

Chapter Review

 ## key terms by topic

Use the CD-ROM disk enclosed with your textbook to hear the pronunciation of the key terms in the chapter.

Inflammation
inflammation, diapedesis, macrophages, phagocytosis

Acute inflammation
cellulitis, abscesses, incision and drainage, fistula, lymphadenitis, leukocytosis, endogenous pyrogens

Chronic inflammation
catabolism, anabolism

Infection
infection, immunosuppression, pathogens, virulence, invasiveness, exotoxins, endotoxins, carriers, colonization, leukopenia

Collaborative care of infections
therapeutic range, bacteriostatic, bactericidal, narrow-spectrum antibiotics, broad-spectrum antibiotics, prophylactic, mutation, superinfection, antibiotics

Infection control
standard precautions, transmission-based precautions

key points

- The body is protected from microorganisms by the skin, physical barriers such as coughing, and chemical defenses.

- Cardinal manifestations of local inflammation are: redness, warmth, pain, edema, and loss of function.

- The chain of infection includes a microorganism, a reservoir, a portal of exit from the reservoir, a mode of transmission from the reservoir, and an entry point into a susceptible host.

- Fever and WBC count greater than 10,000/mm³ may indicate a generalized infection.

- Antibiotics, antiviral, antifungal, and anti-parasitic medications are the common medications used to manage infections.

- Older adults are at greater risk for developing pneumonia, influenza, and urinary tract and skin infections.

- Handwashing is the most important measure in preventing nosocomial infections.

- Two tiers of isolation are (1) standard precautions, and (2) transmission-based precautions.

 ## Medialink

Additional interactive resources for this chapter can be found on the Companion Website at www.prenhall.com/burke. Click on Chapter 12 and "Begin" to select the activities for this chapter.

For NCLEX review questions and an audio glossary, access the accompanying CD-ROM in this book.

for further study

For more on the healing process and wound care, see Chapter 7.

For more on the client receiving corticosteroid medications, see Table 16-4.

For in-depth discussion on septic shock, see Chapter 10.

For more information on immunizations, see Chapter 13.

Critical Thinking Care Map

Caring for a Client Exposed to *Staphylococcus aureus*
NCLEX-PN Focus Area: Reduction of Risk Potential

Case Study: Mr. Fields, age 76, was transferred from a long-term nursing care facility for a mild left-side stroke. He has an intravenous line and Foley catheter in place. Mr. Fields weighs 140 lbs. and is 6′ tall. He shares a hospital room with another client who is diagnosed with *Staphylococcus aureus* pneumonia. Mr. Fields's vital signs are BP 158/90, P 88, R 24, T 99° F.

Nursing Diagnosis: Risk for Infection

COLLECT DATA

Subjective	Objective
_____	_____
_____	_____
_____	_____
_____	_____
_____	_____
_____	_____

Would you report this data? Yes/No

If yes, to: _____

Nursing Care

_____
_____
_____
_____
_____
_____
_____
_____

How would you document this? _____
_____
_____

Data Collected
(use those that apply)

- Roommate with *S. aureus* pneumonia
- Pale coloring
- Weight 140 lbs.
- Urine output 200 mL for shift
- Temperature 99° F
- Dislikes being in the nursing home
- Pressure ulcer on right great toe
- History of Type 2 diabetes

Nursing Interventions
(use those that apply)

- Provide a diet high in protein.
- Place in protective isolation.
- Monitor vital signs every 4 hours.
- Monitor skin for further breakdown.
- Increase fluid intake as tolerated.
- Prevent food from pocketing on the right side of his mouth.

NCLEX-PN Exam Preparation

1. A client, age 82, has been admitted to your surgical unit after 3 days in the intensive care unit. You note that his medical diagnosis is currently status-post left inguinal hernia repair. His vital signs are stable and his urinary bag contains 300 mL of clear yellow urine. Which of the following would be the most important information in determining if the client is at risk for developing a nosocomial infection?
   a. Foley catheter insertion during surgery
   b. use of an antibiotic for one week prior to surgery
   c. weight of 150 lbs.
   d. poor venous circulation in the left leg

2. Your client is scheduled for a routine appendectomy. Which of the following lab values must you report to the physician immediately?
   a. WBC count of 7,000
   b. WBC count of 3,500
   c. WBC count of 15,000
   d. WBC count of 4,500

3. Prior to the administration of aspirin to your client with rheumatoid arthritis, it is most important to assess:
   a. the age of the client
   b. the client's use of alcohol
   c. the expiration date of the medication
   d. the client's allergy history

4. A client has been taking penicillin G for a staph infection. Three days after beginning the drug, she returns to your clinic. She complains of vaginal itchiness and redness. You suspect that the client has developed vaginitis. Your response to the client should be:
   a. "Oh, don't worry about that. It will go away after you finish the medication."
   b. "I will let the doctor know right away."
   c. "Its just vaginitis. We'll give you something for it."
   d. "Okay. Are you having any other problems?"

5. You are planning discharge care for your client who has suffered numerous abrasions sustained in a motor vehicle accident. Which of the following should be included in the discharge instructions?
   a. Discontinue the antibiotics once the redness has subsided.
   b. A slight fever is common and should not be reported.
   c. Drink at least 2 quarts of water per day.
   d. Wash your hands carefully before changing the wound dressings.

6. Which medication treatment would the nurse anticipate for the client with a diagnosis of MRSA?
   a. vancomycin (Vancocin)
   b. erythromycin (E-Mycin)
   c. fluconazole (Diflucan)
   d. acyclovir (Zovirax)

7. A 70-year-old male client was admitted to the medical floor with a diagnosis of left periorbital cellulitis. Based on this diagnosis, which of the following interventions should the nurse include in the client's care plan in order to promote the healing process?
   a. Administer IV antibiotics as ordered.
   b. Maintain bed rest.
   c. Medicate the client around the clock with IM morphine.
   d. Monitor the WBC count.

8. Which of the following conditions indicate that an infection has become systemic?
   a. A fistula forms.
   b. Lymphadenitis is observed.
   c. Abscesses form in the area of infection.
   d. Cellulitus begins to develop.

9. Your AIDS client has been diagnosed with *Pneumocystis carinii*. Your client asks you what type of "bug" causes this illness. You state that *Pneumocystis carinii* is a:
   a. virus
   b. fungus
   c. bacteria
   d. protozoa

10. An elderly woman was admitted on your shift with varicella. You have been delegated to prepare her room. Knowing the transmission of the varicella virus, you obtain the following sign from the infection control nurse:
    a. droplet precautions
    b. contact precautions
    c. airborne precautions
    d. standard precautions

Cultural Care STRATEGIES

Considering Cultural Variations Related to Environmental Control

Mrs. Jones, 43, a white woman from Appalachia, is admitted to a small Appalachian hospital in respiratory distress and reports she has had difficulty getting her breath for the past 3 days. She has a persistent cough, which she reports having had for 8 months. The nurse doing the admission notes that she is emaciated, has ashen color, tires easily, and has a productive cough. When the nurse asks why she has not sought treatment, she responds, "Sickness is God's will. Whatever will be will be. I have tried some herbal remedies but they have not done much good. It is my time to go. I guess I'm ready, although I wish I could stay and see my children get married."

Environmental control refers to the ability of a person to plan activities that control nature. Environmental control also refers to people's perception that they can direct factors in the environment. Feelings of control are an important part of responding to illness and of taking actions to promote health. Thus, it is important to assess each client for beliefs related to locus of control.

Locus of Control

Individuals may be described as having internal or external locus of control (Rotter, 1966). An individual who feels that actions and outcomes are related to *internal control* feels some power over future behaviors and situations. Personal actions are considered to be important in influencing events.

The term *external control* describes the belief that events are unpredictable and are influenced by outside forces such as luck, change, or fate. Individuals who believe in external feelings of control believe that efforts and rewards are not related to each other.

The locus-of-control construct can be applied to a variety of phenomena including the weather, preventive health, curative actions, and feelings of well-being (Giger & Davidhizar, 1999). An individual who believes in internal locus of control is more likely to comply with treatment and to take preventive actions related to future health. On the other hand, an individual who believes that compliance with treatment and health are unrelated will have little motivation to develop behaviors that influence the future or enhance health.

The culturally competent nurse should be aware that people with an Appalachian, Hispanic, or Puerto Rican cultural orientation may have an external locus of control. Northern Europeans or African-Americans may have either an internal or external locus of control (Kluckhohn & Strodtbeck, 1961).

Many North Americans have a strong internal locus of control and believe they are in control of their own destiny. The beliefs of some Native-Americans, Chinese-Americans, and Japanese-Americans do not include the locus-of-control construct, but focus on harmony with nature.

Folk or traditional medicine beliefs and practices may be part of a person's world view and belief about what will influence health. Folk medicine beliefs classify illness or diseases as natural or unnatural. Folk medicine differs from Western medicine in the way in which illness is explained and treated. Alternative and traditional therapies provide options for treatment other than relying on medication or surgery.

Nursing Implications

- **Assess the client for locus of control.** The nurse needs to appreciate that individuals differ, and that actions to seek health care or to promote health may depend on culturally based locus-of-control orientation.
- **Show respect for folklore and folklore practices.** The nurse should appreciate that persons from diverse cultural backgrounds may have deeply ingrained beliefs about how to attain and maintain health. These beliefs may be linked to the natural and supernatural worlds, may adversely affect the physician–client or nurse–client relationship, and may influence the individual's decision to follow or not to follow prescribed treatment recommendations.
- **Try to incorporate folklore practices with Western medicine.** Rather than disregarding folklore practices, it is important to incorporate beliefs of the client with practices of Western medicine. When folk beliefs of the client are respected and incorporated into the nurse's plan of care, the client may be more cooperative and have a better response to nursing interventions.

Self-Reflective Questions

1. What are your beliefs about internal or external locus of control?
2. Can you relate your beliefs to early parental teaching?
3. Do you have any folk beliefs that are outside the scope of Western medicine?
4. What folk beliefs have you encountered in your client interactions?

chapter 13

Caring for Clients
with Altered Immunity

LEARNING outcomes

After completing this chapter, you will be able to:

- Describe the functions of the lymphoid organs and tissues.
- Compare natural and acquired immunity and active and passive immunity.
- List recommended immunizations for adult clients.
- Identify laboratory and diagnostic tests used to diagnose and monitor immune response.
- Describe the nursing implications for medications ordered for clients with altered immunity.
- Teach clients with altered immune responses and their families.
- Use the nursing process to collect data, establish outcomes, provide individualized care, and evaluate responses for the client experiencing altered immunity.
- Identify three ways to prevent the transmission of HIV infection.
- Identify laboratory tests used to diagnose HIV and to monitor HIV progression.
- Provide the nursing management of a client with AIDS, including medications and diet therapy.

MediaLink

 www.prenhall.com/burke

Use the above address to access the free, interactive Companion Website created for this textbook. Get hints, instant feedback, and textbook references to chapter-related multiple choice questions. Link to other interesting sites.

The human body is constantly bombarded by foreign invaders such as bacteria, viruses, parasites, insect venoms, and transfusions. Because the body provides the perfect host environment, microbes try to break through the skin and mucous membrane barriers. The role of the immune system is either to keep out the foreign substances or, once they break through the defenses, to destroy them.

Sometimes the immune system malfunctions causing allergies or autoimmune diseases like rheumatoid arthritis. Newer emerging diseases, such as human immunodeficiency virus (HIV) infection and multiple-drug-resistant tuberculosis, also affect the immune system.

Overview of the Immune System

The immune system is a complex network of cells and organs that protect the body against infection-causing microorganisms, foreign substances, and cancerous cells. Three defense mechanisms provide this protection. The first line of defense involves the skin, mucous membranes, and body secretions. If these defenses are penetrated, the body's inflammatory response is activated within seconds as the second line of defense. It is a nonspecific response in which white blood cells engulf and neutralize any harmful invaders. (See Chapter 12 for more information on inflammation.) A much slower response involves the third line of defense: immunity. The immune response provides specific immunity with T lymphocytes and B lymphocytes.

The immune system can recognize the body's own cells (self) and foreign cells (nonself). Normally, the body's immune defenses coexist peacefully with any cell marked as "self." When any nonself substance (**antigen**) invades the body, the immune system responds. Antigens can be bacteria, viruses, or tissues transplanted from another person. If the immune system perceives transplanted tissues or organs as nonself, they may be rejected. Sometimes, harmless substances such as dog hair or pollen set up an allergic response. This kind of antigen is called an **allergen**. In other circumstances, the immune system mistakes self for nonself and attacks it. The result is autoimmune diseases.

IMMUNE SYSTEM COMPONENTS

The immune system consists of cells and organs that produce the immune response. These components may be involved in the nonspecific inflammatory response, the specific immunologic response, or both.

Leukocytes

Leukocytes, or white blood cells (WBCs), are the primary cells involved in nonspecific and specific immune system responses. Leukocytes start as stem cells in the bone marrow. They move throughout the body by the circulatory system. This mobility allows them to detect, attack, and destroy any foreign invaders at the site of involvement.

The normal number of circulating leukocytes is 4,500 to 10,000 cells per mm^3 of blood as indicated on the WBC count. If an infection develops, additional WBCs are released from the bone marrow, leading to leukocytosis. The WBC differential test identifies the percent of the total number of WBCs for each type of granulocyte.

From the original stem cells, leukocytes develop into three major groups of WBCs: granulocytes, monocytes, and lymphocytes (Table 13-1 ◆). Granulocytes make up the greatest number of normal blood leukocytes. Monocytes are the largest leukocyte. Lymphocytes are subdivided into B-cell lymphocytes, T-cell lymphocytes, and natural killer (NK) cells (Figure 13-1 ◆). T cells and B cells are the basis for the specific immune response and are discussed further in this chapter.

Natural killer cells survey the body for potential foreign invaders such as viruses and malignant cells. Unlike B and T cells, which attack only specific infected cells or malignant cells, natural killer cells can attack any target identified as foreign. They assume a key role in destroying early malignant cells. The functions of all leukocytes are closely interrelated.

Lymphoid Organs and Tissues

The organs and tissues of the immune system are found throughout the body. They are called lymphoid organs because they are home to the lymphocytes. The *lymphoid system* consists of the bone marrow, thymus, spleen, lymph nodes, and lymphoid tissue scattered in the connective tissues and mucosa (Figure 13-2 ◆). The bone marrow and thymus are considered primary or central lymphoid organs. The spleen, lymph nodes, and other peripheral lymphoid tissue (e.g., the tonsils and appendix) are secondary lymphoid organs.

Bone marrow is the soft tissue in the hollow center of all bones. Red bone marrow produces blood cells from the stem cells. In adults, red marrow is located in the ends of the long bones, as well as in the pelvis, skull, sternum, ribs, and vertebrae. Yellow bone marrow is found in the other bones; it stores fat for an energy reserve.

The *thymus gland* is located in the neck area above the heart and behind the sternum. The gland is fully developed at puberty, and gradually decreases in size and function over a person's life span. Its main function is to mature lymphocytes into T cells.

The *spleen,* the largest lymphoid organ, is found in the upper left quadrant of the abdomen. The spleen has both white pulp and red pulp. White pulp contains macrophages, which destroy bacteria in the blood. Red pulp filters out damaged or aged RBCs and stores blood for future use. The spleen is not essential for life. If it is removed, the liver and the bone marrow assume its functions.

The *lymphatic system* includes the lymph nodes, lymphatic vessels, and lymph. *Lymph* is a clear, protein-containing fluid. *Lymphatic vessels* transport lymph to the lymph nodes. *Lymph nodes,* small bean-shaped encapsulated tissues, are distributed

TABLE 13-1

CELLS OF THE IMMUNE SYSTEM

TYPE OF LEUKOCYTE	FUNCTION
Granulocytes	Involved in inflammatory response; make up 60–80% of normal blood leukocytes
▪ Neutrophils	First to appear after an injury; involved in phagocytosis
▪ Eosinophils	Involved in phagocytosis; protect against parasites; part of allergic response
▪ Basophils	Protect mucosal surfaces; secrete histamine during allergic reactions
Monocytes	Involved in inflammatory response; mature into macrophages
	Trap and phagocytize foreign substances and cellular debris
Lymphocytes	Involved in specific immune response; make up 20–40% of circulating leukocytes
▪ T Lymphocytes	Provide cell-mediated immunity: Mature in thymus gland
▪ Helper T Cells (T4)	Turn on immune system function
	Stimulate B cells to produce antibodies
	Release lymphokines to destroy viral infections and cancer cells
	Involved in hypersensitivity reactions and graft tissue rejection
▪ Suppressor T Cells (T8)	Turn off immune system function
▪ Cytotoxic T Cells	Kill tumor cells, viral-infected cells, and foreign tissue
▪ B Lymphocytes	Responsible for humoral immunity; mature in bone marrow
▪ Plasma Cells	Produce antibodies (immunoglobulins)
▪ Memory Cells	Produce specific antibody when reexposed to a specific antigen
▪ Natural Killer Cells	Kill virus-infected and tumor cells

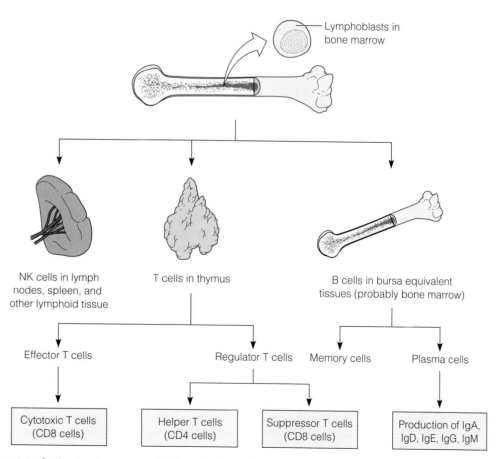

Figure 13-1. ◆ The development and differentiation of lymphocytes from the lymphoid stem cell (lymphoblasts).

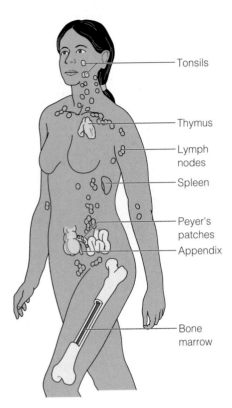

Figure 13-2. ◆ The lymphoid system: the central organs of the thymus and bone marrow, and the peripheral organs, including the spleen, tonsils, lymph nodes, and Peyer's patches.

Labels: Tonsils, Thymus, Lymph nodes, Spleen, Peyer's patches, Appendix, Bone marrow

throughout the body (concentratetd in the neck, axillae, abdomen, and groin). In the lymph nodes, T and B lymphocytes and macrophages filter out and destroy foreign products. The lymph nodes can become tender and palpable when a person develops a systemic infection. Clumps of specialized lymphoid tissue are also located in the tonsils, adenoids, appendix, and Peyer's patches in the intestines. They protect the body from inhaled foreign agents or ingested pathogens.

Recognition of Self

The effectiveness of the immune system depends on whether it can differentiate normal body tissue (self) from foreign tissue (nonself). Each body cell has cell surface markers that are unique to each person. These are known as *human leukocyte antigens (HLA).* A person's HLA characteristics are coded within a large cluster of genes known as the *major histocompatibility complex (MHC).* The possibility of two people having the same HLA is rare except in identical twins. Some siblings may have similar HLA. In organ transplants, matching the HLA as closely as possible tends to decrease rejection.

HUMORAL IMMUNITY AND CELL-MEDIATED IMMUNITY

When antigens enter the body, a specific immune response occurs. The immune system recognizes the particular antigens (viruses, bacteria, or transplanted tissue) and destroys them without harming itself. Unlike a localized inflammatory response, the immune response is systemic. The immune

response also has memory. Repeated exposures to an antigen produce a more rapid response.

A person whose immune system identifies and effectively destroys antigens is said to be **immunocompetent.** When the immune response is altered, health problems such as hypersensitivity (allergy and autoimmune disorders) may occur. Immunodeficiency diseases or malignancies develop when the immune system is incompetent or cannot respond effectively.

Humoral Immunity

B lymphocytes (B cells) are responsible for humoral immunity. When an antigen enters the body, T cells activate B cells, which differentiate into plasma cells and memory cells (Figure 13-3 ◆). Plasma cells produce antibodies or **immunoglobulins** (Ig) that are released into the bloodstream.

An **antibody** is an immunoglobulin molecule that binds to and inactivates a specific antigen. Immunoglobulins make up the gamma globulin portion of the blood proteins. Antibodies fall into five classes of immunoglobulins: IgG, IgM, IgA, IgD, and IgE. Each has a slightly different structure and function (Table 13-2 ◆).

Memory cells remember a prior exposure to a particular antigen even if they have been inactive for years. When exposed to the same antigen, they convert into plasma cells and inactivate the antigen. This rapid response means that either a person avoids the disease or the second infection is milder. Memory cells are responsible for acquired immunity against diseases like measles or chickenpox.

Cell-Mediated Immunity

T lymphocytes (T cells) are the foundation for cell-mediated or cellular immunity (Figure 13-4 ◆). There are three types of T cells: (1) helper T cells, (2) suppressor T cells, and (3) cytotoxic T cells.

Helper T cells, also known as CD4+ cells, are responsible for switching on the immune system. They also recognize antigens such as a virus or transplanted tissue. **Suppressor T cells (CD8 cells)** limit the immune response so that the body does not destroy itself. These cells are important in preventing autoimmune disorders. **Cytotoxic T cells** can destroy cancer cells, cells of transplanted organs, and grafted tissues. They are vital in the control of viral and bacterial infections.

IMMUNE FUNCTION IN THE OLDER ADULT

As immune function declines with aging, there is an increased susceptibility to infections and a diminished immune response. The thymus gland atrophies and, by age 60, thymic hormone secretions stop. Although the total number of T cells remains the same, T cell function and reproduction decrease. T lymphocytes cannot eliminate foreign invaders as well as when the person was younger.

With these changes, cell-mediated immune function declines. Immune memory against such diseases as chickenpox and tuberculosis weakens. In the older person, reactivation of the chickenpox virus leads to herpes zoster (shingles). Immunoglobulins, especially IgG, decrease, followed by a

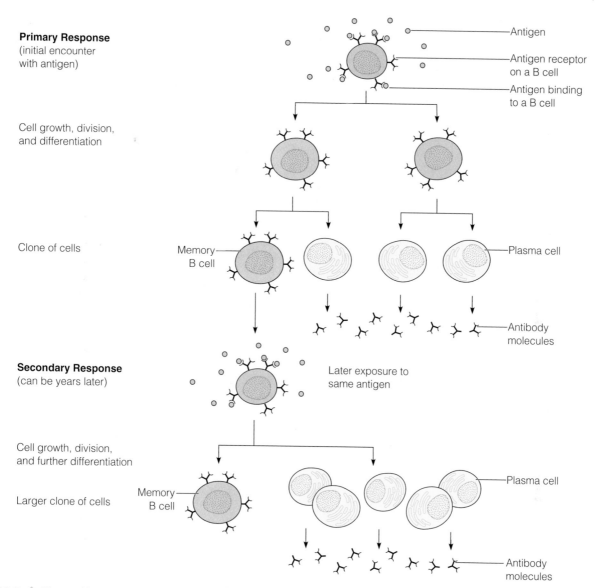

Primary Response (initial encounter with antigen)

Antigen

Antigen receptor on a B cell

Antigen binding to a B cell

Cell growth, division, and differentiation

Clone of cells

Memory B cell

Plasma cell

Antibody molecules

Secondary Response (can be years later)

Later exposure to same antigen

Cell growth, division, and further differentiation

Larger clone of cells

Memory B cell

Plasma cell

Antibody molecules

Figure 13-3. ◆ Humoral immunity. *Primary response:* During first exposure to an antigen, B cells are stimulated to become plasma cells and produce antibodies or memory cells. *Secondary response:* With reexposure to the same antigen, the memory cells respond rapidly with antibody production.

reduced antibody response to influenza, tetanus, and pneumococcus immunizations.

There is also a rise in autoantibody production that may increase the potential for autoimmune diseases. Some autoimmune diseases (such as myasthenia gravis, rheumatoid arthritis, and multiple sclerosis) start in young adulthood or middle age and cause progressive damage.

External factors that may influence immune function include exposure to excessive ultraviolet radiation, environmental pollution, and poor nutrition. An older person's genetic background and history of chronic and past illness may also impair the immune system. Even with all of these influences, some older individuals have an immune system as effective as that of younger persons.

Natural and Acquired Immunity

There are three types of immunity: natural, active, and passive. Immunity results from activating humoral or cell-mediated responses. In the immunocompetent client, the immune response eliminates the antigen and either prevents the disease or promotes recovery.

PATHOPHYSIOLOGY

Natural immunity or innate immunity is a person's resistance to foreign substances, which occurs because of gender, race, heredity, age, or health status. Natural immunity does

TABLE 13-2	IMMUNOGLOBULIN CHARACTERISTICS AND FUNCTIONS	
CLASS	PERCENTAGE OF TOTAL	CHARACTERISTICS AND FUNCTION
IgG	75%	Found in intravascular and interstitial compartments Most abundant Ig; also known as gamma globulin Active against bacteria, bacterial toxins, and viruses Crosses placenta providing immune protection to neonate
IgA	10–15%	Found in saliva, sweat, tears, mucus, bile, colostrum, and vaginal secretions Provides local protection to prevent entry of bacteria and viruses especially through the respiratory and gastrointestinal tracts
IgM	5–10%	High concentrations in the blood; less in the lymph First antibody formed and lasts about 1 week Reacts effectively against bloodborne bacteria and viruses.
IgD	1%	Found on surface of B cells Exact function unknown; may bind antigens to B-cell surface
IgE	< 1%	Found on mast cells and basophils Stimulates release of chemical mediators such as histamine, and bradykinin that cause allergic reactions and hypersensitivity responses such as anaphylaxis Acts in preventing helminth (worm) infections

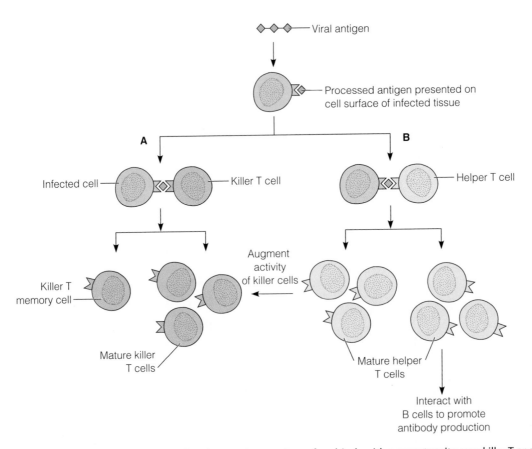

Figure 13-4. ◆ Cellular immunity. (A) An infected cell with an antigen on its surface binds with a receptor site on a killer T or a helper T cell. The killer T cell produces memory cells or mature cytotoxic cells. (B) The helper T cell assists the cytotoxic activity of the killer cells and stimulates B cells to produce antibodies.

not produce an immune response. Individuals are naturally protected because of their physical and chemical barriers.

Active immunity can be *naturally acquired* by actually developing the disease or *artificially acquired* through an immunization. Either way, the body produces plasma and memory cells against specific antigens. Children may naturally acquire active immunity when exposed to mumps or measles. If reexposed later in life, the memory cells should protect them against these diseases. Active immunity can last from years to a lifetime, depending on the disease.

Immunization or vaccination against highly contagious diseases like influenza provides artificially acquired active immunity. Immunizations require the body to actively initiate an immune response. This process can take days to weeks to complete. Vaccines do not produce disease but rather stimulate the B cells to remember a specific disease.

Passive immunity involves injecting serum with ready-made antibodies from other humans or animals. Once these antibodies are used up (a few weeks or months), their protection is lost. For example, human immune globulin or gamma globulin is given to clients when they are exposed to hepatitis A. This is known as *artificially acquired* passive immunity. *Naturally acquired* passive immunity occurs when neonates receive antibodies from their mothers via the placenta.

COLLABORATIVE CARE

Collaborative care focuses on assessing the client's immune status and promoting acquired immunity to prevent disease.

Laboratory and Diagnostic Tests

- *Serum immunoglobulins* measure the level of IgA, IgD, IgE, IgG, and IgM (see Table 13-2). IgG levels are increased during acute infections. Decreased levels of IgG, IgA, and IgM are found in malignancies.

- *Antibody titer testing* may determine whether a client has developed antibodies in response to an infection or immunization. Antibodies for hepatitis, rubella, and infectious mononucleosis can be identified. An elevated titer level indicates the presence of antibodies.

- *Skin testing* can detect impaired cell-mediated immunity. A known antigen such as streptokinase, tuberculin purified protein derivative (PPD), or *Candida albicans* is injected intradermally. The site is assessed in 24 to 48 hours for signs of induration and redness. An induration of 10 mm in diameter is a positive reaction (Figure 13-5 ◆) indicating previous exposure and sensitization to the antigen. No reaction, or **anergy**, indicates depressed cell-mediated immunity.

Immunizations

Immunizations or **vaccines** are suspensions of live, *attenuated* (weakened), or killed microorganisms that promote active immunity against a specific organism. Special treatment makes them incapable of causing disease. Some vaccinations are combined to protect against several diseases. The most common combinations in the United States are MMR (measles, mumps, rubella), and DTP (diphtheria, tetanus, pertussis). (Recommended adult immunizations are found in Table 13-3 ◆.)

Inactivated vaccines are made by killing the disease-producing microorganism with heat or chemicals. For example, each year a new influenza vaccine is made, containing the three strains of influenza most likely to occur in the upcoming winter. These vaccines stimulate a weaker immune response, so yearly influenza immunizations are required.

Live, attenuated vaccines (like the MMR) are made by growing the disease-producing organism under special laboratory conditions. The process causes the organisms to lose their virulence or disease-producing power.

Toxoids contain an inactivated toxin that is produced by a microbe. They are made harmless by exposing them to chemical or heat. Diphtheria and tetanus toxoids are combined into a single immunization (Td for adults, DT for children). New vaccines (such as hepatitis B) are being developed by using recombinant genetic engineering. Some vaccines are made from portions or subunits of the antigen; one such vaccine protects clients against pneumonia caused by *Streptococcus pneumoniae.*

Hepatitis B vaccine is recommended for everyone at high risk for exposure to blood or other body fluids. It is mandated by the Occupational Safety and Health Administration (OSHA) for all health care workers. Other high-risk populations include intravenous drug users, sexual partners of infected individuals, clients on hemodialysis, prison guards, and athletic coaches.

People traveling outside the United States and Canada should receive vaccines against diseases that are found in certain regions of the world. Additional vaccines might include cholera, yellow fever, and typhoid.

Figure 13-5. ◆ Skin testing on the forearm showing induration (hardness) and erythema (redness) typical of a positive response to an antigen.

TABLE 13-3   RECOMMENDED IMMUNIZATIONS FOR ADULTS

VACCINE	TYPE	DOSE	INDICATIONS	PRECAUTIONS AND NURSING IMPLICATIONS
Measles–mumps–rubella (MMR)	Live, attenuated virus	0.5 mL SC	Males born after 1957, females born after 1957 who never had rubella or the rubella vaccine and test seronegative.	Do not administer to pregnant females; pregnancy should be avoided for 3 months after vaccination. Do not give to immunosuppressed clients (AIDS, cancer); those with a history of anaphylaxis or allergy to eggs.
Tetanus and diphtheria toxoids (Td)	Attenuated toxoid	0.5 mL IM	If never immunized, give series of 3 injections; booster every 10 years; after a contaminated wound.	Do not give in 1st trimester of pregnancy or to clients with a history of anaphylaxis reaction to horse serum; give deep IM in deltoid of dominant arm.
Hepatitis B (recombinant) (Recombivax-B)	Inactivated virus	1.0 mL IM (20 mcq/ mL)	Series of 3 doses; initial and at 1 and 6 months.	Do not administer to clients allergic to yeast. Give in deltoid site only.
Influenza (Fluzone)	Inactivated virus	0.5 mL IM	Yearly for clients > 65; in nursing homes; or with chronic pulmonary, renal, or cardiovascular diseases, or diabetes.	Do not give to clients with a history of anaphylactic reaction to eggs or to acutely ill clients.
Pneumococcal (Pneumovax-23)	Bacterial	0.5 mL IM	One dose for clients > 65. 1st dose for age 2–64 with chronic diseases and a booster 5 years after 1st dose.	Do not give to those with hypersensitivity to phenol.

Note: For pediatric clients, please consult a pediatric textbook for recommended immunizations.

When a client has been exposed to a specific disease, immune globulins made from human or animal sources are given to provide passive immunity. Human sources carry less risk for an allergic reaction and are available for hepatitis A and B, tetanus, varicella, rabies, measles, rubella, and respiratory syncytial virus.

Animal immune serums are made by injecting an antitoxin into an animal, allowing antibodies to develop, then withdrawing blood and preparing a serum for human injection. Antitoxins are used against diphtheria, tetanus, rabies, and botulism. Antivenins, another form of passive immunization, are given after a client has been bitten by potentially lethal snakes or spiders.

A *sensitivity test* should be done before the first immunization to determine allergy to horse serum or eggs. The test dose is injected intradermally; if no hives appear after 20 minutes, the selected vaccine is given.

Immunization side effects can range from mild local reactions to anaphylaxis. Local reactions at the injection site include redness, swelling, tenderness, and muscle ache. Giving the vaccine in the dominant arm of the client reduces the local discomfort, because arm movement helps to increase absorption of the solution. Warm compresses may also be beneficial. Sometimes the client may experience systemic manifestations like fever or malaise. Anaphylaxis is most likely with horse serum injections.

NURSING CARE

Nurses have an important role in preventing the spread of communicable diseases. This includes encouraging immunizations. Factors that may prevent active use of immunization programs are religious beliefs, poverty, and unfamiliarity with the health care system (e.g., among immigrants). Also, many people simply neglect routine immunization in adulthood. The result is increased risk for infectious disease among all people.

Before immunizations are given, the nurse should collect assessment data to determine whether immunization is appropriate (Box 13-1).

Nursing care focuses on preventing injury from the vaccination and on providing client education.

RISK FOR INJURY

■ Check the expiration date and the manufacturer's instructions for administration guidelines, dosage, routes, sites, precautions, and contraindications. *Outdated vaccines may not*

provide protection against the specific disease. Some sites have better absorption than others.
■ Do not administer any immunization to a client with an upper respiratory infection or other infection. *Infections can increase the inflammatory reaction from an immunization.*
■ Do not administer oral polio vaccines (OPV) or MMR to immunosuppressed clients or to clients who are in close household contact with an immunosuppressed person. *Live virus vaccines can cause disease in the immunosuppressed client or can transmit disease to close household contacts during the initial postvaccination period.*
■ Observe the client for 20 to 30 minutes following vaccination. *Allergic reactions usually occur within this time frame.*
■ Keep epinephrine 1:1000 readily available when administering immunizations. *Epinephrine causes vasoconstriction and reduces laryngospasm; in acute anaphylaxis, it can be lifesaving.*

Discharge Considerations

Provide instructions in the following areas:

■ Appropriate immunizations and recommended schedules for initial vaccination and boosters.
■ How and where to obtain immunizations. County or public health departments may offer immunization clinics at a lower cost than private physicians or urgent care clinics.
■ Possible side effects of the immunization, as well as the need to observe the client for up to 30 minutes following a vaccine for possible adverse reactions.
■ Self-care measures for side effects such as warm compresses over the injection site and taking acetaminophen (Tylenol) for fever.
■ The need to report immediately any adverse reactions such as fever, rash, itching, or shortness of breath.
■ Importance of maintaining permanent immunization records.

Altered Immune Responses

HYPERSENSITIVITY REACTIONS

Normally, the immune system protects humans against foreign substances, but sometimes it overreacts. **Hypersensitivity** is an altered immune response to an antigen that results in harm to the client. Hypersensitivity responses include hay fever, blood transfusion reactions, and organ transplant rejections. The tissue response to a hypersensitivity reaction may be simply a runny nose or itchy eyes, or it may be life threatening, leading to blood cell hemolysis or anaphylaxis.

There are four types of hypersensitivity reactions (Table 13-4 ◆). Types I, II, and III have an immediate tissue response and are caused by the humoral system. Type IV has a delayed response and results from the cell-mediated system. (See Chapter 10 for substances that may cause anaphylaxis.)

BOX 13-1
ASSESSING CLIENTS: IMMUNE STATUS

SUBJECTIVE DATA
- Present health status:
  - General health status
  - Exposure to any infections? Any fever or infections, especially upper respiratory?
  - Swollen glands in neck, axilla, or groin?
  - Pregnancy status?
  - Any immunosuppressive diseases (e.g., AIDS, cancer), chemotherapy, or radiation therapy?
  - Chronic pulmonary, cardiac, or renal disorders or diabetes?
- Past medical history:
  - History of infectious diseases
  - Immunization history: For which diseases and dates of immunizations? Any adverse effects? Any foreign travel that required immunizations?
  - Allergy to horse serum or eggs?
  - Ever received tetanus toxoid for any wounds?

OBJECTIVE DATA
- Vital signs: Blood pressure, pulse, respirations, temperature
- Height and weight
- Observe client for any signs of infection
- Assess for any skin lesions, rashes, or impaired healing

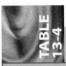

TABLE 13-4 TYPES OF HYPERSENSITIVITY REACTIONS

TYPE	CAUSES	PATHOPHYSIOLOGY	EXAMPLES
I—Immediate hypersensitivity	Pollens, foods, insect bites, animal dander, and drugs	Allergen binds to IgE antibodies that are attached to mast cells in connective tissue, skin, and mucous membranes where they release histamine. Histamine constricts smooth muscle and causes peripheral vasodilation leading to watery, itchy eyes; runny nose; rash; hives; or anaphylaxis.	Allergic asthma, hay fever, insect sting reactions, food allergies, anaphylaxis
II—Cytotoxic hypersensitivity	Incompatible blood	IgG or IgM antibodies bind with an antigen such as ABO or Rh. This triggers an autoimmune destruction of the target cell, causing a systemic reaction.	Blood transfusion reactions, hemolytic disease of the newborn
III—Immune hypersensitivity	Horse antitoxin; extracellular bacteria, fungi, and viruses	IgG or IgM antibody-antigen complexes form in the circulation and begin the inflammatory process.	Serum sickness, systemic lupus erythematosus, rheumatoid arthritis
IV—Delayed hypersensitivity	Chemicals or plants; skin tests with fungi or mycobacteria; foreign tissues	T lymphocytes interact with an antigen and activate the inflammatory response. Reactions may be delayed for 24–72 hours after exposure.	Contact dermatitis, tuberculin skin test; graft or tissue transplant reaction

LATEX ALLERGY

A unique hypersensitivity response is latex allergy. Once the natural rubber latex is removed from the tree, more than 200 chemicals may be added to prevent degradation. Latex allergy results from reaction to the chemicals or to the latex proteins. Latex proteins can enter the body through the skin and mucous membranes, by invasive lines and tubes, or by inhalation. Box 13-2 lists common products of natural rubber latex.

Type I and type IV allergic reactions to latex may occur. Type I response, a reaction to the natural rubber proteins, may occur within minutes of exposure. Symptoms range from mild (hives, itching, and generalized edema) to severe (wheezing, dyspnea, feeling of faintness, laryngospasm, and cardiac arrest). Type IV response results from an allergic reaction to the processing chemicals. Manifestations develop from 1 to 48 hours later and include local redness and itching.

Prevention of adverse reactions is most important. Ask clients about their allergy history, including food allergies. There seems to be a cross-sensitivity between latex allergy and certain foods, such as avocados, bananas, kiwi, pineapples, and chestnuts. Instruct clients with known latex sensitivity to wear a Medic-Alert bracelet.

Since 1998 all medical products must identify that they contain latex. Health care workers with latex allergies should

BOX 13-2
NATURAL RUBBER LATEX PRODUCTS

HOME

- Balloons
- Condoms, diaphragms
- Band-Aids

HEALTH-CARE SETTING

- Ace bandages (brown)
- Jobst elastic stocking
- Bulb syringes
- Blood pressure cuffs and tubing
- Gloves
- Intravenous tubing
- Tourniquets
- Wound drains
- Rubber stoppers in medication vials
- Rubber dams used in dental work
- Stethoscopes
- Urinary catheters
- Mattress covers

investigate their facility's policies, request powder-free gloves, and if necessary, request transfer to a different department. Manufacturers are looking to develop latex-free alternatives that also provide safe barrier protection.

COLLABORATIVE CARE

A key aspect of management is identifying allergens so that exposure is minimized. A complete history of all of the client's allergies is obtained, including medications, foods, animals, plants, and other materials. The type of hypersensitivity response is documented, as are onset, manifestations, and usual treatment. Several tests may be ordered:

- *Radioallergosorbent test (RAST)* measures the amount of IgE to specific allergens. This test is very expensive and takes longer but poses less risk for an anaphylactic reaction.
- *Skin tests* are used to identify specific allergens to which a person may be sensitive. Allergens used for testing are based on the client's history. Test solutions are injected intradermally or by a prick or patch on the back or arms.
  - The *prick test* may be done first to avoid a systemic reaction. A drop of allergenic solution is placed on the skin and the skin is punctured through the drop. A positive test yields a wheal and redness within 15 to 20 minutes.
  - *Intradermal:* A small amount of allergen is injected on the forearm or intrascapular area. Several allergens can be tested by allowing ½- or ¼-inch intervals between injections. A plain diluent is injected opposite the test site. A positive test yields a wheal and redness within 15 to 20 minutes (see Figure 13-5).
  - *Patch:* A 1-inch patch impregnated with the allergen is applied to the skin for 48 hours. Positive responses range from mild redness to severe redness, papules, or vesicles.

Pharmacology

Treatment focuses on avoiding the offending allergen, but sometimes medications provide symptomatic relief. Antihistamines, nasal and oral decongestants, and corticosteroids are usually ordered. Epinephrine is given during an acute anaphylactic reaction (see Chapter 10).

Antihistamines are the major class of drugs for treating symptoms of hypersensitivity responses. (Nursing care for the client receiving antihistamines is outlined in Table 13-5 ◆.)

Nasal decongestants like oxymetazoline (Afrin) and oral decongestants such as pseudoephedrine (Sudafed) may relieve allergy symptoms. Overuse of Afrin may result in decreased effectiveness and rebound nasal congestion. Remind clients to see their health care provider if symptoms last longer than a week. Decongestants should be used for less than 5 days.

Glucocorticoids are used in systemic and topical hypersensitivity responses. They have an anti-inflammatory effect. Short-term corticosteroid therapy is used for severe asthma, allergic contact dermatitis, and some immune-complex disorders. Corticosteroids in topical forms or delivered by inhaler may be used for longer periods of time with few side effects.

Another option is **desensitization,** a form of immunotherapy that involves injecting small doses of the allergen weekly. Over time, antibodies develop to block the allergic IgE response. This process can take years to accomplish symptomatic relief.

NURSING CARE

Nursing care is directed toward prevention of adverse effects and providing prompt, effective treatment. Prior to administering any medication, ask the client's allergy history, includ-

TABLE 13-5	NURSING IMPLICATIONS FOR PHARMACOLOGY: CLIENTS RECEIVING ANTIHISTAMINES		
CLASS/DRUGS	**PURPOSE**	**NURSING RESPONSIBILITIES**	**CLIENT TEACHING**
Antihistamines ■ Diphenhydramine (Benadryl) ■ Clorpheniramine (Chlor-Trimeton) ■ Hydroxyzine (Vistaril)	Antihistamines block H$_1$ histamine receptors to relieve allergic rhinitis and anaphylactic reactions such as urticaria and angioedema.	Give cautiously to older adults who are taking other medications. Monitor for side effects: excessive sedation, dizziness, palpitations, or urinary retention. Encourage a fluid intake of 2,500–3,000 mL/day unless contraindicated. Give Benadryl before blood transfusion or diagnostic tests that use contrast media as ordered.	Take only one antihistamine at a time. If drowsiness occurs, do not drive or operate machinery while taking this medication. Do not drink alcohol. Use hard candy, gum, ice chips, or mouth rinses to relieve dryness. Stop the drug and notify the physician if excessive sedation, dizziness, palpitations, or urinary retention occur.

ing the allergic response and its treatment. If the client experienced rash, hives, or difficulty breathing, check with the physician before giving the drug. If the client is receiving a new medication, observe closely. Even without any past allergic reaction to the drug, the client is still at risk for anaphylaxis. A second exposure increases the risk for a reaction and increases the severity of the reaction. While the client is hospitalized, ask about allergies to latex, skin cleansers, and radiopaque dyes.

When a suspected hypersensitivity reaction occurs, stop the intravenous medication or transfusion immediately. With a type I hypersensitivity response, the first priority is managing the client's airway. The client with a type II hypersensitivity reaction may need aggressive treatment to control bleeding. A type III reaction is treated by removing the antigen and stopping the inflammatory response. Treatment of type IV reactions includes eliminating the antigen and giving anti-inflammatory drugs. Antihistamines may relieve the client's discomfort. (Chapter 10 discusses management of anaphylaxis and transfusion reactions.)

Discharge Considerations

Most hypersensitivity responses can be treated by the client or family with little or no medical intervention. Teaching should include the following points:

- Tell clients to inform health care personnel of all allergens.
- Encourage clients to wear a Medic-Alert bracelet or tag identifying allergies.
- Instruct the client and family members on how to give emergency injections of epinephrine.
- Teach clients to use prescribed and over-the-counter medications as recommended.
- For the client with contact dermatitis, discuss appropriate skin care.

 Autoimmune Disorder

In **autoimmune disorders,** the immune system mistakes self for nonself, and the body reacts against itself. **Autoantibodies** (antibodies made against self-antigens) attack various body tissues, leading to tissue damage and chronic inflammation. Autoimmune disorders can affect any tissue, cell group, or organ. When the inflammatory process involves multiple organs, the client is said to have a systemic autoimmune disorder. Selected autoimmune disorders are listed in Box 13-3.

Certain families have a greater incidence of autoimmunity. Autoimmune disorders are more common in females and the elderly. Clients may develop more than one autoimmune disorder. The onset of an autoimmune disorder is frequently associated with a severe physical or psychological stressor.

BOX 13-3
AUTOIMMUNE DISORDERS

Cell or Organ Specific	Systemic
Blood	Rheumatoid arthritis
Idiopathic	Scleroderma
thrombocytopenia purpura	Systemic lupus
Endocrine System	erythematosus
Graves' disease	
Thyrotoxicosis	
Type 1 diabetes mellitus	
Addison's disease	
Central Nervous System	
Multiple sclerosis	
Muscles	
Myasthenia gravis	
Gastrointestinal System	
Pernicious anemia	
Ulcerative colitis	

PATHOPHYSIOLOGY

It is unclear exactly how autoimmune disorders develop. Several theories have been proposed:

- Trauma, drugs, radiation, and infections alter body tissues so that the body no longer recognizes itself, and autoantibodies are produced.
- Bacteria such as group A beta-hemolytic *Streptococcus* may cross-react with the heart muscle, causing heart damage.
- Viruses may alter tissues that are not usually antigenic. This may be the cause of multiple sclerosis and Type 1 diabetes mellitus.

Manifestations vary according to the tissues or organs affected. Most often, the client shows signs and symptoms of the inflammatory process (pain, fatigue, and fever). Autoimmune disorders are characterized by periods of acute flare-ups followed by no symptoms. As these diseases progress, remission periods become less frequent.

COLLABORATIVE CARE
Laboratory and Diagnostic Tests

Diagnosis of an autoimmune disorder is usually based on the client's clinical manifestations. Serum assays are helpful to identify increased levels of antibodies. Other laboratory and diagnostic tests more specific to the suspected disorder are ordered. Symptoms can be managed, but a cure is unlikely.

- *Antinuclear antibody (ANA)* test is used to screen for systemic lupus erythematosus (SLE). *Lupus erythematosus (LE) cell prep* is also used to detect SLE and monitor its treatment. Like the ANA, the LE cell prep is nonspecific for SLE. Positive results may be seen in rheumatoid arthritis or drug-induced lupus from penicillin, tetracycline, dilantin, and oral contraceptives.

- *Rheumatoid factor (RF)* is an immunoglobulin present in the serum of approximately 80% of clients with rheumatoid arthritis.

Pharmacology

Treatment of autoimmune disorders focuses on relieving symptoms. Because there is chronic inflammation, anti-inflammatory medications such as aspirin, nonsteroidal anti-inflammatory drugs (NSAIDs), and corticosteroids may be prescribed (see Chapters 12 and 16). COX-2 inhibitors such as celocoxib (Celebrex) and rofecoxib (Vioxx) inhibit cyclooxygenase-2 enzymes that are produced during inflammation.

Other slow-acting anti-inflammatory drugs may be added to the treatment plan. Disease-modifying antirheumatics are given to clients with rheumatoid arthritis. These drugs include gold salts, hydroxychloroquine (Plaquenil), and penicillamine. They are discussed further in Chapter 28. Cytotoxic drugs (discussed below) may be used in combination with plasmapheresis in treating many autoimmune disorders.

NURSING CARE

Nursing care is individualized for the client with an autoimmune disorder. Clients are taught stress reduction techniques, good nutrition, and medication uses and side effects. Most clients can be managed in outpatient settings. Interventions for the following nursing diagnoses should be included in the nursing care plan:

- Fatigue related to inflammatory effects of autoimmune disorder
- Acute and Chronic Pain related to inflammation
- Impaired Physical Mobility related to pain and activity intolerance
- Ineffective Coping related to chronic disease process
- Disturbed Body Image related to joint deformity, rashes, and altered body function
- Ineffective Protection related to immune disorder

Discharge Considerations

Because autoimmune disorders are chronic, the client and family need to understand their long-term effects. They must learn about medications and possible side effects. During periods of remission, clients may not appear ill, and it may be difficult for the family to understand their needs. Often, these clients are at risk for unproven remedies and quackery. Nurses can provide psychological support, listening, teaching, and referral to local support groups and state or national agencies.

Organ/Tissue Transplant

At one time, transplants were considered an experimental treatment option. Now they have become fairly common. Skin, cornea, bone, and heart valve transplants are done more frequently and require less extensive tissue matching. Kidney, heart, and liver transplants are no longer considered extraordinary procedures. However, these surgeries cannot be considered lightly. They cost from $40,000 to $250,000. (Medicare will cover the costs of kidney, liver, and heart transplants.) The client must also be able to afford the yearly cost of medications.

Organ and tissue transplants are used when clients with cancer need healthy cells; for example, those with leukemia may need stem cells. They are also used when an organ is about to fail or has irreversible disease, or when part of the body is destroyed as in transplant of skin to a burn victim.

Transplant success is closely tied to matching antibodies of the donor and the recipient. As discussed, HLA antigens are unique to the individual. Although identical twins may have the same HLA type, the chance is reduced to 1 in 4 for siblings, and less than 1 in several thousand for unrelated individuals. Matching the HLA type of the donor and decreases, but does not eliminate, the potential for transplant rejection.

PATHOPHYSIOLOGY

An **autograft** (a transplant of the client's own tissue) is the most successful type of tissue transplant. Skin grafts are the most common examples of autografts. Increasingly, **autologous** (self) bone marrow transplants and blood transfusions are being used to reduce the immune response. When the donor and recipient are identical twins, the term **isograft** is used. These grafts are usually successful, with only mild rejection episodes.

Most often, organ and tissue transplants are **allografts** (grafts between members of the same species). Because of the growing number of transplant candidates, allografts from living donors are needed to fill the shortage of organs. Living donors do not have to be blood relatives. Whole or partial organs are donated (one kidney, the lobe of the liver or lung, and part of the pancreas tail). Bone marrow transplant (BMT) is exclusively from a living donor.

Organs are obtained most often from cadavers. Donors must meet the criteria for brain death; be less than 70 years old; and be free from diabetes, hypertension, cancer, HIV, hepatitis B, and hepatitis C. The organ is removed immediately before or after cardiac arrest and is preserved until transplanted into the waiting recipient. Organ donation is coordinated by United Network for Organ Donation, a federally funded organization (see also Chapter 10).

Xenograft (transplant from an animal species to a human) is the least successful transplant and is seldom used. The one exception is the use of pig skin as a temporary covering for a massive burn.

Tissue typing determines the **histocompatibility** (the ability of cells and tissues to survive transplantation without rejection). Tissue typing identifies HLA type and blood types (ABO, Rh) of the donor and recipient, as well as any preformed antibodies to the donor's HLA antigens.

Transplant rejection is stimulated by humoral and cell-mediated immune responses. It typically begins 24 hours after the transplant, although it may develop immediately. Rejection episodes are characterized as follows (Table 13-6 ◆):

1. *Hyperacute rejection:* The grafted organ initially appears pink and healthy, but then turns soft and white and is usually lost.
2. *Acute rejection:* The client shows signs of the inflammatory process. Manifestations are related to the specific organ, for example, elevated blood urea nitrogen (BUN) and creatinine, liver enzyme and bilirubin elevations, or elevated cardiac enzymes and signs of cardiac failure.
3. *Chronic rejection:* This results from antibodies and complement being deposited in the transplant vessel walls. Narrowing of the vessels causes decreased blood flow and ischemia. The organ eventually fails.

Graft-versus-host disease (GvHD) is a frequent complication of bone marrow transplant. When there is no close match between donor and recipient HLA antigen, immunocompetent cells in the grafted tissue attack other body tissues, especially the skin, liver, and intestine. Acute GvHD occurs within the first 100 days following a transplant. A maculopapular rash begins on the palms of the hands and soles of the feet. The rash may spread over the entire body, eventually causing the epidermis to shed. Intestinal symptoms are abdominal pain, nausea, and bloody diarrhea. Chronic GvHD has a poor prognosis.

COLLABORATIVE CARE

Pre- and post-transplant care focuses on reducing the risk of tissue rejection. Laboratory tests are used to identify a suitable donor and to monitor the immune response to the transplant. Immunosuppressive medications are often the key to successful organ transplants.

Laboratory and Diagnostic Tests

Basic laboratory tests and diagnostic studies are done prior to surgery (complete blood count [CBC] and differential, urinalysis, chemistry panel, coagulation studies, arterial blood gases, an electrocardiogram, and chest x-ray). Other laboratory studies are ordered specifically before organ or tissue transplantation:

- *Blood type* and *Rh factor* of both donor and recipient.
- *Crossmatching* of the client's serum against the donor's lymphocytes to identify preformed antibodies.
- HLA *histocompatibility testing* to identify donors with an HLA type close to that of the recipient.
- *Mixed lymphocyte culture (MLC) assay tests* to determine histocompatibility between the donor and the recipient.

Various diagnostic tests may detect signs of transplant rejection. Ultrasonography or magnetic resonance imaging (MRI) of the transplanted organ can evaluate its size, perfu-

TABLE 13-6	TRANSPLANT REJECTION EPISODES			
TYPE	**CAUSE**	**PRESENTATION**	**TREATMENT**
Hyperacute	Preexisting antibodies (usually associated with previous transplant) immediately react against the ABO and HLA antigens of the donor organ.	Occurs within minutes to hours or days of the transplant. Rapid deteriorization of organ function	Transplant cannot usually be saved. Prevent with crossmatch and by using antimetabolite and anti-inflammatory drugs before surgery.
Acute	Antigens on the donor organ (usually from cadaver) trigger the release of cytotoxic T cells that attack the foreign organ.	Occurs within 4 days to 4 months after the transplant. Signs of inflammation (fever, swelling, redness and tenderness over graft site) and impaired organ function	Most common and treatable type of rejection. Increase immunosuppression using steroids, cyclosporines, monoclonal antibodies, or antilymphocyte globulins.
Chronic	Probably antibody-mediated response; may also involve inflammatory damage to the lining or vessel walls of the transplant.	Occurs 4 months to years after the transplant. Gradual deterioration of organ function	Changing to another immunosuppressive drug may help, but usually transplant is lost, requiring retransplant.

sion, and function. Tissue biopsies of the transplanted organ can provide evidence of tissue rejection.

Pharmacology

Preoperatively, antibiotic and antiviral drugs may be prescribed, such as trimethoprim–sulfamethoxazole (Septra, Bactrim), acyclovir (Zovirax), and ganciclovir (Cytovene).

Postoperatively, a combination of immunosuppressive drugs is given to prevent tissue rejection. Drug selection is based on the transplanted tissue or organ and the preference of the medical center.

Corticosteroids, prednisone (Deltasone) and methylprednisolone (Solu-Medrol) reduce the inflammatory response and decrease the production of T-helper cells and cytotoxic cells. Although beneficial, corticosteroids have numerous side effects: poor wound healing, fluid retention, hypertension, gastrointestinal (GI) distress, increased sodium and glucose levels, and muscle weakness. (Corticosteroids are discussed further in Chapter 16.)

Cytotoxic agents such as azathioprine (Imuran) and cyclosporine (Sandimmune) have been used as immunosuppressants since the 1970s. *Monoclonal antibodies* and *antilymphocyte globulins* are newer agents. (Nursing responsibilities and client teaching for immunosuppressive agents are outlined in Table 13-7 ◆.)

NURSING CARE

The client who has undergone an organ or tissue transplant has immediate and long-term nursing care needs. Immediately after the transplant, the client is transferred to the critical care or transplant unit and is monitored closely. Both physical and psychosocial needs of client and family must be considered.

RISK FOR INFECTION

- Monitor vital signs and temperature frequently. Assess for abnormal wound drainage, changes in body secretions, complaints of pain, or behavior changes. Culture abnormal wound drainage. *Incisions, invasive lines and tubes, nutritional deficits, immunosuppressive drugs, and chronic disease all increase the potential for infection. The client on immunosuppressive therapy is more susceptible to infection, but the usual signs and symptoms may be absent. To prevent life-threatening complications, assess the client constantly and start appropriate interventions immediately.*

- Ensure meticulous handwashing by all caregivers before providing direct care. Use strict aseptic technique for care of invasive lines, incisions, and wounds. *Handwashing provides first-line defense against infection and cross-contamination. Aseptic technique reduces risk of transferring microorganisms to the client.*

- Monitor CBC, especially WBC differential; report changes to the physician. *An elevated WBC count with a shift to the left may be an early indication of infection.* (See Chapter 12.)

- Initiate protective isolation precautions as indicated by facility policy and the client's immune status. Screen staff, family, and visitors for signs of infection. *These procedures further protect the severely immunocompromised client from infection.*

- Encourage deep breathing and coughing. *This mobilizes respiratory secretions and reduces the potential for atelectasis and pneumonia.*

- Provide adequate nutrition with supplementary feedings or parenteral nutrition if necessary. *Adequate nutrition is important for healing and immune system function.*

- Provide frequent mouth care. *Meticulous mouth care reduces oral microorganisms and helps maintain an intact mucous membrane lining.*

- Change intravenous bags and tubing at least every 24 hours, and change peripheral intravenous sites every 48 to 72 hours, unless contraindicated. Remove invasive catheters and lines as soon as possible. *Changing lines and sites helps reduce bacterial contamination. Fewer invasive lines mean fewer sites for bacterial invasion.*

- Monitor for potential adverse effects of medication:
  - Bleeding due to thrombocytopenia
  - Fluid retention with edema and possible hypertension
  - Anorexia, nausea, vomiting, and abdominal pain
  - Decreased urine output from renal toxicity
  - Jaundice from hepatic toxicity
  - Bone or joint pain

Medications used to maintain immunosuppression and to preserve the allograft have many potential adverse effects that can alter normal protective and homeostatic mechanisms.

RISK FOR IMPAIRED TISSUE INTEGRITY: ALLOGRAFT

- Administer immunosuppressive therapy as ordered. *Agents that suppress the immune response reduce transplant rejection.*

- Assess the client for signs of graft rejection: tenderness, redness, and swelling over the site; sudden weight gain, edema, and hypertension; chills and fever; malaise; and an increased WBC count and sedimentation rate. Report any changes immediately. *The risk for transplant rejection is highest in the initial postoperative period, but it is never completely eliminated. The client with a bone marrow transplant has the additional risk of developing graft-versus-host disease. Early identification allows adjustment of medication regimens and may preserve the graft.*

- Monitor tests of organ function. Report changes to the physician. *A decline in function of the transplanted organ (e.g., a rising BUN and creatinine in the renal transplant client) may be an early indication of transplant rejection.*

- In the client who has had a bone marrow transplant, assess for and report signs of GvHD immediately. Look for maculopapular rash, erythema of the skin and possible desqua-

TABLE 13-7 NURSING IMPLICATIONS FOR PHARMACOLOGY: CLIENTS RECEIVING IMMUNOSUPPRESSIVE AGENTS

CLASS/DRUGS	PURPOSE	NURSING RESPONSIBILITIES	CLIENT TEACHING
Cytotoxic Agents ■ Azathioprine (Imuran) ■ Cyclophosphamide (Cytoxan) ■ Cyclosporine (Sandimmune) ■ Methotrexate (Rheumatrex) ■ Mycophenolate (Cellcept) ■ Tacrolimus (Prograf)	Cytotoxic agents treat cancer and prevent tissue or organ rejection reactions.	Use meticulous handwashing to prevent infection. Notify the MD if WBCs fall below 4,000 or platelets below 75,000. Monitor BUN, creatinine, and liver enzymes. Increase fluids to maintain output. Monitor for bleeding gums, bruising, petechiae, or tarry stools. Monitor for oral candidiasis; client may need an antifungal drug.	Follow directions for taking the medications. Avoid large crowds and people with infections. Report signs of infection, any bleeding, reduced urine output, and jaundice. Do not take aspirin or ibuprofen. Use contraception to avoid pregnancy; drugs could harm the fetus. Wear protective clothing and use sunscreens. Wear Medic-Alert tag.
Monoclonal Antibody ■ Muromonab-CD3 or OKT3 (Orthoclone) ■ Basilizimab (Simulect) ■ Daclizumab (Zenapax)	A mouse is injected with an antigen that produces a specific monoclonal antibody. The antibody is harvested from the mouse and given by IV route to prevent organ transplant rejection.	Obtain chest x-ray before therapy starts. Premedicate the client as ordered to reduce potential side effects. Monitor closely for side effects of chills, fever, tremor, dyspnea, chest pain, or wheezing.	Discuss potential side effects and the need to report symptoms promptly. Explain that side effects may occur during the first two doses, requiring close observation at that time.
Antilymphocyte Globulins ■ Antilymphocyte globulin (ALG) ■ Antithymocyte globulin (ATG)	These drugs are given to horses or rabbits to produce antibodies. It is removed from the, animal, refined, and given IV to the client. They are used after an organ transplant to cause immunosuppression.	Before the initial dose, perform skin test to test for allergy to horse serum. Premedicate as ordered. Monitor for anaphylaxis during the infusion. Monitor client's WBC and platelet count daily.	Explain the need for special precautions and close monitoring during the IV infusion. Report any side effects to the nurse immediately.

mation, hair loss, abdominal cramping and diarrhea, jaundice with elevated bilirubin and liver enzymes (aspartate transaminase [AST], alanine transaminase [ALT]). *GvHD is a potentially lethal complication. It requires immediate intervention.*

■ Stress with the client the importance of maintaining immunosuppressive therapy and of reporting signs of graft rejection promptly. *The risk for transplant rejection is never completely eliminated.*

ANXIETY

■ Assess the client's level of anxiety by noting restlessness, tension, apprehension, fear, facial expression, and poor eye contact. *Clients may have difficulty talking about their fears and anxieties about organ rejection. When the transplant comes from a living donor, clients may also worry about the condition of the donor. Nonverbal cues help to identify anxiety.*

■ Use opening statements such as, "Facing an organ transplant must be very stressful." Listen attentively. *Encouragement and active listening help identify issues that can lead to problem solving.*

■ Stay with the client as much as possible. When leaving, tell the client when you will return. Also encourage family members to remain with the client as much as possible. *Time the nurse spends with the client promotes trust. The presence of family helps reduce anxiety.*

■ Provide clear, concise information and directions. *Highly anxious clients have difficulty focusing and retaining information.*

■ Encourage the use of coping behaviors that were useful in the past. If necessary, consult with a mental health specialist. Encourage client and family to meet other transplant recipients. *Past coping mechanisms may work again. A specialist can help the client deal with feelings. Hearing about the success and problems of others can reduce anxiety.*

Discharge Considerations

Thorough client education is necessary before the client with a transplant is discharged. The client and family need to understand the long-term treatment regimen as well as any lifestyle changes. Box 13-4 outlines assessment data to consider when planning for discharge.

Provide verbal and written instructions about the following points:

■ The signs and symptoms of transplant rejection and the importance of notifying the physician should these occur

■ How to monitor temperature, blood pressures, pulse, and weight

■ The importance of following the prescribed medication regimen; understanding interactions with other medications, appropriate OTC drugs, and maintaining a medication record

■ Side effects of immunosuppressive drug therapy. Include management techniques for minor side effects. Indicate which side effects should be reported to the physician.

■ The importance of avoiding exposure to infectious diseases, especially upper respiratory infection (URI), influenza, or pneumonia. Wearing a mask when going outside is helpful. Good handwashing technique is essential.

■ The importance of oral hygiene and regular visits to the dentist

■ Dietary needs and expected changes associated with medications

■ The importance of avoiding damage to the skin. Steroids increase the fragility of the skin. Any injury could allow microorganisms to enter.

BOX 13-4
ASSESSING FOR DISCHARGE

POST-TRANSPLANTATION
Client

• *Self-care:* Ability to perform activities of daily living (ADLs) independently; to plan rest periods; to self-administer prescribed medications; to monitor temperature, blood pressure, and pulse; to weigh daily

• *Knowledge:* Postoperative care; infection prevention; prescription and over-the-counter medications; well-balanced diet; need to obtain laboratory tests or diagnostic studies; physical activity limitations; manifestations of rejection or infection and when to seek medical care

• *Home environment:* Appropriate heating and cooling; access to clean water for drinking and handwashing; safe environment to minimize risk of injury

Family

• Members of household: Individuals with infections; presence of birds or animals

• Caregivers: Availability and willingness to provide care as needed; ability to apply infection control precautions, to give long-term immunosuppressive therapy, to identify manifestations of rejection and infection; to provide wound care and transportation to physician, dentist, and laboratory

• Financial resources: Income; availability of sick leave; resources for drugs and medical care

Community

• Access to health care resources
• Access to transplant clubs or support groups

■ Wearing a Medic-Alert bracelet or tag identifying the client as a transplant patient receiving immunosuppressive drug therapy

■ The importance of follow-up visits to the physician or clinic

Impaired Immune Responses and the Client with HIV

When function of either the B cells or T cells is impaired, the result is an immunodeficiency disorder. Immunodeficiency disorders can be inherited, acquired though infection, or produced unintentionally by immunosuppressive drugs.

Primary immunodeficiency is a rare congenital disorder that is usually found in infants and young children. In addition to a higher risk for infection, these children have more autoimmune diseases and cancer.

Secondary immunodeficiency is acquired and results in impaired immune function. One or more factors can cause immunodeficiency: stress, malnutrition, trauma, age, viral infections, cancer, or drugs. Infection with the human immunodeficiency virus (HIV) may lead to **acquired immunodeficiency syndrome (AIDS),** the final, fatal stage of HIV infection and the most well-known secondary immunodeficiency.

AIDS was first identified in 1981 among homosexual males in Los Angeles and New York who had developed an unusual opportunistic infection. By 1982, the Centers for Disease Control (CDC) acknowledged the presence of a new infection involving immune system deficits and associated opportunistic disorders. In 1985 the **human immunodeficiency virus (HIV)** was isolated as the cause of AIDS.

By December 2000, the CDC estimated that 800,000 to 900,000 people were living with HIV infection, with a third of them unaware of their HIV status. An estimated 40,000 new HIV infections develop each year in the United States. AIDS is the fifth leading cause of death among adults of ages 25 to 44; however, the death rate has been slowly decreasing since 1995.

Among men with new HIV infections, 60% were men who had sex with men (homosexuals, bisexuals, prisoners), 25% injected drugs, and 15% had heterosexual contact. Of the women, 75% were infected through heterosexual contact and the remainder through IV drug use. African American and Hispanic males make up 56% of AIDS cases; women of these ethnic groups represent 78% of cases in females. The number of AIDS cases in women increased from 7% in 1985 to 23% of newly reported cases in 2000 (National Institute of Allergy and Infectious Diseases [NIAID], 2001). Pediatric AIDS cases (children under 13) are also more prevalent in African American and Hispanic families.

AIDS in older adults cannot be overlooked. The number of AIDS cases in clients over age 60 has steadily risen in the past ten years (Lueckenotte, 2000).

By the end of 2000, approximately 36.1 million were living with HIV/AIDS worldwide and in nearly every country (NIAID, 2001). Of this number, 1.4 million were children under the age of 15. The highest incidence is in sub-Saharan Africa and Southeast Asia, especially India and Thailand. In some urban areas of central and eastern Africa, as many as one third of sexually active adults are infected, mostly through heterosexual intercourse.

There are three main routes of transmission: (1) direct person to person through sexual contact; (2) direct injection with contaminated blood, blood products, or needles; and (3) mother to fetus. HIV is transmitted through blood, semen, vaginal secretions, the placenta, and breast milk. It can also be found in saliva, but no known cases have been transmitted by saliva.

Certain behaviors increase the risk for contracting HIV. The most common behavior is intercourse with an infected partner. Sexual relations by anal, oral, or vaginal routes without the use of a condom is the major risk factor. Sharing of needles and other drug paraphernalia is the second leading risk factor for IV drug users. Multiple sexual partners, hetero-

sexual intercourse with an infected drug user, and exchanging sex for drugs or money are major risk factors for women. Hemophiliacs who received intravenous clotting factors and people infected through blood transfusion represent less than 2% of the cases.

Among the general population of the United States, HIV infection is very low. HIV is not transmitted by casual contact such as sneezing, coughing, handshaking, hugging, dry kissing, or sharing eating utensils or linens. There is no evidence that it can be transmitted by vectors such as mosquitoes. Blood donation also poses no risk, because only new, sterile equipment is used.

A small but real occupational risk exists for health care workers. The main exposure routes are needle-stick injuries or nonintact skin and mucous membranes. A needle-stick injury poses a 0.3% to 0.4% risk of becoming HIV positive. Mucosal exposures, such as splashing in the eyes or mouth, pose a much smaller risk.

PATHOPHYSIOLOGY

HIV is a retrovirus, which means it reproduces in a "backward" manner. Instead of reproducing from deoxyribonucleic acid (DNA) to ribonucleic acid (RNA); it uses RNA to make DNA copies. After the virus enters the blood stream, it attaches to CD4+ T-4 helper lymphocytes. CD4 is a receptor antigen on the T-4 helper surface.

Once inside the CD4+ cell, the virus sheds its protein coat and releases an enzyme called *reverse transcriptase* to convert the RNA to DNA (Figure 13-6 ◆). Then the viral DNA inserts itself into the host cell DNA and duplicates during normal cell division. At this point, the virus may remain latent or produce new RNA with the assistance of an enzyme *protease* to form very small virus particles (buds). These buds have the ability to move to other CD4+ cells where they disrupt and eventually destroy the host cell. Billions of HIV buds are produced and destroyed each day along with CD4+ cells. The loss of helper T cells leads to the immunodeficiencies seen with HIV infection. The infection eventually overwhelms the body's immune system (Figure 13-7 ◆).

The virus may remain inactive in infected cells for years. During this stage, B-cell antibodies are produced in a process known as **seroconversion.** These antibodies can be detected 6 weeks to 6 months after the initial infection.

A diagnosis of HIV infection is based on the client's history and risk factors, physical examination, laboratory studies, and manifestations. HIV infection and AIDS in adolescents and adults are classified according to the CDC system. This system uses CD4+ T-cell counts and clinical manifestations to diagnose a client.

Clinical manifestations of HIV infection range from no symptoms (after the initial mononucleosis-like onset), to severe immunodeficiency with multiple opportunistic infections and cancers in the late stages (Box 13-5).

Following the primary infection, clients enter a long-lasting asymptomatic period (usually 8 to 10 years). The virus

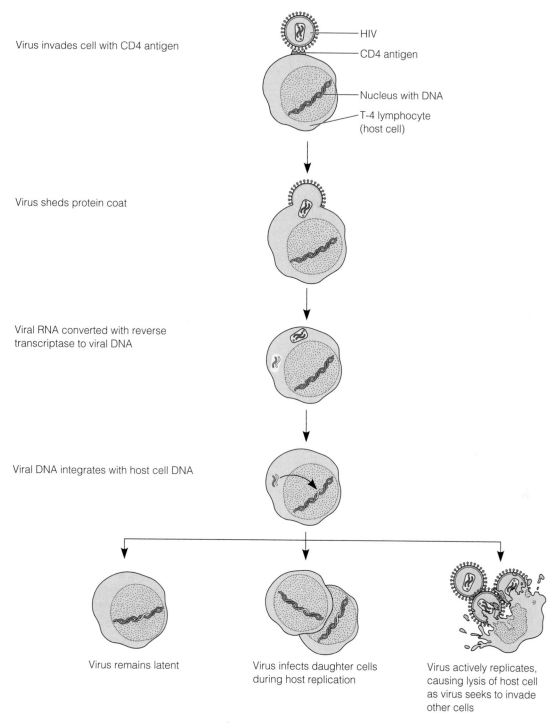

Virus invades cell with CD4 antigen

— HIV
— CD4 antigen
— Nucleus with DNA
— T-4 lymphocyte (host cell)

Virus sheds protein coat

Viral RNA converted with reverse transcriptase to viral DNA

Viral DNA integrates with host cell DNA

Virus remains latent

Virus infects daughter cells during host replication

Virus actively replicates, causing lysis of host cell as virus seeks to invade other cells

Figure 13-6. ◆ How HIV infects and destroys CD4 cells.

can be transmitted to others during this time. The next stage is acute infection, characterized by persistent generalized lymphadenopathy lasting 3 or more months. It is unclear exactly what causes a client to progress from HIV infection to AIDS. However, once clients are diagnosed with AIDS, they are at risk for developing multiple opportunistic infections and cancers. AIDS affects almost all organ systems. The client with AIDS has a poor prognosis, but newer treatments and medications enable clients to live longer.

Opportunistic Infections

Clients with AIDS are more likely to develop opportunistic infections when their CD4+ count falls below 200. These infections mostly affect the respiratory, gastrointestinal, and neurologic systems.

RESPIRATORY SYSTEM

***Pneumocystis carinii* Pneumonia.** *Pneumocystis carinii* pneumonia (PCP) (a fungus-like organism that rarely causes

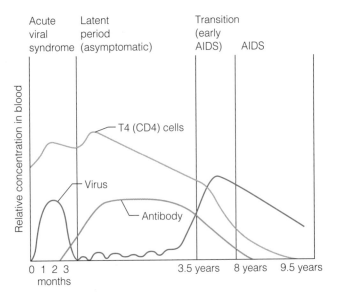

Figure 13-7. ◆ The progression of HIV infection. The primary infection begins shortly after contracting the virus, corresponding with a rapid rise in viral levels. Antibodies are formed and remain throughout the infection. Late in the disease, viral activity increases destroying CD4 (T4) cells. Antibody levels gradually decrease as immune function is impaired.

disease in clients with an intact immune system) affects about 75% of AIDS clients at some point in their disease. It tends to recur and often leads to death without prophylactic treatment.

PCP settles in the lungs and damages the lung alveoli. The client may experience fever, nonproductive cough, shortness of breath, dyspnea, tachypnea, crackles, decreased breath sounds, and cyanosis. Diagnosis is made by chest x-ray or bronchoscopy. A chest x-ray will show diffuse infiltrates. The bronchoscopy is used to obtain sputum for a culture.

Tuberculosis. Tuberculosis (TB) is caused by *Mycobacterium tuberculosis*. It usually invades the lungs but can also be found in the bone, central nervous system, and kidneys. Tuberculosis in AIDS clients is increasing and may contribute to the rising number of tuberculosis cases in the United States. In addition, multidrug-resistant strains are emerging.

TB is diagnosed by the Mantoux test; however, clients with a CD4+ cell count below 200 may not react to it. A follow-up chest x-ray provides a more accurate diagnosis. Persistent cough, night sweats, fever, fatigue, and weight loss are seen in clients with pulmonary tuberculosis.

***Mycobacteria avium* Complex (MAC).** MAC is caused by a bacterial organism found in the food, water, and soil. MAC affects nearly every organ. The most common manifestations are a high fever, diarrhea, abdominal pain, and weight loss.

GASTROINTESTINAL SYSTEM

Candidiasis. Oral candidiasis or *thrush* (a fungal infection caused by *Candida albicans*) occurs in most clients with AIDS. It is characterized by white patches in the mouth that may

BOX 13-5
MANIFESTATIONS OF HIV INFECTION

I. Primary Infection
   • Fever
   • Sore throat
   • Arthralgias and myalgias
   • Headache
   • Rash
   • Nausea, vomiting, and abdominal cramping
II. Asymptomatic Infection
   • None; converts to seropositive status
III. Acute Infection
   • Persistent generalized lymphadenopathy
   • General malaise, fatigue
   • Low-grade fever
   • Night sweats
   • Involuntary weight loss
   • Diarrhea
IV. AIDS and Opportunistic Disorders
   A. Respiratory
      • *Pneumocystis carinii* pneumonia
      • *Mycobacterium tuberculosis*
      • *Mycobacterium avium* complex
   B. Gastrointestinal
      • Candidiasis
      • Cryptosporidiosis
      • Wasting syndrome
   C. Neurologic
      • Cryptococcosis
      • Toxoplasmosis
   D. Other infections
      • Herpes simplex 1 and 2, herpes zoster
      • Cytomegalovirus (CMV)
      • Pelvic inflammatory disease
      • Human papillomavirus
   E. AIDS dementia complex and neurologic effects
   F. Secondary cancers
      • Kaposi's sarcoma
      • Non-Hodgkin's lymphoma

extend to the esophagus and stomach. Clients may complain of mouth soreness and an unpleasant taste. Esophagitis may lead to painful swallowing, an inability to eat, and malnutrition. In women, vaginal candidiasis is frequent and often recurs.

Cryptosporidiosis. A protozoan, *Cryptosporidium,* is normally found in birds, fish, reptiles, and humans. Transmission occurs from ingesting contaminated water or food or from human-to-human contact. The organism settles in the small intestine. AIDS clients experience large watery, nonbloody diarrhea that often causes dehydration, electrolyte imbalances, and malnutrition. Diagnosis is made by sending a stool sample for ova and parasites.

Wasting Syndrome. In the later stages of AIDS, most clients develop wasting syndrome. This is described as an unplanned weight loss of 10% along with chronic diarrhea or an unexplained fever. Fatigue, nausea, vomiting, and oral lesions lead to poor food intake, and chronic diarrhea results in malabsorption of nutrients. The client appears emaciated (Figure 13-8 ◆).

NEUROLOGIC SYSTEM. **Toxoplasmosis** and **cryptococcosis** are parasitic infections with *Toxoplasma gondii* and *Cryptococcus neoformans.* Toxoplasmosis can cause encephalitis. Cryptococcosis settles in the lungs but can travel to the brain or meninges, causing meningitis. Symptoms for both conditions include headache, fever, stiff neck, altered mental status, and seizures.

Other Infections

Herpes simplex 1 and 2 frequently develop in clients with AIDS. Type 1 infections involve the oral cavity, while type 2 infections develop in the genital and anal regions. Large groups of painful lesions form in the affected areas. When the lesions rupture, the virus is easily transmitted to other parts of the body and to caregivers.

Cytomegalovirus (CMV) is part of the herpesvirus family. It can affect the retina, the gastrointestinal tract, or lungs. CMV is the primary cause of blindness in AIDS clients.

Women with AIDS have a high incidence of pelvic inflammatory disease (PID). They seem to contract the human papillomavirus, which increases their risk for cervical cancer.

AIDS Dementia Complex and Neurologic Effects

AIDS dementia complex (ADC) is caused by HIV acting directly on the brain. It results in progressive deterioration of cognitive, motor, and behavioral functioning. Typical manifestations include forgetfulness, difficulty concentrating, con-

fusion, leg weakness, and clumsiness. Clients lose interest in personal hygiene, work, and social activities. In the later stages, the client may develop tremors, incontinence, and paraplegia.

Secondary Cancers

KAPOSI'S SARCOMA (KS). Kaposi's sarcoma is the most common cancer associated with HIV infection. Tumors develop in the lining of small blood vessels, causing reddish-purple lesions on the skin and mucous membranes. Initially, the lesions are painless but may become painful as the disease progresses. Tumors within body organs can disrupt function or cause bleeding. Diagnosis is made by tissue biopsy.

LYMPHOMAS. Lymphomas are malignancies of the lymphocytes, lymph nodes, the spleen, and bone marrow. AIDS clients develop either non-Hodgkin's lymphoma or primary lymphoma of the brain. Symptoms may be vague or reflect brain involvement, such as headache and changes in mental status.

COLLABORATIVE CARE

New treatments are being investigated, but research has not yet found a cure for HIV infection and AIDS. Because an AIDS diagnosis eventually means death, preventive strategies are most important. Clients at risk for HIV infection need help in identifying their HIV status. Once a positive diagnosis is made, they should be taught how to maintain their health and prevent opportunistic infections. Health care workers and support persons play a key role in providing emotional and psychosocial support.

Prevention

To date, no safe immunization to protect against HIV infection has been developed. Education and counseling are the key elements for AIDS prevention.

The nurse first focuses on sex education. All sexually active individuals need to know how HIV is spread. The only safe sex practices are: (1) no sex; (2) long-term monogamous sexual relations between two uninfected people; and (3) mutual masturbation without direct contact. Clients who engage in sexual activity must understand and practice safer sex (Box 13-6).

It is often difficult to find and educate injection drug users. People in this group should never share needles, syringes, or other drug paraphernalia. Needle-exchange programs provide a sterile needle and syringe in exchange for a used one. A fresh solution of household bleach and water in a 1:10 ratio is effective to clean injection paraphernalia when sterile supplies are unavailable. This population also should be taught safe sex practices. Most heterosexual HIV transmission occurs between injection drug users and their partners.

Screening of voluntary blood donors and donated blood supplies has reduced the risk of transmission by transfusion. However, it is possible for HIV to be transmitted during the time between contracting the virus and developing detectable antibodies (the *window period*). The window period usually

Figure 13-8. ◆ Wasting syndrome in a client with AIDS.

BOX 13-6
GUIDELINES FOR SAFER SEX

- Limit the number of sexual partners, preferably to one.
- Do not engage in unprotected sex, especially if HIV status of partner is unknown.
- When entering into a new monogamous relationship, both partners should undergo HIV testing initially. If both are negative, practice abstinence or safer sex for 6 months, followed by retesting.
- Use latex condoms for oral, vaginal, or anal intercourse; avoid natural or animal skin condoms, which allow HIV to pass through.
- For vaginal or anal sex, lubricate the condom with the spermicidal agent nonoxynol-9 for additional protection.
- Do not use an oil-based lubricant (e.g., petroleum jelly), which can damage the condom.
- Store condoms in cool, dry place and prevent damage to condom.
- Apply and remove condom properly; do not reuse condoms.
- Do not swallow urine or semen.
- Women should carry and use a female condom.
- Remember that oral contraceptives provide no protection against HIV.
- Engage in safer sexual practices that are less damaging to sensitive tissues (e.g., mutual masturbation, avoiding anal or oral sex).
- Do not use drugs or alcohol.
- Do not share needles, razors, toothbrushes, sexual toys, or other items that may be contaminated with blood or body fluids.
- If HIV positive:
  a. Do not engage in unprotected sexual activity.
  b. Inform all current and former sexual partners of HIV status.
  c. Inform all health care personnel—primary care providers, physicians, and dentists, in particular—of HIV status.
  d. Do not donate blood, plasma, blood products, sperm, organs, or tissue.
  e. If female, do not become pregnant.

lasts from 6 weeks to 6 months. For this reason, it is important for persons to donate their own blood prior to an anticipated surgery.

Health care workers can prevent most exposures to HIV by using standard precautions. With standard precautions, all body fluids are treated as if they are infectious, and barrier precautions are used to prevent skin, mucous membrane, or percutaneous exposure to them.

Any health care worker who is exposed to blood or receives a needle-stick injury should report it immediately to an employee health department. They should be tested at regular intervals for a year and receive appropriate counseling. The CDC recommends postexposure prophylaxis with azidothymidine (AZT) therapy after a needle-stick injury from an HIV-positive client. Treatment must be started *within 1 hour* after exposure. Research confirms that follow-up treatment with AZT can reduce the rate of infection.

Laboratory and Diagnostic Tests

- *Enzyme-linked immunosorbent assay (ELISA)* is the first screening test used to determine the presence of HIV antibodies (not presence of the virus itself). The client must give informed consent before the test is performed. An infected client may test negative during the window period. If the test is positive, a second test is done to confirm it. When the second test is positive, the Western blot test is done.
- *Western blot antibody testing* is more reliable but more time consuming and more expensive than ELISA. A positive Western blot test indicates that the client is seropositive.
- *HIV viral load* tests measure the amount of HIV viral activity. Viral loads are one of the best predictors of disease progression and response to antiretroviral medications. Levels greater than 5,000 to 10,000 copies/mL indicate the need for treatment.
- *CD4+ cell count* is used to confirm progression from HIV infection to AIDS. The normal range for the CD4+ count is 800 to 1,200 mm^3. AIDS is defined not only by the presence of opportunistic infections but also by a CD4+ count of less than 200/mm^3 or a percentage of CD4 lymphocytes of less than 14%. CD4 counts are recommended every 3 to 6 months for all people with HIV disease.
- *CD4+:CD8+ ratio* measures the ratio of helper T cells to suppressor T cells (normally 2:1). With decreased immune function, the ratio is reversed.
- *CBC* detects anemia, leukopenia, and thrombocytopenia, which are often present in HIV infection.

Tests may be ordered to diagnose secondary cancers and opportunistic infections. *Tuberculin skin testing* can identify tuberculosis infection. *Magnetic resonance imaging (MRI)* and *computed tomography (CT) scan* of brain can identify lymphomas and other opportunistic infections. *Cultures* of urine, blood, stool, spinal fluid, and sputum identify PCP, toxoplasmosis, cryptosporidiosis, cryptococcosis.

Pharmacology

Antiretroviral medications are given (1) to reduce the client's viral load, (2) to maintain CD4+ cell counts above 500, and (3) to treat opportunistic infections and malignancies. Three classes of antiretroviral drugs are used: nucleoside reverse transcriptase inhibitors (NRTIs), non-nucleoside reverse transcriptase inhibitors (NNRTIs), and protease inhibitors. The new treatment protocol known as HAART is the standard for treating HIV infection. Highly active antiretroviral therapy (HAART) combines three or four of the antiretroviral drugs.

(Each drug group, with nursing responsibilities, is discussed in Table 13-8 ◆.)

Before clients begin the HAART protocol, they should understand the benefits and risks as well as the effects on their daily life. They will need to take multiple medications at specific times throughout the day, and the HAART drugs cost more than $15,000 per year. This does not include the cost of other medications to treat or prevent opportunistic infections or cancers. Antiretrovirals cause adverse reactions that affect quality of life. For these reasons, clients with HIV must be fully committed to the treatment plan and be partners in their care.

Treatment is started when the client (1) shows symptoms of HIV infection or (2) shows no symptoms and the CD4+ cell count is less than 500 or the viral load is greater than 20,000 copies. Usually, the client is given two NRTIs and one protease inhibitor. Single drugs are avoided, to prevent drug resistance.

If successful, the drug regimen should reduce the viral load by 99% in four to eight weeks. However, not all clients receive the same results. Some clients cannot tolerate the multiple medications, side effects, or strict dosing schedule. Resulting feelings of despair, depression, and hopelessness may require antidepressants and counseling.

As mentioned above, the client may need medications for opportunistic infections and malignancies associated with HIV infection and AIDS. Many of these disorders cannot be eliminated, but pharmacologic agents attempt to control their devastating effects (Table 13-9 ◆).

TABLE 13-8

NURSING IMPLICATIONS FOR PHARMACOLOGY: CLIENTS RECEIVING ANTIRETROVIRAL AGENTS

CLASS/DRUGS	PURPOSE	NURSING IMPLICATIONS	CLIENT TEACHING
Nucleoside Reverse Transcriptase Inhibitors (NRTIs) ▪ Zidovudine (AZT, Retrovir, ZDV) ▪ Didanosine (ddI, Videx) ▪ Zalcitabine (ddC, HIVID) ▪ Stavudine (d4T, Zerit) ▪ Lamivudine (3TC, Epivir) ▪ Abacavir (ABC, Ziagen) ▪ Zidovudine plus lamivudine (Combivir)	NRTIs inhibit action of reverse transcriptase to prevent HIV reproduction.	Give at the ordered times around the clock. If a dose is missed, call the MD. Assess for bone marrow suppression: anemia, leukopenia, granulocytopenia. Monitor the client's CBC. Give epoetin (Epogen) or filgrastim (Neupogen) to treat anemia and neutropenia. Monitor CD4+ counts and viral load for drug effectiveness.	Take drug at ordered times to maintain serum blood levels. Report all side effects. Have regular blood tests: viral load, CD4+ counts, CBC, kidney or liver to monitor for drug toxicity. Notify physician if any signs of infection occur: sore throat, fever, swollen lymph nodes.
Non-Nucleoside Reverse Transcriptase Inhibitors (NNRTIs) ▪ Nevirapine (Viramune) ▪ Delavirdine (Rescriptor) ▪ Efavirenz (Sustiva)	NNRTIs block HIV reproduction.	Give at the ordered times around the clock. Monitor for skin rash, nausea, and headache. Monitor CD4+ counts and viral load for drug effectiveness.	Take drug at ordered times to maintain serum blood levels. Report side effects. Have regular blood tests: viral load, CD4+ counts, liver to monitor for drug toxicity. Notify physician if any signs of infection occur: sore throat, fever, swollen lymph nodes.
Protease Inhibitors ▪ Indinavir (Crixivan) ▪ Ritonavir (Norvir) ▪ Nelfinavir (Viracept) ▪ Saquinavir (Fortovase) ▪ Amprenavir (Agenerase) ▪ Lopinavir/Ritonavir (Kaletra)	Protease inhibitors block the production of the HIV protease enzyme, which is needed to make mature virions.	Give at the ordered times around the clock. Assess for GI upset: nausea, vomiting, diarrhea. Monitor liver studies for signs of toxicity and CD4+ counts and viral load for drug effectiveness.	Take drug at ordered times to maintain serum blood levels. Have regular blood tests: viral load, CD4+ counts, liver to monitor for drug toxicity. Notify physician if any signs of infection occur.

Many clients at some point need central venous access devices, such as a Groshong catheter, to draw blood and to give medications, transfusions, and parenteral nutrition. (See Chapter 24 for nursing care of the client with an intravenous access device implant.)

The following immunizations are recommended for all HIV-infected clients: pneumococcal, influenza, hepatitis B, and *Haemophilus influenzae b* vaccines. Persons with a positive PPD and negative chest x-ray film are given isoniazid (INH) for one year. When the client's CD4+ cell count falls to less than 200, the client is started on trimethoprim–sulfamethoxazole.

It was hoped that a vaccine would be developed to stop the HIV epidemic. To date, research has not found a successful vaccine, partly because new viral forms emerge constantly. Another roadblock is that so far animal testing has been unsuccessful, and the ethics of human testing has not been resolved. So, the best control method for HIV is prevention.

NURSING CARE

Because HIV and AIDS can affect all body systems, the client needs physical and psychosocial support. Initially, the nurse focuses on prevention, maintaining a health lifestyle, education, and coping with a terminal illness. If the client develops opportunistic infections and malignancies, direct care becomes more important. Nursing care for the AIDS client needs to address such issues as ineffective individual coping, risk for infection, nutrition, skin integrity, fatigue, impaired breathing, and altered thought processes.

Nurses are providing care for clients with HIV infection on medical-surgical, maternal–child, and pediatric units, as well as in hospices, clinics, and home settings. They must respect these clients' right to confidentiality. The nurse should never discuss a client's diagnosis except with the health care team.

ASSESSING

The nurse must collect a database before selecting the appropriate nursing interventions. The database can help determine the extent to which HIV infection and AIDS is affecting the client's life and can identify potential complications (Box 13-7).

DIAGNOSING, PLANNING, AND IMPLEMENTING

Individuals with HIV may require acute and chronic care throughout their illness.

TABLE 13-9

PHARMACOLOGIC TREATMENT OF OPPORTUNISTIC INFECTIONS AND MALIGNANCIES

CONDITION	TREATMENT	POTENTIAL ADVERSE EFFECTS
Infections *Pneumocystis carinii* pneumonia	Trimethoprim–sulfamethoxazole (TMP-SMX, Bactrim) Pentamidine (Septra)	Nausea, anorexia, rashes, fever, hypotension, cough
Tuberculosis	Antitubercular drugs	See Chapter 26
Mycobacterium avium complex	Clarithromycin (Biaxin) Azithromycin (Zithromax) Ciprofloxacin (Cipro)	Diarrhea, hepatotoxicity Headache, nausea, vomiting Nausea, abdominal pain, rash
Candidiasis Oral thrush	Clotrimazole troches (Lotrimin) Nystatin suspension (Mycostatin)	Nausea Nausea, epigastric pain
Recurrent vaginitis	Ketoconazole (Nizoral)	Nausea, hepatotoxicity
Cryptococcosis	Fluconazole (Diflucan)	Jaundice, rash
Herpes simplex	Acyclovir (Zovirax)	Vomiting, diarrhea, headache
Malignancies Kaposi's sarcoma	Chemotherapy with (doxorubicin) bleomycin, and vincristine Radiation therapy Alpha-interferon	Nausea, vomiting, bone marrow supression, alopecia Same as for chemotherapy plus possible radiation burns Mental status changes, chills, fever
Lymphoma	Chemotherapy	Nausea, vomiting, bone marrow suppression, alopecia

BOX 13-7
ASSESSING CLIENTS WITH HIV INFECTION AND AIDS

SUBJECTIVE DATA

- Present health status:
  - General health status
  - Any difficulty swallowing, weight loss, anorexia, abdominal pain, or diarrhea
  - Rashes or lesions on skin or in mouth
  - Complaints of fatigue, weakness, difficult walking
  - Insomnia or night sweats
  - Headaches, confusion, forgetfulness, personality changes, visual changes
  - Fever, nonproductive cough, shortness of breath, difficulty breathing
  - Any swollen lumps in neck, axillae, or groin
  - Drug or alcohol use
- Past medical history:
  - Any screening tests for TB or HIV?
  - Sexual history (unprotected sex, multiple partners, anal intercourse)
  - History of tuberculosis, STDs, hepatitis, or other infectious diseases
  - Use of any immunosuppressive drugs
  - Exposure to blood, blood products, or needles
  - Ever receive a blood transfusion?

OBJECTIVE DATA

- Vital signs: Blood pressure, pulse, respirations, temperature
- Height and weight
- Observe for poor nutritional status: Thinness, sunken eyes, muscle wasting
- Carefully observe client for lethargy, depression, inability to concentrate, memory loss, tremors, slurred speech, aphasia. Manifestations may be due to toxoplasmosis or cryptococcis.
- If possible, have client walk in the room; observe for ataxia and poor coordination
- Inspect oropharynx with penlight and tongue depressor for gray-white patches (Candida)
- Inspect skin for discolorations (KS)
- Inspect genital area for lesions or discharge from candidiasis or STDs
- Palpate lymph nodes in neck, axillae, and groin for swelling or tenderness
- Auscultate lungs for crackles and wheezing

INEFFECTIVE COPING

- Assess the client's support network and coping skills. *Once clients learn of HIV seropositive status, they face an uncertain future and social stigma. They may feel guilty about their chosen* lifestyle and the way the disease was contracted. As the disease progresses, social isolation and body image changes can tax their coping skills. The nurse helps the client identify available people and skills.
- Provide continuity of care. Spend time actively listening to the client. *This promotes trust and a caring atmosphere for the client to express feelings and work through issues related to HIV infection.*
- Support positive coping behaviors, client decisions, actions, and achievements. *As the client's self-esteem is enhanced, coping improves.*
- Promote and support the client's social network. *The client will need others in order to cope with the diagnosis and disease progression.*
- Provide referral to counselors, support groups, and agencies. Include addresses and phone numbers for local and national information resources and hot lines. Encourage the client, family, and significant others to participate in support groups. *Resource persons and groups can provide information and support. Support groups decrease the risk of social isolation and encourage clients to find ways to cope.*

RISK FOR INFECTION

- Wash hands before and after all care. Use standard precautions for all clients. Use aseptic technique when performing invasive procedures. *Handwashing decreases risk of cross-contamination. Standard precautions reduce the risk of disease transmission. Asepsis prevents nosocomial infections in hospitals or long-term care facilities.*
- Monitor for signs of infection (e.g., chills, sweating; burning on urination; shortness of breath; redness, tenderness, or drainage from wounds). Monitor WBC count. *Remember, immunocompromised clients may not have a fever; the nurse must look for other signs of infection.*
- Culture lesions, blood, urine, and sputum as ordered. *Cultures may identify infections or determine the effectiveness of medications.*
- Clean client's nails frequently. *Fungal infections are common under the nails.*
- Administer antiretrovirals and other anti-infective drugs as ordered. *These medications help control the HIV infection and may prevent opportunistic infections.*

IMBALANCED NUTRITION: LESS THAN BODY REQUIREMENTS

- Consult with dietitian to identify client's nutritional needs. *The dietitian can plan appropriate meals, supplements, and the need for parenteral nutrition.*
- Serve small portions of soft foods and avoid hot or spicy foods. Limit fluids before and with meals. *Small portions do not overwhelm the client. Soft foods are easily digested. Very hot or spicy foods can irritate the client's mouth when lesions are present. Excess fluids decrease appetite and food intake.*

■ Provide foods that the client likes. Encourage significant others to bring favorite foods from home. *The client is more likely to eat favorite foods.*

■ Encourage client to sit up for meals. Assist the client with eating as needed. Encourage client to rest before meals. *Fatigue and weakness can prevent the client from eating an adequate diet. An upright position reduces the risk of aspiration.*

■ Provide frequent oral hygiene. *Oral hygiene improves comfort and appetite and reduces the risk of mucosal lesions.*

■ Provide supplementary vitamins and enteral feedings, such as Ensure. *This improves the client's nutritional status and caloric intake.*

■ Give appetite stimulants such as megestrol (Megace) and dronabinol (Marinol) as ordered. *Both drugs may increase appetite and promote weight gain.*

■ Offer topical anesthetics such as Xylocaine viscous to clients with mouth lesions. Give antiemetics prior to meals and antidiarrheals after stools as ordered. *A topical anesthetic may reduce pain and improve oral intake. These medications can increase food intake and improve nutrient absorption.*

■ Monitor weight and albumin levels. *These measures promote early intervention to prevent anemia and wasting syndrome. Albumin levels reflect the client's nutritional status.*

IMPAIRED SKIN INTEGRITY

■ Monitor lesions for signs of infection or impaired healing. *Maintaining skin integrity is important because of the progressive and debilitating nature of AIDS. Infection or poor tissue perfusion not only impairs healing but may lead to further skin breakdown.*

■ Turn the client at least every 2 hours with a turn sheet. *Turning decreases stress over bony prominences, improves circulation, and promotes healing. A turn sheet prevents skin shearing.*

■ Use pressure and eggcrate mattresses, or sheepskin pads for elbows and heels. *These devices reduce pressure on skin.*

■ Wash skin with mild, nondrying soaps and pat dry gently. Apply lotion as needed. *Clean, dry skin is a barrier to infection. Gentle drying prevents skin tears. Lotion reduces skin dryness.*

■ If blisters are present, leave intact, and cover with a transparent film (e.g., Tegaderm). *Covering may prevent bacterial invasion and promote healing.*

■ Trim fingernails regularly. Teach client to avoid scratching. If the client is confused, apply mitts or soft restraints to prevent scratching, and check circulation of hands and fingers frequently. *Scratching with long fingernails can damage skin, increasing risk of infection. Tight or restrictive restraints or mitts may decrease circulation.*

■ Cleanse perianal area with water and oil-based products. Apply A&D ointment afterwards. *These measures prevent skin damage from diarrhea.*

■ Encourage ambulation. If the client is confined to bed, encourage active or passive range-of-motion exercises. *Activity increases circulation, decreases pressure and skin breakdown, and maintains muscle tone.*

FATIGUE

■ Balance activities with rest periods and assist with activities of daily living (ADLs) if necessary. *Fatigue may be related to low energy levels, medication side effects, or the emotional stress of the disease. Establishing realistic activity goals helps the client perform activities when energy levels are the highest, and gives the client a sense of accomplishment.*

■ Provide supplemental oxygen. *Anemia and hypoxemia reduce oxygen to the cells leading to fatigue.*

■ Identify energy-saving techniques (e.g., sitting for a shower; using a cane, walker, or wheelchair). *Energy-saving techniques enable the client to do more activities throughout the day. Assistive devices help conserve energy.*

■ Refer to physical or occupational therapist as needed. *Physical therapy and occupational therapy exercises can increase muscle strength and tone.*

INEFFECTIVE BREATHING PATTERNS

■ Promote coughing and deep breathing. Instruct client to use incentive spirometer. Suction airway as needed. *Thick secretions (as in PCP infection) reduce the flow of oxygen to the tissues. These interventions promote lung expansion and mobilize secretions.*

■ Monitor oxygen levels with pulse oximetry. If less than 90%, give supplemental oxygen. *Oxygen levels should be above 90% to provide adequate oxygen to tissues and cells.*

■ Increase fluid intake as tolerated. *Increased fluids will thin secretions and make them easier to expectorate.*

■ Place client in semi- or high Fowler's position. *Elevating the head of the bed reduces abdominal pressure against the diaphragm and prevents aspiration.*

■ Give anti-infective medications according to culture and sensitivity tests. *Anti-infective medications help control opportunistic infections.*

DISTURBED THOUGHT PROCESSES

■ Use simple, short sentences. Always call client by name. *Cognitive and neurologic functioning may be altered by brain malignancies and HIV infection of the central nervous system. These measures decrease confusion and help the client remain oriented.*

■ Reorient to time and place frequently. Provide calendar, clock, radio, TV, and a room with a window. *Frequent reorientation may be necessary during acute periods of confusion.*

■ Provide quiet room with minimal lights at night. *Excess noise and bright lights confuse the client between day and night.*

■ Apply a bed alarm if client tends to get out or bed unassisted. Move the client closer to the nurses' station or place in a monitored room. *The client may experience confusion and impaired judgment. Bed alarms alert nursing staff to check on client's safety. Staff can monitor the client more easily if the room is close or is a monitored room.*

■ Encourage family and significant others to socialize with the client. *Contacts with familiar persons can maintain reality orientation.*

■ Maintain safe environment by removing excess furniture, placing call bell within client's reach, and padding siderails as needed. *If motor coordination is altered, clients may injure themselves. These measures can decrease the risk for injury.*

OTHER NURSING DIAGNOSES

With a disease such as HIV infection, the list of possible nursing diagnoses is long. Some additional nursing diagnoses to consider are:

■ Powerlessness related to terminal disease
■ Pain related to Kaposi's sarcoma and peripheral neuropathy
■ Risk for Caregiver Role Strain related to care needs of the client with HIV
■ Impaired Home Maintenance related to fatigue and weakness
■ Ineffective Sexuality Patterns related to HIV infection

EVALUATING

Evaluate effectiveness of care by collecting data related to client's overall health, absence of opportunistic infections, laboratory values especially CD4 cell count, and the ability to care for self at home.

Discharge Considerations

Most clients with HIV infection and AIDS are cared for in the home. Box 13-8 outlines assessment to collect when planning discharge. The client and significant other need thorough teaching. They should understand HIV infection and AIDS, disease transmission, and the stages of the disease including opportunistic infections. Provide the client and family with current factual information so they can plan their future. Discuss the myths, misperceptions, and prejudices that accompany this diagnosis.

Teach the client and family how to maintain optimal health. Discuss diet and nutritional intake, balancing rest and exercise, stress reduction, lifestyle changes, and safe sexual practices. Teach them that the client needs a diet high in protein and calories to meet increased metabolic needs and maintain weight. Activity and rest periods should be balanced to prevent unnecessary fatigue.

Provide instruction on handwashing techniques and disinfection procedures for the home. Teach them to clean bathrooms and kitchens daily with disinfectant. Emphasize that all blood spills should be cleaned up immediately by using a 1:10 dilution of bleach and water (½ cup bleach to 5 cups water).

Teach care providers to use gloves when handling the client's secretions or excretions, to wash hands before and after providing direct care, and to wash the client's laundry sepa-

---

BOX 13-8
ASSESSING FOR DISCHARGE

HIV INFECTION AND AIDS
Client

• *Self-care:* Ability to perform ADLs independently; to plan rest periods; to prepare nutritional meals; to self-administer prescribed medications at scheduled times; to monitor temperature; and to practice safe sexual relations
• *Knowledge:* HIV infection and AIDS; routes of disease transmission; ways to avoid infection; prescription and over-the-counter medications; adverse reactions of medications; well-balanced diet and nutritional supplements; food preparation; need to obtain laboratory tests; manifestations of infection and when to seek medical care; vaccinations; precautions to use around birds and cats; and disinfecting bedding, clothes, bathroom, and kitchen
• *Home environment:* Appropriate heating and cooling; access to clean water for drinking and handwashing; free of disease-carrying insects and rodents; and safe environment to minimize risk of injury

Family

• Members of household: Individuals with infections; presence of birds or animals
• Caregivers: Availability and willingness to provide care as needed; ability to reduce infection; restrict visitors with infections; to administer long-term antiretroviral and other medications; ability to identify manifestations of infection; to transport to physician, and laboratory
• Financial resources: Income; availability of sick leave; resources for drugs and medical care needed

Community

• Access to community health care resources
• Access to support groups
• Access to spiritual support
• Access to caregiver respite care

---

rately in hot water with 10% bleach. Teach that separate dishes, glassware, and utensils are not necessary, provided they are washed in hot, soapy water. Inform clients that they can assist with food preparation as long as they are feeling well.

Teach strategies to avoid opportunistic infections. Emphasize the importance of avoiding large crowds and people with infectious diseases. Inform clients of the risks of having birds and cats in the home (they can carry toxoplasmosis, cryptosporidiosis, and MAC). Advise clients to avoid changing cat litter boxes or bird cages. Teach the client to wash all raw fruits and vegetables before eating them; to cook all meat, fish, and eggs; and to avoid unpasteurized milk.

Encourage the client to stop smoking and to eliminate alcohol and recreational or illicit drugs. Provide contact with a social worker for referral to the appropriate clinic or agency.

Teach clients and families the signs and symptoms of opportunistic infections and malignancies. They must report a fever, sore throat, night sweats, cough, dyspnea, chest pain, swollen glands, diarrhea, headaches, and skin lesions. Discuss the need for regular follow-up with their health care provider and routine laboratory testing.

Teach the client and significant others about the use and adverse effects of prescribed medications. Provide guidelines for helping the client adapt to the fixed schedules. Be sure the client understands the importance of complying with the medication regimen.

If necessary, provide information about home health care, hospice, and respite care. Provide referrals to local care providers, home health services, support groups, and social agencies as needed. When the client's disease progresses to the advanced stage, give the caregiver instructions on intravenous nutrition and medication delivery systems.

Nursing Process Case Study
■ CLIENT WITH HIV INFECTION

Sara Lu is a 26-year-old elementary school teacher who lives with her parents and two younger sisters. During her yearly physical exam, she complains of feeling fatigued, a persistent sore throat, intermittent bouts of diarrhea, and mild shortness of breath for about a month. Normally, she is very physically active. She is planning to be married in 6 months. Ms. Lu states that she has had unprotected sexual relations only with her fiancé. Seven years ago she had open heart surgery to repair a mitral valve defect. The physician orders a mononucleosis test, ELISA, Western blot test, CD4 T-cell count, a p24 antigen test, and an erythrocyte sedimentation rate (ESR). She is to return to the office in a week.

Assessment On Ms. Lu's follow-up visit, she tells Carole Kee, RN, that she still has flulike symptoms but has improved somewhat. She is less active than usual and is worried about her health. Her appetite is poor because of a sore mouth, and she has lost 10 lbs. over the past month. She has noted white patches on her tongue and cheeks.

A chest x-ray is normal. The results of her laboratory tests are as follows:

- ELISA: Positive for antibodies against HIV
- Western blot analysis: Positive for antibodies against HIV
- p24 antigen test: Positive for circulating HIV antigens
- ESR: Increased
- CD4 T-cell count: 599/mm^3 (normal range is 800 to 1,200).

Ms. Lu's physical examination reveals that she has enlarged lymph nodes in her neck, white patches on her oral mucosa, and somewhat dehydrated. Vital signs are: BP 100/70; R 20; P 90; T 99.9° F (37.7° C).

Ms. Lu is told the results of her laboratory tests and the medical diagnosis of HIV infection. Ms. Lu is distressed and wants to know how this happened, its meaning, whether she has infected her loved ones, and whether she will get better. She is admitted to the hospital for short-term care.

Diagnosis The following nursing diagnoses are developed for Ms. Lu:

- Imbalanced Nutrition: Less Than Body Requirements related to mouth soreness
- Risk for Deficient Fluid Volume related to decreased fluid intake and diarrhea
- Risk for Infection related to altered immunity
- Anxiety related to diagnosis and fear
- Deficient Knowledge about the HIV disease process

Expected Outcomes The expected outcomes established in the plan of care specify that Ms. Lu will:

- Maintain adequate dietary intake.
- Return hydration status to normal.
- Remain free of infections and any complications.
- Discuss anxiety and fears.
- State ways to prevent HIV transmission to others, including safer sex practices.

Planning and Implementation Ms. Kee plans the following interventions to be implemented:

- Monitor daily weight, intake and output, and hydration status.
- Suggest strategies for decreasing anorexia and nausea.
- Provide a consult with a dietitian.
- Provide oral care before and after meals.
- Monitor serum albumin levels.
- Assess bowel sounds and monitor elimination pattern.
- Administer antiemetic and antidiarrheal medications as ordered.
- Increase fluid to 2,500 mL daily.
- Use strict aseptic technique for all invasive procedures.
- Give antiretroviral and antibiotics as ordered.
- Encourage physical activity as possible.
- Encourage Ms. Lu to discuss her feelings and concerns.
- Avoid false reassurances.
- Suggest testing for her fiancé.
- Teach about HIV/AIDS, a nutritionally balanced diet, adequate fluid intake, avoiding people with infectious diseases, safe sex practices, and ways to prevent HIV transmission.

Evaluation Ms. Lu is eager to learn about her illness. She also wants her fiancé and family to attend the teaching sessions with her. Ms. Lu is taking home an antifungal medication, diet plans, and a schedule for increased exercise. She will return in 1 month for a follow-up physical.

Critical Thinking in the Nursing Process

1. Are the laboratory results for Ms. Lu a true indication that she is HIV positive? What additional tests might be ordered?
2. What is the most likely source of Ms. Lu's infection?
3. Ms. Lu says that her fiancé would like to have a child. How will you counsel her regarding pregnancy and child-bearing?

Nursing Interventions Classification

The following nursing interventions developed by McCloskey and Bulechek (2000) may be appropriate for clients with impaired immunity:

- Coping Enhancement
- Infection Protection
- Self-Care Assistance
- Medication Management
- Dying Care

(*Note:* The bibliography listings for this and all chapters have been compiled at the back of the book.)

Chapter Review

key terms by topic

Use the CD-ROM disk enclosed with your textbook to hear the proununciation of the key terms in the chapter.

Immune system
antigen, allergen, B-cell lymphocytes, T-cell lymphocytes, natural killer (NK) cells

Humoral and cell-mediated immunity
immunocompetent, immunoglobulins, antibody, helper T cells, suppressor T cells, cytotoxic T cells

Immunization
natural immunity, active immunity, passive immunity, anergy, vaccines, hypersensitivity, desensitization

Autoimmune disorders and transplants
autoantibodies, autograft, autologous, isograft, allografts, xenograft, histocompatibility

Client with HIV
acquired immunodeficiency syndrome (AIDS), human immunodeficiency virus (HIV)

key points

- The immune system consists of leukocytes, lymphoid organs (bone marrow, thymus, spleen, lymph nodes), and peripheral lymph tissues such as the tonsils and appendix.

- Active immunity provides long-term immunity either by developing the disease or by an immunization. Passive immunity is short term and involves injecting serum with ready-made antibodies for other humans or animals.

- Hypersensitivity reactions range from mild such as hay fever to severe (e.g., blood transfusion reactions, anaphylaxis, and organ transplant rejections).

- Autoimmune disorders develop when the body fails to identify self from nonself (e.g., rheumatoid arthritis).

- The human immunodeficiency virus (HIV) is the cause of acquired immunodeficiency syndrome (AIDS).

- HIV attacks helper T4 lymphocytes which decreases a person's ability to remain immunocompetent and increases the risk for developing opportunistic infections.

- The ELISA and Western blot tests detect antibodies to identify if a person is infected with HIV.

- The client with HIV is managed with a combination of antiretroviral medications, such as zidovudine (AZT).

- Health teaching focuses on safe sex practices, adverse drug reactions, nutrition, ways to reduce opportunistic infection, to prevent transmission, and to maintain self-care.

Medialink

Additional interactive resources for this chapter can be found on the Companion Website at www.prenhall.com/burke. Click on Chapter 13 and "Begin" to select the activities for this chapter.

For NCLEX review questions and an audio glossary, access the accompanying CD-ROM in this book.

for further study

See Chapter 12 for more in-depth discussion of inflammation.

For substances that may cause anaphylaxis and for management of anaphylactic reactions, see Chapter 10.

For pharmacologic treatment of autoimmune disorders, see Chapters 12 and 16.

For pharmacologic treatment of clients with rheumatoid arthritis, see discussion in Chapter 28.

For more on organ donation, see Chapter 10.

For discussion of elevated WBC count with a shift to the left, see Chapter 12 and Figure 12-5.

See Chapter 24 for nursing care of the client with an intravenous access device implant.

Critical Thinking Care Map

Caring for a Client with *Pneumocystis carinii* Pneumonia
NCLEX-PN Focus Area: Physiological Integrity

Case Study: A 42-year-old male client is admitted to the medical floor with *Pneumocystis carinii* pneumonia. Two years ago he was diagnosed with AIDS and has "felt good" until last week when he started to feel tired. His CD4 T-cell count dropped from 500 to 400/mm^3. The nurse notes a dry cough and hears crackles in the bases. He says, "I get really short of breath when I walk." He complains of being cold, yet the room temperature is normal.

Nursing Diagnosis: Ineffective Breathing Pattern

COLLECT DATA

Subjective   Objective

_____   _____

_____   _____

_____   _____

_____   _____

_____   _____

Would you report this data? Yes/No

If yes, to: _____

Nursing Care

_____

_____

_____

_____

_____

_____

_____

How would you document this? _____

_____

Collect Data
(use those that apply)

• States "Short of breath when I walk"
• BP 140/84
• Crackles in the posterior bases
• T 100.8° F
• Complains of being cold
• Easily fatigued
• Purple spots on both arms
• 4 lb. weight loss in last month
• Dry cough
• RR 28, shallow
• Pulse oximetry = 88%
• Night sweats
• CD4 T-cell count = 400 mm^3

Nursing Interventions
(use those that apply)

• Instruct in use of incentive spirometer.
• Provide quiet room with minimal lights.
• Collect sputum culture.
• Monitor oxygen levels with pulse oximetry.
• Encourage coughing and deep breathing.
• Provide frequent oral hygiene.
• Increase fluid intake as tolerated.
• Place in semi-Fowler's position.
• Monitor weight daily.
• Give nasal oxygen at 3 L/M.

NCLEX-PN Exam Preparation

TEST-TAKING TIP

Review therapeutic communication techniques. Communication that contains barriers will not be the correct answer.

1. A client was given an immunization for influenza B 10 minutes ago. Which of these statements, if made by the client, would indicate that the client has a correct understanding of the discharge instructions?
   a. "I must be having a severe reaction; my arm is red."
   b. "My ride is here. I have to leave now."
   c. "I'll put a heating pad on my arm when I get home."
   d. "I'll be back in 2 weeks to get my second shot."

2. A nursing assistant tells you that she is allergic to pineapples. Your best response should be:
   a. "Make sure you don't eat foods with pineapple as an ingredient."
   b. "I'm allergic to peanuts. What symptoms do you get?"
   c. "You must have a type I hypersensitivity reaction."
   d. "I will order you some latex-free gloves for your client care."

3. A client arrives in the clinic complaining of a swollen lip after being stung by a bee. The nurse's first priority would be to:
   a. assess the respiratory status
   b. ask the client about prior episodes with insect bites
   c. administer epinephrine
   d. explain the allergic reaction pathophysiolgy

4. The physician has ordered Imuran for a post–kidney transplant recipient. Which of the following instructions must be included on the client teaching sheet?
   a. Increase PO fluids to 2,000 mL/day.
   b. Avoid large crowds.
   c. Bed rest must be strictly enforced.
   d. Decreased urine output is expected.

5. When a client diagnosed with HIV says to the nurse, "I guess hugging my little girl is out of the question now," the best response by the nurse would be:
   a. "HIV is not transmitted by casual kissing or hugging."
   b. "I'm sorry, but you don't want to infect your child."
   c. "Perhaps you can show your affection in other ways."
   d. "You're right; you must not share your utensils either."

6. When assessing a client who has recently been diagnosed with HIV, the nurse should expect the client to have which of these symptoms?
   a. diarrhea
   b. *Pneumocystis carinii* pneumonia
   c. sore throat
   d. night sweats

7. Safe sex techniques decrease the transmission rate of HIV and other sexually transmitted diseases. Which of these guidelines should be included in client teaching?
   a. Use oil-based lubricants.
   b. Oral contraceptives are effective in preventing transmission.
   c. Anal sex is acceptable if a condom is used.
   d. Do not reuse condoms.

8. A client reports a persistent cough, night sweats, fever, fatigue, and weight loss. The Mantoux test is assessed at 10 mm. The most likely condition that the nurse expects is:
   a. *Mycobacteria avium* complex
   b. tuberculosis
   c. candidiasis
   d. cryptosporidiosis

9. When caring for a client with AIDS dementia, which of these nursing interventions should be given priority?
   a. Obtain vital signs every 4 hours.
   b. Assess the client's support system.
   c. Serve small portions of soft foods.
   d. Remove excess furniture from the room.

10. A client who is undergoing chemotherapy for Kaposi's sarcoma states, "I'm just too sick to eat." Which of these actions should the nurse take?
    a. Remove the tray of food.
    b. Administer nausea medication prior to meals.
    c. Encourage fluids with meals.
    d. Give appetite stimulants as ordered.

Answers for Review Questions, as well as discussion of Case Study Critical Thinking questions, appear in Appendix V.

chapter

14

Caring for Clients with Skin Disorders

CARING tip

❝Knowledge is power; never stop learning. Take advantage of every opportunity to learn something new.❞

Rhonda L. Brown, RN, BSN • Nursing Instructor • El Paso Community College (Mission Campus) • El Paso, Texas
kdjl

LEARNING outcomes

After completing this chapter, you will be able to:

- Identify the structure and functions of the skin and its appendages.
- Describe skin changes in the older adult, and relate those changes to an increased risk for dry skin, pruritus, skin cancer, and pressure ulcers.
- Compare and contrast the pathophysiology, manifestations, and collaborative care of clients with common skin disorders, infections and infestations of the skin, malignant skin disorders, and pressure ulcers.
- Use the nursing process to collect data and provide interventions for clients with common skin disorders, infections and infestations of the skin, malignant skin disorders, and pressure ulcers.
- Provide client and family teaching appropriate for prevention and self-care of disorders of the skin.

MediaLink

 www.prenhall.com/burke

Use the above address to access the free, interactive Companion Website created for this textbook. Get hints, instant feedback, and textbook references to chapter-related multiple choice questions. Link to other interesting sites.

The skin and its appendages (glands, hair, and nails) make up the integumentary system. The skin provides an external covering for the body, separating the body's organs and tissues from the external environment. The skin contains receptors for touch and sensation, helps regulate body temperature, and assists in fluid and electrolyte balance. It provides cues to racial and ethnic background, conveys emotional responses, and helps determine self-concept, roles, and relationships. (Functions of the skin, glands, hair, and nails are described in Table 14-1 ◆.)

There are many different disorders of the skin. The client with a minor or benign disorder is often treated in a physician's office or outpatient setting. The client with a disorder that involves large areas of the body, is chronic, or is malignant may require inpatient care. The nurse collects data about client needs and implements interventions to meet a wide variety of physical, emotional, and social responses.

Common primary and secondary skin lesions are described and illustrated in this chapter (Table 14-2 ◆). These terms are used throughout this chapter and in Chapter 15. This chapter discusses common disorders of the skin. Chapter 15 discusses burns.

Structure and Function of the Integumentary System

THE SKIN

The skin has a surface area of 15 to 20 square feet and weighs about 9 pounds. It has been estimated that each square inch of skin contains 15 feet of blood vessels, 4 yards of nerves, 650 sweat glands, 100 oil glands, 1,500 sensory receptors, and over 3 million cells that are constantly dying and being replaced.

The skin is composed of two regions: the epidermis and the dermis (Figure 14-1 ◆). The **epidermis** (the surface or outermost part of the skin) is made up of several layers of epithelial cells. The deepest layer of the epidermis contains cells that produce melanin and keratin. *Melanin* forms a shield to protect nerve endings in the dermis from the damaging effects of ultraviolet light. *Keratin* is a fibrous, water-repellent protein that makes the epidermis tough and protective. The outermost layer of the epidermis makes up about 75% of the epidermis's total thickness. It consists of about 20 to 30 sheets of dead cells filled with keratin fragments arranged in "shingles" that flake off as dry skin. The **dermis** (the second, deeper layer of skin) is made up of a flexible connective tissue. This layer is richly supplied with blood cells, nerve fibers, and lymphatic vessels. Most of the hair follicles, sebaceous glands, and sweat glands are located in the dermis.

The color of the skin is the result of varying levels of pigmentation. *Melanin,* a yellow-to-brown pigment, is darker and is produced in greater amounts in persons with dark skin color than in those with light skin. Exposure to the sun causes a buildup of melanin and a darkening of the skin in people with light skin. *Carotene* (a yellow-to-orange pigment) is more abundant in the skins of persons of Asian ancestry, and together with melanin accounts for their golden skin tone. The epidermis in Caucasian skin has very little melanin and is almost transparent. The color of their red blood cells shows through, lending Caucasians a pinkish skin tone.

Skin color is influenced by emotions and illnesses. **Erythema** (a reddening of the skin) may occur with embarrassment (as in blushing), fever, hypertension, or inflammation. It may also result from a drug reaction, sunburn, or other factors. **Cyanosis** (bluish discoloration of the skin and mucous membranes) results from poor oxygenation of hemoglobin.

TABLE 14-1	FUNCTIONS OF THE SKIN AND ITS APPENDAGES	

STRUCTURE	FUNCTIONS
Epidermis	Protects tissues from physical, chemical, and biologic damage. Prevents water loss and serves as a water-repellent layer. Stores melanin, which protects tissues from harmful effects of the ultraviolet radiation in sunlight. Converts cholesterol molecules to vitamin D when exposed to sunlight. Contains phagocytes, which prevent bacteria from penetrating the skin.
Dermis	Regulates body temperature by dilating and constricting capillaries. Transmits messages via nerve endings to the central nervous system.
Sebaceous (oil) glands	Secrete sebum, which lubricates skin and hair and plays a role in killing bacteria.
Eccrine sweat glands	Regulate body heat by excretion of perspiration.
Apocrine sweat glands	Unknown.
Hair	Cushions the scalp. Eyelashes and cilia protect the body from foreign particles. Provides insulation in cold weather.
Nails	Protect the fingers and toes, aid in grasping, and allow for various other activities, such as scratching the skin, picking up small items, peeling an orange, and so on.

TABLE 14-2

PRIMARY AND SECONDARY SKIN LESIONS

Macule, Patch

Flat, nonpalpable change in skin color. Macules are smaller than 1 cm, with a circumscribed border, and patches are larger than 1 cm and may have an irregular border.

Examples Macules: freckles, measles, and petechiae. Patches: mongolian spots, port-wine stains, vitiligo, and chloasma.

Papule, Plaque

Elevated, solid, palpable mass with circumscribed border. Papules are smaller than 0.5 cm; plaques are groups of papules that form lesions larger than 0.5 cm.

Examples Papules: elevated moles, warts, and lichen planus. Plaques: psoriasis, actinic keratosis, and also lichen planus.

Nodule, Tumor

Elevated, solid, hard or soft palpable mass extending deeper into the dermis than a papule. Nodules have circumscribed borders and are 0.5 to 2 cm; tumors may have irregular borders and are larger than 2 cm.

Examples Nodules: small lipoma, squamous cell carcinoma, fibroma, and intradermal nevi. Tumors: large lipoma, carcinoma, and hemangioma.

Vesicle, Bulla

Elevated, fluid-filled, round or oval-shaped, palpable mass with thin, translucent walls and circumscribed borders. Vesicles are smaller than 0.5 cm, bullae are larger than 0.5 cm.

Examples Vesicles: herpes simplex/zoster, early chickenpox, poison ivy, and small burn blisters. Bullae: contact dermatitis, friction blisters, and large burn blisters.

Wheal

Elevated, often reddish area with irregular border caused by diffuse fluid in tissues rather than free fluid in a cavity, as in vesicles. Size varies.

Examples Insect bites and hives (extensive wheals).

Pustule

Elevated, pus-filled vesicle or bulla with circumscribed border. Size varies.

Examples Acne, impetigo, and carbuncles (large boils).

Cyst

Elevated, encapsulated, fluid-filled or semisolid mass originating in the subcutaneous tissue or dermis, usually 1 cm or larger.

Examples Varieties include sebaceous cysts and epidermoid cysts.

Atrophy

A translucent, dry, paperlike, sometimes wrinkled skin surface resulting from thinning or wasting of the skin due to loss of collagen and elastin.

Examples Striae, aged skin.

Erosion

Wearing away of the superficial epidermis causing a moist, shallow depression. Because erosions do not extend into the dermis, they heal without scarring.

Examples Scratch marks, ruptured vesicles.

Lichenification

Rough, thickened, hardened area of epidermis resulting from chronic irritation such as scratching or rubbing.

Example Chronic dermatitis.

Scales

Shedding flakes of greasy, keratinized skin tissue. Color may be white, gray, or silver. Texture may vary from fine to thick.

Examples Dry skin, dandruff, psoriasis, and eczema.

(continues)

TABLE 14-2 CONTINUED

Crust	Dry blood, serum, or pus left on the skin surface when vesicles or pustules burst. Can be red-brown, orange, or yellow. Large crusts that adhere to the skin surface are called scabs. **Examples** Eczema, impetigo, herpes, or scabs following abrasion.	Scar	Flat, irregular area of connective tissue left after a lesion or wound has healed. New scars may be red or purple; older scars may be silvery or white. **Examples** Healed surgical wound or injury, healed acne.
Ulcer	Deep, irregularly shaped area of skin loss extending into the dermis or subcutaneous tissue. May bleed. May leave scar. **Examples** Decubitus ulcers (pressure sores), stasis ulcers, chancres.	Keloid	Elevated, irregular, darkened area of excess scar tissue caused by excessive collagen formation during healing. Extends beyond the site of the original injury. Higher incidence in people of African descent. **Examples** Keloid from ear piercing or surgery.
Fissure	Linear crack with sharp edges, extending into the dermis. **Examples** Cracks at the corners of the mouth or in the hands, athlete's foot.		

Pallor, or paleness of skin, may occur with shock, fear, or anger, or in anemia and hypoxia. **Jaundice** is a yellow-to-orange color visible in the skin and mucous membranes; it most often results from a liver disorder.

Glands of the Skin

The skin has three types of glands: sebaceous (oil) glands, sweat (sudoriferous) glands, and ceruminous glands. Each of these glands has a different function (see Table 14-1).

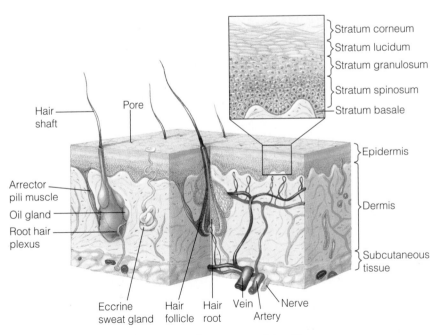

Figure 14-1. ◆ Anatomy of the skin

Sebaceous glands are found all over the body except the palms and soles. These glands secrete an oily substance (*sebum*) that softens and lubricates the skin and hair. Sebum also protects the body from infection by killing bacteria. The secretion of sebum is stimulated by hormones, especially androgens.

There are two types of sweat glands: eccrine and apocrine. The production of sweat is regulated by the sympathetic nervous system and serves to maintain normal body temperature. The secretions from apocrine glands are similar to those of sweat glands. Ceruminous glands are modified apocrine sweat glands that secrete yellow-brown waxy cerumen. This substance provides a sticky trap for foreign materials.

THE HAIR AND NAILS

Hair is distributed and scattered all over the body, except the lips, nipples, parts of the external genitals, the palms of the hands, and the soles of the feet. Hair is produced by a hair bulb, and its root is enclosed in a hair follicle. The visible hair is composed of dead cells. Many factors, including nutrition and hormones, influence hair growth. Hair in various parts of the body has protective functions. A nail is a modified scale-like epidermal structure. Like hair, nails consist mainly of dead cells. Review Table 14-1 for hair and nail functions.

Common Skin Disorders

PRURITUS

Pruritus is a subjective itching sensation producing an urge to scratch. Pruritus may occur in a small, circumscribed area, or it may involve a widespread area; it may or may not be associated with a rash. Pruritus is not a disorder itself but is rather a manifestation of an underlying irritation or condition. Itching is triggered by heat and prostaglandins and is increased by release of histamine and morphine. Almost anything in the internal or external environment can cause pruritus. Insects, animals, plants, fabrics, metals, medications, allergies, and emotional distress are among the most common causes. Pruritus also may occur as a secondary manifestation of systemic disorders, such as certain types of cancer, diabetes mellitus, hepatic disease, and renal failure.

Pruritus is initiated by a stimulation or irritation of receptors in the junction between the epidermis and dermis. The response by the person is to scratch or rub the affected area. This may irritate the skin and cause further inflammation, setting off a cycle of increasingly intense itching and scratching, called the *itch–scratch–itch* cycle.

The secondary effects of pruritus include skin excoriation, erythema, wheals, changes in pigmentation, and infections. Pruritus that persists may interrupt sleep patterns, because the itching sensation is often more intense at night. Long-term pruritus may be debilitating; broken skin also increases the risk of infection.

DRY SKIN

Dry skin (*xerosis*) is most often a problem in the older adult (Box 14-1). In older adults, decreased activity of sebaceous and

BOX 14-1

population
FOCUS

Skin Changes in Older Adults

A variety of normal skin changes are seen in the older adult. Loss of subcutaneous tissue, dermal thinning, and decreased elasticity may cause wrinkles and sagging of the skin. The skin is thinner, and turgor is decreased. Other age-related changes include the following:

- Dry, itchy skin may result from the reduction of sweat and oil glands.
- Overall production of melanocytes decreases, while abnormal localized proliferations of melanocytes may occur in specific areas. This localized hyperpigmentation may lead to the development of senile lentigines, commonly called "liver spots." These flat, brown macules commonly appear on the arms and hands in areas of sun exposure. Keratoses also result from hyperpigmentation. Seborrheic keratoses are dark, raised lesions. Actinic keratoses are reddish, raised plaques on areas of high sun exposure. They may become malignant.
- Skin tags, small flaps of excess skin, are normal in aging skin.
- Both hair and nail growth decrease with aging. Older men may develop coarse hair in the ears and nose and over the eyebrows. Decreased estrogen levels may cause postmenopausal women to develop dark facial hair over the upper lip and under the chin.
- Hair becomes gray due to a reduction of melanocytes.
- Nails may thicken, yellow, and peel.

sweat glands reduces the skin's lubrication and moisture retention. However, dry skin may occur at any age from exposure to environmental heat and low humidity, sunlight, excessive bathing, and a decreased intake of liquids.

The primary manifestation of dry skin is pruritus. Other manifestations include visible flaking of surface skin and an observable pattern of fine lines over the area. If the skin has been excessively dry and pruritic for a long period, the client may have secondary skin lesions and *lichenification* (thickening).

PSORIASIS

Psoriasis is a chronic, noninfectious skin disorder. It is characterized by raised, reddened, round circumscribed plaques of varied size, covered by silvery white scales (Figure 14-2 ◆). The plaques shed thick gray scales. The lesions may appear anywhere on the body. However, they are most commonly found on the scalp, extensor surfaces of the arms and legs, elbows, knees, sacrum, and around the nails. As with any chronic illness, the skin manifestations may disappear and recur throughout life.

The actual cause of psoriasis is unknown, but some evidence suggests it may be an autoimmune disorder. Sunlight, stress, seasonal changes, hormone fluctuations, steroid withdrawal, and certain drugs (such as alcohol, corticosteroids, lithium, and chloroquine) appear to make the disorder worse.

Figure 14-2. ◆ The characteristic lesions of psoriasis are raised, red, round plaques covered with thick, silvery scales.

Figure 14-3. ◆ Atopic dermatitis or eczema.

About one third of clients have a family history of psoriasis. Trauma to the skin (from surgery, sunburn, or excoriation) may also precipitate it.

Pruritus is common over the lesions. If the lesions are located in an *intertriginous zone* (between toes, under breasts, or in the perianal region), the psoriatic scales may soften, allowing painful fissures to form. When psoriasis affects the nails, pitting and a yellow or brown discoloration results. The nail may separate from the nail bed, thicken, and crumble, increasing the risk for infection.

DERMATITIS

Dermatitis is an acute or chronic inflammation of the skin characterized by erythema and pain or pruritus. Various agents or illnesses cause the inflammatory response of the skin. Initial skin responses include erythema, formation of vesicles and scales, and pruritus. Later, irritation from scratching promotes edema, a serous discharge, and crusting. Long-term irritation in chronic dermatitis causes the skin to become thickened, leathery, and darker in color.

Contact (allergic) dermatitis is caused by a hypersensitivity response or chemical irritation. The major sources known to cause contact dermatitis are dyes, perfumes, poison plants (ivy, oak, sumac), chemicals, and metals. Latex dermatitis is a contact dermatitis that is common in the health care field.

Atopic dermatitis is also called *eczema*. The exact cause is unknown, but related factors include depressed cell-mediated immunity, elevated immunoglobulin E (IgE) levels, and increased histamine sensitivity. Clients with atopic dermatitis have a family history of hypersensitivity reactions, such as eczema, asthma, and allergic rhinitis. Characteristic lesions include chronic lichenification, erythema, and scaling, the result of pruritus and scratching. The lesions are usually found on the hands, feet, or flexor surfaces of the arms and legs (Figure 14-3 ◆). Scratching and excoriation increase the risk of secondary infections, as well as invasion of the skin by viruses such as herpes simplex.

Seborrheic dermatitis is a chronic inflammatory disorder that involves the scalp, eyebrows, eyelids, ear canals, nasolabial folds, axillae, and trunk. The cause is unknown. This disorder is seen in all ages, from the very young (called "cradle cap") to the very old. Clients taking methyldopa for hypertension occasionally develop this disorder, and it is a component of Parkinson's disease. Seborrheic dermatitis is also frequently seen in clients with AIDS. The lesions are yellow or white plaques with scales and crusts. The scales are often yellow or orange and have a greasy appearance. Mild pruritus is also present.

Exfoliative dermatitis is an inflammatory skin disorder characterized by excessive peeling or shedding of skin. A preexisting skin disorder (such as psoriasis, atopic dermatitis, contact dermatitis, or seborrheic dermatitis) may be present. Exfoliative dermatitis is also associated with leukemia and lymphoma. Systemic manifestations include weakness, malaise, fever, chills, and weight loss. Scaling, erythema, and pruritus may be localized or involve the entire body. In addition to peeling of skin, the client may lose the hair and nails.

ACNE

Acne is a disorder of the sebaceous glands. These glands empty into the hair follicles and are open to the skin surface through a pore. They produce sebum in response to direct hormonal stimulation by testicular androgens in men and to adrenal and ovarian androgens in women. Most sebaceous glands are on the face, scalp, and scrotum.

Acne lesions are primarily *comedones* (pimples, whiteheads, and blackheads). Whiteheads are pale, slightly elevated papules. Blackheads are plugs of material that accumulate in the sebaceous glands. Inflammatory acne lesions include comedones, erythematous pustules, and cysts (Figure 14-4 ◆). The lesions may itch. The common types of acne are:

- *Acne vulgaris* (common in adolescents and young to middle-aged adults). Many factors once thought to cause acne vulgaris, including high-fat diets, chocolate, infections, and cosmetics, have been disproved (Porth, 1998).
- *Acne rosacea* (chronic facial acne that occurs more often in middle and older adults). The lesions begin with erythema over the cheeks and nose. Over years of time, the skin color changes to dark red, and the pores over the area become enlarged.

Figure 14-4. ◆ Inflammatory acne lesions include comedones, erythematous pustules, and cysts. There lesions often leave scars when they heal.

COLLABORATIVE CARE

Pruritus, dry skin, psoriasis, dermatitis, and acne are most often treated by self-care at home. Treatment focuses on identifying and eliminating or modifying any precipitating factors, providing relief from itching and pain, and reducing the risk of further damage to the skin.

Laboratory and Diagnostic Tests

Culture and sensitivity of skin scrapings and studies for fungal infections are conducted by microscopic examination to distinguish pruritus from psoriasis, dermatitis, and other disorders. Cutaneous scratch or patch testing may be performed if allergic reactions are the suspected cause.

If the client has atypical manifestations, or to differentiate psoriasis from inflammatory or infectious dermatitis, a skin biopsy may be done. Ultrasound tests may be performed to measure skin thickness. Results reveal typical psoriatic changes in the stratum corneum layer of the epidermis and dermal inflammation.

Pharmacology

PRURITUS. If possible, the client discontinues all medications to determine whether the pruritus is due to a drug reaction. Oral medications include antihistamines, tranquilizers, and antibiotics. Antihistamines provide relief from pruritus in some clients. Tranquilizers provide sedation, which may relieve the emotional stress associated with pruritus. Systemic antibiotics are used to treat infection resulting from the scratching and excoriation.

Topical medications that contain corticosteroids are often used to relieve pruritus and inflammation. Topical medications may also be administered through therapeutic baths or

soaks with agents that relieve pruritus, such as cornstarch, baking soda, or coal tar concentrates (see Box 14-2).

PSORIASIS. Topical corticosteroids, tar preparations, and retinoids decrease inflammation and suppress mitotic activity of psoriatic cells. The most effective topical corticosteroids are potent preparations. They are well absorbed through the skin and are used under an occlusive dressing. Corticosteroids may also be taken systemically or injected directly into the lesions.

BOX 14-2
THERAPEUTIC BATHS

AGENTS USED IN THERAPEUTIC BATHS
- Saline or tap water
- Antibacterial agents: Potassium permanganate, acetic acid, hexachlorophene
- Colloid substances: Oatmeal (Aveeno), cornstarch, sodium bicarbonate
- Potassium permanganate
- Emollients: Alpha-Keri, Lubath, mineral oil

Therapeutic baths have a variety of uses in treating skin disorders. Depending on the agent used, therapeutic baths soothe the skin, lower the skin bacteria count, clean and hydrate the skin, loosen scales, and relieve itching.

NURSING RESPONSIBILITIES
- Ensure that the bath water is at a comfortable temperature that is neither too hot nor too cool (usually 110 to 115° F [43 to 46° C]).
- Fill the tub one third to one half full.
- Mix the agent well with the water.
- Assist the client into and out of the tub to prevent falls.
- Dry the client by blotting with the towel.

CLIENT AND FAMILY TEACHING
- Use a bath mat in the tub: The medications may cause the tub to become slippery.
- Keep the bathroom warm but adequately ventilated.
- Follow directions carefully for the amount of medication to use in the bath.
- Fill the bath one third to one half full of water that is at a comfortable temperature.
- Stay in the bath for 20 to 30 minutes, and immerse the areas to be treated.
- Do not get the bathwater in your eyes.
- Dry by blotting (not rubbing) with the towel.
- If the medications cause staining, use old towels or linens.
- If the itching is not relieved or the skin becomes excessively dry, call your health care provider.

Tar preparations, applied topically or in a bath, are effective in some cases. They do have the undesirable side effect of staining. A topical retinoid (Tazarotene [Tazorac]) gel results in longer-lasting remissions, but may cause skin irritation and pruritus. Calcipotriene (Dovonex), a vitamin D analogue, has been shown to be effective and safe in both short and long-term treatment of psoriasis.

Photochemotherapy, using methoxsalen, is a treatment for severe psoriasis. This drug is an antimetabolite that inhibits deoxyribonucleic acid (DNA) synthesis. Exposure to ultraviolet-A (UVA) rays activates methoxsalen. It is administered orally, and the client is exposed to UVA 2 hours later. Treatments are administered 2 to 3 times a week. Usually, 10 to 20 total treatments are given over 1 to 2 months. The eyes are covered by dark glasses during the treatment. Treatment causes tanning, and direct sunlight must be avoided for 8 to 12 hours thereafter. If the client has erythema, the treatments are stopped until the redness and swelling resolve. Photochemotherapy can accelerate aging of exposed skin, induce cataract development, alter immune function, and increase the risk of melanoma.

Ultraviolet-B (UVB) light is often used to treat psoriasis. UVB light decreases the growth rate of epidermal cells. Mercury vapor lights or fluorescent UV tubes provide the UVB light. Fluorescent tubes are often arranged in a cabinet so the client can stand and expose psoriatic lesions more easily. These units may be purchased or constructed to be used in the client's home. The light therapy is administered in gradually increasing exposure times, until the client experiences a mild erythema, like a mild sunburn. Treatments are given daily and are measured in seconds of exposure. The eyes are shielded during the treatment. The erythema response occurs in about 8 hours. Careful assessment is necessary to prevent more severe burning, which could exacerbate the psoriasis.

ACNE. Treatment for acne is based on the type and severity of the lesions. For acne with comedones, tretinoin (retinoic acid, Retin-A) or benzoyl peroxide preparations are prescribed. Azelaic acid (Azelex) may also be used. Benzoyl peroxide preparations are found in over-the-counter medications such as Fostex, Acne-Dome, Desquam-X, Benzagel, Clear By Design, and Xerac BP. These products are keratolytic and loosen the comedones. Inflammatory acne is treated with oral or topical antibiotics, such as tetracycline, erythromycin, and minocycline. Severe forms of inflammatory acne are treated with isotretinoin (Accutane), which is effective but has serious side effects. (Nursing responsibilities for these medications are discussed in Table 14-3 ◆.) The treatment for acne lasts months, and in some cases for the rest of one's life.

Surgery

Dermabrasion of inactive acne lesions can improve the client's appearance, especially if the scars are flat. The skin is first frozen (and anesthetized) with Freon or ethyl chloride. The lesions are carefully abraded with fine sandpaper or abrasive brushes.

NURSING CARE

Nursing care for the client with common skin problems focuses on promoting comfort and decreasing the risk of infection. Because clients care for themselves at home, nursing interventions are primarily educational. Teaching focuses on methods of relieving itching and dry skin and preventing infection. Clients with psoriasis require information about medications and light treatments.

ASSESSING

Assessment data are collected by the nurse to determine the degree of discomfort, the extent to which the skin condition is interfering with the client's activities of daily living and usual lifestyle, and the risk factors for complications. Box 14-3 suggests subjective and objective data to collect.

DIAGNOSING, PLANNING, AND IMPLEMENTING

Although pruritus, dry skin, psoriasis, dermatitis, and acne are not life threatening, they may result in physical and emotional distress. The priority nursing diagnoses are impaired skin integrity, disturbed body image, and deficient knowledge about medication administration.

IMPAIRED SKIN INTEGRITY

- Recommend that the nails be trimmed short, the environmental temperatures be slightly cool, and loose clothing be worn. *These measures relieve pruritus and decrease the risk of infection.*
- Suggest the following strategies to relieve itching:
  - Rub the pruritic area with the surface of the hand rather than scratching with the nails, briefly apply pressure or cold to help relieve pruritus, and wear cotton gloves at night.
  - Use distraction or relaxation techniques.
  - Wash clothing in a mild detergent and rinse twice. Do not use fabric softeners.
  - Avoid using perfumes and lotions containing alcohol, and apply skin lubricants after a bath to help retain moisture.
  These strategies relieve itching and prevent excoriation.
- Demonstrate methods of taking therapeutic baths or treatments. Use warm, not hot, water. Gently rub lesions with a soft washcloth, using a circular motion. *Hot water increases itching. Gentle rubbing reduces the risk of injury to the skin.*
- Dry the skin with a soft towel, using a blotting or patting motion. *Washing or drying the skin with rough linens may excoriate the skin over lesions.*
- Teach the client and family to watch for and report to the health care provider any complications of treatment, such

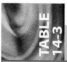

TABLE 14-3			

NURSING IMPLICATIONS FOR PHARMACOLOGY: CLIENTS WITH ACNE

DRUG GROUP/ DRUGS	ACTION/USES	NURSING IMPLICATIONS	CLIENT TEACHING
Antiacne Retinoids ■ Isotretinoin (Accutane) ■ Tretinoin (Retin-A)	These agents are vitamin A metabolites that, depending on the drug, either act as an irritant to decrease comedome formation or decrease sebum production. Baseline lipid levels are measured at the onset of treatment, at 2 weeks, and then monthly during treatment (lipids > 500–800 mg/dL indicates a need to stop the drug to prevent acute pancreatitis). Liver function tests are performed at 2- to 3-week intervals for 6 months and then once a month during treatment.	Do not administer to clients with eczema or who are sensitive to the sun. Do not administer to pregnant women. Assess for side effects of redness, scaling, severe erythema with topical use.	Cleanse affected skin areas well with a bland soap and dry completely before applying drug. Expect redness and peeling of skin. Use only nonmedicated cosmetics, lotions, or shaving lotions and wash them off before applying drug. Use sunscreen and protective clothing when outside. Do not take vitamin A supplements or drink alcohol while using the drugs. Use a reliable contraceptive from 1 month before beginning treatment to 1 month following the end of treatment. A pregnancy test should be conducted within 2 weeks of beginning treatment to rule out pregnancy. Report jaundice, pruritus, and/or dark urine immediately. If visual disturbances, nausea, vomiting, and headache occur, stop the drug at once and report manifestations to the physician.

BOX 14-3
ASSESSING CLIENTS WITH COMMON SKIN PROBLEMS

SUBJECTIVE DATA

- Present health status:
  - Location, duration, and type of itching present
  - Ability to sleep at night
  - Skin oily or dry, amount of sweating
  - Medications used to treat dry skin, itching, or skin lesions
- Past medical history:
  - History of allergies
  - History of exposure to environmental substances
  - Chronic illness, such as thyroid disorders, diabetes mellitus, or liver disease

OBJECTIVE DATA

- Inspect the entire skin for color and lesions
  - Redness, swelling, and pain may indicate a secondary infection from itching, or may follow phototherapy treatments for psoriasis
  - Dry, rough skin with visible flaking indicates severe xerosis
- Palpate the skin for temperature, texture, moisture, and turgor:
  - Increased warmth may indicate infection. Dry skin is rough.
  - Pinch the skin gently over the collarbone or top of the hand; tenting (in which the skin remains in a fold for a few moments) is common in older adults

as excoriation, increased redness, increased skin peeling, or blister formation. *The medications and treatments may cause damage to skin cells through chemical burns or exposure to ultraviolet light. Times and methods of treatment need to be adjusted if these occur.*

DISTURBED BODY IMAGE

- Establish a trusting nurse–client relationship by verbally and nonverbally expressing acceptance. For example, touching the client on the shoulder demonstrates that the lesions and the client's appearance are not offensive. *One's body image is affected not only by self-perception but also by the responses of others. The skin eruptions and lesions, especially chronic ones, often cause clients to isolate themselves from social contacts, withdraw from normal roles and responsibilities, and feel helpless or powerless.*
- Encourage talking about about self-perception and questions about the disease and the treatment. *The client adapts to a changed body image through a process of recognition, acceptance, and resolution. Each person responds individually to changes in body image and loss.*
- Encourage interaction with others through family involvement in care, referral to support groups, and referral to organizations such as the National Psoriasis Foundation. *Acceptance of others is critical to acceptance of self. By becoming involved in care, the family demonstrates love and acceptance. Sharing experiences with others who have the same health problem is a source of strength in adjusting to a visible health problem. Local, state, and national organizations can provide resources and information.*

DEFICIENT KNOWLEDGE: MEDICATION ADMINISTRATION

- Many of the common skin problems are treated with topical medications. Teach the client the following general guidelines for applying these medications:
  - Each time a medication is applied, the skin surface must be clean and dry. Remove creams by washing with tap water. Remove ointments by first washing the skin with mineral oil, and then with mild soap and water.
  - To apply *gels, creams,* and *pastes:* Squeeze about ½ to 1 inch of the medication into the palm of the hand and rub the hands together. Apply with the hands to the affected areas using long strokes until the skin is thinly covered. Exceptions are:
    - *Corticosteroids* are usually applied two or three times a day in small amounts and rubbed directly into the skin. If prescribed, cover with a dressing.
    - Medications containing *tar* are applied in the direction of the hair growth. Do not apply these medications to the face, the genitals, or in skin folds. These medications will stain clothing.
  - To apply *lotions:* Shake the bottle well. Pour a small amount into the palm of the hand and pat the medication on the skin. If the lotion is thin, use a gauze pad.

- To apply *sprays:* Hold the container about 6 inches from the skin and apply the medication in a short spray.
- To apply *medicated shampoo:* Rinse the hair. Apply the shampoo, massage into the hair and scalp. Allow it to remain for the prescribed time. Rinse.
- To apply *pastes:* Use enough paste on an applicator (such as a wooden tongue depressor) to cover the lesion thinly. *Teaching guidelines ensure accurate administration.*

EVALUATING

Collect data to determine the client's understanding of medications and their use, the client's degree of comfort, and any changes in the level of skin integrity or involvement.

 Discharge Considerations

In addition to teaching the client how to administer topical medications, the nurse should provide the following information for self-care.

- Medications and treatments do not cure the disease. They only relieve the symptoms.
- Dry skin increases pruritus, which stimulates scratching. Scratching may in turn cause excoriation, and excoriation increases the risk of infection.
- It may be necessary to change the diet or environment to avoid contact with allergens.

CLINICAL alert

Teach clients using oral corticosteroids to never stop taking the medication abruptly.

Infections and Infestations of the Skin

The skin's resistance to infections and infestations is provided by normal skin flora, sebum, and the immune response. Disorders may occur from a break in the skin surface, a virulent agent, or decreased resistance due to a compromised immune system.

BACTERIAL INFECTIONS

Bacterial infections of the skin arise from the hair follicle, where bacteria can accumulate and grow and cause a localized infection. If the bacteria invade deeper tissues, they can cause a systemic infection, a potentially life-threatening disorder. Most bacterial infections are treated by a primary care provider, and the client remains at home for care. Nosocomial infections of wounds or open lesions in hospitalized clients are often the result of bacterial infections, especially by methicillin-resistant *Staphylococcus aureus* (MRSA). (See Chapter 12.)

Folliculitis

Folliculitis is most often caused by *Staphylococcus aureus.* The infection begins at the skin surface and extends down into the hair follicle. The bacteria release enzymes and chemical agents that cause an inflammation. The lesions appear as pustules surrounded by an area of erythema on the surface of the skin. Folliculitis is found most often on the scalp and extremities, on the face (of bearded men), on the legs of women who shave, and on the eyelids (called a *stye*). Although folliculitis may appear without any apparent cause, contributing factors include poor hygiene, poor nutrition, prolonged skin moisture, and trauma to the skin.

Furuncles

A **furuncle** ("boil") is also an infection of the hair follicle. (A group of infected hair follicles is called a *carbuncle*). It often begins as folliculitis, but the infection spreads down the hair shaft, through the wall of the follicle, and into the dermis. The causative organism is commonly *Staphylococcus aureus.* Contributing factors include poor hygiene, trauma to the skin, areas of excessive moisture (including perspiration), and systemic diseases, such as diabetes mellitus.

A furuncle is initially a deep, firm, red, painful nodule from 1 to 5 cm in diameter. After a few days, the nodule changes into a large, tender cystic nodule. The cysts may contain purulent drainage. Carbuncles have multiple openings onto the skin and may cause fever, chills, and malaise.

Cellulitis

Cellulitis is a localized infection of the dermis and subcutaneous tissue. Cellulitis can occur following a wound or skin ulcer or as an extension of furuncles or carbuncles. The infection spreads as a result of a substance called *spreading factor,* or *hyaluronidase,* which is produced by the causative organism. Hyaluronidase breaks down the fibrin network and other barriers that normally localize the infection.

The area of cellulitis is red, swollen, and painful (Figure 14-5 ◆). In some cases, vesicles may form over the area of cellulitis. The client may also experience fever, chills, malaise, headache, and swollen lymph glands.

FUNGAL INFECTIONS

Fungi are plantlike organisms that live in the soil, on animals, and on humans. The fungi that cause superficial skin infections are called **dermatophytes.** In humans, the dermatophytes live on keratin in the stratum corneum, hair, and nails. Superficial fungal infections of the skin are often referred to as *ringworm* or *tinea.* Fungal disorders are also called *mycoses.*

The organism may be transmitted by direct contact with animals or other infected persons or by inanimate objects such as combs, pillowcases, towels, and hats. The onset and spread of the fungal infection is greatest in moist areas, such as in skin folds, between the toes, and in the mouth. Other factors that increase the risk of a fungal infection include the use of broad-spectrum antibiotics that kill off normal flora and allow the fungi to grow, the presence of diabetes mellitus, immu-

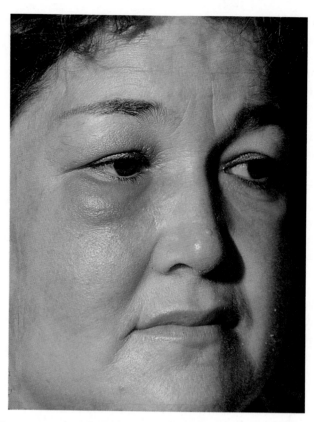

Figure 14-5. ◆ Cellulitis is a bacterial infection localized in the dermis and subcutaneous tissue. The involved area is red, swollen, and painful.

nodeficiencies, nutritional deficiencies, pregnancy, increasing age, and iron deficiency.

Dermatophyte (Tinea) Infections

The dermatophyte *(tinea)* infections are named by the body part affected: Those most common in adults are:

- *Tinea pedis (athlete's foot)* affects the soles of the feet, the space between the toes, and the toenail. The lesions vary from mild scaliness to painful fissures with drainage, and they are usually accompanied by pruritus and a foul odor.
- *Tinea cruris* is an infection of the groin that may extend to the inner thighs and buttocks. Also called "jock itch," it is often associated with tinea pedis and is more common in people who are physically active, are obese, and/or wear tight underclothing.

Candidiasis Infections

Candidiasis infections are caused by *Candida albicans,* a yeast-like fungus. This fungus is normally found on mucous membranes, on the skin, in the vagina, and in the gastrointestinal tract. The fungus becomes a pathogen when certain conditions encourage its growth: an environment of moisture, warmth, or altered skin integrity; systemic antibiotics; pregnancy; birth control pills; poor nutrition; immunosuppression; or diabetes mellitus, Cushing's disease, or other chronic debilitating illnesses.

Candidiasis affects only the outer layers of the skin and mucous membranes. It occurs in the mouth, vagina, uncircumcised penis, nails, and deep skin folds. The first sign of infection is a pustule that often burns and itches. As the infection spreads, a white to yellow curdlike substance covers the infected area.

VIRAL INFECTIONS

Viruses are pathogens that consist of a ribonucleic acid (RNA) or DNA core surrounded by a protein coat. They depend on live cells for reproduction. The viruses that cause skin lesions either increase cellular growth or cause cellular death. An increase in the incidence of viral skin disorders has been attributed to a variety of causes, including some commonly used drugs like birth control medications, corticosteroids, and antibiotics.

Warts

Warts *(verrucae)* are lesions caused by the human papillomavirus (HPV). Warts may be found on skin and mucous membranes. Nongenital warts are benign lesions; genital warts may be precancerous. Warts are transmitted through skin contact. Warts may be flat, fusiform (tapered at both ends), or round, but most are round and raised and have a rough, gray surface. Warts resolve spontaneously when immunity to the virus develops. This response may take up to 5 years. There are many different types of HPV. Those most common are described below:

- A *common wart* may occur anywhere on the skin or mucous membranes. It grows above the skin surface and may be dome-shaped with ragged borders. A flat wart is a small flat lesion, usually seen on the forehead or dorsum of the hand.
- *Plantar warts* occur at pressure points on the soles of the feet. The pressure of shoes and walking prevents these warts from growing outward. They tend to extend deeper beneath the skin surface than common warts, and they are often painful.
- *Condylomata acuminata (venereal warts)* occur in moist areas, along the glans of the penis, in the anal region, and on the vulva. They are usually cauliflower-like in appearance and have a pink or purple color.

Herpes Simplex

Herpes simplex ("fever blister," "cold sore") infections are caused by two types of herpesvirus: HSV I and HSV II. Most infections above the waist (most commonly on lips, face, and mouth) are caused by HSV I. (Genital herpes infections, which result from either HSV I or HSV II, are classified as sexually transmitted diseases and are discussed in Chapter 34). The virus may be transmitted by physical contact, oral sex, or kissing. The virus lives in nerve ganglia and may cause recurrent lesions in response to sunlight, menstruation, injury, or stress.

The infection begins with a burning or tingling sensation, followed by the development of erythema, vesicle formation, and pain. The vesicles progress through pustules, ulcers, and crusting until healing occurs in 10 to 14 days. The initial infection is often severe and accompanied by systemic manifestations, such as fever and sore throat. Recurrences are more localized and less severe.

Herpes Zoster

Herpes zoster ("shingles") is a viral infection of a dermatome section of the skin caused by varicella zoster, the same herpesvirus that causes chickenpox. The infection is believed to result from reactivation of a varicella virus that remains in the sensory dorsal ganglia after a childhood infection of chickenpox. When reactivated, the virus travels from the ganglia to the corresponding skin dermatome area.

Clients with Hodgkin's disease, certain types of leukemia, and lymphomas are more susceptible to an outbreak of herpes zoster. Herpes zoster is more prevalent in people who are immunocompromised (e.g., by HIV), those who are receiving radiation therapy or chemotherapy, and those who have had major organ transplants. In people with HIV infections, the appearance of the lesions may be one of the first manifestations of immune compromise.

The lesions are vesicles with an erythematous base. The lesions usually appear unilaterally on the face, trunk, and/or thorax; continue to erupt for 3 to 5 days; then crust and dry. Recovery occurs in 2 to 3 weeks. The client experiences severe pain before and during eruption of the lesions. The older adult is especially sensitive to the pain and often experiences more severe outbreaks of herpes zoster lesions. In most cases, the disease is benign and localized. Complications of herpes zoster include *postherpetic neuralgia* (a sharp, spasmodic pain along the course of one or more nerves) and visual loss. The neuralgia, described as burning or stabbing, results from inflammation of the root ganglia. Permanent loss of vision may follow occurrence of lesions that arise from the ophthalmic division of the trigeminal nerve.

PARASITIC INFESTATIONS

The skin may be invaded by parasites or insects. Infestations affect people of all social classes but are associated with crowded or unsanitary living conditions. Two of the more common parasites are mites and lice.

Pediculosis

Pediculosis is an infestation with lice. Lice are parasites that ingest blood of an animal or human host. One louse (a 2- to 4-mm oval organism) is capable of laying hundreds of eggs. All species of lice have a similar life cycle. The first stage is an unhatched egg (a *nit*) laid by the female louse on a hair shaft. The nit is a small pearl-gray or brown egg visible to the naked eye. Three types of lice live on human hosts:

- *Pediculosis corporis* is an infestation with body lice. The lice live in clothing fibers and are transmitted primarily by contact with infested clothes and bed linens. The louse bites cause a macule, followed by wheals and papules. Itching is common.

- *Pediculosis capitis* is an infestation with head lice. The lice are most often found behind the ears and nape of the neck, but may spread to other hairy areas of the body. Transmission is by contact with an infected person or object (such as a comb). The infestation causes itching, scratching, and erythema.
- *Pediculosis pubis* is an infestation with pubic lice ("crabs"). The lice are spread through sexual activity or contact with infested clothing or linens. The infestation causes skin irritation and intense itching.

Scabies

Scabies is an infestation caused by a mite. The infestation is found between the fingers, the inner surfaces of the wrist and elbow, the axillae, the female nipple, the penis, the belt line, and the gluteal crease. The lesions are small red-brown burrows, about 2 mm in length, sometimes covered with vesicles that appear as a rash. Pruritus is common, especially at night. Excoriations from scratching predispose the person to secondary bacterial infections.

COLLABORATIVE CARE

Clients with infections and infestations of the skin and mucous membranes are usually diagnosed and treated by their primary health care provider, and then provide self-care at home. Treatment is focused on identifying the causative agent and administering medications to kill the bacteria or eradicate the organism, and preventing secondary infections.

Laboratory and Diagnostic Tests

Bacterial infections are diagnosed by a culture and sensitivity of the drainage from a lesion to identify organisms and to target the most effective antibiotic. If the infection is systemic, a blood culture may be conducted to identify the causative organism.

Fungal infections are diagnosed by various methods. Cultures of skin scrapings, nail scrapings, or hairs are done. Microscopic examination of scrapings may be done to visualize spores and filaments. The affected skin may be inspected under ultraviolet light (called a Wood's lamp); fungal spores fluoresce blue-green.

Laboratory tests may be necessary to differentiate herpes zoster from impetigo, contact dermatitis, or herpes simplex. Cultures of fluids from vesicles and antibody tests are used to identify the herpesvirus types.

When a client has pediculosis, the hair shaft and clothing are inspected, with microscopic examination used for a positive diagnosis. Scabies is diagnosed by skin scrapings and microscopic examination of the mites or their feces.

Pharmacology

BACTERIAL INFECTIONS. The primary treatment for bacterial infections is an antibiotic specific to the organism. The antibiotic is usually administered systemically, but may also be applied topically. Multiple furuncles and carbuncles may be treated with cloxacillin, a penicillinase-resistant penicillin;

the cephalosporins also are often effective. (Antibiotic therapy is discussed in Chapter 12.)

FUNGAL INFECTIONS. Fungal infections are treated by topical or systemic antifungal medications. (Nursing implications for antifungal medications are discussed in Table 14-4 ◆.) Dermatophyte infections are usually treated with topical antifungals. Candidiasis infections are treated with nystatin (Mycostatin) in powder, tablet, or vaginal suppository form. Other medications that may be used include ketoconazole and fluconazole, administered orally.

VIRAL INFECTIONS. Most viral skin infections are treated with antiviral medications, and other medications are used to relieve pruritus and pain in clients with herpes zoster. A common method of wart removal is acid therapy, using a colloidal solution of 16% salicylic acid and 16% lactic acid. The solution is applied to the wart every 12 to 24 hours, and the wart disappears in 2 or 3 weeks. Other methods of eradicating warts are cryosurgery, freezing with liquid nitrogen, and electrodesiccation with an electric cautery. Herpes lesions are treated with acyclovir (Zovirax), an antiviral agent that may be administered topically, orally, or parenterally.

PARASITIC INFESTATIONS. Lice are eradicated with topical agents that kill the parasite, such as medications that contain gamma benzene hexachloride, malathion (Prioderm lotion), or permethrin (NIX). Scabies may be eradicated with a single treatment of lindane lotion or Kwell, applied to the entire skin surface.

NURSING CARE

Nursing care of the client with a skin infection or infestation focuses on preventing the spread of infection and restoring normal skin integrity. Most clients provide self-care at home. If the hospitalized client develops a secondary bacterial infection, isolation procedures should be implemented to limit the spread of infection to others.

One of the most effective methods in reducing the spread of infection in any setting is careful handwashing. Health care providers must wash their hands with soap and water before and after every client contact, even if gloves are worn. All clients, family members, and visitors should be taught how to wash their hands effectively, and the importance of this procedure should be stressed.

ASSESSING

The nurse collects subjective and objective assessment data to identify the manifestations of an infection or infestation, and to determine the degree to which the client is at risk for complications. Ask the client about personal and intimate contact with others who may have been infected or infested, manifestations of increased infection (increased erythema, fever, puru-

TABLE 14-4   NURSING IMPLICATIONS FOR PHARMACOLOGY: CLIENTS WITH FUNGAL INFECTIONS

DRUG GROUP/DRUGS	ACTION/USES	NURSING IMPLICATIONS	CLIENT TEACHING
Antifungal Agents ■ Amphotericin B (Fungizone) ■ Clotrimazole (Mycelex) ■ Fluconazole (Diflucan) ■ Griseofulvin Microsize (Fulvicin-U/F) ■ Ketoconazole (Nizoral) ■ Miconazole (Monistat) ■ Nystatin (Mycostatin)	Some drugs interfere with the fungal cell membrane permeability; others interfere with DNA synthesis. They are prepared in many forms: powders, shampoos, suspensions, troches, oral tablets, and vaginal tablets.	Assess for known hypersensitivity to these agents. Assess for side effects: skin rash, gastrointestinal symptoms, and mental status. Administer ketoconazole with food. Shake suspensions well before administering, and ask clients to swish them around in their mouth before swallowing. Tell clients to let oral tablets dissolve in the mouth.	Treatment continues for a long time, but it is important to complete the full prescription. Take griseofulvin with meals. Avoid alcohol and exposure to sunlight. Continue vaginal applications through the menses, and either refrain from sexual intercourse or have partner wear a condom. Your sexual partner must be treated at the same time or the infection will be passed back and forth.

lent drainage), and living conditions. Include questions about any chronic illnesses, such as diabetes mellitus, immune disorders, and previous viral infections (including having chickenpox as a child). Inspect the skin, hair, and mucous membranes. Note the location, appearance, and size of lesions; type and color of lesions; and nits. Take and record vital signs. Report abnormal findings.

DIAGNOSING, PLANNING, AND IMPLEMENTING

Nursing interventions for most infections and infestations of the skin focus on providing information so the client can perform self-care at home (see Discharge Considerations below). However, the client with herpes zoster may have increased nursing care needs, with such priority nursing diagnoses as Pain, Sleep Pattern Disturbance, and Risk for Infection.

ACUTE PAIN

■ Assess and monitor the location, duration, and intensity of the pain. *Each person experiences and expresses pain differently. Pain tolerance is individualized.*

■ Administer prescribed medications regularly and evaluate their effectiveness. *Regular administration prevents the pain from reaching an intensity at which the medication would be less effective.*

■ Use measures to relieve pruritus. Administer prescribed antipruritic medications. Apply calamine lotion or cool compresses, if prescribed. Keep the room temperature cool. *Pruritus is a common problem for these clients, and it may intensify pain. Scratching increases the risk of secondary infection. Lotions and cool compresses are often effective in decreasing the itch–scratch–itch cycle.*

■ Encourage the use of distraction (such as music) or a specific relaxation technique (such as progressive muscle relaxation or deep breathing). *Noninvasive methods help the client manage the pain and also increase the effectiveness of pain medications.*

DISTURBED SLEEP PATTERN

■ Provide appropriate interventions (above) to relieve pain and pruritus. *The pain and pruritus of herpes zoster are often more intense at night, probably as a result of decreased distraction. Analgesics and noninvasive methods of relief may be necessary before bedtime.*

■ Maintain a cool environment and avoid heavy bed covers. Use a bed cradle if necessary to keep bed linens off the client. *Heat and touch intensify pruritus. Pruritus stimulates scratching, which awakens the client. Pain may then be perceived as being more acute. A cycle is established that interferes with sleep.*

RISK FOR INFECTION

■ Take and record vital signs every 4 hours. Report increased body temperature. Assess skin lesions for increased erythema, formation of pustules, or purulent drainage. Monitor white blood cell (WBC) count. Palpate lymph nodes for enlargement. *Secondary bacterial infections may occur, manifested by fever, changes in lesions or drainage, an increased WBC, or enlarged lymph nodes.*

■ Use interventions to decrease the itch–scratch–itch cycle. *Clients with herpes zoster have increased risk for infection because of pruritus, scratching, and skin excoriation. Excoriations from scratching provide a portal for bacterial infection.*

■ Institute infection control procedures. Maintain strict isolation for immunocompromised clients. Wear gloves and gown if contact with lesions is likely. Instruct pregnant women (visitors and health care providers) to avoid exposure until lesions have crusted over. *Isolation procedures are instituted for the immunocompromised client to protect the client from infection. The client is also contagious to others who did not have chickenpox as a child. The nurse wears gloves and a gown to prevent spreading the infection to self and others. Pregnant women must avoid exposure because the herpesvirus can cross the placental barrier.*

EVALUATING

To evaluate the effectiveness of nursing care for clients with skin infection or infestation, collect assessment data, evaluating for changes in skin integrity and the need for additional measures to protect skin and underlying tissues from injury. Determine the client's understanding of medications and their use, and of how to prevent transmission of the infection or infestation.

Discharge Considerations

Planning and teaching for home care are important nursing responsibilities when caring for the client with a skin infection or infestation. Specific teaching for each type of illness follows.

BACTERIAL INFECTIONS

Teaching focuses on facilitating tissue healing and eliminating the infection. Stress the importance of bathing daily with antibacterial soap, gently washing off crusts during the bath. Warm compresses may be applied to the lesions two or three times a day to increase comfort and decrease swelling. Teach the client to cover draining lesions with a sterile dressing, to handle soiled dressings or linens according to standard precautions, and to wear disposable rubber gloves when changing dressings. Other instructions should be given:

■ Maintain good nutrition.
■ Carefully wash hands before and after dressing changes.
■ Do not share linens and towels. Wash all linens and towels in hot water.
■ Never squeeze or try to open a lesion. Clean the skin and keep it dry, especially in hot weather. Do not pluck nasal hair or pick the nose.
■ Take the full course of prescribed medications until the supply is finished.

FUNGAL INFECTIONS

Many people treat themselves with over-the-counter antifungal medications. It is recommended that the person be diagnosed at the first occurrence. The nurse should provide the following information:

■ Fungal infections are contagious. Do not share linens or personal items with others. Use a clean towel and washcloth each day.
■ Carefully dry all skin folds, including those under the breasts, under the arms, and between the toes. Do not wear the same pair of shoes every day. Wear cotton socks or hose with cotton feet. Do not wear rubber or plastic-soled shoes. Use talcum powder or an antifungal powder twice a day.
■ For vaginal yeast infections: Avoid tight jeans and pantyhose. Wear cotton or cotton-crotch panties. Bathe more frequently, and dry the genital area well. Have your sexual partner treated at the same time you are so you don't pass the infection back and forth.

VIRAL INFECTIONS

The nurse provides the following information:

■ The diseases are usually self-limiting and heal completely.
■ Do not have contact with children or pregnant women until crusts have formed over the blistered areas in clients with herpes zoster.

PARASITIC INFESTATIONS

Client and family teaching is necessary to facilitate treatment at home, to prevent the spread of the infestation, and to dispel the myth that only dirty people have lice. Teach this specific information:

■ Wash clothing and linens in soap and hot water, or have them dry-cleaned.
■ Iron clothing to kill lice eggs.
■ Boil personal care items, such as combs and brushes, to kill parasites.
■ Treat all family members and sexual partners.
■ Do not use combs, brushes, or hats of others.

See Critical Thinking Care Map on herpes zoster at the end of this chapter.

Malignant Skin Disorders

The skin is a common site for malignancy. Many of these lesions are found on skin surfaces that have had long-term exposure to the sun or the environment. Skin cancer is the most common of all cancers. This section of the chapter discusses the various types of malignant skin disorders.

NONMELANOMA SKIN CANCER

The skin is a fragile organ and is subject to damage from ultraviolet radiation and chemicals. Over time, this damage results in alterations in cellular structure and function, and malignancies may occur. The two types of **nonmelanoma skin cancers** (named because they do not arise from melanin-producing cells) are basal cell carcinoma and squamous cell carcinoma.

It is estimated that over 1.3 million new cases of nonmelanoma skin cancer are diagnosed each year, and that about

1,900 deaths will occur (American Cancer Society, 2001). However, the relative survival rate is greater than 99%. Nonmelanoma skin cancer is the most common malignant neoplasm found in fair-skinned Americans. Of the two types of nonmelanoma skin cancer, basal cell carcinoma is the most common, outnumbering squamous cell carcinoma three to one. Men develop nonmelanoma skin cancer more often than do women, probably because of occupational exposures. Adults between the ages of 30 and 60 have the majority of these cancers. The factors involved in the development of nonmelanoma skin cancer include ultraviolet radiation, chemicals, skin pigmentation, and preexisting pigmented skin lesions.

Ultraviolet radiation (UVR) from the sun is believed to be the cause of most nonmelanoma skin cancers. Sun rays are believed to either alter DNA or suppress T-cell and B-cell immunity. People who live in higher altitudes receive greater ultraviolet radiation exposure. The amount of clothing worn, the time of day, and the amount of time in the sun also determine the amount of exposure. Exposure to ultraviolet radiation in tanning booths has been implicated in nonmelanoma skin cancer development.

Certain chemicals have also been associated with nonmelanoma skin cancer. Hydrocarbons, found in mixtures of coal, tar, asphalt, soot, and mineral oils have been linked with skin cancer. Other factors associated with nonmelanoma skin cancer are the use of ionizing radiation, viruses, and physical trauma. Human papillomavirus is implicated in the development of squamous cell carcinoma, as is damage to the skin from burns.

Skin pigmentation affects the development of nonmelanoma skin cancer. The more melanin a person has, the more the skin is protected from damaging ultraviolet rays. Thus, African Americans, Asian Americans, and people of Mediterranean descent have a much lower incidence of nonmelanoma skin cancer than do people who have red hair and fair complexions and who tend to freckle or sunburn easily.

Most people have many pigmented moles or other lesions on their body, and almost all of them are normal. However, a major risk factor in the development of nonmelanoma skin cancer is a change in an existing lesion or the presence of a premalignant lesion, such as actinic keratosis.

BASAL CELL CARCINOMA

Basal cell carcinoma begins in the basal cell layer of the epidermis, usually on sun-exposed areas of the body, especially the head and neck. About 75% of all skin cancers are basal cell carcinomas (American Cancer Society, 2001). They are slow-growing and rarely metastasize, but they can invade nearby areas. They can recur in the same location after treatment.

SQUAMOUS CELL CARCINOMA

Squamous cell carcinoma is a malignant tumor of the squamous epithelium of the skin or mucous membranes. It occurs most often on areas of skin that are exposed to ultraviolet rays and weather, such as the forehead, helix of the ear, top of the nose, lower lip, and back of the hands. Squamous cell carcinoma may also arise on skin that has been burned or has

chronic inflammation. This is a much more aggressive cancer than basal cell cancer, with a faster growth rate and a much greater potential for metastasis if untreated.

Squamous cell carcinoma begins as a firm, flesh-colored or erythematous papule. The tumor may be crusted. As it grows, it may ulcerate, bleed, and become painful. As the tumor extends into the surrounding tissue and becomes a nodule, the area around the nodule becomes *indurated* (hardened) (Figure 14-6 ◆). Recurrent squamous cell carcinoma can be invasive, increasing the person's risk of metastasis.

MELANOMA

Melanoma, also called *cutaneous* or *malignant melanoma,* is a skin cancer that arises from melanocytes, the cells that produce melanin. The incidence of this serious skin cancer is increasing annually; its incidence doubled in the past three decades. Melanoma is the cause of 4% of all skin cancer cases, but accounts for 79% of skin cancer deaths (American Cancer Society, 2001).

The incidence is highest in Caucasians, people who had severe sunburn with blistering during childhood, and in people who live in sunny climates, burn easily, and visit tanning parlors. However, melanoma may arise from lesions that are already present or from skin that is normally covered with clothing. While they are still confined to the epidermis, the lesions are flat and relatively benign. However, when they penetrate the dermis, they mingle with blood and lymph vessels and are capable of metastasizing. At this latter stage, the tumors develop a raised or nodular appearance and often have smaller nodules, called satellite lesions, around the periphery.

The prognosis for survival for people diagnosed with malignant melanoma is determined by several variables, including tumor thickness, ulceration, metastasis, site, age, and gender. Younger clients and women have a somewhat better chance of survival. Tumors on the hands, feet, and scalp have a poorer prognosis. Tumors of the feet and scalp may not be noticed and diagnosed until they grow into the dermis.

Precursor lesions for the development of melanoma are dysplastic **nevi** (moles), congenital nevi, and lentigo maligna. *Dysplastic nevi* (also called atypical moles) appear during child-

Figure 14-6. ◆ As a squamous cell cancer grows, it tends to invade surrounding tissue. It also ulcerates, may bleed, and is painful.

hood and become dysplastic (have abnormal development) after puberty. They most often appear on the face, trunk, and arms but also are seen on the scalp, female breast, groin, and buttocks. They have irregular borders and pigmentation colors. A client with classic dysplastic nevi has more than 100 nevi, at least one of which is larger than 8 mm in diameter, and at least one has the characteristics of melanoma. *Congenital* nevi are present at birth. They are often slightly raised, with an irregular surface and a fairly regular border. *Lentigo maligna* is a tan or black patch on the skin that looks like a freckle. It grows slowly, becoming mottled, dark, thick, and nodular. It is usually seen on one side of the face of an older adult who has had a large amount of sun exposure.

A change in the color or size of a nevus is reported in 70% of people diagnosed with a melanoma. The ABCD rule (American Cancer Society, 1998) is used to assess suspicious lesions:

A = asymmetry (one half of the nevus does not match the other half)

B = border irregularity (edges are ragged, blurred, or notched)

C = color variation or dark black color

D = diameter greater than 6 mm (size of a pencil eraser)

During the initial radial phase, which may last from 1 to 25 years (depending on the type), the melanoma grows parallel to the skin surface. During this phase, the tumor rarely metastasizes and is often curable by surgical excision. However, during the next vertical growth phase, atypical melanocytes penetrate into the dermis and subcutaneous tissue, greatly increasing the risk for metastasis and death. When the lesion enters the vertical growth phase, it grows rapidly, and its color changes from a mixture of tan, brown, and black to a characteristic red, white, and blue color. The lesion also develops irregular borders and often has raised nodules and ulcerations (Figure 14-7 ◆).

COLLABORATIVE CARE

Treatment of all skin cancers focuses on removal of malignant tissue using such methods as surgery, curettage and electrodesiccation, cryotherapy, or radiotherapy. These treatments offer a greater than 90% cure rate. The management of melanoma begins with identification, diagnosis, and tumor staging. Besides surgical excision, melanoma is also treated with chemotherapy, immunotherapy, radiation therapy, and biological therapies (interleukin-2 and interferon, or therapeutic vaccines containing melanoma antigens).

Laboratory and Diagnostic Tests

Skin cancer is diagnosed by microscopic examination of tissue biopsied from any suspicious lesion. The biopsies are usually done as office procedures under local anesthesia. Laboratory and diagnostic tests are also conducted to determine whether a melanoma has metastasized.

Liver function tests are done. The combination of an elevated lactic dehydrogenase (LDH), alkaline phosphatase, and

Figure 14-7. ◆ Malignant melanoma is a serious skin cancer that arises from melanocytes.

serum glutamic oxaloacetic transaminase (SGOT) suggests metastasis to the liver. If liver enzymes are abnormal, a computed tomography (CT) scan of the liver is conducted. A complete blood count is done to determine hematologic abnormalities. Serum blood chemistry tests are conducted to identify electrolyte and mineral abnormalities.

Chest x-rays for possible lung metastasis are taken if the client has respiratory difficulty or hemoptysis. If there is undetermined bone pain, a bone scan is performed. If the client has headaches, seizures, or neurologic deficits, a CT scan or magnetic resonance imaging (MRI) of the brain is conducted.

The systems used to describe the level of invasion of a melanoma and the maximum tumor thickness are called *microstaging*. In the Clark system of microstaging, the vertical growth of the lesion is measured from the epidermis to the subcutaneous tissue. In the Breslow system, the vertical thickness is measured from the granular level of the epidermis to the deepest level of tumor invasion. This determination is important, because as the thickness of the melanoma increases, survival rate decreases. (Staging of malignant tumors is discussed in Chapter 8.)

Surgery

Nonmelanoma skin cancers may be removed through Mohs' micrographic surgery or surgical excision. In Mohs' micrographic surgery, thin layers of the tumor are shaved off horizontally. A frozen section of the tissue is stained at each level to determine tumor margins. This is the most accurate method of assessing the extent of nonmelanoma skin cancer, and it conserves the most normal tissue. Cure rates with Mohs' microscopic surgery are at 99% for primary basal cell cancer and 94% for squamous cell carcinoma. For melanoma, surgical excision is the preferred treatment. A wide excision is used that includes the full thickness of the skin and the subcutaneous tissue.

Curettage and Electrodesiccation or Cryosurgery

Small basal cell cancers may be removed with curettage and electrodesiccation. This procedure provides good cosmetic results and preserves normal tissue. However, healing time is longer, and it is difficult to ensure that all tumor margins have been removed. Cryosurgery is noninvasive; liquid nitrogen is used to freeze and destroy the tumor tissue. The area of the tumor is locally anesthetized. Then, liquid nitrogen is applied to the lesion by either a spray or cryoprobes. Cryosurgery is used for some primary basal cell cancers and for low-risk squamous cell cancers.

Radiation

Radiation is used for lesions that are inoperable because of their location (e.g., on the eyelid, the canthus, or the lip) or their size (between 1 cm and 8 cm). Radiation is also used for clients who are older and of poor surgical risk. The treatment is given over a 3- to 4-week period in a clinical facility. It does not allow control of tumor margins, and may itself cause skin cancer.

Immunotherapy

Immunotherapy is a relatively new treatment for melanoma. The immunologic response was explored because the number of spontaneous remissions in clients with melanoma was higher than with any other adult tumor. Tumor-specific antigen–antibodies have also recently been identified. Agents such as interferons, interleukins, monoclonal antibodies, Calmette–Guérin bacillus (BCG), levamisole, transfer factors, and tumor vaccines have all shown activity in melanoma, with varying response rates. The effectiveness of these agents alone, in combination with chemotherapy, or in combination with each other is under investigation.

NURSING CARE

Surgical excision is the most common form of treatment for skin cancer. Nursing care depends on the treatment employed and on the extent of the procedure.

ASSESSING

The nurse assesses the skin of clients who seek care for many different health problems and may be the first to identify suspicious lesions. Assessment data is collected by the nurse to determine factors in the client's history that may have increased the risk for skin cancer and to identify any skin lesions. Box 14-4 lists subjective and objective data to collect.

DIAGNOSING, PLANNING, AND IMPLEMENTING

The increasing incidence of skin cancer requires that nurses be involved in early detection and in teaching preventive behav-

---

BOX 14-4
ASSESSING CLIENTS WITH SKIN CANCER

SUBJECTIVE DATA

- Present health status:
  - Any change in the size, shape, or color of a mole, wart, birthmark, or scar
  - Bleeding, crusting, itching, or pain of a mole, wart, birthmark, or scar
  - Exposure to hazardous chemicals
  - Use of sunscreen
  - Use of tanning salons
  - Knowledge about and frequency of skin examinations
- Past medical history:
  - Previous removal of skin cancer
  - Family history of treatment for skin cancer
  - Geographic area of residence during lifetime
  - Previous serious sunburn

OBJECTIVE DATA

- Inspect and palpate the entire skin for lesions. Use a good light and stretch the skin tightly as necessary to better view lesions. Pay special attention to areas covered with hair, skin folds (such as under the breasts), the axilla, webs between the fingers and toes, soles of the feet, the area between the buttocks, oral cavity, ear canals, and mucous membranes. Assess for:
  - Obvious lesions
  - Visible swelling
  - Contour, size, and color of moles, warts, birthmarks, and scars
  - Enlarged lymph nodes
  - Discoloring of the skin
  - Areas of ulceration, scaling, crusting, or erosion
- Measure and document all skin lesions on an anatomic chart. If possible, take photographs of any suspicious lesions to use for future comparison.

---

iors in all settings. Information about skin self-examination, suncreens, and skin cancer prevention are discussed in Discharge Considerations.

Wide excision and the high risk of metastasis from melanoma usually require inpatient surgical treatment. The nurse provides care and teaching. The most common nursing diagnoses are Anxiety, Impaired Skin Integrity, and Hopelessness.

ANXIETY

■ Provide reassurance by sitting quietly with the client, speaking slowly and calmly, and conveying empathetic understanding by touch. Support the client's coping mechanisms, such as crying and talking. Use short, simple sentences; focus on the here and now, and provide concise information. *Higher levels of anxiety result in a focus on the present, inability to concentrate, and difficulty understanding verbal communications.*

■ Provide accurate information to the client and family about the illness, treatment, and expected length of recovery. *Accurate information enables a person to make informed decisions.*

■ Encourage discussion of expected physical changes and ways to minimize disfigurement through cosmetics and clothing. Provide the client with strategies for participating in the recovery process. *Coping behaviors differ from person to person and from situation to situation. Surgical incisions to remove melanoma may cause disfigurement. Active participation in care provides the client with some control over the future and is often an effective means of coping with anxiety.*

IMPAIRED SKIN INTEGRITY

■ Monitor the client every 4 hours for fever, tachycardia, and malaise, as well as for incisional erythema, swelling, pain, or drainage that increases or becomes purulent. *These manifestations may indicate infection. Skin cancers not only destroy skin layers but also can invade body structures. Both open lesions (from tumors that ulcerate before diagnosis) and incisions (from biopsy and surgery) increase the risk for secondary infection.*

■ Keep the incision line clean and dry by changing dressings as necessary. *Moisture increases the risk of infection.*

■ Follow principles of medical and surgical asepsis when caring for a client's incision. Teach family members and visitors the importance of careful handwashing. Maintain standard precautions if drainage is present. *Aseptic techniques are necessary when caring for any surgical incision to prevent infection. Careful handwashing helps prevent the spread of infection. Nurses must use precautions with blood and body fluids to protect themselves from exposure to HIV.*

■ Encourage and maintain adequate calories and protein intake in the diet. Suggest a consultation with the dietitian if client does not want to eat. *The client with cancer has increased metabolic needs. If these are not met, healing may be impaired.*

HOPELESSNESS

■ Use active listening, ask open-ended questions, and reflect on the client's statements. Acknowledge and respect the client's feelings of apathy or anger as expressions of distress. Convey an empathetic understanding of the client's fears and concerns. *Hopelessness is a common response to the diagnosis of cancer. Clients who experience hopelessness are often withdrawn, passive, and apathetic. An empathetic listener can help them face their concerns.*

■ Provide opportunities for the client to express hope, faith, a sense of purpose, and the will to live. *The client with melanoma faces the possibility or reality of metastasis; the possibility that the cancer may recur and cause death; and alterations in*

self-concept, roles, and relationships. Inspiring hope in clients during this health crisis is a legitimate nursing action.*

■ Explore the client's perceptions. Provide information, and correct misconceptions if necessary. *Verbalizing feelings, concerns, and goals allows others to validate or correct them, promotes a therapeutic nurse–client relationship, and fosters feelings of self-worth.*

■ Encourage the client to identify support systems and past sources of strength and coping. *Identifying support systems and effective coping strategies from past crises helps the person resolve the current crisis and develop hope.*

■ Encourage the client to participate in self-care, mutual decision making, and goal setting. *Meeting self-care needs and making decisions about one's own care build self-confidence.*

■ Encourage focusing not only on the present but also on the future: Review past occasions for hope, discuss personal meaning of hope, establish and evaluate short-term goals with the client and family, and encourage them to express hope for the future. *Mobilizing the client's resources strengthens motivation, hope, and the will to live.*

EVALUATING

Evaluating the effectiveness of nursing care for the client with skin cancer requires ongoing assessment. Collect data about effectiveness of treatment measures, client's understanding of and compliance with treatments, and effectiveness of medications.

Discharge Considerations

Nurses provide client and family education for prevention and early detection of skin cancer (Box 14-5). Numerous brochures are also available from the American Cancer Society, health education and support agencies, and pharmaceutical companies that manufacture sunscreen. Most of this literature is free of charge.

Teach the client or family who is at risk for, or has been diagnosed with, skin cancer how to conduct a self-examination of the skin. Stress that it should be conducted on the same day of each month. Family members can help with areas that are hard to examine (ears, scalp, back, extremities), or the client can use a mirror. Showing photographs of both normal and cancerous skin lesions may help teach the client and family what to watch for when doing self-examination. Teach about the following changes:

■ Color, especially any lesion that becomes darker or variegated in shades of tan, brown, black, red, white, or blue

■ Size, especially any lesion that becomes larger or spreads out

■ Shape, especially any lesion that protrudes more from the skin or begins to have an irregular outline

BOX 14–5
TEACHING FOR DISCHARGE

PREVENTING SKIN CANCER

It is well known that cumulative sun exposure positively correlates with nonmelanoma skin cancers. Many skin cancers can be prevented by limiting exposure to risk factors. Primary prevention behaviors recommended by the American Cancer Society and the Skin Cancer Foundation follow:

- Minimize exposure to the sun between the hours of 10 A.M. and 3 P.M., when ultraviolet rays are the strongest.
- Cover up with a wide-brimmed hat, sunglasses, long-sleeved shirt, and long pants made of tightly woven material when you are in the sun.
- Use a waterproof or water-resistant sunscreen with a sun protective factor (SPF) of 15 or more before every exposure to the sun. Apply sunscreen not only on sunny but also on cloudy days, when ultraviolet rays can penetrate 70% to 80% of the cloud cover.
- Reapply the sunscreen before the protection time is up. If you are at risk for skin cancer, apply sunscreen daily.
- Use sunscreen and protective clothing when you are on or near sand, snow, concrete, or water, which can reflect more than half of the ultraviolet rays onto the skin.
- Avoid tanning booths; UVA radiation emitted by tanning booths damages the deep skin layers.

- Appearance, especially bleeding, drainage, oozing, ulceration, crusting, scaliness, or development of a mushrooming outward growth
- Consistency, especially any lesion that becomes softer or is more easily irritated
- Surrounding skin—redness, swelling, or leaking of color from a lesion into the surrounding skin
- Sensation—itching or pain

If any of these changes occurs, the client should immediately contact the health care provider for further assessment. If treatment is conducted in an outpatient setting, teach the client and family specific measures for self-care, including how and when to change dressings, the use of aseptic technique and careful handwashing when caring for the wound, symptoms to report (such as bleeding, fever, or signs of wound infection), and how to protect the operative site against trauma and irritations. The client who undergoes extensive surgery will require preoperative and postoperative care (see Chapter 7).

Encourage clients with melanoma to schedule regular medical checkups every 3 months for the first 2 years, every 6 months for the next 5 years, and yearly thereafter. Emphasize that proper self-care combined with regular medical care can help the client lead a fairly normal life. If assistance for home care is necessary, provide referrals to a community health or home care agency. Refer the client to a local cancer support group if the client believes this will be helpful.

Nursing Process Case Study
■ CLIENT WITH MELANOMA

Geoff Sanders, age 69, is retired from the postal service. He has always been an avid participant in outdoor sports. When he was younger he played baseball and tennis, and for the last 10 years he has played golf at least twice a week. He now lives in Connecticut, but as a younger man he lived in Florida for almost 15 years. Mr. Sanders has a variety of warts and moles and has rarely paid attention to them. However, after taking a shower one day he noticed that a mole on his left lower leg looked bigger and darker. Mr. Sanders had just seen a public announcement on television about the dangers of changes in moles. He immediately called his primary health maintenance organization (HMO) physician for an appointment at the dermatology clinic.

Assessment On arriving at the clinic, Mr. Sanders is interviewed and examined by nurse Tom Hall. Following the assessment, Mr. Hall documents the following information.

Mr. Sanders has a family history of skin cancer. His father had several squamous cell carcinomas removed from his face. He has numerous nevi on his body. The one causing concern is located on the medial anterior left leg, 2 inches below the patella. Mr. Sanders states that the mole has been present for years but that he noticed just yesterday that it has become larger and darker. On further questioning, he states that the mole itches sometimes but has never hurt or bled. Mr. Sanders lived in Florida for 15 years and experiences a sunburn early each summer before he tans. The sunburn involves the lower legs because Mr. Sanders wears shorts during his twice-weekly golf game.

A complete skin assessment reveals various freckles, warts, and nevi. With the exception of the nevus that prompted Mr. Sanders to come to the clinic, all lesions appear normal. The nevus in question is raised, 3 cm in diameter, with irregular borders and a nodular surface. It is variegated in color, with various shades of brown. The skin surrounding the nevus is slightly erythematous. Inguinal lymph nodes are not enlarged or painful. A photograph of the lesion is taken with Mr. Sanders's permission.

Mr. Sanders discusses the lesion with a surgeon, who recommends excision. Mr. Sanders is scheduled for a biopsy under a local anesthetic the following morning. Following the biopsy, histologic examination reveals lentigo maligna melanoma. Staging of the tumor reveals no metastasis to regional lymph nodes. Mr. Sanders undergoes a wide excision of the lesion in inpatient surgery the following afternoon and goes home the day after.

Diagnosis The following nursing diagnoses are identified for Mr. Sanders:

- *Impaired Skin Integrity* related to excision of melanoma from the left lower leg
- *Risk for Infection* related to surgical wound on left lower leg
- *Acute Pain* related to wide excision of melanoma on left lower leg
- *Anxiety* related to diagnosis of skin cancer

Expected Outcomes The expected outcomes established in the plan of care specify that Mr. Sanders will:

- Demonstrate complete healing of the incision without manifestations of infection.
- Verbalize fears and concerns about his diagnosis.
- Verbalize relief of pain by the time the incision is healed.

Planning and Implementation The nurses caring for Mr. Sanders implement the following interventions:

- Make the first dressing change, but ensure that Mr. Sanders can safely change the dressing himself prior to discharge the day after surgery.
- On discharge, provide Mr. Sanders with adequate dressings and tape for the first home dressing change. Include in discharge instructions necessary information about where to buy supplies and how many dressing supplies will be needed.
- Review and provide written instructions for prescribed systemic antibiotic and pain medication.
- Provide Mr. Sanders with written instructions for dressing change, manifestations of infection, and phone number of clinic. Stress the importance of calling if any abnormal symptoms occur.
- Discuss diagnosis, positive outlook for treatment, and the client's concerns.
- Stress importance of lifelong regular health care evaluations to identify any recurrence or metastasis.

Evaluation Mr. Sanders returns to the dermatology clinic 1 week after his surgical incision. His incision is well approximated and shows no signs of infection. He is taking his antibiotic 4 times a day as prescribed and reports that his need for pain medications is decreasing. During his clinic visit the following week, the nurse removes the sutures and assesses the wound as healed. Mr. Sanders completed his antibiotics and no longer requires pain medications. He says he is still "scared to death" about having cancer, but he has decided to join a local cancer support group. He also says he had gotten a list of skin safety rules from the American Cancer Society and will be sure to cover up and use sunscreens when he plays golf. Mr. Sanders makes an appointment for follow-up care in 3 months.

Critical Thinking in the Nursing Process

1. Consider reasons why people who notice a change in a skin lesion put off seeking health care. What can nurses do to effect change?

2. What would you say to Mr. Sanders if he called the clinic and said that the antibiotics were making him sick and he didn't think he needed them anyway?

Pressure Ulcers

Pressure ulcers (bedsores, decubitus ulcers) are ischemic lesions of the skin and underlying tissue caused by external pressure that impairs the flow of blood and lymph (Porth, 1998). The ischemia causes tissue necrosis and eventual ulceration. Pressure ulcers tend to develop over a bony prominence (e.g., heels, greater trochanter, sacrum, and ischia), but they may appear on any part of the body that is subjected to external pressure, friction, or shearing forces. Pressure causes more damage when it is applied to a small area than when it is distributed over a large surface.

When a person lies or sits in one position for an extended length of time without moving, pressure on the tissue between a bony prominence and the external surface of the body distorts capillaries and interferes with normal blood flow. If the pressure is relieved, blood flow to the area increases, a brief period of reactive hyperemia occurs, and no permanent damage occurs. However, if the pressure continues, platelets clump in the endothelial cells surrounding the capillaries and form *microthrombi* (very small blood clots). These microthrombi impede blood flow, resulting in ischemia and hypoxia of tissues. Eventually, the cells and tissues of the immediate area and of the surrounding area die and become necrotic.

Alterations in the involved tissue depend on the depth of the injury. Injury to superficial layers of skin results in blister formation. Injury to deeper structures causes the pressure ulcer area to appear dark reddish-blue. As the tissues die, the ulcer becomes an open wound that may be deep enough to expose the bone. The necrotic tissue elicits an inflammatory response. The client experiences fever and pain and has an increased white blood cell count. Secondary bacterial invasion is common. Enzymes from bacteria as well as macrophages dissolve necrotic tissue, resulting in a foul-smelling drainage.

Shearing forces result when one tissue layer slides over another. The stretching and bending of blood vessels cause injury and thrombosis. Clients in hospital beds are subject to shearing forces when the head of the bed is elevated and the torso slides down toward the foot of the bed. Pulling the client up in bed also subjects the client to shearing forces. (For this reason, clients are always lifted up in bed.) In both cases, friction and moisture cause the skin and superficial fascia to remain fixed to the bed sheet, while the deep fascia and bony skeleton slide in the direction of body movement.

Although pressure ulcers may occur in an adult with impaired mobility, those most at risk are older adults with limited mobility, people with quadriplegia, and clients in the critical care setting. Others at risk are clients with fractures of large bones (e.g., hip or femur), and those who have undergone orthopedic surgery or sustained spinal cord injury. Incontinence, nutritional deficit, chronic illnesses (like renal failure and anemia), edema, and infection also create increased risk.

Because of age-related skin changes, the older adult is at increased risk for the development of pressure ulcers. The skin of the older adult has a thicker epidermis, a thinner dermis with decreased vascularity, decreased sebaceous gland activity, and decreased strength and elasticity. The more fragile and less nourished dermal layer is more prone to shear and friction problems. The skin of the older adult responds more slowly to inflammation, and wounds heal more slowly. When pressure ulcers occur, they are more difficult to reverse.

Pressure ulcers are graded or staged to classify the degree of damage. The stages, defined by the Panel for the Prediction and Prevention of Pressure Ulcers in Adults as part of the U.S. Department of Health and Human Services (1992) are listed in Box 14-6.

COLLABORATIVE CARE

If a client is at risk for pressure ulcers, the goal is prevention. Ulcers that are already present require collaborative treatment to promote healing and restore skin integrity.

Laboratory tests are conducted to determine the presence of a secondary infection and to differentiate the cause of the ulcer. If the ulcer is deep or appears infected, drainage or biopsied tissue is cultured to determine the causative organism.

Topical and systemic antibiotics specific to the infectious organism are used to eradicate any infection present and to promote healing (Table 14-5 ◆). Surgical debridement may be necessary if the pressure ulcer is deep; if subcutaneous tissues are involved; or if an *eschar* (a scab or dry crust) has formed over the ulcer, preventing healing by granulation. Large wounds may require skin grafting for complete closure.

NURSING CARE

The client with one or more pressure ulcers not only has impaired skin integrity but also is at increased risk for infection, pain, and decreased mobility; prolonged treatment for other conditions; increased health care costs; and diminished quality of life.

RISK FOR IMPAIRED SKIN INTEGRITY AND IMPAIRED SKIN INTEGRITY

The interventions and rationales below are adapted from the clinical guidelines of the Agency for Health Care Policy and Research (1992) for identifying adults at risk and treating those with stage I pressure ulcers.

- Identify at-risk individuals and the specific factors that place them at risk.
  - Assess bed- and chair-bound clients, as well as those who cannot reposition themselves, for immobility, incontinence, nutritional status, and altered level of consciousness.

- Assess clients on admission to acute care and rehabilitation hospitals, nursing homes, home care programs, and other health care facilities, using a validated risk assessment tool.
- Document all assessments of risk.

Identifying individuals at risk for pressure ulcers allows reduction of risk factors. Clients who cannot reposition themselves or whose activity is limited to bed or chair should be assessed. Using a validated assessment tool ensures systematic evaluation and allows reassessment over time. Accurate and complete documentation ensures continuity of care.

- Conduct a systematic skin inspection at least once a day, paying particular attention to the bony prominences. *Systematic, comprehensive, and routine skin care decreases incidence. Data from skin inspection are used to design interventions to reduce risk and evaluate outcomes.*
- Clean the skin at the time of soiling and at routine intervals, as frequently as the client's need or preference dictates. Avoid hot water, use a mild cleansing agent, and clean the skin gently, applying as little force and friction as possible. *Metabolic wastes and environmental contaminants accumulate on the skin and should be removed regularly. Feces and urine cause chemical irritation. Hot water may cause skin injury. Mild cleansing agents are less likely to remove the skin's natural resistance to injury.*
- Minimize environmental factors leading to skin drying, such as low humidity and exposure to cold. Treat dry skin with moisturizers. *Well-hydrated skin resists mechanical trauma. Low humidity dries the skin, making it less pliable. Severe dryness is associated with fissures and cracks in the stratum corneum. Moisturizers help reduce dryness of skin.*

CLINICAL alert

Do not massage over bony prominences. Evidence suggests that massage may lead to deep tissue trauma in at-risk clients.

- Minimize skin exposure to moisture from incontinence, perspiration, or wound drainage. Use materials that absorb moisture and present a quick-drying surface to the skin. Change underpads and briefs frequently. Do not place plastic directly against the skin. *Factors in urine, perspiration, or wound drainage may irritate the skin. Moisture alone can increase the skin's susceptibility to injury.*
- Minimize friction and shearing forces. Use proper positioning, transferring, and turning techniques. Lubricants (such as cornstarch or creams), protective films (such as transparent dressings and skin sealants), protective dressings (such as hydrocolloids), and protective padding may also reduce friction injuries. *Proper positioning can eliminate most shear injury. Friction injuries to the skin occur from moving across a rough surface (such as bed linens). Any agent that eliminates contact or decreases friction reduces this risk.*

BOX 14-6
PRESSURE ULCER STAGING

STAGE I

Nonblanchable erythema of intact skin; the heralding lesion of skin ulceration. Identification of stage I pressure ulcers may be difficult in clients with darkly pigmented skin. *Note:* Reactive hyperemia can normally be expected to be present for one half to three fourths as long as the pressure occluded blood flow to the area. This should not be confused with stage I pressure ulcer.

STAGE II

Partial-thickness skin loss involving epidermis and/or dermis. The ulcer is superficial and presents clinically as an abrasion, blister, or shallow crater.

STAGE III

Full-thickness skin loss involving damage or necrosis of subcutaneous tissue that may extend down to, but not through, underlying fascia. The ulcer presents clinically as a deep crater with or without undermining of adjacent tissue.

STAGE IV

Full-thickness skin loss with extensive destruction; tissue necrosis; or damage to muscle, bone, or supporting structures (e.g., tendon or joint capsule). Sinus tracts may also be associated with stage IV ulcers.

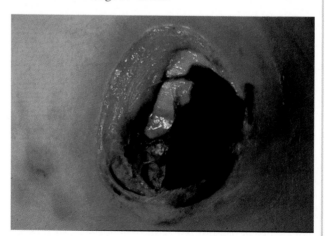

Note: When eschar is present, accurate staging of the pressure ulcer is not possible until the eschar has sloughed or the wound has been debrided.

Text is from Agency for Health Care Policy and Research. (1992). *Pressure Ulcers in Adults: Prediction and Prevention.* Rockville, MD: U.S. Department of Health and Human Services.

TABLE 14-5 PRODUCTS USED TO TREAT PRESSURE ULCERS

STAGE	PRODUCT	PURPOSE
I	Skin Prep Graulex Hydrocolloid dressing (e.g., DuoDerm) Transparent dressing (e.g., Tegaderm)	Toughens intact skin and preserves skin integrity. Prevents skin breakdown, increases blood supply, adds moisture, contains trypsin to aid in removal of necrotic tissue. Prevents skin breakdown and promotes healing without the formation of a crust over the ulcer. Is permeable to air and water vapor; prevents the growth of anaerobic organisms. Prevents skin breakdown; prevents entrance of moisture and bacteria but allows oxygen and moisture vapor permeability.
II	Transparent dressing Hydrocolloid dressing	Enhances healing Enhances healing. *Note:* If infection is present, these types of dressings are contraindicated. A sterile dressing should be applied instead.
III	Wet-to-dry gauze dressing with sterile normal saline Hydrocolloid dressing Proteolytic enzymes (such as Elase)	Allows necrotic material to soften and adhere to the gauze, so that the wound is debrided. Enhances healing Proteolytic enzymes serve as a debriding agent in inflamed and infected lesions.
IV	Wet-to-dry gauze dressing with sterile normal saline Vacuum-assisted closure (VAC)	Enhances healing. *Note:* Transparent or hydrocolloid dressings or skin barriers are contraindicated. Creates a negative pressure to help reduce edema, increase blood supply and oxygenation, and decrease bacterial colonization. Also helps promote moist wound healing and the formation of granulation tissue.

- For inadequate dietary intake of protein or calories, offer nutritional supplements and support the client during mealtimes. If dietary intake remains inadequate, enteral or parenteral feedings may be needed. *Poor dietary intake of protein, calories, and iron has been associated with pressure ulcer development.*
- Maintain the client's current level of activity, mobility, and range of motion. *Frequent turning, repositioning, and movement are essential in reducing risk.*
- Teach clients who can do so to shift their weight every 15 minutes. *Data support that spontaneous movements by older, bedridden clients lower the incidence of pressure ulcers.*
- Reposition all at-risk clients at least every 2 hours. Use a written schedule for systematic turning and repositioning. Avoid leaving clients sitting in a chair or wheelchair. *Fewer pressure ulcers develop in clients who are turned every 2 to 3 hours.*
- For clients on bed rest, use positioning devices, such as pillows or foam wedges, to protect bony prominences. For clients who are completely immobile, use devices that relieve pressure on the heels (the most common method is to raise the heels off the bed). Place any at-risk client on a pressure-reducing device, such as foam, static air, alternating air, gel, or water mattress. Do not use donut-type devices. *Suspending the heels is the best way to redistribute pressure to those areas. Pressure-reducing devices and beds can reduce the incidence of pressure ulcers. Donut cushions may actually contribute to pressure ulcer development.*

- Avoid placing clients in the side-lying position directly on the trochanter.
- Maintain the head of the bed at the lowest degree of elevation consistent with the client's medical condition and other restrictions. Limit the amount of time the head of the bed is elevated. *Proper positioning can reduce pressure on body prominences.*
- Use assistive devices, such as a trapeze or bed linen, to move clients in bed who cannot assist during transfers and position changes. *Lifting, rather than dragging, clients up in bed is less likely to cause friction injury.*

Discharge Considerations

Client and family teaching focuses on prevention of pressure ulcers as discussed. Because many clients at risk for pressure ulcers are older or have other serious illnesses, the nurse may need to teach a caregiver about the following topics:

- Definition, description, and common locations of pressure ulcers
- Risk factors for the development of pressure ulcers
- Skin care
- Ways to avoid injury
- Diet

Depending on the stage of the pressure ulcer, teach the client or caregiver how to care for ulcers that are already present: how to change wet-to-dry dressings, apply skin barriers, and avoid injury and infection. Referrals to a home health agency or community health department can help the family through the lengthy healing process.

Nursing Interventions Classification

The following nursing interventions (McCloskey & Bulechek, 2000) also may be appropriate for the client with common skin disorders:

- Pruritus Management
- Sleep Enhancement
- Distraction
- Infection Protection
- Skin Surveillance

(*Note:* The bibliography listings for this and all chapters have been compiled at the back of the book.)

Chapter Review

key terms by topic

Use CD-ROM disk enclosed with your text-book to hear the pronunciation of the key terms in the chapter.

Structure and function of skin
epidermis, dermis, erythema, cyanosis, pallor, jaundice

Skin disorders
pruritis, psoriasis, dermatitis, acne

Skin infections and infestations
folliculitis, furuncle, cellulitis, dermatophytes, candidiasis, warts, herpes simplex, herpes zoster, parasitic infestations, pediculosis, scabies

Skin malignancy
nonmelanoma skin cancers, basal cell carcinoma, squamous cell carcinoma, melanoma, nevi

Pressure ulcers

key points

- The skin and its appendages provide an external covering for the internal tissues and organs, help regulate body temperature, assist in fluid and electrolyte balance, protect tissues, and convey emotions.

- Common skin disorders include pruritus (itching), dry skin, psoriasis, dermatitis, and acne. The goals of client care are to identify and eliminate precipitating factors, provide relief from itching and pain, and reduce the risk of further damage to the skin.

- The skin may be infected or infested with various agents, including bacteria, fungi, viruses, and parasites. Treatment is provided to identify the causative agent, administer medications to kill or eradicate the organism, and prevent secondary infections.

- Nonmelanoma skin cancers (basal cell carcinoma and squamous cell carcinoma) are the most commonly occurring of all cancers. They are believed to be primarily due to damage from ultraviolet radiation from sun exposure. They do not tend to metastasize and are treated by excision.

- Melanoma skin cancers are serious malignancies that do metastasize. Any change in the shape, border, color, size, consistency, or sensation of a nevus (mole) should be immediately evaluated for transformation into a malignant melanoma.

- Pressure ulcers are ischemic lesions of the skin and underlying tissue. They are caused by external pressure or shearing forces that cause ischemia. The most common sites of development are over bony prominences. Older adults, as well as clients who are immobile, are most at risk for pressure ulcers. Nursing interventions are implemented to reduce risk factors and maintain intact skin.

Medialink

Additional interactive resources for this chapter can be found on the Companion Website at www.prenhall.com/burke. Click on Chapter 14 and "Begin" to select the activities for this chapter.

For NCLEX review questions and an audio glossary, access the accompanying CD-ROM in this book.

for further study

For discussion of the nursing care of burns, see Chapter 15.

For more about treatment of infections, see Antibiotic Therapy in Chapter 12.

For further study of the staging of malignant tumors, see Chapter 8.

For more about surgery in the care of a client with cancer, see Chapter 7.

Critical Thinking Care Map

Caring for a Client with Herpes Zoster
NCLEX-PN Focus Area: Prevention and Health Maintenance

Case Study: Jesus Rivera is a 34-year-old migrant farm worker living in temporary housing in a rural area of southwestern America. He visits a free clinic and reports that he has not felt well for a week, and has had chills and fever. He has painful oozing blisters in a line on his left thorax. His vital signs are T 99° F (37.2° C), P 74, R 22, BP 148/88. He does remember having chickenpox as a child. He is afraid that exposure to pesticides has caused his blisters. The primary health care provider diagnoses Mr. Rivera with herpes zoster and prescribes a topical antiviral medication and an oral pain medication.

Nursing Diagnosis: Risk for Infection

COLLECT DATA

Subjective

Objective

_____   _____
_____   _____
_____   _____
_____   _____
_____   _____
_____   _____
                                 _____

Would you report this data? Yes/No

If yes, to: _____

Nursing Care

_____
_____
_____
_____
_____
_____
_____
_____
_____

How would you document this? _____
_____
_____

Data Collected
(use those that apply)

- Age 34
- Migrant farm worker
- Reports chills and fever
- T 99° F
- BP 148/88
- Open blisters on thorax
- Exposure to pesticides

Nursing Interventions
(use those that apply)

- Provide chickenpox immunization.
- Teach how to apply topical medications.
- Stress importance of avoiding intimate contact with family members.
- Report migrant status to local authorities.
- Discuss need for careful handwashing.
- Teach effects of pain medications.

NCLEX-PN Exam Preparation

1. A client diagnosed with psoriasis is preparing for bed. Which nursing intervention should be given the highest priority at this time?
   a. Prepare the ordered therapeutic bath.
   b. Administer a pain medication.
   c. Teach the client to scratch the lesions to decrease discomfort.
   d. Decrease the temperature in the client's room.

2. The nurse recognizes that which factor in a client's history is most likely to be related to a diagnosis of cellulitis?
   a. cervical cancer
   b. spider bite 5 days ago
   c. surgical repair of an inguinal hernia
   d. measles at the age of 20

3. A client has been receiving antibiotics for 3 days. The nurse should observe for the development of:
   a. furuncles
   b. candidiasis
   c. tinea pedis
   d. folliculitis

4. Topical acyclovir has been ordered for a client with genital herpes. The nurse should teach the client to:
   a. wear gloves when applying the medication
   b. stay out of bright sunlight
   c. use the medication once a week
   d. abstain from sexual intercourse

5. A client diagnosed with pediculosis corporis returns to the clinic on two separate occasions with complaints of itching. The client states that all of the medicine given to treat the condition was taken as directed. The most important question to ask the client at this time is:
   a. "Are other family members affected by the itching?"
   b. "Did you wash all of your bed linen after taking the medicine?"
   c. "Do you have any pets living in your home?"
   d. "Are you having difficulty sleeping at night?"

6. Which information relates directly to a diagnosis of non-melanoma skin cancer?
   a. exposure to ultraviolet radiation
   b. excessive ingestion of alcohol
   c. decreased estrogen levels
   d. appearance of liver spots

7. A client has developed a small basal cell cancer on the forearm and has been scheduled for cryosurgery. The client tells you that life is not worth living now that cancer has been found. An appropriate nursing diagnosis for this client might be:
   a. anxiety
   b. hopelessness
   c. fear
   d. impaired skin integrity

8. The most important instruction given to clients who are at risk for the development of skin cancer should be:
   a. self-examination of skin
   b. the major risk factors for developing skin cancer
   c. treatments for the various types of skin cancer
   d. prognosis for skin cancer

9. Which of these observations would be most significant when assessing the condition of a client who is at risk for a pressure ulcer?
   a. diminished lung sounds
   b. decreased appetite
   c. permanent redness over the sacrum
   d. contracture of the lower extremities

10. Nursing interventions which should be included on the care plan for a client diagnosed with impaired skin integrity are:
    a. massage over the bony prominences
    b. reposition the client every 4 hours
    c. use hot water for bathing
    d. diet high in proteins and calories

Answers for Review Questions, as well as discussion of Case Study Critical Thinking questions, appear in Appendix V.

chapter

15

Caring for the Client with Burns

“Practical Nursing is rooted in a philosophy of human caring . . . don't be afraid to follow your human instincts and show compassion in your relationships with patients and their families.”

Mary Claybon-Watson, RN, EdD(c) • *Practical Nursing Program Administrator* • *Vocational Education and Practical Extension Board* • *Uniondale, New York*

LEARNING outcomes

After completing this chapter, you will be able to:

- Discuss types, classification, extent estimation, and stages of treatment for burns.
- Describe the pathophysiology of a major burn.
- Identify the collaborative care necessary for the client with a major burn, including laboratory and diagnostic tests; pharmacology; fluid resuscitation; respiratory management; nutritional support; wound management; surgery; biologic and biosynthetic dressings; scar, keloid, and contracture prevention; and wound dressings.
- Use the nursing process to collect data and provide interventions for clients with major burns.
- Provide client and family teaching for care of the burn after discharge.

MediaLink

www.prenhall.com/burke

Use the above address to access the free, interactive Companion Website created for this textbook. Get hints, instant feedback, and textbook references to chapter-related multiple choice questions. Link to other interesting sites.

It is estimated that more than 2.5 million burns occur each year in the United States, resulting in about 500,000 emergency room visits and more than 50,000 hospitalizations. The home is the most common site for fire-related burns. Home fires cause 73% of all fire-related deaths, with about 12 people dying in home fires each day. Factors associated with deaths from burns are age (especially children and older adults), careless smoking, alcohol or drug intoxication, and physical and mental disabilities. Occupation is also a factor: electricians and chemical workers are among those at greatest risk (Rutan, 1998).

Burns range from minor loss of the outermost layer of the skin to a complex injury involving all body systems. Treatments vary from simple application of a topical antiseptic agent in an outpatient clinic to an invasive, multisystem, interdisciplinary health team approach in the aseptic environment of a burn center.

Types of Burn Injury

A **burn** is an injury in which a transfer of energy from a heat source to the human body results in tissue loss, damage, or irreversible destruction. Burns may be the result of thermal, chemical, electrical, or radiation damage. Although all four types can lead to generalized tissue damage and multisystem involvement, the causative agents and priority treatment measures are unique to each.

- *Thermal burns* result from exposure to dry heat (flames) or moist heat (steam and hot liquids). They are the most common burns and occur mostly in children and older adults.
- *Chemical burns* are caused by direct skin contact with either acidic or basic agents. More than 25,000 products found in the home or workplace can cause chemical burns.
- The severity of *electrical burns* depends on the type and duration of current and amount of voltage. Electricity follows the path of least resistance, which in the human body tends to lie along muscles, bone, blood vessels, and nerves. Necrosis of the tissue results from impaired blood flow secondary to blood coagulation at the site of the electrical injury.
- *Radiation burns* are usually associated with sunburn or radiation treatment for cancer. These kinds of burns tend to be superficial, involving only the outermost layers of the epidermis.

CLASSIFICATION OF BURN DEPTH

After a burn, tissue damage is determined primarily by the extent of the burn (the percentage of body surface area involved) and the depth of the burn (affected layers of underlying tissue). The American Burn Association uses both the extent and depth of burn to classify burns as minor, moderate, or major. (Characteristics of burns within each classification are summarized in Table 15-1 ◆ and illustrated in Figure 15-1 ◆.)

TABLE 15-1 CHARACTERISTICS OF BURNS BY DEPTH

CHARACTERISTIC	SUPERFICIAL (FIRST DEGREE)	SPLIT OR PARTIAL THICKNESS (SECOND DEGREE)	FULL THICKNESS (THIRD DEGREE)
Skin layers lost	Epidermis	Epidermis and dermis	Epidermis, dermis, and underlying tissues
Skin appearance over burn	Pink-toned; may have local edema	Fluid-filled blisters; bright pink; may appear waxy white with deep partial-thickness burns	Waxy white; dry, leathery, charred
Skin function	Present	Absent	Absent
Pain sensation	Present	Present	Absent
Manifestations at the burn site	Pain; local edema	Severe pain; edema; weeping of fluid	Little pain; edema
Treatment	Regular cleaning Topical agent of choice Mild analgesics	Regular cleaning Topical agent of choice May require skin grafting	Regular cleaning Topical agent of choice Skin substitutes Excision of eschar Skin grafting
Scarring	None; outer layer peels	May occur in deep burns	Occurs in grafted area
Time to heal	3 to 6 days	14 to > 21 days	Requires skin grafting to heal

Full-thickness Partial-thickness Superficial
burn   burn   burn

Epidermis

Dermis

Subcutaneous
tissue

Muscle

Bone

Normal tissue

Figure 15-1. ◆ Burn injury classification according to the depth of the burn.

A **superficial burn** (first-degree burn) involves only the epidermal layer. This type of burn most often results from sunburn, ultraviolet light, minor flash injury (from a sudden ignition or explosion), or mild radiation burn associated with cancer treatment. Because the skin remains intact, this degree of burn is not calculated into the estimates of burn injury. Clients with superficial burns involving large body surface areas may have chills, headache, nausea, and vomiting. Extensive superficial burns, especially in older adults, may require intravenous fluid treatment.

Partial-thickness burns (second-degree burns) may be subdivided into superficial or deep, depending on the depth of the burn.

A *superficial partial-thickness* burn involves the entire dermis. Causes may include a brief exposure to flash flame or dilute chemical agents, or contact with a hot surface. This burn is often bright red, and has a moist, glistening appearance with blister formation. The burned area blanches on pressure. Pain in response to temperature and air is usually severe. Pigment changes are common.

A *deep partial-thickness* burn involves the entire dermis plus hair follicles, but sebaceous glands and epidermal sweat glands remain intact. This level of burn may be caused by hot liquids or solids, flash flame, direct flame, intense radiant energy, or chemical agents (Figure 15-2 ◆). The surface of the burned skin appears pale and waxy and may be moist or dry. Large, easily ruptured blisters may be present. Capillary refill is decreased, but sensation to deep pressure is present. The wound is less painful than a superficial partial-thickness burn, but areas of both pain and decreased sensation may be present. Healing often requires more than 21 days. Necrosis may extend the depth of the wound. Contractures are possible, as are hypertrophic scarring and functional impairment.

A **full-thickness burn** (third-degree burn) involves all layers of skin. The wound may extend into the subcutaneous fat, connective tissue, muscle, and bone. Full-thickness burns

are caused by prolonged contact with flames, steam, chemicals, or high-voltage electric current. Depending on its cause, the burn may appear pale, waxy, yellow, brown, mottled, charred, or nonblanching red. The wound surface is dry, leathery, and firm to the touch. Pain and touch receptors are destroyed.

Estimating the Extent of a Burn

The **"rule of nines"** is a rapid method of estimating extent of partial- and full-thickness burns. It is used during prehospital and emergency care phases (Figure 15-3 ◆). The head, trunk, arms, legs, and perineum, are assigned percentages. For example, a client with burns of the face, anterior right arm, and anterior trunk has burn injury involving 27% of total body surface area (TBSA). On the client's admission to a facility, more accurate methods for estimating the extent of injury are employed.

STAGES OF BURN INJURY TREATMENT

The treatment for the burn client is divided into three, sometimes overlapping, stages. At each stage, different groups of

Figure 15-2. ◆ Partial-thickness burn injury.

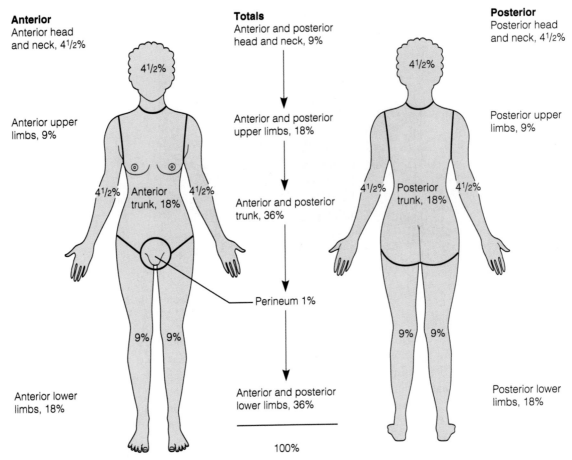

Anterior
Anterior head
and neck, 4¹/2%

Anterior upper
limbs, 9%

4¹/2% Anterior
trunk, 18% 4¹/2%

9% 9%

Anterior lower
limbs, 18%

Totals
Anterior and posterior
head and neck, 9%

Anterior and posterior
upper limbs, 18%

Anterior and posterior
trunk, 36%

Perineum 1%

Anterior and posterior
lower limbs, 36%

100%

Posterior
Posterior head
and neck, 4¹/2%

Posterior upper
limbs, 9%

4¹/2% Posterior
trunk, 18% 4¹/2%

9% 9%

Posterior lower
limbs, 18%

Figure 15-3. ◆ The "rule of nines" is a way to estimate the percentage of TBSA affected by a burn injury. This quick method is useful in emergency situations, but it is not accurate for adults who are short, obese, or very thin.

nurses, physicians, and allied health care specialists collaborate to manage the client's recovery.

Emergent or Resuscitative Stage
This stage lasts from the onset of injury through successful fluid resuscitation. It includes estimating the extent of the burn, instituting initial first-aid measures, and implementing fluid resuscitation therapies. The client is assessed for shock and respiratory distress. Health care workers determine whether the client is to be transported to a burn center.

Acute Stage
The acute stage begins with the start of diuresis and ends with closure of the burn wound. Hydrotherapy and excision and grafting of full-thickness wounds are performed as soon as possible. Enteral and parenteral nutritional interventions are started early to address caloric needs. Topical and systemic antimicrobial agents are administered to combat infection. Narcotic agents must be administered before all invasive procedures to maximize client comfort and to reduce the anxieties associated with wound debridement and intensive physical therapy.

Rehabilitative Stage
This stage begins with wound closure and ends when the client returns to the highest level of health, which may take

years. The primary focus is biopsychosocial adjustment: the prevention of contractures and scars, and the client's successful resumption of work, family, and social roles through physical, vocational, occupational, and psychosocial rehabilitation.

PATHOPHYSIOLOGY OF A MAJOR BURN
The pathophysiologic changes specific to major burns involve all body systems.

Cardiovascular System
Within minutes of the burn, the loss of cell wall integrity at the injury site and in the capillary bed causes a massive amount of fluid to shift into the extravascular spaces. This shifting creates a state of hypovolemic shock called **burn shock**. Fluid leaks from the capillaries at the burn wound site and throughout the body, decreasing intravascular fluid volume. Plasma proteins and sodium escape, further increasing edema formation. Blood pressure falls as cardiac output diminishes. Vasoconstriction occurs as the vascular system attempts to compensate for fluid loss (see Chapter 10). Abnormal platelet aggregation and white blood cell (WBC) accumulation result in ischemia and eventual thrombosis (clotting) in the deeper tissue below the burn. Red blood cells (RBCs) and WBCs remain in the circulation, producing elevated erythrocyte and leukocyte counts secondary to hemoconcentration.

The leakage of fluid into the extracellular spaces compromises the lymphatic system, resulting in intravascular hypovolemia and edema at the burn wound site. Edema impairs peripheral circulation and results in necrosis of the underlying tissue. Potassium ions leave the cells, increasing the risk of cardiac dysrrhythmias.

Burn shock reverses when fluid is reabsorbed from the extracellular spaces into the circulatory system. The blood pressure rises as cardiac output increases, and urinary output improves. Diuresis continues from several days to 2 weeks postburn. During this phase, the extra cardiac workload may predispose the older client or the client with cardiovascular disease to fluid volume overload. Fluid restriction, diuretic therapy, and close monitoring of hemodynamic function are needed to support circulatory function. Even after capillary integrity is restored, fluid losses continue until the burn wound is closed.

Immune System

The capillary leakage that occurs in the early stages of a burn continues throughout the burn shock phase and impairs the active components of both the cell-mediated and humoral immune systems. Serum levels of all immunoglobulins are significantly diminished. Serum protein levels remain persistently low until wound closure is effected. These changes in the immune system create a state of acquired immunodeficiency, which places the burn client at risk for infection for up to 4 weeks following the injury. During this time, infections can develop and cause death despite aggressive antimicrobial therapy.

Integumentary System

The burn injury impairs the normal physiologic functions of the skin (see Chapter 14). If the microcirculation of the skin remains intact during burning, it cools and protects the deeper portions of the skin and cools the outer surface once the heat source is removed. With extensive burn injury, however, the microcirculation is lost, and the burning process continues even after the heat source is removed.

The thickness of the dermis and epidermis varies considerably from one area of the body to another. A temperature that damages the medial aspect of the forearm may not cause damage to the skin covering the same person's back.

Respiratory System

Inhalation injury is a complication that may range from mild respiratory inflammation to massive pulmonary failure. Exposure to asphyxiants, smoke, and heat initiates the pathophysiologic processes.

Carbon monoxide, a common asphyxiant, is a colorless, tasteless, odorless gas that displaces oxygen and binds with hemoglobin. The result is decreased arterial oxyhemoglobin and tissue hypoxia. The manifestations of carbon monoxide poisoning range from mild visual impairment to coma and death.

Smoke inhalation and poisoning result when toxic gases and soot are deposited on the pulmonary mucosa. Inflammation occurs at localized sites within the airways, cells are destroyed, and the bronchial cilia that help clear the lungs are inactivated. Because of this, the client may develop bronchial congestion and infection.

Interstitial pulmonary edema develops secondary to the movement of fluid from the pulmonary blood vessels into the interstitial compartment of the lung tissue. Surfactant is inactivated, and atelectasis may result. Sloughing of the damaged and dead lung tissue occasionally produces debris that may lead to complete airway obstruction.

Upper airway thermal injury results from the inhalation of heated air. Physical findings include the presence of soot, charring, edema, blisters, and ulcerations along the mucosal lining of the oropharynx and larynx. The resulting edema in the airway peaks within the first 24 to 48 hours of injury. Because laryngeal reflexes protect the lower airway, thermal injury below the vocal cords is seldom seen. When it does occur, it is typically associated with the inhalation of steam or explosive gases or the aspiration of hot liquids.

Gastrointestinal System

Curling's ulcer is an acute ulceration of the stomach or duodenum that may form following a burn injury. Abdominal pain, acidic gastric pH levels, hematemesis (vomiting blood), and occult blood in the stool may indicate the presence of gastric ulcer formation.

Paralytic ileus may occur secondary to burn trauma. Lack of intestinal motility leads to gastric distention, nausea, vomiting, and hematemesis.

Urinary System

During the early stages of the burn injury, massive fluid losses occur. These losses lead to dehydration, hemoconcentration, and decreased urinary output. Dark brown concentrated urine may indicate myoglobinuria, which is the result of the release of large amounts of dead or damaged erythrocytes after a major burn. The pigments can occlude the renal tubules and cause renal failure, especially when dehydration, acidosis, or shock is also present.

Metabolism

Two distinct metabolic phases occur as the body responds to the burn injury. The ebb phase, lasting over the first 3 days of the injury, is manifested by decreased oxygen consumption, fluid imbalance, shock, and inadequate circulating volume. These responses protect the body from the initial impact of the injury.

A second phase, the flow phase, occurs when adequate burn resuscitation has been accomplished. This phase is characterized by increased cellular activity and protein catabolism, lipolysis, and gluconeogenesis. The basal metabolic rate (BMR) reaches twice the normal rate. Body weight and heat drop dramatically. Hypermetabolism persists until after wound closure and may reappear if complications occur.

COLLABORATIVE CARE

After stabilization in the emergency department, the client is transferred to the critical care unit or a specialized burn center. In both settings, continuous monitoring of laboratory tests, administration of fluids and pharmaceutical agents, pain control, wound management, and nutrition support therapies are the focus of care.

Laboratory and Diagnostic Tests

Laboratory and diagnostic tests are conducted to assess and monitor the client's response to the burn injury as well as to the treatment prescribed. Cultures of sputum, blood, urine, and wound tissue are done to indicate the presence of infection. Blood is typed and crossmatched upon the client's arrival to the unit, in case transfusions are required.

A urinalysis is done to evaluate renal perfusion and nutritional status. In catabolic states, nitrogen is excreted in large amounts into the urine. Nitrogen loss is measured through 24-hour urine collections for total nitrogen, urea nitrogen, and amino acid nitrogen. Loss of plasma protein and dehydration lead to proteinuria and elevated urine specific gravity.

Many different blood studies are conducted. Hematocrit is elevated secondary to hemoconcentration and fluid shifts from the intravascular compartment. Hemoglobin is decreased secondary to hemolysis. Sodium levels are decreased secondary to massive fluid shifts into the interstitium. Potassium levels initially are increased, but decrease after burn shock resolves, as fluid shifts back to intracellular and intravascular compartments. Protein levels indicate nutritional status during the rehabilitative stage. White blood cells are elevated in the presence of infection. Arterial blood gases are used to monitor oxygen status and acid–base disturbances. The burn-injured client may demonstrate elevated or lowered pH, decreased PCO_2, decreased PO_2, and low-normal bicarbonate levels.

Pulse oximetry allows continuous assessment of oxygen saturation levels. The burn-injured client may have saturation levels below 95%. Chest x-ray studies document changes within the first 24 to 48 hours that may reflect the presence of atelectasis, pulmonary edema, or acute respiratory disease. If an upper airway injury is manifested, a flexible bronchoscopy permits direct visualization. Electrocardiograms (ECGs) are necessary to monitor the development of dysrhythmias, especially those associated with hypokalemia and hyperkalemia.

Pharmacology

Burns often cause excruciating pain. In the early stages of care, intravenously administered narcotics are the best means of managing pain. Once the client has been stabilized, it is appropriate to administer narcotic agents prior to wound care or intensive exercising routines.

To eliminate infection on the surface of the burn wound, topical antimicrobial therapy is used, depending on protocol. There are many antimicrobial agents available. The three most widely used are 0.5% silver nitrate, 1% silver sulfadiazine, and 10% mafenide acetate. The latter two agents are broad-spectrum antibiotics that are supplied in a cream form. Silver nitrate is applied as a wet dressing, which is changed twice daily and soaked every 2 hours. With each dressing change, the nurse carefully assesses the wound for evidence of healing or signs of infection (Table 15-2 ◆).

Other medications that may be used include histamine receptor antagonists and antacids to reduce gastric acidity, and medications to decrease respiratory mucous production.

Fluid Resuscitation

To counteract the effects of burn shock, fluid resuscitation guidelines are used to replace the extensive fluid and electrolyte losses associated with major burn injuries. Fluid replacement is necessary in all burn wounds that involve more than 20% of the TBSA. Colloids, crystalloids, blood, and blood products are used for fluid resuscitation and maintenance. Crystalloid fluids are administered through large-bore peripheral or central lines at rates sufficient to maintain urine output at 30 to 50 mL/h. Lactated Ringer's solution is the intravenous fluid of choice, because it most closely approximates the body's extracellular fluid composition.

Fluid resuscitation rates are adjusted periodically throughout the emergent stage of care. During the fluid resuscitation stage, the client may require invasive hemodynamic monitoring (see Chapter 24). A pulmonary artery catheter monitors cardiac output, cardiac index, and pulmonary artery wedge pressures. All measurements must be maintained within normal limits to effect adequate fluid resuscitation.

Respiratory Management

The client's head is elevated to 30 degrees or more to maximize respiratory efforts. Airways may need frequent suctioning. If airway obstruction occur, the client will require intubation. Oxygen flow rate is based on arterial blood gas results. The client may be placed on a face mask, T-piece, mechanical ventilation with positive end-expiratory pressure (PEEP), pressure support ventilation, or high-frequency jet ventilation. The goal of all therapies is to maintain adequate tissue oxygenation with the least amount of inspired oxygen flow necessary.

Nutritional Support

Oral intake can seldom meet the caloric requirements necessary to reverse negative nitrogen balance and begin the healing process. Enteral feedings are started within 24 to 48 hours of the burn injury to offset hypermetabolism, improve nitrogen balance, and decrease length of hospital stay. A gastrointestinal feeding tube is inserted, with the tip extending past the pylorus to prevent reflux and aspiration. Enteral feeding is contraindicated in Curling's ulcer, bowel obstruction, feeding intolerance, pancreatitis, or septic ileus. When the enteral route cannot be used, a central venous catheter is inserted via the subclavian or jugular vein for the administration of total parenteral nutrition (TPN).

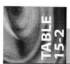

TABLE 15-2 NURSING IMPLICATIONS FOR PHARMACOLOGY: CLIENTS RECEIVING TOPICAL ANTIMICROBIAL AGENTS

DRUGS	ACTION/USES	NURSING RESPONSIBILITIES	CLIENT TEACHING
Mafenide acetate (Sulfamylon)	A synthetic antibiotic that appears to interfere with the metabolism of bacterial cells. Effective against many gram-positive and gram-negative organisms. Used to prevent burn wound infections.	Use with caution in clients with renal or pulmonary disease. Assess for itching, swelling, or blisters on unburned areas, which indicate an allergy to the drug.	When applied, the drug causes pain or burning. Apply one to two times a day until the burn is healed. If symptoms of an allergy develop, stop using the drug and notify your health care provider.
Silver nitrate	A bacteriostatic agent that inhibits many different gram-positive and gram-negative organisms. Used as a 0.5% solution in distilled water to prevent burn wound infections.	Apply the solution to gauze dressings every 2 hours and change dressings completely two times a day. Monitor the client for decreased blood sodium and chloride levels as large amounts of water are absorbed from the dressing site.	Silver nitrate causes the skin and dressings to turn black. Saturate the dressings with the solution every two hours, and change all the dressings two times a day. Report symptoms of infection, swelling, weight gain, or breathing difficulty to your health care provider.
Silver sulfadiazine (Silvadene)	Acts on bacterial cell membranes as a bactericidal. Effective against many gram-negative and gram-positive organisms. Used to prevent burn wound infections.	Monitor for fluid volume overload: abnormal breath sounds, edema. Monitor for dark urine and force fluids to prevent sulfa crystals from forming in the urine.	Apply the drug one to two times a day, completely covering the burn wound. Drink an increased amount of fluids.

WOUND MANAGEMENT

Burn wounds must be cleaned and debrided of necrotic tissue and blisters to promote healing and prevent prolonged inflammation. **Debridement** is the process of removing dead tissue from the wound.

The wound is cleaned with an antimicrobial soap, such as chlorhexidine gluconate (Hibiclens, Hibistat). However, Dial soap or Shurclens is used for facial burns, because chlorhexidine gluconate is toxic to eyes and ears. The area is shaved close to the burn wound before debridement to decrease the risk of infection, and intravenous narcotics are administered during debridement to control pain.

Mechanical debridement is performed during hydrotherapy. In this procedure, loose necrotic tissue is washed with a washcloth or gauze pad to remove dead skin and **eschar** (a hard crust that forms over the burn wound). Blistered skin is grasped with a dry gauze and gently removed. The edges of blisters or eschar are trimmed with blunt scissors. Wounds should be rubbed hard enough to remove debris yet not cause bleeding. Hydrotherapy measures include showering, using a spray table, or immersion in a tub of water. Although tubbing has traditionally been the method of choice, it is currently used less often because of the increased risk of wound infection.

Enzymatic debridement involves the use of a topical agent to dissolve and remove necrotic tissue. Following hydrotherapy, an enzyme of choice is applied in a thin layer directly to the wound and covered with one layer of fine mesh gauze. A topical antimicrobial agent is applied, covered with a bulky wet dressing, and the wound is immobilized with expandable mesh gauze.

Surgery

Various surgical procedures are performed to treat the burn wound. These include:

- *Surgical debridement* is the process of excising tissue from the burn wound to the level of viable tissue. The most common technique is electrocautery. Debridement may also be performed by using a dermatome to slice off thin layers of damaged skin.
- *Escharotomy* is performed by the physician with a scalpel or by electrocautery. A sterile surgical incision is made longitudinally along the extremity or the trunk to prevent constriction, impaired circulation, and possible gangrene.
- *Autografting* is used to effect permanent skin coverage. Early burn wound excision and skin grafting decreases the hospital stay and enhances rehabilitation. Skin is removed from healthy tissue (donor site) of the burn-injured client

and applied to the burn wound (Figure 15-4 ◆). After the autograft is applied, the grafted area is immobilized.

- *Cultured epithelial autografting* is a technique in which skin cells are removed from unburned sites on the client's body, minced, and placed in a culture medium for growth. With this technique, enough skin can be grown over a period of 3 to 4 weeks to cover an entire human body. The cells are prepared in sheets and attached to petroleum jelly gauze backing, which is applied to the burn wound site.

Biologic and Biosynthetic Dressings

Biologic dressing and biosynthetic dressing refer to any temporary material that rapidly adheres to the wound bed, promotes healing, or prepares the burn wound for permanent autograft coverage. Ideally, these kinds of dressings should be easy to apply and remove, inexpensive, elastic, able to reduce pain, able to serve as a bacterial barrier, and able to enhance the natural healing process. The dressings are applied to the burn wound as soon as possible. They help eliminate the loss of water through evaporation, reduce infection, and promote wound healing. Biologic and biosynthetic dressings that are currently in use include Biobrane, Dermagraft, Integra, Alloderm, and TransCyte.

Scar, Keloid, and Contractures

Following a minor burn, the newly formed skin closely resembles its neighboring tissue. The epidermis does not thicken or heighten as a scar. However, when a burn extends into the dermal layer of skin, the skin is repaired through scar formation. Two types of excessive scar may develop. A **hypertrophic scar** is an overgrowth of dermal tissue that remains within the boundaries of the wound. A **keloid** is a scar that extends beyond the boundaries of the original wound. People with dark skin are at greater risk for the formation of hypertrophic scars and keloids. During the healing process, the burn scar shrinks and becomes fixed and inelastic, resulting in **contracture** of the wound (permanent shortening of connective tissue). Once a contracture forms, the tissue resists being stretched, and its inelasticity limits

Figure 15-4. ◆ Skin graft for burn injury (autograft).

body movement. Positioning, splinting, exercise, and constant pressure application help prevent contractures from forming.

Wound Dressings

After the wound has been cleaned and debrided, it may be dressed by the open or closed method. In the open method, the burn wound remains open to air, covered only by a topical antimicrobial agent. This method allows easy wound assessment. However, it can be used only where strict isolation precautions are followed. Topical agents must be reapplied frequently because they tend to rub off onto the bedding.

In the closed method, a topical antimicrobial agent is applied to the wound site, which is covered with gauze or a nonadherent dressing and then gently wrapped with a gauze roll bandage. With the closed method, burn wounds are usually dressed twice daily and as needed. Dressings are applied circumferentially in a distal-to-proximal manner. All fingers and toes are wrapped separately. For wet-to-dry dressings, a thick gauze is applied to maintain moisture and is soaked every 2 hours with the ordered solution.

Splints are used to immobilize body parts and prevent contractures of the joints. They are applied and removed according to schedules established by the physical therapist. Early in the acute phase of care, the physical therapist also prescribes active and passive ROM exercises, which are performed during hydrotherapy and every 2 hours at the bedside. Early ambulation is also part of the plan of care once the client's condition becomes stable.

Applying uniform pressure can prevent or reduce hypertrophic scarring. Tubular support bandages are applied 5 to 7 days postgraft. They maintain a tension ranging from 10 to 20 mm Hg to control scarring. The client wears custom-made elastic pressure garments for 6 months to a year postgraft.

NURSING CARE

The client with a burn may require care ranging from education for self-care at home to complex care planning involving the multidisciplinary team.

ASSESSING

The nurse initially assesses all body systems of the client with a major burn to identify not only actual abnormal findings but also potential problems that may occur as a result of the injury. Chapter 4 discusses the assessment of each body system; Box 15-1 summarizes data to collect when the client is admitted to an emergency department or burn center. This information is necessary to determine fluid resuscitation, causative agent, any on-the-scene treatment, health history, and age. Body weight on admission is necessary to monitor nutritional status during treatment.

**BOX 15-1
INITIAL FOCUSED
ASSESSMENT OF THE
CLIENT WITH A MAJOR BURN**

- Time of the injury
- Cause of the injury
- First-aid treatment
- Past medical history
- Age
- Medications
- Body weight

DIAGNOSING, PLANNING, AND IMPLEMENTING

The priority nursing diagnoses for the client with a major burn are Impaired Skin Integrity, Deficient Fluid Volume, Risk for Infection, Impaired Physical Mobility, Imbalanced Nutrition: Less Than Body Requirements, Acute Pain, and Powerlessness.

IMPAIRED SKIN INTEGRITY

Nursing care for burn injuries focuses on assessing and cleaning the wound and controlling infection.

- Monitor appearance of burn wound, amount and type of drainage, body temperature, and white blood cell count. Report changes from usual condition. *Early signs of infection include increased redness and swelling, increased or purulent drainage, fever and increased WBC.*

CLINICAL alert

monitor
Monitor the laboratory data for an increased WBC.
report
Report any increase in WBC (of more than 10,000/mm3) to the physician or charge nurse.

- Assist with hydrotherapy. Explain the procedure. Administer medications to control pain as prescribed. Keep environment warm. *Hydrotherapy is used to remove topical agents and debride the wound. The procedure is often painful and the client is likely to be easily chilled.*
- Apply topical antimicrobial agents as prescribed. Reapply as necessary. *Controlling infection is an essential component in restoring skin integrity for burn wounds.*
- Provide special skin care to sensitive body areas.
  - Clean burns involving the eyes with normal saline or sterile water. If contracture of the eyelid develops, apply drops or ointment to the eye to prevent corneal abrasion.
  - Gently wipe burns of the lips with saline-soaked pads. Apply an antibiotic ointment as ordered. Assess the

mouth frequently, and perform mouth care routinely. If an oral endotracheal tube is in place, reposition it often to prevent pressure sore formation.
  - Position nasogastric and nasotracheal tubes to prevent excessive pressure.
  - Do not cover ears with dressings. Do not use pillows.
  - Clean burns of the perineum during hydrotherapy. Assess the area for evidence of infection, and rinse thoroughly after toileting.

The eyes, mouth, nose, ears, perineum, and exposed deeper tissues require special interventions.

- Change dressings as prescribed. When the open method is used, follow strict isolation procedures. If the closed method is used, apply in a distal-to-proximal manner. Wrap all fingers and toes separately. *These guidelines are necessary to prevent infection, maintain circulation, and cover all burned areas with dressings.*

DEFICIENT FLUID VOLUME

Massive fluid losses occur immediately following the injury and continue throughout the first 2 to 5 days. During this period, nursing care focuses on restoring fluid losses and continuously assessing hemodynamic parameters.

- Assess vital signs frequently. Note increased and weak pulse, decreasing blood pressure, and increased respiratory rate. Document and report changes. *Vital signs change rapidly when fluid resuscitation is inadequate. Those listed indicate decreased fluid volume.*
- Monitor intake and output hourly. Report urine outputs of less than 50 mL/h. *Urine output less than 50 mL/h indicates decreased circulatory volume and renal perfusion.*
- Weigh daily. *Body weight is used to calculate fluid requirements.*

CLINICAL alert

Monitor the client for fluid volume overload (assess breath sounds, pulse and blood pressure). Older clients and those with underlying cardiac disease may demonstrate symptoms of congestive heart failure during the fluid resuscitation stage.

RISK FOR INFECTION

From the onset of the burn injury, the client is at risk for infection.

- Monitor and record body temperature every 2 hours. Document and report increased body temperature. Monitor WBC counts. *Body temperature increase and increased WBC counts indicate infection.*
- Determine tetanus immunization status. *Clients with burns are at risk for infection caused by* Clostridium tetani.
- Maintain an aseptic environment. *Isolation techniques decrease the risk of secondary infections.*

IMPAIRED PHYSICAL MOBILITY

■ Perform active or passive range-of-motion (ROM) exercises to all joints every 2 hours. Ambulate when stable. *Physical therapy begins in the early stages of treatment. As the burn wound heals and new skin tissue forms, the involved area tends to shrink. Contractures significantly limit mobility, especially at joints. Regular exercise prevents further loss of mobility, restores movement, and improves functional status.*

■ Apply splints as prescribed. Maintain antideformity positions, and reposition hourly. *Splinting and positioning help prevent contractures.*

■ Maintain limbs in functional alignment. *This helps preserve joint mobility.*

IMBALANCED NUTRITION: LESS THAN BODY REQUIREMENTS

Daily calorie requirements are determined by the dietitian. As soon as possible, enteral feedings are started. Parenteral nutrition is reserved for instances in which enteral feedings are contraindicated.

■ Maintain nasogastric/nasointestinal tube placement. *This ensures appropriate absorption of nutrients and prevents aspiration.*

■ Maintain enteral/parenteral nutritional support as prescribed. Observe and report any evidence of feeding intolerance. *Diarrhea, vomiting, excessive gastric residue, abdominal distention, absent bowel sounds, and constipation indicate intolerance to the strength or amount of tube feedings.*

■ Weigh daily. *The client's weight is used to measure the adequacy of the nutritional support.*

ACUTE PAIN

■ Assess level of pain. *With extensive superficial and all partial-thickness burns, the client experiences excruciating pain. Pain tolerance is highly individual.* (Pain and pain management are discussed in detail in Chapter 6.)

■ Anticipate the need for prophylactic analgesia. Determine whether patient-controlled analgesia (PCA) is appropriate. Administer narcotic analgesics as ordered. *Narcotic analgesics are administered regularly to minimize discomfort and also before any painful procedure. An inability to manage pain results in client feelings of despair and frustration. Invasive procedures and exposed nerve endings increase the client's pain.*

■ Explain all procedures and expected levels of discomfort. *Clients who are prepared for painful procedures experience less stress and are better able to manage pain.*

■ Explore noninvasive methods of pain control. *As the client progresses to the rehabilitative stage, non-narcotic analgesia and relaxation techniques are implemented. Methods such as relaxation, distraction, and massage can enhance the therapeutic effects of pain medications.*

POWERLESSNESS

■ Allow as much control over the surroundings and daily routine as possible, such as choosing times for dressing changes. *The client with a major burn injury usually endures a lengthy hospital stay. The burn unit is a strange environment, with hospital personnel and even family wearing sterile masks and gowns at client's bedside, everyone appears different. Feelings of powerlessness during the emergent and acute stages of burn care often pose a challenge to the nurse. Powerlessness results from the belief that one is unable to influence the outcome of a situation.*

■ Keep needed items within reach, such as call light, urinal, water pitcher, and tissues. *These items reinforce the client's feelings of control.*

■ Encourage expression of feelings. *Careful listening, a caring presence, and positive reinforcement can help the client cope.*

■ Help set short-term, realistic goals, such as walking from the bedside to the chair twice daily. *Small gains are easier to achieve and allow for ongoing positive reinforcement.*

■ Help access support systems, such as spiritual/cultural healing, support group consultation, and psychologic intervention. *Support systems help the client cope more effectively.*

EVALUATING

Evaluate the effectiveness of nursing care by collecting data about wound healing, fluid status, absence of infection, adequate nutrition, pain relief, and client's perceptions of ability to control the outcomes of treatment and care. As the burn heals, evaluate effectiveness of exercises and splinting in preventing contractures.

Discharge Considerations

Client and family teaching is an important component of all phases of burn care. As treatment progresses, encourage family members to assume more responsibility in providing care. From admission to discharge, teach them to assess all findings, implement therapies, and evaluate progress.

Early in the plan of care, explain to the client and family the long-term goals of rehabilitation care: to prevent soft tissue deformity, protect skin grafts, maintain physiologic function, manage scars, and return the client to his or her optimal level of independence. The teaching plan focuses on helping the client and family prevent dehydration, infection, and pain; maintain adequate nutrition and skin integrity; and restore mobility and psychosocial well-being.

Teach the client and family how to assess for evidence of fluid volume deficit. Explain the rationale supporting all fluid therapies and emphasize the need to report immediately all signs and symptoms of fluid imbalance: weight loss, scanty urine output, dry mucous membranes.

Explain the rationale about asepsis. Instruct caregivers to protect the client from exposure to people with colds or infections and to follow aseptic technique meticulously when caring for the wound. Ensure that the client and family are able to recognize all signs and symptoms of infection: fever, poor wound healing, purulent drainage, malaise.

Consultation with physical therapy begins early in the treatment plan and continues throughout the long-term rehabilitative process. Explain to the client and family the need for progressive physical activity, and help them establish realistic goals. Explain the rationale supporting the use of splints, pressure support garments, and other assistive devices, and demonstrate how to apply them. Ensure that the client and family understand the importance of reporting any evidence of lack of progress.

Identify and answer all questions related to the client's nutritional therapies and maintaining adequate daily caloric intake. Consult with a nutritionist early in the treatment plan and throughout rehabilitation.

Encourage the client and family to express concerns related to pain management. Explain the causes of pain and discomfort and the rationale supporting the use of analgesia. Instruct them to report inadequate pain control. Teach the client and family alternative pain-control therapies.

Instruct the client and family in the care of the graft and donor sites. Provide the rationale for use of all pressure support garments. Emphasize the need to report any evidence of inadequate wound healing: altered skin integrity, drainage, swelling, redness.

Encourage the client and family to express their fears and concerns, and provide referrals to appropriate community resources. The circumstances surrounding the burn injury are often emotionally charged and challenge the nurse to consider all psychosocial implications. Powerlessness, anger, guilt, anxiety, and feelings of loss are common reactions to burn injury. The goal of psychosocial nursing care is to promote functional adaptation, encourage coping mechanisms and facilitate psychological adjustment. The burn injury can create dramatic changes in the client's self-concept, role function, value system, and interpersonal relationships. Direct the client and family to occupational therapy, social service, clergy, or psychiatric services as appropriate.

Nursing Process Case Study
■ CLIENT WITH A MAJOR BURN

Craig Howard, a 39-year-old truck driver, is admitted to the hospital following an accident in which the cab of his truck caught on fire. He was freed from the truck by a passing motorist, who stayed with him until the rescue team arrived and transported him to a local ED. Mr. Howard's wife, Mary, and twin daughters, Jessica and Jane, age 10, have been notified.

Assessment On his admission to the ED, Mr. Howard is diagnosed with deep split-thickness and full-thickness burns of the anterior chest, arms, and hands. A quick assessment based on the rule of nines estimates the extent of his burn injury at 36% of TBSA. His vital signs are as follows: T,

96.2° F (35.6° C); P, 140; R, 40; BP, 98/60. In the field, the paramedics had inserted a large-bore central line into Mr. Howard's right subclavian vein and started a rapid infusion of lactated Ringer's solution. Mr. Howard is receiving 40% humidified oxygen via face mask. Initial ABGs are as follows: ph, 7.49; PO_2, 60 mm Hg; PCO_2, 32 mm Hg; bicarbonate, 22 mEq/L. Lung sounds indicate inspiratory and expiratory wheezing, and a persistent cough reveals sooty sputum production. A Foley catheter is inserted and initially drains a moderate amount of dark, concentrated urine. A nasogastric tube is inserted and connected to low-intermittent suction. Mr. Howard is alert and oriented and complains of severe pain associated with the burn injuries. The burn unit is notified, and Mr. Howard is prepared for transfer.

Diagnosis On Mr. Howard's arrival to the burn unit, Ana Salazar, LVN, assesses Mr. Howard and assists in establishing the following prioritized nursing diagnoses:

- Risk for Ineffective Airway Clearance related to increasing lung congestion secondary to smoke inhalation.
- Deficient Volume Deficit related to abnormal fluid loss secondary to burn injury.
- Risk for Ineffective Tissue Perfusion related to peripheral constriction secondary to circumferential burn wounds of the arms.

Expected Outcomes The expected outcomes established in Ms. Salazar's plan of care specify that during the emergent phase of care, Mr. Howard will:

- Demonstrate a patent airway, as evidenced by clear breath sounds; absence of cyanosis; and vital signs, chest x-ray findings, and ABGs within normal limits.
- Demonstrate adequate fluid volume and electrolyte balance, as evidenced by urine output, vital signs, mental status, and laboratory findings within normal limits.
- Demonstrate adequate tissue perfusion, as evidenced by palpable pulses, warm extremities, and normal capillary refill (toenails).

Planning and Implementation Ms. Salazar plans and implements the following interventions for Mr. Howard during the emergent phase of care:

- Prepare Mr. Howard for prophylactic nasotracheal intubation to maintain airway patency.
- Initiate fluid resuscitation therapy using the prescribed formula to calculate intravenous fluid rate for the first 24 hours postburn.
- Assist the physician to perform escharotomies of both upper extremities.

Evaluation The nurse anesthetist has inserted a nasotracheal tube and connected Mr. Howard to a T-piece delivering 40% oxygen. His arterial blood gases (ABGs) have significantly improved. Bronchodilators have been parenterally administered and mucolytic agents added to his respiratory treatments. His tracheal secretions have begun to show evidence of clearing. Hourly urine outputs are 60 to 90 mL, and color and concentration have improved. Blood pressure has increased to 100/64 and the pulse rate has decreased to 100. To improve tissue perfusion of both arms, the physician has performed bilateral escharotomies and Ms. Salazar has dressed the wounds using sterile procedure. The extremities have demonstrated improved circulation.

 ## Critical Thinking in the Nursing Process

1. Explain the rationale for the immediate insertion of a Foley catheter and nasogastric tube.
2. What is the rationale supporting the intravenous administration of narcotics to control Mr. Howard's pain?

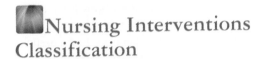
Nursing Interventions Classification

The following nursing interventions (McCloskey & Bulechek, 2000) may be appropriate for the clients with a major burn:

- Airway Management
- Bowel Management
- Caregiver Support
- Gastrointestinal Intubation
- Oxygen Therapy

   (*Note:* The bibliography listings for this and all chapters have been compiled at the back of the book.)

Chapter Review

 ## key terms by topic

Use the CD-ROM disk enclosed with your textbook to hear the pronunciation of the key terms in the chapter.

Types of burn injury
burn, superficial burn, partial-thickness burn, full-thickness burn, "rule of nines"

Major burn
burn shock, debridement, eschar, hypertrophic scar, keloid, contracture

key points

- A burn is an injury resulting from a heat source that results in tissue loss, damage, or irreversible destruction. The heat source may be thermal, chemical, electrical, or radiation.

- Burns are classified as superficial, partial-thickness, or full-thickness. The classification is made based on the depth of the burn.

- The "rule of nines" is often used to estimate the extent of a burn by assigning percentages to different parts of the body.

- The pathophysiology of a burn involves all body systems. One of the most critical is the shift of fluid into the extravascular space, resulting in a type of hypovolemic shock called burn shock. Other pathologic processes include an impaired immune system, disturbed functions of the skin, inhalation injury, gastrointestinal ulcerations and ileus, renal failure, and hypermetabolism.

- The treatment of a major burn includes fluid resuscitation, wound mangement, respiratory management, and nutritional support.

- Nursing care of the client with a burn is provided from initial emergency assessment and treatment through convalescence and rehabilitation. Priority nursing diagnoses focus on skin integrity, fluid volume, infection, physical mobility, nutrition, pain, and powerlessness.

 ## Medialink

Additional interactive resources for this chapter can be found on the Companion Website at www.prenhall.com/burke. Click on Chapter 15 and "Begin" to select the activities for this chapter.

For NCLEX review questions and an audio glossary, access the accompanying CD-ROM in this book.

for further study

For more information on fluid loss in clients experiencing trauma, see Chapter 10.

For more about normal physiologic functions of the skin, see Chapter 14.

For information on fluid resuscitation and hemodynamic monitoring, see Chapter 24.

For further study about assessing each body system, see Chapter 4.

For more about nursing care of pain, see Chapter 6.

Critical Thinking Care Map

Caring for a Client with Major Burns
NCLEX-PN Focus Area: Physiological Integrity: Reduction of Risk Potential

Case Study: Akisha Moore, age 78, was burned over 40% TBSA when her nightgown caught on fire as she was heating coffee in a saucepan. The burns are both partial thickness and full thickness. The partial-thickness burns are covered with large blisters. On admission to the ED, Mrs. Moore is confused. Her blood pressure is 92/62, and her pulse (right wrist is not burned) is 110 and weak. A Foley catheter is inserted, and hourly urine outputs are averaging less than 20 mL per hour. Mrs. Moore is moaning with pain. Her respiratory rate is 36 and shallow and her temperature is 98° F.

Nursing Diagnosis: Risk for Deficient Fluid Volume

COLLECT DATA

Subjective

_____
_____
_____
_____
_____
_____

Objective

_____
_____
_____
_____
_____
_____

Would you report this data? Yes/No

If yes, to: _____

Nursing Care

_____
_____
_____
_____
_____
_____
_____
_____
_____

How would you document this? _____
_____
_____

Data Collected
(use those that apply)

- Age 78
- 40% TBSA burns
- T 98° F
- BP 92/62
- P 110, weak
- R 36, shallow
- Output averages less than 20 mL per hour
- Moans in pain
- Confused

Nursing Interventions
(use those that apply)

- Report and continue to monitor vital signs.
- Report and continue to monitor urine output.
- Report and continue to monitor confusion.
- Report and continue to monitor body temperature.
- Administer morphine intravenously as prescribed.
- Determine body weight.
- Monitor IV fluid flow rate.
- Prepare to debride burned areas.
- Cover with a warm blanket.

NCLEX-PN Exam Preparation

TEST-TAKING TIP

Review the disorders that you had difficulty understanding during school. Include the following: clinical manifestations, etiology, medical treatments, and, most importantly, nursing interventions appropriate for each disorder.

1. During a soccer game, a young student was injured due to a lightning strike. The student began to jerk and speak incoherently. Based on this observation, which body system would be the most affected by the electrical current?
   a. cardiac
   b. pulmonary
   c. urinary
   d. nervous

2. A client was admitted to the intensive care unit with severe burns to the face and chest. The injured skin is dry and leathery, with no pain sensations present. The nurse recognizes that this burn is classified as:
   a. full thickness
   b. partial thickness
   c. superficial
   d. deep partial thickness

3. A client arrives in the emergency room suffering from burns received in a house fire. What assessment data should be obtained first?
   a. pain
   b. respiratory
   c. mobility
   d. urinary

4. An 85-year-old client, diagnosed with third-degree burns to the lower extremities, is complaining of dyspnea. Crackles are heard in all lung fields. The nurse is justifiable in determining that this client may have:
   a. excess intercellular fluid
   b. early stages of congestive heart failure
   c. portal hypertension
   d. increased circulatory volume

5. A silver nitrate dressing is ordered for a client with severe burns. It is important for the nurse to monitor which of these lab studies?
   a. potassium
   b. sodium
   c. magnesium
   d. calcium

6. Excruciating pain is often seen in clients with severe third-degree burns. Which method of administering narcotics is the most effective for these clients?
   a. PO
   b. IM
   c. IV
   d. PR

7. A burn client has developed an ulcer related to the trauma from his injuries. The nurse anticipates that the physician will order which nutrition therapy?
   a. gastrointestinal feeding tube
   b. nasogastric feeding tube
   c. central venous hyperalimentation
   d. peripheral venous hyperalimentation

8. Which of these measures should be included in the nursing care plan for a client with burns to the upper extremities?
   a. meticulous wound care
   b. vital signs every 4 hours
   c. daily weights
   d. range-of-motion exercises

9. A burn client complains of chills and headache. Which nursing intervention should be the highest priority at this time?
   a. Remove the dressings to examine the wound.
   b. Obtain a set of vital signs.
   c. Notify the physician.
   d. Touch the skin to determine temperature.

10. The doctor has ordered silver sulfadiazine for a client with a second-degree burn. The nurse is knowledgeable that the medication may cause:
    a. dehydration
    b. crystalluria
    c. leukocytosis
    d. hemorrhage

Answers for Review Questions, as well as discussion of Case Study Critical Thinking questions, appear in Appendix V.

Cultural Care STRATEGIES

Assessing the Client from Another Culture in a Social Context

Mr. Ararnak, 27, a Saudi man, refused to allow a male lab technician to enter his wife's room to draw blood. She had just had a radical mastectomy. The nurse finally convinced the husband of the need for the blood sample and he reluctantly allowed the technician in the room. However, he made sure his wife was completely covered. Only her arm stuck out from beneath the covers. The nurse was careful to accommodate this request. The nurse knew that for Arab families, honor is one of the highest values. Since family honor is dependent on female purity, many Arabs feel that sexual segregation and extreme modesty must be maintained at all times.

Most clients are part of one or more social organizations, which play an important role in their lives. Thus, the social organizations of which the client is a part and their effect on the client need to be assessed, so culturally appropriate and effective care can be delivered to the client and family.

Family

For many individuals the most significant social organization influencing behavior is the family. However, the primary responsibility for decision making varies among cultural groups (Giger & Davidhizar, 1999). Some individuals, such as those from Appalachia or Mexico, rely heavily on family members for decision making. Some religious groups, such as the Amish, may also want to have the church fellowship involved. On the other hand, many mainstream Americans make decisions for themselves without consulting anyone.

The family structure may be male or female dominated. For example, in some Hispanic families the father is the primary decision maker and controller of the family. The Hispanic female is usually submissive and frequently puts the needs and wants of others above her own. In contrast, in many black American families the female is dominant and has a greater role in decision making.

The family should be viewed in two separate ways (Friedman, 1986). On the one hand, the family is the environment that supports the client and provides values and practices. On the other hand, the family itself should be treated as a client. When an individual is ill, the whole family unit is affected, and care should be delivered to everyone who is part of the family unit.

For some clients, the most important single organization is the nuclear family or the extended family. For others, the family unit may not be composed of blood relatives. The nurse should recognize those individuals who assume the functions customarily provided by blood relatives (Murray, Meili, & Zentner, 1993).

Church or Religious Affiliations

In the United States there are many church types and many major denominations. This is very different from countries like Mexico or Spain, where most people belong to one faith and one church. In the United States some churches are identified with an ethnic group. For example, in the Amish church, religious beliefs are synonymous with the Amish life experience.

Nursing Implications

- **Assess the client–family relationship.** Nurses need to assess the client–family relationship in order to learn their values, the flow of authority, and how decisions are made.
- **Be aware that unrelated persons may provide the functions of a family.** Rules related to "family members" may need to be interpreted flexibly.
- **Involve the family as needed to achieve optimal outcomes.** The person with the decision-making power needs to be included in discussions about treatment options. When client education is done, the individual with the decision-making power should usually be involved. This improves compliance.
- **Respect religious customs.** Personal articles such as statues, shrines, rosaries, amulets, or pictures may have special religious meaning and should be treated with respect.
- **Communicate with health team members if they are unfamiliar with the family's decision-making structure.** The nurse may need to provide insight for team members regarding which family members the client feels need to be included in health care decisions.

Self-Reflection Questions

1. Who made the decisions about health care in your family of origin?
2. When making decisions, do you need or not need input from your family?
3. Do your religious values influence the way you feel about some clients?
4. What conflicts might you have in caring for a client whose religious values differ from your own?
5. What conflicts might you have in dealing with a male physician who is accustomed to male-dominated relationships with women?

chapter **16**

Caring for Clients with Endocrine Disorders

CARING tip

❝Honor your profession by caring for others with integrity, competent practice, and dedication to the standards of nursing.❞

Sandi Emerson, RN, MSN • Associate Professor • Chair, Health Sciences • Director, Nursing Programs • College of the Desert • Palm Desert, California

LEARNING outcomes

After completing this chapter, you will be able to:

- Identify the major endocrine organs and the function of the hormones they secrete.
- Describe the pathophysiology of the common disorders of the pituitary, thyroid, parathyroid, and adrenal glands.
- Contrast the manifestations resulting from hypersecretion and hyposecretion of the hormones from the pituitary, thyroid, parathyroid, and adrenal glands.
- Identify laboratory and diagnostic tests used to diagnose endocrine disorders.
- Discuss the nursing implications for medications and treatments ordered for clients with endocrine disorders.
- Identify the preoperative and postoperative nursing care for a client undergoing either a subtotal thyroidectomy or an adrenalectomy.
- Use the nursing process to care for clients with disorders of the pituitary, thyroid, parathyroid, and adrenal glands.
- Reinforce teaching guidelines for clients receiving long-term hormonal replacement therapy.

MediaLink

   www.prenhall.com/burke

Use the above address to access the free, interactive Companion Website created for this textbook. Get hints, instant feedback, and textbook references to chapter-related multiple choice questions. Link to other interesting sites.

The primary function of the endocrine system is to regulate the body's internal environment. Hormones secreted by endocrine glands regulate growth, reproduction and sex differentiation, metabolism, and fluid and electrolyte balance. The endocrine system helps the body adapt to constant changes in the internal and external environment.

When *hypersecretion* (increase) or *hyposecretion* (decrease) in hormone production occurs, individuals develop an endocrine disorder. Clients with endocrine disorders require care for multiple problems. They often face exhausting diagnostic tests, changes in physical appearance and emotional responses, and permanent alterations in lifestyle. Nursing care focuses on meeting physical and emotional needs and providing education and emotional support for the client and family.

Structure and Function of the Endocrine System

Hormones are chemical messengers of the body. They act on specific target cells causing either an increase or decrease in body function. Hormone levels are regulated by a process called *negative feedback.* Negative feedback acts similar to the way the thermostat in a house regulates temperature. When too much hormone is released, the target cell sends back a message to reduce its hormone release. If too little hormone is released, the target cell sends back a message to increase the hormone to the normal level.

The major endocrine organs are the hypothalamus, pituitary gland, thyroid gland, parathyroid glands, adrenal glands, pancreas, and gonads (reproductive glands) (Figure 16-1 ◆). (Table 16-1 ◆ lists the endocrine organs with their hormones and the primary hormone action.) This chapter focuses on the hypothalamus, pituitary gland, thyroid gland, parathyroid glands, and adrenal glands. (Specific information about the pancreas is found in Chapter 17, and about the gonads in Chapters 32 and 33.)

HYPOTHALAMUS

The hypothalamus is located between the cerebrum and the brain stem. The pituitary gland and the hypothalamus are physically attached. The hypothalamus controls anterior pituitary function by regulating temperature, fluid volume, and growth. It also responds to pain, pleasure, hunger, and thirst stimuli.

PITUITARY GLAND

The pituitary gland (*hypophysis*) is located in the skull beneath the hypothalamus of the brain. It is often called the "master gland" because its hormones regulate many different body functions. The pituitary gland has two parts: the anterior lobe (*adenohypophysis*) and the posterior lobe (*neurohypophysis*). The anterior lobe secretes six different hormones (Figure 16-2 ◆). The posterior lobe releases antidiuretic hormone (ADH) and oxytocin.

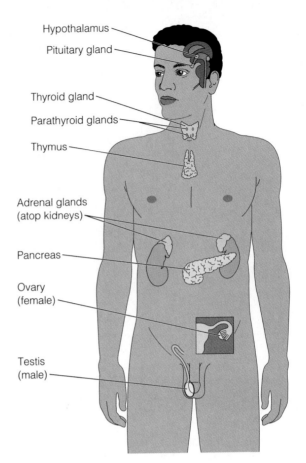

Figure 16-1. ◆ Location of the major endocrine glands.

THYROID GLAND

The thyroid gland is shaped like a butterfly and sits on either side of the trachea. This gland has two lobes connected by a structure called the *isthmus.* The thyroid gland needs an adequate supply of iodine in order to secrete thyroid hormone (thyroxine [T_4] and triiodothyronine [T_3]), which increases metabolism. The thyroid gland also secretes *calcitonin,* a hormone that decreases excess calcium levels in the blood.

PARATHYROID GLANDS

The parathyroid glands (usually four to six) are embedded on the posterior lobes of the thyroid gland. They secrete parathyroid hormone (*PTH,* or *parathormone*). PTH secretion increases calcium levels and decreases phosphorus levels. Normal levels of vitamin D are necessary for calcium absorption in the gut.

ADRENAL GLANDS

The two adrenal glands are pyramid-shaped organs that sit on top of the kidneys. Each gland consists of two parts, an outer cortex and an inner medulla.

Adrenal Cortex

The adrenal cortex secretes several different hormones called *corticosteroids.* They are classified into two groups, *glucocorticoids* and *mineralocorticoids,* and are essential to life. *Cortisol,* a

TABLE 16-1   ENDOCRINE ORGANS, HORMONES, AND FUNCTIONS

ORGAN	HORMONE	FUNCTION
Anterior pituitary	Growth hormone (GH)	Promotes growth
	Thyroid-stimulating hormone (TSH)	Stimulates secretion of thyroid hormone
	Adrenocorticotropic hormone (ACTH)	Stimulates adrenal cortex to secrete glucocorticoids
	Follicle-stimulating hormone (FSH)	Stimulates ovary development and egg and sperm production
	Luteinizing hormone (LH)	Stimulates ovulation and secretion of sex hormones in males and females
	Prolactin	Stimulates breast milk production
Posterior pituitary	Antidiuretic hormone (ADH)	Promotes water retention by kidneys
	Oxytocin	Promotes uterine contractions and milk production
Thyroid gland	Thyroid hormone (TH)	Increases metabolic rate
	Calcitonin	Lowers serum calcium levels
Parathyroid gland	Parathyroid hormone (PTH)	Increases serum calcium levels
Adrenal cortex	Glucocorticoids (Cortisol)	Stimulates gluconeogenesis and increases blood glucose level; anti-inflammatory response
	Mineralocorticoids (Aldosterone)	Regulates blood volume and electrolytes
Adrenal medulla	Epinephrine and norepinephrine	Increases sympathetic nervous system response to stress

glucocorticoid, affects carbohydrate metabolism. The primary mineralocorticoid, *aldosterone,* is released when blood volume or blood pressure falls below normal levels. Also, small amounts of *androgens* (sex hormones) are released by the adrenal cortex.

Adrenal Medulla

The adrenal medulla produces two hormones *(catecholamines)*: epinephrine (also called adrenaline) and norepinephrine (or noradrenaline). Epinephrine and norepinephrine are released during times of stress and initiate the *fight-or-flight response.*

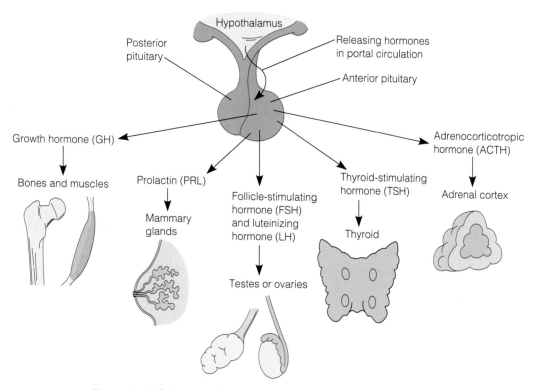

Figure 16-2. ◆ Actions of the major hormones of the anterior pituitary.

Disorders of the Pituitary Gland

The pituitary gland's hormones affect the thyroid, adrenal cortex, ovary, uterus, mammary glands, testes, and kidneys. Disorders result from an excess or deficient production of one or more of the pituitary hormones.

Disorders of the Anterior Pituitary Gland

Hyperpituitarism (hyperfunction of the pituitary gland) is characterized by excess production and secretion of one or more of its hormones. It most commonly causes oversecretion of growth hormone (GH). **Hypopituitarism** (hypofunction of the anterior pituitary gland) results in a lack of one or more of the gland's hormones. Pituitary tumors usually cause both conditions.

PATHOPHYSIOLOGY

Growth hormone is produced by the anterior lobe of pituitary gland. GH stimulates the growth of the epiphyseal plates of the long bones and is necessary for skeletal and muscle growth. Hypersecretion of GH during adulthood results in *acromegaly* (enlargement of bones and connective tissue). Usually, a benign, slow-growing tumor (pituitary adenoma) stimulates the hypersecretion. Because epiphyseal plates close by adulthood, long bones cannot increase in length. However, other bones and connective tissue continue to grow at a very slow rate. Physical changes include enlarged forehead, protruding jaw, and slowly enlarging hands and feet. Manifestations can take as long as 10 to 15 years to develop.

COLLABORATIVE CARE

Diagnosis is confirmed by magnetic resonance imaging (MRI) and computed tomography (CT) scan, which show pituitary gland enlargement and elevated serum growth hormone levels. Acromegaly is treated by **transsphenoidal hypophysectomy** (surgical removal of the pituitary gland through an incision in the roof of the mouth), or irradiation of the pituitary tumor. Drug therapy with bromocriptine mesylate (Parlodel) may decrease growth hormone production but does not reduce tumor size.

NURSING CARE

Nursing care of clients with anterior pituitary disorders focuses on helping them cope with body image changes, and with anxiety about an unknown future following surgery. (See Chapter 29 for nursing care following cranial surgery.) Clients should be taught about the need for lifelong hormone replacement therapy.

Disorders of the Posterior Pituitary Gland

Disorders of the posterior pituitary are caused by too much or too little antidiuretic hormone (ADH). ADH regulates total body water by acting on the kidney to retain or release water. Osmoreceptors in the hypothalamus control the release of ADH in response to serum **osmolarity** (concentration of particles in the blood). When serum osmolarity increases (*hyperosmolarity*), ADH secretion increases, and renal water is reabsorbed, decreasing urine output. *Hypoosmolarity* suppresses the release of ADH, so urine output increases.

DIABETES INSIPIDUS

Diabetes insipidus (DI) is a condition that results from ADH insufficiency. There are two types: neurogenic and nephrogenic. *Neurogenic* DI may occur following head injury or cranial surgery. *Nephrogenic* DI occurs when the kidneys fail to respond to ADH secretion. This condition may be due to renal failure.

Deficient supply of ADH causes a urinary output of 5 to 15 liters per day. The client develops *polydipsia* (excessive thirst). If unable to replace the water loss, the client becomes dehydrated. Additional manifestations are listed in Box 16-1.

BOX 16-1
MANIFESTATIONS OF DIABETES INSIPIDUS

- Extreme thirst
- Polyuria (5–15 L/day)
- Urine specific gravity < 1.005
- Very pale urine
- Weakness
- Dehydration:
  - Tachycardia
  - Poor skin turgor
  - Dry mucous membranes

Collaborative Care

Neurogenic diabetes insipidus is treated by giving additional fluids by mouth or 0.45% normal saline intravenous infusions to replace the lost water. In addition, clients may be given ADH replacement therapy with aqueous vasopressin (Pitressin) or desmopressin (DDAVP). Sodium restriction and thiazide diuretics may be ordered for clients with nephrogenic DI.

NURSING CARE

Nursing care for the client with diabetes insipidus focuses on managing fluid and electrolyte problems.

DEFICIENT FLUID VOLUME RELATED TO DEFICIENCY OF ADH

- Monitor intake and output, urine specific gravity, vital signs, skin turgor, and neurological function every 1 to 2 hours during the acute phase. Monitor daily weight. *Frequent monitoring alerts the nurse to potential complications.*
- Provide adequate fluids. Be sure client is alert and can reach them. *Client needs to drink extra fluids to reduce or prevent dehydration.*
- Give vasopressin or DDAVP as ordered. *Vasopressin is given IM or SQ. DDAVP is given via nasal spray to replace low ADH levels in neurogenic DI. Monitor for side effects of pounding headache and abdominal cramps.*
- Give thiazide diuretics and low-sodium diet as ordered. *These methods are used to treat nephrogenic DI.*

 Discharge Considerations

Teach the client with DI about the disease process, medications, and the need for follow-up care. Instruct clients who need long-term ADH replacement therapy in how to self-administer DDAVP intranasally. Teach them the manifestations of water excess from an overdosage of DDAVP.

SYNDROME OF INAPPROPRIATE ADH SECRETION

Syndrome of inappropriate ADH secretion (SIADH) is a condition that results from excess production of ADH. This disorder may be caused by lung tumors, head injury, pituitary surgery, or the use of barbiturates, anesthetics, or thiazide diuretics.

Excess production of ADH leads to water retention, hyponatremia, and serum hypoosmolarity. The common manifestations of SIADH are decreased urine output and concentrated urine. Neurologic symptoms appear as brain cells swell. No edema is present because water is distributed between the intracellular and extracellular spaces. Manifestations are found in Box 16-2.

BOX 16-2
MANIFESTATIONS OF SYNDROME OF INAPPROPRIATE ADH (SIADH)

- Headache
- Anorexia
- Muscle weakness
- Decreased urine output
- Dark yellow, concentrated urine
- Urine specific gravity > 1.030
- Weight gain without edema

CLINICAL alert

Older adults are at an increased risk for developing hyponatremia. Because geriatric clients take many medications and have decreased kidney function, they should be monitored carefully for signs of SIADH.

Collaborative Care

SIADH is treated by correcting the underlying cause and limiting fluid intake. Diuretics such as furosemide (Lasix) are given along with fluid restriction. Clients with severe hyponatremia may receive intravenous hypertonic saline.

NURSING CARE

EXCESS FLUID VOLUME RELATED TO EXCESS PRODUCTION OF ADH

- Monitor intake and output, vital signs, and level of consciousness frequently. *Frequent monitoring alerts the nurse to potential complications.*
- Monitor daily weight and auscultate lungs. *These measures detect the presence of excess fluid buildup.*
- Restrict fluids as ordered. *Fluid restriction prevents further dilution of the plasma and sodium levels.*
- Provide frequent mouth care. *Oral rinses or sucking on hard candy keeps mucous membranes moist.*
- Give diuretics as ordered. *Diuretics will help to decrease fluid volume excess.*
- Institute seizure precautions. *Dangerously low serum sodium levels can lead to seizures.*

 Discharge Considerations

Teach the client with SIADH about the disease process, and the importance of maintaining water restriction at home. They must know how to weigh themselves daily, and they should learn the number of mL in common beverage containers and how to measure urine output. Discuss medication action and side effects as needed, and stress the need for follow-up care.

Disorders of the Thyroid Gland

Increased or decreased production of thyroid hormone (TH) affects the cardiovascular, gastrointestinal, and neuromuscular systems as well as the metabolic rate. Hyperthyroidism and hypothyroidism are among the most common endocrine disorders.

Hyperthyroidism

Hyperthyroidism (**thyrotoxicosis**) is caused by an excess production of thyroid hormone. It develops more often in women and older adults. The main disorders are Graves' disease, and thyrotoxic crisis.

PATHOPHYSIOLOGY

Hyperthyroidism is caused by many different factors. An autoimmune response leads to Graves' disease. Very large doses of thyroid medication may cause hyperthyroidism. Whatever the underlying cause, increased levels of thyroid hormone increase the metabolic rate. As individuals age, the increased metabolic rate places a strain on the cardiovascular system. If left untreated, this condition can result in cardiac arrhythmias and eventual cardiac failure. With increased metabolism of carbohydrates, proteins, and lipids, the person has an increased appetite, yet loses weight. If the condition is prolonged, nutritional deficiencies occur. (The multisystem manifestations of hyperthyroidism are shown in Figure 16-3 ◆.)

Graves' Disease

Graves' disease is the most common cause of hyperthyroidism. It develops eight times more often in women between the ages of 30 and 50 than in the general population.

Increased production of TH results in a characteristic enlargement of the thyroid gland (Figure 16-4 ◆) and **exophthalmos** (forward protrusion of the eyeballs) (Figure 16-5 ◆). Often, the sclera is visible above the iris. The upper lids may be retracted, and the person has a characteristic unblinking stare. Exophthalmos is usually bilateral, but it may involve only one eye. Inability to close the eyelids completely over the protruding eyeballs increases the risk of corneal dryness, infection, and ulceration. The treatment of Graves' disease does not reverse these eye changes.

Thyrotoxic Crisis

Thyrotoxic crisis (thyroid storm) is an extreme state of hyperthyroidism but rare today. This disorder may result from untreated hyperthyroidism, infection, diabetic ketoacidosis, emotional stress, trauma, or nonthyroid surgery. Thyroid crisis is a life-threatening condition and requires immediate medical attention.

Oversecretion of TH and the release of epinephrine result in a sudden, rapid rise in metabolic rate. The primary manifestations are severe hyperthermia, tachycardia, and hypertension. Restlessness, and tremors are common, progressing to confusion, delirium, coma, and seizures.

Rapid treatment of thyroid crisis is essential to preserve life. The client is admitted to the intensive care unit for close monitoring and treatment. Antithyroid medications are given to reduce thyroid hormone production. An external cooling blanket and acetaminophen are used to lower the severe hyperthermia. The client's cardiovascular status is monitored closely, and treatment is instituted as necessary.

CLINICAL alert

Do not give aspirin during severe hyperthermia because it can increase thyroid hormone levels.

COLLABORATIVE CARE

Treatment of hyperthyroidism focuses on reducing the production of TH and preventing or treating complications. Depending on the client's age and physical status, medications, radioactive iodine therapy, or surgery may be used.

Hyperthyroidism is diagnosed by a thorough history and physical examination. In addition, the following laboratory tests can confirm a diagnosis: elevated serum T_3 and T_4 levels, decreased TSH levels, and an increased radioactive iodine (RAI) uptake.

Pharmacology

Antithyroid medications that reduce TH production are given to treat hyperthyroidism. Because these drugs do not affect already formed thyroid hormone, therapeutic effects

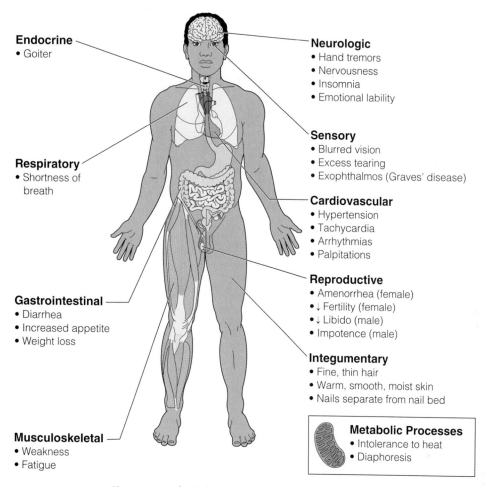

Endocrine
• Goiter

Respiratory
• Shortness of breath

Gastrointestinal
• Diarrhea
• Increased appetite
• Weight loss

Musculoskeletal
• Weakness
• Fatigue

Neurologic
• Hand tremors
• Nervousness
• Insomnia
• Emotional lability

Sensory
• Blurred vision
• Excess tearing
• Exophthalmos (Graves' disease)

Cardiovascular
• Hypertension
• Tachycardia
• Arrhythmias
• Palpitations

Reproductive
• Amenorrhea (female)
• ↓ Fertility (female)
• ↓ Libido (male)
• Impotence (male)

Integumentary
• Fine, thin hair
• Warm, smooth, moist skin
• Nails separate from nail bed

Metabolic Processes
• Intolerance to heat
• Diaphoresis

Figure 16-3. ◆ Multisystem effects of hyperthyroidism.

may not be seen for several weeks. (The commonly prescribed drugs, their actions, and nursing implications are shown in Table 16-2 ◆.)

Radioactive Therapy

Radioactive iodine (I^{131}) is used to destroy thyroid cells so that they produce less thyroid hormone. Usually, this treatment is done in an outpatient setting. Results should begin in 6 to 8 weeks and last a lifetime. After therapy, the client may become hypothyroid and require lifelong thyroid hormone replacement.

Elimination of radioactive iodine (RAI) from the body takes about 2 to 3 days and is excreted in the urine, saliva, and feces. Nurses and family members should avoid prolonged

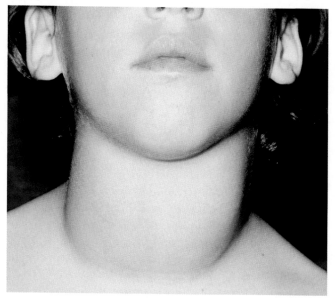

Figure 16-4. ◆ Individual with enlargement of the thyroid gland (goiter).

Figure 16-5. ◆ Exophthalmos in a client with Graves' disease. This is caused by enlargement of muscle and fatty tissue surrounding the eye, which pushes the eyes outward.

	NURSING IMPLICATIONS FOR PHARMACOLOGY: CLIENTS WITH HYPERTHYROIDISM			
CLASS/DRUGS	**PURPOSE**	**NURSING IMPLICATIONS**	**CLIENT TEACHING**	
Antithyroid Drugs ■ Methimazole (Tapazole) ■ Propylthiouracil (Propyl-Thyracil)	Antithyroid drugs inhibit thyroid hormone production.	Give at the same time each day to maintain stable blood levels. Monitor for itching, rash, fever, nausea, loss of taste, and agranulocytosis. Monitor for hypothyroidism: bradycardia, fatigue, weight gain.	Take at the same time each day. Do not take any drugs with iodine. Report signs and symptoms of hypothyroidism to MD. Carry Medic-Alert card stating condition and medications.	
Iodine Sources ■ Potassium iodide, saturated solution (SSKI) ■ Strong iodine solution (Lugol's solution)	Inhibits TH release. Decreases vascularity of thyroid gland to make surgery safer.	Ask about allergies to shellfish. Monitor for hypothyroidism: bradycardia, fatigue, weight gain.	Take at the same time each day. Avoid drugs with iodine and limit iodine-rich foods. Dilute in milk or fruit juice.	
Beta-Adrenergic Blockers ■ Propranolol (Inderal)	Relieves thyrotoxicosis, e.g., heat intolerance, palpitations, nervousness, and tremors.	Do not give to clients with asthma or heart disease. Monitor for side effects of bradycardia, fatigue, and weakness.	Teach patient how to check pulse. Notify physician of side effects: bradycardia, fatigue, and weakness.	

contact with the client for this time period. Fluid intake is increased to aid in flushing RAI from the body. The toilet should be flushed twice after each use. The client should use disposable eating utensils and dishes.

Surgery

When an enlarged thyroid gland causes breathing or swallowing problems, a **subtotal thyroidectomy** (partial removal of the thyroid gland), or **total thyroidectomy** (complete removal) may be indicated. The most common procedure is subtotal; this leaves enough of the gland to produce an adequate amount of thyroid hormone. After a total thyroidectomy (done to treat cancer of the thyroid), the client requires lifelong hormone replacement. However, before surgery, the client should be in as nearly a *euthyroid* (balanced thyroid) state as possible. This is done by giving antithyroid drugs to reduce hormone levels and iodine preparations to decrease the vascularity and size of the gland. Nursing care of the client having a subtotal thyroidectomy is discussed in Box 16-3.

NURSING CARE

Nursing care focuses on the multisystem effects of the disorder. Although each client has different needs, the most com-

mon problems are altered nutrition, fatigue, cardiovascular problems, visual deficits, and body image disturbance.

ASSESSING

Assessment data collected by the nurse can help determine how much hyperthyroidism is interfering with the client's life, and can identify risk factors for complications (Box 16-4).

DIAGNOSING, PLANNING, AND IMPLEMENTING

RISK FOR IMBALANCED NUTRITION: LESS THAN BODY REQUIREMENTS

■ Assess client's daily food intake. Weigh at the same time each day and report losses. *Assessing food intake determines whether food intake is adequate to meet client's needs. The body's inability to meet metabolic demands results in weight loss. Regular monitoring detects continued weight loss.*

■ Encourage client to eat a high-calorie, high-protein diet in six small meals a day. *Increased metabolism causes the body to use protein for energy. Smaller, more frequent meals are easier for clients to increase their daily food intake. This diet can prevent weight loss and muscle breakdown.*

BOX 16-3
NURSING CARE CHECKLIST

CARE OF THE CLIENT HAVING A SUBTOTAL THYROIDECTOMY

Preoperative Care

☑ Review standard preop care in Chapter 7.
☑ Give ordered antithyroid medications and iodine preparations.

Postoperative Care

☑ Review standard postop care in Chapter 7.
☑ Place the client in a semi-Fowler's position; support head and neck with pillows.
☑ Monitor and report the following complications to the physician.

　a. *Hemorrhage.* Assess dressing and the back of the neck for bleeding. Assess tightness of dressing. Monitor blood pressure and pulse for symptoms of hypovolemic shock.

　b. *Respiratory distress.* Assess respiratory rate, rhythm, depth, and effort. Provide humidification. Have suction equipment, oxygen, and a tracheostomy set available for immediate use.

　c. *Laryngeal nerve damage.* Assess for the ability to speak aloud and hoarseness.

　d. *Tetany.* Assess for tingling of toes, fingers, and lips; positive Chvostek's and Trousseau's signs. Keep IV calcium gluconate or calcium chloride at the bedside.

　e. *Thyroid storm.* Assess for high fever, hypertension, and tachycardia.

■ Teach client to avoid high-fiber foods and highly seasoned foods that increase peristalsis or cause diarrhea (apple or prune juice). *Increased gastrointestinal (GI) action and/or diarrhea decreases nutrient absorption.*

FATIGUE

The increased metabolic rate robs the client of energy. The client may be unable to perform normal activities of daily living and may have difficulty concentrating.

■ Take pulse and blood pressure before and after an activity. Note any shortness of breath. *This determines how much the client's activity is affecting the cardiovascular and respiratory systems.*

■ Provide rest periods between activity. *Rest is needed to prevent total energy depletion.*

■ Provide back rubs or cool showers as well as a cool, quiet environment. *This promotes relaxation while decreasing nervous energy. A cool, quiet environment reduces stimuli and stressors.*

BOX 16-4
ASSESSING CLIENTS WITH HYPERTHYROIDISM

SUBJECTIVE DATA

● Any changes in appetite, diet, or weight
● Any palpitations, chest pain, or shortness of breath
● Complaints of nervousness, fatigue, or insomnia
● Any vision changes
● Any changes in emotional status
● Past medical history:
　● Use of thyroid hormones

OBJECTIVE DATA

● Blood pressure, pulse, respirations, and temperature
● Height and weight
● Observe client during interview for nervousness.
● Assess condition of nails and hair.
● Inspect neck for visible signs of masses.

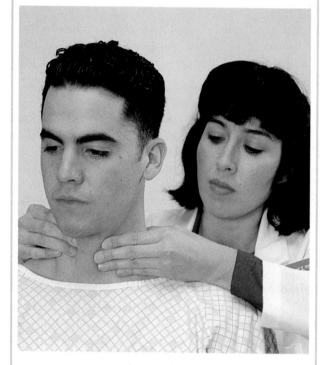

● Inspect eyes for signs of exophthalmos.
● Palpate the skin for moisture.

RISK FOR DECREASED CARDIAC OUTPUT

■ Monitor blood pressure, pulse rate and rhythm, respiratory rate, and breath sounds. Assess for peripheral edema. *Increased heart rate and cardiac output increase the body's oxygen needs. Stress on the heart may result in hypertension, arrhythmias, angina, and congestive heart failure. Clients with a preexisting cardiovascular disorder are at a special risk.*

■ Teach relaxation procedures. *Stress increases circulating catecholamines, which further increase cardiac workload.*

RISK FOR INJURY: CORNEAL ABRASION

If the client is unable to close the eyelids because of exophthalmos, corneal dryness may develop. Without intervention, this could lead to blurred vision or corneal ulceration.

■ Ask the client about feelings of grittiness or eye pain. Assess for incomplete lid closure. *These are signs of corneal abrasion. Prompt intervention is needed to prevent corneal ulceration and loss of visual acuity.*

■ Teach the client measures for protecting the eye from injury and maintaining visual acuity: using tinted glasses or shields as protection; using artificial tears to moisten the eyes; using cool, moist compresses to relieve irritation; covering or taping the eyelids shut at night if they do not close; sleeping with the head of the bed elevated; and promptly reporting any pain or changes in vision. *These measures decrease the risk of injury, provide comfort, and decrease periorbital edema.*

DISTURBED BODY IMAGE

Clients with hyperthyroidism often experience an altered body image due to the physical changes found with this disorder. These changes frighten both the client and family members.

■ Encourage the client to discuss feelings and to ask questions about the illness and treatment. Provide reliable information, and clarify misconceptions. *Body image is very important to clients. They need to understand what is causing the physical changes and whether they will last forever.*

■ Explain the effects of the illness on the client's physical and emotional status. *Family members can be sources of support as the client adapts to the illness. They must understand that changes in appearance and behavior may be disease related and can be controlled with treatment.*

EVALUATING

Evaluate the care for the client with hyperthyroidism by collecting data about the client's weight, energy level, resting pulse, and visual acuity. Determine the client's understanding of medications, diet, and need for rest and sleep.

Discharge Considerations

Clients with hyperthyroidism primarily require self-care at home. Individualized planning and teaching for home care is an important nursing responsibility. Box 16-5 lists the assessment data to consider when planning for discharge.

Teach clients who are taking oral medications that the condition requires lifelong treatment. After a thyroidectomy, provide information about postoperative wound care. Teach clients the importance of regular follow-up with their health care provider. When teaching, focus on the signs and symp-

---

BOX 16-5
ASSESSING FOR DISCHARGE

ENDOCRINE DISORDERS
Client

• Self-care: Ability to perform ADLs independently; to plan adequate rest, nutrition, and physical activity; and to self-administer prescribed medications
• Knowledge: Disease process; prescription medications; special diet and fluid intake; indications for seeking medical care
• Home environment: Appropriate heating and cooling; access to clean water for drinking and handwashing

Family

• Members of household: Individuals with infections
• Caregivers: Availability and willingness to provide care as needed; assist with household chores when client is fatigued
• Financial resources: Income, availability of sick leave; resources for drugs and medical care required

Community

• Access to health care resources

---

toms of hypothyroidism and hyperthyroidism, and tell clients when to seek medical care.

Nursing Process Case Study
■ CLIENT WITH GRAVES' DISEASE

Juanita Manuel is a 33-year-old mother of four small children. For the past 3 months, she is always hungry and eats more than usual, but she has lost 15 lb. Her hands shake, she can feel her heart beating rapidly, and she finds herself laughing or crying for no apparent reason.

Assessment T, 101° F (38.3° C); BP, 162/86; P, 110; R, 24. Her skin is moist and warm, her hair thin and fine. Her eyeballs protrude, and she cannot close her eyelids completely. Her thyroid is enlarged and she has increased T_3 and T_4 levels. Mrs. Manuel is diagnosed with Graves' disease and is started on the antithyroid medication propylthiouracil, 150 mg orally every 8 hours.

Diagnosis The following nursing diagnoses are developed for Mrs. Manuel:

■ Risk for Imbalanced Nutrition: Less Than Body Requirements related to weight loss of 15 lbs.

■ Risk for Injury: Corneal Abrasion related to incomplete eyelid closure

- Deficient Knowledge related to a lack of knowledge about disease process

Expected Outcomes The expected outcomes for the plan of care are that Ms. Manuel will:

- Gain at least 1 lb. per week.
- Maintain normal vision and state ways to protect her eyes.
- State medical treatment and self-care needs.

Planning and Implementation The following nursing interventions are done for Ms. Manuel:

- Ask her to record her weight before breakfast daily.
- Encourage her to eat a high-calorie diet.
- Teach Ms. Manuel how to apply artificial tears.
- Tell her to elevate the head of her bed to 45 degrees at night, and tape eye shields over her eyes before sleep.
- Teach her about Graves' disease, her medications, side effects, and the need for continued medical care.

Evaluation By her next office visit, Mrs. Manuel gained 1 lb. (0.45 kg). She uses her eyedrops, wears the eye shields, and elevates the head of her bed at night. Ms. Manuel states, "I'll always take my medicine. I never want to feel like that again!" She also says that she feels less anxious now.

 Critical Thinking in the Nursing Process

1. Why are Mrs. Manuel's vital signs abnormal?
2. Why should Mrs. Manuel wear eye shields at night?
3. If Ms. Manuel tells you that she plans to stop taking her medications, how would you respond to her?

Hypothyroidism

Hypothyroidism occurs when the thyroid gland produces an insufficient amount of thyroid hormone. It is about 10 times more common in women, and the incidence rises with age. This disorder can occur at any age.

CLINICAL alert

Careful evaluation of symptoms is important in the older adult because manifestations of hypothyroidism may be misdiagnosed as normal manifestations of aging.

Thyroid deficiency may be caused by congenital defects in the gland, antithyroid medications, surgical removal of the gland, or iodine deficiency. The main disorders are goiter, Hashimoto's thyroiditis, and myxedema coma.

PATHOPHYSIOLOGY

The underlying problem in hypothyroidism is failure of the thyroid gland. Hypothyroidism has a slow onset, with manifestations occurring over months or even years. With treatment, the mental and physical symptoms rapidly reverse in

clients of all ages. Unfortunately, thyroid hormone replacement may result in hyperthyroidism.

Because reduced thyroid hormone levels decrease metabolic rate and heat production, the rest of the body systems slow. Many of the manifestations are opposite of those in hyperthyroidism (Figure 16-6).

Goiter

When TH production decreases, the thyroid gland enlarges in an attempt to produce more hormone. This enlargement is called a **goiter** (see Figure 16-4). Iodine is necessary for TH synthesis and secretion, so iodine deficiency can result in hypothyroidism. People living around the Great Lakes, where the soil is deficient in iodine, are more prone to become hypothyroid and develop simple goiter. The use of iodized salt has reduced this risk in the United States.

Hashimoto's Thyroiditis

The most common cause of primary hypothyroidism is Hashimoto's thyroiditis. This disease is classified as an autoimmune disorder because antibodies destroy thyroid tissue. The primary manifestation is the presence of a goiter. It is more common in women between 30 and 50 years old. Clients with a family history of thyroid disease have an increased chance of developing hypothyroidism.

Myxedema Coma

Myxedema coma is a life-threatening form of hypothyroidism requiring immediate medical attention. It may be brought on by exposure to cold temperatures, infection, surgery, trauma, or use of central nervous system depressants (especially narcotics and tranquilizers). This crisis occurs most often in the winter months. Myxedema coma develops frequently in older adults after the age of 60.

The client presents with lethargy quickly progressing to coma and hypothermia. Without adequate thyroid hormone, the respiratory and cardiovascular systems shut down. Clients have bradycardia and decreased respiratory rate. Treatment focuses on maintaining a patent airway; monitoring cardiac function; administering intravenous thyroid hormone (levothyroxine), and treating the underlying cause. The mortality rate is high without prompt recognition and treatment.

COLLABORATIVE CARE

The medical treatment of the client with hypothyroidism focuses on diagnosis, prevention or treatment of complications, and replacement of the deficient thyroid hormone.

Hypothyroidism is diagnosed by a thorough history and physical examination. The presence of hypothyroidism manifestations and a decrease in thyroid hormone, especially T_4, confirms the diagnosis.

Hypothyroidism is treated with thyroid hormone. Drug therapy is started with small doses, which are gradually increased (Table 16-3).

If the hypothyroid client has a goiter large enough to cause respiratory difficulties or dysphagia, a subtotal thyroidectomy may be performed (see Box 16-3).

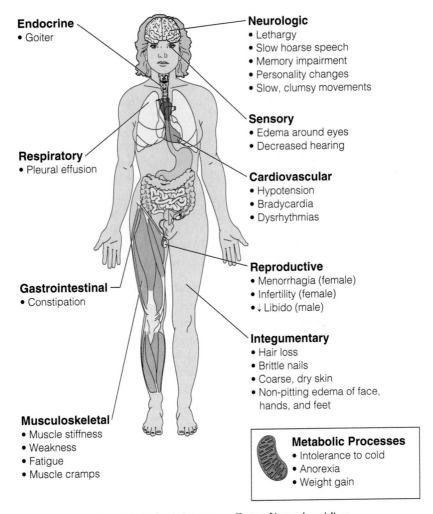

Endocrine
● Goiter

Neurologic
● Lethargy
● Slow hoarse speech
● Memory impairment
● Personality changes
● Slow, clumsy movements

Sensory
● Edema around eyes
● Decreased hearing

Respiratory
● Pleural effusion

Cardiovascular
● Hypotension
● Bradycardia
● Dysrhythmias

Reproductive
● Menorrhagia (female)
● Infertility (female)
● ↓ Libido (male)

Gastrointestinal
● Constipation

Integumentary
● Hair loss
● Brittle nails
● Coarse, dry skin
● Non-pitting edema of face, hands, and feet

Musculoskeletal
● Muscle stiffness
● Weakness
● Fatigue
● Muscle cramps

Metabolic Processes
● Intolerance to cold
● Anorexia
● Weight gain

Figure 16-6. ◆ Multisystem effects of hypothyroidism.

TABLE 16-3

NURSING IMPLICATIONS FOR PHARMACOLOGY: CLIENTS WITH HYPOTHYROIDISM

CLASS/DRUGS	PURPOSE	NURSING IMPLICATIONS	CLIENT TEACHING
Thyroid Preparations ■ Levothyroxine sodium (Synthroid, Levothroid) ■ Liothyronine sodium (Cytomel)	Increases blood levels of thyroid hormone. Older adults usually require lower doses when treatment is first started.	Give 1 hour before breakfast. Check pulse before giving; call MD when resting pulse > 100. Monitor for side effects of insomnia, nervousness, and weight loss. Monitor for bruising or bleeding if also taking anticoagulants. Monitor blood glucose levels closely in diabetics. Thyroid drugs decrease the effects of insulin and oral hypoglycemics. Monitor for chest pain or arrhythmias if taking digitalis.	Take each morning before breakfast. Take pulse daily; call physician when resting pulse > 100. Do not change brands without physician approval. Take the medication for the rest of your life. Report side effects of insomnia, weight loss, and nervousness. If taking an anticoagulant, report any bleeding. Diabetics need to monitor blood glucose levels. You may need extra insulin or oral hypoglycemics. Carry Medic-Alert card.

NURSING CARE

Hypothyroidism affects all organ systems. Nursing care focuses on the most common problems: hypothermia, constipation, activity, and altered thought processes.

ASSESSING

Assessment data collected by the nurse can help determine the extent to which hypothyroidism is interfering with the client's life and can identify risk factors for complications (Box 16-6).

DIAGNOSING, PLANNING, AND IMPLEMENTING

HYPOTHERMIA

- Provide extra clothing and blankets to client. *Clients with hypothyroidism often complain of feeling cold. Extra clothing and blankets will increase the client's comfort.*
- Increase room temperature to avoid chilling; avoid drafts. *Chilling increases metabolic rate and puts increased stress on the heart. Warming the room promotes the client's comfort.*

CONSTIPATION

- Increase fluid intake to 2,000 mL per day and provide low-calorie liquids. *The hypothyroid client usually has a reduced appetite, decreased food intake, lowered activity level, and reduced peristalsis. All of these factors contribute to the client's developing constipation and possibly fecal impaction. Adequate fluids are necessary to maintain soft stool.*
- Provide a high-fiber diet. *Diets high in fiber increase fecal mass and assist moving feces through the intestines.*
- Encourage activity as tolerated. *Activity stimulates peristalsis.*
- Give stool softeners and/or laxatives as ordered. *These stimulate bowel elimination, but their use should be limited.*

ACTIVITY INTOLERANCE

- Monitor blood pressure, pulse rate and rhythm, and respiratory rate before, during, and after activity level. *Thyroid hormone deficit reduces cardiac and respiratory function. Symptoms of cardiac stress include dyspnea, chest pain, palpitations, and dizziness.*
- Alternate activity with rest periods. Ask the client to report any breathing difficulties, chest pain, heart palpitations, or dizziness. *Activity increases demands on the heart and should be balanced with rest, which decreases oxygen demands.*
- Assist client with activities of daily living (ADLs). *Meeting the needs of the client promotes comfort and well-being.*

DISTURBED THOUGHT PROCESSES

- Reorient the client frequently; keep calendar and clock in the room. *Hypothyroidism may slow intellectual processes. Decreased cardiac output reduces cerebral blood flow resulting in impaired memory. Measures provide orientation to time and day.*
- Remove clutter from room. *Deficiency in thyroid hormone produces clumsy movements. Clutter increases risk for injury.*
- Check on client during the night. *Ensures patient safety when they are disoriented.*
- Repeat information as needed. *This allows the client more time to understand the information.*
- Explain to family the relationship between the personality changes and hypothyroidism. *Family will be able to cope with the client's changes if they understand the reasons.*

EVALUATING

Evaluate the care for the client with hypothyroidism by collecting data about the client's elimination patterns, ability to perform ADLs, temperature, and pulse. Determine the client's understanding of medications, diet, and need for rest and sleep.

Discharge Considerations

The lifelong care required for clients with hypothyroidism can be accomplished at home. Teach the client and family about self-care, compliance with prescribed medications, and the need for regular follow-up with health care provider. The older adult may need referrals to social services or community health services, especially if home support is not available.

BOX 16-6
ASSESSING CLIENTS WITH HYPOTHYROIDISM

SUBJECTIVE DATA

- Any weight gain or constant constipation
- Complaints of muscle or joint pain, intolerance to cold, or headaches
- Any change in memory, attention span, personality
- Past medical history:
  - Any preexisting goiter
  - Use of thyroid hormones

OBJECTIVE DATA

- Blood pressure, pulse, respirations, temperature
- Height and weight
- Observe client during interview for sluggishness, memory lapses, decreased attention span, and hoarse voice.
- Inspect neck for visible signs of masses.
- Palpate the skin for dryness and presence of edema.
- Auscultate heart for irregularities and bradycardia.
- Auscultate bowel sounds. Decreased bowel sounds indicate decreased peristalsis.

Review Box 16-5 for assessment data to consider when planning discharge.

Because the client may have altered thought processes, be sure to include the family in any teaching sessions and to provide written instructions. Instruct them about the signs and symptoms of hypothyroidism, hyperthyroidism, and myxedema coma. Teach the importance of a high-fiber, low-calorie diet with adequate fluid intake. Emphasize the need to balance rest and physical activity, and to avoid extreme cold temperature and people with infection. Provide instruction about thyroid preparations as presented in Table 16-3.

 ## Cancer of the Thyroid

Thyroid cancer is relatively rare, with an estimated rate of 13,900 new cases annually. The most consistent risk factor is exposure to external radiation to the head and neck during childhood. The elderly are also at increased risk for thyroid cancer.

Thyroid cancer appears as a small nodule in the thyroid. If undetected, it may grow and press on the esophagus or trachea, causing difficulty in swallowing or breathing. Diagnosis is made by performing a radioisotope scan, performing ultrasound, and by needle biopsy of the nodule.

The usual treatment is subtotal or total thyroidectomy. A radical neck dissection is performed when lymph nodes are involved. Thyroid-stimulating hormone (TSH) suppression therapy with levothyroxine may be given after surgery. Radioactive iodine therapy, external radiation, and chemotherapy are additional therapeutic options. If the tumor has not metastasized, the 5-year survival rate is 96%. (See nursing care for the client with cancer in Chapter 8.)

Disorders of the Parathyroid Glands

Disorders of the parathyroid glands, hyperparathyroidism and hypoparathyroidism, are not as common as those of the thyroid gland. The main alterations in parathyroid function result in hypercalcemia and hypocalcemia (See Hypercalcemia and Hypocalcemia sections in Chapter 5).

 ## Hyperparathyroidism

Hyperparathyroidism is the result of an increase in the secretion of PTH, which regulates normal serum levels of calcium. This disorder occurs more often in older adults and is twice as common in women. It is classified as either primary or secondary. Primary hyperparathyroidism is the most common and usually results from an adenoma in one of the parathyroid glands. Secondary hyperparathyroidism may result from chronic renal failure.

PATHOPHYSIOLOGY

The increase in PTH causes calcium to leave the bones and enter the blood; this condition is known as *hypercalcemia*. Many clients with hyperparathyroidism are asymptomatic. When symptoms occur, they affect the musculoskeletal, renal, and gastrointestinal systems. Release of calcium and phosphorus from the bones results in bone decalcification and possible pathologic fractures. Elevated calcium levels alter neural and muscular activity, causing muscle weakness and atrophy. Kidney function is altered, leading to polyuria and renal *calculi* (stones) formation from calcium deposited in the kidney. The manifestations of hyperparathyroidism are summarized in Box 16-7.

COLLABORATIVE CARE

Elevated levels of serum calcium, PTH, and alkaline phosphatase confirm a diagnosis of hyperparathyroidism. Once the diagnosis is confirmed, bone density studies are conducted to determine whether bone loss has occurred.

Treatment of hyperparathyroidism focuses on decreasing the serum calcium levels. Large amounts (2,000–3,000 mL/day) of oral fluids may be ordered. Diuretics, such as furosemide (Lasix), are given orally or intravenously to increase renal excretion of calcium. The medication Plicamycin (Mithracin) can reduce calcium levels within 48 hours.

The main treatment for primary hyperparathyroidism is surgical removal of the parathyroid glands caused by an adenoma. Nursing care of the client having surgery of the

---

BOX 16-7
MANIFESTATIONS OF HYPERPARATHYROIDISM

- *Musculoskeletal:* Chronic low back pain; pathologic fractures; muscle weakness; decreased muscle tone
- *Renal:* Polyuria; renal calculi
- *Gastrointestinal:* Abdominal pain; anorexia; nausea; constipation; peptic ulcers; pancreatitis
- *Cardiovascular:* Arrhythmias; hypertension
- *Central nervous system:* Depression; impaired memory; psychosis; stupor; coma

parathyroids is essentially the same as that for the client having a thyroidectomy (see Box 16-3).

NURSING CARE

Care focuses on interventions related to impaired physical mobility and risk for injury due to the client's muscle weakness, and altered mentation. The client may also experience pain and altered nutrition intake. (Nursing care of the client with hypercalcemia is discussed in Chapter 5.)

Discharge Considerations

Once the client's condition is stabilized, teach the client and family how to adapt his or her lifestyle at home. Consult a dietitian to discuss a calcium-restricted diet, as well as increased dietary fiber and fluid intake to prevent constipation. The client should contact the health care provider before taking any over-the-counter medications containing calcium.

Teach the client the importance of developing an exercise plan because immobility increases calcium excretion and the risk for kidney stones. Discuss safety hazards and injury prevention guidelines. Review the manifestations of hypercalcemia and hypocalcemia, and stress the importance of keeping annual appointments.

Hypoparathyroidism

Hypoparathyroidism results from inadequate secretion of parathyroid hormone (PTH). The usual cause is accidental damage to or removal of the parathyroid glands during a thyroidectomy. The lack of circulating PTH causes hypocalcemia and an elevated blood phosphate level.

PATHOPHYSIOLOGY

Reduced PTH levels impair kidney regulation of calcium and phosphate. Decreased activation of vitamin D leads to lower calcium absorption by the intestines. The low calcium levels increase neuromuscular activity, especially the peripheral motor and sensory nerves.

Clients with a mild hypoparathyroidism may be asymptomatic. With more acute disease, neuromuscular manifestations result. **Tetany** (a continuous spasm of muscles) is the primary symptom of hypocalcemia. In severe cases, bronchospasms, laryngeal spasms, convulsions, and even death may occur. Nursing assessments for tetany include Chvostek's sign and Trousseau's sign (see Chapter 5). The manifestations of hypoparathyroidism are summarized in Box 16-8.

COLLABORATIVE CARE

Hypoparathyroidism is diagnosed by low serum calcium levels and high phosphorus levels in the absence of renal failure, an absorption disorder, or a nutritional disorder. Tetany usually occurs when serum calcium levels drop below 6 mg/dL.

> **BOX 16-8**
> **MANIFESTATIONS OF HYPOPARATHYROIDISM**
>
> - *Musculoskeletal:* Muscle spasms and tremors, positive Chvostek's and Trousseau's signs
> - *Integumentary:* Hair loss; brittle nails; dry, scaly skin
> - *Gastrointestinal:* Abdominal cramps
> - *Cardiovascular:* Arrhythmias
> - *Central nervous system:* Numbness and tingling in lips, hands, feet; irritability, depression, psychosis

The first priority for treating hypoparathyroidism is to increase calcium levels. Intravenous calcium salts are given immediately to reduce or prevent tetany. Because the client can develop respiratory distress, the nurse must ensure a patent airway. If the client is conscious, instruct him or her to breathe in and out of a paper bag. This rebreathing technique increases acid levels in the blood, which temporarily stabilizes calcium levels.

CLINICAL alert

Keep oxygen, suctioning equipment, and a tracheostomy set at the bedside.

The client needs a calm environment to prevent excessive neuromuscular irritability. Dim lights, reduced noise, and few visitors are recommended. If the client is at risk for seizures, pad the side rails. Placing the client near the nurses' station decreases the client's anxiety and enables the nurse to provide closer observation.

Long-term therapy includes supplemental calcium with oral calcium salts. The client needs a diet high in calcium but low in phosphorus. Vitamin D therapy is given to increase GI absorption of calcium.

NURSING CARE

Nursing care of the client with hypoparathyroidism must consider the client's risk for injury due to tetany. There may be altered thought processes, personality changes and impaired memory. The client's need for a diet high in calcium must be included. (Nursing care for the client with hypocalcemia is discussed in Chapter 5.)

Discharge Considerations

Clients with hypoparathyroidism need instruction for taking calcium and phosphate binders. Teach them the necessity of lifelong medication and dietary modification. Consult a dietitian to identify foods high in calcium and vitamin D and low in phosphorus. (Milk and milk products are restricted because they contain high levels of phosphorus. More appropriate foods include spinach, soybeans, and tofu). Review the

signs and symptoms of hypocalcemia and hypercalcemia with the client and family and stress the importance of regular visits with their health care provider. Teach clients to wear a Medic-Alert bracelet identifying condition and medication therapy.

Disorders of the Adrenal Gland

Disorders of the adrenal gland involve either the adrenal cortex (which secretes steroids) or the adrenal medulla (which releases epinephrine and norepinephrine). Disorders of the adrenal cortex cause physical, psychological, and metabolic alterations that are potentially life threatening. The most common disorders are Cushing's syndrome, Addison's disease, and pheochromocytoma.

Cushing's Syndrome

Cushing's syndrome is a chronic disorder in which the adrenal cortex produces excessive amounts of the hormone cortisol. Cushing's syndrome is more common in women between the ages of 30 and 50 (Figure 16-7 ◆). Several factors may lead to Cushing's syndrome: (a) adrenal tumors causing an increased production of cortisol; (b) a tumor of the pituitary gland increases adrenocorticotropic hormone (ACTH) release which

causes the adrenal cortex to produce cortisol; (c) chronic glucocorticoid therapy; and (d) increased release of ACTH from lung or pancreatic tumors.

PATHOPHYSIOLOGY

With excess production of glucocorticoids, there are changes in carbohydrate, protein, and fat metabolism. There are fat deposits in the abdomen, fat pads under the clavicle, a "buffalo hump" over the upper back, and a round "moon" face. Altered protein metabolism leads to muscle weakness and wasting in the extremities. As thinned skin stretches over the abdomen and buttocks, purple *striae* (stretch marks) appear. Glucose metabolism decreases, and diabetes mellitus frequently results.

Decreased calcium absorption results in osteoporosis and compression fractures of the vertebrae. Mineralocorticoid release promotes sodium and water retention and potassium loss, leading to hypertension.

Figure 16-7. ◆ A woman before and after developing Cushing's syndrome. In the photo at right, notice the swollen facial features.

The inflammatory and immune responses are delayed, so there is a greater risk for infection. Increased gastric acid secretion may lead to peptic ulcers. Emotional changes range from euphoria to depression. In women, increased androgen levels cause **hirsutism** (excessive facial hair), acne, and menstrual irregularities (Figure 16-8 ◆).

Untreated Cushing's syndrome can lead to multiple complications, including hypernatremia, hypokalemia, hypertension, hyperglycemia, and congestive heart failure. Emotional instability may progress to psychoses. Because of suppressed immunity, severe infections can become life threatening.

COLLABORATIVE CARE

The treatment of Cushing's syndrome includes medication, diet, or surgery. Radiation therapy might be considered for inoperable pituitary gland tumors. The most common treatment is surgery.

Laboratory and Diagnostic Tests

Diagnosis of Cushing's syndrome is confirmed by an increased plasma cortisol level and an elevated 24-hour urine test for 17-ketosteroids and 17-hydroxycorticosteroids. Plasma ACTH levels are elevated when Cushing's syndrome is caused by a pituitary gland tumor. Serum sodium and glucose levels are also elevated in Cushing's syndrome.

Pharmacology

Cushing's syndrome caused by inoperable pituitary or adrenal tumors is treated with medications. Although the drugs control symptoms, they do not effect a cure. Commonly prescribed drugs include:

- Mitotane (Lysodren)—suppresses activity of the adrenal cortex
- Metyrapone and aminoglutethimide (Cytaden)—inhibit cortisol synthesis by the adrenal cortex

Clients receiving any of these medications should be monitored closely for side effects of decreased adrenal function.

Radiation Therapy

Radiation therapy may be used in clients with an inoperable pituitary tumor causing Cushing's syndrome. Radioactive isotopes may be implanted into the pituitary gland. If the pituitary gland is destroyed, lifelong replacement of pituitary hormones is necessary.

Surgery

When an adrenal cortex tumor causes Cushing's syndrome, an *adrenalectomy* may be done. Usually, only one adrenal gland is involved. When both adrenal glands are involved, a bilateral adrenalectomy is performed. Removal of both glands requires the client to take lifelong hormone replacement therapy. Following an adrenalectomy, the client is cared for in the intensive care unit because of the risk for adrenal crisis.

Surgical removal of the pituitary gland (*hypophysectomy*) is indicated when Cushing's syndrome is the result of a pituitary tumor. (Nursing care for the client having cranial surgery is discussed further in Chapter 29.)

NURSING CARE

The nurse caring for the client with Cushing's syndrome must consider a wide variety of problems. The most common problems are related to fluid and electrolyte balance, injury, infection, and body image. (For additional information about clients with alterations in fluid and electrolyte balance, see Chapter 5.)

ASSESSING

The nurse must collect assessment data to determine the extent to which Cushing's syndrome is interfering with the client's life. Assessment also identifies risk factors for complications (Box 16-9).

DIAGNOSING, PLANNING, AND IMPLEMENTING

Clients with Cushing's syndrome may need both acute and chronic interventions. When the client is acutely ill, hospital-

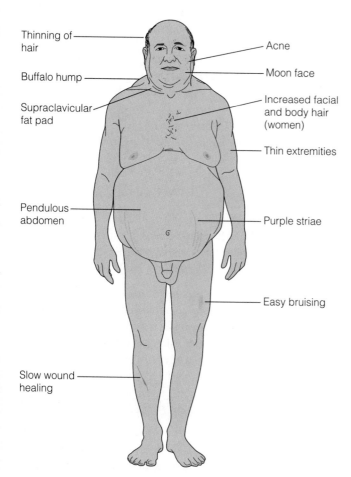

Thinning of hair

Buffalo hump

Supraclavicular fat pad

Pendulous abdomen

Slow wound healing

Acne

Moon face

Increased facial and body hair (women)

Thin extremities

Purple striae

Easy bruising

Figure 16-8. ◆ Major clinical manifestations of Cushing's syndrome.

SUBJECTIVE DATA

- Present health status
- Any changes in weight, increased facial or body hair, poor wound healing, or bruising
- Any increased thirst or urination
- Presence of back pain, muscle weakness, or fatigue
- Any changes in memory, ability to concentrate, or sleep patterns
- Past medical history:
  - Any frequent infections
  - Use of steroids

OBJECTIVE DATA

- Vital signs: Blood pressure, pulse, respirations, temperature
- Height and weight
- Observe client during interview for general body appearance, memory lapses, decreased ability to concentrate.
- Assess for excess body hair and acne; thinning head hair.
- Inspect for thin, fragile skin; bruising; delayed wound healing; purple striae over abdomen; and edema.

ization may be needed. During the chronic phase, the nurse focuses on client teaching for self-management at home.

EXCESS FLUID VOLUME

- Monitor daily weight, and intake and output every 8 hours. *Excess cortisol secretion causes sodium and water retention, which leads to fluid volume excess. The client will have weight gain and edema. Body weight and intake and output are accurate indicators of fluid status.*
- Monitor blood pressure, rate and rhythm of pulse, respiratory rate, and breath sounds. Assess for peripheral edema. *Sodium and water retention is manifested by hypertension and a bounding, rapid pulse. Also, there may be crackles, wheezes, and dependent edema.*
- Limit fluid intake. *This prevents risk of fluid overload.*

RISK FOR INJURY

The client with Cushing's syndrome has muscle weakness and fatigue, increasing the potential for accidental falls. Excess cortisol increases the likelihood of osteoporosis and risk of pathologic fractures.

- Maintain a safe environment. Keep unnecessary clutter and equipment out of the way and off the floor. Ensure ade-

quate lighting, especially at night. *A well-lit, clutter-free environment reduces the risk of injury.*

- Encourage the client to use assistive devices for ambulation or to ask for help if needed. Encourage the use of nonskid slippers or shoes. *Encouraging the client to use assistive devices and nonslip footwear can decrease injury risk.*
- Provide rest between physical activities. *Rest conserves energy so that the client is less likely to fall from fatigue.*

RISK FOR INFECTION

- Place the client in a private room, and limit visitors. *The client with impaired immunity must avoid exposure to infection.*
- Monitor temperature, pulse, and client's feeling of well-being. *Increased temperature and pulse are systemic indicators of infection, but in the client with Cushing's syndrome, a feeling of malaise may be the first indicator.*
- Use sterile technique for invasive procedures. *Aseptic technique reduces the risk of infection in the client with an impaired immune system.*
- Assess wounds for pain, color, odor, and drainage. *Increased cortisol affects protein synthesis, causing delayed wound healing and closure.*

RISK FOR IMPAIRED SKIN INTEGRITY

- Change client's position frequently. *Clients with Cushing's syndrome have thin, fragile skin, which increases the risk for tissue injury. Position changes and massage minimize pressure and improve circulation to keep skin intact.*
- Use mild soap, dry gently and thoroughly, and apply lotion as needed. *Good hygiene promotes healthy skin to prevent bacteria from entering the body.*
- Provide protection by using pillows, pads, foam mattress and so forth. *These measures increase circulation and reduce tissue pressure.*

DISTURBED BODY IMAGE

The abnormal fat distribution, moon face, buffalo hump, striae, acne, and facial hair (in women) disrupts the way clients view themselves. They may be unable to perform usual activities because of their negative feelings about their appearance.

- Encourage the client to express feelings about the physical changes. *Understanding the disease and adapting to changes are the first steps in regaining control of one's own body.*
- Spend time with client and listen carefully. *Each situation affects individuals differently, depending on their coping skills.*

EVALUATING

Collect the following data to evaluate the effectiveness of care for the client with Cushing's syndrome: (a) no edema; (b) no falls or injuries; (c) normal temperature without signs of infection; (d) no skin breakdown; and (e) coping with physical changes.

Discharge Considerations

The client with Cushing's syndrome requires education about self-care at home. Review Box 16-5 for assessment data to consider when planning for discharge.

Teach about safety measures if fatigue, weakness, and osteoporosis are present. Caution the client to avoid extremes of temperature, infections, and emotional stress. Stress can lead to acute adrenal insufficiency, so it is important to teach the client signs and symptoms of urinary tract, upper respiratory, and wound infections. Also, stress the importance of contacting the physician if cuts do not heal.

Instruct the client about prescribed medications; including side effects and adverse reactions. Recommend wearing a Medic-Alert bracelet indicating the client has Cushing's syndrome and listing the medication therapy.

Provide instruction on a diet high in potassium and low in calories, sodium, and carbohydrates. Teach the client and family why fluid intake is restricted. Be sure the client and family understand and are able to perform protective skin measures. Stress the importance of regular visits to their physician.

 # Addison's Disease

Adrenal cortex hypofunction may be *primary* (Addison's disease) or *secondary,* from lack of pituitary ACTH. Addison's disease is the most common form of adrenal cortex insufficiency. It occurs most frequently in women between 30 and 50 years old.

PATHOPHYSIOLOGY

In primary Addison's disease, an autoimmune response destroys the client's own adrenal cortex. This leads to reduced levels of glucocorticoids, mineralocorticoids, and androgens. The onset of Addison's disease is slow, and manifestations develop when more than 90% of the gland is destroyed. The primary manifestations result from elevated ACTH levels and decreased aldosterone and cortisol (Box 16-10).

Complications of Addison's disease include addisonian crisis and the onset of other autoimmune endocrine disorders, such as insulin-dependent diabetes mellitus and thyroid disease.

BOX 16-10
MANIFESTATIONS
OF ADDISON'S DISEASE

- *Integumentary:* Bronze color over knuckles, knees, and elbows
- *Musculoskeletal:* Muscle weakness, joint pain
- *Cardiovascular:* Postural hypotension; weak, irregular pulse
- *Central nervous system:* Dizziness, lethargy, depression
- *Gastrointestinal:* Anorexia, nausea, vomiting, salt craving

---

Addisonian Crisis

Addisonian crisis is a serious, life-threatening response to acute adrenal insufficiency. Major stressors such as surgery, trauma, or severe infections usually precipitate this condition. Addisonian crisis may also occur in clients who are abruptly withdrawn from corticosteroid medications.

The client is monitored for hypotension; rapid, weak pulse; extreme weakness; and confusion resulting from circulatory collapse and shock. Potassium levels can reach dangerously high levels, leading to cardiac arrhythmias. The client is managed in the intensive care unit for intravenous administration of fluids, glucose, sodium, and glucocorticoids. During the crisis stage, the client is kept warm and quiet. Once the crisis has resolved, the client requires teaching and follow-up.

COLLABORATIVE CARE

The client with Addison's disease requires early diagnosis and treatment. Medical treatment involves cortisol replacement therapy. Unfortunately, this can induce Cushing's syndrome.

Laboratory and Diagnostic Tests

Addison's disease is diagnosed through findings of decreased serum levels of cortisol and aldosterone, and urinary 17-ketosteroids. Potassium is increased, and blood glucose and sodium levels are decreased. CT scan and MRI may identify atrophy of the adrenal glands.

Pharmacology

Addison's disease is treated by replacing corticosteroids and mineralocorticoids and by giving a diet high in sodium. Hydrocortisone is given orally to replace cortisol; fludrocortisone (Florinef) is given orally to replace mineralocorticoids. (Nursing implications and client teaching guidelines for these drugs are presented in Table 16-4 ◆.)

 # NURSING CARE

Nursing care of the client with Addison's disease focuses on managing fluid and electrolyte problems, activity intolerance, and altered nutrition.

ASSESSING

Assessment data (Box 16-11) can help determine the extent to which Addison's disease is affecting the client's life and can identify risk factors.

DIAGNOSING, PLANNING, AND IMPLEMENTING

Clients with Addison's disease may require acute and chronic interventions. Acutely ill clients need immediate hospitalization. During the chronic phase, the client needs support and teaching to manage the disease.

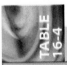

TABLE 16-4 NURSING IMPLICATIONS FOR PHARMACOLOGY: CLIENTS WITH ADDISON'S DISEASE

CLASS/DRUGS	PURPOSE	NURSING IMPLICATIONS	CLIENT TEACHING
Corticosteroids ▪ Cortisone (Cortone) ▪ Hydrocortisone (Cortef, Solucortef) ▪ Prednisone (Deltasone) ▪ Dexamethasone (Decadron) ▪ Prednisolone (Deltacortef) ▪ Methylprednisolone (Solu-Medrol)	Used to replace glucocorticoids in acute and chronic adrenal insufficiency.	Give oral forms of the drug with food to reduce ulcers. Check stools for occult blood; urine for glycosuria. Report increased blood pressure, edema or weight gain, bruising, or weakness (Cushing's syndrome). Assess for impaired wound healing.	Take medications with food; report any gastric distress or dark stools. Never abruptly stop the medication. Take medications for the rest of your life. Eat a diet high in potassium, low in sodium. Weigh yourself daily; report weight gain, edema, or round face (adrenal excess). Use safety measures to avoid accidents. Wear a Medic-Alert bracelet. Avoid exposure to infection; wash hands frequently. Report adrenal insufficiency: dizziness on sitting or standing, nausea and vomiting, pain, thirst, feelings of anxiety, malaise, infections.

DEFICIENT FLUID VOLUME

In the client with Addison's disease, fluid volume deficit results from loss of water and sodium often caused by vomiting and diarrhea. During the crisis phase, acute volume deficit may lead to hypotension and hypovolemic shock.

▪ Monitor intake and output, and assess for signs of dehydration (dry mucous membranes; thirst; poor skin turgor; sunken eyeballs; scanty, dark urine; and weight loss). *Glucocorticoid and mineralocorticoid depletion causes fluid volume deficit.*

▪ Monitor blood pressure (lying, sitting, standing) and strength of peripheral pulses. *Fluid volume deficit may lead to hypotension and a rapid, weak, or thready pulse.*

▪ Increase oral fluids to 3,000 mL per day and increase salt intake. *Fluids and sodium are given to manage fluid volume deficit and hyponatremia characteristic of adrenal insufficiency.*

▪ Teach the client to stand up slowly. *Dehydration causes orthostatic hypotension, increasing the risk for falls.*

ACTIVITY INTOLERANCE

▪ Keep client on bed rest and perform ADLs for client. *This prevents stimulation of an overly stressed adrenal cortex.*

▪ Slowly increase physical activity. *Once adrenal cortex hormones are replaced, the client will be able to regain normal physical activity.*

IMBALANCED NUTRITION: LESS THAN BODY REQUIREMENTS

▪ Provide a high-calorie diet in six small meals. *A high-calorie diet is used to replace lost weight.*

BOX 16-11
ASSESSING CLIENTS WITH ADDISON'S DISEASE

SUBJECTIVE DATA

• Present health status
• Describe skin color changes
• Presence of anorexia, nausea, vomiting, salt craving
• Complaints of muscle weakness, joint pain, dizziness
• Feelings of lethargy or depression
• Past medical history:
  • Use of steroids, adrenal surgery, recent infection

OBJECTIVE DATA

• Vital signs: Blood pressure (standing and sitting), pulse, respirations, temperature
• Height and weight
• Observe client during interview for lethargy or depression.
• Test muscle strength.
• Inspect exposed skin for bronze color.
• Auscultate pulse for irregularities.

■ Auscultate bowel tones and note presence of diarrhea. *Hyperactive bowel sounds and diarrhea indicate an inability to absorb nutrients.*

EVALUATING

Collect the following data to evaluate the effectiveness of care for the client with Addison's disease: (a) no signs of dehydration; (b) activity level increases; and (c) increased dietary intake.

Discharge Considerations

The client with Addison's disease and the family need education about self-care at home. Review Box 16-5 for assessment data to consider when planning for discharge.

Emphasize the need for lifelong treatment and self-care, and the possible complications that can result from not following the treatment plan. Teach clients that regular follow-up with the health care provider is important, and how to recognize the signs and symptoms that require medical attention.

Discuss the relationship between hormone levels and stress. Teach clients and families how to adjust medication doses during times of physical and emotional stress. Instruct them about the manifestations of adrenal hormone excess and insufficiency.

Teach the client and family how to administer steroids. Stress the importance of carrying at all times an emergency kit containing parenteral cortisone and a syringe/needle. Advise the client to wear a Medic-Alert bracelet that identifies both the disease and medication therapy.

Remind the client to increase oral fluid intake and to maintain a diet high in sodium and low in potassium. Stress the importance of not skipping meals.

Disorder of the Adrenal Medulla

Pheochromocytoma is a benign tumor of chromaffin tissues in the adrenal medulla. It occurs in adults between 30 and 50 years old. The tumor erratically produces excessive amounts of catecholamines (epinephrine or norepinephrine). The client may experience mild to severe, continuous to intermittent attacks. Exercise, external pressure on the tumor, or trauma may cause an attack. Usually, the attacks occur suddenly, lasting for a few minutes to hours. Untreated attacks can lead to such life-threatening conditions as myocardial infarction and stroke.

Manifestations are caused by the excess production of epinephrine and norepinephrine that stimulate the sympathetic nervous system. This leads to hypertension with a systolic range of 200 to 300 mm Hg and a diastolic range over 150 mm Hg. Additional symptoms include pounding headache, tachycardia, profuse sweating, flushing, and palpitations.

A pheochromocytoma is diagnosed by increased catecholamine levels in the blood or urine, CT scan, and MRI. Surgical removal of the tumor(s) by adrenalectomy is the treatment of choice.

Nursing care during the acute attack and prior to surgery focuses on stabilizing the client's blood pressure. The client is admitted to the intensive care unit, where constant hemodynamic monitoring and intravenous antihypertensive medications are instituted. Following surgery, the client may require adrenal hormone replacement therapy. Sometimes clients remain hypertensive and require continual follow-up.

Nursing Interventions Classification

Some of the following nursing interventions from the Nursing Interventions Classification Project (McCloskey & Bulechek, 2000) may be useful in planning and implementing care for clients with endocrine disorders:

■ Electrolyte Management
■ Emotional Support
■ Fall Prevention
■ Infection Protection
■ Skin Surveillance

(*Note:* The bibliography listings for this and all chapters have been compiled at the back of the book.)

Chapter Review

key terms by topic

Use the CD-ROM disk enclosed with your textbook to hear the pronunciation of the key terms in the chapter.

Structure and function
hormones

Pituitary gland
hyperpituitarism, hypopituitarism, transsphenoidal hypophysectomy, osmolarity

Thyroid gland
thyrotoxicosis, exophthalmos, thyrotoxic crisis (thyroid storm), thyroidectomy, goiter, myxedema coma

Parathyroid glands
tetany

Adrenal gland
hirsutism, Addison's disease, pheochromocytoma

key points

- Hyposecretion of the posterior pituitary gland can result in diabetes insipidus; hypersecretion can lead to syndrome of inappropriate ADH secretion (SIADH).

- Graves' disease is the most common disorder caused by hyperthyroidism and leads to an increased metabolic rate.

- A life-threatening form of hyperthyroidism is thyroid crisis; it requires immediate medical treatment.

- Hypothyroidism develops when the thyroid gland fails to secrete an adequate amount of thyroid hormones.

- The primary symptom of acute hypoparathyroidism is tetany as manifested by positive Chvostek's and Trousseau's signs.

- Excess production of glucocorticoid hormones by the adrenal cortex can result in Cushing's syndrome.

- Addison's disease is an acute deficiency of glucocorticoid, mineralocorticoid, and androgen hormones.

 ## Medialink

Additional interactive resources for this chapter can be found on the Companion Website at www.prenhall.com/burke. Click on Chapter 16 and "Begin" to select the activities for this chapter.

For NCLEX review questions and an audio glossary, access the accompanying CD-ROM in this book.

for further study

For more information about the pancreas, see Chapter 17.

For more information about the gonads, see Chapters 32 and 33.

For more information about cranial surgery, see Chapter 29.

For more information about cancer, see Chapter 8.

For more information about fluids and electrolytes, hypercalcemia, hypocalcemia, and tetany, see Chapter 5.

Critical Thinking Care Map

Caring for a Client with Hypothyroidism
NCLEX-PN Focus Area: Psychosocial Adaptation

Case Study: Jane Lee is a 60-year-old retiree. She has gained 10 lbs. (4.5 kg) in the past 6 months, even though she is rarely hungry and eats much less than normal. Diagnostic tests reveal decreased serum T_4 level and increased TSH. The medical diagnosis of hypothyroidism is made, and Mrs. Lee is started on levothyroxine 0.05 mg daily.

Nursing Diagnosis: Disturbed Body Image

COLLECT DATA

Subjective   Objective

_____   _____

_____   _____

_____   _____

_____   _____

_____   _____

_____   _____

Would you report this data? Yes/No

If yes, to: _____

Nursing Care

_____

_____

_____

_____

_____

_____

_____

How would you document this? _____

_____

_____

Data Collected
(use those that apply)

• Rarely hungry, eats less than normal
• Yellowish, dry skin
• Eyelids will not close
• Weight gain of 10 lbs. in past 6 months
• Hoarse voice
• Puffy face
• Always cold
• Slurred speech
• No energy to do housework

Nursing Interventions
(use those that apply)

• Teach Mrs. Lee how to increase fluids and fiber in her diet.
• Recommend that Mrs. Lee join a weight reduction class.
• Provide information that helps Mrs. Lee understand why the body changes occurred from hypothyroidism.
• Teach Mrs. Lee about reversible body changes.
• Encourage her to allow her husband and daughter to help with housecleaning and cooking.
• Refer Mrs. Lee for a visual screening.

NCLEX-PN Exam Preparation

1. An assessment of your client reveals the following data: enlarged jaw, protruding brow, abnormally large hands and feet. You suspect that your client will be diagnosed with:
   a. Addison's disease
   b. acromegaly
   c. Cushing's syndrome
   d. Graves' disease

2. In caring for a client who has had a subtotal thyroidectomy, the nurse should assess for which immediate life-threatening complication?
   a. hemorrhage
   b. tetany
   c. dehydration
   d. laryngeal nerve damage

3. A client is admitted with a diagnosis of a goiter. This condition is primarily due to:
   a. hypothyroidism
   b. hyperthyroidism
   c. hypoparathyroidism
   d. hyperparathyroidism

4. Hyperparathyroidism is clinically diagnosed by elevated serum blood calcium levels. Which of the following nursing interventions would best indicate the effect of this increased blood level on kidney function?
   a. Order a renal function panel.
   b. Perform in-and-out catheterizations every 6 hours.
   c. Strain all urine.
   d. Assess the client's level of consciousness.

5. Your client has recently been diagnosed with Cushing's syndrome. Medical treatment with Cytaden was initiated. Which of these nursing diagnoses should be addressed on the care plan?
   a. Fluid Volume Deficiency
   b. Impaired Skin Integrity
   c. Body Image Disturbances
   d. Constipation, Acute

6. The dietary plan for a client with hypoparathyroidism should include foods high in:
   a. phosphorus
   b. calcium
   c. vitamin B_{12}
   d. magnesium

7. Nursing implications for the administration of a beta-adrenergic blocker to a client with hyperthyroidism includes which of the following?
   a. Mix in a full glass of water to disguise the bitter taste.
   b. Observe for tachycardia.
   c. Do not give to clients with asthma.
   d. Monitor weight once a day.

8. Your client with newly diagnosed SIADH is preparing for discharge. Which of the following teaching points should be included in the discharge instructions?
   a. Teach the client how to measure urine output.
   b. Encourage the client to eat a high-protein diet.
   c. Instruct the client to balance rest and activity periods.
   d. Teach client to avoid crowds.

9. Mr. Caruso has been receiving Synthroid (levothyroxine sodium) for 3 months. Which evaluation would indicate a therapeutic response to this drug?
   a. decreased body temperature
   b. noticeable intolerance to cold
   c. decreased cardiac output
   d. weight loss of 5 lbs.

10. A client's MRI revealed a tumor on the adrenal gland. Which clinical sign would the nurse expect to observe?
    a. ECG changes
    b. hyperglycemia
    c. peripheral edema
    d. increased cortisol lab values

chapter

17

Caring for Clients with Diabetes Mellitus

LEARNING outcomes

After completing this chapter, you will be able to:

- Describe the actions of insulin and glucagon.
- Define diabetes mellitus, and explain the pathophysiology of Type 1 and Type 2 diabetes mellitus with the related manifestations.
- Identify the laboratory and diagnostic tests used to diagnose and monitor self-management of diabetes mellitus.
- Discuss the nursing implications for insulin and oral antidiabetic agents ordered for clients with diabetes mellitus.
- Compare and contrast the manifestations and collaborative care of hypoglycemia, diabetic ketoacidosis (DKA), and hyperglycemic hyperosmolar nonketotic syndrome (HHNS).
- Describe the pathophysiology and collaborative care of chronic complications for clients with Type 1 and Type 2 diabetes mellitus.
- Reinforce teaching guidelines to clients with diabetes mellitus regarding self-management of medications, diet, exercise, and foot care.
- Identify specific concerns for young, middle-aged, and older adults with diabetes mellitus.
- Use the nursing process to collect data, establish outcomes, provide individualized care, and evaluate responses for the client with diabetes mellitus.

MediaLink

 www.prenhall.com/burke

Use the above address to access the free, interactive Companion Website created for this textbook. Get hints, instant feedback, and textbook references to chapter-related multiple choice questions. Link to other interesting sites.

Diabetes mellitus is a common chronic disease of adults. It is not a single disorder but a group of metabolic disorders characterized by hyperglycemia (too much glucose in the blood). This condition is due to an insufficient supply of insulin, ineffective insulin action, or both.

Clients with diabetes mellitus face lifelong changes in lifestyle and health status. Depending on the type of diabetes and the client's age, client needs and nursing care may vary greatly. Nursing care is provided in many settings for the diagnosis and care of the disease and treatment of complications.

Structure and Function of the Pancreas

To understand diabetes mellitus, one must first understand the pancreatic hormones and their relationship to maintaining normal blood glucose levels. They are responsible for the cell's use of carbohydrates, proteins, and fats. Without sufficient insulin, a chronic state of excess glucose exists. This state of excess glucose increases the client's risk for developing acute and chronic complications.

PANCREAS

The primary organ involved in diabetes mellitus is the pancreas. It is located behind the stomach between the spleen and the duodenum. The pancreas serves two major functions: (1) acini cells secrete digestive enzymes into the duodenum, and (2) the *islets of Langerhans* release insulin and glucagon into the bloodstream. To prevent **hyperglycemia** (high blood glucose level) or **hypoglycemia** (low blood glucose level), these hormones must be in balance.

INSULIN

Beta cells in the islets of Langerhans produce insulin. Insulin's primary function is to regulate blood glucose levels. This is accomplished through several mechanisms. Insulin eases the active transport of glucose into muscle and fat cells, where it is used as an energy source and for cell functions. It facilitates fat formation, inhibits the breakdown and movement of stored fat, and helps move amino acids into cells for protein synthesis. Excess glucose unused by the cells is stored in fat cells as glycogen or is converted into fat. Insulin release increases when blood glucose levels rise and decreases when blood glucose levels fall. When a person eats food, insulin levels rise in minutes, peak in 30 to 60 minutes, and return to baseline in 2 to 3 hours.

GLUCAGON

Alpha cells in the islets of Langerhans produce glucagon. Glucagon prevents blood glucose from decreasing below a certain level when the body is fasting or is between meals. Glucagon makes new glucose (**gluconeogenesis**), converts glycogen into glucose in the liver and muscles (**glycogenolysis**), and prevents excess glucose breakdown. Usually, glucagon is released when blood glucose falls below about 70 mg/dL. The primary function of glucagon is to decrease glucose oxidation and to increase blood glucose.

BLOOD GLUCOSE HOMEOSTASIS

Normal blood glucose is maintained in healthy people primarily through the balancing actions of insulin and glucagon (Figure 17-1 ◆). However, other hormones (known as counterregulatory hormones) can help increase blood glucose levels during periods of hypoglycemia, stress, growth, or increased metabolic demand. Counterregulatory hormones include epinephrine, norepinephrine, growth hormone, and cortisol.

Definitions of normal blood glucose levels vary in clinical practice, depending on the laboratory that performs the assay. In this chapter, normal blood glucose is defined as 70 to 110 mg/dL.

Overview of Diabetes Mellitus

The American Diabetes Association estimates that approximately 16 million people in the United States have diabetes. Unfortunately, 5.4 million people are undiagnosed. Approximately 798,000 new cases are diagnosed each year. Diabetes varies with race and ethnicity. There is increased prevalence of Type 2 diabetes among older adults, African American women, and Hispanic American women. Diabetes mellitus cannot be cured, but it can be controlled in order to reduce complications, which most often affect the eyes, kidneys, and the nervous and cardiovascular systems.

The term *diabetes,* or DM, when used throughout the chapter, refers to diabetes mellitus.

TYPES OF DIABETES MELLITUS

There are two broad categories of diabetes, Type 1 and Type 2 (Table 17-1 ◆). The type of diabetes that was known as Type I diabetes mellitus, juvenile-onset diabetes mellitus, or insulin-dependent diabetes mellitus (IDDM) is now *Type 1* diabetes. The type of diabetes that was known as Type II non-insulin-dependent diabetes mellitus (NIDDM) or adult-onset diabetes is now known as *Type 2* diabetes.

DIABETES MELLITUS IN THE ADULT CLIENT

Diabetes can affect men and women at any stage, either as a newly diagnosed disease process or as a disease present since childhood or adolescence. The impact of the disease on the adult is discussed here at two developmental levels: diabetes in the young and middle adult, and diabetes in the older adult. (See Chapter 2 for the adult client's developmental stages.)

Diabetes in the Young or Middle Adult

Diabetes in the young and middle adult can disrupt normal physical, emotional, and sociocultural aspects of life and development. Although young and middle adults may have either type of diabetes, Type 1 commonly occurs before age 35, and Type 2 occurs more commonly later. Young and middle adults with diabetes are at risk for developing complications at an earlier age if they do not make necessary lifestyle changes. Teaching healthy behaviors is very important for this age group.

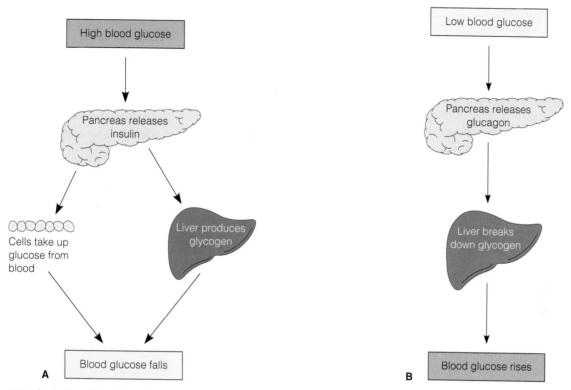

Figure 17-1. ◆ Action of insulin and glucagon on blood glucose levels. (A) High blood glucose is lowered by insulin release. (B) Low blood glucose is raised by glucagon release.

DIET. Young adults who are obese should be placed in a weight management program to prevent cardiovascular disease and hypertension. Dietary recommendations should focus on limiting their intake of salt and saturated fat, especially foods from fast-food restaurants.

CIGARETTE SMOKING. Nicotine constricts small blood vessels, increasing the risk of peripheral vascular and cardiovascu-

lar diseases. Through teaching, referrals, and careful follow-up, nurses should strongly encourage clients with diabetes to stop smoking.

EXERCISE. Exercise helps maintain ideal body weight and cardiovascular health. Moderate exercise should be a regular part of a diabetic management program. In addition to learning how to promote their own good health (see Chapter 2), young

TABLE 17-1

CLASSIFICATION AND CHARACTERISTICS OF DIABETES

CLASSIFICATION	CHARACTERISTICS
I. Type 1 diabetes	State of absolute insulin deficiency Usually occurs before 30 but may occur at any age Autoimmune destruction of beta cells Client prone to developing ketoacidosis Insulin dependent *(If client does not receive insulin, he or she will die.)*
II. Type 2 diabetes	State of sufficient insulin to prevent ketoacidosis but insufficient to lower blood glucose levels Usually occurs after age 30 Most clients are obese May become *insulin-requiring* but not insulin dependent *(If client does not receive insulin, he or she will become ill but will not die.)*
III. Other types	May occur from genetic defects or associated with pancreatitis, trauma, infection, or chemical agents
IV. Gestational	Any degree of glucose intolerance with onset or first recognition of diabetes mellitus during pregnancy

Source: American Diabetes Association. (2000). Report of the Expert Committee on the Diagnosis and Classification of Diabetes Mellitus. *Diabetes Care, 23* (Suppl.), S4–S19.

and middle adults with diabetes must also learn about the disease itself to prevent further illness.

Diabetes in the Older Adult

Most older adults with diabetes have Type 2 DM. Improved management strategies have increased the survival rates for people with Type 1 DM. As people reach age 50, blood glucose levels rise. The normal physiologic changes of aging may mask manifestations of a diabetes onset and may also increase the potential for complications. Box 17-1 presents common problems in the older adult that make the diagnosis and management of diabetes mellitus more difficult.

The older adult with diabetes has multiple and complex health care problems and needs. The following concerns should be considered when working with the older client:

- Chronic illness often interferes with family communication and relationships.
- Dietary restrictions may cause the older adult to avoid social gatherings.
- Physical limitations may interfere with food preparation, activities of daily living, insulin administration and blood glucose testing, foot care, and hygiene.
- Lower fixed incomes and rising costs of medications, blood glucose monitoring equipment, visits to the physician, and hospitalization may be a problem. Even though Medicare pays part of the medical expenses, the client is still responsible for part of the cost.
- Cultural background and ethnic origin may encourage a fatalistic acceptance of illness and its complications or a lack of concern for the future.
- Vision, hearing, or educational deficits may require that the nurse adapt teaching materials and methods.

PATHOPHYSIOLOGY

Although there are various types of diabetes mellitus, the two major types are Type 1 diabetes and Type 2 diabetes. These two major types of diabetes are discussed below.

Type 1 Diabetes Mellitus

Type 1 DM results from an autoimmune reaction. The immune system mistakes proteins made by pancreatic beta cells (the insulin producers) for foreign invaders. The resulting attack destroys beta cells so insulin can no longer be produced. Type 1 DM usually occurs in children and young adults, but it may occur at any age. Insulin deficiency causes hyperglycemia (excess glucose in the blood), a breakdown of body fats and proteins (since cells are being "starved" for energy), and the development of **ketosis**, a toxic accumulation of *ketone bodies* (by-products from the burning of fatty acids).

When blood glucose exceeds the level the kidneys can process, glucose spills into the urine, and **glycosuria** (excess glucose in the urine) occurs. The body's state of hyperglycemia and glycosuria cause the three primary manifestations of Type 1 DM: polyuria, polydipsia, and polyphagia. Hyperglycemia acts as an **osmotic diuretic,** meaning it draws fluid from the

BOX 17-1

population FOCUS

Nursing Implications for Older Adults

Health Problem	Implications for Nursing Care
Urinary incontinence	May be confused with polyuria from diabetes.
Decreased thirst	Polydipsia, a classic symptom of diabetes, is not seen in the elderly.
Decreased hunger and weight loss	May be associated with aging process, medications, depression, or poor nutrition.
Fatigue	Fatigue is a common symptom of diabetes but may be blamed on increased age or anemia.
Blurred or decreased vision	May be confused with cataracts rather than elevated glucose levels. Vision deficits threaten safety, independence, and mobility.
Unsteady gait	May be blamed on aging process or prior stroke.
Peripheral vascular disease	May be related to cardiovascular disease. Impairs ability to climb stairs and walk.
Numbness and tingling in lower extremities	May be blamed on aging process or lack of exercise. If ignored, increases risk of falls and potential for gangrene and amputation.
Confusion and disorientation	May be due to meals or medications omitted or taken inconsistently.
Hypertension	Treatment with diuretics may further impair glucose tolerance tests.
Arthritis	Degree of disability may interfere with self-care. Medications for pain such as nonsteroidal anti-inflammatory drugs (NSAIDs) may interfere with glucose control.
Parkinson's disease	The tremors and rigidity of this disease may interfere with self-care.
Medications	Increased risk for drug interactions from taking multiple medications and decreased renal function.

Data partially collected from Funnell, M. M., & Merritt, J. H. (1996). Diabetes Mellitus and the Older Adult. In D. Haire-Joshu (Ed.), *Management of diabetes mellitus: Perspectives of care across the life span* (2nd ed.) (pp. 755–830). St. Louis, MO: Mosby; Roach, S. (2001). *Introductory gerontological nursing.* Philadelphia: Lippincott; and Ebersole, P. & Hess, P. (2001). *Geriatric Nursing and Healthy Aging.* St. Louis, MO: Mosby.

intracellular spaces into the general circulation. This causes **polyuria** (increased urine output). The increased urinary output leads to dehydration. The mouth becomes dry, and thirst sensors are activated, causing the person to drink increased amounts of fluid (polydipsia).

Because glucose cannot enter the cell without insulin, energy production decreases. This decrease in energy stimulates hunger, and the person eats more food (polyphagia). Despite increased food intake, the person loses weight. Malaise and fatigue accompany the decrease in energy. Manifestations are listed in Box 17-2.

Type 2 Diabetes Mellitus

Type 2 DM is characterized by insufficient insulin production or insulin resistance. Sufficient insulin is produced to prevent the breakdown of fats; therefore, ketosis does not occur. However, the amount of available insulin is inadequate to lower blood glucose levels through the uptake of glucose by muscle and fat cells. While it can occur at any age, Type 2 DM is usually seen in older people. Heredity plays an important role in its transmission. Other risk factors include obesity, increasing age, and belonging to a high-risk ethnic group.

The majority of people with Type 2 DM are overweight. Obesity, especially of the upper body, reduces available insulin receptor sites in the cells of skeletal muscles and adipose tissues and leads to insulin resistance. About three fourths of older adults with Type 2 are overweight. All older adults with Type 2 DM develop insulin resistance. Diabetics who lose weight through diet and exercise can lessen insulin resistance and improve insulin release. Sometimes insulin efficiency can improve enough so that the Type 2 diabetic may no longer require oral hypoglycemic agents.

Unfortunately, Type 2 DM often is undiagnosed for years. People are unaware of its presence until health care is sought for another problem. The hyperglycemia found in Type 2 is less severe than Type 1, so only polyuria and polydipsia are seen. Other manifestations include recurrent infections, blurred vision, fatigue, and paresthesias (see Box 17-2). Accumulated glucose in the tissues provides a breeding ground for bacterial infections. High glucose levels cause a cloudiness of the lens, leading to blurred vision, as well as destruction of peripheral nerves, resulting in paresthesias. Fatigue results from an inadequate amount of glucose available to feed the cells.

BOX 17-2
MANIFESTATIONS OF TYPE 1 AND TYPE 2 DIABETES MELLITUS

Type 1	Type 2
Polyuria	Polyuria
Polydipsia	Polydipsia
Polyphagia	Recurrent infections
Weight loss	Obesity
Fatigue	Fatigue
Malaise	Blurred vision
	Paresthesias

COLLABORATIVE CARE

Treatment of the client with diabetes focuses on maintaining blood glucose at levels as nearly normal as possible through medications, diet, and exercise.

Laboratory and Diagnostic Tests

Three laboratory and diagnostic tests are used to screen for the presence of diabetes mellitus: a plasma glucose (PG) level, fasting blood glucose (FBG), and an oral glucose tolerance test (OGTT). Although any of the three tests may be used, in the clinical setting the FBG is preferred as it is easier to administer, more convenient, and economical.

Diagnostic criteria have been developed by the American Diabetes Association. The criteria are:

1. Classic diabetic symptoms plus *causal* plasma glucose (PG) concentration greater than 200 mg/dL (*causal* is defined as any time of day without regard to when last meal was eaten); or
2. Eight-hour *fasting* plasma glucose (FPG) greater than 126 mg/dL (*fasting* is defined as no food or drink intake for 8 hours); or
3. 2-hour PG greater than 200 mg/dL during an oral glucose tolerance test (OGTT).

It is usually recommended that the diagnostic test be repeated on a subsequent day to confirm the diagnosis of diabetes mellitus.

Because of the risk for developing multisystem complications, routine screening should be done for any person who meets one or more of the following seven risk criteria:

1. Is obese (> 120% of standard body weight)
2. Has a first-degree relative with diabetes
3. Is a member of a high-risk ethnic population (e.g., African American, Hispanic American, Native American, Asian American, Pacific Islander)
4. Has delivered a baby weighing more than 9 lbs. or has been diagnosed with gestational diabetes mellitus
5. Is hypertensive (> 140/90)
6. Has a high-density lipoprotein (HDL) cholesterol level < 35 mg/dL and/or a triglyceride level > 250 mg/dL
7. On previous testing, had impaired glucose tolerance or impaired fasting glucose

Delayed insulin release from the pancreas, decreased tissue sensitivity to insulin, or both lead to decreasing glucose tolerance in older adults. Because of these physiologic changes in persons over age 60, their fasting blood glucose levels may be slightly increased. (The diagnostic tests and expected results used to diagnose and monitor clients with diabetes are summarized in Table 17-2 ◆.)

MONITORING BLOOD GLUCOSE AND KETONES. People with diabetes must monitor their condition daily by testing glucose levels. Two types of tests are available. The first type, direct measurement of blood glucose, is widely used in all types of health care settings and in the home. The second type is urine

TABLE 17-2 DIAGNOSTIC AND MONITORING TESTS FOR DIABETES MELLITUS

TEST	PROCEDURE	RESULT
Fasting blood glucose (FBG)	After 8-hour fast, blood sample drawn	FBG > 126 = hyperglycemia and possible diabetes
2-Hour oral glucose tolerance test (OGTT)	Client eats a high-carbohydrate diet for 3 days; fasts for 12–16 hours before fasting blood and urine samples are taken; then client drinks a special glucose solution. Blood and urine collected at 30 minutes, 1 hour, and 2 hours	2-Hour plasma glucose > 200 = possible diabetes
Glycosylated hemoglobin	Blood sample drawn	Determines average blood glucose level over previous 4 months; > 7.5% considered elevated
Urine test for albuminuria	Collect a urine sample	+ For albumin may indicate early nephropathy

testing for glucose and ketones. Urine testing is less common today.

Self-Monitoring of Blood Glucose. Self-monitoring of blood glucose (SMBG) is a useful method for all people with diabetes to manage their disease. SMBG allows the person with diabetes to monitor and achieve metabolic control. In addition, SMBG is useful when the person is ill or pregnant or has symptoms of hypoglycemia or hyperglycemia.

Type 1 and Type 2 diabetics must be taught some method of monitoring their blood glucose. However, timing of SMBG is highly individualized. Some people may test from four to six times daily and others with good control may test once daily or weekly.

Equipment needed for SMBG includes:

- Some type of device to perform a finger-stick for obtaining a drop of blood (such as an Autolet, Penlet, or Soft Touch).
- A blood glucose measuring machine (e.g., the Glucometer, the Accuchek, or the Ultra) if the most accurate measurement is desired or recommended.
- Test strips that change color when they come into contact with glucose or that can be read by machine (e.g., Glucostix and Chemstrip bG). Usually, the strip is read by comparing its color with a color chart on the side of the container or on an insert.

Blood glucose monitoring machines can provide a single reading or are computerized and/or include a memory of previous glucose readings to show a pattern of control. Each machine has specific operating instructions that must be followed closely. If the timing of the blood on the strip is not exact, or if the strip is overblotted or underblotted, the test will be inaccurate. Also, the machine must be cleaned according to the manufacturer's directions to ensure accuracy. Monitors that use no-wipe technology, thereby improving the accuracy of glucose measurement, are now being marketed.

Urine Testing for Ketones and Glucose. At one time, urine testing for glucose and ketones was the only available method for evaluating diabetic management. Although inexpensive and noninvasive, it has unpredictable results and cannot be used to detect or measure hypoglycemia.

Urine testing should be done in people with Type 1 DM who have unexplained hyperglycemia, during illness, and during pregnancy to monitor for hyperglycemia and ketoacidosis.

To test the urine for ketones:

1. Ask the client to void, discard the urine, and drink a full glass of water.
2. Thirty minutes later, collect a urine sample.
3. For Acidtest tablets: Place the tablet on a white paper towel, place 1 drop of urine on the tablet, and wait 30 seconds. If the tablet turns any shade from lavender to deep purple, the test is positive for ketones.
4. For Ketostix: Dip the reagent stick into the urine sample. Wait 15 seconds, and compare the color of the pad at the end of the stick to an accompanying color chart. Purple indicates **ketonuria.**

To test the urine for glucose:

1. Follow the same procedure to collect a urine sample.
2. Dip the reagent stick into the urine sample, and wait the specified time. Compare the color of the pad on the end of the reagent stick with an accompanying color chart. The glucose is expressed as a percentage (for example, ½%, 1%, 2%). *Remember:* Normally, no glucose is found in the urine, so the presence of glucose indicates hyperglycemia.

Pharmacology

The pharmacologic treatment for diabetes mellitus depends on the type of diabetes. People with Type 1 require lifelong insulin replacement therapy; those with Type 2 are usually able to control glucose levels with an oral antidiabetic medication, but they may require insulin when control is inadequate.

INSULIN. Insulin is derived from pork pancreas or made in the laboratory. Synthetically produced insulin comes either from altered pork insulin or through genetic engineering using strains of *Escherichia coli* to form a biosynthetic human insulin. Insulins are available in rapid-acting, short-acting, intermediate-acting, and long-acting preparations. (The common insulins, times of onset, peak, and duration of action are listed in Table 17-3 ◆.)

CLINICAL alert

Regular and Lantus insulins appear clear. All other insulins appear cloudy.

Insulin is ordered in units. The most common concentration is 100 U/mL (U-100 insulin). U-500 insulin is made for people who need doses in excess of 200 U per day. Insulin is given in sterile, single-use, disposable insulin syringes, marked in units per milliliter. This means that in U-100 insulin, there are 100 U of insulin in 1 mL. Common syringe size is either 0.5 mL (50 U), or 1.0 mL (100 U). The advantage of the 0.5-mL size is that the distance between unit markings is greater so that it is easier to measure the dose accurately. Most insulin syringes are manufactured with the needle permanently attached in a 25- to 26-gauge, 0.5-inch size.

All insulins are given parenterally. Only regular insulin may be given by either subcutaneous or intravenous routes; all others are given only subcutaneously. If the intravenous route is not available, regular insulin may be administered intramuscularly in an emergency situation, but this route is seldom used.

Special Injection Products. Other special injection products are available. These products include insulin pens and jet injectors. Insulin pens use an insulin cartridge with a disposable needle. The insulin pen is useful for people who need only one type of insulin or need to travel away from their home. Jet injectors deliver insulin into the skin under pressure. Different absorption rates and bruising limit their use.

Regular insulin can be delivered through continuous subcutaneous insulin infusion (CSII) devices or insulin pump. CSII device has a small external pump that holds a syringe connected to a subcutaneous needle by tubing. The client places the needle into the subcutaneous tissue, usually the abdomen. This device delivers a constant amount of programmed insulin throughout each 24-hour period. It also can be used to deliver a bolus of insulin manually (e.g., before meals). Blood glucose levels determine the amount of insulin to be delivered. The advantages of CSII include greater lifestyle flexibility and, for some patients, better glucose control. Disadvantages are an increased risk of ketoacidosis from a malfunctioning pump and infection at needle insertion site.

INSULIN INJECTION SITES. Recommended injection sites are the upper arm, the abdomen except for a 2-inch circle around the navel (the umbilicus), the anterior lateral part of the thigh, and the buttocks (Figure 17-2 ◆). Absorption and peak action of insulin differ according to the site. The most rapid absorption site is the abdomen, followed by the arms, thighs, and buttocks.

To administer insulin, gently pinch a fold of skin and inject the needle at a 90-degree angle. If the person is very thin, a 45-degree angle may be required to avoid injecting into muscle. Do not massage the site after giving the injection because this may interfere with absorption. Rotation within injection sites is recommended to give more consistent blood glucose levels and to prevent lipodystrophy. The distance between injections should be about 1 inch. Techniques to minimize painful injections are summarized in Box 17-3.

Lipodystrophy (hypertrophy of subcutaneous tissue) or lipoatrophy (atrophy of subcutaneous tissue) may occur if the same injection sites are used repeatedly. The use of refrigerated synthetic or animal insulin may trigger the development of

TABLE 17-3 ACTION OF INSULIN PREPARATIONS			
TYPE OF INSULIN	**ONSET (HR)**	**PEAK (HR)**	**DURATION (HR)**
Rapid-Acting			
▪ Lispro (Humalog)	0.25	0.5–1.5	4–5
Short-Acting			
▪ Regular	0.5–1	2–4	4–6
Intermediate-Acting			
▪ NPH	1–2	6–12	18–24
▪ Lente	1–3	8–12	18–24
▪ Novolin NPH 70/regular 30	0.5	4–8	Up to 24
Long-Acting			
▪ Ultralente	4–6	18–24	36
▪ Glargine (Lantus)	1.5	Unclear peak	Up to 24

Figure 17-2. ◆ Sites of insulin injection.

tissue hypertrophy or atrophy. These problems rarely occur with the use of human insulins. Lipodystrophy and lipoatrophy alter insulin absorption by delaying its onset. Lipodystrophy usually resolves if the area is unused for a minimum of 6 months.

MIXING INSULINS. People who require more than one type of insulin must mix their insulins to avoid multiple injections per dose. In addition, clients often need different doses of insulin throughout the day to provide adequate blood glucose control. The *procedure* for mixing insulins is described in Procedure 17-1. (Additional nursing implications and guide-

BOX 17-3
TECHNIQUES TO MINIMIZE PAINFUL INJECTIONS

- ☑ Inject insulin that is at room temperature.
- ☑ Make sure no air bubbles remain in the syringe before the injection.
- ☑ Wait until alcohol on the skin dries completely before performing the injection.
- ☑ Teach client to relax muscles in the injection area.
- ☑ Penetrate the skin with the needle quickly.
- ☑ Don't change the direction of the needle during insertion or withdrawal.
- ☑ Don't reuse dull needles.

Source: American Diabetes Association. (2000). Insulin administration. *Diabetes Care, 23* (Suppl. 1), S86–S89.

lines for teaching clients insulin administration techniques are listed in Table 17-4 ◆.)

CLINICAL alert

1. Mix only insulins of like concentration (e.g., regular insulin U-100 with NPH insulin U-100).
2. Regular insulin may be mixed with all other types of insulin.
3. Do not mix human and animal insulins because they will inactivate each other.

INSULIN REGIMENS. Most diabetic clients require two or more insulin injections each day. Usually, they mix short-acting and intermediate-acting insulins. Timing of the injections depends on blood glucose levels, food consumption, exercise, and types of insulin used.

The results of a 10-year Diabetes Control and Complications Trial (DCCT) demonstrated that tight glucose control resulted in fewer long-term complications. This can be achieved through intensive insulin regimen (three or four injections per day) (Table 17-5 ◆). Whether the client needs one or multiple daily injections, the goal is to avoid daytime hypoglycemia while achieving adequate blood glucose control overnight.

ORAL ANTIDIABETIC AGENTS.
Oral antidiabetic agents are used to treat people with Type 2 DM (Table 17-6 ◆).

CLINICAL alert

Clients taking sulfonylureas can develop hyperglycemia or hypoglycemia when taken with the following drugs:

Monitor for Hyperglycemia	Monitor for Hypoglycemia
● Corticosteroids	● Alcohol
● Estrogen	● Coumadin
● Thiazide diuretics	● Aspirin
● Epinephrine	● Beta blockers
	● Ranitidine (Zantac)

Medical Nutrition Therapy

Diabetes management requires a careful balance between nutrient intake, daily expenditure of energy, and the dose and timing of insulin or oral antidiabetic agents. Persons with diabetes must eat a more structured diet in order to prevent hyperglycemia. The American Diabetes Association has established the following dietary goals for adults with diabetes:

1. Maintain as near normal blood glucose levels as possible by balancing food intake with insulin or oral glucose-lowering medications and exercise.
2. Achieve optimal serum lipid levels.
3. Provide adequate calories to maintain or attain reasonable weights and to recover from illness.
4. Prevent and treat acute and chronic complications.

PROCEDURE 17-1 ## Mixing Insulins: 10 Units of Regular and 20 Units of NPH

1. Wash hands.
2. Inspect regular insulin for clarity. *Regular insulin is contaminated if cloudy.*
3. Gently rotate NPH insulin to mix well. *Shaking insulin creates bubbles and prevents accurate dose from being withdrawn.*
4. Wipe off the top of both vials with an alcohol pad. *Prevents contamination of insulin.*
5. Draw 20 U of air into the syringe, and inject air into the NPH vial. Withdraw needle. *Prepares vial by creating pressure.*

A Injecting air into the NPH vial.

6. Draw 10 U of air into the syringe, and inject air into the regular vial. *Prepares vial by creating pressure.*

B Injecting air into the regular insulin vial.

7. Invert the regular insulin vial, and withdraw 10 U of regular insulin. Withdraw the needle. *Withdrawing regular insulin first prevents contaminating regular insulin with NPH insulin.*

C Withdrawing regular insulin.

8. Insert the needle into the NPH vial, and carefully withdraw 20 U of NPH insulin. *Accurate dosage is important for effectiveness.*

D Withdrawing NPH insulin.

9. Administer the insulin.
10. Dispose of the syringe properly and wash hands.

■ **SAMPLE DOCUMENTATION**

10/1/01   07:30am Regular insulin 10 units and NP.H insulin 20 units given sub-q in right upper arm.
_____ R. Perry, LPN.

TABLE 17-4   NURSING IMPLICATIONS FOR MONITORING AND CLIENT TEACHING

NURSING IMPLICATIONS	CLIENT/FAMILY TEACHING
▪ Discard vials of insulin whose expiration has passed. ▪ Discard any vial that is discolored or contains clumps, granules, or solid deposits on the sides. ▪ Check client's blood glucose level 30 minutes before giving an insulin injection. ▪ When drawing up insulin dose, always check type and dose with another nurse. ▪ If a client's meal is delayed, hold administration of rapid-acting insulin. ▪ Monitor and maintain a record of blood glucose readings before each meal and at bedtime or as ordered. ▪ Monitor food intake; notify physician when client eats an inadequate diet. ▪ Inspect injection sites for signs of lipodystrophy. ▪ Monitor for signs and symptoms of hypoglycemia or hyperglycemia and take appropriate action.	▪ Know the manifestations of diabetes mellitus. ▪ Store opened insulin vials in a cool place for up to 4 weeks; avoid exposure to extreme temperatures (36° to 46° F) or sunlight. ▪ Refrigerate unopened extra insulin vials; do not freeze them. ▪ Refrigerated insulin should be brought to room temperature before using it. ▪ Demonstrate self-administration of insulin (review procedure steps in Procedure 17-1). ▪ Know how to mix two types of insulin. ▪ Discard outdated or discolored insulin. ▪ Keep a regular insulin vial available for emergencies. ▪ Check blood glucose before meals, at bedtime, and as prescribed. ▪ If breakfast is delayed, also delay giving rapid-acting insulin. ▪ Know the signs of hypoglycemia and hyperglycemia. ▪ Keep candy or sugar source available to treat hypoglycemia. ▪ Avoid alcoholic beverages to prevent hypoglycemia. ▪ Observe injection site for hardness, dimpling, or sunken areas; develop a plan for rotating injection sites.

Early in the diagnosis of diabetes, clients should be referred to a certified diabetic educator and registered dietitian for meal planning and teaching. The dietary plan should consider food preferences, food habits, age, and other medical conditions (Table 17-7 ◆).

MEAL PLANNING. Several different systems for meal planning are available to the person with diabetes. The two primary systems are the Food Guide Pyramid and the exchange lists. Regardless of the system selected, the dietitian must consider the person's usual eating habits, diet history, food values, and special needs. Altering foods and meal patterns is one of the most difficult parts of diabetes management. Careful consideration of individual preferences promotes dietary compliance.

Food Guide Pyramid. The Diabetes Food Guide Pyramid adapts the basic Food Guide Pyramid (see Figure 18-4), and lists the recommended number of servings for each group. The largest group (at the bottom) contains grains, beans, and starchy vegetables and should be eaten more than the top group, which contains fats, sweets, and alcohol.

Exchange Lists. The exchange list diet is based on the person's ideal (or reasonable) weight, activity level, age, and occupation. These factors determine the total kilocalories (kcal) that the person may consume each day. After the calories have been determined, the proportions of carbohydrates, proteins, and fats are calculated, using the guidelines established by the American Diabetes Association and the American Dietetic Association (see Table 17-7).

The distribution of foods throughout the day is based on the exchange lists. There are six main exchange lists: bread/starch, vegetable, milk, meat, fruit, and fat. Foods are grouped into each exchange list according to their composition. Portion sizes are specified so that each serving within the list has approximately the same number of carbohydrates, protein, fat, and calories. Standard household measurements are used to determine portion sizes. The number of servings is based on the calorie count needed by the client. A food item on the list can be substituted ("exchanged") for another with very little difference in calories or amount of carbohydrates, proteins, and fats. The meal plan prescribes how many exchanges are allowed for each food group per meal and snacks (Table 17-8 ◆).

NUTRITIONAL CONCERNS FOR OLDER ADULTS. An obese older adult with Type 2 DM may need a diet, exercise, and weight reduction program. To improve the likelihood of following diet modifications, the nurse should consider the following factors: dietary likes and dislikes, eating habits, meal preparation skills, cooking facilities, age-related changes in taste and smell, and dental health. In addition, most older adults live on a fixed income that may limit their diet to canned meat, fruits, and vegetables. Co-existing illnesses and the use of multiple medications can decrease appetite and reduce their energy to plan, cook, or eat. If possible, encourage older adults to eat their meals with others. Socialization with others usually increases appetite.

Exercise

Exercise is extremely important for diabetic clients. It reduces blood glucose levels by increasing glucose use by the muscles. This potentially decreases the need for insulin. Exercise also decreases cholesterol and triglycerides, reducing the risk of

TABLE 17-5

INSULIN REGIMENS

REGIMEN	INSULIN TYPE*	GENERAL INFORMATION
One injection per day	NPH or NPH with regular before breakfast	One injection of either NPH or NPH with regular is used to cover all meals. This is a simple regimen, it is often difficult to control FBG levels, and afternoon hypoglycemia may result from increases in NPH.
Two injections per day	NPH or NPH with regular or premixed (N and R) before breakfast and dinner	This regimen aims to mimic normal pancreatic function, but the client must have a fairly rigid schedule of food intake and exercise.
Three or four injections per day	R before each meal; NPH at dinner or bedtime	This regimen more closely mimics normal pancreatic function; it allows greater choice in mealtimes and exercise. However, each premeal dose of R must be determined by blood glucose tests.

*Insulin types are abbreviated as follows: NPH = intermediate-acting, R = regular, rapid-acting.

- - - - - = Regular

———— = NPH

cardiovascular disorders. People with diabetes should consult their primary health care provider before beginning or changing an exercise program. The ability to maintain an exercise program is affected by fatigue and glucose levels.

The nurse should assess the client's lifestyle before determining the type of exercise program. Lifestyle factors to consider are the client's usual exercise habits, living environment,

and community programs. The type of exercise the person usually enjoys is probably the one that he or she will continue throughout life. Whatever exercise the client chooses, it must be done on a regular basis.

Clients with diabetes should follow the recommendations of the American Diabetes Association when exercising: Use proper footwear, inspect the feet daily and after exercise,

TABLE 17-6

NURSING IMPLICATIONS FOR PHARMACOLOGY: CLIENTS RECEIVING ORAL ANTIDIABETIC AGENTS

CLASS/DRUGS	PURPOSE	NURSING RESPONSIBILITIES	CLIENT TEACHING
Sulfonylureas ■ Glimepiride (Amaryl) ■ Glipizide (Glucotrol, Glucotrol XL) ■ Glyburide (Dia Beta)	Increases release of insulin from pancreas and increases the number and action of receptor cells to maintain blood glucose levels within normal range.	Assess for allergy to sulfonamides. Observe for signs and symptoms of hypoglycemia (sweating, hunger, weakness, dizziness, tremor, tachycardia, anxiety). Test client's blood glucose level before giving drug. Assess for side effects of nausea, heartburn, or diarrhea.	Take at the same time each day. Take 30 minutes before meals, except Glucotrol XL, which must be taken with food. Know the signs and symptoms of hypoglycemia. Drink a glass of orange juice or eat hard candy if hypoglycemia develops. Test blood glucose level before taking drug. Continue with prescribed diet and exercise program.
Biguanides ■ Metformin (Glucophage)	Reduces liver glucose production and improves glucose use in skeletal muscle to maintain blood glucose levels within normal.	Monitor renal function, especially in clients at risk for kidney disease. Monitor glucose levels throughout therapy. Discontinue 48 hours before injection with any radiocontrast dye. Call physician if fatigue, weakness, muslce pain, or stomach upset occurs. These are early signs of lactic acidosis.	Take at the same time each day; breakfast and/or dinner as ordered. If a dose is missed, do not double doses. Monitor blood glucose levels as ordered. Call physician if fatigue, weakness, muscle pain, or stomach upset occurs. These are early signs of lactic acidosis.
Alpha-Glucoside Inhibitors ■ Acarbose (Precose) ■ Miglitol (Glyset)	Slows digestion and absorption of carbohydrates to maintain normal blood glucose levels.	Assess for intestinal disorders; acarbose will worsen these conditions.	Take with the first bite of a meal. May cause gas, abdominal pain, and diarrhea; tends to decrease with continued therapy.
Meglitinides ■ Repaglinide (Prandin) ■ Nateglinide (Starlix)	Stimulates mealtime insulin secretion.	Monitor for hypoglycemia because it acts like sulfonylureas.	Monitor for hypoglycemia.
Thiazolinediones ■ Rosiglitazone (Avandia) ■ Pioglitazone (Actos)	Increases insulin sensitivity at receptor sites on liver, muscle, and fat cells.	Assess for signs of **liver toxicity** (e.g., anorexia, jaundice, or dark urine).	Call physician if anorexia, jaundice, or dark urine develops.

avoid exercise in extreme heat or cold, and avoid exercise during periods of poor glucose control. The client over age 35 should have an exercise-stress electrocardiogram prior to beginning an exercise program. (See Chapter 22). General exercise guidelines for clients with Type 1 and Type 2 diabetes are listed in Box 17-4.

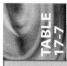

TABLE 17-7

NUTRIENT RECOMMENDATIONS FOR ADULTS WITH DIABETES

NUTRIENT	RECOMMENDED DAILY INTAKE
Calories (kcal)	Amount needed to attain and maintain as close as possible the desired body weight.
Carbohydrates	Individualized, based on client's individual eating habits and glucose and lipid goals.
Sweeteners	Non-nutritive sweeteners such as saccharin (Sweet & Low) or aspartame (Nutrisweet) contain few kcal and produce little or no changes in blood glucose levels. Nutritive sweeteners including sorbitol are often contained in foods labeled "sugar-free." They contain fewer kcal than sugar but must be counted as carbohydrate.
Protein	Approximately 10% to 20% of the daily caloric intake; should be from both animal and vegetable sources. Clients with nephropathy need lower protein intake.
Saturated fat and cholesterol	Less than 10% of the daily calories should be from saturated fats, with dietary cholesterol limited to ≤ 300 mg/day.
Fiber	20–35 g of dietary fiber each day from a wide variety of food sources.
Sodium	The same as for the general population; no more than 2,400–3,000 mg/day.
Vitamins and minerals	Sufficient to meet daily requirements.
Alcohol	For Type 1 diabetics, limit alcohol intake to no more than two alcoholic beverages per day. Alcohol should be ingested with a meal to decrease the risk of hypoglycemia and counted in the meal plan (one alcoholic beverage equals 12 ounces of beer, 5 ounces of wine, or 1.5 ounces of distilled spirits). Alcohol abstention is advised for people with a history of alcohol abuse, during pregnancy, and for those with pancreatitis or neuropathy.

Source: American Diabetes Association. (2000). Nutrition recommendations and principles for people with diabetes mellitus. *Diabetes Care, 23*(Suppl. 1), S43–S46.

COMPLICATIONS OF DIABETES MELLITUS

The person with diabetes mellitus, regardless of type, is at increased risk for acute and chronic complications involving multiple body systems (Figure 17-3 ◆). Altered blood glucose levels affect the vascular and nervous systems and cause an increased susceptibility to infection. Figure 17-3 shows the progression from early manifestations to acute complications to chronic multisystem complications. A discussion of each of these complications with related collaborative care and nursing care follows.

Acute Complications

Diabetic ketoacidosis, hyperglycemic hyperosmolar nonketotic syndrome, and hypoglycemia are the primary acute complications of diabetes mellitus. These can be life threatening and require immediate medical treatment.

DIABETIC KETOACIDOSIS. Diabetic Ketoacidosis (DKA) is a life-threatening illness occurring in Type 1 diabetics and is characterized by hyperglycemia and coma. DKA occurs in a client with untreated Type 1 DM. It also may occur during

TABLE 17-8

SAMPLE LUNCH MENUS BASED ON EXCHANGE LISTS

EXCHANGES	SAMPLE LUNCH #1	SAMPLE LUNCH #2
2 starch	2 slices whole-wheat bread	Hamburger bun
3 meat	2 oz. sliced chicken breast and 1 oz. low-fat cheese	3-oz. lean beef patty
1 vegetable	Lettuce, tomato	Green salad
1 fat	1 tsp. mayonnaise	1 tbsp. salad dressing
1 fruit	1 small banana	⅓ small cantaloupe
Free items (optional)	8 oz. unsweetened iced tea 1 dill pickle	1 cup decaffeinated unsweetened coffee Mustard, onion, and relish

population
FOCUS

Exercise Guidelines for Clients with Type 1 and Type 2 DM

1. Include a warm-up and cool-down period in your exercise program.
2. Perform aerobic exercises that use large muscles (walking, biking, swimming) and increase heart rate to 60–80% of maximum.
3. Consume adequate fluids before, during, and after exercise.
4. Monitor blood glucose before and after exercise.
5. Always carry quick-acting carbohydrate (Life-Savers or 5-g glucose tablets).
6. Always carry diabetic ID card and wear ID bracelet.

Type 1	Type 2
• Exercise within 30–60 minutes of eating.	• Exercise at least three times per week.
• Avoid exercise if fasting blood glucose is > 250 mg/dL and ketosis is present.	• If taking sulfonylureas, eat a snack before exercising.
• Inject insulin into abdomen for fastest absorption.	

Sources: American Diabetes Association. (2000). Diabetes mellitus and exercise. *Diabetes Care, 23*(Suppl. 1), S50–S54; and Goldberg, J. M. (2001). *Nutrition and exercise. RN, 64*(7), 34–39.

periods of excessive physical or emotional stress, illness, infection, or in anyone who decreases or omits insulin doses. One or more of these events lead to hyperglycemia. Hyperglycemia causes **osmotic diuresis** (extracellular volume depletion) resulting in dehydration and sodium loss.

Because the Type 1 diabetic client lacks insulin, the fat stores break down, resulting in continued hyperglycemia and burning of fatty acids with **ketosis.** When more ketones are produced than the cell can use and the kidneys can excrete, *ketoacidosis* develops, causing metabolic acidosis. In addition, the increased buildup of ketones depresses the central nervous system (CNS) leading to coma and death if left untreated (Figure 17-4 ◆). The manifestations of DKA are listed in Box 17-5.

Treatment of Diabetic Ketoacidosis. DKA is the most serious metabolic disturbance of people with Type 1 DM. Hospital admission may be required when the person has a blood glucose of greater than 250 mg/dL and ketones in the urine (**ketonuria**).

DKA is treated with fluids (for dehydration), insulin (to reduce hyperglycemia and acidosis), and correction of electrolyte imbalances. If the client is alert and conscious, fluids may be given orally. Unconscious clients require intravenous fluids. The nurse should be prepared to administer a 0.9% normal saline solution to replace the sodium losses. After 2 to 3 hours, the intravenous (IV) solution is changed to 0.45% normal saline to prevent hypernatremia. When the blood glucose levels reach 250 mg/dL, dextrose is added to prevent hypoglycemia. Potassium may be added to an IV solution if the client's laboratory values show a deficit. Regular insulin is used to treat the client's hyperglycemia. The degree of hyperglycemia and ketosis determines whether insulin is given by the subcutaneous or IV route. Typically, a continuous insulin infusion is started and maintained until the ketoacidosis is resolved.

CLINICAL alert

Only regular insulin may be given by the intravenous route.

HYPERGLYCEMIC HYPEROSMOLAR NONKETOTIC SYNDROME (HHNS). Hyperglycemic hyperosmolar nonketotic syndrome (HHNS) occurs in people with Type 2 DM. It is characterized by severely elevated blood glucose levels, extreme dehydration, and an altered level of consciousness. This condition usually develops slowly over several hours to days. It is a serious, life-threatening medical emergency that has a higher mortality rate than DKA. Infection, surgery, and dialysis are a few factors that can trigger HHNS.

The state of extreme hyperglycemia leads to osmotic diuresis and results in severe dehydration, especially of the brain. The manifestations result from the effects of hyperglycemia and dehydration (see Box 17-5). Ketosis does not occur like it does in DKA, because the Type 2 DM client has sufficient insulin.

Treatment of Hyperglycemic Hyperosmolar Nonketotic Syndrome. Treatment is similar to that of DKA, namely, correcting fluid and electrolyte imbalances and providing insulin to lower hyperglycemia. Intravenous fluids of 0.9% normal saline are given, followed by 0.45% normal saline to correct the fluid and sodium losses. Insulin is administered to reduce the severe hyperglycemia. When blood glucose levels reach 250 mg/dL, the insulin is discontinued because, in contrast to DKA, ketosis is not present.

Whether caring for the client with DKA or HHNS, the nurse is responsible for measuring the client's vital signs, monitoring the level of consciousness, monitoring IV infusions, monitoring fluid status through intake and output, and notifying the physician of the client's response to treatment.

HYPOGLYCEMIA. Hypoglycemia can occur in people with Type 1 DM and people with Type 2 DM who are treated with oral antidiabetic agents. It may be caused by *hyperinsulinism* (too much insulin), overdose of oral antidiabetic agents, too

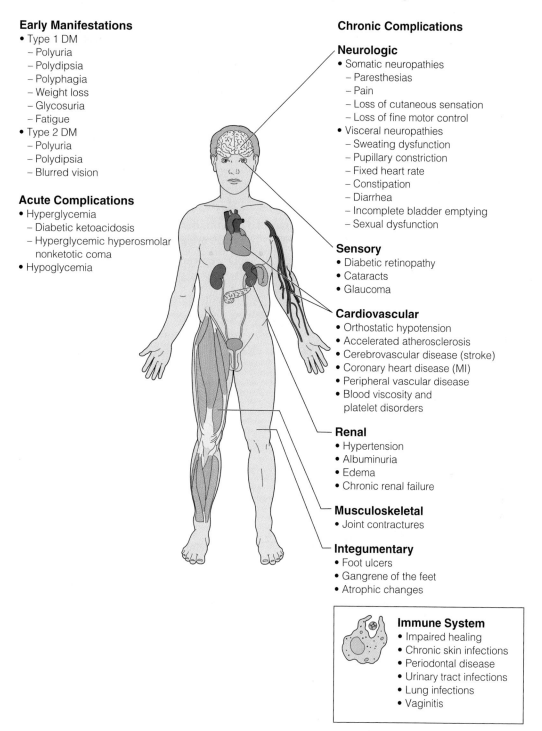

Early Manifestations
- Type 1 DM
  - Polyuria
  - Polydipsia
  - Polyphagia
  - Weight loss
  - Glycosuria
  - Fatigue
- Type 2 DM
  - Polyuria
  - Polydipsia
  - Blurred vision

Acute Complications
- Hyperglycemia
  - Diabetic ketoacidosis
  - Hyperglycemic hyperosmolar nonketotic coma
- Hypoglycemia

Chronic Complications

Neurologic
- Somatic neuropathies
  - Paresthesias
  - Pain
  - Loss of cutaneous sensation
  - Loss of fine motor control
- Visceral neuropathies
  - Sweating dysfunction
  - Pupillary constriction
  - Fixed heart rate
  - Constipation
  - Diarrhea
  - Incomplete bladder emptying
  - Sexual dysfunction

Sensory
- Diabetic retinopathy
- Cataracts
- Glaucoma

Cardiovascular
- Orthostatic hypotension
- Accelerated atherosclerosis
- Cerebrovascular disease (stroke)
- Coronary heart disease (MI)
- Peripheral vascular disease
- Blood viscosity and platelet disorders

Renal
- Hypertension
- Albuminuria
- Edema
- Chronic renal failure

Musculoskeletal
- Joint contractures

Integumentary
- Foot ulcers
- Gangrene of the feet
- Atrophic changes

Immune System
- Impaired healing
- Chronic skin infections
- Periodontal disease
- Urinary tract infections
- Lung infections
- Vaginitis

Figure 17-3. ◆ Multisystem effects of diabetes mellitus.

little food, or excess physical activity. The onset is sudden, and blood glucose is usually less than 50 mg/dL.

The brain requires a constant supply of glucose, so a hypoglycemic episode alters brain function. The manifestations of hypoglycemia (Box 17-6) result from activation of the autonomic nervous system (ANS) and from impaired cerebral function. People who experience frequent hypoglycemic episodes during which the blood glucose level drops below 20 mg/dL may develop decreased cerebral function. Severe untreated hypoglycemia may lead to death.

CLINICAL alert

As the body ages, the autonomic nervous system becomes less responsive. The elderly may not experience the manifestations caused by the autonomic nervous system.

Treatment of Hypoglycemia. Although hypoglycemia may occur at any time, it most often occurs during exercise, 8 to 24 hours after strenuous exercise, and in the middle of the night.

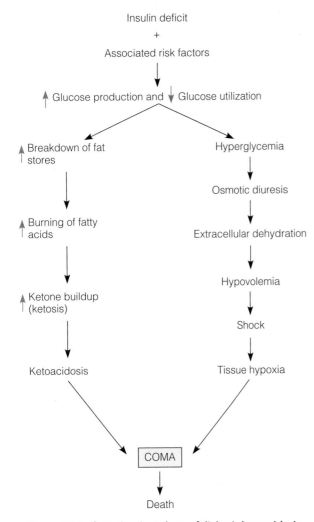

Insulin deficit
+
Associated risk factors

↑ Glucose production and ↓ Glucose utilization

↑ Breakdown of fat stores

Hyperglycemia

↑ Burning of fatty acids

Osmotic diuresis

↑ Ketone buildup (ketosis)

Extracellular dehydration

Ketoacidosis

Hypovolemia

Shock

Tissue hypoxia

COMA

Death

Figure 17-4. ◆ Pathophysiology of diabetic ketoacidosis.

Mild hypoglycemia is usually recognized and self-managed, but severe hypoglycemia requires treatment by health care providers.

MILD HYPOGLYCEMIA. When mild hypoglycemia occurs, immediate treatment is necessary. People experiencing hypoglycemia should take about 15 g of a rapid-acting sugar. Examples of fast-acting glucose are:

- 3 glucose tablets
- ½ cup of fruit juice or regular soda
- 8 oz. of skim milk
- 6 to 8 Life Savers candies
- 2 to 3 tsp of sugar or honey

Sugar should not be added to fruit juice, because it could cause a rapid rise in blood glucose. The resulting hyperglycemia would require additional treatment.

If the manifestations continue, the 15/15 rule should be followed: Wait 15 minutes, then monitor blood glucose; if it is low, eat another 15 g of carbohydrate. This procedure can be repeated until blood glucose levels return to normal. People with diabetes should always carry a rapid-acting carbohydrate

BOX 17-5
MANIFESTATIONS OF DIABETIC KETOACIDOSIS (DKA) AND HYPERGLYCEMIC HYPEROSMOLAR NONKETOTIC SYNDROME (HHNS)

DKA	HHNS
Dehydration (from hyperglycemia)	**Dehydration**
Thirst	Extreme thirst
Warm, dry skin with poor turgor	Warm, dry skin with poor turgor
Dry mucous membranes	Dry mucous membranes
Rapid, weak pulse	Rapid, weak pulse
Hypotension	Hypotension
Soft eyeballs	
Metabolic Acidosis (from Ketosis)	**Neurologic Manifestations**
Nausea and vomiting	Depressed level of consciousness to coma
Lethargy to coma Ketone (fruity, alcohol-like) breath odor	Grand mal seizures
Other Manifestations	**Other Manifestations**
Abdominal pain	Abdominal discomfort may be present
Kussmaul's respirations (rapid, deep respirations; a compensatory response to prevent a further decrease in pH)	Rapid, shallow breathing
Laboratory Findings	
Blood glucose: > 250 mg/dL	> 600 mg/dL
Blood and urine ketones: Positive	Negative
Arterial blood pH: < 7.3	Normal (7.35–7.45)
Serum osmolality: < 340 mOsm/L	> 340 mOsm/L

source. Clients experiencing frequent hypoglycemic episodes should consult their health care provider.

SEVERE HYPOGLYCEMIA. Diabetic clients with severe hypoglycemia are often hospitalized. If the client is conscious and alert, 10 to 15 g of an oral carbohydrate may be given. If the client has a

BOX 17-6
MANIFESTATIONS
OF HYPOGLYCEMIA

CAUSED BY RESPONSES OF THE AUTONOMIC NERVOUS SYSTEM

Hunger	Shakiness
Nausea	Irritability
Anxiety	Rapid pulse
Pale, cool skin	Hypotension
Sweating	

CAUSED BY IMPAIRED CEREBRAL FUNCTION

Strange or unusual feelings	Blurred vision
Headache	Decreasing levels of
Difficulty in thinking	consciousness
Inability to concentrate	Seizures
Change in emotional behavior	Coma
Slurred speech	

LABORATORY FINDINGS

Blood glucose	< 50 mg/dL
Blood and urine ketones	Negative
Plasma pH	Normal
Serum osmolality	Normal

decreased level of consciousness, parenteral glucose or glucagon is given.

Intravenous glucose is administered as a 25% to 50% solution followed by intravenous infusion of 5% dextrose in water (D_5W). Intravenous glucose acts the fastest to raise blood glucose levels. When it is unavailable, glucagon 1 mg may be given by the subcutaneous or intramuscular route to stimulate the release of glycogen. Because glucagon has a short action period, an oral or intravenous carbohydrate should be administered following the glucagon to prevent a recurrence of hypoglycemia. Glucagon should be included in the emergency supplies for diabetic clients. Family members or other support persons should be taught how and when to administer it.

OTHER ALTERATIONS IN BLOOD GLUCOSE LEVELS

Somogyi Phenomenon. Somogyi phenomenon is a morning rise in blood glucose to hyperglycemic levels following an episode of nighttime hypoglycemia. The morning hyperglycemia is thought to be caused by the release of counterregulatory hormones.

Clients with Somogyi phenomenon should be taught to monitor their blood glucose levels and assess for manifestations of nocturnal hypoglycemia: tremors, night sweats, and restlessness. The treatment focuses on increasing the bedtime snack or decreasing the evening dose of intermediate-acting insulin.

Dawn Phenomenon. Dawn phenomenon is a rise in blood glucose between 5 A.M. and 8 A.M. The exact cause is unknown

but may be related to nighttime release of growth hormone. Treatment may include increasing the insulin dose or changing the injection time of the intermediate-acting insulin from dinnertime to bedtime.

Chronic Complications

Chronic complications of diabetes mellitus result from consistently high glucose levels in the body. The longer the client has been diagnosed with diabetes, the greater the chance of developing one or more of these complications. The complications are categorized as macrovascular disease, microvascular disease, and neuropathy.

In a landmark study the Diabetes Control and Complications Trial (DCCT), people who kept their blood glucose levels close to normal reduced their risk for development and progression of complications involving the eyes, the kidneys, and the nervous system. This was accomplished by frequent blood glucose monitoring, several daily insulin injections, exercise, and a healthier diet.

MACROVASCULAR COMPLICATIONS.
The macrocirculation (the large blood vessels) in people with diabetes undergoes changes due to atherosclerosis. Atherosclerosis has an increased incidence and earlier age of onset in people with diabetes. Macrovascular complications include coronary artery disease, stroke, and peripheral vascular disease.

Atherosclerotic coronary artery disease is a major risk factor in the development of myocardial infarction in the Type 2 diabetic. These people also have high cholesterol and triglyceride levels. Coronary artery disease is the most common cause of death in people with Type 2 diabetes. Persons who have a myocardial infarction are more prone to develop congestive heart failure as a complication of the infarction. They are also less likely to survive in the period immediately following the infarction. (Myocardial infarction is fully discussed in Chapter 22.)

Stroke is two to six times more likely to occur in the Type 2 diabetic. Although the exact cause is unknown, hypertension plays a major role in its development. The manifestations of impaired cerebral circulation are often similar to hypoglycemia and warrant immediate medical attention.

Peripheral vascular disease of the lower extremities accompanies both types of diabetes mellitus, but the incidence is greater in Type 2 DM. Diabetes-induced arteriosclerosis of the lower legs is usually bilateral, develops at an earlier age, progresses more rapidly, and develops equally in men and women. Occlusions can form in the large vessels below the knee, causing impaired peripheral circulation. Decreased arterial circulation can lead to lower leg ulcers and **gangrene** (necrosis or tissue death). Gangrene from diabetes is the most common cause of nontraumatic amputations of the lower leg. Manifestations of peripheral vascular disease are summarized in Box 17-7. (Peripheral vascular disease is discussed in Chapter 23.)

MICROVASCULAR COMPLICATIONS.
Microvascular complications involve alterations in the microcirculation (the smaller

> ### BOX 17-7
> ### MANIFESTATIONS OF PERIPHERAL VASCULAR DISEASE
>
> - Loss of hair on lower leg, feet, and toes
> - Atrophic skin changes: Shininess and thinning
> - Cool to cold feet
> - Legs become red when dependent, legs become white when elevated
> - Thick toenails
> - Diminished or absent peripheral pulses
> - Intermittent claudication—pain with walking
> - Pain at rest, usually at night

blood vessels and capillaries). Microvascular disease is sometimes called microangiopathies. Altered microcirculation can affect all body tissues but is seen primarily in the eyes and the kidneys.

Diabetic retinopathy is the collective name for the destructive retinal changes that occur in the person with diabetes. Changes in the retinal capillaries cause decreased blood flow to the retina, leading to retinal ischemia and possible retinal hemorrhage or detachment. Retinopathy has three stages: nonproliferative, preproliferative, and proliferative. Varying degrees of visual impairment can occur at any stage. Retinopathy is the leading cause of blindness in people between ages 25 and 74. In addition, Type 1 and Type 2 diabetics have a greater risk for developing cataracts (opacity of the lens) as a result of increased glucose levels within the lens. Yearly eye exams by an ophthalmologist are recommended for these clients.

Diabetic nephropathy is a disease of the kidneys characterized by the presence of albumin in the urine, hypertension, edema, and progressive renal insufficiency. This disorder is the most common cause of renal failure requiring dialysis or transplantation in the United States. Nephropathy occurs in 20% to 30% of people with diabetes mellitus within 10 to 20 years after diagnosis.

Changes in the glomerular capillaries in the kidney result in glomerulosclerosis (fibrosis of the glomerular tissue). This condition severely impairs the filtering function of the glomerulus so that albumin is lost in the urine.

Microalbuminuria (small amounts of albumin in the urine) may be diagnosed during a 24-hour urine collection. With the presence of microalbuminuria, usually the client progresses to end-stage renal disease or renal failure. (Renal failure is discussed in Chapter 21.) Early in the diagnosis of nephropathy, clients may be treated with angiotensin-converting enzyme (ACE) inhibiting drugs such as captopril (Capoten).

Diabetic Neuropathies. *Peripheral and autonomic neuropathies* are disorders of the peripheral nerves and the autonomic nervous system. Diabetic neuropathies cause one or more of the

following problems: sensory and motor impairment, postural hypotension, delayed gastric emptying, diarrhea, and impaired genitourinary function.

Peripheral neuropathies are bilateral sensory disorders. The manifestations appear first in the toes and feet and then eventually progress upward to involve the fingers and hands. Initial manifestations include **distal paresthesia** (a subjective feeling of numbness or tingling); pain described as aching, burning, or shooting; and feeling of cool to cold feet. People with peripheral neuropathy lose feeling, touch, and position sense, which increases their risk for falling. In addition, they may experience foot injuries due to impaired temperature and pain sensation. There is no specific treatment for peripheral neuropathy. Collaborative management focuses on controlling the neuropathic pain with tricyclic antidepressants or a topical cream called capsaicin (Zostrix).

Autonomic neuropathies occur in numerous organ systems. Some of the individual systems with the related manifestations are:

- Cardiovascular: Fixed, slightly rapid heart rate and postural hypotension
- Gastrointestinal: Delayed gastric emptying, resulting in irregular blood glucose control, constipation, and diarrhea
- Genitourinary: Neurogenic bladder (inability to empty the bladder completely), leading to urinary retention and an increased risk of urinary tract infections; sexual dysfunction in men and women

The Diabetic Foot. People with diabetes mellitus experience more problems with their feet and subsequent amputations because of macrovascular disease, neuropathy, and infection. Often, they experience some type of foot trauma without knowing it. Because they have lost their perception of pain, an injury may go unattended for days or weeks. Common sources of foot trauma are cracks and fissures caused by dry skin or infections such as athlete's foot, blisters from ill-fitting socks and shoes, ingrown toenails, and direct trauma (cuts, bruises, or burns).

Foot lesions usually begin as a superficial injury, then progress into an ulceration (Figure 17-5 ◆). In time, the ulcer extends deeper into muscles and bone and can lead to abscess or osteomyelitis. Infections commonly occur in the traumatized or ulcerated tissue. Dry gangrene is manifested by cold, dry, shriveled, and black tissues of the toes and feet. If untreated, the whole foot eventually becomes gangrenous and requires amputation. Treatment consists of bed rest, antibiotics, and debridement. Additional foot care guidelines are discussed later in the chapter under Discharge Considerations.

Increased Susceptibility to Infection. The person with diabetes has an increased risk of developing frequent bacterial and fungal infections. Normally, glucose is used efficiently throughout the body, but in people with diabetes, glucose accumulates in the epidermal layer of the skin. Moisture tends

Figure 17-5. ◆ Ulceration following trauma to the foot of a person with diabetes.

to collect under the armpits, breasts, groin, or genitalia. The higher-than-normal concentration of glucose in the skin coupled with the moisture creates a perfect breeding area for microorganisms. When the skin appears beefy red to violet red, an infection should be suspected. Fungal infections can develop under the nails, giving them a thick, yellow, crumbly appearance. Treatment focuses on prevention of infection.

SPECIAL CONCERNS

Sick-Day Management. When the person with diabetes is sick, blood glucose levels increase, even though food intake decreases. The person mistakenly alters or omits the insulin dose or oral hypoglycemic agent, causing further problems. Dietary guidelines during illness focus on preventing dehydration and providing nutrition for promoting recovery. The nurse teaches the following sick-day management:

- Monitor blood glucose every 4 hours throughout the illness.
- Test urine for ketones if the blood glucose level is greater than 250 mg/dL.
- Continue to take the usual insulin dose or oral hypoglycemic agent.
- Drink 8 to 12 oz. of fluid each waking hour.
- Eat 10 to 15 g of carbohydrate every 1 to 2 hours such as:
  - ½ cup regular Jello
  - 1 whole popsicle
  - ½ cup regular soft drink
  - ½ cup pure fruit juice
  - ½ cup applesauce
  - 1 cup Gatorade
- Call the physician if you are unable to eat for more than 24 hours or if vomiting and diarrhea last for more than 6 hours.

Surgery Management. Surgery is a stressor that releases excess counterregulatory hormones, causing hyperglycemia and insulin resistance. Protein stores are decreased. In addition, diet and activity patterns change, and medication types and dosages vary. As a result, surgical clients with diabetes are at a

greater risk for postoperative infection, delayed wound healing, fluid and electrolyte imbalances, hypoglycemia, and DKA.

For clients with Type 2 DM, oral hypoglycemia agents are usually withheld 1 to 2 days before surgery, and clients are given regular insulin. Clients with Type 1 DM follow a carefully prescribed insulin regimen to meet their specific needs.

The surgical procedure should be scheduled for early in the morning to decrease the fasting time. If there is no food intake after surgery, intravenous dextrose should be given, accompanied by subcutaneous regular insulin every 6 hours. The dose should be adjusted to blood glucose levels. Although intake is decreased postoperatively, stress can increase insulin requirements. Glucose control is also affected postoperatively by nausea and vomiting, anorexia, and gastrointestinal suction.

During the postoperative period, the client with Type 2 DM may continue to require insulin or may resume oral medications, depending on glucose levels. The client with Type 1 DM may require reduced insulin as healing progresses and stress-induced hyperglycemia diminishes. Regular blood glucose monitoring is essential, as are assessments for hypoglycemia.

Sometimes postsurgical clients require enteral tube feedings or total parenteral nutrition to meet their dietary needs. Both nutritional supplements contain glucose. Diabetic clients receiving these supplements must be monitored closely for hyperglycemia. Often, they need additional insulin to prevent acute hyperglycemia complications.

Pancreas Transplantation. Surgical management of persons with Type 1 diabetes involves replacing or transplanting the pancreas. Pancreas transplantation may be accompanied by kidney transplant when end-stage renal disease exists. Before clients can be considered transplant candidates, they must participate in a physical and emotional evaluation as well as meet the hospital's transplant criteria.

NURSING CARE

Nursing care differs for the person with newly diagnosed diabetes, the person with long-term diabetes, and the person with acute complications. Clients with DM require lifelong collaborative care. Nursing care focuses on maintaining and promoting health status related to nutrition, skin care, and prevention of complications. A primary focus is teaching the client self-management strategies.

ASSESSING

Assessment data collected by the nurse can determine the extent to which DM is affecting the client's life, identify risk factors for complications, and suggest guidelines for medical treatment or self-care (Box 17-8).

BOX 17-8
ASSESSING FOR DIABETES MELLITUS

SUBJECTIVE DATA

- Present health status:
  - Presence of hyperglycemia manifestations: Polyuria, polydipsia, polyphagia
  - Weight loss or gain; changes in appetite
  - Changes in vision
  - Muscle weakness and fatigue
  - Fainting spells or dizziness
  - Presence of numbness and/or tingling or burning in feet
  - Presence of slow healing wounds
  - Pain or burning with urination
  - Problems of vulvular itching in females
- Family history for Type 1 or Type 2 diabetes mellitus
- Use of insulin or oral hypoglycemic medications
- Any recent surgery

OBJECTIVE DATA

- Vital signs (blood pressure—standing and lying, pulse, respirations, temperature)
- Weight and height
- Assess for DKA, HHNS, and/or hypoglycemia.
- Assess visual acuity.
- Assess sensations of touch and position, pain, and temperature.
- Observe mental status for signs of confusion or disorientation; slurred speech.
- Observe gait patterns, use of assistive devices for walking, and abnormal wear patterns on shoes.
- Test range of motion and strength.
- Inspect oral cavity for bad breath, bleeding, red gums, and tooth pain.
- Inspect skin for dryness or excessive perspiration; presence of hair on lower extremities.
- Inspect the skin for lesions, fissures between toes, corns, calluses, plantar warts, ingrown or overgrown toenails, redness over pressure points, blisters, cellulitis, or gangrene.
- Palpate skin turgor and temperature.
- Palpate peripheral pulses for decrease or absence.
- Palpate lower extremity for capillary refill, color and temperature of skin, lesions, and edema.
- Auscultate bowel sounds.

DIAGNOSING, PLANNING, AND IMPLEMENTING

IMBALANCED NUTRITION

- Monitor blood glucose levels regularly and report values below 60 mg/dL or above 200 mg/dL. *Clients with diabetes are at risk for hypoglycemia or hyperglycemia.*

- Encourage client to eat all of the prescribed diet. *Anorexia, gastric fullness, and abdominal pain can reduce oral intake. To prevent hypoglycemia, the client must consume the amount of food included in the diet plan.*
- Monitor percentage of meals and snacks that client eats. *Monitoring of nutritional intake helps to determine the need for a dietary consult.*
- Identify food preferences, including ethnic/cultural needs. *Clients are more likely to eat food they like and that meets their ethnic/cultural requirements.*
- Provide meals and snacks on time. *Glucose and insulin control is more effective when meals are eaten on time.*
- Give insulin and/or oral hypoglycemic agents as ordered. *To prevent hyperglycemia, insulin and/or oral hypoglycemic agents must be given on time. Altered times might be necessary when food is delayed or diagnostic procedures are being done.*

IMPAIRED SKIN INTEGRITY

- Perform meticulous foot care. Wash feet daily with lukewarm water and mild hand soap; pat dry, especially between the toes. Apply a thin film of lubricating lotion except between the toes. *Proper hygiene decreases the chance of infection. Check water temperature with a bath thermometer to prevent burns.*
- Use alternating pressure mattresses, elbow and heel protectors, and foot cradle as ordered. *These devices reduce pressure on the skin to prevent skin breakdown.*
- Encourage fluid intake of at least 2,500 mL/day unless cardiac complications exist. *Adequate fluid intake prevents dry skin and the risk for skin breakdown. However, clients with cardiac disease may develop fluid overload with an excess intake.*
- Discuss the importance of not smoking. *Nicotine in tobacco causes vasoconstriction and decreases blood supply to the feet.*
- If skin breakdown occurs, notify the physician immediately. *Immediate intervention is needed to prevent the development of deep wounds and infection.*
- Rotate insulin injection sites. *Site rotation prevents lipodystrophy.*
- Conduct foot care teaching sessions as often as necessary (Box 17-9). *Foot care is a priority in diabetes management to prevent serious problems.*

RISK FOR INFECTION

- Assess for manifestations of infection: fever; chills; tachycardia; abnormal breath sounds; vaginal discharge; cloudy, foul-smelling urine; or redness, pain, swelling, or discharge at injury site. *The types of infections seen in clients with diabetes mellitus include urinary tract and nail infections, osteomyelitis, vaginal yeast infections, chronic gingivitis, and pyorrhea. Early diagnosis and treatment of infections can control their severity and decrease possible complications.*

BOX 17-9
SAMPLE FOOT CARE TEACHING SESSION

BUYING AND WEARING SHOES AND STOCKINGS

- Shoes that allow ½ to ¾ inch of toe room are best; there should be room for toes to spread out and wiggle. The lining and inside stitching should be smooth, and the insole soft. The sole should be flexible and cushion the foot. The heel should fit snugly, and the arch support should give good support.
- Do not wear open-toed shoes, sandals, high heels, or thongs; they increase the risk of trauma.
- Buy shoes late in the afternoon, when feet are at their largest; always buy shoes that feel comfortable and do not need to be "broken in."
- Shoes made of natural materials (leather, canvas) allow perspiration to escape.
- Check the shoes before each wearing for foreign objects, wrinkled insoles, and cracks that might cause lesions.
- Stockings made of wool or cotton allow perspiration to dry.
- Do not wear garters, knee stockings, or panty hose; they may interfere with circulation.
- Wear insulated boots in the winter.
- Avoid constrictive clothing as it reduces peripheral circulation.

INSPECTING THE FEET

- Check the feet daily for red areas, cuts, blisters, corns, calluses, or cracks in the skin. Check between the toes for cracks or reddened areas.
- Check the skin of the feet for dry or damp areas.
- Use a mirror to check each sole and the back of each heel.
- If you are unable to inspect the feet daily, be sure that someone else does so.

CARE OF TOENAILS

- Cut the toenails after washing, when they are softer and easier to trim.
- Cut the nails straight across with a clipper, and smooth edges and corners with an emery board.
- Do not use razor blades to trim the toenails.
- If you are unable to see well or to reach the feet easily, have someone else trim the nails. If the nails are very thick or ingrown, if the toes overlap, or if circulation is poor, get professional care.

GENERAL INFORMATION

- Never go barefoot. Wear slippers when leaving the bed during the night.
- Do not use commercial corn medicines or pads, chemicals (such as boric acid, iodine, or hydrogen peroxide), or over-the-counter cortisone medications on the feet.
- Do not put heating pads, hot water bottles, or ice packs on the feet. If the feet become cold at night, wear socks or use extra blankets.
- Do not allow the feet to become sunburned.
- Do not put tape on the feet.
- Do not sit with the legs crossed at the knees or ankles.

- Obtain specimens and send for culture and sensitivity test as ordered. *Before antibiotic therapy is begun, specimens must be sent for culture and sensitivity to identify the causative organism and appropriate antibiotic.*
- Use and teach meticulous handwashing. *Handwashing is the best method for preventing the spread of infection.*
- Keep the skin clean and dry, using mild soap and lukewarm water. *Clean, intact mucous membranes are the first line of defense against infection.*
- Provide catheter and perineal care. Teach female client to wipe from front to back after elimination. *Clients with diabetes are prone to developing urinary tract infections.*
- Maintain meticulous sterile technique when performing wound care or any invasive procedure. *These measures prevent infection in existing wounds or introduction of bacteria into the body.*
- Turn client and encourage coughing, deep breathing, and activity as tolerated. *Sedentary clients are prone to developing atelectasis and/or pneumonia.*
- Encourage adequate nutrition and fluid intake. *Maintaining satisfactory food and fluid intake reduces susceptibility to infection.*

- Assist client with oral hygiene. Brush teeth with a soft toothbrush and fluoridated toothpaste at least twice a day and floss. *Proper oral hygiene reduces the risk of periodontal disease.*
- Teach female diabetics the symptoms and preventive measures of vaginitis caused by *Candida albicans*:
  - Symptoms are an odorless, white or yellow, cheeselike vaginal discharge and itching.
  - Preventive measures include not douching, wiping from front to back after voiding, wearing cotton underwear, and avoiding tight jeans and nylon pantyhose.
  - Sexual transmission is unlikely, but discomfort may cause the client to avoid sexual activity. *Diabetes is a predisposing factor for* Candida albicans *vaginitis. Poor personal hygiene and use of clothing that keeps the vaginal area warm and moist increase the risk of vaginitis.*

RISK FOR INJURY

- Reduce environmental hazards in the health care facility.
  - Orient the client to new surroundings on admission.

- Keep the bed at the lowest position; raise side rails at night if needed.
- Keep the floors free of objects and wipe up spills immediately.
- Use a night-light.
- Teach the client to wear shoes or slippers when getting out of bed.
- Monitor for side effects of prescribed medications, such as dizziness or drowsiness. *Strange environments increase the risk of falls.*
- Teach about safety in the home and community.
  - Use a night-light, preferably one with a soft, nonglare bulb. (*Note:* Red light is better, because the eyes adjust more quickly.)
  - Turn the head away when switching on a bright light.
  - Avoid looking directly into headlights when driving at night.
  - Conduct a daily foot inspection.
  - Wear shoes and slippers with nonskid soles.
  - Do not use throw rugs.
  - Provide handgrips in the tub and shower and next to the toilet.
  - *Environmental hazards increase the risk of falls or other accidents. Glare is often responsible for falls when visual deficits exist.*
- Assist the client with tasks requiring finger and hand dexterity. *Clients with neuropathies may lose their ability to grip handles of cups or sharp objects.*
- Assist client during ambulation; provide ambulatory aids as needed. Do not rush the client. *These interventions decrease the potential for falls.*
- Advise client to get out of bed slowly. *Autonomic neuropathy can cause postural hypotension. When a client rises too quickly, there is a risk for dizziness and falls.*
- Monitor for DKA in the client with Type 1 DM and for HHNS in the client with Type 2 DM. Teach the client and family to recognize and seek care for the manifestations of DKA or HHNS. *DKA and HHNS can be life threatening. Immediate medical treatment is required.*
- Monitor for hypoglycemia in clients with either Type 1 or Type 2 DM. Teach the client and family to recognize and seek care for manifestations. *The person should carry some form of a rapid-acting sugar source at all times.*
- Recommend that clients wear a Medic-Alert bracelet or necklace identifying themselves as having diabetes. *In case of sudden illness or accident, a Medic-Alert tag alerts health professionals about the client's diagnosis so that appropriate medical attention can be begun.*

INEFFECTIVE COPING

- Assess the client's perception of the current situation. *This establishes how the client feels about his or her diagnosis.*
- Assess the client's emotional resources and support sources. *Chronic illness affects all dimensions of a person's life as well as those lives of family members.*

- Provide an atmosphere of trust and support. *A positive emotional environment helps clients feel comfortable about discussing their concerns.*
- Explore with client and family the effects of the diagnosis and treatment on finances, occupation, energy levels, and relationships. *Failure to cope successfully can lead to noncompliance and poor blood glucose control. Common frustrations associated with diabetes are the disease itself, the treatment modalities, and the health care system.*
- Provide information about support groups and community resources. *Support groups offer opportunities for mutual support and problem solving. Community resources may help the client and family with other methods for coping with diabetes.*

EVALUATING

To evaluate the effectiveness of care for a client with DM, collect data related to the presence of chronic complications such as frequent infections, unhealed wounds, decreased vision, altered kidney function, peripheral neuropathy, and hypertension. In addition, identify the frequency that the client has experienced DKA or HHNS, and hypoglycemia.

Discharge Considerations

Teaching the client and family involves all aspects of diabetes management. The nurse's role is to reinforce teaching completed by other health care providers such as registered nurses, certified diabetes educators, or dietitians. Because diabetes mellitus is a chronic disease, clients must be able to self-manage their disease at home. Box 17-10 lists assessment data to consider when planning for discharge.

During hospitalization, teaching should begin on admission. Before the actual teaching session starts, the nurse assesses the client's and the family's knowledge and learning needs, educational level, preferred learning methods and style, life experiences, and support systems. In addition, the nurse determines past diabetes management practices and identifies physical, emotional, and sociocultural needs.

It is important that the nurse and client establish mutual goals based on the assessment data. Responsibility for daily management lies with the client. Family members must understand that their primary role is support. However, they must know how to provide physical care for the client if necessary.

If the client is newly diagnosed, the teaching first focuses on basic skills, then progresses to lifelong management strategies. Clients with a long-standing history of DM should not be overlooked. Often, they need a review of basic management strategies.

A variety of teaching methods may be used, including demonstration, return demonstration, audiovisual aids, pamphlets, and written lists. The method selected is based on how

BOX 17-10
ASSESSING FOR DISCHARGE

DIABETES MELLITUS
Client

- Self-care: Ability to perform activities of daily living (ADLs) independently; perform glucose monitoring; self-administer insulin or oral antidiabetic; perform foot care
- Knowledge: Recommended diet, exercise, skin, dental, and foot care; insulin or oral antidiabetic agents and their side effects; early manifestations of hypoglycemia and hyperglycemia; monitoring blood glucose; safety precautions; sick-day management; indications for seeking medical care
- Home environment: Appropriate heating and cooling; access to clean water for drinking and handwashing; cooking and refrigeration facilities; safety precautions

Family

- Members of household: Willingness to provide support to client
- Caregivers: Availability and knowledge to provide care as needed; assist with ADLs, shopping, and transportation; knowledge and willingness to assist in maintaining diabetic diet
- Financial resources: Income; resources for drugs, equipment (self-monitoring glucose machine, syringes), and medical care required; affect on employment

Community

- Diabetes education classes
- Access to health care resources

the client learns best. In addition to teaching how a procedure is done, the nurse must be sure to include the reasons why a method or step is used. Below are some general guidelines for the nurse on teaching clients with diabetes mellitus:

- Listen to the client's concerns and priorities. Anxiety about keeping one's job may be more important than knowing how to administer an insulin injection.
- Listen to questions and provide information about common myths regarding diabetes.
- Present information in small segments.
- Speak in simple terms. Explain medical terms so that the client understands their meaning.
- Be specific about what the client needs to know.
- Teach in a well-lighted area that is free from distraction.
- Be nonjudgmental.
- Use positive reinforcement.
- Repeat and reinforce information as many times as necessary.
- Validate the person's knowledge and skills.

- Adapt teaching to the special needs of the older adult. Considerations for teaching the older person with diabetes include the following:
  - Diet changes may be difficult to implement. Favorite foods are hard to give up. Balanced meals at regular times may not have been part of the client's lifestyle. Purchasing, storing, and preparing foods may be a problem. Dentures may not fit well. Changes in taste sensation may cause the client to use more salt and sugar. A decreased thirst mechanism must lead to dehydration.
  - Exercise of any type may not have been part of the activities of daily living. Exercise must be individualized to accommodate physical limitations caused by arthritis, Parkinson's disease, chronic respiratory diseases, and/or cardiovascular diseases.
  - A chronic illness diagnosis threatens independence and self-worth. After years of taking care of themselves, older adults who have to depend on others may withdraw from social situations. Distance from family or death of a spouse may cause depression.
  - Money to purchase medications and supplies or visit health care providers must be taken out of a fixed income.
  - Visual and fine motor skill deficits can make insulin administration, blood glucose monitoring, food preparation, exercises, and foot care difficult or impossible.

Box 17-11 summarizes the knowledge and skills needed for self-management of DM.

Multiple resources are available to provide information on all aspects of self-management. Most hospitals or outpatient settings offer diabetes educational programs and support groups. Blood glucose screenings are often provided at little or no cost as part of community health promotion activities. Restaurants and airlines provide diabetic meals on request. Encourage clients to explore resources in their own communities.

Nursing Process Case Study
■ CLIENT WITH TYPE I DM

James Meligrito, 24 years old, is a first-year nursing student at a local community college. He attends school full time and works 20 hours a week as a campus student security guard. He works from 8 P.M. to 12 midnight, 5 nights a week. Mr. Meligrito dislikes cooking and usually eats "whatever is handy." He was diagnosed with Type 1 diabetes mellitus when he was 12. Currently, he takes a total of 32 units of insulin each day, 10 units of NPH, and 6 units of regular insulin each morning and evening. He monitors his blood glucose about three times a week. He feels that he is too busy for a regular exercise program and that he gets enough exercise in clinicals and in weekend sports activities. He has not seen a health care provider for over a year.

BOX 17-11
TEACHING FOR DISCHARGE

CLIENT SELF-MANAGEMENT OF DIABETES

The nurse reinforces teaching and skills for clients with DM. The content of a teaching plan includes the following points:

- Information about normal glucose metabolism and how diabetes changes metabolism
- Dietary plan: How diet helps keep blood glucose in normal range; number of kcal required and why; why they should eat complex carbohydrates and foods high in fiber but limit the intake of sugar, fat, sodium, and alcohol; concerns regarding meal preparation; how to read food labels for sugar, fat, and protein; integrating personal food preferences; eating meals away from home; relationships between diet, exercise, and medication. Fluid intake should be encouraged, because the thirst mechanism may be impaired.
- Exercise: How it helps lower blood glucose; the importance of regular exercise program; types of exercise; and integrating personal exercise choices
- Glucose levels: Self-monitoring of blood glucose; how to perform the tests accurately; how to care for equipment; what to do for high or low blood glucose.
- Medications:
  - Insulin type, dosage, mixing instructions (if necessary); times of onset and peak actions; how to get and care

for equipment; how to give injections; where to give injections; timing of insulin injections and mealtimes
- Oral agents: Type, dosage, side effects, interaction with other drugs
- Complications:
  - Factors that cause diabetic ketoacidosis or HHNS; manifestations of each; what to do when they occur.
  - Factors that cause hypoglycemia; manifestations; what to do when they occur
- Safety precautions: Identify family to contact in an emergency; carrying ID card and tag; carrying rapid-acting glucose; carrying insulin and glucagon kit
- Hygiene: Skin, dental, foot care
- Vision: Yearly exam, sources for vision aids such as magnifying sleeve for insulin syringe or large-print instructions
- Sick days: What to do about food, fluids, and medications
- Communication and follow-up:
  - What signs and symptoms to report; whom to contact; when to report
  - Importance of keeping follow-up appointments
  - Resources such as American Diabetes Association, diabetic education classes, diabetic support groups, weight loss programs, and publications like *Diabetes Forecast;* whom to contact for answers to questions

---

One day during a 6-hour clinical, Mr. Meligrito notices that he is urinating frequently, is thirsty, and has blurred vision. He is very tired but blames all his symptoms on working too much and studying for school. He forgot to take his morning insulin and realizes he must have hyperglycemia but decides that he will be all right until he gets home in the afternoon. Around noon, he complains of abdominal pain, weakness, and a rapid pulse. When he reports his physical symptoms to his clinical instructor, she takes him immediately to the hospital emergency room.

Assessment In the ER his blood glucose level is 300 mg/dL. Urine shows the presence of ketones. His electrolytes are normal, with a pH of 7.1. Vital signs are: T 99° F (37.2° C); P 140; R 28; BP 102/52. An IV of 1,000 mL 0.9% normal saline with 40 mEq KCl is started at a rate of 400 mL/h. He receives 10 units of regular insulin IV. Three hours later, his blood glucose level is 160, with normal vital signs. He is sent home with an appointment the next morning with the hospital's diabetes clinical specialist, Carole Traci.

Diagnosis The following nursing diagnoses are identified for Mr. Meligrito:

- Powerlessness related to a perceived lack of control of diabetes due to demands on his time
- Deficient Knowledge regarding self-management of diabetes
- Ineffective Therapeutic Regimen Management related to difficulty in modifying his personal habits.

Expected Outcomes The expected outcomes for the plan of care are that Mr. Meligrito will:

- Identify those aspects of diabetes that can be controlled and participate in making decisions about self-managing care.
- Demonstrate an understanding of diabetes self-management through planned medication, diet, exercise, and blood glucose self-monitoring activities.
- Verbalize ways to modify his personal habits.

Planning and Implementation Ms. Traci plans and implements the following nursing interventions for Mr. Meligrito during the diabetes education program:

- Develop short-term and long-term goals for Mr. Meligrito's self-management of control of blood glucose.
- Discuss Mr. Meligrito's personal habits and ways to modify them.

- Provide positive reinforcement for increasing his involvement in self-care activities.
- Review insulin administration, dietary management, exercise, self-monitoring of blood glucose, and healthy lifestyle.

Evaluation After participating in weekly diabetes classes for 2 months, Mr. Meligrito has increased his understanding of and compliance with managing his diabetes. He states that he finally understands how insulin, food, and exercise affect his body, having previously thought they were "just things I should do when I wanted to." Mr. Meligrito developed a workable meal schedule and weekly grocery list. Mr. Meligrito and a friend have arranged to walk 2 to 3 miles three times a week on a community hiking trail. To gain a sense of control over his illness, Mr. Meligrito has also worked out a schedule that allows time for school, health care, and himself.

Critical Thinking in the Nursing Process

1. What factors caused Mr. Meligrito's diabetic ketoacidosis?
2. Explain why this client received an intravenous infusion of 0.9% NS and intravenous insulin?

3. Consider that you are teaching Mr. Meligrito and another client, Mr. McDaniel (age 75, newly diagnosed with Type 2 DM). What components of your teaching plan would be the same and what components would be different?

Nursing Interventions Classification

The following nursing interventions (McCloskey & Bulechek, 2000) may be appropriate for the client with diabetes mellitus:

- Foot Care
- Medication Management
- Pressure Ulcer Care
- Pressure Ulcer Management
- Skin Care: Topical Treatments

(*Note:* The bibliography listings for this and all chapters have been compiled at the end of the book.)

Chapter Review

key terms by topic

Use the CD-ROM disk enclosed with your textbook to hear the pronunciation of the key terms in the chapter.

Clients with DM
diabetes mellitus

The pancreas
hyperglycemia, hypoglycemia, gluconeogenesis, glycogenolysis

Diabetes mellitus
ketosis, glycosuria, osmotic diuretic, polyuria, polydipsia, polyphagia, ketonuria

Complications
diabetic ketoacidosis (DKA), osmotic diuresis, ketosis, ketonuria, hyperglycemic

hyperosmolar nonketotic syndrome (HHNS), Somogyi phenomenon, dawn phenomenon, gangrene, diabetic retinopathy, diabetic nephropathy, microalbuminuria, diabetic neuropathies, distal paresthesia

key points

- Diabetes mellitus (DM) is a metabolic disorder of the pancreas that results from insulin deficiency.

- The classic manifestations of Type 1 diabetes include polydipsia, polyuria, polyphagia, weight loss, and fatigue. Type 2 diabetes is characterized by polyuria, polydipsia, obesity, recurrent infections, and fatigue.

- Diabetes is diagnosed by fasting blood glucose, glycosylated hemoglobin, and oral glucose tolerance test.

- Type 1 diabetes is managed with insulin, diet, and exercise. Type 2 diabetes may be managed with oral antidiabetic drugs, diet, and exercise.

- Diabetic ketoacidosis (DKA) can occur in Type 1 DM while hyperglycemia hyperosmolar nonketotic syndrome develops in Type 2 DM; both of which are life-threatening complications.

- DKA is treated with a combination of intravenous fluid and electrolyte solutions, and insulin.

- Clients who develop hypoglycemia must be treated immediately with 15 g of a rapid-acting sugar to prevent prolonged neurologic damage.

- Clients with long-term diabetes have a greater incidence of chronic complications especially affecting vision, the kidneys, renal and nerve function, and lower extremities.

- Nursing management focuses on maintaining normal blood glucose levels, preventing acute and chronic complications, maintaining skin integrity, teaching self-management, and increasing coping skills.

Medialink

Additional interactive resources for this chapter can be found on the Companion Website at www.prenhall.com/burke. Click on Chapter 17 and "Begin" to select the activities for this chapter.

For NCLEX review questions and an audio glossary, access the accompanying CD-ROM in this book.

for further study

For the Food Guide Pyramid, see Figure 18-4.

For more information about exercise-stress electrocardiograms, and discussion of myocardial infarctions, see Chapter 22.

For more about peripheral vascular disease, see Chapter 23.

For more information on renal failure, see Chapter 21.

For more brief review of adult developmental stages, see Chapter 2.

Critical Thinking Care Map

Caring for a Client with Diabetes Mellitus
NCLEX-PN Focus Area: Health Promotion and Maintenance

Case Study: Mrs. Yontz, age 64, has Type 2 diabetes mellitus and is visiting her physician for a 6-month checkup. As she walks to the exam, the nurse notices that she walks with a slight limp. She is helped to remove her shoes, and the nurse notices several red spots over the top of the toes on her right foot and a blister on her left heel. Mrs. Yontz tells you that she does not know how this happened. "I never saw these red spots on my toes or the blister on my heel." She also says that she bought a new pair of shoes last week and has been wearing them every day.

Nursing Diagnosis: Impaired Skin Integrity

COLLECT DATA

Subjective

Objective

Would you report this data? Yes/No

If yes, to: _____

Nursing Care

How would you document this? _____

**Data Collected
(use those that apply)**

- Weight 160 lbs.
- Red spots on top of the toes on her right foot
- Fasting blood glucose 160 mg/dL
- Blister on the left heel
- Does not complain of any discomfort in her feet
- Says she uses a hot water bottle on her feet at night
- Complains of tingling in both feet

**Nursing Interventions
(use those that apply)**

- Discuss changes in her diet.
- Cleanse feet with normal saline.
- Discuss the importance of not smoking.
- Apply lubricating lotion to her feet and between the toes.
- Teach her to wear new shoes for a short period of time each day.
- Instruct client in proper foot care.
- Teach her to monitor red areas for signs of skin breakdown.

NCLEX-PN Exam Preparation

1. A client is instructed to check his blood glucose qid and administer insulin according to a sliding scale. The nurse will teach him to use which type of insulin?
   a. Humulin N
   b. Humulin R
   c. Lente
   d. Humulin 70/30

2. A client with diabetes mellitus experiences hypoglycemia during the night followed by episodes of hyperglycemia when the blood glucose is assessed in the morning. The nurse recognizes these symptoms as:
   a. dawn phenomenon
   b. diabetic ketoacidosis
   c. Somogyi phenomenon
   d. hyperglycemic hyperosmolor nonketotic syndrome

3. A female client with a history of diabetes mellitus visits her physician because of flulike symptoms. Which of the following indicates a need for further teaching when she discusses her sick-day care:
   a. "I will check my blood glucose every 4 hours."
   b. "I will hold my daily insulin dose until I stop vomiting."
   c. "I will check my urine ketones if my blood glucose is above 250 mg/dL."
   d. "I will consume 10 to 15 grams of carbohydrates every 1 to 2 hours."

4. A client with diabetes mellitus asks if he must stop smoking because diabetes mellitus increases his risk of lung disease. The nurse's response is based on the knowledge that:
   a. diabetics are at greater risk for lung cancer
   b. diabetics are at greater risk for emphysema
   c. nicotine in tobacco causes arterial vasodilatation
   d. nicotine in tobacco leads to arterial vasoconstriction

5. A 16-year-old girl is diagnosed with diabetes mellitus. Which of her following statements indicates a need for further instruction?
   a. "I will be able to stop my insulin and take pills for my diabetes when my blood sugar is stable."
   b. "I will rotate my insulin injection sites."
   c. My blood glucose should be maintained between 70 and 110 mg/dL."
   d. "I will complete foot care and inspect them daily."

6. A client with diabetes received Humulin N 40 units at 7:30 A.M. The MOST LIKELY time the nurse would expect him to experience hypoglycemia is:
   a. 8:00 A.M.
   b. 9:30 A.M.
   c. 11:00 A.M.
   d. 12:30 P.M.

7. The nurse instructs a client to mix Humulin N and Humulin R insulin. Which of the following, during the return demonstration, indicates that the client understands the procedure?
   a. She shakes both vials prior to mixing.
   b. She injects air into the Humulin R vial first.
   c. She withdraws the Humulin R first.
   d. She withdraws the Humulin N first.

8. A client is admitted to the nursing unit with a diagnosis of diabetic ketoacidosis. Which of the following assessment findings would the nurse expect?
   a. cool, clammy skin
   b. blood glucose above 250 mg/dL, large urine ketones
   c. arterial blood pH of 7.45
   d. radial pulse 70, bounding

9. A client's blood glucose is 450 mg/dL on admission. The physician prescribes 20 units of insulin intravenously. The nurse expects to administer which type of insulin?
   a. Humulin N
   b. Humulin 70/30
   c. Humulin R
   d. Humalog

10. The nurse instructs a diabetic client on foot care. Appropriate instruction would include:
    a. open toe shoes are acceptable if they are soft leather
    b. have a family member check heating pads or hot water bottles before applying
    c. apply lotion or oil generously between the toes
    d. cut the toenails straight across with a clipper, and use an emery board to smooth edges

chapter 18

Caring for Clients with Nutritional and Upper GI Disorders

CARING tip

"Always put yourself in the patient's place. How would you want to be cared for if you were that patient?"

Verna R. Myers, RN MSN • Clinical Instructor • HMI Regency School • Washington, DC

LEARNING outcomes

After completing this chapter, you will be able to:

- Describe the structure and function of the upper gastrointestinal (GI) tract.
- Identify sources of various nutrients, including vitamins.
- Collect assessment data related to digestion and nutritional status.
- Describe the causes, pathophysiology, and manifestations of common nutritional and upper GI disorders.
- Discuss the nursing implications of diagnostic tests and treatment for clients with nutritional and upper GI disorders.
- Use the nursing process to provide nursing care for clients with nutritional and upper GI disorders.

MediaLink

 www.prenhall.com/burke

Use the above address to access the free, interactive Companion Website created for this textbook. Get hints, instant feedback, and textbook references to chapter-related multiple choice questions. Link to other interesting sites.

Nutrition is the process of ingesting, absorbing, using, and eliminating food in the body. The digestive organs involved in these processes are the gastrointestinal (GI) tract and the accessory digestive organs. The GI tract includes the mouth, pharynx, esophagus, stomach, small intestine, and large intestine (Figure 18-1 ◆). The accessory digestive organs (see Chapter 19) include the liver, gallbladder, and pancreas. The large intestine is primarily an organ of elimination. (See Chapter 20 for its structure and function.) Clients with problems affecting nutrition, eating, or digestion require holistic nursing care that addresses nutritional needs, education, and psychosocial factors.

Structure and Function of the Upper Gastrointestinal Tract

The gastrointestinal (GI) tract is a continuous hollow tube. Once foods are ingested, they are broken down into products that can be absorbed as they move through the GI tract.

MOUTH, PHARYNX, AND ESOPHAGUS

The *mouth,* the upper opening of the GI tract, is lined by mucous membranes. In the mouth, the teeth chew and grind food into smaller parts. *Saliva* (produced by the salivary glands) moistens food for tasting, chewing, and swallowing. The digestive process starts in the mouth as enzymes in saliva (*amylase* and *lysozyme*) begin to break down food. The tongue mixes food with saliva, forms the food into a mass (*bolus*), and initiates swallowing. Muscles in the pharynx move food to the esophagus. The esophagus carries food to the stomach through

peristalsis (alternating waves of contraction and relaxation). The esophagus enters the stomach through the *cardiac* or *lower esophageal sphincter.* This sphincter, normally closed except during swallowing, keeps food in the stomach.

STOMACH

The *stomach,* connected to the esophagus at the upper end and to the small intestine at the lower end, can expand to hold up to 4 L of food and fluid (Figure 18-2 ◆). The stomach continues the digestive process. Mechanical digestion in the stomach mixes partially digested food with gastric juices to produce **chyme.** Four to five liters of gastric juices are produced by specialized cells in the stomach lining every day:

- *Parietal cells* secrete hydrochloric acid and intrinsic factor. Hydrochloric acid is vital to protein digestion; intrinsic factor is necessary for vitamin B_{12} absorption.
- *Chief cells* produce pepsin, the primary enzyme in gastric juice, which digests protein.
- *Mucous cells* produce alkaline mucus that protects the lining of the stomach from gastric juices.
- *Enteroendocrine cells* secrete hormones that help regulate digestion.

The nervous system also controls gastric secretion. Seeing, smelling, or tasting food stimulates the parasympathetic nervous system to send signals via the vagus nerve that increase gastric secretion. Emotions such as anxiety or stress, on the other hand, inhibit gastric secretion and motility.

The *pyloric sphincter* controls emptying of the stomach into the duodenum. The stomach empties completely within 4 to 6 hours after a meal.

SMALL INTESTINE

The small intestine is about 20 ft. (6 m) long but only about 1 in. (2.5 cm) in diameter. It hangs in coils in the abdomen, suspended by folds of peritoneal membrane and surrounded by

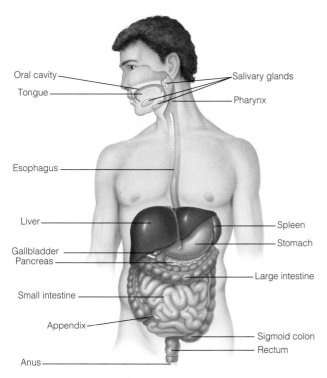

Figure 18-1. ◆ Organs of the gastrointestinal tract and accessory digestive organs.

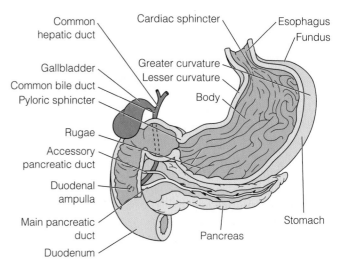

Figure 18-2. ◆ Structures of the stomach and duodenum, including the common bile duct, pancreatic duct, pancreas, and gallbladder.

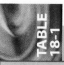

TABLE 18-1 NUTRIENTS, FOOD SOURCES, AND FUNCTION

NUTRIENT	COMMON FOOD SOURCES	FUNCTION	EFFECT OF EXCESS OR DEFICIT
Carbohydrates ■ Composed of simple or complex sugars ■ *Recommended intake: 125–175 g/day*	Simple sugars: Milk, sugar cane, sugar beets, honey, fruits Complex starches: Grains, legumes, root vegetables	Converted to glucose, used by cells to make ATP Excess glucose converted to glycogen or fat for storage	Excess: Obesity, dental caries, elevated serum triglycerides Deficit: Tissue wasting (protein breakdown), metabolic acidosis (fat breakdown)
Proteins ■ Composed of amino acids ■ *Recommended intake: 0.8 g/kg body weight*	Complete proteins (contain all the essential amino acids): Eggs, milk, milk products, and meat, fish, and poultry Plant (or *complementary*) proteins: Legumes, nuts, grains, cereals, and vegetables	Vital for body structure and function *Nitrogen balance* maintained by intake equal to that needed for protein synthesis, preventing breakdown of body proteins	Excess: Obesity Deficit: Weight loss, tissue wasting, thin, sparse hair, edema, anemia
Fats (Lipids) ■ Composed of triglycerides, phospholipids, sterols ■ *Recommended intake: 30% or less of total daily caloric intake; saturated fat, 10% or less of total daily caloric intake*	Saturated fats: Animal fats, cocoa butter, palm and coconut oils; hydrogenated (solid) vegetable fats (stick margarine, vegetable shortening) Unsaturated fats: Liquid vegetable oils, soft margarines	Triglycerides: Fuel supply, insulation; essential fatty acids help form cell membranes and hormones; carry fat-soluble vitamins A, D, E, and K Phospholipids: Cell membranes Sterols: Bile, sex hormones, adrenal hormones, vitamin D, and cholesterol	Excess: Obesity, increased risk of heart disease Deficit: Weight loss; skin lesions
Vitamins ■ Organic, essential nutrients; includes fat soluble A, D, E, K; water-soluble B complex, C, niacin, biotin, folic acid ■ *Recommended intake: Varies by specific vitamin*	Found in a variety of foods, including fruits, vegetables, grains, and animal products	Specific functions that promote growth, reproduction, maintenance of health	Selected effects of deficits: Nails: Iron—soft, spoon-shaped Hair: Zinc—dry, dull, sparce Skin: Vitamins A, B—flaky, dry; niacin—cracks; vitamin K—easy bruising; vitamin C—delayed healing Eyes: Vitamin A—poor night vision; iron—pale conjunctiva
Minerals ■ Inorganic elements; includes sodium, potassium, calcium, magnesium, chloride, phosphorus ■ *Recommended intake: Varies by mineral*	Found in a variety of foods, including fruits, vegetables, grains, and animal products	Specific regulatory functions (see Chapter 5)	Nervous system: Thiamine—↓ deep tendon reflexes, peripheral neuropathies, confusion, apathy Musculoskeletal: Thiamine—calf pain; vitamin C—joint pain GI: Vitamin B complex—*cheilosis,* stomatitis, glossitis

(continues)

TABLE 18-1	NUTRIENTS, FOOD SOURCES, AND FUNCTION (CONTINUED)		
NUTRIENT	**COMMON FOOD SOURCES**	**FUNCTION**	**EFFECT OF EXCESS OR DEFICIT**
Water ■ *Recommended intake:* 1,500 to 2,000 mL/ day as fluid	Water Other liquids such as fruit juices, milk, coffee, tea, soft drinks Foods such as gelatin	Body structure and form Transport and exchange medium Medium for metabolic reactions within cells Insulation and temperature regulation Lubricant	Deficit: Thirst, weakness, weight loss, ↓ BP, orthostatic hypotension, ↑ heart rate, poor skin turgor Excess: ↑ BP, ↑ heart and respiratory rates, shortness of breath, weight gain, edema

the large intestine. The small intestine has three regions: the duodenum, the jejunum, and the ileum. The *duodenum* begins at the pyloric sphincter and extends for about 10 in. (25 cm). Pancreatic enzymes and bile from the liver enter the small intestine at the duodenum (see Figure 18-2). The *jejunum,* the middle region, is about 8 ft. (2.4 m) long. It connects with the *ileum,* the distal 12 ft. (3.6 m) of small bowel, which meets the large intestine at the ileocecal valve.

Food is chemically digested, and most of it is absorbed, as it moves through the small intestine. Enzymes in the small intestine break down carbohydrates, proteins, and fats. Buffers produced by the pancreas neutralize the acid from the stomach. *Microvilli* (tiny cell projections), *villi* (fingerlike projections of the mucosa), and deep folds of the mucosal layers increase the surface area of the small intestine to enhance absorption of food. Almost all food products and water, as well as vitamins and minerals, are absorbed through the intestinal mucosa into the blood or lymph. Only indigestible fibers, some water, and bacteria enter the large intestine.

METABOLISM

After nutrients are ingested, digested, absorbed, and transported to the cells, they are metabolized to produce energy. **Metabolism** is the term for biochemical reactions that occur in the cells. Metabolism involves two basic processes. *Catabolism* breaks down complex structures into simpler forms, like carbohydrates into adenosine triphosphate (ATP)—the fuel for cell processes. *Anabolism* combines simpler molecules to build more complex structures (e.g., amino acids into proteins). Water and carbon dioxide are waste products of metabolism. The energy produced by foods is measured as *kilocalories (kcal).*

NUTRIENTS

Nutrients are substances in foods that are used by the body for growth, maintenance, and repair. They include carbohydrates, proteins, fats, vitamins, minerals, and water (Table 18-1 ◆).

Nutritional Disorders

Nutritional disorders are major causes of illness and disability. The major nutritional disorders in the world today are obesity and undernutrition (malnutrition). Developmental, sociocultural, psychological, and physiologic factors contribute to these disorders. Regardless of their cause, nutritional disorders affect many body functions and often lead to serious health problems.

Obesity

Obesity is body weight more than 20% above the ideal for gender and height. *Morbid obesity* is body weight of more than

100% over ideal weight. *Overweight* is more than the ideal weight but less than 20% over the ideal. Obesity occurs when excess calories are stored as fat. It is one of the most prevalent, preventable health problems in the United States. Obesity is associated with an increased risk for many serious problems and diseases (Box 18-1) and an increased mortality rate.

PATHOPHYSIOLOGY

Body weight is regulated by a complex set of factors. Overeating and physical inactivity do contribute to obesity, but they are not the entire cause of the problem.

BOX 18-1
PROBLEMS ASSOCIATED WITH OBESITY

- Cancers of the breast, uterus, prostate, and colon
- Cholecystitis and cholelithiasis
- Coronary heart disease
- Heart failure
- Hiatal hernia
- Hypertension
- Muscle strains and sprains
- Osteoarthritis
- Peripheral vascular disease
- Postoperative complications
- Stress incontinence

Appetite is regulated by the central nervous system and by emotional factors. Appetite may have little relationship to hunger: People sometimes eat to relieve depression or anxiety. Several *hormones* are involved in regulating obesity, including thyroid hormone, insulin, and leptin (a peptide produced by fatty tissue that suppresses appetite and increases energy expenditure). Some studies suggest that leptin resistance is a cause of obesity. There is a strong link between *heredity* and obesity. A person with one obese parent has a 40% chance of becoming obese; one with two obese parents has an 80% chance. *Physical inactivity* is probably the most important factor contributing to obesity. Inactive people may consume fewer calories than active people and continue to gain weight due to lack of energy expenditure. *Fat intake* also contributes to obesity: People who eat more fat have a higher body fat content than people who consume less fat and more complex carbohydrates and fiber. *Environmental and sociocultural influences*—such as an abundant and readily accessible food supply, rewarding behavior with food, and spending significant amounts of time watching television—play a role in the prevalence of obesity in the United States.

COLLABORATIVE CARE
Because obesity is caused by many factors, its treatment is complex. Most experts recommend an individualized program combining exercise, diet, and behavior modification to meet the client's specific needs.

Diagnostic Tests
- *Standard height–weight tables* (Table 18-2 ◆) may be used to determine a person's ideal weight.
- The *body mass index (BMI)* can be calculated using the following formula: BMI = weight in kg/height in m². A BMI of 19 to 24 is considered healthy for adults.
- *Fat-fold measures* (Figure 18-3 ◆) provide an estimate of total body fat and its distribution.
- *Waist circumference* is used to evaluate abdominal fat. Abdominal obesity is associated with a higher risk of heart

TABLE 18-2   HEALTHY WEIGHTS FOR ADULTS

HEIGHT	WEIGHT RANGE IN POUNDS[a]
4'10"	91—119
4'11"	94—124
5'0"	97—128
5'1"	101—132
5'2"	104—137
5'3"	107—141
5'4"	111—146
5'5"	114—150
5'6"	118—155
5'7"	121—160
5'8"	125—164
5'9"	129—169
5'10"	132—174
5'11"	136—179
6'0"	140—184
6'1"	144—189
6'2"	148—195
6'3"	152—200
6'4"	156—205
6'5"	160—211
6'6"	164—216

Note: The higher weights in the ranges generally apply to men; the lower weights more often apply to women.
[a] Without shoes or clothing.

Figure 18-3. ◆ With calipers, measure the thickness of a fold of skin on the back of the arm or below the shoulder blade.

disease, brain attack (stroke), diabetes, high blood pressure, and some types of cancer.

Other diagnostic tests may be done, such as a *thyroid profile* (see Chapter 16), *serum glucose* and *cholesterol,* and *lipid profile.* An *electrocardiogram (ECG)* may be ordered to evaluate effects of obesity on the heart.

Diet and Exercise

Treatment of obesity focuses on changing both eating and exercise habits. A pound of body fat is equivalent to 3,500 kcal. To lose 1 pound, therefore, a person must increase activity to burn these calories or reduce daily caloric intake by 250 kcal for 14 days.

Exercise is critical to weight loss and maintenance. After consulting their health care providers, clients should engage in aerobic exercise for 30 minutes a day, 3 to 5 days a week. This will reduce *adipose* (fatty) tissue, increase lean body mass (which burns more calories), and promote weight loss and long-term weight control.

The diet should be low in kilocalories and fat and contain adequate nutrients, minerals, and fiber. The Food Guide Pyramid is a valuable guide (Figure 18-4 ◆) to proper nutrition. Regular meals with small servings are recommended. Weight loss should be gradual, no more than 1 to 2 pounds per week. This usually means a diet of 1,000 to 1,500 kcal per day. Fewer than 1,200 kcal each day may lead to nutritional deficiencies and loss of lean tissue.

Behavior modification is a critical part of successful weight management. Keeping food records and identifying cues that create a desire to eat can help the dieter gain self-control. Weight loss and weight maintenance are separate but related issues. Most dieters regain lost weight within 2 years. Long-term weight management requires a lifelong commitment to changing food and eating habits, activity and exercise routines, and lifestyle. Box 18-2 outlines strategies for weight management.

Social support and group programs (Weight Watchers, Overeaters Anonymous, and Take Off Pounds Sensibly) provide weight-loss strategies and peer support. Most programs charge a fee; this may also encourage compliance.

Pharmacology

Drugs may be helpful for people with morbid obesity. However, tolerance, addiction, and side effects may occur. Appetite suppressants such as sibutramine (Meridia) may be prescribed for limited periods of time (no more than 3 months). Sibutramine also may increase the metabolic rate, promoting weight loss. Orlistat (Xenical) has a different mechanism of action: It reduces the absorption of fat from the GI tract, leading to weight loss. It has the added benefit of lowering blood glucose and cholesterol. These products must be used in combination with diet and exercise to be successful.

Surgery

Surgery to treat obesity generally is reserved for morbidly obese individuals. *Lipectomy* (removal of adipose tissue) and *liposuction* (suctioning of adipose tissue from under the skin) remove fat deposits. However, fat can be regenerated in affected areas after these procedures. *Gastric bypass* and *gastroplasty* reduce GI capacity, prompting the client to eat and absorb less food. Side effects of these procedures include persistent nausea and vomiting, vitamin deficiencies, and gastrointestinal scarring.

NURSING CARE

ASSESSING

Ask about eating habits, and have the client describe food intake for a typical day. Identify activity and exercise patterns

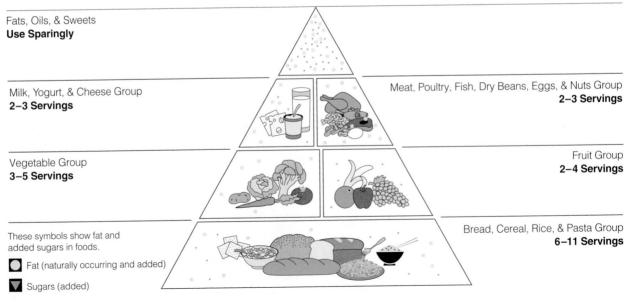

Figure 18-4. ◆ The Food Guide Pyramid.

BOX 18-2
TEACHING FOR DISCHARGE

BEHAVIOR STRATEGIES FOR WEIGHT LOSS

Control the Environment

- Purchase low-calorie foods, shopping from a prepared list and on a full stomach.
- Keep all foods in the kitchen or pantry. Store them in opaque containers out of sight.
- Prepare exact portions of food to eliminate leftovers.
- Eat all foods in the same place, avoiding the kitchen.
- Do not eat while watching television or reading.
- Reduce frequency of eating out at restaurants, parties, and picnics.

Control Physical Responses to Food

- Eat a salad or drink a hot beverage before a meal.
- Eat slowly; take small bites and chew each thoroughly. Allow 20 minutes for a meal.
- Put eating utensils or food down between bites.
- Concentrate on the eating process; savor the food.
- Stop eating with the first feelings of fullness.

Control Psychosocial Responses to Food

- Make eating a pleasant experience, using attractive dinnerware and a formal setting.
- Use small plates and cups to make servings of food look larger.
- Concentrate on conversations and socialization during the meal.
- Use nonfood rewards for meeting a goal.
- Acknowledge small successes and improvements in all behavior.
- Substitute other pleasurable activities for eating (e.g., reading, exercise, hobbies).

- Establish realistic weight-loss goals. *Success is more likely with small, reasonable goals (losing 1 to 2 pounds per week) and a longer-term goal of losing 10% of current body weight.*
- Assess knowledge and provide teaching about well-balanced diet plans. *Knowledge empowers the client to make appropriate diet choices.*
- Help develop an exercise plan that fits into the client's lifestyle and includes enjoyable activities. Encourage 30 minutes of sustained activity daily. *A realistic, enjoyable exercise plan promotes participation and self-esteem.*
- Explore ability and willingness to make changes in daily patterns of diet, exercise, and lifestyle. *This provides assessment data for setting realistic goals with the client.*
- Help identify behavior-modification strategies and support systems to promote weight loss and maintenance. *Lifestyle patterns that motivate the client to continue exercising and eating sensibly promote success. Family and social support are critical to sticking with the plan.*
- Refer the client to a dietitian, nutritional counselor, or weight-loss support program. *Professionals and support groups provide additional resources to help achieve and maintain weight loss.*
- Help plan strategies to deal with "stress" eating or relapses to previous eating patterns. *Overeating or not exercising can cause a sense of failure and lead to further overeating. Identifying strategies ahead of time helps the client accept and deal with relapses.*

CHRONIC LOW SELF-ESTEEM

Obese clients often experience "fat prejudice" in their family, workplace, or community. These experiences, coupled with the difficulty of finding attractive clothing or a chair large enough to sit on, can affect the client's self-esteem. Hospitalized obese clients may be subject to frequent comments about their physical condition.

- Set small goals with the client and offer positive feedback and encouragement. *Small goals provide more opportunities for success. Positive feedback and encouragement help develop self-esteem.*
- Explore the possibility of psychological counseling with the client. *Many clients benefit from counseling for issues related to self-esteem.*

EVALUATING

To evaluate the effectiveness of nursing care, monitor weight, looking for a slow, progressive weight loss. Ask about eating and exercise patterns. Assess knowledge and willingness to consume a nutritionally sound diet. Discuss the client's sense of success and self-image.

for a typical weekday and weekend. Ask about prior weight-loss efforts and discuss whether the client is satisfied with current weight and appearance. Inquire about recent changes in appetite or weight. Ask about any medical problems such as cardiovascular disease and diabetes. Assess height and weight, and compare actual weight to ideal body weight (see Table 18-2). Using a caliper, obtain fat-fold measurements (see Figure 18-3). Measure waist circumference at the level of the umbilicus.

DIAGNOSING, PLANNING, AND IMPLEMENTING

IMBALANCED NUTRITION: MORE THAN BODY REQUIREMENTS

- Encourage identification of factors that contribute to excess food intake. *Identifying cues to eating helps the client eliminate or reduce these cues.*

Discharge Considerations

The client is ultimately responsible for managing and maintaining weight loss. Teaching and planning must therefore be individualized. Tailor teaching and weight-loss strategies to address co-existing health problems. (For example, teach the overweight client with diabetes about a diabetic, calorie-restricted diet. Develop an individualized exercise program for the overweight client with heart disease.) Provide information about community or hospital-based programs and resources. Discuss strategies for incorporating exercise into the client's daily schedule.

Undernutrition

Undernutrition occurs when calorie or nutrient intake is not enough to meet the needs for growth, development, or function. Undernutrition can lead to **malnutrition,** a condition in which long-term deficiencies of nutrients or calories cause health problems. Undernutrition affects all body systems and increases the risk of disease and death. Undernutrition is common in hospitalized clients, often leading to poor wound healing and lower resistance to infection.

Other groups at risk for undernutrition include the young, poor, elderly, homeless, low-income women, and ethnic minorities. Clients may be undernourished because of poor food choices. Disorders like *anorexia nervosa* (an eating disorder marked by a disturbed body image and fear of gaining weight) and *bulimia* (episodic binge eating and self-induced vomiting) are a serious concern, especially among teenagers and young adults. Fad diets may also result in nutritional deficiencies. Gastrointestinal problems such as nausea or vomiting, altered digestion, or impaired absorption can lead to undernutrition, as can other illnesses (Box 18-3).

PATHOPHYSIOLOGY

Inadequate protein and calorie intake can lead to *protein–calorie malnutrition (PCM)*. Glucose and glycogen stores, the energy sources in the body, are depleted within 12 to 24 hours of no food intake. When adequate calories are not available to meet energy needs, the body then turns to its proteins (in muscle and organs) and fats (in subcutaneous tissue). Protein synthesis is impaired, delaying wound healing. Serum albumin levels fall, leading to edema. Immune function is impaired, increasing the risk of infection. The cardiovascular and GI systems also are impaired by malnutrition.

CLINICAL alert

Approximately half of all hospitalized adults are malnourished or at risk for PCM. Carefully assess your client's food and fluid intake, and alert the charge nurse or physician when poor appetite, nausea, or NPO status interfere with intake.

Manifestations of undernutrition vary, depending on the nutrient deficit (see Table 18-1; see also Table 8-5, Signs of Nutritional Status). Weight loss and loss of subcutaneous fat are evident. Clients may have a wasted appearance, dry and

BOX 18-3
CONDITIONS ASSOCIATED WITH UNDERNUTRITION

- Aging
- AIDS
- Alcoholism
- Burns, trauma
- Cancer
- Chronic diseases (COPD, renal disease)
- Eating disorders (anorexia, bulimia)
- Gastrointestinal disorders, short bowel syndrome
- Neurologic disorders
- Surgery

brittle hair, pale mucous membranes, peripheral edema, and a sore, smooth tongue.

COLLABORATIVE CARE

Laboratory studies can provide additional assessment data to evaluate the effects of undernutrition on the client. Clients with PCM have low *serum albumin* levels. On complete blood count (CBC), the *lymphocyte count, hemoglobin,* and *hematocrit* often are decreased due to iron deficiencies. *Serum electrolyte levels* also may be altered.

The goal of treatment is to restore the undernourished client to ideal body weight and replace necessary nutrients and minerals. In severe undernutrition, food and fluids are reintroduced gradually. Oral feedings and supplements to replace fluid and nutrients are preferred. Small, around-the-clock feedings are generally tolerated best. Energy- and protein-rich foods or commercially available nutritional supplements (Carnation Instant Breakfast, Ensure, etc.) may be ordered. Intravenous solutions may be used to replace fluids and electrolytes. Vitamin replacements are ordered based on specific needs.

Enteral Feedings

Enteral or *tube feedings* may be used to meet all or part of the nutritional needs in clients who are unable eat. Tube feedings are usually administered through a soft, small-caliber nasogastric or nasoduodenal tube with a weighted tip. Procedure 18-1 outlines the procedure for inserting a nasogastric tube. Enteral feedings also can be administered through a gastrostomy or jejunostomy tube, discussed under Stomach Cancer later in the chapter.

A number of tube-feeding formulas are commercially available. All are nutritionally complete. Some formulas have added fiber to reduce the incidence of diarrhea, a common side effect of enteral feedings. Others have specific formulations for clients with chronic diseases such as chronic obstructive pulmonary disease (COPD) or kidney disease. Formulas may be diluted to half strength for the first day of therapy. If tolerated, they are given at three-fourths strength on the sec-

PROCEDURE 18-1   Inserting a Nasogastric Tube

- Gather all supplies.
- Provide for privacy.
- Explain the procedure, using nonthreatening terms. Inserting the tube may be uncomfortable, but once the tube is in place, little or no discomfort should be felt. Emphasize the need to follow instructions to swallow during tube insertion.
- Follow standard precautions; wear clean gloves.
- Place client in Fowler's or high-Fowler's position with a towel or disposable pad on the chest.
- Occluding one nares at a time, ask the client to breathe. Use the nares with the better airflow for insertion.
- Measure the tube: Hold the tip of the tube at the client's nose, extend the tube to the tip of the earlobe and then to the tip of the sternum (see photo). If the tube is to be placed in the duodenum, add 8 to 10 inches (20 to 25 cm) to the measurement. Mark the tube.

Measuring the appropriate length for nasogastric tube insertion.

- Provide a glass of water with a straw if allowed.
- For a small-bore tube, insert the guidewire or stylet into the tube.
- Using water-soluble lubricant, lubricate 3 to 4 inches of the tube tip.
- Gently insert the tube into the selected nares, directing it along the floor of the nares toward the ear. Use a smooth, continuous motion. Have the client tip the head forward, chin to chest, and ask the client to sip and swallow on command. Advance the tube 3 to 4 inches (7 to 10 cm) with each swallow until the point marked on the tube is at the opening of the nares.
- Pause briefly if the client gags (do not withdraw the tube); have the client take a few breaths through the mouth, then resume advancing the tube. If gagging continues, check the mouth. If the tube is curled in the mouth, withdraw it until the tip is in the oropharynx before resuming.
- If the client coughs and is unable to speak, withdraw the tube until the tip is in the oropharynx. Have the client tip the head further forward and swallow to prevent this from occurring.
- Verify that the tube is correctly placed. Withdraw a small amount of fluid from the tube and check the pH of the fluid. If the pH is 5 or lower, the tube is very likely in the stomach. If the pH is 6 or higher, confirm tube placement with an X-ray.
- Secure the tube with tape.
- Initiate feeding or gastric suction as ordered.
- Reposition the client and provide mouth and nose care as indicated.

■ SAMPLE DOCUMENTATION

> 1030:   8 Fr. Dobbhoff gastric feeding tube inserted via R nares. Small amount green drainage obtained, pH 4. Tolerated procedure well.
> ─────────────── S. Williams, LPN.

ond day and at full strength thereafter. Fluid and electrolyte status is monitored carefully, and additional water is given to meet the client's specific needs. The volume of feedings is gradually increased, with a maximum feeding of 240 to 360 mL every 2 to 4 hours, or 2 L for a 24-hour period, based on the client's caloric needs. Formulas may be administered as a bolus feeding, by continuous drip, or on a cyclic schedule (Procedure 18-2). To prevent aspiration, elevate the head of the bed at least 30 degrees during feeding and for at least 1 hour after feeding.

PROCEDURE 18-2 Enteral Feedings

- Obtain ordered formula and all supplies. Use standard precautions.
- Elevate the head of the bed to at least 30 degrees during and for at least 1 hour after the feeding.
- Provide mouth care.
- Explain the procedure.
- Check residual stomach contents prior to intermittent feedings or every 4 hours if continuous. Reinstill the aspirated formula.
- Withhold the feeding and notify the charge nurse or physician if more than 100 mL (gastrostomy tube) or 200 mL (nasogastric tube) residual is obtained.
- Fill the feeding bag with the ordered amount of formula and water. Clear the tubing of air and/or attach it to a feeding pump.

- Attach the tubing to the feeding or gastrostomy tube. Set the flow rate by drip or on the pump and begin feeding.

■ SAMPLE DOCUMENTATION

1000:	340 mL Sustacal with 100 mL water administered via gastric feeding tube. 75 mL residual obtained prior to feeding; reinstilled. Tolerated well with no evidence of aspiration.
	_____ S. Williams, LPN.

Parenteral Nutrition

Total parenteral nutrition (*TPN* or *hyperalimentation*) is the intravenous administration of a solution that meets all the client's nutritional needs (except for fiber). TPN is used for both short- and long-term management of nutritional deficiencies when the client is unable to eat or use enteral feedings. Clients who have undergone major surgery or trauma, or who are seriously undernourished, are often candidates for TPN. Many clients are discharged to home with TPN and are monitored by home health nurses.

TPN formulas have high concentrations of dextrose, protein (amino acids), electrolytes, vitamins, minerals, and fat emulsions. They are usually administered through a central vein, such as the subclavian vein. To initiate therapy, the physician usually inserts a triple-lumen catheter that permits medications and other intravenous solutions to be given at the same time. Nursing responsibilities related to TPN are outlined in Box 18-4.

NURSING CARE

ASSESSING

Ask about eating habits and typical food intake for a day. Ask about recent weight changes and factors contributing to weight change. Assess for other factors such as anorexia, nausea, medications, or inability to buy and prepare food for meals. Ask about medical problems such as chronic lung or heart disease, thyroid problems, or kidney disease. Look at psychosocial factors affecting nutrition, such as body image, loneliness, depression, and economic status. Determine food preferences. Assess height, weight, and fat-fold measurements (see the section on obesity earlier in the chapter). Wearing gloves, evaluate the mouth, looking for inflammation, gum disease, dental caries, or poorly fitting dentures. Assess ability to swallow liquids, semisolid, and solid foods.

BOX 18-4
NURSING CARE CHECKLIST

PARENTERAL NUTRITION

☑ Use aseptic technique at all times. Do not add any medication to the solution or administer medications or other IV solutions through the catheter lumen into which TPN is being administered.

☑ Use an infusion pump to ensure the correct rate of infusion.

☑ Keep accurate intake and output records for clients receiving TPN.

☑ Check blood glucose by finger stick and administer insulin as ordered.

☑ Monitor and record vital signs, including temperature, reporting any changes to the charge nurse or physician.

☑ Carefully assess respiratory status. Report changes to the charge nurse or physician.

☑ Monitor for signs of infection such as fever, malaise, or redness, swelling, or drainage at the catheter insertion site. Report these signs if noted.

DIAGNOSING, PLANNING, AND IMPLEMENTING

IMBALANCED NUTRITION: LESS THAN BODY REQUIREMENTS

- Monitor and record weight. Note the amount and type of foods eaten at meals and snacks. *This data is important to evaluate the effectiveness of nutritional therapy.*
- Consult with the dietitian, client, family, and caregivers to plan a nutritionally complete diet. *The best diet plan will not achieve its objective if the client cannot or will not eat it or if the caregivers will not prepare it.*
- Provide mouth care before and after meals, eliminate foul odors, and offer frequent, small meals including foods the client prefers. *Oral hygiene and a pleasant environment make food more appetizing. Small meals are generally more appealing and less overwhelming to a client with anorexia.*
- Provide a rest period before and after meals. *Eating requires energy, and the undernourished client may have decreased physical strength.*

RISK FOR INFECTION

- Monitor and record temperature; report any elevation to the charge nurse or physician. Note and report chills, malaise, confusion, local inflammation, or elevated WBC. *Early detection of infection may prevent complications.*
- Maintain standard precautions and sterile technique for procedures as indicated. *Handwashing is the best strategy to prevent the spread of infection. Sterile technique is required for procedures such as changing dressings.*

RISK FOR DEFICIENT FLUID VOLUME

The client with undernutrition is at risk for fluid volume deficit due to inadequate fluid intake, concentrated enteral feeding solutions, or hypertonic parenteral nutrition.

- Monitor oral mucous membranes, skin turgor, urine output and specific gravity, level of consciousness, and laboratory results (see Fluid Volume Deficit in Chapter 5). *Dry mucous membranes, poor skin turgor, decreased urine output, and increased specific gravity may indicate dehydration. Dehydrated clients may have a decreased level of consciousness. Laboratory studies such as serum osmolality, electrolytes, and hematocrit also provide data about fluid balance.*
- Weigh daily at the same time, on the same scale, and with the same clothing. Monitor intake and output. Document carefully. *Daily weights and intake and output records help monitor fluid balance.*
- If fluids are allowed, offer them often in small amounts, considering the client's preferences. *Small amounts are tolerated best; frequent drinking promotes adequate intake.*

RISK FOR IMPAIRED SKIN INTEGRITY

- Frequently assess the skin, noting areas of redness, abrasions, or other lesions. Record and report any abnormal findings or changes from previous assessments to the charge nurse or physician. *Skin integrity depends on adequate nutrition. Early identification of pressure areas or lesions allows intervention to prevent further breakdown or complications.*
- Turn and reposition every 2 hours. Encourage passive and active range-of-motion exercises. *Pressure areas are at high risk for decreased circulation and breakdown. These measures reduce pressure and promote oxygenation of cells.*
- Keep skin dry and clean, and minimize shearing forces. Keep linens smooth, clean, and dry. Provide therapeutic beds, mattresses, or pads. *These measures promote comfort and reduce the risk of skin breakdown.*

BOX 18-5
ASSESSING FOR DISCHARGE

UNDERNUTRITION
Client

- Self-care: Ability to perform ADLs independently; obtain, prepare, and eat prescribed diet or manage enteral or parenteral feedings
- Knowledge: General nutrition; recommended diet or feeding regimen; importance of monitoring weight and intake; indications for seeking medical care
- Psychosocial: Self-concept and body image; support network or significant others; willingness to follow dietary plan for weight gain
- Home environment: Facilities for food storage and preparation; access to clean water for drinking and handwashing; atmosphere conducive to eating

Family and Caregivers

- Members of household: Responsibilities for obtaining and preparing food; other members with nutritional deficits or special diets
- Caregivers: Availability, willingness, and knowledge to provide nutritional care and support as needed, assist with shopping, transportation, and management of enteral or parenteral feedings
- Financial resources: Income; resources for food, nutritional support, and medical care

Community

- Access to health care resources such as home health agencies or home IV therapy services; access to grocery stores or home-delivered groceries
- Availability of communal meals or home-delivered meals
- Financial support options such as Women, Infants, and Children (WIC) programs

EVALUATING

Collect the following data to evaluate the effectiveness of nursing interventions for the client with undernutrition: consuming prescribed diet; evidence of weight gain; stable intake and output; laboratory values improving; remains free of infection or skin breakdown.

Discharge Considerations

Diet therapy (including enteral or parenteral nutrition) often is continued in the home setting. Box 18-5 lists assessment data to collect when planning for discharge. Box 18-6 describes strategies for older adults with undernutrition.

Teach the client and care providers about the importance of handwashing and proper food and supplement storage. If enteral or parenteral nutrition will continue at home, instruct the client, family, and caregivers how to: (a) prepare and handle enteral or parenteral solutions; (b) add solutions to either the feeding tube or central line; (c) manage infusion pumps; (d) care for the feeding tube or central catheter; and (e) recognize and manage problems and complications. Teach the client how and when to notify the home health agency or health care provider of problems. Document all teaching and the learners' understanding of what has been taught. Assess compliance with the treatment plan on a continuing basis, especially when psychosocial factors contribute to undernutrition.

population FOCUS

Promoting Nutrition in the Older Adult

Changes that occur with aging can affect nutrition and the enjoyment of food in the older adult. The ability to taste salty and sweet flavors declines, and the sense of smell is reduced. Less saliva is produced, making it more difficult to swallow. Increased problems with teeth and gums or ill-fitting dentures affect eating. The lower esophageal sphincter relaxes, increasing the incidence of gastroesophageal reflux and heartburn. Less gastric acid is produced, impairing absorption of some nutrients. Peristalsis and digestion slow, often causing the older adult to feel full after eating small amounts. Medications taken for chronic diseases can lead to anorexia. Functional limitations may impair the ability to shop and cook. Psychosocial issues such as a fixed income, depression, social isolation, and loneliness contribute to the risk of nutritional problems. Older adults who eat alone often do not eat as well as those who share meals with companions.

To promote nutrition in older adults:

- Suggest congregate meals (usually offered through senior centers) and programs such as Meals-on-Wheels (for people who are homebound and physically unable to prepare meals).
- Discuss a well-balanced diet that includes whole grains, fresh fruit, and vegetables.
- Advise clients to avoid processed foods and foods high in fat, to drink adequate fluids, and to exercise regularly.
- Assist clients to shop wisely to get the most value for their money.

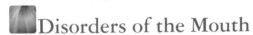

Upper GI Disorders

Disorders of the Mouth

Inflammations of the mouth and oral cancer affect the ability to eat and nutrition. Although oral problems affect many adults, they often are unrecognized and untreated.

STOMATITIS

Stomatitis, inflammation of the oral mucosa, is a common problem that affects eating. Clients with stomatitis may experience pain, difficulty eating, and body image disturbances. Stomatitis frequently develops secondarily to conditions such as cancer, dental disease, and acquired immune deficiency syndrome (AIDS).

Stomatitis may be caused by viral infection (herpes simplex) or fungal infection (*Candida albicans*). Clients on prolonged antibiotic therapy are at risk for candidiasis (thrush). Other causes include mechanical trauma (e.g., cheek biting) and irritants such as tobacco. Chemotherapy or radiation therapy also can cause stomatitis. *Aphthous ulcers* (canker sores) are a type of stomatitis. These ulcers are usually less than 1 cm in diameter and can last weeks to months.

The manifestations of stomatitis vary, depending on the cause. Herpes lesions are clustered and painful, usually occurring on the lips and oral mucosa. Candidiasis (thrush) causes painful white patches with a red base. Other manifestations of stomatitis include red and swollen oral mucosa, pain, and possible ulcerations.

Treatment is directed at both the cause and the symptoms of stomatitis. Lesions may be cultured or scrapings examined to determine the cause of stomatitis. Table 18-3 ◆ lists nursing implications and client teaching for selected drugs used to treat stomatitis.

Suspect stomatitis in a client who refuses to eat or who complains about mouth pain. Wearing gloves, inspect the mouth and oropharynx. Document any visible lesions, as well as the general condition of mucous membranes, teeth, and gums. Note the client's breath. Foul breath odor may be noted in clients with stomatitis. Assess ability to chew and swallow, as well as food and fluid intake.

Assist with mouth care as needed after eating and at bedtime. If the client is unable to tolerate a toothbrush, use sponge or gauze toothettes or a water pick with gentle pressure. Avoid alcohol-based mouthwashes. Encourage a high-calorie, high-protein diet tailored to the client's likes and dislikes. Offer soft, lukewarm, or cool foods or liquids (eggnog, milkshakes, nutritional supplements, popsicles, and puddings) frequently in small amounts. Avoid spicy or irritating foods. Use straws or feeding syringes as needed to promote intake.

To evaluate the effectiveness of nursing interventions, monitor the client's weight, food intake, comfort, and healing. Assess the client's understanding of the problem and its treatment.

For discharge, provide clear and easily understood instructions for oral care. Instruct the client to avoid alcohol, tobacco, and spicy or irritating foods. Discuss nutritional needs and strategies to minimize discomfort when eating. Teach the client and family about prescribed medications, including how and when to use and possible side effects. Discuss signs and symptoms to report to the physician.

ORAL CANCER

An estimated 30,000 new cases of oral cancer are diagnosed annually in the United States. The incidence is twice as high in men as in women, and it is seen more often in men over 40. The major risk factor for oral cancer is tobacco use (both smoking and smokeless tobacco). Alcohol consumption and

TABLE 18-3			
NURSING IMPLICATIONS FOR PHARMACOLOGY: CLIENTS WITH STOMATITIS			
AGENTS/DRUGS	**PURPOSE**	**NURSING RESPONSIBILITIES**	**CLIENT TEACHING**
Topical Anesthetics/Anti-inflammatory Agents ▪ Orajel ▪ Viscous lidocaine ▪ Ambesol ▪ Triamcinolone acetonide	Provide temporary pain relief. Triamcinolone has an anti-inflammatory effect.	Assess for adverse or hypersensitivity reactions. Notify the primary care provider if they occur. Provide mouth care after eating and at bedtime.	Apply every 1 to 2 hours or as directed. Brush teeth after eating and at bedtime. Contact primary care provider if symptoms worsen or do not heal within 1 week after starting treatment.
Topical Antifungal Agents ▪ Clotrimazole ▪ Nystatin	Used to treat candidiasis. Effect is local rather than systemic.	These drugs are contraindicated in pregnancy. Instruct client to dissolve troches or lozenges in mouth. For oral suspension, instruct client to swish the solution throughout the mouth for at least 2 minutes, then either expectorate or swallow as directed.	Use the medication as prescribed. Do not eat or drink for 30 minutes after the medication. Contact your primary care provider if symptoms worsen or do not improve. Brush teeth after eating and at bedtime. Remove dentures at bedtime and cleanse well.
Antiviral Agent ▪ Acyclovir (Zovirax)	Reduces the severity and duration of herpes lesions. May reduce frequency of outbreaks.	Administer with food or on an empty stomach.	Begin taking the medication at the first sign of an outbreak. Take as ordered. Contact your primary care provider if symptoms worsen.

prolonged exposure to sunlight also are significant risk factors.

Most oral cancers are squamous cell carcinomas. Tobacco and alcohol damage cells lining the mouth and oropharynx. These damaged cells grow more rapidly to repair the damage, increasing the risk for malignancy. Oral cancer may develop anywhere on the oral mucosa, including the lips, tongue, or pharynx. (Figure 18-5 ◆). Box 18-7 lists manifestations of oral cancer.

Biopsy is done to determine whether an oral lesion is benign or malignant. Treatment for oral cancer depends on the stage of the tumor.

Eliminating risk factors (tobacco and alcohol) is vital. Early lesions without cancerous cells may heal when exposure to these substances is eliminated. Early cancers may be treated with radiation therapy (external beam or implants), resection of the tumor, or both. Advanced oral cancers may require extensive surgery. Chemotherapy is used as adjunctive treatment when the tumor has metastasized beyond the local area.

Oral cancer and its treatment can affect airway clearance, food intake and nutrition, communication, and the client's body image. Assess airway patency and respiratory status, particularly if the client has undergone surgery to remove the tumor. Place the client in Fowler's position, and assist with turning, coughing, and using the incentive spirometer. Maintain adequate hydration to help loosen respiratory secretions and promote airway clearance.

Enteral feedings or parenteral nutrition may be necessary for clients with oral cancer. Monitor weight daily and food and nutrient intake. If the client is able to eat, offer a soft, bland diet with enriched foods or dietary supplements. Offer small, frequent feedings, making mealtimes pleasant. Consider a dietary consultation to assess diet and plan appropriate supplements.

Provide a magic slate, flash cards, or picture or alphabet board as needed to facilitate communication. Allow ample time for communication, and do not answer for the client. Observe nonverbal communications to supplement verbal efforts. If the client is unable to speak clearly, use yes/no questions and simple phrases. Keep the call light within easy reach and respond promptly. Alert all staff if the client is unable to

> ### BOX 18-7
> ### MANIFESTATIONS
> ### OF ORAL CANCER
>
> - A sore or lesion in the mouth that does not heal
> - *Leukoplakia:* Irregular white patches on the lips, tongue, gums, tonsil, or oral mucosa
> - *Erythroplakia:* Slightly raised, irregular red patches that bleed easily when scraped
> - Visible or palpable masses of the lips, cheek, or tongue
> - Sore throat or a feeling of something caught in the throat
> - Difficulty chewing, swallowing, or moving the jaw or tongue
> - Asymmetry of the head, face, jaws, or neck
> - Loosening of teeth, or dentures that no longer fit properly
> - Swollen lymph nodes
> - Blood-tinged sputum

respond verbally over the intercom system. Consult with a speech therapist as needed.

Radical surgery of the head or neck can seriously affect the client's body image. Assess coping, self-perception, and responses to surgery. Encourage the client to express feelings regarding body image changes, and provide emotional support.

Teach all clients about the relationship between alcohol and tobacco use (especially smokeless tobacco) and oral cancer. Provide referrals to smoking cessation classes and Alcoholics Anonymous or alcohol treatment agencies as appropriate. Teach the early signs of oral cancer, demonstrating how to check tissues of the mouth. For clients with oral cancer, teach about the cancer, its treatment, and any specialized care. As needed, teach caregivers how to change dressings and to provide tube or gastrostomy feedings, tracheostomy care, or central line care. Provide referrals to home health agencies as appropriate, and discuss support groups for cancer survivors or clients who have had head and neck surgery. If the client and family have decided not to pursue treatment, support their decision and refer them to cancer support groups or hospice care.

Disorders of the Esophagus

The esophagus, essential for ingesting food and fluids, may be affected by inflammatory, mechanical, or cancerous disorders. The symptoms of these disorders may mimic other illnesses.

GASTROESOPHAGEAL REFLUX DISEASE

Gastroesophageal reflux is the backward movement of gastric contents into the esophagus. When the reflux of gastric contents causes inflammation and tissue damage to the esophagus, it is known as *gastroesophageal reflux disease (GERD)*.

Figure 18-5. ◆ Oral cancer.

The lower esophageal sphincter normally prevents gastric contents from entering the esophagus. However, if the sphincter does not function effectively or gastric emptying is delayed, gastric contents may *reflux* (back up) into the lower esophagus. Corrosive gastric fluids lead to tissue inflammation and may cause erosions, ulcers, or *strictures* (narrowing) of the esophagus. Heartburn that increases after meals and is aggravated by bending over or lying down is the primary symptom of GERD. The client also may have a sore throat, pain with swallowing, or chest pain.

GERD is managed with a combination of lifestyle changes and medications. Histamine-2 receptor blockers and proton pump inhibitors are often ordered to suppress acid secretion in the stomach and promote esophageal healing. Table 18-4 later in the chapter discusses the nursing implications and client teaching for these drugs.

Nursing care for clients with GERD focuses on teaching. Instruct clients to avoid lying down within 3 hours after meals and to elevate the head of the bed on 6-inch blocks or use a foam wedge when sleeping. Discuss the need to avoid using alcohol and tobacco. Provide information about smoking cessation and support groups as needed. Weight loss, smaller meals, and avoiding bending may help to relieve symptoms. Discuss diet changes, such as avoiding acidic foods (such as orange juice), and foods that affect the lower esophageal sphincter or gastric emptying (fatty foods, peppermint, and chocolate).

HIATAL HERNIA

A *hiatal hernia* occurs when part of the stomach protrudes through the opening of the diaphragm into the chest cavity. Hiatal hernias usually occur with aging or because of increased intra-abdominal pressure. Most people have no symptoms.

With a *sliding hernia* (the more common type), part of the stomach slides through the opening of the diaphragm when the client reclines and moves back into place when the client stands. With a *paraesophageal hernia,* part of the stomach protrudes through the opening beside the esophagus (Figure 18-6 ◆). Upper GI bleeding or erosive esophagitis may complicate hiatal hernias.

The same medical, life-style, and pharmacologic interventions used for GERD are usually prescribed for clients with hiatal hernia. If the hernia becomes trapped, impairing blood flow to the hernia, surgery may be necessary. Nursing care for the client undergoing hiatal hernia surgery is similar to that for a client undergoing other abdominal or thoracic surgery (see Chapter 7 for care of the surgical client).

ESOPHAGEAL CANCER

Cancer of the esophagus is relatively uncommon in the United States. Cigarette smoking and alcohol consumption, particularly in combination, are the major risk factors for esophageal cancer.

Most tumors affect the middle or lower third of the esophagus. The most common symptom, which often does not develop until late in the disease, is **dysphagia** (difficulty or

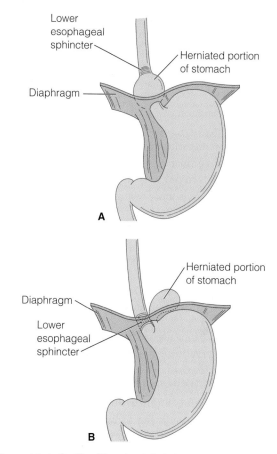

Figure 18-6. ◆ Hiatal hernias. (A) Sliding. (B) Paraesophageal.

pain in swallowing). Later symptoms include reflux, weight loss, regurgitation, and blood loss.

Treatment may involve surgery, radiation therapy, and/or chemotherapy. (See Chapter 8 for more information about cancer treatments.) Controlling dysphagia is essential; many clients with esophageal cancer are undernourished because of dysphagia. TPN or enteral (tube) feedings may be needed to maintain weight and nutrition (see Procedure 18-2 and Box 18-4). A gastrostomy tube may be inserted.

Following surgery, the client is at high risk for aspiration and airway problems. Assess level of consciousness and respiratory status at least every hour after surgery. Encourage coughing and deep breathing every 1 to 2 hours and as needed.

Teach the client, family members, and caregivers about the diagnosis and prescribed treatment, including wound care and follow-up care. If tube feedings or TPN will be continued at home, have the client and caregivers demonstrate skills required to perform the procedure. Refer the client to home health services or hospice as indicated.

Disorders of the Stomach and Upper Intestinal Tract

The stomach and upper intestinal tract (duodenum and jejunum) are responsible for the majority of food digestion.

Gastritis, peptic ulcer disease, and cancer of the stomach are the major disorders affecting digestion. Nurses provide both acute care for the hospitalized client and teaching for the client who will manage these conditions at home.

GASTRITIS

Gastritis, inflammation of the stomach lining, is a common stomach disorder. *Acute gastritis,* the most common form, is usually caused by ingesting irritants like aspirin, alcohol, caffeine, or foods contaminated with certain bacteria. *Chronic gastritis,* however, leads to progressive and irreversible changes in the gastric mucosa. It is more common in the elderly, chronic alcoholics, and cigarette smokers.

Pathophysiology

Normally, the stomach is protected from the digestive substances it secretes—namely hydrochloric acid and pepsin—by the mucosal barrier (Figure 18-7 ◆). When this barrier is disrupted, the gastric mucosa becomes irritated and inflamed.

ACUTE GASTRITIS. In acute gastritis, a local irritant disrupts the mucosal barrier, allowing gastric juices to come into contact with the gastric tissue. This causes irritation, inflammation, and superficial erosions. The gastric mucosa rapidly regenerates, and healing occurs within several days.

Acute gastritis often is caused by drugs such as aspirin or other nonsteroidal anti-inflammatory drugs (NSAIDs), corticosteroids, and chemotherapy. Bacterial toxins in contaminated food can cause an abrupt, severe gastritis. Ingestion of a strong alkali (such as ammonia) or acid severely damages the stomach, and may lead to perforation, hemorrhage, and peritonitis. *Erosive* or *stress-induced gastritis* (a severe form of acute gastritis) is a potential complication of conditions such as shock, severe trauma, or major surgery. Decreased blood flow

to the gastric mucosa leads to superficial erosions and a significant risk for bleeding.

The client with acute gastritis may have few symptoms. Possible manifestations are listed in Box 18-8. Gastric bleeding may occur, causing **hematemesis** (vomiting of blood) or **melena** (black, tarry stool that contains blood).

CLINICAL alert

Clients with stress gastritis often have no symptoms until signs of severe bleeding, shock, or an *acute abdomen* (severely painful, rigid, boardlike abdomen) develop.

CHRONIC GASTRITIS. Chronic gastritis is a progressive disorder in which the gastric mucosa thins and atrophies, and the mucosal barrier becomes less effective. Chronic gastritis is associated with colonization of the gastric mucosa by *Helicobacter pylori (H. pylori),* the bacteria that cause peptic ulcer disease. Chronic alcohol use, cigarette smoking, and exposure to toxins such as lead may also contribute to chronic gastritis.

Chronic gastritis is often asymptomatic until digestion and gastric emptying are affected. The client may complain of vague gastric distress after eating or ulcerlike symptoms.

Collaborative Care

Acute gastritis is often diagnosed by the client's history and symptoms. It usually is treated in a community-based setting unless severe vomiting or bleeding occurs. Chronic gastritis may require lifelong therapy.

DIAGNOSTIC TESTS. The following diagnostic tests may be ordered:

- *Gastric analysis* to assess hydrochloric acid secretion. A nasogastric tube is passed into the stomach, and drug is given to stimulate hydrochloric acid secretion.
- *Hemoglobin* and *hematocrit* are used to identify possible anemia due to bleeding.

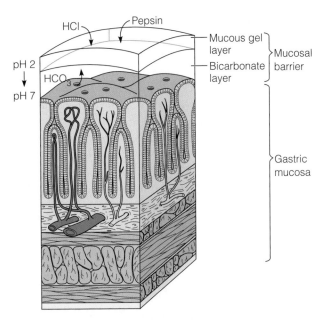

Figure 18-7. ◆ The gastric mucosa and the mucosal barrier. The mucous gel and bicarbonate of the mucosal barrier protect the gastric mucosa from damage by gastric secretions.

BOX 18-8
MANIFESTATIONS OF ACUTE AND CHRONIC GASTRITIS

ACUTE GASTRITIS

- Anorexia
- Nausea and vomiting
- Abdominal pain or discomfort
- Hematemesis (vomiting blood)
- Melena (black, tarry stool)

CHRONIC GASTRITIS

- Vague discomfort after eating
- Anemia
- Fatigue

■ *Endoscopy* may be done to inspect the gastric mucosa, evaluate for *H. pylori* infection, and obtain tissue for biopsy. Areas of bleeding may be treated directly. Box 18-9 describes nursing care of the client having an endoscopy.

PHARMACOLOGY. Antiemetics and antacids are used in acute gastritis to control gastric distress and vomiting. If nausea and vomiting are severe, intravenous fluids and electrolyte replacement are ordered.

Antacids and histamine-2 (H$_2$)-receptor antagonists (such as cimetidine or famotidine) may be ordered for clients with chronic gastritis. Sucralfate (Carafate) may also be used. It works locally to prevent acid and pepsin from damaging gastric tissue. If *H. pylori* infection is found, treatment to eradicate the infection is initiated (see the section on peptic ulcer disease that follows). Table 18-4 ◆ outlines the nursing implications and client teaching for these drugs.

OTHER THERAPIES. For *acute gastritis,* 6 to 12 hours of GI tract rest is prescribed. Food and fluids are slowly reintro-duced, beginning with clear liquids (broth, tea, gelatin, carbonated beverages), followed by heavier liquids (cream soups, puddings, milk) and finally solid foods.

When acute gastritis results from ingesting a poisonous or corrosive substance (acid or strong alkali), the substance must immediately be diluted and removed. Vomiting is not induced because it might further damage the esophagus and trachea. Instead, *gastric lavage* (irrigation or washing out of the stomach) is performed (Procedure 18-3).

COMPLEMENTARY THERAPIES. Complementary therapies such as herbal remedies or aromatherapy may be appropriate to recommend for clients with gastritis. Refer the client to a health care provider trained in natural and herbal remedies or to an aromatherapist for an individualized treatment plan. Recommendations may include:

■ Chamomile tea or the essential oil used in aromatherapy
■ Garlic; one clove chopped fine and taken daily at bedtime
■ Ginger, powdered, capsules, or made into a tea taken before or after meals
■ Mint oil aromatherapy via a diffuser, in a bath, or diluted with a carrier oil and used for a soothing massage

NURSING CARE

ASSESSING

Collect data regarding the onset, duration, and nature of the client's symptoms. Ask specifically about foods, fluids, and other substances (such as aspirin or other drugs) that have been taken recently. Inquire about evidence of bleeding in emesis or stools. Note appearance and any visible distress. Assess vital signs, including orthostatic blood pressures. Inspect the abdomen and auscultate bowel sounds. Measure abdominal girth, and lightly palpate for tenderness. Measure and document the color and character of any emesis or stools.

DIAGNOSING, PLANNING, AND IMPLEMENTING

DEFICIENT FLUID VOLUME

Nausea, vomiting, and abdominal distress are the primary manifestations of acute gastritis. Fluid and electrolyte imbalances may develop as a result.

■ Frequently monitor vital signs, including orthostatic vital signs. *Tachycardia and orthostatic hypotension may indicate fluid volume deficit. Electrolyte imbalances may affect heart rate and rhythm, as well as blood pressure.*
■ Monitor and record intake and output. Weigh daily. *Intake and output records and daily weights provide important data about fluid balance.*
■ Provide meticulous skin and mouth care frequently. *Clients with fluid volume deficit are at high risk for impaired skin and mucous membrane integrity.*

BOX 18-9
NURSING CARE CHECKLIST

UPPER ENDOSCOPY
Before the Procedure

☑ Provide routine preoperative care as ordered (see Chapter 7).
☑ Assess knowledge and understanding of the procedure, reinforcing teaching as needed. Conscious sedation often is used during the procedure, which requires 20 to 30 minutes to complete.
☑ Remove dentures and check for loose teeth prior to the procedure. Provide mouth care. Remove eyewear, jewelry, hairpins, and combs.

After the Procedure

☑ Provide routine postoperative care as ordered (see Chapter 7).
☑ Monitor for evidence of complications: bleeding, abdominal or back pain, dyspnea, dysphagia, or fever.
☑ Withhold all food and fluids until gag and swallow reflexes have returned. Place in semi-Fowler's position with the head to side to allow drainage of saliva from mouth.
☑ Provide tissues for the client to expectorate into.
☑ Tell the client that a sore throat, hoarseness, abdominal bloating, belching, and flatulence are common after the procedure. Warm saline gargles or throat lozenges may help relieve discomfort.
☑ Ensure that the client is not discharged alone.
☑ Instruct the client to notify the physician immediately if any of the following develop: persistent difficulty swallowing; epigastric, substernal, or shoulder pain; vomiting blood; black, tarry stools; or fever.

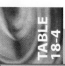

TABLE 18-4 NURSING IMPLICATIONS FOR PHARMACOLOGY: CLIENTS WITH GERD, GASTRITIS, AND PEPTIC ULCER DISEASE

AGENTS/DRUGS	PURPOSE	NURSING RESPONSIBILITIES	CLIENT TEACHING
Proton Pump Inhibitors ▪ Lansoprazole (Prevacid) ▪ Omeprazole (Prilosec)	These drugs significantly reduce gastric acid secretion and the amount of acid in the stomach between and following meals. They are used to heal and prevent recurrence of peptic ulcers and for GERD.	Administer at bedtime or before breakfast. Do not open or crush omeprazole capsules. Lansoprazole capsules can be opened and the granules given via NG or gastrostomy tube by mixing with apple juice. Flush the tube after giving the medication. These drugs may slow the elimination of diazepam, warfarin, and phenytoin; monitor for adverse effects.	Take at bedtime or before breakfast. Omeprazole capsules should be swallowed whole. If you have difficulty swallowing, lansoprazole capsules may be opened and the granules sprinkled on pudding, applesauce, or yogurt, or mixed with a small amount of juice and taken immediately. Adverse effects are rare with these drugs but should be reported to your physician.
H$_2$-Receptor Blockers ▪ Cimetidine (Tagamet) ▪ Famotidine (Pepcid) ▪ Nizatidine (Axid) ▪ Ranitidine (Zantac)	H$_2$-receptor blockers reduce stomach acid by blocking the acid-stimulating effects of histamine. This reduces the volume and concentration of hydrochloric acid in the stomach.	Should not be taken during pregnancy and lactation. Administer 30 minutes before meals and at bedtime or as ordered. Do not administer antacids within 1 hour before or after these drugs to ensure absorption. When given intravenously, do not mix with other drugs. Administer in 20–100 mL of solution over 15 to 30 minutes.	Take as directed, even after pain and gastric discomfort are relieved. Avoid taking antacids for 1 hour before and 1 hour after taking H$_2$ blockers. Report any of the following to the physician: Diarrhea, confusion, rash, fatigue, malaise, or bruising.
Antacids ▪ Aluminum hydroxide (Amphojel, AlternaGEL) ▪ Magnesium hydroxide (Milk of Magnesia) ▪ Calcium carbonate (Tums) ▪ Magnesium hydroxide and aluminum hydroxide (Maalox, Mylanta, Gelusil)	Antacids buffer or neutralize gastric acid, generally by a local action. They help relieve pain and prevent further damage to the gastric mucosa.	Antacids interfere with absorption of many drugs; separate dosage times by at least 2 hours. Monitor for constipation or diarrhea. Notify the physician should either occur; a different antacid may be prescribed. Monitor for electrolyte imbalances in clients taking high doses of antacids.	Do not use sodium bicarbonate as an antacid because of its local and systemic effects. Take as prescribed; to work effectively, the antacid must be in the stomach. Avoid taking the antacid for approximately 2 hours before and after taking other medication. Report diarrhea or constipation to the physician. Continue taking the antacid for the duration prescribed; mucosal healing takes 6–8 weeks.

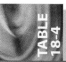

TABLE 18-4	NURSING IMPLICATIONS FOR PHARMACOLOGY: CLIENTS WITH GERD, GASTRITIS, AND PEPTIC ULCER DISEASE (CONTINUED)		
AGENTS/DRUGS	**PURPOSE**	**NURSING RESPONSIBILITIES**	**CLIENT TEACHING**
Sucralfate	Sucralfate creates a protective barrier against gastric juices. It does not neutralize gastric acid or affect its secretion.	Give sucralfate on an empty stomach 1 hour before meals and at bedtime or as ordered. Sucralfate may interfere with absorption of other drugs; separate administration times by at least 2 hours.	This drug has few side effects. Constipation may rarely develop. If you have difficulty swallowing the tablets, an oral suspension is available.
Bismuth Compounds ■ Bismuth subsalicylate (Pepto-Bismol) ■ Ranitidine bismuth citrate (Tritec)	Bismuth has a local antibiotic effect on *H. pylori;* it also may help prevent the bacteria from adhering to the gastric mucosa.	Do not give bismuth subsalicylate if fecal impaction is suspected. This drug is contraindicated for clients who are allergic to aspirin.	This drug may cause stools to turn dark or appear black. Do not take this drug if you are allergic to aspirin. Do not give this drug to children who have chickenpox or another viral illness.
Misoprostol (Cytotec)	Misoprostol is a synthetic prostaglandin used to prevent ulcers in clients who require long-term NSAID therapy.	Do not give during pregnancy as it may cause abortion of the fetus. Administer with meals and at bedtime.	Stress the importance of avoiding this drug during pregnancy. May cause diarrhea, abdominal pain, spotting, and uterine cramps. Report these effects to the doctor.

■ Report significant changes or deviations from normal laboratory values for electrolytes and acid-base balance. *Significant changes in electrolyte or acid–base balance may occur as a result of vomiting and poor food and fluid intake.*

■ Provide fluids by mouth or parenterally as ordered. *Oral fluids are gradually reintroduced when the client is no longer vomiting. Intravenous fluids restore or maintain hydration until adequate oral intake is resumed.*

■ Administer antiemetic and other medications as ordered to relieve nausea and vomiting. *Medications can help prevent or relieve vomiting and can promote oral intake.*

■ Provide for the safety of clients with orthostatic hypotension: Place the signal light within reach, put up the side rails, instruct the client not to get up or walk without assistance. *Orthostatic hypotension may lead to fainting or falls.*

IMBALANCED NUTRITION: LESS THAN BODY REQUIREMENTS

The client may become fearful of eating or may reduce food intake to the point of becoming undernourished.

■ Monitor and record food and fluid intake and any abnormal losses (such as vomiting). *Careful monitoring provides valuable information about nutritional status.*

■ Weigh daily at the same time. *Weight changes occurring over days to weeks are an indicator of nutritional status.*

■ Arrange for dietary consultation. *Clients with chronic gastritis may have specific food intolerances and preferences that need to be considered.*

■ Provide nutritional supplements between meals or frequent small feedings as needed. *Many clients with chronic gastritis tolerate small, frequent feedings better than three large meals per day.*

EVALUATING

Collect the following data to evaluate the effectiveness of nursing care: indicators of fluid and electrolyte balance, such as thirst, skin turgor, weight, intake and output, mental status, and laboratory values; appetite and food intake; skin condition, color, and other indicators of nutritional status.

Discharge Considerations

Teaching is a vital component of nursing care for clients whose gastritis is managed at home. Teach clients with acute gastritis how to identify and avoid causative factors, manage acute symptoms, reintroduce fluids and foods, and when to contact the physician (unrelieved vomiting, severe weight loss, changes in mental status or lack of urine output).

PROCEDURE 18-3 Gastric Lavage

- Obtain all supplies.
- Provide for privacy.
- Use standard precautions.
- Explain the procedure. Instruct client to report any pain, difficulty breathing, or other problems during the procedure.
- Document baseline vital signs, abdominal girth, and bowel sounds.
- Place in semi-Fowler's or Fowler's position. If hypotension is present, place in left side-lying position.
- Insert a nasogastric (NG) tube (14 to 16 French, unless otherwise indicated) if one is not already in place, and verify placement. (See Procedure 18-1.)

■ CLOSED SYSTEM IRRIGATION

Connect irrigating solution to NG tube with Y connector. Attach drainage or suction tube to other arm of connector. Empty the stomach, clamp drain tube or turn off suction, and allow 50 to 200 mL of solution to run into stomach by gravity. Stop solution and allow to drain or suction out. Repeat until ordered amount has been used or desired results are obtained. Measure the drainage, subtracting the amount of irrigant instilled, to obtain gastric output.

Wall suction unit

Normal saline irrigating solution

Kelly clamp

Y connector

A client with a closed system gastric lavage.

■ INTERMITTENT OPEN SYSTEM

Empty the stomach using suction or a 50-mL catheter-tip syringe. Measure and discard the aspirate. Using the syringe, draw up approximately 50 mL of irrigation solution, and instill it using gentle pressure. Withdraw and discard the solution into a measuring container. Continue until the desired amount of irrigant or desired results have been obtained.

- Monitor vital signs, respiratory status, and client tolerance during the procedure.
- Notify the charge nurse or physician if the procedure is ineffective or the client is unable to tolerate it.

■ SAMPLE DOCUMENTATION

1030:	Gastric lavage with 750 mL normal saline. Irrigant returned clear; no bleeding noted. 50 mL gastric contents returned with irrigant. Tolerated procedure well with no abdominal or respiratory distress.
	_____ S. Williams, LPN.

Teach clients with chronic gastritis how to manage their condition. Provide information on maintaining nutritional status, helpful dietary modifications, known gastric irritants, use of prescribed medications, and complementary therapies. Refer clients to smoking-cessation classes or programs to treat alcohol abuse if appropriate. In all cases, document teaching and referrals.

Peptic Ulcer Disease

A **peptic ulcer** is a break in the mucous lining of the stomach or duodenum where it comes in contact with gastric juice. *Peptic ulcer disease (PUD)* is a chronic health problem that primarily affects adults (often duodenal ulcers in young and middle adults, and gastric ulcers in older adults). Chronic *H. pylori* infection, aspirin, and other NSAIDs are the major risk factors. Cigarette smoking doubles the risk of PUD.

Pathophysiology

The mucosal barrier protects the gastric mucosa. It is maintained by (a) bicarbonate secreted by epithelial cells, (b) mucous gel produced in response to prostaglandins, and (c) an adequate blood supply to the mucosa. Ulcers develop when the mucosal barrier is unable to prevent damage by gastric digestive juices.

The mucosal barrier can be impaired by poor circulation, decreased mucus, or reflux of bile or pancreatic enzymes into the stomach or duodenum. Aspirin and other NSAIDs inhibit prostaglandins and mucous gel production. About three fourths of the people with PUD have *H. pylori* infection. This bacterium secretes substances that break down mucous gel and also appears to stimulate acid production in the stomach. It also causes an inflammatory response in the lining of the stomach. Cigarette smoking contributes by inhibiting bicarbonate secretion.

Ulcers may develop in the esophagus, stomach, or duodenum. In the stomach, the lesser curvature and area closest to the pylorus are most often affected (Figure 18-8 ◆). Ulcers may be superficial or deep, affecting all layers of the mucosa.

Epigastric pain is the classic symptom of PUD. The pain is often described as gnawing, burning, aching, or hunger-like. It occurs when the stomach is empty (2 to 3 hours after meals and in the middle of the night) and is relieved by eating. It may radiate to the back. The client may complain of heartburn or regurgitation and vomiting. Older adults with PUD may have no symptoms, or complain of vague discomfort, chest pain, or dysphagia. Weight loss or anemia may be present.

COMPLICATIONS. The complications of PUD include hemorrhage, obstruction, and perforation. *Hemorrhage* results from ulceration and erosion into blood vessels of the gastric mucosa. Erosion into small blood vessels may cause slow bleeding and black, tarry stools. Erosion into a larger vessel can lead to sudden, severe bleeding with hematemesis or *hematochezia* (red blood with clots in the stool), and signs of shock. Box 18-10 lists the manifestations of PUD complications.

BOX 18-10
MANIFESTATIONS OF PUD COMPLICATIONS

HEMORRHAGE
- Occult or obvious blood in the stool
- Hematemesis
- Fatigue, weakness, dizziness
- Orthostatic hypotension
- Shock

OBSTRUCTION
- Feeling of epigastric fullness
- Nausea and vomiting

PERFORATION
- Severe upper abdominal pain, radiating to the shoulder
- Rigid, boardlike (acute) abdomen
- Absent bowel sounds
- Signs of shock: Diaphoresis, tachycardia, rapid and shallow respirations
- Fever

Peptic ulcer disease can cause *obstruction* of the upper GI tract. This usually occurs gradually. If the obstruction becomes complete, vomiting occurs.

Perforation of the ulcer through the mucosal wall is the most dangerous complication of PUD. When perforation occurs, gastric or duodenal contents enter the peritoneum, causing inflammation and *peritonitis*. Chemical peritonitis from GI secretions develops immediately; bacterial peritonitis from contamination of the normally sterile peritoneal cavity follows. When an ulcer perforates, the client develops immediate manifestations of an acute abdomen, with pain, guarding, and absent bowel sounds. Signs of shock may be present. Older adults may have less specific manifestations of perforation; pain may be absent.

Collaborative Care

Treatment of PUD focuses on relieving symptoms, healing ulcers, and preventing complications and ulcer recurrence.

DIAGNOSTIC TESTS

- *Upper endoscopy (gastroscopy)* is done to inspect the mucosa of the upper GI tract and obtain samples for biopsy and *H. pylori* testing. (Review Box 18-9 for nursing care related to an upper endoscopy.)
- A *urea breath test* may be done to detect *H. pylori* infection. An enzyme produced by the bacteria converts radioactive urea to ammonia and CO_2. The CO_2 then can be detected as it is exhaled by the lungs.
- *CBC* to assess for anemia.
- *Stool* for occult blood.

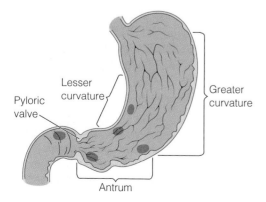

Figure 18-8. ◆ Sites commonly affected by peptic ulcer disease.

PHARMACOLOGY. Drug therapy is used to eradicate *H. pylori* and heal existing ulcers. A combination of a proton-pump inhibitor and two antibiotics is commonly prescribed to treat *H. pylori* infection. Amoxicillin, metronidazole (Flagyl), and clarithromycin (Biaxin) are commonly used antibiotics for this therapy. (See Chapter 12 for nursing responsibilities and client teaching related to antibiotic therapy.)

Proton pump inhibitors and H_2-receptor antagonists are used to reduce gastric acid production, to promote healing, and to prevent stress gastritis and ulcers in at-risk clients. Agents that protect the mucosa (sucralfate, bismuth, antacids, and prostaglandin analogs) also may be prescribed. Review Table 18-4 for nursing implications and client teaching related to drugs used to treat PUD.

DIET. No special diet is prescribed for PUD. Encourage clients to eat a well-balanced diet with meals at regular intervals. Bland or restrictive diets are no longer recommended. Mild alcohol intake is not harmful. Discourage smoking because it slows the rate of healing and increases the frequency of relapses.

TREATMENT OF COMPLICATIONS. Clients with complications of PUD require additional treatment measures.

In *hemorrhage* associated with PUD, restoring and maintaining circulation is the priority of care. Intravenous solutions are administered to restore intravascular volume. Whole blood or red blood cell concentrate (packed cells) may also be given to restore the oxygen-carrying capacity of blood.

When the client is stable, an endoscopy is done to identify and treat the bleeding site. A vasoconstricting agent may be injected at the site or the vessel may be cauterized. Most clients can be discharged within 72 hours following endoscopy for bleeding.

If *obstruction* is suspected, a nasogastric tube is inserted to relieve pressure and vomiting. The obstruction is visualized by endoscopy, and balloon therapy may be used to dilate the obstruction. Surgery may be required to relieve the obstruction.

Perforation requires immediate intervention. The client is kept NPO; intravenous fluids are administered. To minimize peritoneal contamination, gastric contents are removed by nasogastric tube connected to suction. The client is placed in Fowler's or semi-Fowler's position so that peritoneal contaminants will pool in the pelvis. Intravenous antibiotics are given to treat bacterial infection by intestinal flora. Many perforations seal spontaneously, but some require closure by laparoscopic surgery.

SURGERY. When drug therapy and lifestyle management cannot control the symptoms or complications of PUD, surgery may be necessary. Acute perforation or massive hemorrhage may require emergency surgery. A *total* **gastrectomy** (removal of the entire stomach) is rarely done because of its impact on digestion and nutrition. Extensive gastric cancer may require it. In a total gastrectomy, an **anastamosis** (surgical connec-

tion) connects the esophagus to the duodenum or jejunum. More commonly, surgery involves *partial gastrectomy,* removal of a portion of the stomach (usually the distal half to two thirds). Table 18-5 ◆ illustrates and describes the surgical procedures most likely to be performed and the advantages and disadvantages of each. Nursing care of the client having gastric surgery is outlined in Box 18-11.

Complications of Surgery. *Dumping syndrome* is the most common problem following a partial gastrectomy. After pyloric resection or bypass, concentrated chyme may enter the small bowel rapidly. Water is pulled from the vascular system into the intestine, decreasing blood volume and dilating the intestine. Early symptoms of dumping syndrome occur within 5 to 30 minutes after eating; they include nausea and possible vomiting, epigastric pain, cramping, **borborygmi** (loud, hyperactive bowel sounds), and diarrhea. Systemic symptoms from decreased blood volume include tachycardia, orthostatic hypotension, dizziness, flushing, and diaphoresis. The rapid entry of undigested carbohydrates into the jejunum stimulates the pancreas to release excess insulin, and the client develops symptoms of hypoglycemia 2 to 3 hours later.

Dumping syndrome is managed primarily by altering dietary intake to delay gastric emptying and allow smaller boluses of undigested food to enter the intestine. Meals are small and more frequent. Liquids and solids are taken at separate times instead of together. Proteins and fats in the diet are increased, because they exit the stomach more slowly than carbohydrates; carbohydrates, especially simple sugars, are reduced. The client is taught to rest in a recumbent or semirecumbent position for 30 to 60 minutes after meals.

After gastric surgery, clients are at risk for nutritional deficiencies because of reduced absorption and inability to eat large meals. Nearly 50% of clients who undergo gastric surgery experience significant weight loss due to insufficient calorie intake.

NURSING CARE

ASSESSING

Collect the subjective and objective data identified in Box 18-12. Ask the client specifically about pain, carefully assessing each episode. Do not make assumptions about cause and severity. Document all complaints of pain, and notify the charge nurse or physician if pain becomes severe or changes in character or timing.

CLINICAL alert

Pain may indicate a complication of PUD, or may be related to another process (e.g., coronary heart disease, gallbladder disease).

TABLE 18-5

SURGICAL PROCEDURES USED FOR PEPTIC ULCER DISEASE OR GASTRIC CANCER

PROCEDURE	DESCRIPTION	ADVANTAGES/DISADVANTAGES
Billroth I (Gastroduodenostomy) Duodenal anastomosis Portion of stomach removed Body Duodenum	Removal of the distal portion of the stomach with anastomosis to the duodenum. Vagotomy often done at the same time.	**Advantages:** Removes damaged mucosa; reduces number of gastrin and acid-producing cells; reduces ulcer recurrence **Disadvantages:** Decreases size of the stomach, causing problems with absorption and emptying
Billroth II (Gastrojejunostomy) Portion of stomach removed Duodenal stump Jejunal anastomosis Jejunal loop	Removal of the distal portion of the stomach with anastomosis to the proximal jejunum. Vagotomy done at the same time.	Same as Billroth I
Pyloroplasty Pylorus Longitudinal incision 1 2 Transverse suture 3	Surgical enlargement of the pylorus or gastric outlet. Done to improve gastric emptying in clients with obstruction or who have had a vagotomy that interferes with emptying.	**Advantages:** Relief of obstruction and improved gastric emptying; relatively easy procedure with low surgical risk **Disadvantages:** May contribute to dumping syndrome; does not inhibit ulcer recurrence

(continues)

TABLE 18-5 SURGICAL PROCEDURES USED FOR PEPTIC ULCER DISEASE OR GASTRIC CANCER (CONTINUED)		
PROCEDURE	**DESCRIPTION**	**ADVANTAGES/DISADVANTAGES**
Vagotomy Esophagus Vagus nerve Truncal — Selective Highly selective (proximal parietal cell) Stomach Duodenum	Severs vagal innervation to the stomach to remove the autonomic stimulus that causes parietal cells to produce hydrochloric acid.	**Advantages:** Reduces gastric acid production **Disadvantages:** May cause delay in gastric emptying; increased risk of diarrhea and gallstone formation

BOX 18-11
NURSING CARE CHECKLIST

GASTRIC SURGERY

Before Surgery

☑ Provide routine preoperative care and teaching (see Chapter 7).

After Surgery

☑ Provide routine postoperative care as outlined in Chapter 7.

☑ Assess position and patency of NG tube, connecting it to low suction. Unless contraindicated, gently irrigate with sterile normal saline if tube becomes clogged.

☑ Assess color, amount, and odor of gastric drainage, noting any changes, the presence of clots, or bright bleeding. Chart all assessments and notify the charge nurse or physician of clots or bright bleeding.

☑ Monitor bowel sounds and abdominal girth.

☑ Maintain intravenous fluids while nasogastric suction is in place.

☑ Resume oral food and fluids as ordered. Initial feedings are clear liquids, progressing to full liquids and then frequent small feedings of regular foods. Monitor bowel sounds and for abdominal distention frequently during this period.

☑ Begin discharge planning and teaching. Consult with a dietitian for diet instructions and menu planning; reinforce teaching. Teach the client how to recognize and prevent potential postoperative complications, such as infection, dumping syndrome, postprandial hypoglycemia, or pernicious anemia.

If the client is being admitted with a possible complication such as bleeding, obstruction, or perforation, determine the duration and severity of symptoms. Carefully observe the client's general appearance, watching for signs of acute distress. Focus interview questions and physical assessment to collect data quickly.

BOX 18-12
ASSESSING CLIENTS WITH PEPTIC ULCER DISEASE

SUBJECTIVE DATA

- Pain: Location, character, intensity, duration, and timing; relationship to meals; measures that relieve or aggravate pain
- Complaints of nausea, vomiting, heartburn, indigestion, or abdominal pain
- Color, consistency, and amount of any emesis
- Color and consistency of feces, any recent changes
- Current or previous treatment (prescribed or over-the-counter); compliance with treatment regimen
- Use of tobacco, alcohol, nonsteroidal anti-inflammatory drugs (NSAIDs), or other medications

OBJECTIVE DATA

- Check vital signs, including orthostatic blood pressures.
- Inspect abdomen, observing shape, contour, and appearance.
- Auscultate bowel sounds in all four quadrants; note frequency.
- Palpate for tenderness and guarding.
- Test any emesis and stool for the presence of occult blood.

PAIN

- Assess pain, reporting any changes in intensity or character to the charge nurse or physician. *A change in the nature or severity of pain may indicate a complication of PUD or a separate problem.*

- Administer medications as ordered. *Medications for PUD help prevent pain and promote healing. Administration at bedtime helps prevent nighttime ulcer pain that typically occurs between 1:00 and 3:00 A.M.*

- Limit food intake after the evening meal; eliminate bedtime snacks. *Eating before bed can stimulate gastric acid and pepsin production, increasing the chance of nighttime pain.*

IMBALANCED NUTRITION: LESS THAN BODY REQUIREMENTS

- Assess diet, including pattern of food intake, eating schedule, and foods associated with pain. *This step increases client awareness and identifies whether nutrient intake is adequate.*

- Arrange consultation with a dietitian. *A dietitian can help plan meals that meet the client's nutritional needs and preferences. Foods that increase pain should be avoided. Providing six small meals per day generally helps increase food tolerance and decrease discomfort after meals.*

- Document and report complaints of anorexia, fullness, nausea, vomiting, or symptoms of dumping syndrome. *Problems with gastric emptying may be associated with PUD or surgery to treat PUD. It is important to monitor and report symptoms, because a change in therapy or food intake may be necessary.*

DECREASED CARDIAC OUTPUT

Acute bleeding or dumping syndrome can cause hypovolemia and a fall in cardiac output.

- Frequently monitor and record vital signs until stable. Closely monitor urinary output. Weigh daily. *Careful monitoring is essential to identify possible shock and to intervene at an early stage.*

- Monitor stools and gastric drainage for overt and occult blood. Assess gastric drainage (vomitus or from a nasogastric tube) to estimate the amount and rate of hemorrhage. *Drainage is bright red with possible clots in acute hemorrhage; dark red or the color of coffee grounds when blood has been in the stomach for a period of time. Hematochezia (stool containing red blood and clots) is present in acute hemorrhage; melena (black, tarry stool) indicates less acute bleeding.*

- Maintain intravenous infusions and assist with blood administration as needed. *Intravenous fluids and blood products are administered to maintain or restore blood volume. Whole blood and packed cells provide additional oxygen-carrying capacity to meet cell needs.*

- Insert a nasogastric (NG) tube and maintain its position and patency. Initially, measure and record gastric output hourly, then every 4 to 8 hours. *NG suction is used to remove blood from the GI tract, and prevent vomiting and possible aspiration. Gastric output is replaced with a balanced electrolyte solution to maintain homeostasis.*

- Prepare for possible endoscopy. *Endoscopy can identify bleeding sites and allow direct treatment of the erosion.*

- Monitor hemoglobin and hematocrit, serum electrolytes, blood urea nitrogen (BUN), and creatinine. Report abnormal findings. *Hemoglobin and hematocrit are low in clients with acute or chronic GI bleeding. Electrolytes are lost through vomiting, gastric drainage, and diarrhea. Digestion and absorption of blood in the GI tract may cause elevated BUN and creatinine levels.*

- Assess abdomen, including bowel sounds, girth, and tenderness every 4 hours and record findings. *Borborygmi and abdominal tenderness are common in clients with acute GI bleeding. Increased abdominal girth, absent bowel sounds, or extreme tenderness with a rigid, boardlike abdomen may indicate perforation.*

- Maintain bed rest with the head of the bed elevated and side rails up; ensure safety. *Loss of blood volume may cause orthostatic hypotension with syncope or dizziness upon standing.*

In order to evaluate the effectiveness of nursing care for a client with peptic ulcer disease, collect data regarding pain, weight, nutritional status (including food intake), fluid balance, and circulation (vital signs, peripheral pulses and capillary refill, mental status, and urinary output). Frequently monitor for and promptly report any manifestation of complications of the disease or gastric surgery.

Discharge Considerations

Because PUD is a chronic disease, it is managed primarily by the client at home. Teach clients about treatment measures and counter common misconceptions and myths (e.g., drinking milk or cream every 2 hours "to coat the stomach" is no longer part of the treatment plan). Provide written and verbal instruction about medications, including the importance of continuing therapy even when symptoms are relieved. Teach clients taking metronidazole to eradicate *H. pylori* infection to avoid alcohol in any form while taking the drug and for a minimum of 48 hours after discontinuing the medication. Discuss the relationship between peptic ulcers and factors like smoking. If indicated, refer the client to a smoking-cessation clinic. Stress the importance of avoiding aspirin and other NSAIDs, as well as the need to read the labels of over-the-counter medications to identify the presence of aspirin.

Discuss the manifestations of PUD complications, such as abdominal pain or distention, vomiting, black or tarry stools, light-headedness, or fainting. Reinforce stress and lifestyle management techniques that may help prevent flare-ups. Refer the client to resources for stress management, such as classes, counseling, and formal or informal groups.

Nursing Process Case Study
■ CLIENT WITH PEPTIC ULCER DISEASE

Sean O'Donnell is a 47-year-old policeman. He has had "heartburn" and epigastric pain for years but thought it went along with his job. Last year, after becoming weak, light-headed, and short of breath, he was found to be anemic and was diagnosed as having a duodenal ulcer. He took famotidine and ferrous sulfate for 3 months before stopping both, saying he had "never felt better in his life." Sean has now been admitted to the hospital with active upper GI bleeding.

Assessment Mr. O'Donnell is alert and oriented, though very apprehensive about his condition. Skin pale and cool; BP 136/78 and pulse 98. Abdomen distended and tender with extremely active bowel sounds. NG tube inserted; 200 mL bright red blood obtained. Laboratory results include hemoglobin 8.2 g/dL and hematocrit 23%. An endoscopy is done to control Mr. O'Donnell's bleeding, and he receives two units of packed red blood cells as well as intravenous fluids to replace his lost blood volume.

Diagnosis The following nursing diagnoses are identified for Mr. O'Donnell:

- Deficient Fluid Volume related to acute upper GI bleeding
- Impaired Tissue Integrity: Gastrointestinal related to active peptic ulcer disease
- Ineffective Therapeutic Regimen Management related to lack of understanding of the need for continued treatment

Expected Outcomes The expected outcomes for the plan of care specify that Mr. O'Donnell will:

- Regain homeostasis with stable vital signs and normal hemoglobin and hematocrit
- Remain free of further bleeding and other potential complications of peptic ulcer disease
- Demonstrate knowledge and understanding of prescribed treatment measures
- Identify ways to promote ulcer healing and prevent recurrence
- State manifestations to report to his primary care provider

Planning and Implementation The nurse plans and implements the following interventions for Mr. O'Donnell:

- Monitor and document vital signs, mental status, intake and output, and abdominal assessment every 4 hours until stable, then every 8 hours.
- Maintain intravenous fluids and blood replacement as ordered.

- Monitor laboratory values (hemoglobin, hematocrit, serum electrolytes), reporting abnormal values to the charge nurse or physician as indicated.
- Explain PUD and ulcer healing, clarifying misconceptions.
- Discuss the importance of following the treatment plan to ensure healing and prevent further ulcers from developing.
- Discuss the effect of smoking, aspirin, and NSAIDs on PUD. Provide information about other over-the-counter analgesics.
- Provide written and verbal instructions about prescribed medications.
- With the client, plan a medication schedule that fits his lifestyle.
- Discuss stress-reduction strategies such as exercise, meditation, controlled breathing, and other relaxation exercises.

Evaluation Mr. O'Donnell is discharged after 72 hours. He has had no further bleeding, and is eating a normal diet. His hemoglobin and hematocrit levels have improved; other blood values are within normal limits. His physician has prescribed omeprazole (Prilosec), amoxicillin, and clarithromycin for 2 weeks to eradiate *H. pylori* infection confirmed during the endoscopy. He will continue to take the omeprazole daily at bedtime for another 6 weeks. He verbalizes an understanding of the need for these medications, when to take them, and what side effects he should report. He had used aspirin and ibuprofen regularly for tension headaches, but says he is willing to try acetaminophen and relaxation techniques to "avoid ending up in here again!" He states that the hardest part of going back to work will be not drinking six to ten cups of coffee a day, as he used to do.

Critical Thinking in the Nursing Process

1. What is the likely reason Mr. O'Donnell developed another peptic ulcer and hemorrhage after having been treated for a previous episode?
2. Discuss the relationship between aspirin and NSAIDs and peptic ulcer disease.
3. What additional life-style changes would you recommend for Mr. O'Donnell?

Cancer of the Stomach

Except for skin cancer, cancer of the stomach is the most common cancer in the world, but it is less common in the United States. Its incidence is highest in Hispanics, African Americans, and Asian Americans; men are affected twice as often as women. Chronic *H. pylori* gastritis is the major risk factor for gastric cancer.

Gastric carcinomas usually develop in the distal portion of the stomach. Half of all gastric cancers occur in the antrum or pyloric region (see Fig. 18-8). Lesions spread by direct extension to tissues surrounding the stomach, particularly the liver. Lymph node involvement and metastasis occur early due to the rich blood and lymphatic supply to the stomach. Metastatic lesions are often found in the liver, lungs, ovaries, and peritoneum.

Early symptoms of gastric cancer are vague (early satiety, anorexia, indigestion, and possibly vomiting). There may also be ulcerlike pain, typically occurring after meals and unrelieved by antacids. As the disease progresses, weight loss occurs, and the client may be *cachectic* (very thin and malnourished). An abdominal mass may be palpable, and there may be occult blood in the stool. The diagnosis is confirmed with an endoscopy and biopsy of the lesion.

When gastric cancer is diagnosed before metastases develop, a partial or total gastrectomy is done. Radiation, chemotherapy, or both may be used to reduce the risk of spread. For the client with more advanced disease, treatment is palliative and may include surgery and chemotherapy. These clients may require a gastrostomy or jejunostomy feeding tube. Gastrostomy tubes are inserted into the stomach through a stoma in the epigastric region (Figure 18-9 ◆). The tube may initially be connected to low suction or plugged. Tube feedings may be restarted shortly after the procedure. Box 18-13 describes nursing care of the client with a gastrostomy tube.

Because gastric cancer is often advanced by the time of diagnosis, the prognosis is poor. The 5-year survival rate of all clients treated for gastric carcinoma is 10%.

Nursing and home care for the client with gastric cancer depends on the stage of the disease and the treatment planned. If surgery is performed, provide pre- and postoperative care as outlined in Box 18-11. *Imbalanced Nutrition: Less than Body Requirements* is a priority nursing diagnosis for clients with gastric cancer because of the effects of the cancer, surgery, and other treatments such as chemotherapy or radiation therapy. Total parenteral nutrition may be necessary to maintain weight and nutrition. Refer to home health services as needed for assistance with dressing changes, tube feedings, or TPN.

Because disease is usually advanced at the time of diagnosis, provide grief counseling and refer the client and family to cancer support groups or hospice services as appropriate.

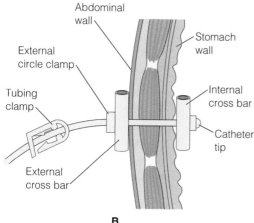

Figure 18-9. ◆ (A) Gastrostomy tube placement. (B) The tube is held in place by cross bars.

BOX 18-13
NURSING CARE CHECKLIST

GASTROSTOMY TUBE
Nursing Care

- ☑ Use standard precautions.
- ☑ Assess tube placement by aspirating stomach contents and checking the pH of aspirate (see Procedure 18-1 for expected pH readings for the stomach and small intestine).
- ☑ Inspect skin around the stoma for healing, redness, swelling, and any drainage. If drainage is present, note the color, amount, consistency, and odor. Document findings and report to charge nurse or physician.
- ☑ Assess the abdomen for distention, bowel sounds, and tenderness; document.
- ☑ Until the stoma is well healed, use sterile technique for dressing changes and site care. Clean technique is appropriate for use once healing is complete.
- ☑ Cleanse the site with antiseptic swabs or soap and water. A well-healed stoma site may be cleansed in the shower with the tube clamped or plugged. Allow to air dry. Apply a protective barrier cream as needed.
- ☑ Redress the wound using a stoma dressing or folded 4 × 4 gauze pads.
- ☑ Irrigate the tube with 30 to 50 mL of water; clean the tube inside and out as indicated or ordered. A special brush may be used to clean the inside of soft gastric tubes.
- ☑ Provide mouth care or remind the client to do so.
- ☑ If the client is to be discharged with a gastrostomy tube, teach the client and family how to care for the tube and feedings. Refer to a home health agency or visiting nurse for support and reinforcement of learning.

Nursing Interventions Classification

Some of the following nursing interventions from the Nursing Interventions Classification Project (McCloskey & Bulechek, 2000) may also be useful in planning and implementing care for clients with nutritional and upper GI disorders:

- Eating Disorders Management
- Diet Staging

- Nutrition Management
- Weight Reduction Assistance/Weight Gain Assistance
- Fluid Management
- Bleeding Reduction: Gastrointestinal
- Blood Products Administration

(*Note:* The bibliography listings for this and all chapters have been compiled at the back of the book.)

Chapter Review

 ## key terms by topic

Use the CD-ROM disk enclosed with your textbook to hear the pronunciation of the key terms in the chapter.

Structure and function of the upper GI tract
chyme, metabolism, nutrients

Nutritional disorders
obesity, malnutrition, enteral, total parenteral nutrition

Disorders of the mouth and esophagus
stomatitis, gastroesophageal reflux, dysphagia

Disorders of the stomach and upper intestinal tract
gastritis, hematemesis, melena, peptic ulcer, gastrectomy, anastamosis, borborygmi

key points

- Nutritional disorders such as obesity and malnutrition are major causes of illness and disability. These disorders may be caused by a wide variety of factors, including diseases or their effects, problems of access to adequate food and nutrients, or by eating disorders such as anorexia nervosa. Protein-calorie malnutrition (PCM) is now recognized as a major problem in hospitalized clients.

- Tobacco and alcohol use contribute to a number of upper GI disorders, including GERD, oral and esophageal cancers, and peptic ulcer disease. Encourage all clients to stop smoking or using smokeless tobacco and to consume alcohol in moderate amounts if at all to reduce their risk of these disorders.

- Both esophageal and gastric cancer often are diagnosed late in the disease because their symptoms may be vague. Encourage all clients with complaints of dyphagia, a sensation of gastric fullness, or heartburn to seek medical evaluation.

- While acute gastritis is generally benign and self-limited, stress gastritis can lead to unexpected gastric hemorrhage. Chronic gastritis, especially when associated with *H. pylori* infection, is a risk factor for gastric cancer.

- *H. pylori* infection also is the primary cause of peptic ulcer disease. Effectively treating the infection can reduce or eliminate the risk of future exacerbations of PUD.

- Promptly report a change in the nature of abdominal pain in a client with PUD, especially if the pain is accompanied by vomiting, guarding of the abdomen, or a change in bowel sounds. These manifestations could indicate an obstruction or perforation into the peritoneal cavity.

 ## Medialink

Additional interactive resources for this chapter can be found on the Companion Website at www.prenhall.com/burke. Click on Chapter 18 and "Begin" to select the activities for this chapter.

For NCLEX review questions and an audio glossary, access the accompanying CD-ROM in this book.

for further study

For more information on the liver, gallbladder, and pancreas, see Chapter 19.

For more on the structure and function of the large intestine, see Chapter 20.

For more information on the thyroid, see Chapter 16.

For further information on fluid volume deficit, see Chapter 5.

For more information on care of the surgical client, see Chapter 7.

For more information about cancer treatments, see Chapter 8.

For nursing responsibilities and client teaching related to antibiotic therapy, see Chapter 12.

Critical Thinking Care Map

Caring for a Client with Altered Nutrition
NCLEX-PN Focus Area: Prevention and Health Maintenance

Case Study: Sam Elliott has gained 30 pounds since retiring 2 years ago, and now the most active thing he does each day is "walk to the end of the driveway to get the mail." He reports having juice, oatmeal, a muffin, and coffee with cream for breakfast and meeting friends midmorning for doughnuts and coffee. Lunch is usually a bologna-and-cheese sandwich with chips and a root beer. He has cheese, crackers, and wine before a dinner of meat, potatoes, vegetables, and dessert. He tells the nurse, "I have never had to diet. I just don't know how to get this weight off."

Nursing Diagnosis: Imbalanced Nutrition: More than Body Requirements

COLLECT DATA

Subjective

Objective

_____   _____
_____   _____
_____   _____
_____   _____
_____   _____
_____   _____
_____   _____

Would you report this data? Yes/No

If yes, to: _____

Nursing Care

_____
_____
_____
_____
_____
_____
_____
_____

How would you document this? _____
_____
_____

Data Collected
(use those that apply)

• Height 5'10" (178 cm)
• Easily fatigued
• Weight 201 lbs. (91.2 kg)
• "Needs to lose weight"
• Shortness of breath with activity
• LDL 180 mg/dL
• BP 138/90
• Fasting blood glucose 103 mg/dL
• Reports feeling hungry most of the time
• Cholesterol 240 mg/dL
• Stool negative for occult blood

Nursing Interventions
(use those that apply)

• Instruct client to lose 30 pounds in 60 days.
• Discuss Food Guide Pyramid.
• Discuss role of exercise in weight loss and control.
• Instruct client to jog 45 minutes a day.
• Suggest food substitutions that will reduce fat intake.
• Provide a list of local support groups and weight-loss programs.
• Instruct client to exercise at least three times a week, gradually increasing time.

NCLEX-PN Exam Preparation

1. Which of the following would be an expected finding when assessing a client who has morbid obesity?
   a. Weight 310 lbs., height 5'10".
   b. Serum cholesterol 180 mg/dL.
   c. The client states that he exercises regularly.
   d. The client's parents are obese.

2. When planning care for a client who has a diagnosis of malnutrition, the nurse would include which of these goals?
   a. Will gain 1 to 2 lbs. per week.
   b. Will consume a 1,200-kcal diet.
   c. Will state need to exercise 60 minutes five times per week.
   d. Will limit fat intake to less than 15% of total kcal.

3. When planning care for a client who has stomatitis, the nurse should give priority to which of these treatment measures?
   a. Provide a quiet environment to aid digestion.
   b. Administer viscous lidocaine prior to each meal.
   c. Assess the client's gag reflex.
   d. Encourage the client to use a mouthwash after each meal.

4. During the initial assessment, you discover that your client has a small, painless, dark-colored lesion on his tongue. Your client states that the sore has been in his mouth for several months. Which of the following interventions should be your next priority?
   a. Document your findings and notify the health care provider.
   b. Tell the client to report any changes in the size or color of the lesion.
   c. Prepare the client for a biopsy of the lesion.
   d. Immediately notify the charge nurse.

5. Your client has been diagnosed with candidiasis. Which of the following would you most likely observe during the oral assessment?
   a. Painful, small, round ulcerations
   b. Areas of fluid-filled blisters on the lips
   c. Dark, painless ulceration on the tongue
   d. White patches on the tongue

6. A 58-year-old male is admitted to your unit with the diagnosis of esophageal cancer with erosion to the middle portion of the esophagus. Which of the following is most important to immediately report?
   a. Aspiration pneumonia
   b. Uncontrolled bleeding from the mouth
   c. Weight loss
   d. Difficulty swallowing

7. During the insertion of a nasogastric tube, your client begins to gag. Your next action should be to:
   a. withdraw the tube completely
   b. briefly halt the insertion
   c. have the client sip water to assist the tube to advance
   d. check for placement

8. Your client is to receive a tube feeding of Ensure (240 mL/can) at a rate of 60 mL/hr. You pour one can into the feeding bag and set the machine rate. You can anticipate that the bag will empty in:
   a. 2 hours
   b. 1 hour
   c. 4 hours
   d. 6 hours

9. Your client's physician has prescribed an antibiotic for your client with a peptic ulcer. He asks you why this type of medication is being given. Your response should be:
   a. "This medication will help reduce the gastric acid in your stomach."
   b. "The antibiotic will help to rid the stomach of the *H. pylori* bacteria."
   c. "It will increase the production of mucus in the stomach."
   d. "It is used only as a prophylactic to prevent colonization of bacteria in the stomach."

10. You must develop a nursing care plan for a client who will be undergoing a partial gastrectomy. You are focusing on the dumping syndrome. Which of the following should be included for client teaching?
    a. Diet low in protein and fats
    b. Taking a walk before each meal
    c. Eating three meals a day
    d. Resting in a semirecumbent position after eating

Answers for Review Questions, as well as discussion of Case Study Critical Thinking questions, appear in Appendix V.

Cultural Care STRATEGIES

Integrating Cultural Diversity in Client Education

Judith Lightfoot, a 29-year-old Native American, comes in to see the nurse about her diet for diabetes. While the nurse and Judith are talking, Judith says, "I really can't follow the diabetic diet you gave me. You see, on our Indian reservation everybody shares what we have. We don't have much food at our house, so if I have special food I can't save it for the week. I need to share it with anybody in the house who is hungry. Of course, that means that some days we don't have anything to eat. But things usually work out. It is part of our culture to be generous with what we have and we will worry about tomorrow when the times comes."

When a client is from a different culture, the nurse should be alert for cultural barriers that may interfere with the treatment regimen or effective client education. Initial assessment is necessary to determine whether the client understands the language being spoken. If necessary, an interpreter should be obtained to serve as translator. When interpreters are not available at an agency, a telephone translator service may be an option. In some cases, a bilingual family member can help. Children should be avoided as interpreters, since the child may not be able to translate medical information adequately, and in some cultures getting information from a child is not acceptable (Davidhizar & Brownson, 2000).

Differences in Dialect

It is important for nurses to be aware that there can be significant contrasts within cultural groups. For example, there are 10 Hispanic/Latino groups, over 20 Asian-American/Pacific Islander groups, and over 500 Native American tribal groups. In addition, census-defined African-Americans may come from non-African countries such as Haiti, Jamaica, and Panama. Significant differences in language and dialects within a culture may exist. Thus, even though an interpreter may speak the language of the client—for example, Spanish—communication may not be clear.

Differences in Communication Variables

It is important to assess not only language but also the essential elements of communication of the language including dialect, style (language and social situations), volume (silence), use of touch, context of speech (emotional tone), and kinetics (gesture, stance, and eye behavior). If the nurse always associates a soft voice with timidity, lack of assertiveness, and incompetence, the cultural reasons for this behavior may be ignored. If the nurse always associates loudness with aggressiveness, while in the client's culture loudness has a different meaning, behavior may be misinterpreted.

Even when individuals speak the same language, communication may be difficult. The meaning of words and how facts are presented may vary based on life experiences and cultural context. For example, "That person is a real dog" may have a positive meaning in one cultural setting while having a negative meaning in another.

Differences in Gender and Family Member Roles

Gender and gender roles can significantly influence attitudes about health and health education. Taboos related to sexual behavior have special significance for client education. In male-dominated societies (Arab, Hispanic, and many Asian societies), information and decision making must be given to the male. Women are expected to be modest and submissive. Thus, education about sexual matters needs to take into account who should be present in the room and who is appropriate (Davidhizar & Brownson, 2000).

Literacy/Educational Handouts

Many English-speaking people have difficulty understanding medical terminology. If English is a second language, medical terminology is even more challenging. When written instructions are used, the language, the literacy, and the reading level of the client should be evaluated. Written handouts should match the client's reading level.

Nursing Implications

- **Before teaching, assess the client's understanding of English.** If the nurse and the client do not speak the same language, an interpreter may be necessary in order to provide effective teaching. If the client and family can speak English but either speaks English as a second language or is from another culture, the nurse should be aware that there may be obstacles to communication.
- **Match client education materials to the literacy level of the client.** If a client is from another culture, both literacy level and understanding of medical terminology should be assessed. Select appropriate educational materials that can be understood.

Self-Reflection Questions

1. Are you an effective teacher?
2. If your client cannot understand English, what translating services are available to assist in client teaching?
3. What teaching materials are available that can assist in client education?

chapter 19

Caring for Clients with Gallbladder, Liver, and Pancreatic Disorders

CARING tip

"Learn all you can about diabetes. It often causes or complicates many other diagnoses."

Nettie Seale, RN, MS • Instructor of Practical Nursing • Kiamichi Technology Center • Stigler Campus • Stigler, Oklahoma

LEARNING outcomes

After completing this chapter, you will be able to:

- Identify the major structures and functions of the accessory digestive organs: the liver, gallbladder, and pancreas.
- Describe the pathophysiology, manifestations, and management of commonly occurring disorders of the gallbladder, liver, and exocrine pancreas.
- Discuss nursing implications for dietary and pharmacologic interventions related to the gallbladder, liver, and exocrine pancreas.
- Provide appropriate nursing care for the client who has surgery of the gallbladder, liver, or pancreas.
- Use the nursing process to assess, plan, provide, and evaluate care for clients with disorders of the gallbladder, liver, or exocrine pancreas.

MediaLink

 www.prenhall.com/burke

Use the above address to access the free, interactive Companion Website created for this textbook. Get hints, instant feedback, and textbook references to chapter-related multiple choice questions. Link to other interesting sites.

Disorders of the accessory digestive organs, the gallbladder, liver, and exocrine pancreas may present as solitary problems or may be related to other disease processes. One organ's functioning frequently affects that of another. Duct inflammation or obstruction as well as changes in the multiple functions of the gallbladder, liver, and exocrine pancreas are some of the problems that can adversely affect a person's health.

Clients who have a gallbladder, liver, or exocrine pancreatic disorder may experience severe pain, altered body image, and a host of metabolic and nutritional disturbances. Nursing care addresses the client's and family's physiologic and psychosocial needs through attention to individualized care planning.

Structure and Function of the Accessory Digestive Organs

LIVER AND GALLBLADDER

The liver is the largest gland in the body, weighing about 3 lbs. (1.4 kg) in the average-sized adult. It is located in the right side of the abdomen, inferior to the diaphragm and anterior to the stomach (see Figure 18-1). The liver has four lobes: right (the largest), left, caudate, and quadrate. It is encased in a fibrous capsule and covered by a layer of visceral peritoneum.

Each lobe contains many **lobules,** the basic functional units of the liver. Within each lobule, plates of **hepatocytes** (liver cells) are arranged like the spokes of a wheel out from a central vein (Figure 19-1 ◆). Each lobule receives oxygen-rich blood from a branch of the hepatic artery and nutrient-rich venous blood from the digestive tract via the portal vein. Arterial and venous blood flows through enlarged capillaries *(sinusoids)* into the central vein. The sinusoids are lined with

macrophages called *Kupffer cells,* which remove debris, such as bacteria and aged blood cells, from the blood.

Hepatocytes produce bile and perform many metabolic functions. Bile is a greenish, watery solution containing bile salts, cholesterol, bilirubin, electrolytes, water, and phospholipids. Bile is necessary to emulsify and absorb fats. The bile flows out through tiny channels called *canaliculi* to the bile ducts.

The liver's primary activities can be categorized as metabolic, hematologic, and digestive. It performs many different functions essential to life:

- Metabolizes carbohydrates, proteins, and fats
- Eliminates old blood cells, cellular debris, and bacteria
- Inactivates toxins and foreign substances such as alcohol and drugs
- Synthesizes plasma proteins and enzymes
- Metabolizes or inactivates hormones
- Stores blood, vitamins, and minerals
- Produces and excretes bile

Liver cells make from 700 to 1,200 mL of bile every day. When bile is not needed for digestion, the *sphincter of Oddi* (located at the point at which bile enters the duodenum) is closed, and the bile backs up the cystic duct into the gallbladder for storage.

Bile is concentrated and stored in the *gallbladder,* a small sac on the inferior surface of the liver (Figure 19-2 ◆). When food containing fats enters the duodenum, hormones stimulate the gallbladder to secrete bile into the cystic duct. The cystic duct joins the hepatic duct to form the common bile duct, from which bile enters the duodenum.

PANCREAS

The pancreas, a gland located between the stomach and small intestine, produces enzymes necessary for digestion. It extends across the abdomen, with its tail next to the spleen and its head next to the duodenum (see Figure 18-1). The body and tail of the pancreas lie behind the stomach and the peritoneal membrane *(retroperitoneal).* The pancreas is actually two organs in one, having both exocrine and endocrine structures and functions. The exocrine portion secretes alkaline pancreatic juice into the pancreatic duct. The pancreatic duct joins with the common bile duct just before it enters the duodenum (Figure 19-2). The pancreas also has endocrine functions (see Chapter 17).

Every day, the pancreas produces 1 to 1.5 L of pancreatic juice containing bicarbonate to neutralize the acidic chyme as it enters the duodenum. The increased pH promotes digestion in the small intestine. Pancreatic secretion is controlled by the vagus nerve and the hormones secretin and cholecystokinin. Pancreatic juice contains enzymes that can digest all categories of foods: *Lipase* promotes fat breakdown and absorption; *amylase* completes starch digestion; and *trypsin, chymotrypsin,* and *carboxypeptidase* are responsible for half of all protein digestion. *Nucleases,* which digest nucleic acids, are also present in pancreatic juice.

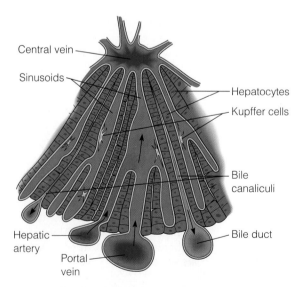

Figure 19-1. ◆ A liver lobule with plates of hepatocytes, the central vein, bile duct, portal vein, and hepatic artery.

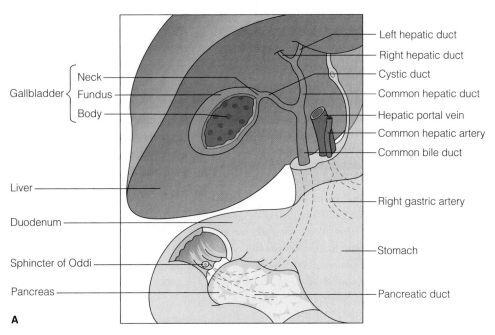

Figure 19-2. ◆ The gallbladder, common bile duct, and sphincter of Oddi.

Gallbladder Disorders

Cholelithiasis and Cholecystitis

Cholelithiasis is the formation of stones *(calculi)* within the gallbladder or biliary duct system. Gallstone formation is the most common cause of obstructed bile flow into the small intestine.

PATHOPHYSIOLOGY

Most gallstones are formed in the gallbladder. Gallstones usually contain cholesterol, bile pigments, and small amounts of other materials, such as calcium salts. Risk factors for cholelithiasis include middle age, female gender, obesity, pregnancy, and use of oral contraceptives or estrogen therapy.

CLINICAL alert

Use the 4 Fs to remember the risk factors for gallstones: Fat, forty, female, and fertile.

Cholecystitis is inflammation of the gallbladder. It usually results from stones obstructing the cystic or common bile duct (Figure 19-3 ◆). The obstruction causes increased pressure and ischemia of the gallbladder, as well as chemical irritation from the bile. The gallbladder becomes acutely inflamed as a result. The inflammation causes edema and further obstruction

of bile flow. Chronic cholecystitis is caused by repeated attacks of acute cholecystitis.

If the common bile duct is obstructed, bile backs up into the liver and possibly the pancreas, producing jaundice, pain, possible hepatic damage, pancreatitis (discussed later in this chapter), or sepsis.

MANIFESTATIONS

Cholecystitis is classified as either acute or chronic. *Acute cholecystitis* is characterized by severe epigastric or upper right quadrant pain radiating posteriorly to the scapular region.

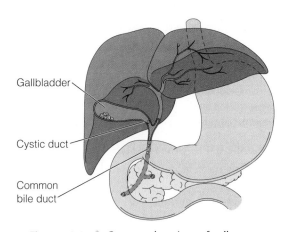

Figure 19-3. ◆ Common locations of gallstones.

This spasmodic pain results from contraction of the ducts and is usually initiated by a high-fat meal. *Chronic cholecystitis* generally has a more moderate presentation. See Box 19-1 for the manifestations of acute and chronic cholecystitis.

Perforation of the gallbladder and peritonitis are possible complications of cholecystitis. Other complications include infection, pancreatitis, fistula formation, and cancer.

COLLABORATIVE CARE

Gallstones often are diagnosed through a right upper quadrant *abdominal ultrasound.* This test is noninvasive and requires no special preparation, except the caution that the conductive gel used during the exam is cold. An *oral cholecystogram* is performed in nonacute situations. In this study, an oral dye is used to assess the gallbladder's ability to concentrate and excrete bile. *Gallbladder scans,* also called liver-biliary scans, use nuclear medicine techniques to assess acute cholecystitis. Laboratory tests may show elevated white blood cell (WBC), serum bilirubin, alkaline phosphase, alanine transaminase (ALT), and aspartate transaminase (AST) levels.

Because dietary fat stimulates gallbladder contraction, clients are usually placed on a low-fat diet. Examples of foods to avoid are listed in Box 19-2. Clients who are obese are encouraged to lose weight to reduce surgical risks. All food and fluids may be withheld during an attack of acute cholecystitis; total parenteral nutrition may be used to maintain the client's nutritional status.

Pharmacology

Clients who do not have complications from gallstones or for whom surgery would pose a high risk (e.g., a frail older adult) may be treated with oral bile acids to dissolve stones. Ursodeoxycholic acid (UDCA) or chenodiol (Chenix) may be used to treat small cholesterol stones. Nurses need to monitor liver enzymes and watch for possible diarrhea in clients taking

> ## BOX 19-2
> ## HIGH-FAT FOODS TO AVOID IN CHOLELITHIASIS
>
> - Whole milk products (e.g., cheese, cream, ice cream)
> - Deep-fried foods and pastries (e.g., donuts, French fries, batter-fried fish)
> - Avocados
> - Sausage, bacon, hot dogs
> - Gravies made with fat or cream
> - Most nuts
> - Snack foods (e.g., potato chips, tortilla chips)
> - Peanut butter
> - Chocolate

these drugs. Several years of therapy may be required, and stones frequently recur after treatment is stopped. *Extracorporeal shock wave lithotripsy (ESWL),* a procedure in which stones are fragmented by shock waves, may be used in conjunction with drug treatment.

If infection is suspected, antibiotics may be prescribed. Parenteral narcotic analgesics such as morphine may be necessary to relieve the pain.

Surgery

Most clients with symptomatic gallbladder disease are treated with *laparoscopic cholecystectomy.* This minimally invasive surgery allows a hospital stay of 24 hours or less, and the client often is able to return to work within a week. See Box 19-3 for nursing care of the client having laparoscopic cholecystectomy.

> ## CLINICAL alert
>
> During laparoscopic cholecystectomy, the abdomen is inflated with carbon dioxide. This can cause shoulder pain after surgery. Carefully assess the client's pain and provide adequate analgesia. Inform the client that as the gas is absorbed, the pain will be relieved.

Nursing care for clients who require a traditional cholecystectomy is similar to that required by any client having abdominal surgery. (See Chapter 7 for more information about care of the surgical client.) Coughing, deep breathing, and early ambulation are vital to prevent respiratory complications because of the upper abdominal incision.

Clients may return from surgery with a T-tube (Figure 19-4 ◆). Inserted after common bile duct exploration, a T-tube keeps the duct open and promotes bile flow until edema decreases. Excess bile is collected in a drainage bag secured below the surgical site. Nursing care of a client with a T-tube is outlined in Box 19-4.

> ## BOX 19-1
> ## MANIFESTATIONS OF CHOLECYSTITIS
>
> ### ACUTE CHOLECYSTITIS
> - Epigastric or right upper abdominal pain; may radiate to back
> - Pain precipitated by high-fat meal
> - Right upper quadrant guarding and tenderness
> - Nausea and vomiting
> - Fever
> - Possible jaundice
>
> ### CHRONIC CHOLECYSTITIS
> - Fatty food intolerance
> - Belching
> - Vague gastric symptoms
> - Pain after eating

BOX 19-3
NURSING CARE CHECKLIST

LAPAROSCOPIC CHOLECYSTECTOMY

Before Surgery

☑ Reinforce preoperative teaching, including the procedure, postoperative care, and pain management.

☑ Provide routine preoperative care as outlined in Chapter 7.

After Surgery

☑ Monitor vital signs every 15 minutes for 2 hours or until stable, then every 4 hours until discharge.

☑ Provide routine postoperative care.

☑ Assess location and severity of pain; provide analgesia as needed.

☑ Assist out of bed and with ambulation as ordered.

☑ Reinforce and provide postoperative and discharge teaching:
   ☑ Wound care
   ☑ Pain management
   ☑ Diet and activity
   ☑ Medications
   ☑ Follow-up appointments and care

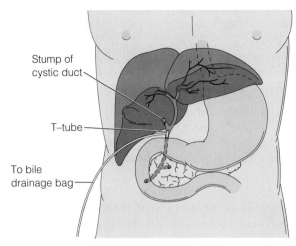

Figure 19-4. ◆ T-tube placement in the common bile duct. Bile flows by gravity into a collection device placed below the level of the abdomen.

Labels: Stump of cystic duct; T–tube; To bile drainage bag

■ Administer prescribed antiemetics. *Giving antiemetic medication before meals and procedures helps promote food intake and prevent vomiting.*

■ Promptly remove noxious items and odor-producing substances (e.g., food, commodes). *The sight or smell of food and noxious substances can stimulate or aggravate nausea.*

■ Provide oral care and clean bedding (as needed) after each emesis. *This reduces nausea stimuli.*

NURSING CARE

ASSESSING

Assessment data to collect on clients with suspected gallbladder disease is outlined in Box 19-5.

DIAGNOSING, PLANNING, AND IMPLEMENTING

ACUTE PAIN

■ Teach clients to avoid fat in their diets. *Fat initiates gallbladder contractions and is a stimulus for pain.*

■ Administer narcotic analgics as ordered for severe pain. *Severe pain can cause muscle spasm and increased GI symptoms. Parenteral analgesia may be required.*

■ Place in Fowler's position. *Fowler's position decreases pressure on the inflamed area and may help relieve pain.*

NAUSEA

■ Monitor complaints of nausea. Document amount, color, and consistency of any emesis. Monitor food and fluid intake. *Nausea may result from cholecystitis or be caused by pain. Nausea increases the risk of a nutritional deficit; vomiting can lead to fluid volume deficit.*

BOX 19-4
NURSING CARE CHECKLIST

T-TUBE CARE

☑ Connect T-tube sterile container; keep the tube below the level of the surgical wound.

☑ Monitor color and consistency of drainage; record amount on output record. Up to 500 mL of drainage is expected in the first 24 hours after surgery, decreasing to under 200 mL in 2 to 3 days; thereafter, drainage is minimal. Initial drainage may be blood tinged, changing to green-brown. Report excessive drainage to the charge nurse or physician immediately (after 48 hours, drainage greater than 500 mL is considered excessive).

☑ Place in Fowler's position to promote drainage.

☑ Assess skin for bile leakage during dressing changes; apply a protective skin barrier if necessary.

☑ Teach client how to manage tube when turning, ambulating, and performing activities of daily living.

☑ Clamp the T-tube only as ordered by the physician.

☑ If indicated, teach the client care of the T-tube, how to clamp it, and signs of infection.

BOX 19-5
ASSESSING CLIENTS WITH GALLBLADDER DISEASE

SUBJECTIVE DATA

- Pain: Location, character, radiation; frequency and timing, relationship to meals and foods; aggravating factors, relief measures and their effectiveness
- Nausea and vomiting; relationship to pain, meals, foods
- Epigastric upset or heartburn
- Usual diet and effect of symptoms on diet
- Previous diagnosis of gallbladder disease and its treatment

OBJECTIVE DATA

- Observe:
  - General appearance; apparent nutritional status
  - Color, consistency, and amount of any emesis
  - Color and consistency of feces
  - Color of skin and sclera, presence of jaundice
- Inspect abdomen for distention.
- Auscultate bowel sounds.
- Palpate abdomen (especially right upper quadrant) for tenderness and guarding.

- Withhold food and fluids during episodes of nausea and vomiting. Offer cold, low-fat or fat-free foods and foods with little odor in small quantities when the client is able to eat. *Attempting to eat when nauseous may precipitate vomiting. Cold, low-fat foods are better tolerated, as are small quantities rather than large meals.*

RISK FOR IMPAIRED GAS EXCHANGE

- Assist the client who has had an open (traditional) cholecystectomy to turn, deep breathe, and cough at least every 2 hours; use incentive spirometry every hour while awake, and ambulate at least four times daily. *These interventions help expand the lungs and prevent accumulation of secretions in the lungs following a traditional cholecystectomy. Clients may have difficulty ventilating all lung areas because of the high abdominal incision.*
- Assist with splinting the incision during coughing and deep breathing. *Splinting the incision with a blanket or pillow reduces the discomfort of deep breathing and coughing.*
- Monitor temperature every 4 hours; promptly report elevations to the charge nurse or physician. *An elevated temperature may indicate infection.*

EVALUATING

To evaluate the effectiveness of nursing interventions, collect data related to level of comfort, ability to consume the ordered diet and fluids, respiratory status, and freedom from infection.

Discharge Considerations

Clients with cholelithiasis may manage their disease at home with medical interventions, or they may require prompt surgical intervention. Reinforce teaching about the disease, prescribed medications, diagnostic procedures, and treatment options. Discuss the relationship of food intake to episodes of acute cholecystitis, and the importance of maintaining a low-fat, low-kilocalorie diet if indicated. Explain the role of bile and the function of the gallbladder in terms that the client and family can understand.

Provide preoperative teaching, discussing what to expect before and after surgery. Discuss measures to reduce discomfort, promote healing, and prevent complications.

After surgery, prepare the client for discharge and home care. Discuss pain control, monitoring for and preventing infection, and T-tube care. Include instructions about activities, diet, and returning to work. Inform about signs or symptoms to report to the physician.

Refer to a dietitian to review low-fat foods; include the person preparing foods. Most clients start with a low-fat diet and gradually add fatty foods as tolerated. Refer the client to home care services as indicated.

Nursing Process Case Study
■ CLIENT WITH CHOLELITHIASIS

Joyce Red Wing is a 44-year-old member of the Chickasaw tribe. Recently, she has noticed a dull pain in her upper abdomen that gets worse after eating fatty foods; the pain is accompanied by nausea. She remembers having similar pain after the birth of her last child. The diagnosis of cholelithiasis is made, and Ms. Red Wing is admitted for a laparoscopic cholecystectomy.

Assessment Ms. Red Wing's admission history reveals that her usual diet consists of fatty foods, particularly tacos or fried bread and biscuits with gravy for breakfast. She reports "not wanting to eat much of anything lately." She states she has never had surgery before and hopes "everything goes well." She has a good understanding of the procedure to be done. Physical assessment findings: T 100° F (37.7° C); BP 130/84; P 88; R 20. Weight 130 lbs. (59 kg), a 5-pound weight loss from her usual; 5'3" (160 cm) tall. Abdomen tender to palpation in the upper right quadrant. No jaundice, chills, or other evidence of complications noted.

Diagnosis The following nursing diagnoses are identified for Ms. Red Wing:

- Anxiety related to concerns about surgery
- Acute Pain related to surgery

- Deficient Knowledge: Low Fat Diet related to lack of nutritional information

Expected Outcomes The expected outcomes specify that Ms. Red Wing will:

- Verbalize reduced anxiety related to undergoing surgery.
- Maintain adequate pain control postoperatively.
- Follow prescribed diet postoperatively.

Planning and Implementation The following interventions are planned and implemented:

- Teach about the gallbladder and the function of bile.
- Discuss pre- and postoperative care, including plans for discharge, pain management, wound care, activities, and follow-up.
- Provide analgesia as needed.
- Review specific high-fat foods to avoid and ways to maintain weight.

Evaluation Ms. Red Wing is discharged the morning following surgery. She has no signs of infection and is able to care for her incisions. She identifies the importance of eating a low-fat diet and keeping her weight stable, as well as gradually resuming activities. Ms. Red Wing states that she "is glad it is over, but it wasn't as bad as I thought it would be at first." She has an appointment to see her surgeon in 1 week.

 Critical Thinking in the Nursing Process

1. What is the rationale for a low-fat diet with cholelithiasis? Discuss nutritional practices as they relate to cholelithiasis and Ms. Red Wing's culture.
2. Why would it be important to place Ms. Red Wing in Fowler's position after surgery?
3. List five areas to cover in predischarge teaching for Ms. Red Wing.

Cancer of the Gallbladder

Gallbladder cancer is rare, primarily affecting people over 65. Women are more likely to develop the disorder. Clients with cancer of the gallbladder complain of intense pain in the right upper quadrant of the abdomen; a mass may be palpated in the region. Jaundice and weight loss usually accompany the pain. Most gallbladder cancers metastasize via the blood, lymph system, or through direct extension; the liver is most commonly affected. Most cancers of the gallbladder cannot be treated surgically unless they are found at an early stage incidental to another surgical procedure. Most clients with primary cancer of the gallbladder die within 1 year.

 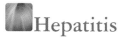

Liver Disorders

When liver function is impaired by inflammation, cell damage, or cancer, the function of all other body systems is affected.

Hepatitis

Hepatitis is inflammation of the liver. It usually is caused by a virus, but also may be caused by alcohol, toxins (such as drugs), or gallbladder disease. Acute and chronic forms of hepatitis exist. Cirrhosis, discussed in the next section, is a possible consequence of hepatic cell damage resulting from hepatitis.

PATHOPHYSIOLOGY

Although the underlying pathophysiology of hepatitis varies, the general manifestations are similar. Much depends on the degree of liver damage and the client's concurrent health status.

Viral Hepatitis

At least six different viruses (designated by letters of the alphabet) can cause hepatitis. Hepatitis A virus (HAV) and hepatitis B virus (HBV) are the most common, although the incidence of hepatitis C (HCV) is increasing. Viral infection causes liver cell injury and necrosis. The liver cell damage may be directly caused by the virus or may occur as a result of the body's immune response to the virus. The manifestations of viral hepatitis are similar for all types, but other characteristics of the disease vary. Table 19-1 ◆ compares the onset, incubation, mode of transmission, and other characteristics of different types of viral hepatitis.

Hepatitis A causes epidemics and sporadic cases of hepatitis. Transmitted by the fecal–oral route, it frequently occurs in crowded, unsanitary living conditions. Contaminated food, water, or shellfish often are responsible for outbreaks of hepatitis A.

Hepatitis B is usually transmitted by blood transfusion or contaminated needles, but also may be spread by sexual contact and from an infected mother to her fetus. *Carriers* can transmit HBV while having no symptoms of the disease. The risk of liver cancer is significant in clients infected with hepatitis B. Health care workers are at risk for hepatitis B. Following standard precautions and obtaining hepatitis B immunization are important preventive strategies.

TABLE 19-1 TYPES OF VIRAL HEPATITIS

	HEPATITIS A (HAV)	HEPATITIS B (HBV)	HEPATITIS C (HCV)	HEPATITIS D (HDV OR DELTA HEPATITIS)	HEPATITIS E (HEV)	HEPATITIS G (HGV)
INCUBATION (IN WEEKS)	2–6	8–24	5–12	3–13	3–6	Unknown
ONSET	Abrupt	Slow	Slow	Abrupt	Abrupt	Abrupt or slow
TRANSMISSION	Fecal–oral	Blood and body fluids; perinatal	Blood and body fluids	Blood and body fluids; possible perinatal	Fecal–oral	Blood
COMMUNICABLE	1 week before onset; minimal after onset of jaundice	1–2 months before symptoms; when HBsAg present in blood	When HCV present in blood	When HDVAg present in blood	Rarely spread person to person	Unknown
CARRIER STATE	No	Yes	Yes	Yes	Yes	Probable
POSSIBLE COMPLICATIONS	Rare	Chronic hepatitis, cirrhosis, liver cancer	Chronic hepatitis, cirrhosis, liver cancer	Chronic hepatitis, cirrhosis, fulminant hepatitis	May be severe in pregnant women	Chronic viremia
LABORATORY FINDINGS	Anti-HAV antibodies	Positive HBsAg; anti-HBV antibodies	Anti-HCV antibodies	Positive HDVAg early; anti-HDV antibodies later	Anti-HEV antibodies	Anti-HGV antibodies
PREVENTION	Hepatitis A vaccine (primary dose + booster in 6–12 months)	Hepatitis B vaccine (HBV) (primary dose + second 1–2 months later + third 2–5 months after second)	None	HBV vaccine	None	None
PROPHYLAXIS	Standard immune globulin before or within 2 weeks of exposure	Hepatitis B immune globulin (HBIG) within 1–2 days of exposure; second dose 28–30 days after exposure	None	See hepatitis B prophylaxis	None	None

Hepatitis C is nearly always transmitted by blood and contaminated needles. This type of viral hepatitis affects African Americans and Mexican Americans more frequently than whites. It often leads to chronic liver disease, and is the most common indication for liver transplant. A vaccine has been developed, but is not commonly administered.

The *hepatitis delta virus (HDV)* causes infection only in people who have active hepatitis B. It causes more severe infection, and may lead to *fulminant hepatitis* with widepread liver necrosis and failure.

Chronic Hepatitis

Chronic hepatitis can be classified as persistent or active. *Chronic persistent hepatitis* does not seriously affect liver function. It may follow either HBV or HCV hepatitis infections. The client has mild, nonspecific symptoms such as general malaise and fatigue, as well as an enlarged liver. *Chronic active hepatitis,* by contrast, progresses rapidly to cirrhosis and liver failure. Again, the most common cause of chronic active hepatitis is HBV or HCV infection.

Noninfectious Hepatitis

Alcoholic hepatitis is acute or chronic inflammation of the liver caused by alcohol. While it often is reversible, alcoholic hepatitis can lead to necrosis of liver cells. It is the most common risk factor for cirrhosis (discussed in the next section of this chapter) in the United States. Many drugs (e.g., acetaminophen and tetracyclines) and other toxins (such as poisonous mushrooms, heavy metals, and carbon tetrachloride) can damage the liver, leading to inflammation and necrosis *(toxic hepatitis)*. Interruption of normal bile flow due to cholelithiasis and blockage of the bile duct also can lead to inflammation of the liver, a condition known as *hepatobiliary hepatitis*.

MANIFESTATIONS

The manifestations of hepatitis range from asymptomatic infection to a rapidly fatal disease. The course of acute viral hepatitis generally follows three phases.

The *preicteric* (before jaundice) or *prodromal phase* may have an abrupt or insidious onset. The *icteric (jaundice) phase* of the disease develops after 5 to 10 days. Early manifestations may worsen when jaundice develops, then begin to improve. **Jaundice** occurs when serum bilirubin levels are high, causing the skin, mucous membranes, and sclera of the eyes to appear yellow. The *posticteric* or *convalescent phase* is characterized by an increasing sense of well-being, return of appetite, and the disappearance of jaundice. Box 19-6 summarizes the manifestations of each phase of hepatitis.

COLLABORATIVE CARE

There is no specific treatment for hepatitis. Prevention, early identification of the disease, and teaching are vital.

Diagnostic Tests

■ Blood is drawn to assess for *viral antigens* (e.g., hepatitis B surface antigen [HBsAg]) or *antibodies* to the viral agents that cause hepatitis (see Table 19-1).

BOX 19-6
MANIFESTATIONS OF ACUTE VIRAL HEPATITIS

PREICTERIC OR PRODROMAL PHASE
- "Flulike" symptoms: Malaise, fatigue, headache, muscle aches, nasal discharge, sore throat
- Gastrointestinal: Anorexia, nausea, vomiting, diarrhea or constipation
- Joint pain
- Mild and constant right upper abdominal pain

ICTERIC PHASE
- Jaundice
- Pruritus
- Clay-colored stools, dark urine

POSTICTERIC OR CONVALESCENT PHASE
- Well-being improves, energy increases
- Jaundice resolves

■ *Liver function tests,* including serum *ALT, alkaline phophatase (ALP), AST, gamma glutamyl transferase (GGT),* and *lactic dehydrogenase (LDH)* are measured. Serum levels of these enzymes increase when the liver is inflamed or damaged.

■ *Serum bilirubin* levels also are measured. Total bilirubin usually is elevated, as are both direct (conjugated) and indirect (unconjugated) bilirubin levels. Unconjugated bilirubin rises because the liver does not effectively metabolize it; conjugated bilirubin increases because excretion is impaired.

■ *Prothrombin time* may be prolonged if the liver is not able to manufacture the protein needed for blood coagulation.

Prevention

Vaccines and immune globulin injections are available to prevent hepatitis A and B. Vaccines are recommended for people who are at increased risk for exposure to the disease. Immune globulin is used for postexposure prophylaxis, to prevent the disease after known or suspected contact with the virus. Table 19-1 lists recommended immunizations.

Hepatitis A vaccine is recommended for adults travelling internationally, homosexual men, drug users, and people with clotting disorders, hepatitis C, or an occupational risk. It also is recommended for children over the age of 2 who live in areas where the incidence of hepatitis A is high.

When exposure to hepatitis A virus has occurred, illness often can be prevented by a single dose of immune globulin (IG) given within 2 weeks of exposure. IG is recommended for people in close contact with someone who has hepatitis A, for childcare workers where a case of hepatitis A has been identified, and for restaurant patrons where a food handler has developed hepatitis A.

population
FOCUS

People Who Should Receive Hepatitis B Vaccine

- People at risk for sexual transmission: Homosexual or bisexual men, prostitutes, people with multiple partners or recently diagnosed sexually transmitted disease
- Injection drug users
- Male prison inmates
- People on hemodialysis
- Health care workers
- Clients and staff of institutions for the developmentally disabled
- High-risk populations: Alaska Natives, Pacific Islanders, and immigrants from HBV endemic areas
- Household members and partners of HBV carriers
- International travelers to HBV endemic areas
- Recipients of certain blood products such as clotting factors

Hepatitis B vaccine is recommended for all infants, adolescents who have not been immunized, and adults at risk for exposure to hepatitis B. All health care workers including nurses should be vaccinated. Box 19-7 summarizes who should receive hepatitis B vaccine.

Following exposure to hepatitis B, both hepatitis B vaccine and hepatitis B immune globulin (HBIG) are given to prevent infection. With perinatal exposure, infants are given both HBIG and the vaccine within 24 hours of birth.

Treatment

There currently is no cure for viral hepatitis. Clients are encouraged to get adequate rest, maintain nutritional intake, and avoid strenuous activity, alcohol, and agents that are toxic to the liver. Bed rest is necessary only when symptoms are severe. Intravenous fluids may be given if nausea and vomiting interfere with intake. Interferon may be ordered for clients with hepatitis B or C. Potential complementary therapies for hepatitis B and C are discussed in Box 19-8. In most cases, clinical recovery takes 3 to 16 weeks.

NURSING CARE

ASSESSING

Clients with acute hepatitis often present with an abrupt onset of classic manifestations of hepatitis. However, clients who have chronic hepatitis may have more vague manifestations. Assessment data to collect for clients with confirmed or suspected hepatitis is presented in Box 19-9.

DIAGNOSING, PLANNING, AND IMPLEMENTING

RISK FOR INFECTION (TRANSMISSION)

- Use standard precautions and meticulous handwashing. *One of the most important goals when caring for clients with acute viral hepatitis is preventing the spread of infection. Proper aseptic technique can stem transmission of the viruses.*
- For clients with hepatitis A, use standard precautions and contact isolation if fecal incontinence is present. *The fecal–oral route is the primary mode of transmission of hepatitis A.*
- Encourage at-risk clients to obtain hepatitis A or hepatitis B immunizations, or both. *Prevention is a key strategy for reducing the incidence and long-term consequences of viral hepatitis.*

ACTIVITY INTOLERANCE

- Encourage to rest as needed to relieve fatigue. *Fatigue and possible weakness are common in clients with hepatitis. Adequate rest promotes optimal immune function and recovery.*
- Plan nursing care activities that promote rest, allowing gradual resumption of activities. *As the client recovers, fatigue and activity tolerance improve.*

COMPLEMENTARY THERAPIES

Hepatitis

Herbalists in Europe have used milk thistle to treat liver disease for over 2,000 years. Silymarin is believed to be the active ingredient in milk thistle. Silymarin helps prevent complications and promote more rapid recovery. It also benefits clients who have liver damage due to toxins, cirrhosis, and alcoholic liver disease. It appears that silymarin:

- Promotes liver cell growth
- Is a powerful antioxidant
- Blocks toxins from entering and damaging liver cells
- Reduces inflammation in the liver

Licorice root also may be used by herbalists to treat hepatitis. Licorice root has both antiviral and anti-inflammatory effects, but long-term use may lead to hypertension and affect fluid and electrolyte balance.

Other herbal remedies may help relieve the adverse effects of interferon (flulike symptoms, fatigue, dizziness, anorexia, nausea, diarrhea, and cough). These include ginger for nausea and St. John's wort for depression. Refer clients interested in complementary therapies for hepatitis to a certified herbalist.

BOX 19-9
ASSESSING CLIENTS WITH HEPATITIS

SUBJECTIVE DATA

- Known or possible exposure to hepatitis virus: Recent travel; close contact with someone who has hepatitis; a high-risk occupation or behaviors; eating where a food handler has been diagnosed with hepatitis; injection drug use
- Recent flulike illness
- Anorexia, nausea, vomiting; change in bowel habits; color of feces and urine
- Pain: Location and character, frequency and timing, aggravating factors
- Change in color of skin or sclera; itching
- History of hepatitis vaccine or prophylaxis

OBJECTIVE DATA

- Observe:
  - General appearance; apparent nutritional status
  - Color of skin and sclera, presence of jaundice
  - Color and consistency of feces; color of urine
- Inspect abdomen for distention.
- Auscultate bowel sounds.
- Palpate abdomen for tenderness.

IMBALANCED NUTRITION: LESS THAN BODY REQUIREMENTS

- Encourage the client to eat smaller, more frequent meals. *Clients with hepatitis often experience significant anorexia and possible nausea. Smaller meals are frequently better tolerated.*
- Help the client select a palatable diet with adequate calories. Suggest supplements such as Ensure as needed to maintain intake. Low-fat diets are sometimes better tolerated. *Sufficient energy is required for healing.*
- Encourage eating more food when nausea and anorexia are minimal. *Many clients with acute hepatitis are nauseated in the afternoon and evening hours.*
- If nausea and vomiting persist, give intravenous fluids as ordered. Monitor fluid and electrolytes, and assess for signs of dehydration. *Prompt assessment of fluid and electrolyte imbalance allows early treatment to maintain homeostasis.*

EVALUATING

To evaluate the effectiveness of nursing care, collect data such as the following:

- Household members remain free of infection.
- Client can verbalize appropriate measures to prevent spreading the disease.
- Client gets adequate rest.
- Weight remains stable.

Discharge Considerations

Most clients with acute viral hepatitis are cared for at home and in community-based settings. Box 19-10 outlines assessment data to collect when evaluating the client's home and community setting for care.

Teach the client, family members, and members of the household how to prevent spread of the disease. Instruct the client with hepatitis A not to prepare food for other members of the family until he or she is no longer infectious. Include instructions for cleaning eating utensils and soiled linens. Emphasize the importance of not sharing toothbrushes, razors, or dirty needles, and the need to abstain from sexual activity until the client is no longer infectious. Discuss the need to undergo follow-up evaluation and to avoid hepatotoxins, such as alcohol and acetaminophen.

BOX 19-10
ASSESSING FOR DISCHARGE

VIRAL HEPATITIS
Client

- Self-care: Ability to perform activities of daily living (ADLs); to prepare and eat a nutritionally sound diet
- Knowledge: Understanding of disease process and spread; preventing spread to others; diet and activity recommendations; liver toxins to avoid; indications for seeking further medical care
- Psychosocial: Willingness to abstain from alcohol, other toxins, and behaviors that place others at risk (e.g., sexual intercourse, sharing needles)
- Home environment: Running water and handwashing facilities; food storage and preparation facilities; access to clean drinking water; atmosphere conducive to eating

Family and Caregivers

- Members of household: People at risk for contracting disease; immunization or protection status; willingness to obtain prophylaxis; ability and willingness to help with food preparation and family responsibilities
- Financial resources: Income; resources for food, dietary supplements, hepatitis prevention, and medical care

Community

- Home health services and community resources for immunizations and prophylaxis
- Financial support options
- Community water and sanitation services

Cirrhosis

Cirrhosis is a chronic liver disease that destroys the structure and function of liver lobules. Because the liver performs so many functions, cirrhosis has devastating effects and often leads to death.

Alcoholic liver disease (*Laënnec's* or *alcoholic cirrhosis*) is the most common type of cirrhosis. Cirrhosis also may result from viral hepatitis or toxic liver damage from drugs or chemicals *(postnecrotic cirrhosis)*, from heart failure, or from obstructed bile flow *(biliary cirrhosis)*.

PATHOPHYSIOLOGY

In cirrhosis, hepatocytes are destroyed and replaced by scar tissue that disrupts blood and bile flow within the liver. Impaired blood flow through the liver increases pressure in the portal venous system, leading to portal hypertension. Obstructed bile outflow damages liver cells. Loss of functioning liver lobules ultimately leads to liver failure.

The manifestations and complications of cirrhosis result both from impaired liver function and from altered blood flow through the portal venous system (Figure 19-5 ◆).

Portal hypertension is elevated blood pressure in the portal vein that carries venous blood from the gut through the liver. Higher pressure forces fluid out of the vessels, contributing to the formation of ascites and congestion of veins in the esophagus, rectum, and abdomen.

Ascites is an accumulation of serous fluid in the peritoneal cavity. Portal hypertension is the primary cause of ascites. Impaired liver function causes a decline in plasma protein production (like albumin), reducing plasma osmotic pressure (see Chapter 5). This allows fluid to escape from blood vessels, leading to ascites and peripheral edema. Fluid and electrolyte imbalances also contribute to edema and ascites.

Splenomegaly (enlargement of the spleen) develops as blood is shunted from the portal system into the splenic vein. Splenomegaly can lead to anemia and low platelet and WBC counts. Low platelets *(thrombocytopenia)* and decreased clotting factor production by the liver lead to increased risk for bleeding. Infection is a risk due to low WBC counts *(leukopenia)*.

Esophageal varices are enlarged, overdistended veins in the distal esophagus that result from portal venous congestion. Clients with esophageal varices are at high risk for bleed-

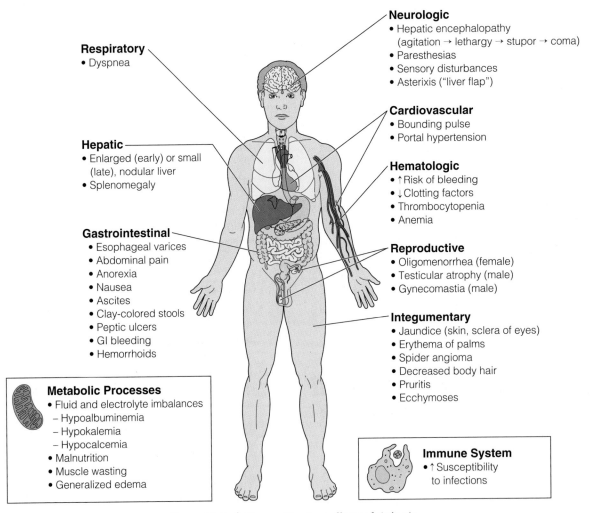

Respiratory
• Dyspnea

Hepatic
• Enlarged (early) or small (late), nodular liver
• Splenomegaly

Gastrointestinal
• Esophageal varices
• Abdominal pain
• Anorexia
• Nausea
• Ascites
• Clay-colored stools
• Peptic ulcers
• GI bleeding
• Hemorrhoids

Metabolic Processes
• Fluid and electrolyte imbalances
  – Hypoalbuminemia
  – Hypokalemia
  – Hypocalcemia
• Malnutrition
• Muscle wasting
• Generalized edema

Neurologic
• Hepatic encephalopathy
  (agitation → lethargy → stupor → coma)
• Paresthesias
• Sensory disturbances
• Asterixis ("liver flap")

Cardiovascular
• Bounding pulse
• Portal hypertension

Hematologic
• ↑Risk of bleeding
• ↓Clotting factors
• Thrombocytopenia
• Anemia

Reproductive
• Oligomenorrhea (female)
• Testicular atrophy (male)
• Gynecomastia (male)

Integumentary
• Jaundice (skin, sclera of eyes)
• Erythema of palms
• Spider angioma
• Decreased body hair
• Pruritis
• Ecchymoses

Immune System
• ↑Susceptibility to infections

Figure 19-5. ◆ The multisystem effects of cirrhosis.

ing. Even high-roughage foods can lead to hemorrhage of these fragile vessels. *Upper gastrointestinal bleeding* is a frequent complication of cirrhosis. Bleeding, which can be massive, may result from varices, gastritis, or peptic ulcer.

As the liver is progressively destroyed, its ability to metabolize proteins is impaired. Ammonia and toxic nitrogenous wastes accumulate in the blood. These substances affect the central nervous system. *Hepatic encephalopathy* is characterized by altered levels of consciousness, cognition, and motor function. *Hepatorenal syndrome* (renal failure associated with end-stage liver disease) also may develop. Its cause is unknown, and treatment generally is ineffective.

COLLABORATIVE CARE

The goals of cirrhosis treatment are to prevent further liver damage and manage the effects and complications of cirrhosis. It is vital to include the family in the plan of care, particularly if alcohol abuse is the cause.

Diagnostic Tests

A number of laboratory and diagnostic tests may be ordered:

- A *complete blood count (CBC)* is done evaluate possible anemia, leukopenia, and thrombocytopenia.
- *Blood chemistries,* including liver function tests, serum electrolytes and glucose, protein, albumin, and ammonia levels are done to evaluate liver function and its effects.
- *Coagulation studies* are ordered to evaluate the client's risk for bleeding.

Liver
Diaphragm
Lung
6th rib

A   **B**   **C**

Figure 19-6. ◆ Liver biopsy. (A) The client exhales completely and holds breath, bringing the liver and diaphragm to their highest position. The needle is inserted between the 6th and 7th ribs. (B) A small amount of saline is injected to clear the needle of blood and tissue. (C) A tissue sample is aspirated into the needle. The needle is then withdrawn and pressure is applied to the site.

- A *liver ultrasound* is performed, and a *liver biopsy* (Figure 19-6 ◆) may be ordered to determine the type and severity of cirrhosis. Nursing implications for the procedure are found in Box 19-11.
- An *upper endoscopy* may be done to assess for esophageal varices. (See Box 18-9 for nursing care related to upper endoscopy.)

Dietary and Fluid Management

Abstinence from alcohol is vital for clients with cirrhosis. Dietary support also is essential. The diet should be palatable and include adequate protein and calories. If serum ammonia levels are high or the client has signs of hepatic encephalopathy, dietary protein is restricted. Sodium intake is restricted to

---

BOX 19-11
NURSING CARE CHECKLIST

LIVER BIOPSY

Before the Procedure

☑ Reinforce teaching about the procedure and its purpose.

☑ Keep NPO as ordered, usually 4 to 6 hours before the procedure.

☑ Assess and record baseline vital signs.

☑ Review prothrombin time (PT) and platelet count; administer vitamin K as ordered.

☑ Have the client empty bladder immediately before the test.

☑ Place client in supine position on far right side of bed; turn head to left and extend right arm above head for better visualization of the biopsy site.

During the Procedure

☑ Help client hold breath following expiration to keep diaphragm and liver high in the abdominal cavity during needle insertion (see Figure 19-6).

☑ Obtaining biopsy tissue usually requires only 10 to 15 seconds.

☑ Some pain or discomfort may be experienced during the procedure.

After the Procedure

☑ Apply direct pressure to the site immediately after the needle is removed.

☑ Position client on right side.

☑ Frequently assess site and vital signs for evidence of bleeding; report immediately.

☑ Advise that pain may occur in the right shoulder as the anesthetic loses effect.

☑ Keep NPO for 2 hours (or as ordered), then resume usual diet.

☑ Instruct to avoid coughing, lifting, or straining for 1 to 2 weeks.

less than 2 g/day. Fluids may be limited as needed to control ascites, edema, and heart failure. Clients who are NPO may require total parenteral nutrition. Vitamin and mineral supplements may be ordered, particularly thiamine, folate, and B$_{12}$. The fat-soluble vitamins, A, D, and E, may need to be given in a water-soluble form. Clients with alcohol-induced cirrhosis may also need a magnesium supplement.

Pharmacology

Substances that are toxic to the liver, such as alcohol, barbiturates, sedatives, hypnotics, and acetaminophen, must be avoided. Doses of other medications may need to be adjusted, because metabolism may be altered by impaired liver function. *Diuretics* are prescribed to reduce edema and ascites. Spironolactone (Aldactone), a potassium-sparing diuretic, or the potent loop diuretic furosemide (Lasix) may be used.

Medications to reduce ammonia absorption from the bowel frequently are used, particularly when blood ammonia levels are high. Two drugs used for this purpose are lactulose and neomycin (see Table 19-2 ◆).

Beta-adrenergic blockers such as propranolol or nadolol may be given to manage portal hypertension. *Vitamin K* is given to promote clotting. *Platelets* and other blood products such as *fresh frozen plasma* or *salt-poor albumin* may be administered to restore blood cells and replenish plasma proteins. *Histamine-2 antagonists* or *antacids* are ordered to manage associated gastritis and upper gastrointestinal bleeding.

Surgical Procedures

Various surgical procedures may be used to manage the effects and complications of cirrhosis. *Liver transplant* is the only definitive treatment, and is not appropriate for all clients with

TABLE 19-2

NURSING IMPLICATIONS FOR PHARMACOLOGY: CLIENTS WITH CIRRHOSIS

AGENTS/DRUGS	PURPOSE	NURSING RESPONSIBILITIES	TEACHING
Diuretics ■ Spironolactone (Aldactone) ■ Furosemide (Lasix)	Spironolactone is a potassium-sparing diuretic that reduces ascites by increasing urine output and decreasing aldosterone levels. Furosemide is a loop diuretic that promotes the excretion of potassium. These drugs may be given in combination.	Monitor vital signs and serum electrolytes and osmolality. Report changes to the charge nurse or physician. Weigh daily. Monitor and record intake and output.	Take diuretics in the morning and early afternoon to avoid sleep disruption caused by increased urine output. Report increases in weight or edema to your physician. Keep scheduled appointments for laboratory testing and with your physician.
Laxatives ■ Lactulose (Cephulac, Chronulac)	Lactulose inhibits ammonia aborption from the bowel and promotes its excretion in feces. It also is an osmotic laxative that pulls water into the bowel lumen, softening stool and stimulating peristalsis. The drug may be given orally or rectally.	Assess bowel sounds and abdominal girth. Maintain accurate stool chart. Adjust dose to achieve two to three soft stools per day as ordered. Monitor electrolytes and hydration status.	Mix with fruit juice, water, or milk to make more palatable. Drink adequate fluids. Report diarrhea to your physician. If this drug causes nausea, take it with a soda or crackers. Do not stop the medication.
Anti-infective Agents ■ Neomycin sulfate (Neo Tabs)	Neomycin sulfate is a gastrointestinal antibiotic that is used to destroy intestinal bacteria and decrease ammonia production in the bowel. It may be given as an oral or rectal preparation.	Assess and monitor hearing, kidney, and neurologic functions before and during treatment. Monitor intake and output. Monitor blood urea nitrogen (BUN) and creatinine levels. Monitor digitalis levels as indicated.	Report dizziness, tinnitus (ringing in ears), hearing loss, headaches, tremors, or visual alterations immediately. Keep follow-up appointments. Maintain fluid intake; avoid dehydration.

cirrhosis (e.g., clients who continue to abuse alcohol). Nursing care of the client having a liver transplant is outlined in Box 19-12.

Paracentesis (removal of fluid from the peritoneal cavity) may be done if ascites is severe (Figure 19-7 ◆). Excess fluid in the peritoneal cavity puts pressure on the diaphragm, increasing the work of breathing. Removing this fluid improves breathing, but fluid will reaccumulate unless the underlying cause of ascites is corrected. Albumin may be given after paracentesis; it increases the intravascular oncotic pressure and slows the development of ascites. Nursing implications for paracentesis are listed in Box 19-13.

Figure 19-7. ◆ Position of the client during paracentesis.

A *transjugular intrahepatic portosystemic shunt (TIPS)* may be used to relieve portal hypertension for some clients. The shunt directs venous blood from the portal vein to the hepatic vein, allowing it to bypass the liver (Figure 19-8 ◆). It can be inserted in a vascular catheterization lab, avoiding the need for surgery. Following the procedure, observe the client closely for evidence of bleeding, either at the insertion site (the jugular

---

BOX 19-12
NURSING CARE CHECKLIST

LIVER TRANSPLANT
Before Surgery

☑ Reinforce preoperative teaching provided by the transplant team.
☑ Provide psychological support.
☑ Provide routine preoperative care and teaching as outlined in Chapter 7.
☑ Prepare the client for returning from surgery to the intensive care unit.

After Surgery

☑ Provide routine postoperative care as indicated by postoperative day.
☑ Manage pain and promote respiratory function through coughing, deep breathing, incentive spirometry, and early ambulation.
☑ Administer drugs to prevent rejection (e.g., cyclosporine A, corticosteroids, and azathioprine) as ordered.
☑ Carefully monitor for infection as these drugs suppress the immune response.
☑ Monitor renal function and blood glucose levels.
☑ Monitor for signs of rejection: Increasing temperature (an early sign), discomfort over transplant site, anorexia, decreased bile drainage from drain, arthralgia (joint pain), abnormal liver function tests. Promptly report abnormal assessment data to the charge nurse or physician.
☑ Provide discharge teaching:
  ☑ Avoiding infections, signs of infection, and the importance of reporting all fevers.
  ☑ Recognizing signs of rejection.
  ☑ Verbal and written instructions and a schedule for all prescribed medications. Stress importance of reporting adverse effects and maintaining regular follow-up appointments.
  ☑ Prepare for potential body image changes associated with steroid use and for psychological effects of receiving a transplanted organ.

BOX 19-13
NURSING CARE CHECKLIST

PARACENTESIS
Before the Procedure

☑ Verify informed consent for the procedure.
☑ Reinforce teaching and clarify questions about the procedure.
☑ Weigh the client, and obtain baseline vital signs.
☑ Have client void immediately prior to the test to avoid bladder puncture.
☑ Place in a sitting position, either on the side of the bed or in a chair, with the feet supported.

During the Procedure

☑ Explain procedure. Following cleansing and local anesthesia, a needle or trocar is inserted through a small abdominal incision to withdraw fluid. The trocar is connected to tubing and a collection bottle; specimens may be sent to laboratory.
☑ Monitor blood pressure.

After the Procedure

☑ Put a small dressing over the puncture site; monitor drainage.
☑ Send specimens with completed requisitions to the laboratory for analysis as ordered.

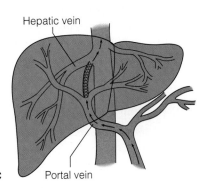

Figure 19-8. ◆ Transjugular intrahepatic portosystemic shunt (TIPS). (A) A catheter inserted via the internal jugular vein is guided into the hepatic vein. From there, a new route connecting the hepatic and portal veins is created through liver tissue. (B) An expandable metal stent is positioned between the portal and hepatic veins. (C) The catheter and guidewire are removed, leaving the stent in place.

vein) or internally. Monitor vital signs, color, and level of consciousness frequently, and report changes to the charge nurse or physician.

Bleeding esophageal varices may be treated with *endoscopic sclerotherapy* or *endoscopic band ligation*. Once the varices have been identified, a sclerosing agent is injected into the enlarged vessel, causing an inflammatory reaction and clotting. In band ligation, the bleeding vessel is obstructed with a latex band or clip. (Review Box 18-9 for nursing care of clients having an upper endoscopy.) In an acute situation, a multiple-lumen gastrointestinal tube such as a Sengstaken– Blakemore tube may be inserted to *tamponade* (place pressure on) the bleeding varices (Figure 19-9 ◆).

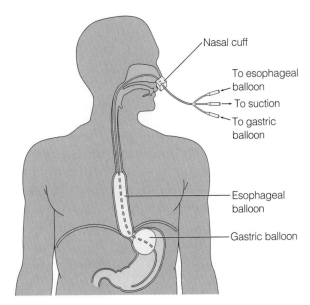

Figure 19-9. ◆ A triple-lumen nasogastric (Sengstaken–Blakemore) tube used to control bleeding esophageal varices.

NURSING CARE

Nursing care of the client with cirrhosis presents many challenges because liver dysfunction affects many body systems. Psychosocial aspects of care are as vital as the physical care needs of the client.

ASSESSING

Clients with cirrhosis may have vague symptoms or be acutely ill with bleeding, respiratory distress, or neurologic manifestations of hepatic encephalopathy. The extent of assessment data collected depends on the situation (Box 19-14).

DIAGNOSING, PLANNING, AND IMPLEMENTING

EXCESS FLUID VOLUME

- Weigh daily. Monitor intake and output. *Impaired salt and water regulation caused by cirrhosis can lead to problems such as peripheral edema, ascites, and heart failure. Changes in daily weight are an accurate indicator of fluid balance, as is monitoring intake and output.*
- Assess for neck vein distention and peripheral edema. *Neck vein distention and peripheral edema are indicators of excess fluid.*
- Measure abdominal girth daily. With the client supine, position the measuring tape around the abdomen at the level of the umbilicus. Mark the skin with indelible marker. *This ensures consistent, accurate measurements about the presence and amount of ascites.*
- Provide a low-sodium diet (500 to 2,000 mg/day) and restrict fluids as ordered. *Sodium causes water retention, which clients with cirrhosis need to avoid.*

BOX 19-14
ASSESSING CLIENTS WITH CIRRHOSIS

SUBJECTIVE DATA

- Risk factors for cirrhosis: Alcohol use (amount per day or week, duration), chronic hepatitis, exposure to drugs or toxic chemicals, gallbladder disease
- Current manifestations such as anorexia, nausea, indigestion; malaise; upper right abdominal pain; change in bowel habits; color of feces and urine
- Change in color of skin or sclera; itching
- History of complications such as ascites, upper GI bleeding, or mental changes
- Current diet and fluid intake

OBJECTIVE DATA

- General appearance; apparent nutritional status
- Level of consciousness, mental status, and cognition
- Color of skin and sclera, ecchymoses (bruising) or spider nevi (branching, dilated capillaries resembling a spider); dryness of skin, evidence of scratching
- Color and consistency of feces, presence of frank blood or melana; color of urine
- Color and consistency of emesis; evidence of GI bleeding
- Inspect abdomen for distention, ascites, dilated, visible veins.
- Auscultate bowel sounds.
- Palpate abdomen for tenderness.

DISTURBED THOUGHT PROCESSES

- Avoid unnecessary medications that can affect the central nervous system (CNS). *Careful use of medications can help avoid worsening manifestations of encephalopathy.*
- Assess level of consciousness and mental status. Monitor for changes in behavior, handwriting, speech, and development of *asterixis* (a flapping tremor of the hands). Notify the charge nurse or physician of changes. *Accumulated nitrogenous waste products affect the CNS and thinking processes. Early identification of problems allows prompt intervention—subtle changes in neurologic functioning are important!*
- If possible, have the same nurses care for client. *Consistent care may allow early recognition of neurologic changes.*
- Provide a low-protein diet as prescribed; teach the family the importance of maintaining diet restrictions. *Nitrogenous by-products from dietary protein increase serum ammonia levels.*
- Administer medications as ordered to prevent gastrointestinal bleeding and reduce gastrointestinal production of nitrogenous waste products. Give laxatives and stool softeners as needed to avoid constipation. *These measures help decrease ammonia production in the bowel and serum ammonia levels.*

- Orient to time, place, and person; provide simple explanations for care at the client's level of understanding. Maintain a calm environment; minimize external stimuli. *These measures help prevent agitation and anxiety when thinking is impaired.*

INEFFECTIVE PROTECTION

- Monitor vital signs. *Increased pulse and decreasing blood pressure may indicate hemorrhage.*
- Institute bleeding precautions. (See Box 19-15 for specific interventions.) *Preventive measures can decrease the incidence of active bleeding.*
- Monitor coagulation studies and platelet count. *The results determine the need to continue bleeding precautions and to administer vitamin K as ordered.*

RISK FOR SUFFOCATION

Clients with a Sengstaken–Blakemore or other multiple-lumen nasogastric tube (Figure 19-9) for bleeding esophageal varices have special care needs. These clients usually are in intensive care units for close monitoring.

- Secure and maintain the original position of the tube. Use soft wrist restraints as needed to prevent the client from pulling on the tube. *If the tube is dislodged while the esophageal balloon is inflated, the airway can be obstructed.*
- Place in Fowler's position. Suction the oropharynx as needed. *The esophageal balloon impairs the ability to swallow oral secretions. Elevating the head of the bed reduces the risk of aspiration and promotes gas exchange.*
- Monitor and release balloon pressures as ordered. *The gastric balloon helps keep the distal end of the tube in the stomach, preventing the esophageal balloon from obstructing the airway. The inflated balloons place pressure on gastric and esophageal tissues; they may be periodically deflated to reduce the risk of tissue necrosis.*

BOX 19-15
BLEEDING PRECAUTIONS

- Prevent constipation.
- Avoid rectal temperatures or enemas.
- Avoid injections; if needed, use small-gauge needle and apply pressure.
- Assess for bruises or purpura (hemorrhage into the skin).
- Apply pressure to bleeding sites.
- Apply direct pressure to venipuncture sites for at least 5 minutes.
- Use only a soft toothbrush.
- Avoid blowing nose.
- Assess oral cavity for bleeding gums.
- Administer H_2 blockers or antacids as ordered to prevent gastrointestinal bleeding.

CLINICAL alert

Always deflate the esophageal balloon before deflating the gastric balloon.

- Frequently check the nares for tissue damage. Keep the nasal cuff (a small piece of foam) in place. *Pressure sores can develop on the nares through which the tube is inserted.*

INEFFECTIVE BREATHING PATTERN

- Place in high-Fowler's position with feet elevated; assist to chair as tolerated. Avoid supine position when possible. *The sitting position permits full expansion of the lungs and allows gravity to pull fluid and abdominal organs away from the diaphragm.*
- Monitor respirations, lung sounds, and oxygen saturation levels. Report abnormal findings or changes in status. *Continuing respiratory assessments are important to prevent problems from impaired ventilation and oxygenation.*
- Administer oxygen as ordered. *Oxygen therapy may be necessary to prevent hypoxia.*

IMPAIRED SKIN INTEGRITY

- Use warm water rather than hot water when bathing. *Hot water can dry the skin further and increase itching.*
- Avoid soap for bathing, apply an emollient or lotion without alcohol to moisten skin, and do not rub the skin. *These measures help prevent dry skin and pruritus.*
- Apply mittens or mitts to hands as needed to prevent scratching. *Clients with encephalopathy may not understand why they should not scratch.*
- Turn at least every 2 hours, use an alternating pressure mattress, and assess skin for breakdown. *Position changes relieve pressure and promote tissue oxygenation.*

EVALUATING

To evaluate the effectiveness of nursing care, collect data related to outcomes for the identified nursing diagnoses. For example:

- Are the weight and abdominal girth stable?
- Is behavior and mental status normal for the client?
- Has the client remained free of bleeding?
- Is the client's respiratory status improved?
- Does the skin remain intact?

Discharge Considerations

Home care for the client with cirrhosis requires a coordinated team effort that includes the client, family, physician, nurses, and social services. Box 19-16 outlines assessment data to consider in planning for discharge.

BOX 19-16
ASSESSING FOR DISCHARGE

CIRRHOSIS
Client

- Self-care: Ability to perform ADLs; to prepare and eat the prescribed diet
- Knowledge: Understanding of disease and its progression; preventing complications; diet and fluid restrictions; toxins to avoid; when to contact the physician
- Psychosocial: Support network and significant others; willingness to abstain from alcohol and other drugs; ability to cope with long-term effects or with liver transplant; evidence of grieving
- Home environment: Factors affecting the client's ability to abstain from alcohol (e.g., roommates, type and location of housing)

Family and Caregivers

- Members of household: Ability and willingness to help with food preparation, family responsibilities, and care
- Financial resources: Income; resources for food, dietary supplements, and medical care; effect of long-term illness on family unit

Community

- Home health and social services
- Support groups and Alcoholics Anonymous meetings or other alcohol treatment options

Include family members in all teaching, particularly when alcohol abuse and hepatic encephalopathy are considerations. Consistently reinforce teaching; repeat explanations as needed. Reinforce teaching about the prescribed diet and any fluid restrictions. If necessary, refer to a dietitian for diet planning. Provide written and verbal instructions about all medications and when to contact the physician. Teach follow-up care and any home care considerations following procedures such as liver biopsy or transjugular intrahepatic portosystemic shunt (TIPS) placement. Stress the importance of avoiding all substances toxic to the liver, including alcohol and over-the-counter medications containing acetaminophen. If the client is in end-stage liver disease, refer for hospice care as appropriate.

Nursing Process Case Study
■ CLIENT WITH ALCOHOLIC CIRRHOSIS

Richard Wright is a 48-year-old man who has alcoholic cirrhosis. He is admitted to the hospital with ascites and malnutrition. He has had three previous admissions for cirrhosis, the most recent being 6 months ago.

Assessment Mr. Wright is lethargic but responds appropriately to verbal stimuli. He complains of "spitting up blood the past week or so" and says, "I just don't feel hungry." He has lost 20 lbs. (9 kg) since his previous admission. He is jaundiced and has petechiae and ecchymoses on his arms and legs. His admitting nurse notes 3+ pitting edema of his ankles and feet. His abdomen is distended and tight, with distended superficial veins. Vital signs are: T 100° F (37.7° C); BP 110/70; P 110; R 24.

Laboratory test results include: RBC 4.0 million/mm^3, WBC 3,700/mm^3, platelets 75,000/mm^3; elevated serum ammonia, total bilirubin, and serum sodium levels; low serum potassium, total protein and albumin levels.

The diagnosis of alcohol-induced cirrhosis with gastritis is made. Mr. Wright is started on Aldactone, Riopan, lactulose, an 800-mg sodium, low-protein diet, and fluid restriction of 1,500 mL/day.

Diagnosis The following nursing diagnoses are identified for Mr. Wright:

- Excess Fluid Volume related to electrolyte imbalance and low serum albumin
- Imbalanced Nutrition: Less Than Body Requirements related to anorexia and possible alcohol abuse
- Disturbed Thought Processes related to high ammonia levels
- Ineffective Protection related to low platelets and malnutrition

Expected Outcomes The expected outcomes for the plan of care specify that:

- Abdominal girth will decrease by 1 to 2 cm per day; peripheral edema will decrease to no more than 1+.
- Weight will increase by 1 lb. (0.45 kg) per week while losing excess fluid.
- Will be alert and oriented to time, place, and person.
- No further active bleeding will occur.

Planning and Implementation The following nursing interventions are implemented:

- Weigh daily before breakfast.
- Consult dietitian to plan a low-salt, low-protein, high-calorie diet.
- Frequently assess mental status; promptly report changes.
- Measure abdominal girth every shift.
- Institute bleeding precautions.
- Keep head of bed elevated; assist to chair with legs elevated tid as tolerated.
- Refer to home health and community agencies for discharge follow-up.

Evaluation Mr. Wright is discharged after 7 days. His weight has decreased by 4 lbs., but decreased peripheral edema (now 1+) and abdominal girth indicate that this is due to loss of excess fluid. He does not experience any further bleeding. His serum ammonia levels return to normal. Lactulose will be continued on discharge.

Mr. Wright and his teenage children have made contact with Alcoholics Anonymous and Al Anon; they also have appointments to meet with a psychiatric social worker and primary caregiver.

 Critical Thinking in the Nursing Process

1. Why was Mr. Wright lethargic on admission? Why does bleeding into the gastrointestinal tract increase serum ammonia levels?
2. Discuss the relationship between portal hypertension, low serum protein levels, and ascites.
3. Outline a 1-day meal plan for Mr. Wright that is low in protein, high in calories, and low in salt.

Cancer of the Liver

Primary liver cancer is uncommon in the United States, but metastases to the liver from other primary sites are relatively frequent. The prognosis for primary hepatic cancer is poor, in part because the disease often is not diagnosed before it reaches an advanced stage. Metastases to the lungs are common.

Most primary liver cancers arise from the liver's **parenchymal** (essential, functional) cells; about 10% develop in the bile duct. Regardless of where the cancer develops, the progress of the disease is similar. Chronic hepatitis B or hepatitis C and alcohol-induced cirrhosis are the primary risk factors for liver cancer in the United States.

Manifestations of liver cancer include malaise, painful mass in the right upper quadrant, epigastric fullness, weight loss, anorexia, and fever. Clients may present with ascites, jaundice, or signs of liver failure. Liver biopsy establishes the diagnosis. Magnetic resonance imaging (MRI), ultrasound, and computed tomography (CT) scans can aid in diagnosis, as can tests for serum markers such as alpha-fetoprotein (AFP).

Partial hepatectomy is possible when the cancer is limited and has not spread beyond the liver. Liver transplantation is a potential option. Radiation therapy is used to shrink the tumor, decreasing pressure on surrounding organs and reducing pain. Chemotherapy may be used as adjunctive treatment for liver cancer.

Preventive nursing care focuses on teaching about the causes of liver cancer and their prevention. Avoiding alcohol, particularly in excess, also is a preventive measure. For the client with liver cancer, pain control is a priority. Refer clients with inoperable liver cancer to hospice services and cancer support groups.

Liver Trauma

Liver trauma can be caused by blunt trauma or penetrating injury to the abdomen. Automobile crashes, stab or gunshot wounds, and iatrogenic sources, such as liver biopsy, are possible causes of liver trauma. Because the liver is highly vascular, hemorrhage is a significant risk in liver trauma.

Preventing and treating hypovolemic shock are priorities of care for clients with liver trauma. Intravenous fluids and blood products may be given to maintain blood volume and cardiac output. Surgery may be necessary to locate and control bleeding. Postoperative nursing care focuses on preventing pulmonary complications and monitoring for signs of infec-

tion or additional bleeding. Keeping family members informed is an important aspect of care, especially until the client's condition stabilizes.

Exocrine Pancreatic Disorders

The pancreas is both an exocrine and an endocrine gland. As an exocrine gland, it produces enzymes that empty through ducts into the small intestine. As an endocrine gland, it produces hormones that enter the bloodstream directly. Disorders of the exocrine pancreas affect the secretion of digestive enzymes and may affect its endocrine functions as well. (*Diabetes mellitus,* a disorder of the endocrine pancreas, is discussed in Chapter 17.)

 Pancreatitis

Pancreatitis (inflammation of the pancreas) may be either acute or chronic. *Acute pancreatitis* usually develops in middle life; gallstones and alcoholism are the primary risk factors for acute pancreatitis. Alcoholism also is the primary risk factor for *chronic pancreatitis,* a disease that eventually leads to pancreatic insufficiency. Clients with pancreatitis often are acutely ill, and they may require lifelong treatment.

PATHOPHYSIOLOGY
Acute Pancreatitis
Acute pancreatitis occurs when the pancreas is damaged or the duct is blocked, allowing pancreatic enzymes to accumulate within the pancreas itself. Obstruction of the outflow of pancreatic enzymes or a backup of bile or duodenal contents into the pancreatic duct are believed to be common causes. Outflow may be obstructed by a stone in the duct or by tissue edema. When this happens, a self-destructive process known as *autodigestion* begins. Pancreatic tissue bleeds and becomes necrotic, and secondary bacterial infection can lead to abscess formation.

Some clients recover completely from acute pancreatitis. Others have recurrent attacks or develop chronic pancreatitis.

The onset of acute pancreatitis is often sudden. The client experiences continuous severe epigastric and abdominal pain. This pain commonly radiates to the back and is relieved somewhat by sitting up and leaning forward. The onset of pain often occurs after a fatty meal or excessive alcohol consumption. Other manifestations are listed in Box 19-17.

Clients with acute pancreatitis may develop hypovolemic shock due to vasodilation and a fluid shift into the small bowel (see Chapter 5). Bleeding into the retroperitoneal space may occur, as evidenced by bruising in the flanks (*Turner's*

sign) or around the umbilicus (*Cullen's sign*). A *pancreatic pseudocyst* (a collection of blood, fluid, and pancreatic secretions in the abdominal cavity) may develop. If the pseudocyst ruptures, peritonitis results. *Pancreatic abscess* (a collection of secretions and necrotic products within the pancreas) may be fatal. These complications usually occur 2 to 3 weeks after the onset of pancreatitis.

Chronic Pancreatitis
Chronic pancreatitis may follow acute pancreatitis or may have no identified cause. In chronic pancreatitis, small ducts of the pancreas are blocked by calcified proteins. This initiates an inflammatory process in which normal pancreatic tissue is destroyed and replaced by fibrous scar tissue. Chronic pancreatitis is progressive and irreversible. It ultimately leads to pancreatic insufficiency, which in turn leads to malabsorption and diabetes mellitus (from destruction of endocrine cells). The manifestations of chronic pancreatitis are listed in Box 19-17.

BOX 19-17
MANIFESTATIONS OF PANCREATITIS

ACUTE PANCREATITIS
- Acute severe epigastric pain; may radiate to back
- Nausea, vomiting
- Abdominal distention, decreased bowel sounds
- Low-grade fever
- Tachycardia, hypotension
- Cool, clammy skin
- Elevated WBC, serum amylase, and lipase
- Low serum calcium and magnesium

CHRONIC PANCREATITIS
- Persistent or recurring episodes of upper abdominal pain radiating to the back
- Anorexia, nausea, vomiting, weight loss
- Flatulence and constipation
- Steatorrhea (fatty, frothy, foul-smelling stools)
- Elevated serum amylase and lipase
- Elevated glucose levels

TABLE 19-3   LABORATORY TESTS FOR PANCREATIC DISORDERS

TEST	NORMAL VALUE	SIGNIFICANCE
Serum amylase	25–125 U/L	Elevated in acute pancreatitis and acute episodes of chronic pancreatitis; may be elevated in pancreatic cancer
Serum lipase	20–180 IU/L	
Urine amylase	4–370 U/L/2hr	Elevated in acute pancreatitis
Blood glucose	70–110 mg/dL	May be elevated in chronic pancreatitis and pancreatic cancer
Serum calcium	8.5–10 mg/dL	Decreased in acute pancreatitis
Serum magnesium	1.6–2.6 mg/dL	
White blood cells (WBCs)	4,500–10,000/mm^3	Elevated in acute pancreatitis
Carcinoembryonic antigen (CEA)	< 2.5 ng/mL	Elevated in pancreatic cancer

COLLABORATIVE CARE
Diagnostic Tests

■ Laboratory tests may be ordered to confirm the diagnosis of pancreatitis (Table 19-3 ◆).

■ *Abdominal x-ray* or *abdominal ultrasound* may show inflammatory changes or the presence of gallstones in acute pancreatitis.

■ *CT scans* help differentiate acute and chronic pancreatitis.

■ *Endoscopic retrograde cholangiopancreatography (ERCP)* is used to diagnose chronic pancreatitis.

Treatment

Treatment of acute pancreatitis focuses on eliminating its causes (such as gallstones or alcohol abuse), minimizing additional damage to the pancreas by reducing pancreatic secretions, relieving pain, and preventing complications. The client initially is given nothing by mouth. A nasogastric tube may be inserted and connected to suction, and intravenous fluid therapy or total parenteral nutrition (TPN) is initiated. These measures decrease pancreatic enzyme production while maintaining hydration and nutrition. Oral food and fluids are resumed when serum amylase levels return to normal, bowel sounds are present, and pain has disappeared. Intake begins with clear liquids and progresses to a low-fat diet as tolerated.

Parenteral narcotic analgesics may be required for pain relief. Antibiotics may be ordered to prevent or treat infection. Once the acute episode resolves, a laparoscopic cholecystectomy is done to reduce the risk of future episodes.

Treatment for chronic pancreatitis includes pain management, nutritional support, and replacement of deficient enzymes and hormones. Narcotic analgesics are avoided if possible, because the risk of addiction is high. Alcohol is forbidden; it may precipitate an attack. Pancreatic enzyme supplements (Table 19-4 ◆) are given to manage *steatorrhea* (fat in stools).

Omeprazole (Prilosec), ranitidine (Zantac), or a similar drug is prescribed to reduce gastric acidity (which stimulates pancreatic enzyme production). Diabetes resulting from chronic pancreatitis is treated (see Chapter 17). Surgery may be performed to drain persistent pseudocysts or to dilate an obstructed duct.

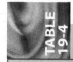

TABLE 19-4   NURSING IMPLICATIONS FOR PHARMACOLOGY: CLIENTS WITH CHRONIC PANCREATITIS

AGENTS/DRUGS	PURPOSE	NURSING RESPONSIBILITIES	CLIENT TEACHING
Pancreatic Enzyme Replacement			
■ Pancrelipase (Lipancreatin)	Pancrelipase promotes starch and fat digestion by replacing the pancreatic enzymes protease, amylase, and lipase. It improves nutrition and decreases the number of bowel movements.	Monitor frequency and consistency of stools. Weigh every other day. Record weights. Administer with meals. Monitor for side effects: Rash, hives, respiratory difficulty, hematuria, gout, or joint pain.	Take the drug with meals or snacks. If medicine is enteric coated, do not crush, chew, or mix with foods such as milk or ice cream. Be sure to follow prescribed diet.

NURSING CARE

ASSESSING

Assessment data focuses on identifying the onset of symptoms and risk factors for pancreatitis. Ask the client to describe the pain: its onset, intensity using a standardized pain scale (see Chapter 6), character (steady, boring, stabbing, radiating), duration, relieving and aggravating factors, and any associated symptoms such as sweating, nausea, or vomiting. Ask about any history of previous attacks or a history of gallbladder disease. Inquire about alcohol use (number of drinks per day or per week, most recent alcohol consumption). Ask about food intake for the day prior to the onset of the pain.

Observe for nonverbal cues of pain: restlessness or rigid stillness; tense facial features; clenched fists; rapid, shallow breathing; tachycardia; diaphoresis. Listen for bowel sounds and gently palpate the abdomen for tenderness. Report assessment data to the charge nurse or physician.

DIAGNOSING, PLANNING, AND IMPLEMENTING

ACUTE PAIN

- Administer ordered narcotic analgesics on a regular schedule or teach the client to use patient-controlled analgesia (PCA). Assess the effectiveness of analgesia. *Severe, established pain is difficult to control. Unrelieved pain may increase secretion of pancreatic enzymes.*
- Maintain nothing by mouth (NPO) status and nasogastric tube patency as ordered. *Gastric secretions stimulate pancreatic secretion, aggravating pain. Withholding food and maintaining nasogastric suction reduce gastric secretions, and help relieve nausea and vomiting.*
- Maintain client on bed rest in a calm, quiet environment. *Reducing physical movement and mental stimulation decreases metabolic rate, gastrointestinal secretion, and resulting pain.*
- Provide comfort measures:
  - Provide oral and nasal care every 1 to 2 hours.
  - Assist to a comfortable position, such as a side-lying with knees flexed and head elevated 45 degrees.
  - Encourage relaxation techniques and guided imagery to decrease pain.
  - Explain all procedures and care; listen carefully to concerns and evaluation of pain relief.
    The client who is NPO needs frequent mouth care for comfort. Inflammation and stretching of the peritoneum causes pain. Sitting up, leaning forward, or lying in a fetal position tends to decrease the pain. Alternative pain relief measures help reduce anxiety and help the client gain a sense of control (see Chapter 6 on pain).
- Ask the family and visitors to avoid bringing food into the client's room. *The sight of food may stimulate pancreatic secretions.*

RISK FOR IMBALANCED NUTRITION: LESS THAN BODY REQUIREMENTS

- Weigh daily at the same time. *Decreasing weight may indicate poor nutritional status.*
- Maintain stool chart; include frequency, color, odor, and consistency of stools. *Pancreatitis affects fat absorption, so undigested fats are excreted in the stool. Steatorrhea may indicate an increase in the severity of pancreatitis.*
- Regularly assess bowel sounds. *Nasogastric suction usually is discontinued within 24 to 48 hours after the return of bowel sounds indicates that the client is regaining bowel motility.*
- Administer intravenous fluids and TPN as prescribed. *Inflammation increases metabolism and nutritional needs. TPN may be ordered to maintain nutritional status while the client is NPO (see Chapter 18).*
- When eating resumes, provide small, frequent feedings and a high-carbohydrate, low-protein, low-fat diet. Avoid caffeine (coffee, tea, colas), spicy foods, or gas-producing foods. *Small, frequent feedings are better tolerated. A low-protein, low-fat diet minimizes pancreatic enzyme secretion, reducing inflammation and pain. Caffeine and spicy or gas-producing foods may increase pancreatic secretion and pain.*

RISK FOR INJURY

- Assess vital signs (including orthostatic blood pressures), peripheral pulses, skin color, temperature, and turgor every 1 to 2 hours until stable, then every 4 hours. Record data and report abnormal findings to the charge nurse or physician. *Frequent assessment of cardiovascular and fluid volume status is important because fluid losses associated with vomiting, diaphoresis, thrid-space shifts, and nasogastric suction can affect cardiac output and tissue perfusion.*
- Monitor respiratory status including breath sounds. Encourage to cough and deep breathe hourly. *Abdominal pain causes shallow respirations and impaired ventilation, increasing the risk of atelectasis (see Chapter 26) or pneumonia. Coughing and deep breathing improve ventilation and mobilize secretions.*
- Measure urine output hourly; maintain accurate intake and output. Report output of less than 30 mL/hr to the charge nurse or physician. *A drop in urine output may be an early indication of decreased cardiac output, which increases the risk of acute renal failure.*
- Frequently assess mental status, level of consciousness, and behavior. *Impaired mental status may indicate poor cerebral oxygenation, alcohol withdrawal, or other complications of acute pancreatitis.*

EVALUATING

When evaluating the effectiveness of nursing care for a client with acute pancreatitis, collect data such as pain level, weight, ability to resume eating, and stability of cardiovascular and respiratory status.

Discharge Considerations

When appropriate, teach the client and family members about the disease and how to prevent further attacks. Discuss specific risk factors and needs, such as:

- Alcohol abstinence is vital to prevent future attacks of acute or chronic pancreatitis. (Refer as needed to community agencies, support groups such as Alcoholics Anonymous, or individual counseling.)
- Smoking and stress stimulate the pancreas and should be avoided.
- Possible treatment for gallstones if appropriate, including options such as laparoscopic cholecystectomy.
- Instruct to take pancreatic enzymes and insulin as ordered. Refer to a diabetes educator as appropriate.
- Advise to maintain a low-fat diet, and to avoid crash dieting or binge eating, which can bring on attacks. Discuss foods to avoid, such as spicy foods, caffeinated beverages, and gas-forming foods. Refer to a dietitian or nutritionist as needed for diet planning and teaching.
- Instruct to report signs of infection promptly (a fever of 102° F [38.8° C] or higher, pain, rapid pulse, malaise) to the physician. An abscess may form months after the initial attack, necessitating further intervention.
- Refer to a community or home health agency as needed for home care.

Pancreatic Cancer

While cancer of the pancreas is not common, its incidence is increasing in the United States. Older adults, African Americans, and men have a greater risk of developing pancreatic cancer. Smoking is a major risk factor for pancreatic cancer. Its incidence is twice as high in smokers as in nonsmokers. The prognosis for pancreatic cancer is poor because the disease often is advanced at the time of diagnosis.

Early manifestations of pancreatic cancer include anorexia, nausea, weight loss, flatulence, and dull epigastric pain. The pain increases in severity as the tumor grows. Cancer of the head of the pancreas, which is the most common site, often obstructs bile flow through the common bile duct, causing jaundice, clay-colored stools, dark urine, and pruritus. Late manifestations include a palpable abdominal mass and ascites.

With early diagnosis, surgery may be done to resect the tumor. If the head of the pancreas is affected, a pancreatoduodenectomy (*Whipple's procedure*) is done to remove the head of the pancreas, the duodenum, the distal third of the stomach, a portion of the jejunum, and part of the common bile duct. The common bile duct is then sutured to the end of the jejunum, and the remaining pancreas and stomach are sutured to the side of the jejunum (Figure 19-10 ◆). Radiation and chemotherapy are often used in addition to surgery.

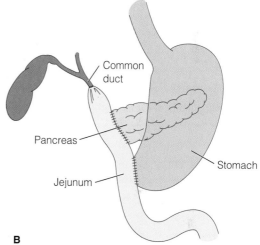

Figure 19-10. ◆ Whipple's procedure. (A) Areas of resection. (B) Appearance following resection.

Postoperative nursing care of the client undergoing Whipple's procedure is similar to that of the client undergoing intestinal surgery (see Chapter 18). The client with pancreatic cancer has multiple problems that require nursing care. (Chapter 8 discusses nursing care for clients cancer.) The nursing diagnoses and interventions discussed for the client with pancreatitis are also appropriate for the client with pancreatic cancer.

Nursing Interventions Classification

When planning and implementing care for clients with disorders of the gallbladder, liver, and pancreas, the following Nursing Interventions (McCloskey & Bulechek, 2000) also should be considered:

- Anxiety Reduction
- Bleeding Reduction: Gastrointestinal
- Fluid/Electrolyte Management
- Gastrointestinal Intubation

- Infection Control
- Nutrition Management
- Pain Management

- Substance Use Treatment: Alcohol Withdrawal
- Tube Care: Gastrointestinal

(*Note:* The bibliography listings for this and all chapters have been compiled at the back of the book.)

Chapter Review

key terms by topic

Use the CD-ROM disk enclosed with your textbook to hear the pronunciation of the key terms in the chapter.

Structure
lobules, hepatocytes

Gallbladder disorders
cholelithiasis, cholecystitis

Liver disorders
hepatitis, jaundice, cirrhosis, portal hypertension, ascites, esophageal varices, paracentesis, parenchymal

Exocrine pancreatic disorders
pancreatitis

key points

- Alcohol abuse is a significant risk factor for the liver and pancreatic disorders discussed in this chapter. Prevention, early identification, and treatment of alcohol abuse reduces the risk of these disorders.

- Hepatitis usually is a viral disease and therefore cannot be cured at this time. Preventing the spread of hepatitis is an important nursing responsibility.

- Some types of viral hepatitis, most notably hepatitis B and C, can lead to a carrier state in which the infected client has no symptoms of the disease, but can spread it to others.

- Hepatitis B and C also can become chronic and ultimately lead to liver failure.

- The complications of cirrhosis, including portal hypertension, ascites, esophageal varicies, and hepatic encephalopathy affect multiple body systems.

- Bleeding from esophageal varices may be massive, and requires prompt control to maintain cardiac output.

- Acute pancreatitis often develops as a complication of gall stones, whereas chronic pancreatitis is more frequently related to alcohol abuse.

Medialink

Additional interactive resources for this chapter can be found on the Companion Website at www.prenhall.com/burke. Click on Chapter 19 and "Begin" to select the activities for this chapter.

For NCLEX review questions and an audio glossary, access the accompanying CD-ROM in this book.

for further study

See Chapter 18 for an illustration of the spleen, liver, and gallbladder (Figure 18-1), and for nursing care related to upper endoscopy (Box 18-9).

For further study about plasma osmotic pressure, see Chapter 5.

For more on diabetes mellitus, see Chapter 17.

See Chapter 10 for more information about hypovolemic shock.

For more information about impaired ventilation, see Chapter 26.

For nursing care related to Whipple's procedure, see Chapter 18.

Critical Thinking Care Map

Caring for a Client with Pancreatitis
NCLEX-PN Focus Area: Physiological Adaptation

Case Study: Rose Schliefer, 59 years old, is home following a 2-month hospitalization for acute pancreatitis. The pancreatitis was caused by gallstones. Mrs. Schliefer spent 3 weeks in intensive care and underwent surgery for the gallstones and to drain a pseudocyst. At discharge she was on a soft, low-protein, low-fat diet and was able to walk in the hall. She has been referred for home health services.

Nursing Diagnosis: Imbalanced Nutrition: Less Than Body Requirements

COLLECT DATA

Subjective

_____
_____
_____
_____
_____
_____

Objective

_____
_____
_____
_____
_____
_____

Would you report this data? Yes/No

If yes, to: _____

Nursing Care

_____
_____
_____
_____
_____
_____
_____

How would you document this? _____

_____
_____

Data Collected
(use those that apply)

- Thin, appears anxious and tired
- States she lost 30 lbs. (13.6 kg) in the hospital
- Weight 102 lbs. (46 kg), height 66 in. (168 cm)
- Vital signs within normal limits
- Well-healed upper abdominal scar and two stab wounds on sides of abdomen noted; scabs present on stab wounds
- Skin cool and dry, poor turgor
- Alert and oriented, responds appropriately
- Blood glucose 80 mg/dL
- States main problems are lack of energy and lack of appetite
- Family expresses concern about ability to provide care

Nursing Interventions
(use those that apply)

- Explain causes of fatigue.
- Help Mrs. Schliefer develop activity goals and identify steps to achieve goals.
- Plan daily rest periods, especially before meals.
- Discuss dietary restrictions and how to adapt to usual diet.
- Assist family to plan six small meals a day.
- Obtain a shower chair.
- Assist family to identify and divide responsibilities for care.
- Encourage client to identify strengths and concerns.

NCLEX-PN Exam Preparation

TEST-TAKING TIP

The practical/vocational nurse is expected to provide care to clients with acute, chronic, or life-threatening conditions. The nurse must develop an understanding of the effects of disease processes on the body systems and be able to initiate appropriate nursing interventions when unexpected responses occur.

1. A client diagnosed with cholelithiasis requests medication for pain relief. Which of the following medications is the physician most likely to prescribe?
   a. acetaminophen (Tylenol)
   b. morphine sulfate
   c. codeine
   d. ibuprofen (Motrin)

2. A client returns to his room following a cholecystectomy. He has a T-tube in place attached to a drainage bag. The nurse would report which of the following assessments to the charge nurse or physician?
   a. There is less than 50 mL output from the T-tube each 8-hour shift.
   b. Client experiences nausea and vomiting 30 minutes after eating.
   c. T-tube drainage decreases after 24 hours.
   d. Client requires pain medication every 4 to 6 hours.

3. A client will manage her cholelithiasis at home using medical interventions. The nurse prepares discharge teaching to include which of the following?
   a. Sleep in prone position to decrease pain.
   b. Report episodes of pain that occur before meals.
   c. Use a heating pad for pain relief.
   d. Adhere to a low-fat, low-calorie diet.

4. A client who was diagnosed with hepatitis A (HAV) states he was told by the nursing assistant that his disease could be transmitted only through blood contact. The appropriate action by the nurse would be to:
   a. provide the correct information to the client and nursing assistant
   b. take no further action because the information is correct
   c. remove all precautions because hepatitis A cannot be transmitted
   d. place a sign on the client's door stating "Blood Precautions"

5. A client is diagnosed with hepatitis B (HBV). Which of the following information, if obtained during the admission assessment, would indicate a risk factor?
   a. She ate in a restaurant 2 weeks ago.
   b. She has been in a monogamous relationship for 7 years.
   c. She is an intravenous drug user.
   d. She has never received a blood transfusion.

6. A client with cirrhosis is scheduled for discharge. The LPN/LVN recognizes the need for further teaching if the client states:
   a. "I will use a soft toothbrush for oral hygiene."
   b. "I will maintain a low-protein diet."
   c. "I will report increased difficulty breathing to my physician."
   d. "I will limit alcohol intake to two servings per day."

7. The nurse evaluates a 54-year-old client with cirrhosis for improvement in her ascites. Which of the following assessment findings may indicate improvement?
   a. weight loss of 3 pounds in the past 72 hours
   b. weight gain of 3 pounds in the past 72 hours
   c. urinary output of 20 mL per hour
   d. urine that is tea colored

8. A 45-year-old client with liver disease is prescribed lactulose (Chronulac) 30 mL every 6 hours. The LPN/LVN explains the action of this medication is to:
   a. promote diuresis
   b. decrease ammonia absorption
   c. decrease fat metabolism
   d. promote reabsorption of potassium

9. A client is admitted to the nursing unit with a diagnosis of acute pancreatitis. The client complains of severe pain. In addition to medication administration, which action by the nurse may provide comfort for the client?
   a. Place in Semi-Fowler's position.
   b. Place the head of the bed flat and encourage the client to remain supine.
   c. Place the head flat and elevate the feet 8 to 12 inches.
   d. Place in a side-lying position with knees flexed and elevate the head of the bed 45 degrees.

10. The nurse is caring for a client with acute pancreatitis. Which nursing assessment should receive the highest priority?
    a. Assess intake and output.
    b. Assess cardiovascular status and fluid volume status.
    c. Assess for pain.
    d. Assess mental status.

chapter

20

Caring for Clients with Bowel Disorders

CARING tip

❝You can do it. You can be the one to make a difference in this world of indifference as you touch lives each day. You can make that difference with one word or one caring act.❞

Janis Grimland, RN, BSN • Program Director • Hill College • Clifton, Texas

LEARNING outcomes

After completing this chapter, you will be able to:

- Identify the major structures and functions of the small and large intestines.
- Describe the physiologic processes involved in bowel elimination.
- Discuss the pathophysiology, manifestations, and management of bowel absorption and elimination disorders.
- Discuss the nursing implications for and teaching related to measures used to manage bowel disorders.
- Provide appropriate nursing care for the client undergoing intestinal surgery.
- Discuss the care of clients with a colostomy or ileostomy.
- Use the nursing process to assess and provide individualized care to clients with disorders of bowel absorption and elimination.

MediaLink

 www.prenhall.com/burke

Use the above address to access the free, interactive Companion Website created for this textbook. Get hints, instant feedback, and textbook references to chapter-related multiple choice questions. Link to other interesting sites.

Structure and Function of the Intestines

Bowel elimination is the end process in digestion; after foods are eaten and broken down into usable elements, nutrients are absorbed and indigestible materials are eliminated.

SMALL INTESTINE

The *small intestine* begins at the pyloric sphincter and ends at the ileocecal valves at the entrance of the large intestine (Figure 18-1 on page 394). The small intestine is about 20 ft. (6 m) long, but only about 1 in. (2.5 cm) in diameter. It hangs in coils in the abdominal cavity, suspended by the mesentery and surrounded by the large intestine.

The small intestine has three regions. The *duodenum,* the shortest segment, extends from the pyloris to the *jejunum* (middle region). The *ileum* is the terminal portion, which meets the large intestine.

Food is chemically digested and mostly absorbed as it moves through the small intestine. Pancreatic enzymes and bile released into the duodenum work with intestinal enzymes to break down starches, proteins, and fats for absorption. Villi (fingerlike projections of cells in the intestinal lining) and deep folds in the intestinal mucosa increase the surface area of the small intestine. Nutrients are absorbed through the mucosa into blood or lymph. Although up to 10 L of food, liquids, and secretions enter the gastrointestinal (GI) tract each day, less than 1 L reaches the large intestine.

LARGE INTESTINE

The *large intestine,* or colon, begins at the *ileocecal valve* and terminates at the *anus* (Figure 20-1 ◆). It is about 5 ft. (1.5 m) long. The first part of the large intestine, the *cecum,* includes the *appendix.* The colon is divided into *ascending, transverse,* and *descending* segments. The descending colon ends at the S-shaped *sigmoid colon.* The sigmoid colon terminates at the rectum.

The *rectum* has transverse folds that help retain feces while allowing flatus to pass. The anorectal junction separates the rectum from the *anal canal,* which terminates at the anus. The *anus,* a hairless, dark-skinned area, is the end of the digestive tract. It has an internal involuntary sphincter and an external voluntary sphincter (Figure 20-2 ◆). The sphincters are usually open only during defecation.

The major function of the large intestine is to eliminate indigestible food residue from the body. It absorbs water, salts, and vitamins from the semiliquid chyme that passes through the ileocecal valve, forming it into *feces (stool).* Feces is moved along the intestine by *peristalsis,* waves of alternating contrac-

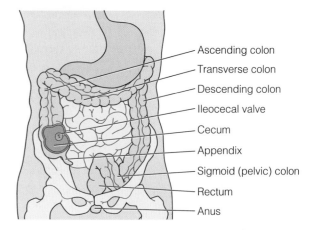

Figure 20-1. ◆ **Anatomy of the large intestine.**

tion and relaxation. Goblet cells lining the large intestine secrete mucus that lubricates the feces, helping it move.

When feces enter the rectum and stretch the rectal wall, the *defecation reflex* causes the walls of the sigmoid colon to contract and the anal sphincters to relax. The reflex can be suppressed by voluntary control of the external sphincter. Defecation can be assisted by closing the glottis and contracting the diaphragm and abdominal muscles to increase intra-abdominal pressure *(Valsalva's maneuver).*

Inflammation, obstructions, disorders of absorption, or changes in structure can alter bowel elimination. Some disorders can severely impair the client's health, cause intense pain, or require surgical intervention. Nursing care focuses on meeting the client's physiologic needs, providing emotional support, and teaching about lifestyle changes.

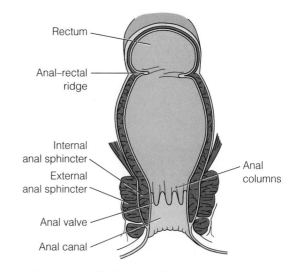

Figure 20-2. ◆ **Structure of the rectum and anus.**

Disorders of Intestinal Motility and of Absorption

"Normal" patterns of defecation vary widely, from two to three stools per day to as few as three stools per week. Few body functions respond as readily to both internal and external factors as the process of defecation. Factors like food and bacteria directly affect the GI tract and the number and consistency of stools. Indirect factors (psychological stress or voluntary postponement of defecation) also affect elimination patterns.

 ## Diarrhea

Diarrhea is an increase in the frequency, volume, and water content of stool. Diarrhea is a symptom, not a primary disorder. Causes of diarrhea include bacterial toxins, infections, malabsorption syndromes, medications, systemic diseases, and psychogenic factors (e.g., preexamination diarrhea).

PATHOPHYSIOLOGY

Diarrhea can result either from impaired water absorption or from increased water secretion into the bowel. Impaired water absorption occurs when the rate of peristalsis increases, or when the absorptive surface of the bowel decreases. Increased water secretion into the bowel may occur by osmosis, from infection (e.g., cholera, *Escherichia coli*), from unabsorbed fat, and from some drugs. Inflammatory disorders cause plasma, blood, and mucus to accumulate in the bowel.

Clients with diarrhea may have several large, watery stools per day or very frequent small stools containing blood, mucus, or pus. The manifestations depend on the cause, duration, and severity of the diarrhea, as well as the area of bowel affected.

Diarrhea can have devastating results as water and electrolytes are lost in the stool. Clients, particularly very young or older, debilitated clients, can become dehydrated. Hypovolemic shock may occur with rapid fluid losses. Potassium, magnesium, and bicarbonate loss may lead to electrolyte deficiencies and metabolic acidosis. (See Chapter 5 for further discussion of the effects of these imbalances.)

COLLABORATIVE CARE

Care of the client with diarrhea focuses on identifying and treating the underlying cause. The diarrhea itself may need to be treated for comfort and to prevent complications.

A *stool specimen* may be ordered to look for blood, pus, mucus, or excess fat. Microscopic examination is done to identify blood cells and parasites. Because parasites may not be in the stool at all times, a series of three stool specimens, spaced 2 to 3 days apart, is obtained when parasitic infection is suspected. *Stool culture* is ordered when an infection is suspected. Blood is drawn to assess for fluid, electrolyte, and acid–base imbalances.

A *sigmoidoscopy* is done to allow direct examination of the bowel mucosa. The preparation and teaching for a client undergoing sigmoidoscopy are outlined in Box 20-1.

Dietary Management

Fluid replacement is most important for clients with diarrhea. If the client is able to take oral fluids, a glucose-balanced electrolyte solution is used (e.g., Pedialyte, Gatorade). Food is withheld during the first 24 hours of acute diarrhea to provide bowel rest. Then frequent, small meals can be added. Milk and milk products are added last. Raw fruits and vegetables, fried foods, bran, whole-grain cereals, condiments, spices, coffee, and alcoholic beverages are avoided during recovery. Clients with chronic diarrhea may need to eliminate certain foods and nonfood substances that can aggravate diarrhea (Table 20-1 ◆). These clients need a diet that is high in calories and nutritional value. Vitamin supplements may be necessary, particularly the fat-soluble vitamins (A, D, E, and K). Parenteral nutrition (see

---

BOX 20-1
NURSING CARE CHECKLIST

SIGMOIDOSCOPY
Before the Procedure

☑ Verify a signed informed consent for the procedure.
☑ Withhold food and fluids as ordered. Clear liquids may be allowed.
☑ Administer enemas or rectal suppositories as ordered.

Client and Family Teaching
Before Procedure
☑ The procedure takes approximately 15 minutes.
☑ You may be positioned in the knee–chest position or on the left side.
☑ Breathe deeply and slowly as the scope is inserted and advanced.
☑ Air may be injected into the bowel to improve visualization.
☑ Specimens of stool or tissue may be obtained during the procedure.

After Procedure
☑ Report any abdominal pain, fever, chills, or rectal bleeding.
☑ If a polyp is removed, avoid heavy lifting for 7 days, and avoid high-fiber foods for 1 to 2 days.

TABLE 20-1 FOODS THAT MAY AGGRAVATE CHRONIC DIARRHEA	
FOODS	**REASON**
Milk, ice cream, yogurt, soft cheeses, cottage cheese	Contain lactose, which requires enzyme lactase to digest; lactase deficiency common
Apple juice, pear juice, grapes, honey, dates, nuts, figs, fruit-flavored soft drinks	Contain fructose, which can draw fluid into the bowel when consumed in large quantities
Table sugar	Contains sucrose, which requires enzyme sucrase to digest
Apple juice, pear juice, sugarless gums and mints	May contain sorbitol, a sugar that is not absorbed and can pull fluid into intestine
Antacids	Magnesium-containing antacids increase peristalsis and can draw fluid into the bowel
Coffee, tea, cola drinks, over-the-counter analgesics	Contain caffeine, which can increase peristalsis

Chapter 18) may be required. A balanced electrolyte intravenous solution may be required to replace fluid losses.

Pharmacology

Antidiarrheal medications may not be used until the cause of diarrhea has been identified, because they could worsen or prolong the disease. Opium derivatives and absorbents such as Pepto-Bismol are commonly used to treat acute diarrhea (Table 20-2 ◆). Opium derivatives also may be used with caution for clients with chronic diarrhea. A potassium supplement may also be prescribed.

NURSING CARE

Nursing care of the client with diarrhea is directed toward identifying the cause, relieving the symptoms, preventing complications, and, if the cause is infectious, preventing the spread of infection to others.

ASSESSING

The client's history and physical examination often provide enough information to identify the cause of diarrhea. Box 20-2 provides assessment data to collect from clients with complaints of diarrhea.

DIAGNOSING, PLANNING, AND IMPLEMENTING

DIARRHEA

- Monitor and record the frequency and characteristics of bowel movements. *This provides a measure of the effectiveness of treatment.*
- Measure abdominal girth and auscultate bowel sounds every shift as indicated. *These indicate the effectiveness and possible complications of treatment such as constipation.*
- Administer antidiarrheal medications as prescribed. *These medications promote comfort and prevent excess fluid loss.*
- Limit food intake for acute diarrhea, slowly reintroducing solid foods in small amounts. *Limiting food allows the bowel to rest and lets the mucosa heal.*

RISK FOR DEFICIENT FLUID VOLUME

- Record intake and output; weigh daily; assess skin turgor, mucous membranes, and urine specific gravity every 8 hours. *These assessments help monitor fluid volume status.*
- Monitor vital signs, including orthostatic vitals, every 4 to 8 hours. *A drop in blood pressure of more than 10 mm Hg on moving from lying to sitting or from sitting to standing indicates orthostatic hypotension and possible fluid volume deficit. The pulse rate typically increases as well.*

TABLE 20-2 NURSING IMPLICATIONS FOR PHARMACOLOGY: CLIENTS RECEIVING ANTIDIARRHEAL MEDICATIONS

AGENT/DRUGS	PURPOSE	NURSING IMPLICATIONS	CLIENT TEACHING
Absorbants and Protectants ▪ Kaolin and pectin (Kaopectate) ▪ Charcoal ▪ Bismuth subsalicylate (Pepto-Bismol)	Absorbant preparations act in the intestines to bind substances that can cause diarrhea. They are safe drugs that are generally available over-the-counter. Bismuth subsalicylate is used to prevent and treat traveler's diarrhea because it has an antimicrobial effect as well.	Assess for contraindications, such as chronic inflammatory bowel disease. If fever is present, check with physician before giving the drug. Give at least 1 hour before or 2 hours after other oral medications; they may interfere with the absorption of other drugs. Observe for potential constipation while using these drugs.	Take at the onset of diarrhea and after each loose stool. Do not use any of these drugs for more than 48 hours. If diarrhea persists, contact your doctor. Chew bismuth tablets, rather than swallowing them whole, for maximal effectiveness. This medication may cause the tongue and stool to darken. If you are allergic to aspirin, do not use bismuth subsalicylate; avoid taking aspirin while taking bismuth subsalicylate.
Opium and Opium Derivatives ▪ Camphorated tincture of opium (Paregoric) ▪ Tincture of opium (laudanum, opium tincture) ▪ Difenoxin (Motofen) ▪ Diphenoxylate (Lomotil, Lotrol, others) ▪ Loperamide hydrochloride (Imodium)	Opium and related drugs act on the CNS to slow peristalsis and allow more water absorption. They also decrease the sensation of a full rectum and increase anal sphincter tone. Paregoric and tincture of opium are controlled prescription drugs. Opium derivatives have few narcotic or abuse-promoting effects and are more commonly used.	Assess for contraindications and drug interactions prior to giving these drugs. Administer paregoric undiluted with water. Observe for increased effects of other CNS depressants, such as alcohol, narcotic analgesics, or barbiturate sedatives. Report abdominal distention to the charge nurse or physician.	Take as recommended at the onset of diarrhea and after each loose stool. These drugs may be habit forming; use for no more than 48 hours. Avoid using alcohol and over-the-counter cold preparations while taking these drugs. These drugs may cause drowsiness; avoid driving or operating machinery while taking them.
Synthetic Hormone ▪ Octreotide acetate (Sandostatin)	Octreotide stimulates fluid and electrolyte absorption from the GI tract and slows intestinal motility. It is primarily used to treat chronic diarrhea associated with certain tumors and HIV disease.	Do not use solution if it is discolored or has particulates. Administer room temperature solution slowly by SC injection. Refrigerate vials for long-term storage; use room temperature solution within 24 hours.	Rotate injection sites, using the hips, thighs, or abdomen. Administer between meals and at bedtime to minimize nausea and diarrhea. Do not use this medication if you are pregnant.

▪ Remind the client to ask for help when getting up. *The client with orthostatic hypotension may become dizzy or lightheaded on rising.*

▪ Provide fluid and electrolyte replacement solutions as indicated. Ensure ready access to fluids. Assist the debilitated client with fluid intake. *If tolerated, oral fluids are encouraged to prevent dehydration. Fluids may be replaced intravenously if necessary. A fluid intake of 3,000 mL or more per day may be necessary to replace losses.*

RISK FOR IMPAIRED SKIN INTEGRITY

■ Provide good skin care. Frequently reposition, and protect pressure areas. *Poorly hydrated skin is at increased risk for breakdown.*

■ Assist with perianal cleaning as needed. Use warm water and soft cloths. Apply protective ointment. *These measures help prevent tissue irritation, trauma, and breakdown.*

EVALUATING

To evaluate the effectiveness of nursing interventions for clients with diarrhea, collect data related to stool frequency, nutritional status, weight, fluid volume status, and skin integrity.

Discharge Considerations

Teach about the causes of diarrhea and preventive measures such as food and water safety. Discuss measures to prevent the spread of bacteria, especially good handwashing after every bowel movement. Stress the importance of seeking medical intervention if diarrhea continues, or is severe or prolonged. Instruct clients planning travel outside the United States or to wilderness areas how to purify water for drinking and cooking.

Discuss the importance of maintaining fluid intake to replace lost water and electrolytes. Encourage use of Gatorade or a similar product rather than water for fluid replacement. A solution of 1 quart (1 L) of water, 1 teaspoon (5 mL) each of table salt and baking soda, 4 teaspoons (20 mL) of granulated sugar, and desired flavoring (such as lemon extract or juice) can be made at home to replace water and electrolytes.

Explain that food intake is not vital or recommended during episodes of acute diarrhea. If an antidiarrheal drug is used, review its precautions and limitations. For the client with chronic diarrhea, provide information on foods to avoid (see Table 20-1) and foods to include to maintain adequate nutritional status.

Constipation

Constipation is defined as infrequent or difficult passage of stools. Clients may complain of constipation when they have less than one stool per day, even if feces are of normal consistency and are not difficult to expel. The term *constipation* is appropriate only when the client has two or fewer bowel movements weekly, or when defecation is excessively difficult or requires straining.

Constipation affects older adults more often than younger people. Although intestinal transit times slow with aging, more significant factors include general health, medications, and activity levels (Box 20-3).

PATHOPHYSIOLOGY

Acute constipation may be due to an organic cause such as a tumor or partial bowel obstruction. Lifestyle and psychogenic factors (such as ignoring the urge to defecate or feeling the need to defecate on schedule) are the most frequent causes of chronic constipation. Other common causes of constipation are listed in Table 20-3 ◆. The client with significant constipation may develop a *fecal impaction* (hardened stool). Small amounts of watery mucus or liquid stool may pass around the impaction. The client has a full sensation in the rectal area and abdominal cramping.

TABLE 20-3   COMMON CAUSES OF CONSTIPATION

FACTOR	RELATED CAUSE
Activity	Lack of exercise; impaired mobility; bed rest
Dietary	Highly refined, low-fiber foods; inadequate fluid intake
Drugs	Antacids containing aluminum or calcium salts; narcotic analgesics; many antidepressants, tranquilizers, and sedatives; antihypertensives; iron salts
Large bowel	Diverticular disease, inflammatory disease, tumor, obstruction; changes in rectal or anal structure or function
Systemic	Advanced age; pregnancy; neurologic conditions (like stroke); endocrine and metabolic disorders (like hypothyroidism)
Psychogenic	Voluntary suppression of urge; perceived need to defecate on schedule; depression
Other	Chronic laxative or enema use

COLLABORATIVE CARE

On examination, the abdomen may appear distended, and bowel sounds may be reduced. Digital examination of the rectum in the client with an impaction reveals a palpable hard or puttylike fecal mass.

Simple or chronic constipation is best treated with education and modification of diet and exercise routines. If the problem is acute or does not resolve, diagnostic studies such as *serum electrolytes* and *thyroid function tests* may be ordered. A *barium enema* or *flexible colonoscopy* may be done to identify structural lesions of the colon. (See the section on colon cancer later in this chapter for nursing care related to a colonoscopy.) Nursing care for clients having a barium enema is outlined in Box 20-4. Table 20-4 ◆ provides nursing implications for commonly prescribed bowel preparations.

Dietary Management

Foods that have a high fiber content are recommended. Review Box 20-3 for recommended foods and strategies.

CLINICAL alert

Bulk-forming agents, such as methylcellulose, are the only safe laxatives for long-term use. They increase the bulk of the feces and draw water into the bowel to soften it. At least 6 to 8 glasses of water should be consumed daily when using these (or any) laxatives.

BOX 20-4
NURSING CARE CHECKLIST

BARIUM ENEMA
Before the Procedure

☑ Verify signed consent for the procedure.
☑ Withhold food and fluids as ordered (usually liquids only the day before and NPO for 8 hours before the procedure).
☑ Administer laxatives, enemas, or suppositories as ordered the evening before and morning of the procedure.

Client and Family Teaching
Before Procedure

☑ Do not eat or drink anything for 8 hours before the exam.
☑ The procedure takes approximately 1 hour.
☑ You will be asked to turn to different positions during this procedure.
☑ You will feel a full sensation and the urge to defecate as the barium is instilled.
☑ The bowel will be examined as it fills with barium, and x-rays will be taken.
☑ You will expel the barium in the bathroom.

After Procedure

☑ You will be given a laxative to help expel the barium.
☑ Your stools may be white for the next 1 to 2 days.

Pharmacology

Laxatives and cathartics were among the earliest drugs. Milder preparations are generally known as *laxatives; cathartics* have a stronger effect. Most laxatives are appropriate only for short-term use. Cathartics and enemas interfere with normal bowel reflexes and should not be used for simple constipation. Commonly ordered laxatives are listed in Table 20-4.

CLINICAL alert

Laxatives should *never* be given if a bowel obstruction or impaction is suspected, nor to people with abdominal pain of unknown cause. Administering laxatives or cathartics when the bowel is obstructed may damage the bowel and lead to perforation.

Enemas

Significant or chronic constipation or a fecal impaction may require the administration of an enema. They may also be prescribed to prepare the bowel for diagnostic testing or examination. They are never used when there may be obstruction or

TABLE 20-4 NURSING IMPLICATIONS FOR PHARMACOLOGY: CLIENTS RECEIVING BOWEL PREPARATION CATHARTICS AND LAXATIVES

AGENT/DRUGS	PURPOSE	NURSING IMPLICATIONS	CLIENT TEACHING
Bowel Preparation Cathartics			
Magnesium Citrate ▪ Citrate of magnesia ▪ Citro-Nesia ▪ Citroma *Polyethylene Glycol and Electrolytes* ▪ Colyte ▪ GoLYTELY ▪ X-Prep	These laxatives often are used as bowel preparation prior to colon x-ray studies or colonoscopy. They promote bowel evacuation by drawing fluid into the bowel. As fluid accumulates, it distends the colon and stimulates peristalsis, causing diarrhea, which rapidly cleans the bowel. Electrolytes may be added to the solution to minimize electrolyte imbalance with their use.	Chill the solution to enhance palatability. Administer in early evening to reduce sleep disturbance. Evacuation begins within 1 hour and continues until stool is clear and free of solid matter. Magnesium Citrate ▪ Administer on an empty stomach followed by a full glass of water. Polyethylene Glycol ▪ Administer 8 ounces of solution every 10 minutes.	Expect some degree of abdominal cramping. Do not eat solid food 3 to 4 hours prior, nor within 2 hours of, ingesting polyethylene glycol solution. Do not use this medication for routine treatment of constipation.
Laxatives			
Bulk-Forming Agents ▪ Bran ▪ Calcium polycarbophil (Fibercon) ▪ Methylcellulose (Citrucel) ▪ Psyllium hydrophilic mucilloid (Metamucil, Effer-Syllium)	Bulk-forming agents contain indigestible vegetable fiber. This natural fiber creates bulk and draws water into the intestine, softening the stool mass.	Mix the agent with a full glass of cool liquid just prior to administering. Do not administer to clients with possible impaction or bowel obstruction.	These agents may be mixed with water, milk, or fruit juice. Take in the morning or with meals. To reduce the risk of impaction, do not take at bedtime. With these and all laxatives, drink at least 6 to 8 glasses of water daily.
Stool Softeners ▪ Docusate (Colace, Surfak, Doxidan, others)	Stool softeners draw water into the stool and form an emulsion of fat and water, softening the stool. They are used to prevent straining and reduce the discomfort of expelling hard stools.	Administer with ample fluids. Stool softeners may affect drug absorption. Do not give within 1 hour of other oral medications. Do not crush or open caplets; a liquid form is available for clients with difficulty swallowing.	Do not use for longer than 1 week. Take in the morning or evening; avoid taking it at the same time as other medications.
Osmotic and Saline Laxative/ Cathartics ▪ Lactulose (Rhodialose) ▪ Sorbitol ▪ Magnesium hydroxide (Milk of Magnesia) ▪ Magnesium citrate ▪ Polyethylene glycol (Klean-Prep)	These laxatives contain poorly absorbed salts or carbohydrates that draw water into the intestine to increase stool volume, decrease its consistency, and stimulate peristalsis. These drugs also may stimulate peristalsis by irritating the bowel mucosa. They are used to relieve acute constipation and should be limited to acute, short-term use; chronic use may suppress normal bowel reflexes.	Assess for contraindications, such as bowel obstruction, fluid or electrolyte imbalances, heart failure, or renal failure. Administer with a full glass of liquid, preferably in the morning to avoid sleep disturbance. Monitor fluid and electrolyte status; skin turgor; mucous membranes; intake and output; daily weight; and serum electrolytes.	Do not use these drugs on a regular basis to treat or prevent constipation. Notify your doctor if you develop abdominal pain, bloody stool, excessive skin or mucous membrane dryness, rapid weight loss, dizziness, or other unusual symptoms. These agents work in 3 to 6 hours; take them in the morning to avoid sleep disturbance.

TABLE 20-4   NURSING IMPLICATIONS FOR PHARMACOLOGY: CLIENTS RECEIVING BOWEL PREPARATION CATHARTICS AND LAXATIVES (CONTINUED)

AGENT/DRUGS	PURPOSE	NURSING IMPLICATIONS	CLIENT TEACHING
Irritant or Stimulant Laxatives ■ Bisacodyl (Dulcolax, Bisco-Lax, Carter's Liver Pills, Codylax, others) ■ Phenolphthalein (Evac-U-Gen, Evac-U-Lax, Feen-A-Mint, Phenolax, others) ■ Cascara sagrada ■ Senna (Senna laxative, Fletcher's Castoria) ■ Castor oil	These laxatives stimulate intestinal motility and secretions. They cause watery stool, often accompanied by abdominal cramping and pain. They are used as a secondary measure to relieve constipation and for bowel preparation prior to diagnostic testing.	Assess for contraindications such as abdominal pain and cramping, nausea and vomiting, anal or rectal fissures. Food may affect absorption; give on an empty stomach. Do not crush enteric-coated bisacodyl tablets. This may hasten their dissolution in the stomach, leading to gastric distress.	Do not use this type of laxative, even in over-the-counter preparations, for initial treatment of constipation. Do not use for more than 1 week as these drugs can be habit forming. Do not use if you are pregnant or lactating. Laxatives that contain phenolphthalein may turn urine pink or red. Stop taking the drug and contact your doctor if you develop difficulty breathing, dizziness or light-headedness, or a rash.
Lubricants ■ Mineral oil	Mineral oil forms an oily coat on feces, preventing water reabsorption, and softening stool. Mineral oil reduces absorption of the fat-soluble vitamins A, D, E, and K and may damage the liver and spleen; pneumonia may develop from aspiration of oil droplets into the lungs.	Do not give with wetting agents or stool softeners, as these may increase systemic absorption and the effects of the mineral oil. Administer in the evening before bedtime to reduce the effect on vitamin absorption and minimize the risk of aspiration. Assess the manifestations of vitamin deficiency.	Long-term use of mineral oil is not recommended. Do not use mineral oil if you have hemorrhoids or rectal lesions; oil leakage may cause itching and interfere with healing. Suck on a lemon or orange slice after taking mineral oil to reduce the oily aftertaste.

risk of perforation. The following types of enemas may be prescribed:

■ A *saline enema* using 500 to 2,000 mL of warmed normal saline solution is the least irritating to the bowel.

■ *Tap-water enemas* use 500 to 1,000 mL of water to soften feces and irritate the bowel mucosa, stimulating peristalsis and evacuation.

■ *Soap-suds enemas* consist of a tap-water solution to which soap is added as a further irritant.

■ *Phosphate enemas* (e.g., Fleet) use a hypertonic saline solution to draw fluid into the bowel and irritate the mucosa, leading to evacuation.

■ *Oil-retention enemas* instill mineral or vegetable oil into the bowel to soften the fecal mass. The instilled oil is retained overnight or for several hours before evacuation.

Excess enema use, especially of tap-water or phosphate enemas, can impair bowel function and cause fluid and electrolyte imbalances.

NURSING CARE

CONSTIPATION

■ Assess and document pattern of defecation, including time of day, amount, and stool consistency. *Information about bowel habits helps identify physiologic versus perceived constipation. Whether real or perceived, constipation disrupts daily activities and life satisfaction.*

■ Assess diet, fluid intake, and activity. Evaluate for other contibuting factors, such as use of narcotic analgesics, prescribed bed rest, painful hemorrhoids, and perianal surgery. *These provide clues about possible causes of constipation. The client may require a bulk laxative or stool softener while contributing factors are present.*

■ Assess abdominal shape and girth, bowel sounds, and tenderness. If impaction is suspected, examine the rectum digitally, using a lubricated, gloved finger. *Constipation may cause abdominal distention, reduced bowel sounds, and some abdominal tenderness. Digital removal of stool impacted in the rectum may be required.*

■ Provide additional fluids to maintain an intake of at least 2,500 mL per day. *Adequate hydration facilitates normal bowel elimination.*

■ Encourage drinking of a glass of warm water before and after breakfast. Provide time and privacy following breakfast for bowel elimination. *Warm water provides mild stimulation of bowel peristalsis. Privacy helps encourage a pattern of natural elimination.*

■ Consult with the dietitian to increase dietary fiber (unless contraindicated). Provide foods such as natural bran, prunes, or prune juice. *Natural fiber adds bulk to the stool and has a mild stimulant effect.*

■ Encourage activity. *Activity stimulates peristalsis and strengthens abdominal muscles, facilitating elimination.*

■ If indicated, obtain an order for a stool softener, laxative, or enema. *Pharmacologic agents may be necessary to relieve acute constipation. Clients with restricted mobility or diet restrictions may need a bulk-forming laxative to prevent constipation.*

Discharge Considerations

Education is key, because the measures to relieve constipation are often the same as those to prevent it. Discuss the importance of maintaining a diet high in natural fiber, including foods such as fresh fruits, vegetables, whole-grain products, and bran. Encourage reduced consumption of meats and refined foods, which are low in fiber and can be constipating. Stress the need to maintain a high fluid intake, particularly when hot weather or exercise increases fluid loss. Discuss the relationship between exercise and bowel regularity. Encourage the client to engage in some form of exercise, such as walking, daily.

Provide information about the range of normal bowel habits. Encourage the client to respond to the urge to defecate when it occurs. Suggest setting aside a time, usually following a meal, for elimination. Discuss restricting the use of laxatives and enemas, and stress that bulk-forming laxatives are the only safe preparations for long-term use. Teach the client that straining to have a bowel movement can lead to hemorrhoids and tissue damage. Suggest abdominal massage to reduce discomfort and promote elimination.

 Irritable Bowel Syndrome

Irritable bowel syndrome is a motility disorder characterized by alternating periods of constipation and diarrhea. It affects up to 20% of people in Western civilization.

Intestinal motility can be affected by eating, stress, hormones, and drugs. Motility of both the small and large intestine are often affected in irritable bowel syndrome. Excess

---

mucus may be secreted in the colon as well. Stress may increase the manifestations of irritable bowel syndrome but does not cause them. The client with irritable bowel syndrome may experience a change in the frequency or consistency of stools, straining, urgency, or a sensation of incomplete evacuation. Other manifestations of the disorder are listed in Box 20-5.

COLLABORATIVE CARE

The diagnosis of irritable bowel syndrome is based on the client's history, the pattern of symptoms and elimination, and physical examination. A *small bowel series* (also known as an upper GI series with small bowel follow-through) and barium enema may be ordered. For the small bowel series, the client is given an oral barium preparation, and the small intestine is examined under fluoroscopy. The entire GI tract may demonstrate increased motility. Box 20-6 outlines nursing care of the client undergoing a small bowel series.

Management is directed toward relieving the symptoms and reducing or eliminating precipitating factors. Stress reduction, exercises, or counseling may benefit the client. Although no specific diet is recommended, reduced milk intake may benefit some clients. Restricting gas-forming foods, fruits and berries, or caffeinated drinks may also be helpful. Addition of dietary fiber reduces the incidence of both loose diarrheal stools and hard, constipated stools.

NURSING CARE

When clients with irritable bowel syndrome are seen in the acute care setting, the disorder usually is a secondary condition. The previous sections on diarrhea and constipation provide selected nursing interventions for clients experiencing these manifestations.

When teaching, emphasize that the symptoms are real, believed, and not "all in the mind." Discuss related factors, such as stress, anxiety, and depression. Assist the client to explore any relationship between mental stress and bowel manifestations. Teach stress- and anxiety-reduction techniques, such as exercise and progressive relaxation. Refer to a counselor for assistance in dealing with psychological factors.

Help identify possible dietary influences on elimination patterns, and suggest changes such as increased water and fiber intake that may help relieve symptoms. Encourage changes in exercise and dietary patterns and use of stress-reduction techniques to gradually eliminate the need for prescribed medications.

Stress the importance of notifying the primary care provider if symptoms change, because the manifestations of irritable bowel syndrome may mask symptoms of an organic problem, such as a tumor.

Fecal Incontinence

Fecal incontinence, the loss of voluntary control of defecation, is an infrequent but distressing problem. Clients often do not reveal this problem when discussing health concerns. Physiologic and psychological factors, as well as age-related changes, can contribute to fecal incontinence (Box 20-7).

Management of fecal incontinence is directed at its cause. Medications to relieve diarrhea or constipation may be ordered. Dietary changes, ample fluids, and regular exercise may be helpful. Kegel exercises to improve sphincter and pelvic floor muscle tone may help. A bowel training program to establish a regular pattern of elimination is often effective. The client is taught to establish a regular time of day for elimination, usually 15 to 30 minutes after breakfast. A stimulant, such as a cup of coffee or a rectal suppository, may be given to prompt defecation.

> **BOX 20-7**
> **SELECTED CAUSES**
> **OF FECAL INCONTINENCE**
>
> - Diarrhea
> - Stool impaction
> - Pelvic floor relaxation or loss of sphincter tone
> - Tumors
> - Local trauma (obstetric tears, anorectal injury, or surgery)
> - Spinal cord injury, head injury, stroke
> - Degenerative neurologic disease
> - Diabetic neuropathy
> - Depression or dementia

NURSING CARE

For the alert client, fecal incontinence can lead to a loss of self-esteem and social isolation.

BOWEL INCONTINENCE

- Teach caregivers to place the client on a toilet or commode and provide for privacy at a certain time of day. *Placing the client in a normal position to defecate at a consistent time of day helps reestablish a pattern of stool evacuation.*
- If necessary, insert a glycerine suppository 15 to 20 minutes before placing on the toilet or commode. *This helps to stimulate evacuation. Once a regular elimination pattern is established, it may be possible to discontinue suppository use.*
- Maintain a caring, nonjudgmental manner. Provide room odor control with deodorizer tablets, sprays, or other devices. *These measures help the client feel accepted and help reduce embarrassment when caregivers or visitors enter the room.*

RISK FOR IMPAIRED SKIN INTEGRITY

- Clean skin thoroughly with soap and water after each bowel movement. Apply a skin barrier cream or ointment. *Irritation of perianal and perineal skin by fecal material can lead to tissue breakdown and pressure ulcers. Toilet tissue may increase irritation and is less effective than soap and water for removing fecal material.*
- If incontinence pads or briefs are used, check frequently for soiling, and change promptly when soiled. *Although these help protect bedding and clothing, they can contribute to skin breakdown if they are not checked and changed frequently.*

Discharge Considerations

Managing fecal incontinence is challenging for both the client and caregivers. Stress that incontinence is never normal (i.e., not a result of aging) and often is treatable. Provide teaching as for constipation (p. 462). Provide bowel training instructions. Stress the importance of good skin care.

Malabsorption

Malabsorption is a condition of ineffective intestinal absorption of nutrients. It commonly occurs with disorders of the small intestine.

Two major causes of malabsorption are celiac disease and lactose intolerance. *Celiac disease* (or nontropical sprue) is a hereditary disorder characterized by sensitivity to *gluten* (a cereal protein found in wheat, rye, barley, and oats). In celiac disease, absorption of nutrients, particularly fats, is impaired. *Lactose intolerance* is caused by deficient lactase, the enzyme required to digest milk and milk products. Lactase deficiency affects up to 90% of Asians and 75% of African Americans and Indians, as well as many Jewish Americans and Hispanics.

Resection of the small intestine *(short bowel syndrome)* also can lead to malabsorption. The severity of the disorder depends on the amount and location of bowel resected. Whatever the cause, manifestations result from impaired absorption of food and nutrients (see Box 20-8).

With any malabsorptive disorder, the first focus is finding the cause. *Stool samples* are examined for fat content. A *D-xylose absorption test* or *xylose tolerance test* is used to evaluate intestinal absorption. A *lactose breath test* or a *lactose tolerance test* may be ordered. Numerous laboratory tests for nutrient deficiencies may be ordered to evaluate the effects of malabsorption.

Treatment focuses on the underlying disorder. A gluten-free diet is ordered for clients with celiac disease (Box 20-9). Clients with lactose intolerance may need to eliminate all milk and milk products. Lactase enzyme preparations may be given to improve milk tolerance. Frequent, small, high-calorie, high-protein feedings are prescribed for short bowel syndrome. All clients may require vitamin and mineral supplements.

Nursing care focuses on the effects of the disorder on nutrition and on bowel elimination. Document nutritional status, including weight, fat-fold measurements, laboratory values, and dietary intake. Supplement intake with enteral feedings as ordered. Maintain central lines and total parenteral nutrition, if required. Assess intake and output, daily weights, skin turgor, and condition of mucous membranes to monitor hydration. For diarrhea, document the number and character of stools. Administer antidiarrheal medications as ordered. Provide good skin care of the perianal region.

Discuss day-to-day management of the disorder, including the recommended diet and medication regimen. Provide a detailed list of foods to include and to eliminate from the diet. Teach to read labels and lists of ingredients to identify hidden sources of the nutrient to which they are sensitive.

Emphasize the importance of adequate fluid intake, increasing intake for hot weather or increased exercise. Teach to regularly monitor weight and report changes. Address manifestations that should be reported to the physician. Refer to a dietitian or counselor for additional dietary teaching and coping strategies.

Inflammatory and Infectious Disorders

The gastrointestinal tract is constantly exposed to the external environment, making it particularly vulnerable to inflammation and infection. Most pathogens that affect it are ingested

in food or water. With acute disorders such as appendicitis and peritonitis, bacteria normally residing in the GI tract infect damaged or normally sterile tissue.

Appendicitis

Appendicitis (inflammation of the appendix) is the most common reason for emergency abdominal surgery in the United States. The appendix is in the right lower quadrant region at *McBurney's point* (Figure 20-3 ◆). Its function is not fully understood, but it regularly fills with and empties digested food. Appendicitis is most common in adolescents and young adults and slightly more common in males than females.

PATHOPHYSIOLOGY

The appendix can become obstructed by a *fecalith* (hard mass of feces). As a result, the appendix becomes distended and its blood supply is impaired. This leads to inflammation, edema, ulceration, and infection. Within 24 to 36 hours, the tissue becomes necrotic and perforates if treatment is not initiated.

Appendicitis is classified by the stage of the process. In *simple appendicitis*, the appendix is inflamed but intact. In *gangrenous appendicitis*, the appendix has areas of tissue necrosis and microscopic perforations. With a *perforated appendix*, the appendix has ruptured, contaminating the peritoneal cavity.

Generalized or upper abdominal pain often is the initial symptom of acute appendicitis. The pain gradually intensifies and localizes in the right lower quadrant of the abdomen. It is aggravated by moving, walking, or coughing. Localized and rebound tenderness are noted at McBurney's point. *Rebound tenderness* is demonstrated by relief of pain during palpation followed by pain on release of pressure. Extension of the right hip increases the pain. Less acute pain and local tenderness may delay diagnosis in pregnant women and older adults. The client may have a low-grade fever, anorexia, nausea, and vomiting.

Perforation is the major complication of acute appendicitis. Perforation is manifested by increased pain and a high fever. It can result in a small, localized abscess, local peritonitis, or significant generalized peritonitis.

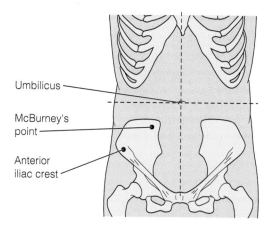

Figure 20-3. ◆ McBurney's point, located midway between the ubilicus and the anterior iliac crest in the right lower quadrant.

Labels: Umbilicus; McBurney's point; Anterior iliac crest

COLLABORATIVE CARE

Because the acutely inflamed appendix can perforate within 24 hours, prompt diagnosis and treatment are important. Diagnostic testing and preoperative treatment are limited. The *white blood count (WBC)* is elevated in appendicitis. An *abdominal ultrasound* may be done to confirm the diagnosis if symptoms are atypical. The client is admitted to the hospital, and intravenous fluids are initiated. Oral food and fluids are withheld until a diagnosis is confirmed.

The treatment of choice for acute appendicitis is an *appendectomy,* surgical removal of the appendix. The appendectomy may be performed through a **laparotomy** (surgical opening of the abdomen) or by **laparoscopy** (exploration of the abdomen using an endoscope). *Laparoscopic appendectomy* requires three very small incisions, and recovery is rapid. Antibiotic therapy is initiated prior to surgery and continues for at least 48 hours postoperatively.

NURSING CARE

Assessment of the client with suspected appendicitis focuses on describing the pain, as well as its onset, severity, and duration. Ask about recent food or fluid intake, allergies, and current medications. Ensure that an informed consent has been signed prior to surgery. Explain why food and fluids are not permitted during this time. If time allows, teach postoperative turning, coughing, deep breathing, and pain management.

INEFFECTIVE TISSUE PERFUSION: GASTROINTESTINAL

- Monitor for signs of perforation and peritonitis preoperatively. *A primary goal of care is to prevent complications. Perforation may be signaled by a sudden relief of pain as the appendix ruptures, followed by increased generalized pain and abdominal distention.*
- Monitor vital signs. *An elevated pulse and rapid shallow breathing may indicate perforation of the appendix with infection and peritonitis. The temperature may be elevated. If sepsis develops, the blood pressure may fall.*
- Maintain intravenous fluids until the client is able to drink adequate amounts postoperatively. *Intravenous fluids help maintain fluid and electrolyte balance and vascular volume.*
- Postoperatively, monitor wound, abdominal girth, and pain. *Swelling of the wound, increased abdominal girth, or increased pain may indicate infection or peritonitis.*

PAIN

- Assess pain, including its character, location, severity, and duration. Report any unexpected changes in description of pain. *Careful pain assessment can provide important clues about diagnosis and possible complications. For example, generalized abdominal pain with guarding of abdominal muscles may indicate peritonitis.*

- Administer prescribed analgesics. *Preoperatively, pain medication can be given after a diagnosis is established. Postoperatively, provide analgesics to promote comfort and enhance mobility.*
- Assess effectiveness of medication after administration. If pain is not relieved, contact the charge nurse or physician. *Pain unrelieved by analgesics may indicate a complication.*
- Provide alternative methods of pain relief, including distraction, therapeutic touch, massage, meditation, or visualization. *These techniques can enhance comfort and the effectiveness of analgesics.*

Discharge Considerations

Following an uncomplicated appendectomy, the client is usually dismissed from the health care setting either the day of surgery or the day following surgery. Teach wound or incision care. Instruct to report swelling, redness, drainage, bleeding, or warmth at the operative site to the surgeon. If a dressing is present, teach proper handwashing and dressing change procedures. Instruct the client to report any fever or increased abdominal pain.

Discuss activity restrictions. Heavy lifting may be restricted for up to 6 weeks. Depending on the surgery, driving and return to work may be allowed within 1 to 2 weeks. Community health or home health care nurses may be required if the client has a preexisting illness or has trouble performing activities of daily living (ADLs) and self-care.

Peritonitis

Peritonitis is inflammation of the peritoneum, a double-layered membrane that lines the walls and organs of the abdominal cavity. It is a serious complication of many acute abdominal disorders. Peritonitis results when the normally sterile, potential space between the layers of the peritoneum is contaminated. A perforated appendix or gastric ulcer, traumatic injury such as a gunshot wound, or contamination during abdominal surgery can lead to peritonitis.

PATHOPHYSIOLOGY

Chemical peritonitis develops immediately following perforation of a peptic ulcer, as gastric juices (hydrochloric acid and pepsin) enter the peritoneal cavity. *Bacterial peritonitis* results when bacteria that are normally confined within the bowel enter the peritoneal cavity. Normal defense mechanisms may effectively eliminate small numbers of bacteria or localize the infection. Massive or continued contamination, however, leads to generalized inflammation of the peritoneal cavity. The inflammatory process causes a fluid shift into the peritoneal space *(third-spacing)*. Peristalsis slows or stops **(paralytic ileus)** due to the inflammation.

The signs and symptoms of peritonitis depend on the severity and extent of the infection, as well as the age and gen-

eral health of the client. Both abdominal and systemic manifestations are present (Box 20-10). The client often presents with evidence of an *acute abdomen*.

CLINICAL alert

The older, chronically debilitated, or immunosuppressed client may have few of the classic signs of peritonitis. Increased confusion and restlessness, decreased urinary output, and vague abdominal complaints may be the only manifestations.

Complications of peritonitis may be life threatening and either localized or systemic. Formation of an *abscess* is the most common complication. *Septicemia* may develop. Without prompt treatment, shock may result from hypovolemia or sepsis. Shock (see Chapter 10) requires immediate, aggressive treatment to prevent multiple organ failure and death. *Adhesions* or bands of scar tissue may develop after peritonitis and subsequently cause a bowel obstruction.

COLLABORATIVE CARE

Care of the client with peritonitis focuses on identifying and treating both the peritonitis and its cause.

The WBC is significantly elevated in peritonitis. *Blood cultures* are obtained to identify possible *bacteremia* (bacterial invasion of the blood), which often precedes septicemia. A *paracentesis* may be done to obtain peritoneal fluid for analysis (see Box 19-13 for nursing care of a client having a paracentesis).

Intestinal decompression is initiated to relieve abdominal distention. A nasogastric or long intestinal tube (Figure 20-4 ◆) is inserted and connected to continuous drainage. Suction is maintained and the client is NPO until peristalsis returns (bowel sounds are heard and flatus is being passed). Intravenous fluids and electrolyte replacements are provided. Total parenteral nutrition is given until oral intake resumes. The client is placed

---

BOX 20-10
MANIFESTATIONS OF PERITONITIS

ABDOMINAL
- Diffuse or localized pain, usually severe
- Tenderness with rebound
- Boardlike rigidity or guarding of abdominal muscles
- Diminished or absent bowel sounds
- Progressive distention
- Anorexia, nausea, and vomiting

SYSTEMIC
- Fever, malaise
- Tachycardia, tachypnea
- Restlessness, confusion
- Oliguria

Figure 20-4. ◆ A Cantor tube used for intestinal decompression. The weighted end of the tube is drawn into the small intestine by peristalsis.

on bed rest in Fowler's position to help localize the infection and to make breathing easier. Oxygen is often ordered.

A broad-spectrum antibiotic is prescribed until the infecting organism has been identified. Then antibiotic therapy is modified to the specific organism(s). (Nursing implications for common antibiotics are outlined in Table 12-5.) The client may receive narcotic analgesics and sedatives to promote comfort and rest.

A laparotomy may be done to close a perforation, remove damaged and inflamed tissue, or remove an abscess. *Peritoneal lavage* (washing of the peritoneal cavity with warm isotonic fluid) may be done during surgery. Peritoneal lavage may be continued for up to 3 days after surgery. The solution is infused into the upper portion of the peritoneal cavity and removed via drains in the pelvis. Careful attention to fluid and electrolyte status and strict aseptic technique are necessary.

Clients who have had laparotomy for peritonitis often return from surgery with drains such as a Jackson-Pratt. In some cases, the incision may be left unsutured. The abdomen may be closed temporarily with mesh containing a nylon zipper or Velcro to allow repeated exploration of the abdomen and drainage of infectious sites.

NURSING CARE

Peritonitis is a serious illness. Clients require intensive nursing and medical interventions to recover fully.

ASSESSING

Nursing assessment of clients with peritonitis focuses on monitoring their current status, progress of recovery, and identifying possible complications. Continuing assessments for clients with peritonitis are listed in Box 20-11.

DIAGNOSING, PLANNING, AND IMPLEMENTING

PAIN

- Place in Fowler's or semi-Fowler's position with the knees and feet elevated. *This position helps minimize stress on abdominal structures and facilitate respirations, promoting comfort.*

BOX 20-11
ASSESSING CLIENTS WITH PERITONITIS

SUBJECTIVE DATA

- Pain: Type or character, location, severity
- Anxiety and coping

OBJECTIVE DATA

- Assess mental status and level of consciousness every 4 to 8 hours. Report changes to the charge nurse or physician.
- Check vital signs (including temperature and measurements such as central venous pressure as ordered) hourly or as indicated.
- Check urine output every 1 to 2 hours. Report output less than 30 mL/hr.
- Assess drainage from gastrointestinal tube and surgical drains such as Jackson-Pratt every 4 hours or as ordered. Record color, odor, and type of drainage; report changes.
- Assess intake (intravenous and oral) every 8 hours or as indicated.
- Weigh daily. Report changes.
- Assess skin turgor, color, temperature; mucous membrane color and moisture every 8 hours.
- Measure abdominal girth with the same measuring tape at the umbilicus every 8 hours.

- Administer analgesics as ordered on a routine basis or using patient-controlled analgesia (PCA). Frequently evaluate response to analgesics. *Routine administration of analgesics helps maintain pain control, facilitating healing and movement. Decreasing effectiveness of the medication may indicate a complication.*
- Teach and assist to use alternative pain management techniques along with analgesics. *Meditation, visualization, massage, and progressive relaxation augment analgesics and increase comfort.*

DEFICIENT FLUID VOLUME

- Record vital signs, intake and output, weight, moisture of skin and mucous membranes as indicated. Measure or estimate fluid losses through abdominal drains and on dressings. *Fluid losses occur through third-spacing, gastrointestinal suction, and drainage from surgical wounds and drains. This can lead to hypovolemia.*
- Monitor laboratory values, such as hemoglobin and hematocrit, urine specific gravity, and serum electrolytes. Report changes to the physician. *These values provide information about the client's fluid and electrolyte status.*
- Maintain intravenous fluids and electrolytes as ordered. *Gastrointestinal drainage may be replaced milliliter for milli-*

liter with a balanced electrolyte solution. In addition, fluid intake must be maintained intravenously while the client is NPO.

■ Provide good skin care and frequent oral hygiene. *Fluid loss increases the risk of skin breakdown and ulceration of mucous membranes.*

INEFFECTIVE PROTECTION

■ Monitor for signs of infection, including fever, tachycardia, redness and swelling around incisions and drain sites, increased or purulent drainage, and cloudy, malodorous, or scant urine. *Surgical interventions and stress on immune defenses increase the risk for further infection.*

■ Obtain cultures of purulent drainage from any site. *Early identification allows appropriate intervention to be instituted.*

■ Practice meticulous handwashing before and after providing care. Use strict aseptic technique for dressing changes and wound or peritoneal irrigations. *Handwashing reduces transient bacteria on the skin and remains the most important method of controlling infection. Interruption of the skin barrier increases the risk for infection.*

■ Maintain fluid balance and adequate nutrition through either enteral or parenteral feedings, as indicated. *Adequate nutrition and fluid balance are necessary for optimal immune system function.*

ANXIETY

■ Assess the client's and family's anxiety level and coping skills. *This provides a basis on which to plan interventions.*

■ Present a calm, reassuring manner. Encourage the client and family to express their concerns; listen carefully, and acknowledge their validity. *This helps establish trust.*

■ Minimize changes in caregiver assignments. *Consistency of nursing care and care providers helps reduce anxiety. Complex wound care and irrigation procedures are best performed by people who are very familiar with prescribed techniques.*

■ Explain all treatments, procedures, tests, and examinations. Reinforce and clarify information provided by physicians. *Understanding what is being done helps reduce anxiety and promote acceptance.*

■ Teach and assist with relaxation techniques such as meditation, visualization, and progressive relaxation. *These measures promote positive coping skills and reduce physical manifestations of anxiety.*

EVALUATING

Collect the following data to evaluate the effectiveness of nursing care for the client with peritonitis: level of pain and effectiveness of analgesics; weight, urine output, and other indicators of fluid volume status; temperature, wound healing and drainage, and other indicators of infection; and indicators of anxiety and effective coping.

Discharge Considerations

Teaching is vital throughout hospitalization and prior to discharge. Assessment data collected prior to discharge helps individualize teaching to the client and family (Box 20-12).

Begin teaching for home care prior to discharge. Provide verbal and written instructions for wound care, dressing changes, and irrigation procedures. Allow the client and family members to practice and demonstrate procedures before discharge. Include information on where to obtain necessary supplies. Discuss medications, including the name and purpose of the drug and potential adverse effects and their management.

Describe the signs and symptoms of further infection (redness, heat, swelling, purulent drainage, chills, and fever) and other potential complications. Emphasize the need to report adverse responses promptly to the primary care provider. Reinforce instructions about activity restrictions. Discuss the importance of consuming a diet with adequate

BOX 20-12
ASSESSING FOR DISCHARGE

PERITONITIS
Client

● Self-care: Ability to independently perform ADLs; to manage wound care and medications; to prepare and eat a nutritionally sound diet
● Knowledge: Wound care needs and medications, diet recommendations and activity limitations, follow-up care; signs of complications to report to physician
● Psychosocial: Ability to cope with continued care needs and economic effects; acceptance of altered body image and roles/relationships
● Home environment: Access to clean running water, handwashing and cooking facilities; clean area in which to perform wound care

Family and Caregivers

● Members of household: Ability and willingness to assist with ADLs, wound care, central line management, and other care needs
● Financial resources: Income; resources for dressings, supplies, food supplements; effect of extended recovery period on roles and relationships, stability of family unit

Community

● Water and sanitation services
● Availability of home health and social support services

calories and protein to promote healing and optimal immune function. Provide a referral to home health services for assessment, wound care, and further teaching, as needed.

Nursing Process Case Study
■ CLIENT WITH A PERFORATED APPENDIX

Jamie Lynn, a 19-year-old college student, presents at the emergency department complaining of general lower abdominal pain that started the previous evening. The pain has localized to the right lower quadrant and became severe about 6 hours ago. She reports nausea and has vomited twice.

Assessment Physical assessment data for Ms. Lynn includes: T 102.6° F (39.2° C); P 96; R 24; BP 110/70. Her skin is warm to the touch. Her abdomen is flat, with marked tenderness in right lower quadrant. Guarding is present throughout. Her WBC is 15,400/mm^3. The diagnosis of acute appendicitis with possible perforation is made, and Ms. Lynn is transferred to surgery for an exploratory laparotomy. In surgery, Ms. Lynn's ruptured appendix is removed and her peritoneal cavity is flushed with warmed saline before her incision is closed.

Diagnosis Following surgery, the nurses caring for Ms. Lynn identify the following diagnoses:

■ Impaired Skin Integrity related to laparotomy
■ Pain related to surgical intervention
■ Risk for Infection related to contamination of peritoneal cavity by bowel contents
■ Anxiety related to situational crisis

Expected Outcomes The expected outcomes specify that Ms. Lynn will:

■ Have normal healing of abdominal incisions.
■ Relate pain level of 3 or less on a scale of 1 to 10.
■ Demonstrate no further signs of infection.
■ Express decreased anxiety.

Planning and Implementation Nursing interventions planned and implemented for Ms. Lynn include:

■ Assess pain every 2 hours and provide analgesics as needed.
■ Assess wound every 8 hours; change dressing as needed using aseptic technique.
■ Teach postdischarge wound care.
■ Discuss activity limitations after discharge, such as refraining from heavy lifting and not driving until approved by the physician.
■ Instruct Ms. Lynn to report temperature elevation and warmth, redness, or drainage from the incision to the physician.
■ Discuss pain management and importance of continuing prescribed antibiotic treatment after discharge.

Evaluation Ms. Lynn is discharged 3 days after surgery. Her incision is healing well, and she shows no further evidence of infection. Her bowel sounds are active, and she is taking food and fluids without nausea. She will return to the physician's office for a follow-up visit in 5 days.

 Critical Thinking in the Nursing Process

1. Why was Ms. Lynn's WBC elevated?
2. Outline a teaching plan to give to clients for home care following a laparotomy.
3. Develop a care plan for Ms. Lynn for the nursing diagnosis Anxiety related to a situational crisis.

Gastroenteritis

Gastroenteritis is inflammation of the stomach and intestines. It usually is caused by a bacterial, viral, or parasitic infection, or by a toxin. Bacterial and viral infections are often termed *food poisoning,* because contaminated food is often the route of entry. Clients experience diarrhea, abdominal discomfort, and often anorexia, nausea, and vomiting.

PATHOPHYSIOLOGY

Bacterial or viral infection of the GI tract produces inflammation, tissue damage, and symptoms by two primary mechanisms:

1. *Production of enterotoxins.* Many bacteria produce and excrete a toxin that damages and inflames the GI tract. Enterotoxins impair intestinal absorption and can cause electrolytes and water to be secreted into the bowel, leading to diarrhea and fluid loss.
2. *Invasion and ulceration of the mucosa.* Other bacteria invade intestinal mucosa, causing ulceration, bleeding, fluid exudate, and water and electrolyte secretion.

Manifestations of bacterial and viral enteritis vary by organism but have several common features (Box 20-13). Excess fluid in the bowel and increased bowel motility causes

---

**BOX 20-13
MANIFESTATIONS
OF GASTROENTERITIS**

GASTROINTESTINAL
• Anorexia, nausea, and vomiting
• Abdominal pain and cramping
• Borborygmi (excessively loud, hyperactive bowel sounds)
• Diarrhea

GENERAL
• Malaise, weakness, muscle aches
• Dry skin and mucous membranes, poor turgor
• Orthostatic hypotension, tachycardia
• Elevated temperature

diarrhea with frequent, watery stools. Lost fluids and electrolytes can lead to dehydration, hypovolemia, and manifestations of fluid and electrolyte or acid–base imbalances.

Severe vomiting may lead to metabolic alkalosis. With diarrhea, metabolic acidosis is more likely. Hypokalemia and hyponatremia may also occur. The specific effects of certain GI infections are summarized in Table 20-5 ◆.

COLLABORATIVE CARE

Identifying the cause, managing symptoms, and preventing complications are the primary goals of care. The client's history and symptoms provide valuable clues about the cause. A *stool specimen* may be obtained for culture, ova and parasites, and leukocyte count.

Fluid and electrolyte replacement is the primary focus of care. Oral rehydration is optimal. An oral glucose–electrolyte solution is often well tolerated in sips, even by the client who is vomiting. Commercial or homemade preparations may be used. Intravenous fluids such as glucose in normal saline, Ringer's, or lactated Ringer's may be ordered when vomiting and diarrhea are severe.

An antidiarrheal drug may be prescribed to promote comfort and reduce fluid loss. Nursing measures related to the use of antidiarrheal agents are outlined in Table 20-2.

Gastric lavage and catharsis—to "wash out" the stomach and intestines—may be ordered if botulism is suspected and if the food has been recently ingested. Botulism antitoxin is administered as soon as possible when botulism is suspected.

TABLE 20-5 SELECTED CAUSES OF GASTROENTERITIS

DISEASE AND ORGANISM	INCUBATION	SOURCE	MANIFESTATIONS
Traveler's diarrhea *Escherichia coli*	24–72 hours	Contaminated food or water	Abrupt onset of diarrhea; vomiting rare
Staphylococcal food poisoning	2–8 hours	Contaminated food—meats and fish, dairy products	Severe nausea and vomiting; abdominal cramping and diarrhea; headache and fever
Botulism *Clostridium botulinum*	1.5–8 days	Improperly preserved foods such as home-canned vegetables, smoked meats, vacuum-packed fish	Diplopia, blurred vision; dry mouth, dysphagia; progressive muscle weakness and paralysis; possible nausea, vomiting, abdominal cramps
Cholera *Vibrio cholerae*	1–3 days	Water or food contaminated by feces; endemic in parts of Asia, Middle East, and Africa	Asymptomatic or severe diarrhea with watery grey, odorless stool; vomiting; thirst, oliguria, muscle cramps; weakness; dehydration
Hemorrhagic colitis *E. coli 0157:H7*	1–3 days	Undercooked beef; unpasturized milk or apple juice	Severe cramping, watery to grossly bloody diarrhea; fever; complications of acute renal failure and thrombotic thrombocytopenic purpura
Salmonellosis *Salmonella*	8–48 hours	Raw or improperly cooked meat, poultry, eggs, and diary products	Diarrhea with cramping, nausea, and vomiting; low-grade fever, chills, weakness
Shigellosis (bacillary dysentery) *Shigella*	1–4 days	Fecal-contaminated food, fomites (inanimate objects), and vectors (such as fleas)	Watery diarrhea with blood, mucus, and pus; severe abdominal cramping and urgency of defecation; lethargy; dehydration
Giardiasis *Giardia lamblia*	1–3 weeks	Fecal–oral spread through contaminated food or water; direct contact	Diarrhea, mild or severe; anorexia, nausea, vomiting; epigastric pain, cramping; flatulence and belching; may be asymptomatic
Amebiasis *Entamoeba histolytica*	2–4 weeks	Fecal–oral spread through contaminated food or water; direct contact	Usually asymptomatic; diarrhea with blood and mucus; abdominal cramping, tenderness, colic, tenesmus, and flatulence; nausea and vomiting; fever, fatigue, weight loss

It can prevent paralysis from progressing but does not affect existing paralysis. Epinephrine is kept at the bedside because the antitoxin can cause anaphylaxis. The client is observed closely for signs of respiratory distress. Respiratory support with endotracheal intubation and mechanical ventilation may be required (see Chapter 26).

CLINICAL alert

Antidiarrheal agents are not used when botulism is suspected. To remove the toxin from the bowel, cathartics may be ordered for these clients.

NURSING CARE

Few clients with acute gastroenteritis require hospitalization. Assessment, education, and support of self-care measures are major nursing responsibilities related to these disorders.

Ask about the onset of diarrhea and other symptoms such as nausea, vomiting, and abdominal pain. Inquire about recent travel, changes in diet or water supply, or activities such as picnics or pot-luck meals. Ask about others in the family or household who also may be experiencing symptoms. Ask about the frequency and severity of vomiting and diarrhea and the nature of diarrheal stools. Ask about other manifestations such as abdominal pain or cramping. Inquire about measures taken to relieve the symptoms and the ability to take in and retain fluids.

Emphasize that fluid replacement is more important than eating while diarrhea is severe. Advise use of a glucose–electrolyte solution. (See directions for making a rehydrating solution in the Discharge Considerations section for Diarrhea earlier in the chapter.) Discuss manifestations of dehydration or hypovolemia that require a physician's care.

Teach the importance of good handwashing to prevent spread of infection to others. Instruct to wash hands thoroughly with soap and running water for at least 10 seconds after each defecation. Wash contaminated clothing and linens separately in hot water and detergent. Emphasize the need to keep toilet areas clean and to maintain good personal hygiene. Advise avoiding rectal contact during sexual activity.

For specific interventions to manage diarrhea, see the preceding section of this chapter.

Discharge Considerations

Teach clients in all settings the following food and water safety measures:

- Maintain proper food temperatures. Promptly refrigerate cooked meats, dairy products, eggs and egg products.
- Do not drink unpasteurized milk.

- Do not eat raw meat products. Cook hamburger until no redness remains.
- Follow directions precisely when home-canning foods; use a pressure canner when processing nonacidic foods, such as vegetables, mushrooms, meats, and fish.
- Boil home-canned foods for 10 to 15 minutes after opening to destroy any potential toxin.
- Destroy, without touching or tasting, any food that is discolored or comes from a container that has been punctured, is cracked or bulging, or does not have a tight seal.
- When using untreated water, boil, filter, or treat it with water purification tablets.
- Where water is untreated or sanitation is poor, avoid foods that cannot be peeled or cooked.
- When traveling out of the country, consume only bottled water unless local water supplies are clearly safe.

Inflammatory Bowel Disease

Ulcerative colitis and Crohn's disease are two conditions categorized as *inflammatory bowel disease (IBD)*. These conditions are similar in many ways:

- Their cause is unknown.
- Both affect primarily young adults.
- Both are chronic and recurrent.
- Diarrhea is the predominant symptom of each.
- Both may have associated manifestations, such as arthritis.

ULCERATIVE COLITIS

Ulcerative colitis is a chronic inflammatory bowel disorder of the mucosa and submucosa of the colon and rectum. It affects primarily the young, although it also is seen in people between ages 50 and 70. It is more common in whites than in people of color.

Ulcerative colitis is thought to be an *autoimmune disorder,* in which the individual's own antibodies attack the colon. Factors such as infection, diet, and environment (e.g., smoking) may contribute to development of ulcerative colitis. Stress and psychological factors affect, but do not cause, ulcerative colitis.

PATHOPHYSIOLOGY

Ulcerative colitis usually begins in the rectal area. It may progress proximally along the colon, involving the bowel in a continuous pattern. The mucosa becomes inflamed and edematous and bleeds easily. The mucosa ulcerates, sloughs, and is lost in the feces. As scar tissue forms, the bowel wall thickens and shortens. In most people, only the rectum and sigmoid colon are affected. Less commonly, the entire colon may be involved.

A gradual onset of diarrhea with intermittent rectal bleeding and mucus is common. Acute attacks last 1 to 3 months and occur at intervals of months to years. Diarrhea is the chief symptom. In mild cases, the client may have fewer than four stools per day with intermittent rectal bleeding and mucus, and few systemic manifestations. Clients with severe ulcerative colitis may have more than six to ten bloody stools per day, extensive colon involvement, dehydration, and malnutrition. Rectal inflammation causes fecal urgency and *tenesmus* (straining). Left lower quadrant cramping relieved by defecation is common. Systemic manifestations include fatigue, anorexia, and weakness. Clients with severe disease may develop a related arthritis.

Complications of ulcerative colitis include *colon perforation,* the leading cause of death in these clients. *Toxic megacolon* is characterized by paralysis of the colon with significant distention, usually in the transverse segment of the large bowel. Manifestations of toxic megacolon include fever, tachycardia, hypotension, dehydration, abdominal tenderness, and cramping. An acute decrease in diarrhea stools may signal toxic megacolon. Clients with ulcerative colitis have a high risk for developing colon cancer.

CROHN'S DISEASE

Crohn's disease *(regional enteritis)* is a chronic, relapsing inflammatory disorder of the GI tract. Crohn's disease usually begins between ages 10 and 30. Genetic and environmental factors, infectious agents, and autoimmune processes may contribute to its development. It is more common in urban settings, among residents of the northern United States, and among Ashkenazi Jews.

Crohn's disease can affect any part of the GI tract from the mouth to the anus, but it usually affects the terminal ileum and ascending colon.

Pathophysiology

Crohn's disease causes inflammatory lesions of the bowel mucosa that may extend into all layers of the bowel wall. These inflammatory lesions are localized, surrounded by normal gut. Ulcers and deep fissures develop, and fistulas may form between loops of bowel or between the bowel and other organs. Inflammation and scarring cause the bowel to narrow and become partially or fully obstructed (Figure 20-5 ◆). Over time, the bowel wall thickens and loses flexibility, and looks somewhat like a rubber hose. Malabsorption and malnutrition may develop as inflammation and ulcers prevent absorption of nutrients, especially vitamin B_{12} and bile salts.

Most people with Crohn's disease experience continuous or episodic diarrhea. Stools are liquid or semiformed and typically do not contain blood. Clients have abdominal pain and tenderness, and a mass may be palpable in the right lower quadrant. Many clients with Crohn's disease develop anorectal lesions, such as fissures, ulcers, fistulas, and abscesses. Systemic manifestations such as fever, malaise, and fatigue are common.

Intestinal obstruction, abscess, and fistula are so common that they are considered part of the disease process. Intestinal obstruction causes abdominal distention, cramping pain, borborygmi, and sometimes nausea and vomiting. When an abscess forms, the client develops chills and fever, a tender abdominal mass, and leukocytosis. Fistulas may be asymptomatic, particularly if they occur between loops of small bowel.

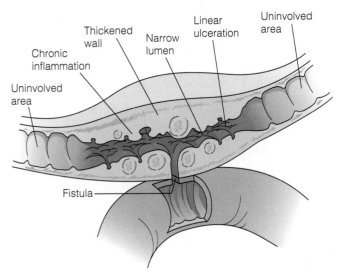

Figure 20-5. ◆ An illustration of the major characteristics of Crohn's disease in the small intestine.

A fistula between the small bowel and colon may increase diarrhea, weight loss, and malnutrition. When a fistula involves the bladder, recurrent urinary tract infections occur. Long-standing Crohn's disease increases the risk of cancer of the small intestine or colon by five to six times.

COLLABORATIVE CARE

There is no specific treatment for IBD. Medical therapy is directed toward managing the symptoms and controlling the disease process. Supportive care measures include rest, stress reduction, drugs, and nutritional support. When the disease does not respond to treatment or complications develop, surgery may be required.

Diagnostic testing is used to establish the diagnosis of IBD. A *stool specimen* is examined for blood and mucus and is sent for culture to rule out infectious causes. A *complete blood count (CBC), serum albumin level,* and serum levels of multiple vitamins are drawn to evaluate nutritional status. *Sigmoidoscopy* or *colonoscopy* is performed to visualize the bowel mucosa and collect tissue for biopsy. (Nursing implications of these diagnostic tests are presented in Boxes 20-1 and 20-17.) Harsh bowel preparations are avoided because they may exacerbate the disease. Instead, a clear liquid diet is ordered for 2 to 3 days prior to endoscopic examination. An *upper GI series with small bowel follow-through* and a *barium enema* (see Boxes 20-4 and 20-6) may be done for x-ray examination of the GI tract.

Pharmacology

Drugs are prescribed to terminate acute attacks of IBD and reduce the incidence of relapse. Locally acting and systemic anti-inflammatory drugs are used to manage IBD.

Sulfasalazine (Azulfidine) and related drugs are poorly absorbed from the GI tract and act as local anti-inflammatory agents on the bowel mucosa. For an acute episode, corticosteroids may also be used to reduce inflammation (Table 20-6 ◆). Immunosuppressive drugs may be prescribed to maintain remission for some clients with inflammatory bowel disease.

Antidiarrheal agents, such as loperamide and diphenoxylate, may be given to slow GI motility and reduce diarrhea. These drugs are not given during acute attacks of ulcerative colitis because they may cause toxic megacolon.

Dietary Management

A well-balanced diet is recommended. Dietary supplements such as Ensure may be added to promote weight gain and nutritional status. Lactose intolerance is common in clients

TABLE 20-6 NURSING IMPLICATIONS FOR PHARMACOLOGY: CLIENTS WITH INFLAMMATORY BOWEL DISEASE

AGENT/DRUGS	PURPOSE	NURSING IMPLICATIONS	CLIENT TEACHING
Local Anti-inflammatory Agents ▪ Sulfasalazine (Azulfidine) ▪ Mesalamine (Rowasa) ▪ Olsalazine (Dipentum)	These drugs have a local anti-inflammatory effect on intestinal mucosa. The drug inhibits prostaglandin production in the bowel. Prostaglandin is an important mediator of the inflammatory process; blocking its production reduces inflammation. These drugs may be administered by rectal suppository, by enema, or by mouth.	Do not give to clients who are pregnant or allergic to sulfonamides or salicylates. Suppositories or retention enemas may be administered at bedtime. Give oral forms with a full glass of water. Monitor for adverse effects: a. Rash, dermatitis, hives, or pruritus b. Bleeding, easy bruising, fever c. Low blood cell counts d. Changes in urine output or renal function studies e. Evidence of hepatitis or myocarditis	Take oral preparations after meals to decrease GI effects. Drink at least 2 quarts of fluid per day. Use sunscreen to prevent sunburns. Do not take aspirin, vitamin C, or any other over-the-counter medications containing aspirin or vitamin C without consulting with your doctor. Oral contraceptives may be less effective; use alternative methods of contraception. Notify your doctor if you develop a rash or hives, sore throat or mouth, bleeding gums, joint pain, easy bruising, or fever.
Corticosteroids ▪ Methylprednisolone (Medrol, Solu-Medrol) ▪ Prednisone	Glucocorticoids have potent anti-inflammatory effects and are used to treat acute episodes of IBD. They can be given by enema, by mouth, or by IV infusion. Because of their multiple and significant side effects, they are used for short periods only.	Notify the physician if the client has peptic ulcer disease, glaucoma or cataracts, diabetes, or a psychiatric disorder. Monitor vital signs, weight, and intake and output during therapy. Assess for edema. Administer in the morning as ordered. Give oral forms with meals. Monitor for adverse effects: a. Infection b. Hyperglycemia c. Hypokalemia d. Fluid retention e. Peptic ulcers or gastritis f. Mental status changes	Take as prescribed, do not take additional doses. Do not stop the drug abruptly. Notify your doctor if you develop adverse effects. Take with food or meals. Monitor weight. Contact your doctor if you gain more than 5 pounds. Moderate salt intake and avoid high-sodium foods and snacks. Increase intake of foods high in potassium, such as fruits, vegetables, and lean meats. Carry a card or wear a tag identifying corticosteroid use.

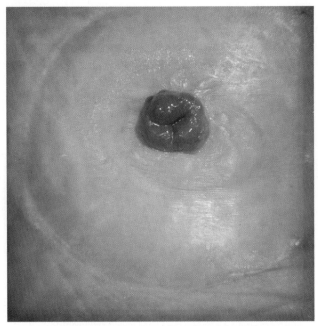

Figure 20-6. ◆ A healthy-appearing stoma.

Figure 20-8. ◆ Ileoanal anastomosis with reservoir.

with IBD, so milk and milk products may be eliminated. When the disease primarily affects the colon, increasing dietary fiber may reduce diarrhea. Clients with obstruction or small-bowel narrowing, however, need a low-roughage diet (no raw fruits and vegetables, popcorn, nuts, etc.).

During an acute exacerbation, the client is usually kept NPO. Total parenteral nutrition (TPN) is administered to maintain nutritional status. As the episode resolves, an elemental diet that contains all essential nutrients in a residue-free formula (like Ensure) may be ordered. These measures reduce intestinal motility and allow the bowel to rest.

Surgery

Surgical removal of the colon cures ulcerative colitis. Most clients, however, choose surgery only when other treatments are ineffective or manifestations of the disease interfere with ADLs. Surgery may also be indicated for complications of Crohn's disease, such as bowel obstruction, fistulas, or abscesses.

Figure 20-7. ◆ Kock's (continent) ileostomy.

Clients with ulcerative colitis may undergo a total **colectomy,** surgical removal of the colon. When the colon is removed, the terminal ileum may be brought to the surface of the abdomen to form an **ostomy,** an opening that allows elimination of fecal material. The surface opening of the ostomy is called a *stoma* (Figure 20-6 ◆). The precise name of the ostomy depends on the location of the stoma (e.g., an **ileostomy** is an ostomy made in the ileum of the small intestine). A permanent ileostomy may allow feces to drain directly (and constantly) through the stoma. The surgeon may create an internal pouch from the terminal ileum to collect feces until the client drains it with a catheter (Figure 20-7 ◆). A nipple valve prevents leakage of the stool between catheterizations.

A pouch formed from the terminal ileum also may be sutured to the anal canal (Figure 20-8 ◆). This procedure allows more normal bowel elimination and helps preserve body image. The client may return from surgery with a temporary ileostomy, which is later closed.

Nursing care of the client having bowel surgery is outlined in Box 20-14. (Nursing care of the client with an ostomy is described later in this chapter in Box 20-18 and Procedures 20-1 and 20-2.)

NURSING CARE

ASSESSING

Assessment for clients with IBD focuses on their current health status, presence of complications, and psychosocial factors related to the disease. Assessment data to collect for clients with inflammatory bowel disease are included in Box 20-15.

BOX 20-14
NURSING CARE CHECKLIST

BOWEL SURGERY

Before Surgery

☑ Provide routine preoperative care and teaching as outlined in Chapter 7.

☑ Assess understanding and clarify information as indicated.

☑ Reinforce preoperative teaching: Pain management, expected tubes, etc.

☑ Insert a nasogastric tube if ordered preoperatively.

☑ Perform bowel preparation procedures as ordered.

After Surgery

☑ Provide routine care for the surgical client (see Chapter 7).

☑ Monitor bowel sounds and abdominal distention.

☑ Assess nasogastric tube position and patency; connect to low suction. If the tube becomes clogged, gently irrigate with sterile normal saline.

☑ Assess color, amount, and odor of drainage from surgical drains and the ostomy (if present), noting any changes or the presence of clots or bright bleeding. Initial ostomy drainage may be bright red and then become dark and finally clear or greenish yellow over the first 2 to 3 days. Report significant changes in color, amount, or odor.

☑ If an abdominoperineal resection has been performed, alert all personnel to avoid rectal temperatures, suppositories, or other rectal procedures.

☑ Maintain intravenous fluids as ordered.

☑ Provide antacids, H$_2$-receptor blockers, and antibiotic therapy as ordered.

☑ Reintroduce oral intake with clear liquids, gradually progressing to frequent small feedings of regular foods. Monitor bowel sounds and abdominal distention frequently during this period.

☑ Encourage ambulation to stimulate peristalsis.

☑ Begin discharge planning and teaching. Consult with a dietitian for diet instructions and menu planning; reinforce teaching. Teach about potential complications, such as abdominal abscess or bowel obstruction, their manifestations, and prevention.

BOX 20-15
ASSESSING CLIENTS WITH INFLAMMATORY BOWEL DISEASE

SUBJECTIVE DATA

- Disease history: Onset, course, and severity; precipitating and relieving factors, including timing and circumstances
- Current manifestations: Abdominal pain or cramping, timing, character (constant or intermittent), factors that aggravate or relieve it; number of stools per day, blood or mucus in the stool; tenesmus; abdominal distention, anorexia, nausea, vomiting; general malaise, fatigue; joint pain or other symptoms; recent weight changes
- Previous surgeries or treatments for the disease; date of most recent colonoscopy
- Current medications, usual diet and current food intake
- Knowledge and understanding of the disease; ability to deal with the ostomy and drainage devices (if present); effect on roles, family relationships, sexuality; ability to cope with disease and its effects

OBJECTIVE DATA

- General appearance, including apparent state of health or distress, weight for height; skin color and condition
- Vital signs, including orthostatic vital signs if indicated
- Weight, height, fat-fold measurements
- Inspect abdomen, noting shape, presence of surgical scars or stomas, and any apparent distention; auscultate bowel sounds; palpate for tenderness, guarding, or masses.
- If indicated, obtain a stool specimen for examination and culture.

■ Administer anti-inflammatory and antidiarrheal medications as ordered. *Anti-inflammatory medications can reduce the severity and manifestations of the disease. Unless contraindicated, antidiarrheals reduce fluid loss and increase comfort.*

■ Assess perianal area for irritated or denuded skin from the diarrhea. Use or provide gentle cleansing agents (Periwash, Tucks, or cottonballs saturated with witch hazel) and zinc oxide–based cream to use after bowel movements. *Digestive enzymes in the stool are very corrosive to the skin.*

RISK FOR DEFICIENT FLUID VOLUME

■ Maintain accurate intake and output records, including emesis and diarrheal stools. *The client with IBD can experience significant fluid losses during an acute exacerbation of the disease. Accurate records help determine fluid replacement needs.*

DIAGNOSING, PLANNING, AND IMPLEMENTING

DIARRHEA

■ Monitor the appearance (including presence of mucus and occult or bright bleeding) and frequency of bowel movements using a stool chart. *The severity of diarrhea often correlates well with the severity of the disease and the need for fluid replacement. Large amounts of bright or dark blood may indicate a complication of the disease.*

- Document vital signs every 4 hours. *Elevated pulse and respiratory rates may indicate fluid volume deficit.*
- Weigh daily. Assess for other indications of fluid deficit. *Weight loss may indicate dehydration from persistent diarrhea. Warm, dry skin; poor skin turgor; dry, shiny mucous membranes; weakness; lethargy; and complaints of thirst are manifestations of dehydration.*
- Maintain fluid intake by mouth or intravenously as indicated. *Adequate fluid replacement is vital. If enteral supplements or TPN is ordered, additional fluids may be necessary to meet the client's needs.*
- Provide good skin care. *A fluid deficit increases the risk for skin breakdown.*

IMBALANCED NUTRITION: LESS THAN BODY REQUIREMENTS

- Carefully monitor food intake. *Accurate assessment of food intake provides a way to estimate the client's calorie intake in relation to nutritional needs.*
- Provide a high-calorie, high-protein diet with nutritional supplements as ordered. Consider food preferences as allowed. Arrange for dietary consultation. *Calories and protein are important to replace lost nutrients and meet metabolic needs. Nutritional supplements help restore losses and promote intake. A dietary consultant can design a diet to meet the client's specific needs and food preferences.*
- Provide parenteral nutrition as necessary. *Parenteral nutrition can help reverse nutritional deficits and promote weight gain when the client is unable to consume adequate amounts of food.*
- Engage family members, especially the primary food preparer, in dietary teaching. *Families can reinforce teaching, encourage intake, and help the client follow the recommended diet.*
- Monitor hemoglobin and hematocrit, serum electrolytes, and serum albumin levels. *Laboratory values provide information about specific nutrient losses as well and the client's overall nutritional status.*

DISTURBED BODY IMAGE

The inability to control, or even predict, fecal elimination, can interfere with the client's body image and self-concept.

- Encourage discussion about the effect of the disease or treatment on the client's feelings, self-perception, and relationships (including intimate). Accept the client's feelings and perceptions; do not discount them. *This demonstrates understanding and acceptance, and gives the client an opportunity to express his or her thoughts and feelings.*
- Discuss possible effects of treatment options openly and honestly. Encourage the client to make choices and decisions about care. *Open discussion allows the client to make more informed decisions and increases the client's sense of control.*
- Involve the client in care. Teach coping strategies (odor control, dietary modifications, etc.), and support their use. *This encourages and facilitates independence and healthy adaptation to the disease.*

- Provide care in an accepting, nonjudgmental manner. *Acceptance of the client despite potential embarrassment about odors or diarrhea enhances self-esteem.*
- Arrange for interaction with others who have IBD or ostomies. *People who have experienced a similar problem can understand the client's feelings better.*

EVALUATING

Collect data related to the following to evaluate the effectiveness of nursing interventions for the client with IBD: number of diarrheal stools per day, maintenance of skin integrity, hydration status, weight, ability to consume an adequate diet, and apparent coping with current situation.

Discharge Considerations

Teaching is a vital component of care for the client with IBD, as it is the client who manages the disease on a day-to-day basis. Teach about the disease process, short- and long-term effects, and the relationship of stress to exacerbations of the illness. Talk about risks and benefits of various treatment options. Present information on stress management. Provide information about prescribed medications (names, desired effects, adverse reactions and their management, and schedules for tapering doses if ordered). Discuss manifestations of potential complications and their management. Discuss the increased risk for colorectal cancer and the need for periodic medical follow-up.

Give verbal and written instructions about the recommended diet, and refer to a dietitian as necessary. Emphasize the need to consume a diet of good nutritional value, and note any specific restrictions (e.g., milk and milk products with lactose intolerance). Discuss use of nutritional supplements as needed. Emphasize the need to maintain a fluid intake of at least 2 to 3 quarts per day to replace fluids lost through the stool. Instruct to drink more fluid in hot weather, during exercise or strenuous work, or when feverish. Explain possible indications of malabsorption and impaired nutrition, self-care measures, and when to seek medical intervention. If home parenteral nutrition is planned, teach catheter care and troubleshooting, as well as TPN administration. Have the client and a family member demonstrate catheter care techniques and initiation of feedings prior to discharge.

If surgery is planned, instruct about the surgery and follow-up care. Contact an enterostomal therapy (ET) nurse to meet with the client and family. Teach ostomy care as indicated. Provide resources for obtaining ostomy supplies. Discuss the use of enteric-coated and timed-release drugs that may not be absorbed adequately before elimination through an ileostomy. Provide a list of local ostomy support groups, such as the Foundation for Colitis and Ileitis and the United Ostomy Association. Refer for home care as needed after discharge.

Nursing Process Case Study
■ CLIENT WITH ULCERATIVE COLITIS

Cortez Lewis is 42 years old and has had ulcerative colitis for 18 years. She has been treated with prednisone and sulfasalazine. During her most recent exacerbation, she had abdominal pain, cramping, frequent bloody diarrhea stools, and a 20 lb. (9 kg) weight loss. A recent colonoscopy showed that her colon is extensively involved. On admission, Mrs. Lewis states, "I'm tired of fighting this disease. I am a prisoner in my home because of the diarrhea." She is admitted for a total colectomy and ileostomy.

Assessment The nursing assessment on admission reveals that Mrs. Lewis weighs 115 lbs. (52.2 kg). Her vital signs are BP 104/72; T 98° F (36.6° C); P 72; R 20. Her skin is cool and pale. Her hemoglobin and hematocrit are low, as is her serum albumin at 2.4 g/dL (normal: 3.5 to 5 g/dL).

Diagnosis The following nursing diagnoses are established for Mrs. Lewis:

■ Imbalanced Nutrition: Less Than Body Requirements related to impaired absorption
■ Risk for Deficient Fluid Volume related to abnormal fluid losses
■ Risk for Impaired Tissue Integrity related to drainage from ileostomy
■ Pain related to surgical intervention
■ Risk for Sexual Dysfunction related to presence of ileostomy
■ Risk for Situational Low Self-Esteem related to presence of ileostomy

Expected Outcomes The expected outcomes are that Mrs. Lewis will:

■ Tolerate prescribed diet.
■ Maintain adequate fluid balance, as demonstrated by assessment data, vital signs, and laboratory results.
■ Demonstrate appropriate ostomy care.
■ Report pain at 3 or less on a scale of 1 to 10.
■ Verbalize feelings about sexuality and discuss issues with her husband.
■ Return to work and social activity in 6 weeks following surgery.

Planning and Implementation The nurses plan and implement the following nursing interventions for Mrs. Lewis:

■ Discuss dietary modifications related to ileostomy, including foods to avoid and the need to limit high-fiber foods and to chew them well.
■ Teach the importance of maintaining a high fluid intake and how to assess its adequacy. Review manifestations of dehydration.
■ Teach to empty and change either a one-piece or two-piece ostomy pouch.
■ Teach to assess her stoma and peristomal skin with each pouch change.
■ Refer to the local United Ostomy Association.
■ Provide names of local medical supply companies that sell ostomy appliances.

Evaluation On discharge, Mrs. Lewis is independently caring for her ileostomy appliance. The ET nurse has given her written and verbal instructions on ileostomy care. Mrs. Lewis verbalizes her understanding of the recommended diet and medications that should be avoided (timed-release forms). The ET nurse has also discussed sexual aspects of having an ileostomy and has given Mrs. Lewis a booklet, "Sex and the Female Ostomate," available through the United Ostomy Association.

 Critical Thinking in the Nursing Process

1. Why is the client with an ileostomy at risk for dehydration? What assessments can Mrs. Lewis use at home to monitor her fluid volume status?
2. Why would Mrs. Lewis's hemoglobin and hematocrit be low on admission?

 # Structural and Obstructive Disorders

 ## Colorectal Cancer

Colorectal cancer, malignancy of the colon or rectum, is the second leading cause of cancer deaths in Western countries. In the United States, about 130,200 new cases of colorectal cancer are diagnosed annually, and 56,300 people die from this disease. The specific cause of colorectal cancer is unknown. A number of risk factors have been identified (Box 20-16), but only about one fourth of clients diagnosed with colorectal cancer fall into a high-risk group. Therefore, screening for the disease is important.

PATHOPHYSIOLOGY

Nearly all colon cancers begin as *polyps,* benign precancerous lesions of the large intestine. The tumor typically grows

> ### BOX 20-16
> ### RISK FACTORS FOR
> ### COLORECTAL CANCER
>
> - Age over 50 years
> - Personal or family history of colorectal cancer
> - Polyps of rectum or colon
> - Inflammatory bowel disease
> - History of ovarian, endometrial, or breast cancer
> - Physical inactivity (possibly)
> - High-fat, low-fiber diet; inadequate fruit and vegetable intake

undetected in the rectum or sigmoid colon (Figure 20-9 ◆). By the time symptoms occur, the disease often has spread into deeper layers of the bowel tissue and adjacent organs. Colorectal cancer spreads by direct extension to involve the entire bowel wall. It may extend into neighboring structures (liver or genitourinary tract). It may "seed" other areas of the peritoneal cavity through the bowel wall or during surgery. Metastasis to regional lymph nodes is common, although sometimes distal nodes contain cancer cells while regional nodes remain normal. Cancerous cells may also spread through the lymphatic or circulatory system to the liver, lungs, brain, bones, and kidneys.

Bowel cancer usually grows slowly. There may be 5 to 15 years of growth before symptoms occur. Manifestations depend on tumor location, type and extent, and complications. Bleeding is often what prompts clients to seek care. A change in bowel habits is another early symptom. In advanced disease, pain, anorexia, and weight loss occur, and a palpable abdominal or rectal mass may be present. Occasionally, anemia from occult bleeding is the presenting symptom.

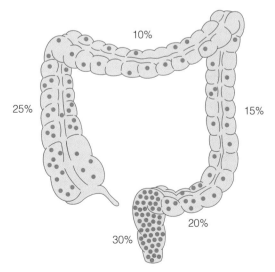

Figure 20-9. ◆ The distribution and frequency of colorectal cancer.

The prognosis for colon cancer depends most on the stage of the disease at diagnosis and initial treatment. Over half of all people diagnosed with colorectal cancer survive 10 years.

Bowel obstruction due to tumor growth is the primary complication associated with colorectal cancer. Bowel wall perforation and tumor spread to adjacent organs may also occur.

COLLABORATIVE CARE

Because colorectal cancer is often a silent disease and treatment at an early stage has a high cure rate, the American Cancer Society recommends routine screening:

- Annual *digital rectal examination* for all people over age 50
- Annual *fecal occult blood test* for people over age 50
- Flexible *sigmoidoscopy* or *colonoscopy* at age 50 and every 5 to 10 years thereafter.

Screening exams should be early and frequent for clients with IBD, a history of polyps, or a strong family history of colorectal cancer.

The client with suspected colorectal cancer may undergo extensive diagnostic procedures. A *barium enema* may detect the presence and location of a tumor. A *sigmoidoscopy* or *colonoscopy* is done to detect and visualize tumors, and to collect

> ### BOX 20-17
> ### NURSING CARE CHECKLIST
>
> #### COLONOSCOPY
> #### Client Preparation
>
> - ☑ Verify signed consent for the procedure.
> - ☑ Withhold food and fluids as ordered. Intake is limited to clear liquids for 1 to 2 days, then NPO for 8 hours before the procedure.
> - ☑ Administer or instruct the client to perform bowel preparation procedures as ordered.
> - ☑ Administer sedation as ordered.
>
> #### Client and Family Teaching
>
> **Before Procedure**
> - ☑ Explain dietary restrictions and their purpose.
> - ☑ The procedure takes 30 minutes to 1 hour. You will be sedated but able to breathe on your own.
> - ☑ The scope is inserted through the anus to visualize the entire large bowel.
> - ☑ Air may be instilled into the bowel during the procedure.
> - ☑ A biopsy may be taken. Polyps may be removed.
> - ☑ Discomfort is minimal.
>
> **After Procedure**
> - ☑ Report any abdominal pain, chills, fever, rectal bleeding, or purulent discharge.
> - ☑ If a polyp has been removed, avoid heavy lifting for 7 days, and avoid high-fiber foods for 1 to 2 days.

tissue for *biopsy.* See Box 20-17 for nursing care of the client undergoing colonoscopy. Tumors typically appear as raised, red, centrally ulcerated, bleeding lesions.

A *complete blood count (CBC)* is done to evaluate for anemia. *Carcinoembryonic antigen (CEA,* a protein found in colorectal cancers) levels are measured. CEA levels are used primarily to predict prognosis and to detect tumor recurrence following surgery.

A *chest x-ray* is obtained to detect tumor metastasis to the lung. *Computed tomography (CT) scans, magnetic resonance imaging (MRI),* or *ultrasound examinations* may identify involvement of other organs.

Surgery

Surgical resection of the tumor, adjacent colon, and regional lymph nodes is the treatment of choice for colorectal cancer. Small, localized tumors may be excised by laser endoscopy, eliminating the need for abdominal surgery. Most clients with colorectal cancer undergo a *colectomy* (surgical resection of the colon with anastomosis of remaining bowel). Most tumors of the ascending, transverse, descending, and sigmoid colon can be resected. Whenever possible, the anal sphincter is preserved and *colostomy* (ostomy made in the colon) is avoided. Tumors of the rectum, however, usually require an *abdominoperineal resection,* in which the sigmoid colon, rectum, and anus are removed through both abdominal and perineal incisions. A permanent *colostomy* is created for elimination of feces. Nursing care of the client having bowel surgery was described in Box 20-14.

A colostomy may be created if the bowel is obstructed by the tumor or as a temporary measure to promote healing of anastomoses. Colostomies take the name of the portion of the colon from which they are formed (Figure 20-10 ◆). In a *double-barrel colostomy,* two separate stomas are created (Figure 20-11 ◆). The distal colon is not removed, but feces are diverted through the proximal stoma. A double-barrel colostomy usually

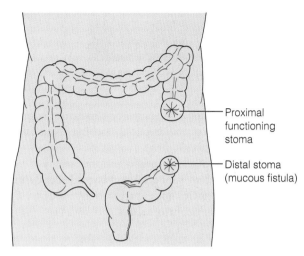

Figure 20-11. ◆ A temporary, double-barrel colostomy. The proximal stoma expels feces; the distal stoma expels mucus from the distal colon.

is temporary but may be permanent. Nursing care of the client with a colostomy is outlined in Box 20-18.

Adjunctive Therapy

Radiation and chemotherapy often are used in conjunction with surgery to treat colorectal cancers. Pre- or postoperative radiation therapy is used to reduce the recurrence of rectal tumors in the pelvic area. Chemotherapeutic agents are also used postoperatively as adjunctive therapy for colorectal cancer. (Further discussion about radiation and chemotherapy and their nursing implications is included in Chapter 8.)

NURSING CARE

Nursing care for the client with colorectal cancer is aimed at providing emotional support, teaching, and addressing the surgical client's needs.

PAIN

The client with colorectal cancer may experience pain from surgical incisions, "phantom" rectal pain, and tumors pressing on nerves and other organs. Postoperatively, patient-controlled analgesia (PCA) and regularly administered analgesics are used to manage pain. If the tumor is inoperable, continuous analgesia delivery (CAD) systems may also be used. (See Chapter 6 for more information on caring for clients with pain.)

■ Assess frequently for pain, using a standard pain scale. Document intensity, location, and character of the pain. *Pain is a subjective experience; careful assessment improves pain management. Controlling pain facilitates healing and recovery.*

■ Assess the effectiveness of pain medications and monitor for adverse effects. *The prescribed dose may need to be increased or decreased based on the client's response.*

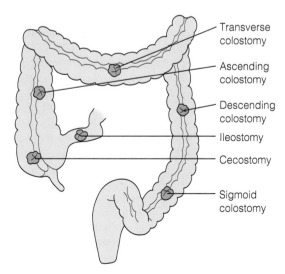

Transverse colostomy

Ascending colostomy

Descending colostomy

Ileostomy

Cecostomy

Sigmoid colostomy

Figure 20-10. ◆ The location of different types of colon and small intestinal ostomies.

BOX 20-18
NURSING CARE CHECKLIST

ILEOSTOMY OR COLOSTOMY

Before Surgery

☑ Contact enterostomal therapy nurse to mark stoma placement and to provide initial teaching about ostomy care and appliances.

☑ Discuss concerns about surgery and the ostomy.

☑ Refer to an ostomy support group as needed or desired.

☑ Provide preoperative bowel preparation as ordered (cathartics, enemas, preoperative antibiotics).

After Surgery

☑ Assess stoma location and appearance. A healthy stoma appears pink or red and moist (Figure 20-6). It should protrude approximately 2 cm from the abdominal wall. Report dark or white color, prolapse, or *retraction* (indentation) of the stoma to the charge nurse or physician.

☑ Position a collection bag or drainable pouch over the stoma. (Application of ostomy pouches is described in Procedure 20-1.) Monitor and record color and consistency of ostomy output.

☑ Empty a drainable pouch or replace the colostomy bag when it is no more than one-third full. Measure the drainage, and record as output.

☑ Assess skin surrounding the stoma, and protect with caulking agents, such as Stomahesive or karaya paste, and a skin barrier wafer as needed. Change the bag or pouch if leakage occurs or the client complains of burning or itching skin.

☑ A small needle hole high on the colostomy pouch will allow flatus to escape. For odor control, this hole may be closed with a Band-Aid and opened only while the client is in the bathroom.

☑ Report abnormal assessment findings such as a rash, purulent drainage, ulcerated skin, or bulging around the stoma to the charge nurse or physician.

☑ Prior to discharge, teach ostomy care, pouch management, skin care, and irrigation (as indicated). Allow time for practice.

☑ Emphasize the importance of adequate fluid intake, particularly for clients with an ileostomy or proximal colostomy.

☑ Discuss dietary concerns. A low-residue diet (Table 20-7 ◆) may initially be recommended. Foods that may cause excessive odor or gas (e.g., vegetables such as asparagus or cabbage, dried beans, beer and carbonated drinks, or dairy products) are typically avoided, as are foods that can cause a blockage (e.g., popcorn, corn, nuts, caraway seeds, cucumbers, celery, fresh tomatoes, and berries).

TABLE 20-7 LOW-RESIDUE DIET

FOOD GROUP	ALLOWED
Breads and cereals	Products made from refined flours (e.g., white bread) or finely milled grains
Desserts	Gelatins, puddings; ice cream without fruit or nuts
Fruits	Juices and strained fruits; cooked or canned fruits; bananas
Meats and other proteins	Roasted, baked, or broiled meat, poultry, or fish; smooth peanut butter; cream and mild cheeses; milk
Potatoes, rice, and pasta	Peeled potatoes; white rice; most pasta products
Vegetables	Juices and strained vegetables; cooked or canned vegetables
Other	Coffee, tea, carbonated beverages; cream sauce and plain gravy

■ Assess abdomen for distention, tenderness, and bowel sounds; incision for inflammation or swelling; and drainage catheters and tubes for patency. *Poorly controlled pain may indicate an infection, impaired tube drainage, or a complication such as bleeding, peritonitis, or paralytic ileus.*

■ Administer analgesics prior to an activity or procedure. *The analgesic can help prevent discomfort with movement or ambulation.*

■ Provide nonpharmacologic relief measures, such as positioning, diversion, guided imagery, and relaxation techniques. *These techniques can enhance the effects of analgesia.*

■ Splint incision with a pillow, and teach how to self-splint when coughing and deep breathing. *Splinting the incision*

reduces discomfort associated with muscle contraction and allows more effective coughing and deep breathing.

ANTICIPATORY GRIEVING

■ Work to develop a trusting relationship with the client and family. Demonstrate respect for cultural, spiritual, and religious values and beliefs. *Providing support during the initial stages of grieving can improve physical recovery, psychological coping, and eventual adaptation. This increases your effectiveness in helping clients work through the grieving process.*

■ Encourage expression of fears and concerns and discussion about the potential impact of loss on individual family

PROCEDURE 20-1 Changing a One- or Two-Piece Ostomy Pouch

■ BEFORE THE PROCEDURE

- Collect all supplies.
- Provide for privacy.
- Explain the procedure.

■ PROCEDURE

- Use standard precautions.
- Remove soiled pouch (and the skin barrier flange if present).
- Empty the pouch; discard in a plastic bag. Save the tail closure (clamp).
- Rinse and reuse pouch from a two-piece system if desired.
- Cleanse skin and stoma with warm water and skin cleanser or mild soap. Rinse and pat dry.
- Assess stoma and skin condition.
- Use a measuring guide or previous pattern to check size of stoma. Trace stoma size onto the back of the pouch flange, and cut the opening no more than ⅛ inch larger than stoma.

A guide to measure the stoma.

- Apply skin prep to peristomal skin and allow to dry.
- Remove backing from pouch or flange.

- Apply a bead of skin barrier paste around the base of stoma or around the opening of the pouch or flange. Allow the paste to air dry for 1 to 2 minutes.
- Center the pouch or flange over the stoma, and press to adhere.

Applying a disposable pouch.

- For a two-piece pouch, snap the pouch onto skin barrier flange.
- Place deodorizing tablets or a few drops of liquid pouch deodorizer in the pouch. Apply clamp.
- "Picture frame" the pouch with tape for extra security as needed.

■ SAMPLE DOCUMENTATION

| 11/12/02 | Ileostomy pouch changed. 250 mL yellowish brown liquid stool emptied. Stoma bright pink, moist; skin pink and intact with no evidence of breakdown or excoriation. |
| | Karen Leah, LPN. |

---

members, as well as family structure and function. *Sharing concerns with one another provides support and helps family members develop coping strategies.*

■ Help the client and family identify strengths, support systems, and successful coping mechanisms used in past experiences. *These resources can help in dealing with the current situation.*

■ Refer to cancer support groups, social services, or counseling as appropriate. *These provide additional resources for support in the grieving process.*

RISK FOR SEXUAL DYSFUNCTION

Sexual function may be impaired by surgery, radiation therapy, chemotherapy, or medications prescribed after surgery. In addition, clients with an ostomy may feel undesirable and fear rejection. They may be concerned about odors or pouch leakage during sexual activity.

■ Provide opportunities for client and family to express their feelings about the ostomy. *By doing this, the nurse acknowl-*

edges that feelings of anger and depression are normal responses to this change in body function.

■ Provide consistent, secure colostomy care. *An accepting attitude and consistent care that controls odor and leakage instill confidence in the client.*

■ Encourage expression of sexual concerns within the client's comfort zone. Provide reassurance that sexual function often improves with healing. *Sexuality is a very private concern, and most people will discuss it only with someone they trust. Many people think an initial decrease in libido means that sexual activity will never be possible again.*

■ Refer to social services or a family counselor for further interventions. *Clients are often discharged from acute care settings before concerns about sexual activity begin to surface. Ongoing counseling provides a continuing resource.*

■ Arrange for a visit by a member of the United Ostomy Association. *A person who is living successfully with an ostomy is a valuable source of information and support, and often can address questions the client hesitates to ask.*

Discharge Considerations

Primary prevention of colorectal cancer is an important nursing issue. Teach all clients about American Cancer Society dietary recommendations, including decreasing intake of fat, refined sugar, and red meats and increasing intake of dietary fiber, fresh fruits, and vegetables.

Stress the importance of regular health examinations, including screening by digital rectal exam, fecal occult blood tests, and colonoscopy after age 50. Also stress the need to seek medical treatment if blood is noted in or on the stool. Teach clients that change in bowel habits may be a warning sign for bowel cancer.

Teach about various tests and preparation for diagnostic procedures including bowel preparation and food and fluid restrictions. Discuss postprocedure care and potential adverse effects.

Teach care of the ostomy and possible complications to report. (See Procedures 20-1 and 20-2.) Provide a list of resources for ostomy supplies. Refer to the local ostomy association or group. Discuss management of adverse effects if radiation and chemotherapy are planned.

If the cancer is advanced, provide information about pain and symptom management. Discuss the hospice philosophy and available services. Provide referrals as needed.

See the Interactive Care Map at the end of this chapter for an opportunity to apply the nursing process for a client with colorectal cancer.

Bowel Obstruction

A *bowel obstruction* occurs when intestinal contents fail to move through the bowel. An obstruction can occur in any portion of the intestinal tract. The small intestine (especially the ileum) is the most common site.

PATHOPHYSIOLOGY

A bowel obstruction may be either mechanical or functional. With a *mechanical obstruction,* the bowel is obstructed by a physical barrier like scar tissue or a tumor. *Adhesions* (bands of scar tissue) are the most common cause of mechanical bowel obstruction. Adhesions usually result from previous abdominal surgery or inflammation. They may cause partial or complete obstruction. With *functional obstruction (paralytic ileus),* the bowel lumen remains patent, but peristalsis stops. Paralytic ileus is common in acutely ill clients. It is associated with gastrointestinal surgery, peritoneal inflammation, and certain drugs such as narcotic analgesics.

When obstruction occurs, gas and fluid collect in the bowel proximal to the obstruction, stretching its lumen. Extracellular fluid and electrolytes are drawn into the bowel lumen, producing further distention. The increased pressure may cause ischemia and necrosis of the bowel wall. Hypovolemia and shock may result from fluid trapping within the intestine.

The manifestations of a small-bowel obstruction depend on how fast the obstruction develops and where it occurs (Box 20-19).

Hypovolemic shock with multiple organ failure and death can result from bowel obstruction. The mortality rate for small bowel obstruction is approximately 10% (mostly in older adults). Strangulation of the bowel significantly increases the risk of death.

COLLABORATIVE CARE

Management of the client with a bowel obstruction focuses on relieving the obstruction and providing supportive care. Restoration and maintenance of fluid and electrolyte balance is vital to prevent complications.

Abdominal x-rays are used to confirm the diagnosis of a bowel obstruction. In addition to plain films, contrast media may be used. Evaluation for iodine or seafood allergies prior to the exam is important, as the contrast medium used may contain iodine.

BOX 20-19
MANIFESTATIONS OF BOWEL OBSTRUCTION

- Abdominal pain: Cramping or colicky; may be intermittent; increasing intensity; tenderness to palpation; severe, continuous pain may indicate bowel ischemia and possible perforation
- Vomiting; may smell of feces
- Borborygmi and high-pitched, tinkling bowel sounds; diminished or absent bowel sounds
- Abdominal distention; visible peristaltic waves
- Signs of hypovolemia and shock: Orthostatic hypotension, tachycardia, tachypnea; decreased urine output

PROCEDURE 20-2 Colostomy Irrigation

■ BEFORE THE PROCEDURE

- Collect all supplies.
- Provide for privacy.
- Explain the procedure.
- If ambulatory, place client on toilet or commode. Position client confined to bed on right side with bedpan in front.

■ PROCEDURE

- Follow standard precautions.
- Fill irrigation or enema bag with prescribed amount of warm water or saline. Clear the tubing of air.
- Remove ostomy pouch and discard.
- Attach an irrigation sleeve over stoma using the belt. Place the bottom of sleeve into the toilet, commode, or bedpan.
- Lubricate the cone and insert tip into the stoma. Hold securely to prevent backflow of water.
- Instill irrigating solution into the colon from a height of no greater than 12 to 18 inches.
- Allow fluid and feces to flow into the toilet or bedpan. Allow about 15 minutes for drainage.
- Cleanse the bottom of the sleeve, clamp, and allow client to resume activities.

- After approximately 30 to 45 minutes, drain the sleeve and remove.
- Clean the stoma and peristomal skin.
- Apply a clean ostomy pouch.

■ AFTER THE PROCEDURE

- Wash and dry all equipment before storing. Irrigation sleeves are reusable.

■ SAMPLE DOCUMENTATION

11/12/02   0930 Colostomy irrigated with 500 mL NS. Moderate amount of formed brown stool returned with irrigant. Tolerated procedure well with minimal abdominal cramping and no pain. Stoma pink and moist; skin intact without signs of breakdown.

_____Mary Alaha, LPN.

Gastrointestinal Decompression

Most partial and functional small bowel obstructions are successfully treated with gastrointestinal decompression using a nasogastric tube or long intestinal tube. An intestinal tube (see Figure 20-4) may be inserted through the nose or via gastrostomy. A balloon or weighted tip draws the tube from the stomach into the intestine by peristalsis. Low suction removes fluid and gas until persitalsis resumes or the obstruction is relieved.

Surgery

Surgery may be required to relieve bowel obstruction. Prior to surgery, a nasogastric or intestinal tube is inserted to relieve vomiting and distention and to prevent aspiration. Intravenous fluids and electrolytes are given to restore fluid and electrolyte balance. Intravenous antibiotics are administered prophylactically. Nursing care of the client having bowel surgery was described in Box 20-15.

NURSING CARE

Nurses can help identify bowel obstructions early in older adults, homebound clients, or long-term care residents, thus significantly reducing morbidity. Assess all clients who com-

plain of abdominal pain or who stop eating. Inspect the abdomen for distention, listen for bowel sounds, and notify the charge nurse or physician of abnormal findings.

In clients with a suspected or confirmed bowel obstruction, frequent assessment for complications such as fluid and electrolyte imbalance, acid–base imbalances, hypovolemic shock, perforation, and peritonitis is necessary. The nurse cares for the client undergoing surgery.

DEFICIENT FLUID VOLUME

- Monitor vital signs and central venous pressure (CVP) hourly. *Tachycardia, a drop in blood pressure, and tachypnea may indicate hypovolemia. The CVP is an effective measurement of fluid volume status.*
- Measure urine output hourly and nasogastric output every 2 to 4 hours. Maintain intravenous fluids and blood replacement as ordered. *Urine output less than 30 mL/hr indicates decreased cardiac output and hypovolemia. Nasogastric output is measured as a guideline for fluid replacement. Intravenous fluids are given to meet current needs and replace losses.*
- Measure abdominal girth every 4 to 8 hours. Mark the area to be measured on the abdomen. *A reference mark allows con-*

sistent, accurate measurements. Increased abdominal girth indicates increasing intestinal distention.

■ Notify the charge nurse or physician of changes in status. *Changes can indicate the need for immediate surgery.*

INEFFECTIVE BREATHING PATTERN

Abdominal distention from a bowel obstruction can place pressure on the diaphragm. Pain from abdominal surgery may lead to shallow breathing. Aspiration of GI contents during vomiting is also a risk in the client with bowel obstruction.

■ Assess respiratory rate, pattern, and lung sounds every 2 to 4 hours. Monitor pulse oximetry levels. *Diminished breath sounds or crackles in the lung bases indicate poor ventilation. Tachypnea, shortness of breath, dyspnea, or fall in pulse oximetry readings (<90% to 92%) may indicate respiratory compromise. Notify the charge nurse or physician.*

■ Elevate the head of the bed. *This reduces pressure on the diaphragm.*

■ Provide a pillow or folded bath blanket to use in splinting the abdomen while coughing postoperatively. *The ease and effectiveness of coughing are improved when abdominal muscles and incisions are splinted.*

■ Maintain the patency of nasogastric or intestinal suction. *Suction prevents further abdominal distention or aspiration of intestinal contents during vomiting.*

■ Encourage use of incentive spirometry or other assistive devices. *Assistive devices help the client open distal airways and prevent atelectasis.*

■ Contact respiratory therapy as indicated. *Additional measures to maintain pulmonary status may be available.*

■ Provide good oral care at least every 4 hours. *Dehydration and nasogastric suction lead to dry mouth and throat, increasing the risk of bacterial growth. Many respiratory infections are the result of aspirated organisms.*

  ## Discharge Considerations

Instruct the client and family about wound care, activity level after discharge, return to work, and any other recommended restrictions or procedures. If a temporary colostomy has been created, teach the client and family about its care. For the client with recurrent obstructions, discuss cause, early identification of symptoms, and preventive measures.

Hernia

A *hernia* is a protrusion of an organ or structure through a defect in the muscular wall of the abdomen. Hernias may contain loops of bowel or other internal organs. They may be congenital or acquired. Acquired hernias are associated with weakening of the normal musculature. They may be related to surgery, trauma such as heavy lifting, or gradual increases in intra-abdominal pressure caused by pregnancy, obesity, or ascites.

PATHOPHYSIOLOGY

Hernias are classified by their location (Figure 20-12 ◆). Most hernias occur in the groin and are known as *inguinal hernias.* Inguinal hernias are usually caused by improper closure of the tract that develops as the testes descend into the scrotum before birth. They often do not become apparent until increased intra-abdominal pressure causes abdominal contents to enter the channel in adulthood. In older adults, weakness of the posterior inguinal wall can also lead to an inguinal hernia. Inguinal hernias often produce no symptoms and are discovered during routine physical examination. A lump, swelling, or bulge in the groin may be noted with lifting or straining. The client may complain of pain that radiates into the scrotum.

Umbilical and ventral *(incisional)* hernias occur in the abdominal wall. *Umbilical hernias* may be congenital or acquired; pregancy, obesity, and ascites are common risk factors. *Ventral hernias* result from inadequate healing of a surgical incision.

If a hernia is *reducible,* contents of the sac return to the abdominal cavity when intra-abdominal pressure is reduced (as with lying down) or with manual pressure. When the contents of a hernia cannot be returned to the abdominal cavity, it is said to be *irreducible* or *incarcerated.* Contents of an incarcerated hernia are trapped, usually by a narrow opening to the hernia. *Obstruction* occurs when the lumen of the bowel contained within the hernia becomes occluded, much like the crimping of a hose.

A *strangulated hernia* occurs when the blood supply to tissue within the hernia is compromised. This can lead to infarction of affected bowel with severe pain and perforation. Manifestations of a strangulated hernia include abdominal pain and distention, nausea, vomiting, tachycardia, and fever.

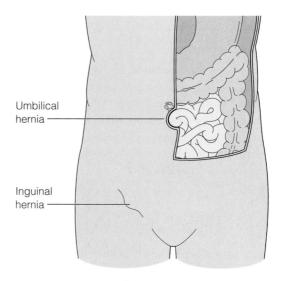

Figure 20-12. ◆ Two types of hernia.

COLLABORATIVE CARE

The diagnosis of a hernia is made by examining the client in a supine and sitting or standing position. A bulge may be seen or felt when the client coughs or bears down. No laboratory or diagnostic testing is usually required, unless bowel obstruction or strangulation is suspected.

All types of hernia are surgically repaired (*herniorrhaphy*) unless specific contraindications to surgery exist. Heavy lifting and heavy manual labor are restricted for approximately 3 weeks after surgery. When surgery is not an option, the client may be taught to reduce the hernia by lying down and gently pushing down against the mass. A binder or truss may be worn to prevent or control the protrusion.

NURSING CARE

The client undergoing a herniorrhaphy has few acute nursing care needs apart from preoperative assessment and immediate postoperative care. Operative nursing care is similar to care of a client with an appendectomy.

RISK FOR INEFFECTIVE TISSUE PERFUSION: GASTROINTESTINAL

■ Assess comfort. Notify the primary care provider if the hernia becomes painful or tender. Promptly report an acute increase in abdominal, groin, perineal, or scrotal pain. *Pain or tenderness of the hernia may indicate incarceration. An abrupt increase in pain may indicate bowel ischemia due to strangulation. Rapid identification of the problem is vital to prevent major complications like peritonitis.*

■ Assess bowel sounds and abdominal distention at least every 8 hours. *A change in bowel sounds—either cessation of sounds or hyperactive, high-pitched sounds—and increasing abdominal girth may indicate obstruction.*

■ If signs of possible obstruction or strangulation occur, place the client in supine position with the hips elevated and knees slightly bent. Keep NPO, and begin preparations for surgery. *This position helps relax abdominal muscles and may facilitate reduction of the hernia. Strangulation or obstruction require immediate surgical intervention.*

Discharge Considerations

Most teaching related to hernias is done during routine health examinations. Teach clients what hernias are and the risk factors for their development. Reassure clients that surgical intervention is generally without complications, even in older adults, and carries a lower risk than not repairing the hernia. Teach clients how to reduce hernias if necessary, and stress the importance of seeking immediate medical intervention if signs of strangulation or obstruction occur. When surgery is planned, instruct the client to notify the physician should he or she develop an upper respiratory infection and cough, because forceful coughing is not recommended postoperatively. Reinforce postoperative teaching about pain management and activity restrictions following surgery.

Diverticular Disease

Diverticula are acquired saclike projections of bowel mucosa through the muscular layer of the colon (Figure 20-13 ◆). They occur most often in the sigmoid colon. Diverticular disease affects millions, but few people have symptoms. A diet of highly refined and fiber-deficient foods is a major risk factor for diverticula.

PATHOPHYSIOLOGY

Diverticula form when increased pressure within the bowel causes the mucosa to herniate through defects in the wall. *Diverticulosis* is the presence of diverticula and is usually asymptomatic. Clients may experience episodic left lower quadrant pain, constipation, and diarrhea. **Diverticulitis** is inflammation and perforation of a diverticulum, usually in the sigmoid colon. Infection occurs when undigested food becomes trapped in a diverticulum, and its blood supply is impaired, allowing bacterial invasion. Perforation results from ischemia and necrosis of the mucosa.

Pain is a common manifestation of diverticulitis. It is usually left sided and may be mild to severe and either steady or cramping. Constipation or diarrhea, nausea, vomiting, and low-grade fever may occur. Complications include hemorrhage, peritonitis, abscess or fistula formation, and bowel obstruction.

COLLABORATIVE CARE

Management of diverticular disease ranges from no prescribed intervention to surgical resection of affected colon. In addition to the history and physical exam, a *flexible sigmoidoscopy* or *colonoscopy* or a *CT scan* may be performed to establish the diagnosis.

A diet high in fiber is prescribed for clients with diverticulosis (Table 20-8 ◆). The client may be advised to avoid

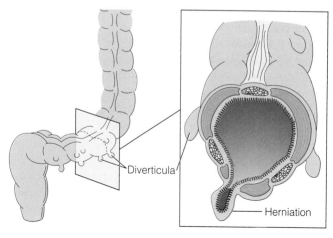

Figure 20-13. ◆ Diverticula of the colon.

TABLE 20-8 HIGH-FIBER, HIGH-RESIDUE DIET	
FOOD GROUP	**RECOMMENDED FOODS**
Cereals and grains	Wheat or oat bran; cooked whole-grain cereals; dry cereals such as bran flakes, corn flakes, shredded wheat; whole-grain breads or crackers; brown rice
Fruits	Unpeeled raw apples, peaches, and pears; oranges
Vegetables	Dried beans (black, red, pinto, or kidney), lima beans; broccoli; peas; corn; squash; raw vegetables such as carrots, celery, and tomatoes; potatoes with skins

foods with small seeds (such as popcorn, caraway seeds, figs, or berries), which could obstruct diverticula.

Bowel rest and antibiotic therapy are prescribed during an acute episode of diverticulitis. The client initially may be NPO with intravenous fluids and total parenteral nutrition. Feeding is resumed gradually, progressing from clear liquids to a soft, low-roughage diet with daily added psyllium seed to soften stool and increase its bulk. The high-fiber diet is resumed following full recovery. Surgery may be required if the client develops an abscess or peritonitis. Review Box 20-14 for nursing care of the client having bowel surgery.

NURSING CARE

The nurse's role for diverticulosis is mainly educational. Teach clients in all settings about the benefits of a high-fiber diet in preventing diverticular disease, bowel cancer, and other disorders. In residential or foster care settings, work with dietary staff and care providers to increase the amount of fiber in residents' diets, unless contraindicated.

Emphasize the importance of maintaining a high-fiber diet to reduce the incidence of complications of diverticulosis. Discuss how to increase dietary fiber, and refer to a dietitian as needed. Provide instruction about complications of the disease and their manifestations.

For the client with acute diverticulitis, explain prescribed treatment and food and fluid limitations. Explain why dietary fiber is limited during acute inflammation but increased for chronic management. Provide discharge instruction for clients undergoing surgery. Refer to community health care agencies as needed.

Anorectal Disorders

Anorectal conditions include hemorrhoids, as well as lesions like fissures, fistulas, abscess, and pilonidal disease.

Hemorrhoids

When pressure on the veins of the anus and anal canal is increased or venous return is impaired, the veins weaken and distend, forming *hemorrhoids* (or *piles*). Virtually all adults have hemorrhoids, usually asymptomatic.

Straining to defecate is the most common cause of hemorrhoids. Pregnancy increases intra-abdominal pressure and also is an important cause of hemorrhoids. Contributing factors include prolonged sitting, obesity, chronic constipation, and a low-fiber diet.

Internal hemorrhoids develop above the mucocutaneous junction of the anus (Figure 20-14 ◆). They rarely cause pain, and usually present with bright red bleeding that is unmixed with stool. It can vary from streaks on toilet tissue to enough to color the water in the toilet. The client may experience a feeling

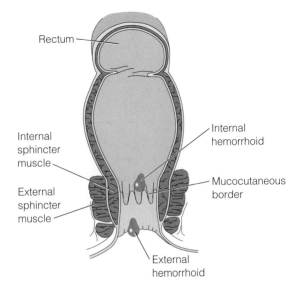

Figure 20-14. ◆ The location of internal and external hemorrhoids.

of incomplete stool evacuation. As they enlarge, hemorrhoids may *prolapse* or protrude through the anus.

External hemorrhoids develop below the mucocutaneous junction. Bleeding is rare with external hemorrhoids. Anal irritation, a feeling of pressure, and difficulty cleaning the anal region may be manifestations of external hemorrhoids.

"Normal" hemorrhoids are not painful. Prolapsed hemorrhoids may become strangulated, leading to thrombosis (clotting). Thrombosed hemorrhoids cause extreme pain. Internal hemorrhoids associated with portal hypertension and liver disease may rupture and bleed profusely.

COLLABORATIVE CARE

Management of hemorrhoids is conservative unless complications occur. Internal hemorrhoids are diagnosed by *anoscopic* exam. A sigmoidoscopy or colonoscopy may be done to rule out colorectal cancer, which can produce similar manifestations.

A high-fiber diet and increased water intake to increase stool bulk, improve its softness, and reduce straining is effective for most clients with internal or external hemorrhoids. Bulk-forming laxatives (e.g., Metamucil) or stool softeners like docusate sodium may be prescribed. Suppositories and local ointments (e.g., Preparation H, Nupercaine) have an anesthetic and astringent effect that reduces discomfort and irritation of surrounding tissues. They have little or no effect on the hemorrhoid itself. Warm sitz baths, bed rest, and local astringent compresses may be recommended to shrink edematous prolapsed hemorrhoids after digital reduction.

Prolapsed or thrombosed hemorrhoids may require additional treatment. *Sclerotherapy* involves injecting a chemical irritant into tissues surrounding the hemorrhoid to cause inflammation and scarring. *Rubber band ligation* involves placing a rubber band snugly around the hemorrhoid and surrounding mucosa, causing the tissue to necrose and slough within 7 to 10 days. Repeat treatments may be necessary. In *hemorrhoidectomy,* hemorrhoids are surgically excised.

 NURSING CARE

Most clients with hemorrhoids are treated in outpatient settings. Nurses have frequent opportunities to teach preventive measures for hemorrhoids. Stress the importance of dietary fiber, liberal fluid intake, and regular exercise to maintain stool bulk, softness, and regularity. Discuss the need to respond to the urge to defecate rather than postpone it. Discuss constipation management, including use of bulk-forming laxatives. Stress that stool softeners should be used only for short-term relief. Discuss appropriate use of over-the-counter preparations for hemorrhoid symptom relief.

Discuss signs of possible complications, such as chronic bleeding, prolapse, and thrombosis. Discuss the link between manifestations of hemorrhoids and colorectal cancer. Urge the client to seek medical care for persistent, unresolved, or progressive symptoms.

When a hemorrhoidectomy is performed, the client requires more direct nursing care. Postoperative care of the client with perianal surgery is outlined in Box 20-20. Anal packing may be left in place for 24 hours after surgery. Closely observe for bleeding when it is removed. Postoperative pain can be significant because of rich innervation of the anal region and possible muscle spasms.

 Anorectal Lesions

ANAL FISSURE

An *anal fissure* is an ulcer on the anal margin. Irritating diarrheal stools, childbirth trauma, habitual cathartic use, and anal intercourse may cause anal fissures. Tissues surrounding the fissure become chronically inflamed. Pain and small amounts of bright red bleeding occur with defecation. Anticipated pain may lead to constipation, which further aggravates symptoms. Treatment involves increased fluid and dietary fiber intake, as well as bulk-forming laxatives. A topical agent such as hydrocortisone cream may be prescribed.

ANORECTAL ABSCESS

Bacterial invasion of tissue around the anus can lead to *anorectal abscess*. Pain, which may be aggravated by sitting or walking, is the primary manifestation of an anorectal abscess. External swelling, redness, heat, and tenderness are apparent

---

BOX 20-20
NURSING CARE CHECKLIST

PERIANAL SURGERY (POSTOPERATIVE)

☑ Monitor vital signs and urinary output every 4 hours.
☑ Inspect rectal dressing every 2 to 3 hours; observe closely for bleeding.
☑ Assist to position of comfort, usually side-lying.
☑ Provide analgesics as ordered and before first bowel movement.
☑ Apply ice packs over rectal dressing as ordered.
☑ Assist with sitz bath three to four times per day, providing a rubber ring or donut device for comfort.
☑ Provide a flotation pad for sitting.
☑ Give stool softeners as ordered.
☑ Encourage fluid intake of at least 2,000 mL per day.

Client and Family Teaching

☑ Take sitz bath after each bowel movement for 1 to 2 weeks after surgery.
☑ Drink at least 2 quarts of fluid per day.
☑ Eat adequate dietary fiber, and exercise moderately.
☑ Take stool softeners as prescribed.
☑ Report to the physician the following symptoms: Rectal bleeding, continued pain on defecation, a temperature greater than 101° F (38.3° C), purulent rectal drainage.

on examination. If the abscess does not drain spontaneously, an incision and drainage (I&D) is performed. Anorectal abscesses rarely resolve with antibiotic therapy alone.

ANORECTAL FISTULA

A *fistula* is a tunnel or tubelike tract with openings at each end. Anorectal fistulas have one opening in the anal canal and the other usually in skin around the anus. A fistula may develop spontaneously or result from an anorectal abscess or Crohn's disease. Drainage is intermittent or constant and may be purulent. It may be accompanied by local itching, tenderness, and pain with defecation. The fistula may heal spontaneously, or a *fistulotomy* may be performed. The primary opening of the fistula is closed, and the tract is opened to allow healing by secondary intention, from the inside out.

PILONIDAL DISEASE

Pilonidal disease is an acute abscess or chronic draining sinus in the sacrococcygeal area. Beneath the abscess or sinus is a cyst that often contains hair tufts. Pilonidal disease usually affects young hirsute (hairy) males; it is probably caused by trapping of hair in deep tissues. It may be congenital. The cyst is generally asymptomatic unless it becomes infected. Infection causes pain, tenderness, redness, heat, and swelling of the affected area. Purulent discharge may be noted. Pilonidal disease is treated with incision and drainage. The sinus tract and underlying cyst are excised and closed.

NURSING CARE

Teach the client with a perianal lesion to maintain a high-fiber diet and liberal fluid intake to decrease discomfort with defecation. Stress the importance of responding to the urge to defecate to prevent constipation.

Following surgical treatment of any of these disorders, teach the client to avoid soiling the dressing with urine or feces during elimination. Instruct to keep the perianal region clean and dry, gently cleansing the area with soap and water after a bowel movement. Encourage sitz baths for cleaning and comfort. Suggest taking an analgesic prior to defecation, but caution that some analgesics may promote constipation. Teach signs and symptoms of infection or other possible complications to report to the physician.

Nursing Interventions Classification

Consider using the following nursing interventions (McCloskey & Bulechek, 2000) to plan and provide care for clients with bowel disorders:

- Bowel Irrigation
- Bowel Management
- Constipation/Impaction Management
- Diarrhea Management
- Ostomy Care
- Perineal Care
- Sexual Counseling
- Teaching: Prescribed Diet
- Tube Care: Gastrointestinal

(*Note:* The bibliography listings for this and all chapters have been compiled at the back of the book.)

Chapter Review

key terms by topic

Use the CD-ROM disk enclosed with your textbook to hear the pronunciation of the key terms in the chapter.

Disorders of motility and absorption
diarrhea, constipation, malabsorption, borborygmi

Inflammatory and infectious disorders
appendicitis, laparotomy, laparoscopy, peritonitis, paralytic ileus, gastroenteritis, steatorrhea, colostomy, ileostomy

Structural and obstructive disorders
diverticulitis

key points

- Diarrhea is a manifestation of many bowel disorders. When prolonged or severe, diarrhea can lead to serious fluid and electrolyte imbalances, as well as excoration of perianal tissues.

- Constipation, another disorder of bowel motility, often is a functional disorder caused by inadequate fluid intake, lack of dietary fiber, or voluntary retention of stool. Encourage all clients (unless specifically contraindicated) to consume generous amounts of water and a diet high in fiber.

- Most laxatives are appropriate for short-term use (1 week or less) only. Bulk-forming laxatives may be used for longer periods if necessary.

- Clients with early manifestations of appendicitis need to be evaluated promptly to reduce the risk of perforation of the inflamed appendix and contamination of the peritoneal cavity.

- A rigid, boardlike abdomen and severe abdominal pain usually indicates acute inflammation of the peritoneum and a need for immediate medical intervention.

- Rectal bleeding may indicate hemorrhoids (a common, benign condition) or colorectal cancer. All clients with rectal bleeding should undergo testing (e.g., colonoscopy) for colorectal cancer.

- Advise all clients over the age of 50 to undergo yearly digital rectal exam and testing for occult blood in the stool. A colonoscopy should be done at age 50 and every 5 to 10 years thereafter. Clients with inflammatory bowel disease have a significantly increased risk for colorectal cancer, and should begin screening exams at an earlier age.

- Early manifestations of a bowel obstruction include high-pitched, tinkling bowel sounds. Later manifestations include absent bowel sounds, abdominal distention, and possible vomiting.

- A warm sitz bath is an appropriate nursing measure for clients with an anorectal disorder such as hemorrhoids (unless contraindicated by specific procedures performed).

Medialink

Additional interactive resources for this chapter can be found on the Companion Website at www.prenhall.com/burke. Click on Chapter 20 and "Begin" to select the activities for this chapter.

For NCLEX review questions and an audio glossary, access the accompanying CD-ROM in this book.

for further study

For more information on fluid imbalances, see Chapter 5.

For more about parenteral nutrition, see Chapter 18; nursing care for the client having paracentesis is in Box 19-13.

For an in-depth discussion of shock, see Chapter 10.

For nursing implications for common antibiotics, see Table 12-5.

For more on endotracheal intubation and mechanical ventilation, see Chapter 26.

For more information on radiation and chemotherapy, see Chapter 8.

Critical Thinking Care Map

Caring for a Client with Colorectal Cancer
NCLEX-PN Focus Area: Reduction of Risk Potential

Case Study: William Cunningham is a 65-year-old man who has noticed small amounts of blood in his stools for the past 3 months. His physician finds a palpable mass on digital rectal exam, and orders a colonoscopy. A large rectal lesion is found; biopsy shows it to be adenocarcinoma. Mr. Cunningham is scheduled for an abdominoperineal resection and sigmoid colostomy.

Nursing Diagnosis: Risk for Impaired Skin Integrity

COLLECT DATA

Subjective

_____
_____
_____
_____
_____
_____

Objective

_____
_____
_____
_____
_____
_____

Would you report this data? Yes/No

If yes, to: _____

Nursing Care

_____
_____
_____
_____
_____
_____
_____
_____

How would you document this? _____
_____
_____

Data Collected
(use those that apply)

- Sense of pressure in rectum
- Intermittent constipation
- BP 118/78; T 98.4° F (36.9° C); P 82; R 18
- Height 5'10" (178 cm), weight 185 lbs. (84 kg)
- States "I really don't want a colostomy, but if that is what it takes to keep me well, I'm ready to get it over with."

Nursing Interventions
(use those that apply)

- Provide analgesia as ordered, evaluating its effectiveness.
- Frequently assess stoma and peristomal skin condition.
- Discuss foods that cause odor and gas.
- Teach colostomy care.
- Maintain consistent nursing personnel assignment to facilitate trust.
- Refer to the local United Ostomy Association.
- Provide a list of local resources for ostomy supplies.
- Provide for privacy when teaching and discussing concerns about ostomy.

NCLEX-PN Exam Preparation

1. Your client has had a surgical resection of the small intestine. Which function is most likely to be affected?
   a. absorption of nutrients
   b. elimination of indigestible food residue
   c. formation of chyme
   d. no effect

2. A client admitted for a cerebrovascular accident (CVA) has lost control of the external sphincter of the anus. Which elimination pattern is most likely to occur?
   a. constipation
   b. tarry stools
   c. diarrhea
   d. fecal incontinence

3. As an acute care nurse, you are admitting a client with the chief complaint of severe diarrhea. Which of the following would be your first priority?
   a. Prevent skin breakdown from stool coming in contact with skin.
   b. Establish measures for fluid replacement.
   c. Administer an antidiarrheal medication.
   d. Obtain a thorough client history.

4. A client with irritable bowel syndrome states: "If it wasn't for my job I wouldn't be here." Your best response would be:
   a. "I think you should discuss this with a trained counselor."
   b. "Usually, this disease is related to stress. I'll get an educational video for you to watch."
   c. "You must have some strong feelings about your job. Do you want to talk about it?"
   d. "I will ask the physician for an antianxiety medication as soon as possible."

5. A client has been admitted with severe diarrhea. The nurse bases his decision whether to administer the prescribed antidiarrheal medication on the understanding that antidiarrheal medication:
   a. should not be used until the cause of diarrhea has been determined
   b. should be administered upon manifestation of diarrhea to prevent losses of fluids and electrolytes
   c. should be withheld until stool cultures and samples have been obtained
   d. should not be administered until fluid and electrolyte status has been established

6. Your client is recovering from a small-bowel resection. To monitor the client's nutritional status you would:
   a. monitor food intake and fecal output
   b. evaluate fluid intake/output record

   c. obtain an order for gluten-free diet
   d. teach the client and family how to read food labels to determine nutrient content

7. When a client is prescribed a low-residue diet, which of the following menu plans indicates an understanding of food restrictions?
   a. sirloin steak, baked potato, carrot sticks, sugar-free lemon meringue pie
   b. steamed fish, baked potato, green beans, fresh fruit cup
   c. broiled chicken breast, mashed potatoes, whipped squash, angel food cake
   d. fried breaded chicken, mashed potatoes, corn, angel food cake

8. A client admitted with abdominal pain is being observed on your unit. Which of the following assessment findings should be immediately reported?
   a. active bowel sounds
   b. a flat, soft abdomen
   c. complaints of anorexia but no nausea or vomiting
   d. increased pain with a rigid, boardlike abdomen

9. A client recovering from bowel surgery is asking for regular food. The nurse's most appropriate response would be:
   a. "When your bowel sounds have returned sufficiently, it will be safe to introduce foods again."
   b. "When you no longer require narcotic pain medication, it can safely be planned to introduce food."
   c. "The IV fluids you are receiving are adequate nourishment."
   d. "When you are able to ambulate, introducing food will be considered."

10. You have been asked to give a lecture within the community, addressing the need to prevent development of colon cancer. Which of the following would be appropriate to include in the presentation?
    a. When you have reached the age of 50, you should have an annual digital rectal exam and a flexible sigmoidoscopy or colonoscopy every 5 years.
    b. If you have inflammatory bowel disease, you need to have a flexible sigmoidoscopy or colonoscopy every 5 years after age 50 to allow for early detection of polyps.
    c. When you have reached the age of 50, you need to have a lab test called carcinoembryonic antigen (CEA) to determine the need for colonoscopy.
    d. When you have reached the age of 50, you need to have annual checks due to the rapid growth of bowel tumors.

chapter

21

Caring for Clients with Renal and Urinary Tract Disorders

CARING tip

"You need to possess the following skills:

- Communication

- Time management

- Critical thinking

- Being a team player

- Being flexible and accountable."

Zenny C. Pancho, RNC, MA • Vocational Nursing Instructor • Long Beach City College • Long Beach, California

LEARNING outcomes

After completing this chapter, you will be able to:

- Identify and describe the structures and functions of the urinary system.
- Describe the pathophysiology of common disorders of the kidneys and urinary tract.
- Provide appropriate nursing care for clients undergoing diagnostic tests to identify these disorders.
- Compare and contrast the manifestations of common disorders of the kidneys and urinary tract.
- Discuss the nursing implications of medications prescribed for clients with these disorders.
- Provide appropriate nursing care for the client having surgery of the kidneys or urinary tract.
- Use the nursing process as a framework for providing individualized care to clients with disorders of the kidneys or urinary tract.

MediaLink

 www.prenhall.com/burke

Use the above address to access the free, interactive Companion Website created for this textbook. Get hints, instant feedback, and textbook references to chapter-related multiple choice questions. Link to other interesting sites.

Structure and Function of the Urinary System

The urinary system includes the paired kidneys and ureters, the urinary bladder, and the urethra (Figure 21-1 ◆). The urinary system is important in maintaining and regulating the body's internal environment. The urinary system excretes metabolic wastes. It also excretes or conserves water and solutes, as needed. The kidneys help regulate acid–base balance and blood pressure. Because these are vital functions, any disorder of the urinary system can affect the entire body.

KIDNEYS

The two kidneys sit behind the peritoneum (*retroperitoneal* space) on either side of the spine. They are partially protected by the rib cage. These highly vascular, bean-shaped organs are about the size of a closed fist. On the inner *(concave)* surface of each kidney is a notch known as the *hilum,* where the ureter, renal artery, renal vein, lymphatic vessels, and nerves enter or exit. The *renal fascia,* a layer of dense connective tissue, protects and anchors the kidney.

Each kidney has three distinct regions: the cortex, medulla, and pelvis (Figure 21-2 ◆). The outer region, or *renal cortex,* contains the **glomeruli,** small clusters of capillaries. The glomeruli are part of the **nephrons,** the functional units of the kidney (Figure 21-3 ◆). Each kidney contains approximately one million nephrons, which process the blood to make urine.

In the *renal medulla,* or inner portion of the kidney, nephrons form the *renal pyramids.* These pyramids channel urine into branches of the innermost region, the *renal pelvis.* These branches are known as *calyces* (singular, *calyx*). Urine is channeled from the pelvis through the ureter and into the bladder for storage.

URETERS

The *ureters* are bilateral tubes about 10 to 12 inches (25 to 30 cm) long. They move urine from the kidney to the bladder by peristaltic waves. The ureters contain smooth muscle and are innervated by the autonomic nervous system.

URINARY BLADDER

The urinary bladder is a hollow, muscular organ that lies behind the symphysis pubis. The ureters enter the bladder at its base, an area known as the *trigone* (Figure 21-4 ◆). The urethral opening is at the third point of this triangular region. Bladder muscle tone in this area prevents a backflow of urine from the bladder into the ureters.

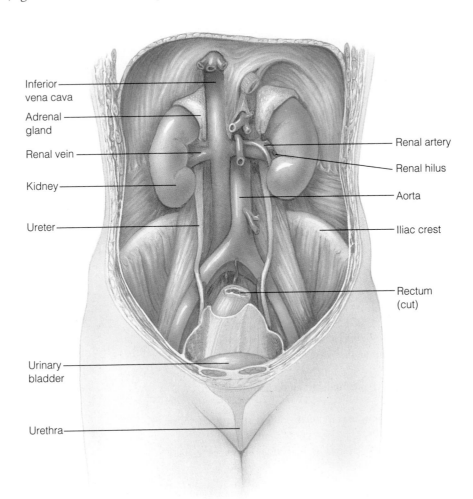

Inferior vena cava
Adrenal gland
Renal vein
Kidney
Ureter
Urinary bladder
Urethra
Renal artery
Renal hilus
Aorta
Iliac crest
Rectum (cut)

Figure 21-1. ◆ Anterior view of the urinary system.

Figure 21-2. ◆ Internal anatomy of the kidney.

The bladder is lined with epithelial mucosa. The muscle (*detrusor muscle*) is arranged in layers that allow the bladder to expand or contract. Healthy adults usually feel the urge to void when the bladder contains 300 to 500 mL of urine. However, the bladder can hold more than twice that amount if necessary. The *internal urethral sphincter* relaxes in response to a full bladder, signaling the need to urinate. A second *external urethral sphincter* formed by skeletal muscle is under voluntary control.

URETHRA

The *urethra* is a thin-walled muscular tube that channels urine out of the body. It extends from the base of the bladder to the *urinary meatus (opening)*. In females, the urethra is approximately 1.5 inches (3 to 5 cm) long; the urinary meatus is anterior to the vagina. In males, the urethra is about 8 inches (20

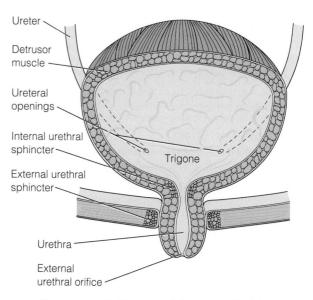

Figure 21-4. ◆ Structure of the urinary bladder.

cm) long; it serves as a channel for semen as well as urine. The prostate gland encircles the urethra at the base of the bladder in males. The male urinary meatus is at the end of the glans penis.

URINE FORMATION

The kidneys process about 180 liters (47 gallons) of filtrate each day. Of this, only 1% is excreted as urine; the rest is returned to the circulation. Urine is formed by the processes of glomerular filtration, tubular reabsorption, and tubular secretion.

Glomerular Filtration

Glomerular filtration is a passive process in which fluid and solutes move from the blood in the glomerulus into Bowman's capsule. The amount of fluid filtered from the blood into the capsule per minute is called the **glomerular filtration rate (GFR)**. Normal GFR in adults is 120 to 125 mL/min. The blood pressure and volume are the primary factors controlling GFR. A drop in blood pressure or blood volume cause the GFR and urine output to fall.

The GFR is regulated by a number of mechanisms. Afferent (incoming) arterioles constrict or dilate in response to blood pressure changes. Specialized cells in the afferent arteriole and distal convoluted tubule (the *juxtaglomerular apparatus*), respond to changes in blood flow by releasing renin, an enzyme that affects systemic blood pressure. Glomerular filtration also is affected by the sympathetic nervous system.

Tubular Reabsorption

Tubular reabsorption begins as the filtrate enters the proximal tubules. In healthy kidneys, virtually all organic nutrients such as glucose and amino acids are reabsorbed. Water and electrolyte reabsorption is continuously regulated and adjusted to maintain homeostasis. Reabsorption occurs by both active and passive mechanisms.

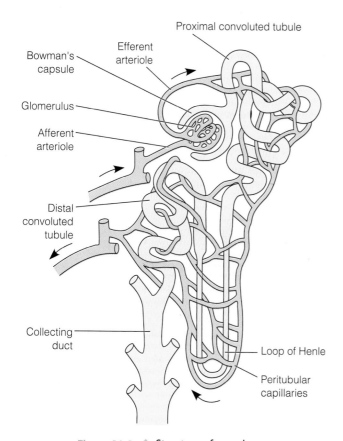

Figure 21-3. ◆ Structure of a nephron.

Tubular Secretion

Through the process of *tubular secretion,* excess potassium and waste products such as hydrogen ion (H⁺), creatinine, and ammonia are eliminated from the body. Both passive and active mechanisms work to eliminate waste products and regulate acid–base balance.

Urine Concentration

In the loop of Henle, urine is concentrated, and further wastes are excreted through reabsorption and secretion. In the distal tubule, antidiuretic hormone (ADH) determines the final dilution or concentration of urine (see Chapter 5). When ADH is secreted, water is reabsorbed in the distal convoluted tubule and collecting duct, and urine is more concentrated. When ADH is not secreted, water cannot be reabsorbed and the urine is more dilute.

Urine is composed, by volume, of about 95% water and 5% solutes. Solutes normally excreted in the urine include urea, sodium, potassium, phosphate, sulfate, creatinine, uric acid, calcium, magnesium, and bicarbonate. The characteristics of normal urine are listed in Table 21-1 ◆.

Renal Clearance

Two substances found in the blood are routinely used to evaluate renal function. *Urea* is formed in the metabolism of dietary and body proteins. *Creatinine* is produced in relatively constant quantities by muscle cell metabolism. Both these substances are eliminated from the body by the kidneys by filtration and secretion; neither is reabsorbed. For this reason, *blood urea nitrogen (BUN)* and *serum creatinine* levels in the blood are effective indicators of renal function. (See Table 21-5 for normal BUN and serum creatinine levels.) The GFR can be evaluated by determining the amount of blood plasma cleared of creatinine during a specific period of time. This is known as the *creatinine clearance test,* explained later in this chapter.

ENDOCRINE FUNCTION OF THE KIDNEYS

Besides producing urine, the kidneys produce renin and erythropoietin, and they activate vitamin D. The enzyme *renin,* produced by the juxtaglomerular apparatus, converts the

TABLE 21-1	CHARACTERISTICS OF NORMAL URINE ON URINALYSIS
Color	Pale yellow to deep amber; clear
Odor	Aromatic
Specific gravity	1.005–1.030
pH	4.5–8.0
Protein	Negative to trace
Glucose	Negative
Ketones	Negative
RBC	0–5/high power field (HPF)
WBC	0–5/HPF
Casts	Negative to occasional
Bacteria	Negative

plasma protein angiotensinogen to angiotensin I. Angiotensin I is converted in the lungs to angiotensin II. Angiotensin II, a potent vasoconstrictor, raises blood pressure. It also stimulates the adrenal cortex to release aldosterone, which promotes sodium and water retention. The net effect of the *renin–angiotensin–aldosterone* system is to raise the blood pressure and blood volume (see Chapter 5).

Erythropoietin is produced by the kidneys in response to hypoxia of renal cells. Erythropoietin stimulates the bone marrow to produce red blood cells.

Vitamin D is important for calcium regulation in the body. It is inactive when it enters the body either through the diet or by exposure to ultraviolet light (sunlight). It is activated in two steps by the liver and then the kidneys.

AGE-RELATED CHANGES IN KIDNEY FUNCTION

Nephrons are lost with aging, reducing kidney mass and the GFR. By age 80, the GFR may be less than half of what it was

TABLE 21-2	NURSING IMPLICATIONS OF AGE-RELATED CHANGES IN KIDNEY FUNCTION	
CHANGE	**EFFECT**	**NURSING IMPLICATIONS**
Decreased GFR	Decreased excretion of drugs primarily eliminated by the kidneys; increased risk of drug toxicity	Monitor clients carefully for signs of toxicity, especially when giving digoxin, certain antibiotics, cimetidine, and chlorpropamide.
Decreased number of nephrons; changes in aldosterone levels and response to ADH	Decreased ability to conserve water and sodium; increased risk of fluid, electrolyte, and acid–base imbalances	Monitor for fluid, electrolyte, and acid–base imbalances. Promote fluid intake of up to 2,500 mL/day unless contraindicated.
Decreased number of functional nephrons	Increased risk of kidney failure	Avoid nephrotoxic drugs if possible; monitor urine output and for signs of renal failure.

at age 30. The kidneys are less able to concentrate urine in the older adult. This fact, combined with diminished thirst in older adults, increases the risk for dehydration. Potassium excretion may be decreased in older adults, increasing the risk of fluid and electrolyte imbalances. (See Table 21-2 ◆.)

Voiding Disorders

Voiding disorders are common, although often unreported. Modesty, embarrassment, difficulty discussing the genitals and elimination, and fear of changes in function often interfere with the client's willingness to seek help.

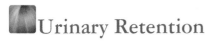Urinary Retention

Normal bladder emptying may be disrupted by an obstruction to urine flow or by a functional problem. When the bladder cannot empty, it becomes overstretched. This, in turn, affects detrusor muscle contraction and further impairs urination.

Benign prostatic hypertrophy (*BPH,* or enlargement of the prostate) is a common cause of *urinary retention.* Difficulty initiating and maintaining urine flow is often the presenting complaint in men with BPH. Acute inflammation associated with infection or trauma of the bladder, urethra, or perineal tissues may also interfere with the ability to urinate. Scarring caused by repeated urinary tract infections can narrow the urethra and obstruct output.

Surgery, particularly abdominal or pelvic surgery, can affect detrusor muscle function, leading to acute urinary retention. Medications also may affect bladder contraction. Drugs with anticholinergic effects may cause urinary retention. These include antianxiety drugs, antidepressant drugs, and many common over-the-counter cough, cold, allergy, and sleep-promoting drugs. Neurologic diseases or trauma may interfere with normal mechanisms of bladder emptying (*neurogenic bladder*). Voluntary urinary retention (particularly common among nurses) may lead to overfilling of the bladder and a loss of detrusor muscle tone.

The client with urinary retention is unable to empty the bladder completely. Overflow voiding or incontinence may occur (see Table 21-3). Assessment reveals a firm, distended bladder that may be displaced to one side of midline.

Acute or chronic urinary retention can lead to complications such as hydronephrosis (distention of the kidney with urine), acute renal failure, and urinary tract infection. These conditions are discussed in subsequent sections of this chapter.

COLLABORATIVE CARE

For the client with a mechanical obstruction to urine flow, retention is treated by removing or repairing the obstruction. The prostate gland may be resected in the client with BPH. Cholinergic medications such as bethanechol chloride (Urecholine) may be ordered to promote bladder emptying. Modifying the client's medication regimen may be necessary.

Techniques to stimulate reflex voiding and promote complete bladder emptying are used for neurogenic bladder. These include using trigger points, for example, stroking or pinching the abdomen, inner thigh, or glans penis. Pulling pubic hairs or tapping the suprapubic region can also stimulate urination.

The *Credé method* (applying pressure over the symphysis pubis with the fingers of one or both hands) may promote complete bladder emptying. Applying manual pressure to the abdomen and using the *Valsalva maneuver* (bearing down while holding one's breath) also promotes bladder emptying.

Intermittent straight catheterization following surgery can prevent overdistention of the bladder. Intermittent catheterization is less likely to cause a urinary tract infection than an indwelling catheter, and so is preferred. Clients with chronic urinary retention may perform intermittent self-catheterization every 3 to 4 hours (see Procedure 21-1).

NURSING CARE

Careful nursing assessment can identify clients with problems of urinary retention. Note intake and output, paying close attention to voiding patterns as well as total output. Notify the charge nurse or physician if it has been 8 or more hours since the client has voided. Gently palpate the lower abdomen just above the symphysis pubis for tenderness and firm distention. Percussing the lower abdomen may be helpful; a full bladder has a dull percussion tone.

Measures to promote urination can be helpful. Place the client in normal voiding position (sitting for females and standing for males) and provide privacy. Run water in the sink or shower, place the client's hands in warm water, pour warm water over the perineum, or provide a warm sitz bath as additional measures. Provide adequate time for voiding; allow up to 10 minutes.

When catheterization is necessary, use strict sterile technique. Nursing care related to catheterization is listed in Box 21-1.

PROCEDURE 21-1   Client Self-Catheterization Checklist

- Wash hands before and after the procedure, and clean the urinary meatus with soap and water.
- Attempt to void. If urine is not of sufficient quantity (at least 100 mL) or if you cannot void at all, do self-catheterization.

■ FEMALE

- While sitting, locate the urethra by looking in a mirror, or feeling it with a fingertip.
- Lubricate the meatus with a water-soluble lubricant.
- Take a deep breath and insert the catheter tip 2 to 3 inches or until urine flows.

■ MALE

- While sitting, hold the penis with slight upward tension and extend it to its full length.
- Lubricate the catheter from the tip to about 6 inches downward.
- Take a deep breath and insert the catheter 6 to 7 inches or until urine flows.

■ BOTH

- Hold the catheter securely and allow urine to drain until the flow stops.
- Withdraw the catheter and wash it with soap and water. Store in a clean container.

Discharge Considerations

Assess the client's ability to provide self-care. Determine understanding of the problem, ability to recognize manifestations of urinary retention, and ability to perform maneuvers to stimulate voiding. If intermittent catheterization is required, assess vision, ability to see the urinary meatus, and motor skills for inserting the catheter. Assess access to water and facilities for handwashing and cleaning the catheter. Discuss the manifestations of acute urinary retention and urinary tract infection, and stress the importance of notifying a health care provider if these develop.

Urinary Incontinence

Urinary incontinence, or involuntary urination, is a common problem, especially among older adults. Incontinence can cause physical problems (e.g., skin breakdown, infection, and rashes), as well as embarrassment, isolation and withdrawal, feelings of worthlessness and helplessness, and depression.

PATHOPHYSIOLOGY

Urinary continence requires a bladder that is able to expand and contract, and sphincters that can maintain a higher pressure in the urethra than that in the bladder. When bladder pressure is higher than urethral resistance, urine can escape. Any condition causing increased bladder pressures or lowered urethral resistance can cause incontinence. Pelvic muscle relaxation, impaired neural control, and bladder problems are common contributing factors.

Incontinence is commonly categorized as stress incontinence, urge incontinence, overflow incontinence, reflex incontinence, and functional incontinence (Table 21-3 ◆).

Urinary Incontinence in Older Adults

Incontinence should *never* be considered a normal part of aging. However, age-related changes contribute to its devel-

BOX 21-1
NURSING CARE CHECKLIST

URINARY CATHETERIZATION

- ☑ Use standard precautions.
- ☑ Use sterile technique for catheter insertion.
- ☑ If possible, use intermittent catheterization instead of an indwelling catheter to reduce the risk of infection.
- ☑ Use appropriate size catheter; a small catheter may leak; a large catheter may traumatize tissues.
- ☑ Provide perineal care before catheterization and for clients with an indwelling catheter. Use soap and water, rinsing carefully. Avoid pulling on an indwelling catheter.
- ☑ Do not drain more than 750 to 1,000 mL from the bladder at one time.
- ☑ Assess amount, color, clarity, and odor of urine. Collect a urine specimen as needed.
- ☑ Monitor intake and output.
- ☑ Secure tubing of an indwelling catheter to prevent trauma.
- ☑ Maintain gravity drainage; prevent loops of tubing or elevation of the drainage container higher than the bladder.

	TABLE 21-3	TYPES OF URINARY INCONTINENCE		
TYPE	**DESCRIPTION**	**PATHOPHYSIOLOGY**	**CONTRIBUTING FACTORS**
Stress	Loss of small amounts of urine when intra-abdominal pressure increases (sneezing, laughing, lifting)	Pelvic muscle relaxation; weakness of urethra and surrounding tissues decreases urethral resistance	Multiple pregnancies Decreased estrogen levels (menopause) Prostate surgery
Urge	Inability to stop urine flow long enough to reach toilet after need to void is felt	Overactive detrusor muscle increases bladder pressure, causing inability to inhibit voiding	Decreased bladder capacity Bladder irritation CNS disorders
Overflow	Urinary retention with bladder overdistention and frequent loss of small amounts of urine (25–50 mL)	Outlet obstruction or impaired detrusor muscle activity leads to overfilling and increased pressure	Neurologic disorders or trauma Enlarged prostate Fecal impaction Anticholinergic drug effects
Reflex	Involuntary loss of moderate amount of urine occurring with warning	Altered spinal cord activity causing hyperreflexia of the detrusor muscle	Neurologic disorders or trauma
Functional	Inability to get to toilet facilities to urinate	Self-care deficit that interferes with ability to respond to urge to void	Physical disability or impaired mobility, neurologic disorders Diuretic therapy or sedation Lack of facilities, privacy, or caregiver assistance

opment. Bladder capacity usually declines with age, and involuntary bladder muscle contractions are more common. In women, decreased estrogen levels and pelvic muscle relaxation cause urethral resistance to decrease, so stress incontinence may occur. Decreased estrogen also may lead to dysuria and urgency. Other risk factors in older adults include immobility, chronic degenerative diseases or dementia, medications, diabetes, and stroke. Incontinence increases the risk for falls, fractures, pressure ulcers, urinary tract infection, and depression. It contributes to caregiver stress, and may be a major factor in institutionalizing the client.

COLLABORATIVE CARE

The focus of collaborative care is to identify and correct the cause if possible. If the underlying problem cannot be corrected, techniques may be taught to manage urine output.

Evaluation begins with a complete history, including the duration, frequency, volume, and associated circumstances of incontinence. A voiding diary (Figure 21-5 ◆) is often used to provide detailed information. The history includes any chronic or acute illnesses, previous surgeries, and current medications, prescription and over-the-counter.

Physical assessment includes abdominal, rectal, and pelvic exams, as well as evaluation of mental and neurologic status, mobility, and dexterity. Women with incontinence often have weak abdominal and pelvic muscle tone, protrusion of the bladder or urethral wall into the vagina (cystocele or

urethrocele), and thin vaginal tissues. In men, an enlarged prostate gland is commonly identified.

Diagnostic tests to identify the cause of urinary incontinence may include a *postvoid residual urine* measurement (Box 21-2) to determine how completely the bladder empties with voiding. Less than 50 mL of residual urine is expected; when 100 mL or more of residual urine is present, further tests are done. Additional studies may include *cystometrography* to evaluate bladder pressures and *uroflowmetry* to evalute voiding patterns.

Urge incontinence may be treated with drugs to inhibit detrusor muscle contractions and increase bladder capacity. These may include tolterodine (Detrol) and oxybutynin (Ditropan). The anticholinergic effects of these drugs may cause dry mouth and eyes, constipation, confusion, and urinary retention.

When incontinence is associated with postmenopausal atrophic vaginitis, estrogen therapy may be effective. Both systemic estrogens and local creams are used.

When incontinence is associated with a cystocele or urethrocele, or is due to an enlarged prostate gland, surgery may be performed. *Bladder neck suspension* is used to treat urethrocele. Nursing care of the client having a bladder neck suspension is outlined in Box 21-3.

Prostatectomy is indicated when an enlarged prostate gland obstructs urine outflow. (See care of the client with a prostatectomy in Chapter 32.)

DATE ___4/15/02___

Please complete this chart prior to your visit. Choose a 24-hour period when it is convenient for you to measure and record the following: The amount of fluid you void (urinate), the amount of fluid you drink and type of beverage, the time, when leakage episodes occur, whether or not you have an urge to void just prior to leaking, and the activity you are doing when you leak or need to void.

VOIDING DIARY

DIARY.URO

Void Amount (oz.)	Fluid Intake Amount (oz.)	Time	Leak?	Urge prior to leak?	Activity
14 oz.		6:23 am	yes	yes	Awakening
8 oz.	14 oz. coffee	6:35			
		8:05	yes	yes	reading
	16 oz. coffee	8:30			
10 oz.		9:10	yes	yes	watch TV
10 oz.		9:30	"	"	"
12 oz.	8 oz. water	10:17	"	"	"
6 oz.		11:40	yes	yes	washing dishes
8 oz.	12 oz. coke	2:12 pm	yes	yes	Lunch
	16 oz. water	6:30			Dinner
10 oz.		8:00	yes	yes	Laundry
6 oz.		9:55	yes	yes	folding clothes
	8 oz. water	11:25			Bed time
6 oz.		1:30 am	—	yes	sleeping
8 oz.	—	5:05	—	yes	sleeping
5 oz.		6:30	—	yes	Awakening
		TOTAL			

Figure 21-5. ◆ A sample voiding diary.

NURSING CARE

ASSESSING

Collect subjective assessment data by asking about problems with urine loss, its frequency, and any contributing factors. Inquire about frequency, urgency, and burning on urination. Identify current medications and their timing. Assess patterns of fluid intake and output. Assess the abdomen for evidence of bladder distention or tenderness. Perform a mental status examination if indicated.

DIAGNOSING, PLANNING, AND IMPLEMENTING

When planning care for clients with incontinence, consider mental and neurologic status, mobility, and motivation. Behavioral techniques require long-term commitment, as well as the physical and mental ability to implement them. Nursing interventions such as scheduled toileting, bladder training, and prompted voiding combined with praise can

BOX 21-3
NURSING CARE CHECKLIST

BLADDER NECK SUSPENSION
Before Surgery
☑ Provide routine preoperative care and teaching as outlined in Chapter 7.
☑ Instruct to avoid straining and the Valsalva maneuver postoperatively.

After Surgery
☑ Provide routine postoperative care as outlined in Chapter 7.
☑ Frequently assess vaginal drainage or dressing. Notify the charge nurse or physician of bright red bleeding on dressing, from vagina, or in urine.
☑ Monitor and record quantity, color, and clarity of urine. Pink urine should gradually clear.
☑ Tape urinary catheters in position to prevent dislodging or pulling on incisions.
☑ Encourage activity and ambulation.
☑ Carefully monitor urine output following catheter removal.
☑ If a urethral or suprapubic catheter is in place at discharge, teach appropriate care.
☑ Stress importance of keeping scheduled appointments and contacting the physician if signs of a urinary tract infection or other complications develop.

BOX 21-4
TEACHING FOR DISCHARGE

PELVIC FLOOR (KEGEL) EXERCISES
• Identify the pelvic muscles by:
  a. Attempting to stop the flow of urine during voiding and holding for a few seconds.
  b. Tightening the muscles of the vagina around a gloved finger or tampon.
  c. Tightening the muscles around the anus as though trying to avoid passing flatus.
• Perform exercises: Tighten pelvic muscles, hold for 10 seconds, and relax for 10 to 15 seconds. Continue the sequence (tighten, hold, relax) for 10 repetitions.
• Keep abdominal muscles and breathing relaxed while performing exercises.
• Initially, exercises should be performed twice per day, working up to four times a day.
• Exercise at a specific time each day or in conjunction with another daily activity (such as bathing or watching the news). Establish a routine, because these exercises should be continued for life.

reduce the need for diapers, incontinence pads, and indwelling catheters in institutionalized clients.

IMPAIRED URINARY ELIMINATION

■ Monitor patterns of fluid intake and urination, including voluntary voiding and wetting accidents. *These data help identify the type and pattern of incontinence.*

■ Teach pelvic floor muscle exercises, called Kegel exercises (Box 21-4). Instruct to consciously tighten pelvic muscles and relax the abdomen when the need to void is perceived. *Improved pelvic muscle strength helps prevent stress incontinence and decrease urge incontinence.*

■ Reduce delays in toileting. Ensure that the call light is within reach. Place a bedside commode in the room or provide clear access to the bathroom. Dress in loose-fitting clothing with elastic waistbands or Velcro closures. *These actions reduce the risk of wetting accidents.*

■ After the evening meal, limit beverages, especially those that irritate the bladder, such as caffeine, Nutri-Sweet, and citrus juices. *Limiting evening fluid intake and bladder irritants reduces the risk of nighttime incontinence.*

■ Administer diuretic drugs in the morning and midafternoon. *This timing allows the peak effect of the medication to occur while the client is awake and more able to respond to the urge to void.*

TOILETING SELF-CARE DEFICIT

In institutions, functional incontinence (see Table 21-3) can be a significant problem in previously continent people. With functional incontinence, the primary problem is an outside factor that interferes with the ability to respond to the urge to void.

■ Assess physical and mental capabilities and limitations, usual pattern of voiding, and ability to assist with toileting. *A thorough assessment helps address specific needs.*

■ Provide assistive devices such as raised toilet seats, grab bars, a bedside commode, or night-lights. *Assistive devices help maintain independence.*

■ Plan a toileting schedule to achieve approximately 300 mL of urine output with each voiding. *Allowing the bladder to fill until the urge to void is felt helps maintain normal bladder capacity.*

■ Position for ease of voiding—sitting for females, standing for males—and provide for privacy. *Normal positioning and privacy enhance the ability to void.*

■ Provide the majority of fluids during times of day when the client is most able to remain continent. *Unless restricted, maintain a fluid intake of at least 1.5 to 2 liters per day.*

SOCIAL ISOLATION

The client with any form of urinary incontinence is at risk for social isolation due to embarrassment, fear of not having ready access to a bathroom, body odor, or other factors.

- Refer for urologic examination and evaluation of incontinence. *Clients who assume that urinary incontinence is a normal part of aging may not be aware of treatment options.*
- Explore alternative coping strategies with client, significant others, staff, and other health team members. *Protective pads or shields, good perineal hygiene, scheduled voiding, and clothing that does not interfere with toileting can enhance continence.*

EVALUATING

To evaluate the effectiveness of nursing actions for the client with incontinence, keep a voiding diary of fluid intake, voidings, and wetting accidents. Identify wetting episodes that occur because of delayed toileting or difficulty manipulating clothing. Assess the client's willingness to participate in social activities.

Discharge Considerations

Appropriate home care and teaching can help keep the client in the home, reduce caregiver stress, and reduce the risk of institutionalization. Assess the home environment (whether in the community or a residential living facility) for possible barriers to urinary elimination such as:

- Inadequate lighting, particularly at night
- Narrow doorways that may interfere with access to the toilet
- Inadequate toilet facilities

Teach the client with urinary incontinence to keep a voiding diary to help identify factors contributing to incontinent episodes. Instruct to maintain a generous fluid intake of 1.5 to 2 quarts of fluid per day. Advise restricting fluid intake after the evening meal. Discuss bladder irritants such as caffeine, citrus juices, and artificial sweeteners, and advise limiting their use. Teach Kegel exercises. Discuss the potential risks and benefits of hormone replacement therapy, surgery, and physical therapy with women. Encourage overweight clients to lose weight.

Discuss scheduled voiding and bladder training techniques with caregivers. Suggest taking the client to the toilet every 2 to 4 hours. To increase bladder capacity, the time between voidings may be gradually increased. Provide a list of resources for assistive devices such as a bedside commode, urinal, grab bars, or raised toilet seat.

Infectious and Inflammatory Disorders

Urinary Tract Infection

Urinary tract infections (UTIs) affect up to 20% of adult women; they are much less common in men until age 50. Their incidence increases with aging in both sexes. Unfortunately, *nosocomial* (hospital-acquired) infections are among the most common UTIs.

UTIs can affect any portion of the urinary tract and are broadly classified according to the region and primary site affected. *Lower urinary tract infections* include *urethritis* (inflammation of the urethra), *prostatitis* (inflammation of the prostate gland), and *cystitis* (inflammation of the bladder). The most common *upper urinary tract infection* is *pyelonephritis* (inflammation of the kidney and renal pelvis).

PATHOPHYSIOLOGY

The urinary tract is normally sterile above the urethra. The most important mechanisms to maintain its sterility are adequate urine volume, unimpeded urine flow, and complete bladder emptying. Other defenses include acid urine, ureteral peristalsis, bacteriostatic properties of the urinary tract, and a *ureterovesical junction* (where the ureters enter the bladder) that prevents backflow of urine toward the kidneys. In males, a long urethra and the antibacterial effect of zinc in prostatic fluid are also important.

Bacteria from the intestines (most commonly *Escherichia coli*) often infect the urinary tract by ascending from the perineal area into the lower urinary tract. Box 21-5 lists risk factors for UTI. Changes in the urinary tract associated with aging further increase the risk for UTI in older adults. These changes are summarized in Box 21-6.

Cystitis

Cystitis (inflammation of the urinary bladder) is the most common UTI. The bladder mucosa becomes inflamed and congested with blood. Pus may form, and the mucosa may bleed. The inflammatory process causes the classic manifestations of cystitis (Box 21-7). Older adults with UTIs may be asymptomatic, or may present with nocturia, incontinence, confusion, behavior change, lethargy, anorexia, or "just not feeling right."

Although cystitis is generally uncomplicated and often resolves spontaneously, the infection can ascend to involve the

---

> ## BOX 21-5
> ### RISK FACTORS FOR UTI
>
> - Instrumentation of the urinary tract (e.g., catheterization, cystoscopy)
> - Structural abnormalities, obstructions, or strictures
> - Incomplete bladder emptying
> - Chronic diseases such as diabetes
>
> #### FEMALES
>
> - Short, straight urethra
> - Proximity of urinary meatus to the vagina and anus
> - Tissue trauma and possible contamination during sexual intercourse
> - Use of a diaphragm for birth control
> - Personal hygiene practices
> - Voluntary urinary retention
>
> #### MALES
>
> - An enlarged prostate gland

> ## BOX 21-7
> ### MANIFESTATIONS OF CYSTITIS
>
> - **Dysuria**—difficult or painful urination
> - Frequency
> - Urgency—a sudden, compelling need to urinate
> - **Nocturia**—voiding two or more times at night
> - Pyuria—presence of pus in the urine (cloudy appearance, foul odor)
> - **Hematuria**—blood in the urine
> - Suprapubic discomfort

kidneys. In older adults or people with impaired immune responses, bacteremia, sepsis, and shock are possible serious complications.

Pyelonephritis

Pyelonephritis is an inflammatory disorder affecting the renal pelvis and *parenchyma* (the functional portion of the kidney tissue). It may be acute, caused by a bacterial infection; or chronic, associated with other disorders.

Bacteria usually enter the kidney from the lower urinary tract. Risk factors include pregnancy (because of slowed ureteral peristalsis), obstruction, and congenital malformation. *Vesicoureteral reflux* (a condition in which urine moves from the bladder back toward the kidney) is a common risk factor in children. It may occur in adults when bladder outflow is obstructed.

E. coli is responsible for most cases of acute pyelonephritis. The infection spreads from the renal pelvis to the cortex.

> ## BOX 21-6
>
> # population
> ## FOCUS
>
> ### Risk Factors for UTI Associated with Aging
>
> - Urine pH increases, promoting bacterial growth
> - Higher incidence of diabetes leading to glucosuria (glucose in the urine provides a good culture medium for bacteria)
> - Incomplete bladder emptying and urinary retention
> - Changes in vaginal pH in women and decreased prostatic secretions in men

The inflamed kidney becomes edematous. Localized abscesses may form, and kidney tissue can be destroyed by the inflammatory process.

The onset of acute pyelonephritis is typically rapid, with chills and fever, malaise, and vomiting, as well as localized manifestations of flank pain and costovertebral tenderness. The client also may have symptoms of cystitis. As with cystitis, older adults may present with a change in behavior, confusion, incontinence, or a general deterioration in condition.

Chronic pyelonephritis leads to fibrosis and scarring of the renal pelvis and calyces. The tubules are gradually destroyed. Chronic renal failure and end-stage renal disease are possible consequences.

COLLABORATIVE CARE

Treatment of UTI focuses on eliminating the cause, preventing relapse or reinfection, and identifying and correcting any contributing factors.

A *urinalysis* is ordered to identify blood cells and bacteria in the urine. A midstream, clean-catch urine specimen should be used (Box 21-8). If necessary, urine may be obtained by a straight catheterization or "mini-cath," using aseptic technique. A urine *culture and sensitivity* also may be done to identify the causative organism. A *complete blood count (CBC) with differential* is done to assess for systemic responses to infection.

In men and in adult females with recurrent UTIs, more extensive diagnostic testing may be done. An *intravenous pyelogram (IVP)* is used to examine the kidneys, ureters, and bladder for abnormalities that may contribute to UTIs. *Voiding cystourethrography* allows assessment of bladder and urethral abnormalities. *Cystoscopy* (direct visualization of the urethra and bladder using an endoscope) is used to diagnose conditions that may contribute to UTIs such as an enlarged prostate, urethral strictures, bladder stones, tumors, and congenital abnormalities. The nursing implications of an IVP and cystoscopy are included in Box 21-9.

Pharmacology

Uncomplicated UTI is treated with a single dose, a 3-day course, or a 7- to 10-day course of antibiotics. Drugs such as sulfonamides, trimethoprim–sulfamethoxazole (TMP-SMZ, Bactrim, Septra), and fluoroquinolones such as ciprofloxacin

BOX 21-8
NURSING CARE CHECKLIST

COLLECTING A MIDSTREAM CLEAN-CATCH URINE SPECIMEN

☑ Explain the purpose of the procedure and specimen.

☑ If alert and ambulatory, provide instructions and supplies for the client to obtain the specimen:

  ☑ Clean the genital and perineal area with soap and water.

  ☑ Use each antiseptic towelette one time as follows:

    ☑ Female clients: Cleanse front to back.

    ☑ Male clients: Use a circular motion to clean the meatus. If uncircumcised, retract the foreskin before cleaning.

  ☑ Start urine flow, then place the container into urine stream to collect the specimen.

  ☑ Tightly cap the container, and, if necessary, rinse and dry the outside.

☑ If the client requires assistance:

  ☑ Obtain all supplies; use standard precautions.

  ☑ Provide perineal care.

  ☑ Position on bedpan, commode, or toilet.

  ☑ Cleanse perineal area with antiseptic towelettes as instructed above.

  ☑ Ask to begin voiding. Place the specimen container into the stream of urine, taking care to avoid touching perineal tissues or hair. Collect 30 to 60 mL of urine.

  ☑ Cap container, avoiding contamination of the inside of the cap.

☑ Label container and send with requisition to the laboratory.

☑ Document specimen collection and any pertinent information.

---

often are used. Treatment often is started before culture results are obtained, because these drugs are effective against the usual organisms. Compliance is better with a single-dose or 3-day course of treatment; however, these are not used for clients with recurrent infections or acute pyelonephritis.

Acute pyelonephritis usually requires 10 to 21 days of antibiotic therapy. Intravenous antibiotics may be necessary if the infection is severe or nausea and vomiting are present. For resistant or recurrent UTI, therapy with urinary anti-infectives may last from 2 weeks to 6 or 12 months (Table 21-4 ◆).

NURSING CARE

ASSESSING

It is important to collect both subjective and objective assessment data from clients with suspected or confirmed UTI. These data provide information that can be used to help the

---

client recover fully from the infection and prevent future UTIs.

Ask the client to describe the symptoms, including their onset and duration. Specifically ask about associated symptoms such as abdominal or back pain, fever, nausea, or vomiting. Ask about UTIs, their frequency, and the effectiveness of treatment. Inquire about birth control method used and the possibility of pregnancy. Have the client identify any chronic diseases, medications, or recent lifestyle changes (e.g., recent marriage or a new sexual relationship). Finally, inquire about hygiene practices such as perineal cleansing after elimination and the use of feminine hygiene sprays or bubble baths.

Assess vital signs, including temperature. Note general appearance and apparent state of health. Palpate the lower abdomen for tenderness and percuss the costovertebral angle. Obtain a clean-catch midstream urine specimen.

DIAGNOSING, PLANNING, AND IMPLEMENTING

IMPAIRED URINARY ELIMINATION

■ Monitor urinary output and color, clarity, and character of urine, including odor. *The client with a UTI often experiences dysuria, frequency, urgency, and nocturia. Urine may appear rusty or blood-tinged, cloudy, and malodorous. Urine normally returns to clear yellow within 48 hours. If it does not, report to the charge nurse or physician.*

■ Provide for easy access to a bedpan, urinal, commode, or bathroom. Make sure lighting is adequate and pathways are clear. *Frequency, urgency, and nocturia increase the risk of urinary incontinence and injury due to falls.*

■ Encourage fluid intake unless contraindicated. Tell the client to avoid caffeinated drinks. *Increased fluid dilutes urine, reducing irritation of the inflamed bladder and mucosa. Caffeine can increase bladder spasms and mucosal irritation.*

NONCOMPLIANCE: PRESCRIBED ANTIBIOTIC REGIMEN

■ Work with the client to develop a plan for taking medications, such as taking them with meals (unless contraindicated) or setting out all doses for the day in the morning. *Missed doses of antibiotic can result in subtherapeutic blood levels and reduced effectiveness, and development of drug-resistant bacteria. Taking medication in association with a regular daily activity such as meals helps clients to remember doses.*

■ Instruct to complete the full course of antibiotic therapy even though symptoms resolve rapidly. Explain that noncompliance can lead to recurrent infection and potential long-term problems. *Although symptoms may be relieved within 1 to 2 days, this may not be adequate time to eliminate bacteria from the urinary tract.*

■ Instruct to keep appointments for follow-up and urine culture. *Follow-up urine culture, scheduled 1 to 3 days after single-dose therapy and 7 to 14 days after conventional therapy, is vital*

BOX 21-9
NURSING CARE CHECKLIST

IVP AND CYSTOSCOPY

Intravenous Pyelography

Client Preparation

☑ Assess and clarify understanding of the procedure.

☑ Inquire about allergies to seafood, iodine, or x-ray contrast media. Notify the physician or radiologist of any known allergies.

☑ Verify signed consent for the procedure.

☑ Instruct or administer preprocedure laxatives as ordered. Allow clear liquids only for 8 hours before the test.

☑ After IVP, monitor vital signs and urinary output. Report signs of reaction to contrast media such as dyspnea, tachycardia, itching, hives, or flushing. Check injection site for redness, pain, and warmth. Apply warm packs to the site if indicated.

Client and Family Teaching

☑ IVP uses x-rays to show the structures of the kidney, ureters, and bladder by injecting a dye that is rapidly excreted in the urine. The test takes about 30 minutes.

☑ As the dye is injected, you may experience transient flushing or burning, nausea, and a metallic taste.

☑ Immediately notify the physician if you develop a rash, difficulty breathing, rapid heart rate, or hives.

☑ Increase fluid intake after the test is completed.

Cystoscopy

Client Preparation

☑ Assess and clarify understanding of the procedure and its purpose.

☑ Verify signed consent for the procedure.

☑ Teach or assist with bowel preparation as ordered.

☑ Withhold food and fluids for 8 hours before the procedure as ordered.

☑ Administer sedation and other medications as ordered.

Client and Family Teaching

☑ The procedure takes about 30 to 45 minutes and is performed in a special cystoscopy room. Local or general anesthesia is used.

☑ You may feel pressure or an urge to urinate as the scope is inserted.

☑ Do not attempt to stand up without assistance after the procedure as you may feel dizzy or faint.

☑ Burning on urination for a day or two after the procedure is considered normal.

☑ Contact your physician immediately if your urine remains bloody or you experience bright bleeding, low urine output, abdominal or flank pain, chills or fever.

☑ Warm sitz baths, analgesics, and antispasmodic medications help relieve discomfort.

☑ Increase fluid intake to decrease pain and difficulty voiding and reduce the risk of infection.

☑ Laxatives may be prescribed after the procedure to prevent constipation and straining.

---

to ensure complete eradication of bacteria and to prevent relapse or recurrence.

Discharge Considerations

Because both upper and lower urinary tract infections are usually managed in the community, teaching is the most important nursing intervention. Teach clients and their families about the risk factors that contribute to UTI. Discuss measures to prevent future UTI:

■ Empty bladder at least every 2 to 4 hours while awake. Avoid voluntary urinary retention.

■ Maintain intake of 2 to 2.5 quarts or 8 to 10 glasses of fluid per day.

■ Complete the prescribed treatment and keep follow-up appointments. Failure to do so increases the risk of unresolved and recurrent infections.

■ Unless contraindicated, maintain acidic urine (e.g., drink two glasses of cranberry juice per day; take vitamin C); avoid excess intake of milk products, other fruit juices, and sodium bicarbonate (baking soda). Box 21-10 lists complementary health care practices to prevent UTI.

■ For women:
  ■ Cleanse perineal area front to back after voiding and defecating.
  ■ Void before and after sexual intercourse.
  ■ Avoid bubble baths, feminine hygiene sprays, and douches.
  ■ Wear cotton briefs; avoid nylon.

Like many infectious processes, urinary tract infection often occurs when immune defenses are low. Inform that lack of adequate rest, poor nutrition, and high levels of emotional stress are often associated with UTI. Discuss possible lifestyle changes to reduce future risk for UTI. Teach clients to identify the early manifestations of UTI, and stress the importance of seeking medical intervention promptly.

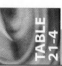

TABLE 21-4

NURSING IMPLICATIONS FOR PHARMACOLOGY: CLIENTS WITH UTI

AGENTS/DRUGS	PURPOSE	NURSING RESPONSIBILITIES	CLIENT TEACHING
Sulfonamides ▪ Sulfisoxazole (Gantrisin) ▪ Sulfamethoxazole (Gantanol) ▪ Trimethoprim–sulfamethoxazole (TMP–SMZ, Bactrim, Septra)	Sulfonamides are effective and inexpensive for treating UTI. They are the drug of choice for most UTI. They may be given alone or in combination with another antibiotic or with a urinary analgesic.	Assess for allergies to sulfa drugs. Stop the drug and notify the physician if a rash develops. Administer on an empty stomach, 1 hour before or 2 hours after meals, with a full glass of water. Assess for bruising, bleeding, fever, and signs of systemic infection. Assess for other drugs that may interact with sulfonamides. Closely monitor diabetic clients receiving oral hypoglycemic agents for hypoglycemic reactions.	Take all of the medication as ordered. If you miss a dose, take it as soon as you can. Drink at least 8 full glasses of water per day. Avoid cranberry juice. Notify your doctor if you are taking any other medications. If you are diabetic, monitor blood glucose closely. Don't take if you are pregnant or breast-feeding. Use sunscreen to reduce the risk of sunburn. Your urine may turn orange. This is harmless.
Urinary Anti-Infectives ▪ Methenamine, (Mandelamine, Hiprex) ▪ Nalidixic acid (NegGram) ▪ Nitrofurantoin (Furadantin, Macrodantin) ▪ Trimethoprim (Proloprim, Trimpex)	Urinary anti-infectives are often used to prevent UTI in clients with chronic infections. They also may be used if the client is allergic or sensitive to commonly used antibiotics.	Ensure fluid intake of 1,500 to 2,000 mL/day. Give drug with meals to minimize GI side effects. Monitor liver and renal function studies. Monitor closely for adverse effects. Do not administer to pregnant clients. These drugs interact with many other medications. Monitor closely for adverse effects.	Continue taking these drugs even after symptoms have cleared. Drink 6 to 8 glasses of water or fluid per day. Take with meals or food to minimize gastric upset. Do not take if you are pregnant or could become pregnant. Use sunscreen to prevent sunburn. Your urine may turn brown; this is not harmful.
Urinary Analgesic ▪ Phenazopyridine (Pyridium)	Phenazopyridine is a urinary analgesic that may be used to relieve pain, burning, frequency, and urgency associated with UTI. It does not treat the infection and must be used along with antibiotic therapy.	Phenazopyridine stains the urine reddish orange. Yellow-tinged sclera or skin may indicate toxicity. Stop the drug and notify the physician. Do not give to clients with impaired renal function; monitor liver and kidney function tests.	Protect your clothing to prevent staining. Do not use for more than 24 to 48 hours. If symptoms continue, contact your doctor. If your skin or eyes appear yellow, stop taking the drug and notify the physician. Take the drug after meals to minimize gastric upset.

The client with an indwelling urinary catheter is at continued risk for UTI. Provide information about alternatives such as scheduled toileting, incontinence pads or diapers, and external catheters. Teach the client with urinary retention or a family member to perform straight catheterization every 3 to 4 hours using clean technique (see Procedure 21-1). If no alternative to an indwelling catheter is feasible, teach clients and their families how to care for the catheter. This includes perineal care, managing and emptying the collection bag, maintaining a closed system, and bladder irrigation or flushing if ordered. Stress the importance of maintaining a generous fluid intake and sup-

Preventing UTI

Blueberries have been shown to contain a compound that prevents bacteria from attaching to the bladder wall to cause cystitis. Bilberry (a relative of the blueberry) also is recommended and is available as an herbal extract in capsules. Saw palmetto is another herbal urinary anti-infective used primarily by men with prostatic enlargement. Bromelain (an enzyme derived from pineapple) may increase the effectiveness of antibiotic therapy for treating UTI. Vitamin C supplements can help treat and prevent UTI. Dietary changes to prevent UTI include reduced intake of sugar, alcohol, and fat.

porting immune function to prevent upper urinary tract infection.

Glomerulonephritis

Disorders and diseases involving the glomerulus are the leading cause of chronic renal failure in the United States. **Glomerulonephritis** is an inflammatory condition that primarily affects the glomerulus. It may be acute or chronic, and may primarily affect the kidney or be secondary to a systemic disease like systemic lupus erythematosus.

PATHOPHYSIOLOGY

Glomerulonephritis affects both the structure and function of the glomerulus. It damages the capillary membrane, allowing blood cells and proteins to escape from the vascular compartment into the filtrate. *Hematuria* (blood in the urine) may be either gross or microscopic. **Proteinuria** (protein in the urine) increases progressively with increased glomerular damage. Loss of plasma proteins in the urine causes *hypoalbuminemia* (low levels of albumin in the blood). Edema develops as a result, caused by reduced osmotic draw within blood vessels.

When glomerular filtration is disrupted, the GFR falls and **azotemia** (increased blood levels of nitrogenous wastes, including urea and creatinine) occurs. This activates the renin–angiotensin–aldosterone system, leading to salt and water retention and hypertension (Figure 21-6 ◆).

Acute Glomerulonephritis

Acute glomerulonephritis usually follows an infection with group A beta-hemolytic streptococcus, such as strep throat. Immune complexes are trapped in the glomerular membrane, causing an inflammatory response. Inflammation damages the glomerular capillary walls and makes them more porous. Plasma proteins and blood cells escape into the urine. Both kidneys are involved. This is primarily a disease of childhood, but it can affect adults.

Manifestations of acute glomerulonephritis typically develop abruptly, 10 to 14 days after the initial infection (Box

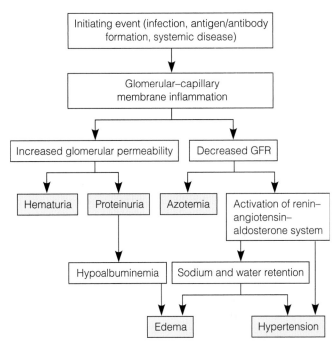

Figure 21-6. ◆ The pathophysiology of glomerulonephritis.

21-11). Older adults may show less characteristic manifestations. Nausea, malaise, arthralgias, and proteinuria are common manifestations; hypertension and edema are seen less often in older adults.

The symptoms may subside spontaneously within 10 to 14 days. Most people recover completely, but some may develop chronic glomerulonephritis with persistent impaired renal function.

Chronic Glomerulonephritis

Chronic glomerulonephritis usually is the end stage of kidney damage by a systemic disease such as diabetes. In many cases, however, no previous kidney disease has been recognized. Chronic glomerulonephritis is characterized by slow, progressive destruction of the glomeruli and gradual loss of entire nephrons. The kidneys decrease in size and their surfaces become granular or rough as nephrons are destroyed.

> **BOX 21-11**
> **MANIFESTATIONS OF ACUTE GLOMERULONEPHRITIS**
>
> - Hematuria; cola- or coffee-colored urine
> - Proteinuria
> - Edema: Periorbital and facial; dependent (upper extremities in particular)
> - Hypertension
> - Fatigue
> - Anorexia, nausea, vomiting
> - Headache
> - Elevated BUN and serum creatinine

Symptoms develop slowly, and the disease is often not recognized until signs of renal failure are evident. Renal failure may develop years to decades after the disease is diagnosed.

Diabetic nephropathy is common in the later stages of diabetes mellitus. Microproteinuria may be seen 10 to 15 years after the onset of diabetes. Overt proteinuria and nephropathy develop within 15 to 20 years of the initial diagnosis. The glomerular membrane becomes scarred and thickened, impairing glomerular filtration.

Systemic lupus erythematosus (SLE) is a disorder that affects the connective tissue of the body. Most people with SLE develop *lupus nephritis*, inflammatory lesions of the supportive tissues of the glomerulus. Both the glomerulus and the renal tubule may be affected. Clients with lupus nephritis have hematuria and proteinuria. Renal failure ultimately may develop.

COLLABORATIVE CARE

Care of the client with acute or chronic glomerulonephritis focuses on identifying and treating the underlying disease process and preserving kidney function. In most cases there is no specific treatment to achieve a cure.

Diagnostic Tests

Laboratory tests may help determine the cause of glomerulonephritis and evaluate its effects on kidney function. An *antistreptolysin-O (ASO) titer* identifies antibodies to group A beta-hemolytic streptococci. The *erythrocyte sedimentation rate (ESR)* is a general indicator of inflammation, and may be elevated in acute glomerulonephritis.

The *BUN* and *serum creatinine* levels increase in kidney disease. The *creatinine clearance,* a very specific indicator of renal function and the GFR, falls (Table 21-5 ◆). *Serum electrolytes* show the effect of impaired kidney function on fluid and electrolyte balance.

BOX 21-12
NURSING CARE CHECKLIST

24-HOUR URINE SPECIMEN

- ☑ Note any diet or medication changes required during the collection period.
- ☑ Obtain specimen container with preservative (if indicated). Label with identifying data, the test, time started, and time of completion.
- ☑ Obtain a clean urine-collection device and place it in the room.
- ☑ Post notices—on chart, in Kardex, on the door, over the bed, and over the toilet—alerting all personnel that all urine is to be saved.
- ☑ At start time, have client empty bladder completely and *discard* urine.
- ☑ Save all urine for next 24 hours in the container, refrigerating as indicated.
- ☑ At end of collection time, have client empty the bladder completely and save this urine in the container. Take entire specimen with requisition to the lab.
- ☑ Chart appropriately.

Teaching

- ☑ Save all your urine for the 24 hours.
- ☑ Urinate (and save) before moving bowels. Do not put any toilet tissue in the urine container.

A *urinalysis* is done to identify blood cells and protein in the urine. A 24-hour urine specimen may be ordered to measure protein and creatinine in the urine. Box 21-12 identifies nursing responsibilities for 24-hour urine specimens.

TABLE 21-5

CHANGES IN LABORATORY VALUES ASSOCIATED WITH KIDNEY DISEASE

TEST	NORMAL VALUE	CHANGE IN GLOMERULONEPHRITIS
Blood urea nitrogen (BUN)	5–20 mg/dL; slightly higher in older adult	20–50 mg/dL or higher
Creatinine, serum	Female: 0.5–1.1 mg/dL Male: 0.6–1.2 mg/dL Slightly lower in older adult	Elevated; levels > 4 mg/dL indicate significantly impaired renal function
Creatinine clearance	Female: 88–128 mL/min Male: 97–137 mL/min Values lower in older adult	Reduced levels indicate impaired GFR and renal function
Serum albumin	3.2–5 g/dL; 3.2–4.8 g/dL in older adult	Decreased due to proteinuria
Urine creatinine	Female: 600–1,800 mg/24 hr Male: 800–2,000 mg/24 hr	Decreased
Urine protein	Resting: 50–80 mg/24 hr Ambulatory: < 150–250 mg/24 hr	Increased
Urine red blood cells	< 2–3/HPF; no RBC casts	Present in glomerulonephritis

In addition, an abdominal x-ray known as a *KUB (kidney, ureter, bladder)* may be done to evaluate kidney size. A *kidney scan* or *biopsy* also may be ordered. The nursing implications for a kidney scan and biopsy are included in Box 21-13.

Pharmacology

There is no specific drug treatment for glomerulonephritis. Glucocorticoids (such as prednisone) or other immunosuppressive drugs may be given for acute glomerulonephritis to reduce the risk of renal failure. Penicillin or other antibiotics may be ordered for the client with poststreptococcal glomerulonephritis to kill any remaining bacteria. Antihypertensives and diuretics may be prescribed to lower blood pressure and reduce edema.

Plasmapheresis

Plasmapheresis removes harmful antibodies in the plasma by passing the blood through a blood cell separator and reinfusing the red blood cells (RBCs) with an equal amount of albumin or plasma. It may be used to treat acute glomerulonephritis. This procedure is usually done in a series, rather than a one-time-only treatment. Informed consent is required for this procedure.

Dietary Management

Sodium intake may be restricted. Dietary proteins may be increased when protein is being lost in the urine. However, if azotemia is present, dietary protein is restricted. When proteins are restricted, those included should be complete proteins like meat, fish, eggs, soy, or poultry. These proteins supply all the essential amino acids required for growth and tissue maintenance.

NURSING CARE

ASSESSING

Assessment data provide valuable clues about the cause and effects of glomerulonephritis on the client. Subjective data to collect include the onset and duration of manifestations such

---

BOX 21-13
NURSING CARE CHECKLIST

DIAGNOSTIC TESTS: RENAL SCAN AND RENAL BIOPSY

Kidney (Renal) Scan

Client Preparation

☑ Informed consent is required. Clarify and reinforce teaching.
☑ Obtain weight.
☑ Provide 2 to 3 glasses of water before the procedure and encourage fluids after.
☑ Have client void prior to the procedure.
☑ Instruct to flush toilet immediately after voiding and to wash hands thoroughly to minimize exposure to radioactivity.
☑ No pregnant personnel should care for client for 24 hours after the procedure.

Client and Family Teaching

☑ Increase fluid intake before and after the renal scan.
☑ No special diet or other preparation is required.
☑ The test takes 1 to 4 hours.
☑ No anesthesia is required, and there will be no pain or discomfort other than that associated with remaining still for a period of time.

Renal Biopsy

Client Preparation

☑ Informed consent is required. Clarify and reinforce teaching.
☑ Withhold food and fluids for 8 hours before the procedure.

☑ After the procedure, apply pressure dressing and position supine to maintain pressure on the biopsy site.
☑ Monitor closely for bleeding during the first 24 hours after the procedure:
  a. Check vital signs frequently. Report tachycardia, hypotension, or other signs of shock.
  b. Monitor the biopsy site for bleeding.
  c. Check hemoglobin and hematocrit, comparing with preprocedure values.
  d. Report complaints of flank or back pain, shoulder pain, pallor, light-headedness.
  e. Monitor urine output. Initial hematuria should clear within 24 hours.
☑ Report manifestations of abdominal pain, guarding, and decreased bowel sounds.
☑ Encourage fluids.

Client and Family Teaching

☑ Local anesthesia is used. The procedure may be uncomfortable but should not be painful.
☑ When the needle is inserted, you will be instructed to hold your breath.
☑ The entire procedure takes about 10 minutes.
☑ Avoid coughing for 24 hours after the procedure. Avoid strenuous activity such as heavy lifting for about 2 weeks after the procedure.
☑ Report manifestations of complications to the physician.

as changes in urine output, weight gain or edema, and other symptoms such as nausea and vomiting. Ask about recent sore throat or other infection and its treatment. Note any history of previous kidney disorders, UTIs, or chronic diseases such as diabetes or lupus. Inquire about current medications.

Obtain the vital signs and weight. Note any edema, particularly of the face, around the eyes, or of the upper extremities. Inspect the throat and skin for evidence of infection. Obtain a urine specimen, and note the color, clarity, and character of the urine.

DIAGNOSING, PLANNING, AND IMPLEMENTING

EXCESS FLUID VOLUME

- Monitor vital signs, including blood pressure, apical pulse, respirations, and breath sounds, at least every 4 hours. Report any significant changes. *Excess fluid volume increases the workload of the heart and the blood pressure. Tachycardia or dysrhythmias may be present. Tachypnea, dyspnea, and crackles may be noted.*
- Record intake and output (I&O) every 4 to 8 hours, or more frequently as indicated. *Accurate I&O records help determine fluid volume status.*
- Weigh daily under consistent conditions. *Daily weights are an accurate indicator of fluid volume status.*
- Assess location and degree of edema. *Edema associated with glomerulonephritis often affects low-pressure tissues such as the face, around the eyes, and the upper extremities.*
- Restrict fluids as ordered, offering ice chips (in limited and measured amounts) and frequent mouth care to relieve thirst. Develop a fluid intake schedule with the client. *Ice chips and frequent mouth care help relieve thirst while maintaining the integrity of oral tissues.*
- Carefully monitor intravenous infusions. Include any fluid used to dilute medications as intake. *Significant "hidden" fluid intake can result from multiple intravenous medications.*
- Arrange dietary consultation to plan the diet when sodium is restricted and when proteins are either restricted or increased. *Providing appealing foods can help maintain adequate nutrition despite anorexia and nausea.*
- Provide frequent position changes and good skin care. *Tissue perfusion may be altered by edema, increasing the risk of skin breakdown.*

FATIGUE

- Provide for rest by scheduling procedures and activities. Assist with activities of daily living (ADLs) as needed. *Rest reduces fatigue and improves the client's ability to tolerate and cope with treatments and activities. The goal is to conserve limited energy reserves.*
- Teach the client and family about the relationship between fatigue and the disease process. Limit visitors and visit length. *Understanding the cause of fatigue helps the client and family to cope with reduced energy and comply with prescribed rest.*

INEFFECTIVE PROTECTION

- Monitor temperature, pulse, and mental status every 4 hours. *Fever, elevated pulse, increasing lethargy, or confusion may be early signs of infection.*
- Assess frequently for other signs of infection such as purulent wound drainage, productive cough, abnormal breath sounds, and red or inflamed lesions. Monitor for indications of UTI such as dysuria, frequency and urgency, and cloudy, foul-smelling urine. *Infection may be masked by the prescribed drugs. Frequent assessment allows early identification.*
- Practice good handwashing. Provide a private room and restrict ill visitors. *Drugs used to treat acute glomerulonephritis may reduce the ability to resist infection.*

INEFFECTIVE ROLE PERFORMANCE

Activity may be limited to minimize proteinuria. Fatigue and muscle weakness may limit physical and social activities. In addition, facial edema affects self-concept and may lead to isolation.

- Encourage self-care and participation in decision making. *Increased autonomy helps to restore self-confidence and reduce powerlessness.*
- Support coping measures, helping identify personal strengths. Whenever possible, enlist the support of family, other clients, and friends. *This support helps the client gain confidence and provide physical, psychological, emotional, and social support.*
- Discuss the effect of the disease and treatments on roles and relationships. Help the client and family develop a plan to deal with potential changes and maintain usual roles to the extent possible. *Planning ahead reduces stress and helps the client and family maintain a sense of control.*
- Refer to social services and support groups as needed. *Groups can help the client and family cope with and adapt to the disease.*

EVALUATING

To evaluate the effectiveness of nursing care for the client with glomerulonephritis, collect data such as:

- Weight, presence of edema, and skin integrity; freedom from infection
- Ability to follow, prepare, and consume the prescribed diet
- Planning for additional rest and modification of usual roles and relationships

 Discharge Considerations

Glomerulonephritis may be self-limiting or progressive. Its course ranges from weeks to years. Self-management is essential, and the key to self-management is a good understanding of the disorder and treatment regimen.

Teach about the disease process and prognosis. Discuss the prescribed treatment, including activity and diet restrictions. Provide information about the use and potential effects, both beneficial and adverse, of all prescribed medications. Discuss the importance of contacting the physician prior to taking any other medications. It is vital to avoid drugs that are potentially toxic to the kidneys. Discuss the risks, manifestations, prevention, and management of complications such as edema and infection. Because the client and family may be monitoring kidney status to a certain extent themselves, teach the signs, symptoms, and implications of improving or declining renal function.

Nursing Process Case Study
■ CLIENT WITH ACUTE GLOMERULONEPHRITIS

Jung-Lin Chang is a 23-year-old graduate student who goes to the university health center when he notices that his urine is brown and foamy. The physician admits him to the infirmary and orders a throat culture, ASO titer, CBC, BUN, serum creatinine, and urinalysis.

Assessment Connie King, the admitting nurse, notes that Mr. Chang's history is negative for past kidney or urinary problems. He states that he had a "pretty bad" sore throat a couple of weeks ago. He took a few antibiotics he had left from a previous bout of strep throat, increased his fluids, and did not see a doctor. The sore throat resolved, and he felt well until noticing the change in his urine. He thought the puffiness around his eyes was due to lack of sleep and fatigue. He has eaten little the past 2 days.

Assessment findings include: BP 136/90, P 98, R 18, and T 98.8° F (37.1° C) PO; weight 165 pounds (75 kg), up from his normal of 160 lb (72.5 kg); and moderate periorbital edema and edema of his hands and fingers.

Lab results show a negative throat culture but high ASO titer. His CBC is normal, BUN 42 mg/dL, and serum creatinine 2.1 mg/dL. Urinalysis shows protein, red blood cells, and RBC casts. A subsequent 24-hour urine contains 1,025 mg of protein, compared to the normal of 30 to 150 mg/24 hours.

Mr. Chang is diagnosed with acute poststreptococcal glomerulonephritis. His orders include bed rest with bathroom privileges, fluid restriction (1,200 mL/day), and a low-sodium and low-protein diet.

Diagnosis
- Excess Fluid Volume related to plasma protein loss and sodium and water retention
- Risk for Imbalanced Nutrition: Less Than Body Requirements related to anorexia
- Anxiety related to prescribed activity restriction
- Deficient Knowledge: Glomerulonephritis related to lack of information

Expected Outcomes The expected outcomes for the plan of care are that Mr. Chang will:
- Maintain blood pressure within normal limits.
- Return to usual weight with no evidence of edema.
- Consume adequate calories following prescribed dietary limitations.
- Verbalize less anxiety regarding ability to continue with his program of study.
- Demonstrate an understanding of acute glomerulonephritis and his prescribed management regimen.

Planning and Implementation
- Monitor vital signs every 4 hours. Notify the physician of significant changes.
- Record intake and output every 8 hours.
- Schedule fluids: 650 mL day shift, 450 mL evening shift, and 100 mL night shift.
- Weigh daily.
- Arrange for dietary consultation.
- Provide small meals with high-carbohydrate snacks.
- Encourage Mr. Chang to talk about his condition and its potential effects.
- Enlist friends and family to listen and provide support.
- Teach about acute glomerulonephritis and prescribed management regimen.
- Instruct in the appropriate use of antibiotics.

Evaluation Mr. Chang is released from the infirmary after 4 days. He decides to return to his parents' home for the 6 to 12 weeks of convalescence prescribed by his doctor.

Mr. Chang's renal function gradually returns to normal with no further azotemia and minimal proteinuria after 4 months. Mr. Chang verbalizes an understanding of the relationship between the episode of strep throat, his inappropriate use of antibiotics, and the glomerulonephritis. He says, "I may not always remember to take every pill on time in the future, but I sure won't save them for the next time again!"

Critical Thinking in the Nursing Process

1. How did Mr. Chang's use of "a few" previously prescribed antibiotics to treat his sore throat affect his risk for developing poststreptococcal glomerulonephritis?
2. What additional risk factors did Mr. Chang have for developing glomerulonephritis?

Nephrotic Syndrome

Nephrotic syndrome is not a disease but a group of symptoms. It results from damage to glomerular membranes and severe protein loss in the urine. A number of disorders cause nephrotic syndrome. *Minimal change disease* is the most common cause in children. In adults, nephrotic syndrome may result from primary kidney disorders or from systemic diseases such as diabetes or lupus.

Clients with nephrotic syndrome have significant proteinuria, low serum albumin levels, high blood lipids, and edema. Edema may be severe, affecting the face and periorbital area as well as dependent tissues (Figure 21-7 ◆). *Thromboemboli* (mobilized blood clots) are a relatively common complication of nephrotic syndrome. Peripheral veins and arteries, pulmonary arteries, and renal veins may be occluded.

Nephrotic syndrome usually resolves without long-term effects in children. Adults are less likely to recover completely. Many have persistent proteinuria and progressive renal impairment that may lead to renal failure.

Clients with nephrotic syndrome are placed on a low-sodium diet, often with a moderate protein restriction. Diuretics and angiotensin-converting enzyme (ACE) inhibitors are prescribed to reduce the edema and protein loss. Drugs such as glucocorticoids (e.g., prednisone) may be given to induce remission. Nonsteroidal anti-inflammatory drugs (NSAIDs) also may be ordered.

Figure 21-7. ◆ Severe edema in a client with nephrotic syndrome.

Obstructive Disorders

Urinary Calculi

Urolithiasis (development of stones within the urinary tract) is the most common cause of obstructed urine flow. *Nephrolithiasis* indicates stone formation within the kidney. The stone (or *calculus*) may develop and cause obstruction at any point within the urinary tract (Figure 21-8 ◆). In the United States, kidney stones are the most common. Males are affected more often than females by a 4:1 ratio.

PATHOPHYSIOLOGY

Calculi (stones) are masses of crystals formed from materials normally excreted in the urine. Most are made of calcium. Risk factors for renal calculi include personal or family history of urinary stones; dehydration; excess calcium, oxalate, or protein intake; gout; hyperparathyroidism; or urinary stasis. Stones form when a poorly soluble salt crystallizes. When the concentration of the salt in the urine is very high, very little stimulus is needed to start crystallization. A meal high in the mineral or decreased fluid intake, as occurs during sleep, may start stone formation. When fluid intake is adequate, no stone growth occurs. Lithiasis is also affected by the pH of the urine and compounds that inhibit stone development.

Calcium stones often are associated with hypercalcemia. Risk factors for calcium stones include hyperparathyroidism (see Chapters 5 and 16) and immobility, as well as alkaline urine and dehydration.

Manifestations of urinary calculi are due to obstructed urine flow, distention, and tissue trauma from the rough-edged stone. They vary by stone location (Box 21-14). Stones

Figure 21-8. ◆ Potential locations of calculi within the urinary tract.

BOX 21-14
MANIFESTATIONS OF URINARY STONES

KIDNEY PELVIS
- May be asymptomatic
- Dull, aching flank pain

URETER
- **Renal colic:** Acute, severe, intermittent flank pain on affected side
- Pain radiating to suprapubic region, groin, and scrotum or labia
- Nausea, vomiting
- Pallor; cool, clammy skin
- Microscopic hematuria

BLADDER
- May be asymptomatic
- Dull suprapubic pain
- Microscopic or gross hematuria

at any level may cause manifestations of UTI, including chills and fever, frequency, urgency, and dysuria.

Urinary tract obstruction by renal calculi may cause few symptoms if it develops slowly. Acute obstruction causes severe pain in the flank region, possibly radiating to the genitals. If the obstruction is unrelieved, the kidney may be damaged. Urine production continues; however, the obstruction blocks its outflow. This leads to increased pressure and distention of the urinary tract behind the obstruction. *Hydronephrosis* (discussed in the next section of this chapter) and *hydroureter* (distention of the ureter with urine) may result. Urinary stasis increases the risk of infection as well.

COLLABORATIVE CARE
Diagnostic tests are used to confirm the diagnosis and determine the type of stone. A *urinalysis* is done to detect hematuria. Any stones passed are analyzed to identify their composition. The nurse often is responsible for retrieving stones. All urine is strained and may be saved. Any visible stones or sediment are sent for analysis.

A *KUB (kidneys, ureters, and bladder) x-ray* is done to identify the presence of calculi in the kidneys, ureters, and bladder. *IVP, renal ultrasound, CT scan,* or *MRI* may be used to locate calculi and identify hydroureter or hydronephrosis. *Cystoscopy* is used to visualize and possibly remove calculi from the urinary bladder and distal ureters. Review Box 21-9 for nursing implications for these studies.

Pharmacology
Pain relief is vital for acute renal colic. Narcotic analgesics are used to provide analgesia and relieve ureteral spasms. Analgesics often are administered intravenously for rapid pain

relief. Indomethacin (an NSAID) in suppository form can reduce the amount of narcotic analgesia required.

After stone analysis, medications may be prescribed to prevent further stone formation. Thiazide diuretics are frequently ordered for calcium stones. They reduce urinary calcium excretion and can prevent future stones.

Dietary Intervention
The diet may be modified to prevent further lithiasis. Fluid intake is increased to 2½ to 3 liters per day to prevent concentration of stone-forming salts. Intake should be spaced throughout the day and evening. The client may be advised to drink one to two glasses of water at night to maintain dilute urine during sleep.

Foods that contributed to stone formation are limited in the diet. For calcium stones, dietary calcium and vitamin D–enriched foods are restricted. Because calcium stones form more readily in alkaline urine, the diet is modified toward foods that lower the urinary pH (Table 21-6 ◆).

Surgery
Stones that are too large to be passed spontaneously (> 5 mm in diameter) may require removal. Bladder stones may be crushed and removed by *cystoscopy.* Cystoscopy also may be used to advance a catheter or basket catheter into a ureter to remove a stone. A laser may be used to disintegrate a ureteral stone via a ureteroscope. Stone fragments are then flushed out with fluid.

Stones in the renal pelvis or calices may require nephrostomy for removal. A small incision is made in the flank, and a nephroscope is inserted to visualize the renal pelvis. The stones may then be removed or crushed.

TABLE 21-6	FOODS TO CONSUME OR AVOID TO PREVENT UROLITHIASIS
Foods that acidify urine	Cheese, cranberries, eggs, grapes, meat and poultry, plums and prunes, tomatoes, whole grains
Foods that alkalinize urine	Green vegetables, fruit (except those noted above), legumes, milk and milk products, rhubarb
Foods high in calcium	Beans and lentils, chocolate and cocoa, dried fruits, canned or smoked fish except tuna, flour, milk and milk products
Foods high in oxalate	Asparagus, beer and colas, beets, cabbage, celery, chocolate and cocoa, fruits, green beans, nuts, tea, tomatoes
Foods high in purines	Goose, organ meats, sardines and herring, venison; moderate in beef, chicken, crab, pork, salmon, veal

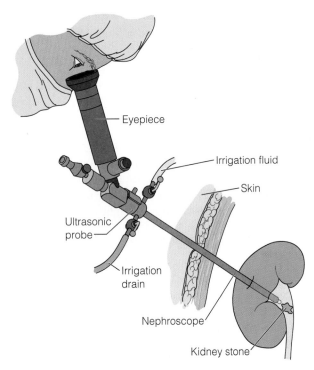

Figure 21-9. ◆ Percutaneous lithotripsy. A nephroscope is inserted through the skin into the renal pelvis, and the stone is fragmented using ultrasonic waves or laser.

Lithotripsy (crushing of renal calculi using sound or shock waves) may be done by laser or using an external lithotriptor device. With *percutaneous lithotripsy,* a nephroscope is inserted through a small incision to crush kidney stones (Figure 21-9 ◆). Fragments are removed by irrigation and suction. In *extracorporeal shock-wave lithotripsy (ESWL),* shock waves generated outside the body travel harmlessly through soft tissue. The shock waves pulverize the stone into fragments that are small enough to be eliminated in the urine. Box 21-15 outlines nursing care for clients having a lithotripsy.

Nephrolithotomy may be required to remove a *staghorn calculus,* which invades the calices and renal parenchyma. If kidney damage has been severe, a partial or total *nephrectomy* (removal of the kidney) may be necessary. (See Box 21-22 which follows for nursing care of clients having kidney surgery.)

NURSING CARE

ASSESSING

The client with a urinary stone often is in acute distress when seeking medical help. The nursing assessment is brief and focused. Ask about the onset, character, intensity, location, and radiation of pain, as well as associated symptoms such as nausea and vomiting. Inquire about previous episodes of pain or a history of kidney stones. Ask about most recent food and fluid intake, and any factors that may have contributed to

---

BOX 21-15
NURSING CARE CHECKLIST

LITHOTRIPSY

Before Surgery

☑ Clarify and reinforce teaching as needed.
☑ Provide routine preoperative care as outlined in Chapter 7.

After Surgery

☑ Frequently monitor vital signs. Report changes to the charge nurse or physician.
☑ Monitor amount, color, and clarity of urine output. Expect hematuria for 12 to 48 hours following surgery.
☑ Anchor ureteral catheters or nephrostomy tubes securely. Irrigate gently if ordered.
☑ Teach catheter and operative site care.
☑ Instruct client to report: Drainage of urine from incision for more than 4 days, symptoms of infection, pain, bright hematuria.

---

dehydration (such as physical labor on a hot day). Be sure to ask about known allergies to medications or foods (seafood in particular).

DIAGNOSING, PLANNING, AND IMPLEMENTING

PAIN

■ Administer analgesia as ordered. *Pain control is vital to reduce anxiety and stress, and to facilitate healing after surgery.*

■ Unless contraindicated, increase fluid intake and encourage ambulation. *Increased fluids and ambulation increase urinary output, help to move the stone through the ureter, and decrease pain.*

■ Check urinary output, catheters, incision, and wound drainage. *Increased pain may indicate a blocked catheter, infection, or bleeding.*

IMPAIRED URINARY ELIMINATION

■ Measure urine output; document hematuria, dysuria, frequency, urgency, and pyuria. *Low urine output is a possible indicator of obstruction. Hematuria is often associated with calculi and with procedures for stone removal. A change in the degree of hematuria may indicate stone passage or a complication. Dysuria, frequency, urgency, and cloudy urine are symptoms of urinary tract infection, and may indicate the need for antibiotic treatment.*

■ Strain all urine for stones, saving recovered stones for laboratory analysis. *Analysis of recovered stones helps direct treatment to prevent further stone formation.*

■ Maintain patency of all catheters. Secure catheters well, label as indicated. Use sterile technique for all irrigations or other procedures. *A kinked or plugged catheter obstructs urine flow, increasing the risk of further urinary system damage. Labeling catheters prevents mistakes, such as inappropriate irrigation or clamping. Aseptic technique minimizes the risk of infection.*

EVALUATING

Collect data about pain level and urine output (amount, color, character) to evaluate the effectiveness of nursing care for the client with urinary stones.

 # Discharge Considerations

Because a history of lithiasis increases the risk of future stone formation, teaching is essential. Assess level of understanding and previous learning. Clarify all diagnostic and therapeutic procedures. Clients whose pain can be managed with oral analgesics may be managed at home. Teach the client to:

■ Collect and strain all urine, saving any stones.
■ Report stone passage to the physician and bring the stone in for analysis.
■ Observe the amount and character of urine, reporting any changes to physician.

Discuss factors that increase the risk of urinary stones and how to minimize this risk. Emphasize the importance of drinking 2.5 to 3 quarts of fluid per day, following dietary recommendations, and taking medication as prescribed. Discuss the relationship between urolithiasis and urinary tract infection. Teach prevention, recognition, and management of UTIs.

When the client is discharged with dressings, a nephrostomy tube, or a catheter, teach dressing changes, tube care, and assessment of the wound and skin. Emphasize the need to keep tubes and catheters patent. Teach how to empty drainage bags, assess urine output, and when to contact the physician.

 ## Hydronephrosis

Hydronephrosis (abnormal dilation of the renal pelvis and calyces) can result from urinary tract obstructions or from *vesicoureteral reflux* (backflow of urine from the bladder to the ureters). Pressure in the renal pelvis increases, and it dilates. The nephrons and collecting tubules may be damaged, affecting renal function. The manifestations of hydronephrosis depend on how rapidly it develops. (Box 21-16). If both kidneys are affected, symptoms of acute renal failure may develop.

Hydronephrosis is diagnosed by *ultrasound* or *CT scan.* Other tests, such as *cystoscopy,* may be done to determine the

---

> ### BOX 21-16
> ### MANIFESTATIONS OF HYDRONEPHROSIS
>
> #### ACUTE
> • Colicky flank pain; may radiate into groin
> • Hematuria, pyuria
> • Fever
> • Nausea, vomiting, abdominal pain
>
> #### CHRONIC
> • Intermittent, dull flank pain
> • Hematuria, pyuria
> • Fever
> • Palpable mass

cause. Prompt treatment is vital to preserve renal function. Immediate treatment involves reestablishing urine flow from the affected kidney. A nephrostomy tube, ureteral stent, or indwelling catheter may be required.

Ureteral stents (small, specialized catheters) are used to keep ureters open and promote healing. Stents can be positioned during surgery or cystoscopy. One or both ends of the stent may be pigtail or J-shaped to keep it in place (Figure 21-10 ◆). A stent may be temporary, or it may be used for longer periods with ureteral obstruction due to tumors, strictures, or other causes. Box 21-17 describes nursing care for a client with a ureteral stent.

Nursing care focuses on preventing hydronephrosis and ensuring urinary drainage. Monitoring intake, urine output, and bladder emptying helps identify impaired urine outflow. Monitoring urine output is vital for clients with risk factors such as pelvic or abdominal tumors, urinary calculi, adhesions

Figure 21-10. ◆ Stent

BOX 21-17
NURSING CARE CHECKLIST

URETERAL STENT

☑ Label all drainage tubes and stents for easy identification. Secure positions.

☑ Attach each catheter and stent to a separate closed drainage system.

☑ Monitor for infection or bleeding: Fever, tachycardia, pain, hematuria, and cloudy or malodorous urine.

☑ Encourage fluids, especially those that acidify urine, such as apple and cranberry juice.

☑ For an indwelling stent, teach follow-up care and recognition and prevention of complications.

and scarring from previous surgeries, or neurologic deficits. Ensuring urinary drainage is also vital in the client with a ureteral stent, nephrostomy, or surgical intervention for hydronephrosis. Label catheters and drainage tubes clearly, and measure outputs separately. Prevent kinking or obstruction. Irrigate tubes only as ordered by the physician.

Polycystic Kidney Disease

Polycystic kidney disease is a hereditary disease characterized by cyst formation and massive kidney enlargement. It is a relatively common disease that affects both children and adults.

PATHOPHYSIOLOGY

Renal cysts develop in the nephron. These fluid-filled sacs can range in size from microscopic to several centimeters in diameter. Both kidneys are affected. As the cysts fill, enlarge, and multiply, the kidneys also enlarge (Figure 21-11 ◆). The cysts gradually destroy functional kidney tissue. Cysts also may develop elsewhere (e.g., liver, spleen, pancreas). Cardiac and vascular abnormalities also may be present.

Figure 21-11. ◆ A polycystic kidney.

Polycystic kidney disease is slowly progressive, with symptoms usually noticed in the thirties or forties. Common manifestations include flank pain, microscopic or gross hematuria, proteinuria, and polyuria and nocturia. Urinary tract infection and stones are common. Most clients develop hypertension. The kidneys become enlarged, palpable, and knobby. Eventually, signs of renal failure develop.

COLLABORATIVE CARE

Management of adult polycystic kidney disease is supportive. A *renal ultrasound* is done to diagnose polycystic kidney disease. This test is noninvasive and can be done at the client's bedside.

Care is taken to avoid further renal damage by nephrotoxins, urinary tract infection, obstruction, or hypertension. A fluid intake of 2,000 to 2,500 mL per day is encouraged to help prevent UTI and lithiasis. ACE inhibitors or other antihypertensive agents are prescribed to manage hypertension. Ultimately, clients with polycystic kidney disease require hemodialysis or kidney transplantation. The section on chronic renal failure later in this chapter gives more information about dialysis and kidney transplants.

NURSING CARE

Although each client has individual nursing care needs, the following nursing diagnoses may be appropriate for the client with polycystic kidney disease:

- Excess Fluid Volume related to impaired renal function
- Anticipatory Grieving related to potential loss of kidney function
- Deficient Knowledge related to lack of information about how to maintain kidney function
- Ineffective Coping related to the potential for transmitting an inherited disorder to offspring

 ## Discharge Considerations

Teach about polycystic kidney disease and how to maintain good kidney function. Instruct to drink about 2,500 mL of fluid per day. Include additional information about preventing urinary tract infection, such as hygiene measures. Discuss early manifestations of UTI, and stress the importance of seeking prompt treatment to prevent further kidney damage. Advise avoiding medications that are potentially toxic to the kidneys and checking with the primary care provider before taking any new drug.

Offspring of clients with adult polycystic kidney disease have a 50% chance of inheriting the disorder. Discuss genetic counseling and screening of family members, especially if renal transplantation is likely and family members are potential donors.

Kidney Trauma

The kidneys are relatively well protected by the rib cage and back muscles but may be injured by blunt force (most common) or penetrating injury. Falls, motor vehicle accidents, and sports injuries can all result in kidney damage. Renal contusion or a small hematoma may result, or, more seriously, a laceration or other damage. Gunshot wounds, knife wounds, impalement injuries, and fractured ribs can cause penetrating damage. Because the kidney is a vascular organ, trauma can lead to hemorrhage and possible shock.

The primary manifestations of renal trauma are hematuria (gross or microscopic), flank or abdominal pain, and oliguria or **anuria** (absence of urine). There may be localized swelling, tenderness, or *ecchymoses* (bruising) in the flank region. Signs of shock may be present, including tachycardia, hypotension, tachypnea, cool and pale skin, and decreased level of consciousness.

Treatment of minor kidney injuries is generally conservative, including bed rest and observation. Bleeding is usually minor and self-limiting. Immediate treatment for major or critical trauma focuses on controlling hemorrhage and treating or preventing shock. Surgery may be required to stop the bleeding. (See Box 21-21 in the section on Kidney Tumors for nursing care of the client undergoing kidney surgery.)

Tumors of the Kidney and Urinary Tract

Any part of the urinary tract can be affected by a tumor, but the most common site is the bladder. Tumors of the urinary tract may lead to obstruction, renal failure, hemorrhage, and invasion of surrounding tissues.

Bladder Cancer

Bladder cancer is the tenth leading cause of cancer deaths. People living in heavily industrialized states are more likely to be affected than those living in agricultural states. People in northern regions have a higher risk than people in southern regions.

Bladder cancer usually affects people over age 50. It is diagnosed in men two to four times more often than in women. Many clients with bladder cancer have more than one tumor at the time of diagnosis.

PATHOPHYSIOLOGY

The major risk factors for bladder cancer are carcinogens in the urine and chronic inflammation or infection of bladder mucosa. Chemicals from cigarette smoke and other chemicals such as those used in the plastics industry, by leather finishers, spray painters, and hair dressers are carcinogenic (cancer producing). They are excreted in the urine and stored in the bladder, increasing the risk of abnormal cell growth.

Bladder tumors begin as cell changes that develop into superficial or invasive lesions. Most are papillomas, with a polyp-like structure attached by a stalk to the bladder mucosa (Figure 21-12 ◆). The prognosis for a full recovery is good. When metastasis occurs, the pelvic lymph nodes, lungs, bones, and liver are most commonly involved.

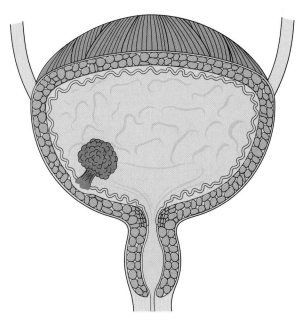

Figure 21-12. ◆ A papillary lesion with minimal invasion of the bladder wall.

Painless hematuria is the most common initial manifestation of bladder cancer. Frequency, urgency, and dysuria are other manifestations of bladder cancer.

COLLABORATIVE CARE

When *urinalysis* shows hematuria, a *urine cytology* may be done to assess for cancer cells. A *cystoscopy* is done to visualize and biopsy the lesion. Review Box 21-9 for nursing implications of a cystoscopy.

Pharmacology

Chemotherapeutic drugs may be instilled into the bladder as the primary treatment for bladder cancer or to prevent recurrence of the tumor after surgery. Bacillus Calmette–Guérin (BCGLive, TheraCys) causes a local inflammatory reaction that eliminates or reduces superficial tumors. Other chemotherapeutic drugs also may be used. Bladder irritation, frequency, dysuria, and contact dermatitis are possible adverse reactions to *intravesical* (within-bladder) chemotherapy.

Surgery

Surgery for bladder tumors ranges from simple resection of noninvasive tumors to removal of the bladder and surrounding structures (Table 21-7 ◆). In a total or radical **cystectomy**, the bladder and adjacent muscles and tissues are removed. In men,

the prostate and seminal vessels are also removed, resulting in impotence. In women, the uterus, fallopian tubes, and ovaries are removed, resulting in sterility. A *urinary diversion* is created for urine collection and drainage. The most common urinary diversion is the *ileal conduit;* a *continent urinary diversion* also may be created (Figure 21-13 ◆). Box 21-18 describes nursing care of the client undergoing a cystectomy and urinary diversion.

NURSING CARE

ASSESSING

Painless hematuria is the most common early manifestation of bladder cancer. Direct any client with blood in the urine to seek medical evaluation and care.

DIAGNOSING, PLANNING, AND IMPLEMENTING

IMPAIRED URINARY ELIMINATION

■ Monitor amount, color, and clarity of urine output from all catheters, stents, and tubes hourly for the first 24 hours postoperatively, then every 4 to 8 hours. *Output of less than*

TABLE 21-7

NURSING IMPLICATIONS FOR PROCEDURES USED TO TREAT BLADDER CANCER

PROCEDURE	DESCRIPTION	NURSING CONSIDERATIONS
Transurethral resection of bladder tumor (TURBT)	Tumor removal via cystoscope inserted through urethra	Maintain continuous bladder irrigation as ordered, ensure catheter patency. Monitor for excessive bleeding. Encourage fluids up to 2,500–3,000 mL/day. Give stool softeners to prevent straining.
Partial cystectomy	Resection of the tumor and a portion of the bladder wall	Maintain urethral and/or suprapubic catheter patency to reduce pressure on suture lines. Monitor for excessive bleeding.
Complete or radical cystectomy	Removal of the entire urinary bladder and surrounding tissues	Permanent urinary diversion required. Maintain stent position and patency. May have urethral catheter to drain pelvic cavity.
Cutaneous ureterostomy	One or both ureters brought to abdominal wall; urine drains via stoma	Requires urinary drainage appliance. Small stoma may make tight seal difficult. Risk of skin irritation from contact with urine. Increased risk of UTI due to direct access from skin to kidney.
Ileal conduit	Portion of ileum formed into pouch; ureters inserted into pouch and open end is brought to surface to form stoma	Continuous urine drainage requires appliance. Risk of infection is significant. Good skin care is vital due to constant contact with urine.
Continent internal ileal reservoir or continent ileal bladder conduit (Kock's pouch)	Pouch created from ileum; nipple valves formed by telescoping tissue where brought to skin and where ureters attach prevent urine leakage and reflux	Drainage-collection device is not necessary. Client must be willing and able to perform clean intermittent self-catheterization every 2 to 4 hours to drain pouch.

A

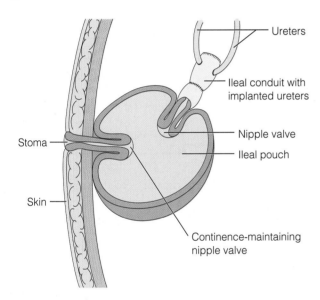

B

Figure 21-13. ◆ Urinary diversion procedures. (A) Ileal conduit. (B) A continent urinary diversion.

30 mL per hour may indicate low blood volume, impaired kidney function, or impaired drainage. A change in urine color or clarity may indicate infection or other complication.

■ Label all catheters, stents, and their drainage containers. Maintain separate closed gravity drainage systems for each. *Clear labeling of tubes can prevent errors in irrigating and calculating outputs. Separate closed systems minimize the risk of infection.*

■ Secure catheters and stents with tape; prevent kinking or occlusion; maintain gravity flow by keeping drainage bags lower than the kidneys. *Impaired urine flow can lead to kidney damage or place pressure on suture lines.*

■ Encourage fluid intake of 3,000 mL per day. *Increased fluid intake reduces the risk of infection and dilutes urine, which is less irritating to the skin around the stoma site.*

■ After removal of any stents or ureteral catheters, monitor urine output closely for 24 hours. *Edema or stricture of ureters may impede output.*

BOX 21-18
NURSING CARE CHECKLIST

BLADDER TUMOR SURGERY
Before Surgery

☑ Contact the enterostomal therapist to determine the stoma site(s).

☑ Provide routine preoperative care as ordered (see Chapter 7).

After Surgery

☑ Monitor intake and output. Assess urine output hourly for the first 24 hours, then every 4 hours or as ordered. Notify the charge nurse or physician if less than 30 mL/hour.

☑ Assess urine color and consistency. Expect pink or bright red urine to clear by third postoperative day. Urine may be cloudy due to mucus produced by bowel mucosa, but excessive cloudiness or malodorous urine may indicate infection.

☑ Assess stoma and surrounding skin every 2 hours for the first 24 hours, then every 4 hours for 48 to 72 hours. Notify the charge nurse or physician if the stoma blanches when touched or is pale, gray, or cyanotic.

☑ Irrigate ileal diversion catheter with 30 to 60 mL sterile normal saline every 4 hours or as ordered.

☑ Teach stoma and urinary diversion care, including odor management, skin care, increased fluid intake, pouch application and leakage prevention, self-catheterization for clients with continent reservoirs, and signs of infection and other complications.

■ Encourage activity. *Ambulation promotes urine drainage and helps prevent calcium loss from bones, which could lead to urinary calculi.*

RISK FOR IMPAIRED SKIN INTEGRITY

■ Assess skin surrounding the stoma for redness, excoriation, or signs of breakdown. Assess for urine leakage from catheters, stents, or drains. Keep the skin clean and dry. *Urine irritates the skin, increasing the risk of breakdown. Meticulous skin care can prevent breakdown.*

■ Ensure gravity drainage of urine-collection device or empty bag every 2 hours. Change urine-collection appliance as needed, removing any mucus from stoma. See the checklist in Procedure 21-2 for care of a urostomy. *Overfilling may damage the seal, allowing leakage and urine contact with skin.*

DISTURBED BODY IMAGE

■ Use active listening and respond to concerns. *Surgical procedures and adjunctive cancer treatments can significantly affect the client's body image. Grieving is a normal response.*

PROCEDURE 21-2   Urinary Stoma Care Checklist

- Gather all supplies. Provide for privacy.
- Assess client's knowledge, ability, and willingness to assist; explain procedure as needed.
- Use standard precautions.
- Remove existing pouch, pulling gently away from skin. Warm water or adhesive solvent may be used to loosen the seal if necessary.
- Assess the stoma. Report a dark purple, black, or very pale stoma to the physician.
- Prevent urine flow during cleaning by placing a rolled gauze square or tampon over the stoma opening.
- Cleanse peristomal skin with soap and water, rinse, and pat or air dry.
- Use stoma guide to determine the correct size for the bag opening and/or protective ring seal. Trim the bag or seal as needed.
- Apply the skin barrier; allow to dry.

- Apply the bag with an opening no more than 1 to 2 mm wider than stoma; prevent wrinkles or creases in bag seal.
- Connect bag to urine-collection device.
- Chart, including the appearance of the stoma and the response of the client.

■ SAMPLE DOCUMENTATION

7/20/02   1400 Urinary stoma bag changed.
Stoma bright pink and moist.
Surrounding skin slightly pink but intact.
Protective gel applied. Urine output yellow
with mucous shreds noted, not malodorous.
—————————— Lynn Jones, LVN.

- Encourage the client to look at, touch, and care for the stoma and appliance as soon as possible. Allow to proceed gradually, providing support and encouragement. *A willingness to provide self-care indicates adaptation to the changed body image.*
- Discuss concerns about resuming usual activities, perceived changes in relationships, and sexual relations. Refer to a support group or a person who has successfully adjusted to a urinary diversion. *If a radical cystectomy has been done, the client will no longer be able to bear children, and may experience erectile dysfunction. Clients and families may be reluctant to ask about sexual topics. Support groups allow open discussion of concerns and anxieties.*

EVALUATING

When evaluating the effectiveness of nursing care, collect data regarding urinary output, skin integrity, and the client's and family's acceptance of and ability to care for any urinary diversion or catheters.

Discharge Considerations

For many clients, surgery for bladder cancer means a lifelong change in urinary elimination. Prior to discharge, assess the client's and family's knowledge and understand-

ing of the cancer diagnosis and recommended treatment plan. When the tumor has been resected, stress the importance of regular follow-up care and monitoring for tumor recurrence.

Teach the client who has had a urinary diversion to care for the stoma and surrounding skin. Discuss strategies to prevent urine reflux and infection. Teach signs and symptoms of UTI and renal calculi. If a continent urinary diversion has been created, teach self-catheterization using clean technique.

Stress the importance of follow-up care and of notifying the physician promptly if signs of a complication develop. Refer the client and family to a cancer support group, and, as appropriate, discuss hospice care.

Nursing Process Case Study
■ CLIENT WITH BLADDER CANCER

Ben Hussain is a 61-year-old man who became alarmed when his urine became bright red. Even though he had no other symptoms, he called his doctor. Urinalysis and cytology showed gross hematuria and abnormal cells. A cystoscopy and biopsy confirmed an invasive bladder tumor. He is admitted to the hospital for a radical cystectomy and ileal diversion.

Assessment Mr. Hussain's admission history indicates that he has lost 10 to 15 pounds over the last few months. He has smoked two to three packs of cigarettes per day for 40 years, but he cut back to a pack a day about a year ago. Mr. Hussain says he is "a little nervous about surgery and what they're going to find." Ms. Mills, the admitting nurse, notes that he fidgets and talks rapidly throughout their interview. He is concerned how he will handle the pain after surgery, because he has never been hospitalized before his cystoscopy. Physical assessment findings include BP 154/86; P 84; R 18; T 98.2° F (36.7° C) PO. He has scattered crackles throughout his lung fields. Mr. Hussain's urine is clear and bright pink. The remainder of his assessment is essentially normal.

Diagnosis The following nursing diagnoses are identified for Mr. Hussain:

- Anxiety related to undetermined extent of disease and fear of pain
- Deficient Knowledge related to lack of information about ileal diversion
- Impaired Urinary Elimination related to cystectomy and ileal diversion
- Risk for Impaired Gas Exchange related to smoking history and effects of anesthesia

Expected Outcomes The expected outcomes of the plan of care for Mr. Hussain are that he will:

- Verbalize a decrease in anxiety.
- Demonstrate ability to manage patient-controlled analgesia (PCA) for postoperative pain control.
- Report pain at a level of 3 or less on a scale of 1 to 10 postoperatively.
- Demonstrate care for his ileostomy stoma, surrounding skin, and collection appliance prior to discharge.
- Maintain urine output with acceptable color and clarity and no signs of infection.
- Maintain adequate gas exchange as evidenced by good skin color, O$_2$ saturation greater than 95%, and clear lung sounds upon auscultation.

Planning and Implementation The following nursing interventions are planned and implemented for Mr. Hussain:

- Allow time to answer questions and verbalize fears pre- and postoperatively.
- Provide written as well as verbal explanations as needed.
- Maintain PCA or epidural infusion postoperatively. Monitor effectiveness of pain relief.
- Explain all procedures related to stoma and appliance care as they are being performed.
- Encourage Mr. and Mrs. Hussain to look at the stoma and touch it when ready.
- Teach stoma, skin, and appliance care, emphasizing techniques to prevent skin irritation and urinary tract infection.

- Monitor urine output, color, clarity, and consistency hourly for 24 hours, then every 4 hours for 24 hours, then every 8 hours. Report output less than 30 mL/hr, bright bleeding, and excessively cloudy or malodorous urine.
- Assist to use an incentive spirometer hourly while awake. Ambulate as soon as possible. Assess lung sounds every 4 hours, reporting increased crackles or diminished breath sounds.
- Refer to a local stoma group on discharge.

Evaluation On discharge, Mr. Hussain has helped clean the stoma and surrounding skin several times. His wife is able to empty the drainage bag and change the appliance, cutting the opening to fit. His urine is pale yellow and slightly cloudy. Mr. Hussain is ambulating independently and using oxycodone (Percocet) twice a day for pain relief. His lungs are clear, and he is very proud of having "survived" 7 days without a cigarette. He says, "Now I'm going to shoot for 7 weeks, then 7 months, then 7 years without a smoke!" A home health referral is made to continue teaching Mr. Hussain to care for his diversion and appliance.

 Critical Thinking in the Nursing Process

1. How does cigarette smoking contribute to the increased risk of urinary tract tumors?
2. How would you respond if Mr. Hussain said "I'm not only giving up on cigarettes, I'm also giving up on sex from here on"?

 # Kidney Tumors

Primary tumors of the kidney are uncommon. Renal cell carcinoma is the most common primary tumor. The highest incidence occurs in people over age 55. Men are affected twice as often as women. Smoking, obesity, and renal calculi are risk factors. Other primary cancers also may metastasize to the kidney.

Renal cancer is often silent, with few signs or symptoms. Hematuria, often microscopic, is the most consistent manifestation. Other symptoms include flank pain, palpable abdominal mass, fever, fatigue, weight loss, and anemia or polycythemia (elevated RBCs). Renal tumors may produce hormones or other substances that can cause such manifestations as hypercalcemia, hypertension, and hyperglycemia.

Renal cancer is often diagnosed by a *renal ultrasound* or *computed tomography (CT) scan*. A *kidney biopsy* is done to identify the presence of cancer cells. (Review Box 21-13 for the nursing implications for a kidney biopsy.)

Radical nephrectomy (removal of the affected kidney and surrounding tissue) is performed if the cancer is limited to the kidney. Box 21-19 describes nursing care of a client having kidney surgery. If the cancer has spread beyond the kidney, chemotherapy or radiation therapy may be prescribed (see Chapter 8).

BOX 21-19
NURSING CARE CHECKLIST

PARTIAL OR TOTAL NEPHRECTOMY
Before Surgery
☑ Assess understanding and reinforce teaching.
☑ Provide routine preoperative care and teaching as ordered (see Chapter 7).

After Surgery
☑ Provide routine postoperative care as described in Chapter 7.
☑ Assess urine output hourly for the first 24 hours then every 4 to 8 hours.
☑ Label and secure all catheters, stents, nephrostomy tubes, or drains. Irrigate only as ordered by the physician.
☑ Monitor for signs of hemorrhage or infection.
☑ Frequently monitor respiratory status and assist with respiratory care.

☑ Support grieving process and adjustment to the loss of a kidney.
☑ Teach home care, including:
  a. Maintain fluid intake of 2,000 to 2,500 mL/day.
  b. Gradually increase exercise to tolerance, avoiding heavy lifting for a year after surgery. Avoid contact sports to reduce the risk of injury to the remaining kidney.
  c. Care of the incision and any remaining drainage tubes, catheters, or stents.
  d. Prescribed medications, including their purpose, dose, scheduling, and potential side effects.
  e. Signs and symptoms of UTI and other complications to report to the physician.

Renal Failure

Renal failure is a condition in which the kidneys are unable to remove accumulated waste products from the blood. Renal failure may be acute or chronic. It is characterized by azotemia (a buildup of nitrogenous waste products in the blood), and leads to fluid, electrolyte, and acid–base imbalances.

Acute Renal Failure

Acute renal failure (ARF) is a rapid decline in renal function with an abrupt onset. It is often reversible with prompt treatment. It is relatively common, affecting at least 10,000 people

in the United States every year. Major trauma or surgery, infection, hemorrhage, severe heart failure, and lower urinary tract obstruction are risk factors. *Iatrogenic* causes of ARF include nephrotoxic medications and contrast dye used in x-rays. Older adults are at particular risk.

PATHOPHYSIOLOGY
The most common causes of ARF are *ischemia* (poor perfusion) of the kidney, and **nephrotoxins** (agents that damage the kidney tissue). Causes of ARF can be classified as prerenal, intrarenal, and postrenal (Table 21-8 ◆).

TABLE 21-8

CAUSES OF ACUTE RENAL FAILURE

CATEGORY	CAUSE	EXAMPLES
Prerenal failure	Impaired blood supply to kidney	Fluid volume deficit, hemorrhage, heart failure, shock
Intrarenal failure	Acute damage to renal tissue and nephrons or *acute tubular necrosis (ATN):* Abrupt decline in tubular and glomerular function due to either prolonged ischemia and/or exposure to nephrotoxins	Acute glomerulonephritis, malignant hypertension, ischemia; nephrotoxic drugs or substances; red blood cell destruction (e.g., hemolytic transfusion reaction); muscle tissue breakdown due to trauma, heatstroke
Postrenal failure	Obstruction of urine outflow	Urethral obstruction by enlarged prostate or tumor; ureteral or kidney pelvis obstruction by calculi

Hypovolemia is a common *prerenal* cause of ARF. It is readily reversible if promptly recognized and treated. If it is not, it can lead to acute tubular necrosis and intrarenal ARF. *Intrarenal* failure results from acute damage to the nephrons by inflammation (e.g., acute glomerulonephritis), by vascular disorders (like severe hypertension), or by exposure to nephrotoxins. The risk for *acute tubular necrosis (ATN)* is particularly high when ischemia and exposure to a nephrotoxin occur at the same time. Obstruction of urine outflow can lead to *postrenal* ARF.

Acute renal failure is generally identified by *oliguria* (urine output < 400 mL/day) and rising BUN or serum creatinine levels. The GFR falls, tubular cells become necrotic and slough, and the nephron is unable to eliminate wastes effectively (Figure 21-14 ◆). The course of acute renal failure includes three phases: initiation, maintenance, and recovery.

1. The *initiation phase* begins with the initiating event and often is recognized only after the client has moved into the maintenance phase.
2. The *maintenance phase* of ARF begins within hours of the initiating event and typically lasts 1 to 2 weeks. Oliguria develops and the kidney cannot efficiently eliminate metabolic wastes, water, electrolytes, and acids. Azotemia can cause confusion and disorientation. Salt and water retention lead to fluid volume excess and edema. Hypertension and heart failure may develop. Hyperkalemia causes muscle weakness, nausea and diarrhea, and dysrhythmias. Metabolic acidosis results from inadequate elimination of hydrogen ions by the kidneys. In this phase, anemia may develop and immune function is impaired, increasing the risk for infections. Toward the end of the maintenance phase, urine output gradually increases, but the serum creatinine and BUN remain high.
3. The *recovery phase* of ARF is characterized by improving kidney function, urine output, and blood values. It lasts for up to 1 year.

Chronic Renal Failure

Chronic renal failure (CRF) is a slow, insidious process of kidney destruction. It may go unrecognized for years as nephron units are destroyed and renal mass is reduced. When the kidneys are no longer able to excrete metabolic wastes and regulate fluid and electrolyte balance adequately, the client is said to have *end-stage renal disease (ESRD),* the final stage of CRF.

End-stage renal disease is increasing in incidence in all age groups, with a particularly sharp increase in people over age 70. The incidence of ESRD is highest in African Americans, followed by Native Americans, Asians, and European Americans. Diabetic nephropathy and hypertension are the leading causes of chronic renal failure in the United States. Among African Americans, hypertension is the leading cause.

PATHOPHYSIOLOGY

As nephrons are destroyed by the disease process, remaining nephrons hypertrophy to compensate for the lost renal mass. The increased demand on these nephrons increases their risk for destruction.

Chronic renal failure progresses over months to many years. In the early stage of *decreased renal reserve,* unaffected nephrons do the work of the lost nephrons, and the client remains free of symptoms. As kidney function is further reduced, BUN and serum creatinine levels begin to rise, and manifestations of *renal insufficiency* may be seen. Any further insult to the kidneys at this stage (infection, exposure to nephrotoxins) can precipitate *end-stage renal failure.* At this stage the GFR is less than 20% of normal, and serum creatinine and BUN levels rise sharply (Figure 21-15 ◆). At this stage, **uremia** (which literally means "urine in the blood") develops.

Chronic renal failure often is not identified until uremia develops. Early manifestations of uremia include nausea, apathy, weakness, and fatigue. As it progresses, the client may experience frequent vomiting, increasing weakness, lethargy, and confusion. The multisystem effects of uremia are illustrated in Figure 21-16 ◆.

COLLABORATIVE CARE

Preventing acute renal failure is a goal in the care of all clients, especially for those in high-risk groups. Maintaining blood volume, cardiac output, and blood pressure is vital to preserve kidney perfusion. Nephrotoxic drugs are avoided if possible. When a nephrotoxic drug must be used, keeping the client well hydrated and avoiding additional nephrotoxins help reduce the risk of renal failure. Care for the client with chronic

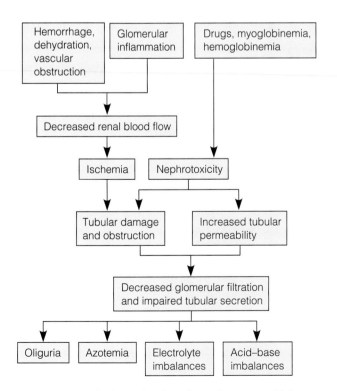

Figure 21-14. ◆ The pathophysiology of acute renal failure.

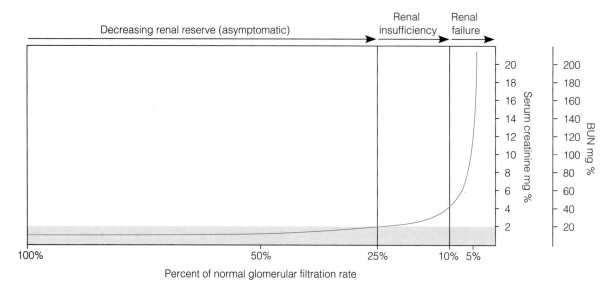

Figure 21-15. ◆ The relationship of renal function to BUN and serum creatinine in the course of chronic renal failure.

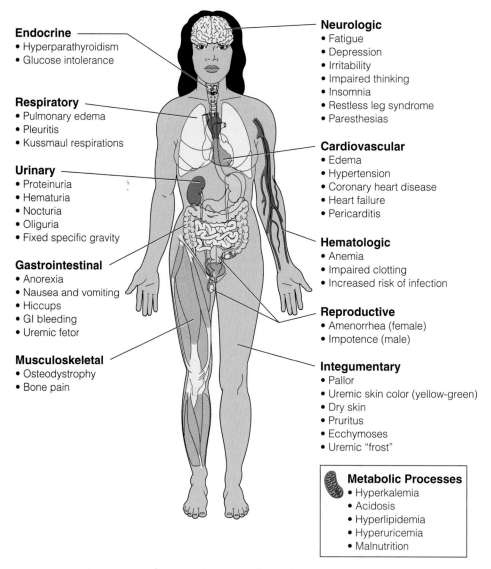

Figure 21-16. ◆ The multisystem effects of uremia.

renal failure focuses on eliminating factors that may further decrease renal function and on slowing the progress of the disease to ESRD.

Serum creatinine and *BUN* are monitored to evaluate the disease progress and the effectiveness of treatment. *Creatinine clearance* is monitored to evaluate GFR and renal function. (Review the normal values for renal function tests in Table 21-5.) *Serum electrolytes, arterial blood gases,* and *CBC* also are frequently monitored. *Urinalysis* may show a fixed specific gravity at 1.010, and abnormal components such as protein, blood cells, and cell casts. *Casts* are protein and cellular debris molded in the shape of the tubular lumen. A *kidney biopsy* may be done to identify the underlying disease process (see Box 21-13).

Diet and Fluid Management

When the kidneys cannot effectively regulate fluid and electrolyte balance and eliminate metabolic waste products, intake of these substances must be regulated. Fluid and sodium intake is restricted. The daily fluid intake is calculated by allowing 500 mL for insensible losses (respiration, perspiration, bowel losses) and adding the amount of urine output (or lost in emesis or diarrhea) during the previous 24 hours. For example, if the client has 325 mL of urine output, intake for the next day is restricted to 825 mL, including both oral and intravenous fluids. Accurate weights and I&O records are essential. Clients with chronic renal failure should notify the physician of any weight gain of more than 5 pounds (2 to 2.5 kg) over a 2-day period. Sodium and potassium intake is regulated. Salt substitutes containing potassium are avoided.

The client with renal failure needs adequate nutrients and calories to prevent tissue breakdown. Proteins are limited to minimize azotemia and should be complete proteins (i.e., meat, fish, poultry, cheese, eggs, milk, or soy). Carbohydrates are increased to maintain adequate calorie intake. Total parenteral nutrition may be ordered if the client is unable to eat.

Pharmacology

The fact that most medications are excreted by the kidney is a major consideration in drug therapy for clients with renal failure. All nephrotoxic drugs (such as NSAIDs) are avoided or used with extreme caution. Drug dosages may be adjusted because excretion is slowed and half-life is prolonged.

Diuretics such as furosemide (Lasix) may be ordered to reduce fluid volume, lower blood pressure, and lower serum potassium levels. Other antihypertensive drugs such as ACE inhibitors are prescribed to maintain the blood pressure within normal levels.

Sodium bicarbonate or calcium carbonate may be used to manage the electrolyte imbalances and acidosis accompanying renal failure. When serum potassium levels are dangerously high, a potassium-binding exchange resin such as sodium polystyrene sulfonate (Kayexalate, SPS Suspension) may be ordered by oral or rectal route. Intravenous insulin and glucose also may be given to lower serum potassium levels.

Folic acid and iron supplements are used to combat anemia. A multiple-vitamin preparation is also often prescribed, because anorexia, nausea, and dietary restrictions may limit nutrient intake.

Dialysis

When conservative management is no longer effective to maintain fluid and electrolyte balance and prevent uremia, dialysis is considered. **Dialysis** is diffusion of solutes across a semipermeable membrane from an area of higher concentration to one of lower concentration. In dialysis, a semipermeable membrane separates the blood from an isotonic dialyzing solution. Water and solutes such as urea, creatinine, and electrolytes diffuse across this membrane, but proteins do not. Dialysis compensates for the kidneys' inability to eliminate excess water and solutes.

The decision to start dialysis is not an easy one. Like insulin therapy for a diabetic, dialysis manages symptoms but does not cure the disease. Dialysis requires a daily commitment. Clients on dialysis may have difficulty maintaining employment. Many families fall apart with the day-to-day stress. Even with dialysis, clients may have constant flulike symptoms and feel controlled by their illness. In the end, clients may choose to discontinue treatment, preferring death over continued dialysis.

HEMODIALYSIS. In *hemodialysis,* electrolytes, waste products, and excess water are removed from the body by diffusion and filtration (see Chapter 5). The client's blood is pumped to a dialyzing membrane unit (Figure 21-17 ◆), where it moves past a semipermeable membrane. *Dialysate* (a solution similar to normal extracellular fluid) is warmed to body temperature and passed along the other side of the membrane. Solutes (electrolytes and waste products) diffuse through the membrane into the dialysate. Medications can be added to the dialysate to diffuse into the blood. Excess water is removed from the blood by creating a higher fluid pressure on the blood side of the membrane. Clients typically undergo two or three sessions of hemodialysis per week for a total of 9 to 12 hours. Hemodialysis can be done at home but usually occurs in an outpatient dialysis center.

An arteriovenous (AV) fistula (Figure 21-18 ◆) is commonly created for vascular access. Often the radial artery and cephalic vein are joined. A functional AV fistula has a palpable pulsation and a *bruit* (audible murmur) on auscultation. Box 21-20 outlines nursing care for the client undergoing hemodialysis.

CLINICAL alert

Do not take blood pressures or allow blood draws or IV starts on the nondominant arm of clients in renal failure, to avoid damaging blood vessels. If a fistula is in place, avoid blood pressures and venipunctures on the arm with the fistula.

Figure 21-17. ◆ A hemodialysis system.

Clients on hemodialysis may experience both systemic and fistula complications. Hypotension is the most frequent complication occurring during hemodialysis. Bleeding may occur due to altered clotting and the use of heparin during dialysis. Infection is a significant risk. Dialysis dementia is a progressive, potentially fatal neurologic complication that may affect clients on long-term hemodialysis.

AV fistula problems include infection and clotting or thrombosis. These complications may cause fistula failure and require development of a new site. AV fistula failure can have a psychological impact, resulting in depression and an altered self-concept.

Continuous venovenous hemofiltration (CVVH) and *continuous arteriovenous hemofiltration (CAVH)* are forms of hemodialysis used for selected clients. Venous or arterial blood is heparinized and filtered, allowing excess water and solutes to drain into a collection device. The blood is then rediluted with a balanced electrolyte and nutrient solution and returned to the circulation (Figure 21-19 ◆). The slower process of CVVH and CAVH reduces adverse effects associated with hemodialysis but may require prolonged immobilization.

PERITONEAL DIALYSIS. In *peritoneal dialysis,* the highly vascular peritoneum serves as the dialyzing membrane. Warmed dialysate is instilled into the peritoneal cavity through a peritoneal catheter. Metabolic waste products and electrolytes diffuse into the dialysate while it remains in the abdomen. Excess water is drawn into the dialysate by osmosis. The fluid is then drained by gravity out of the peritoneal cavity into a sterile bag. Peritoneal dialysis is significantly less costly than hemodialysis, but is used by fewer people with renal failure in the United States.

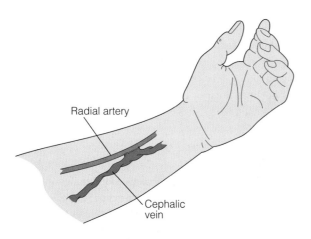

Figure 21-18. ◆ An arteriovenous fistula.

BOX 21-20
NURSING CARE CHECKLIST

HEMODIALYSIS

Before Dialysis

☑ Use standard precautions at all times.

☑ Document vital signs [including orthostatic blood pressures (lying and sitting), apical pulse, respirations], lung sounds, and weight.

☑ Assess vascular access site for a palpable pulsation or vibration, an audible bruit, and signs of inflammation.

☑ Alert all personnel to avoid using the arm with the vascular access site (or the nondominant arm if a site has not yet been established) for blood pressure or venipuncture.

After Dialysis

☑ Document vital signs, weight, and vascular access site assessment. Monitor for orthostatic hypotension, tachycardia, and weight loss.

☑ Monitor BUN, serum creatinine, serum electrolytes, and hematocrit.

☑ Report possible adverse effects of dialysis such as muscle cramping, headache, nausea and vomiting, altered level of consciousness, seizures, or hypertension.

☑ Assess for bleeding at the access site or elsewhere.

☑ If a transfusion was given during dialysis, report manifestations of transfusion reaction, such as chills and fever; dyspnea; chest, back, or arm pain; and urticaria or itching.

☑ Provide psychological support; listen actively for feelings of grief, hopelessness, or anger.

☑ Refer for social services and counseling as indicated.

Figure 21-19. ◆ Continuous arteriovenous hemofiltration (CAVH).

Continuous ambulatory peritoneal dialysis (CAPD) is the most common form of peritoneal dialysis used today. Two liters of dialysate are instilled into the peritoneal cavity, and the catheter is sealed. The client can then continue normal daily activities, emptying the peritoneal cavity and replacing the dialysate every 4 to 6 hours. No special equipment is needed. A variation of CAPD is continuous cyclic peritoneal dialysis (CCPD). CCPD uses a delivery device during nighttime hours and a continuous dwell during the day. CAPD can be performed anywhere, and CCPD allows for home treatment at night, leaving the client free during the day. See Box 21-21 for nursing care of the client having peritoneal dialysis.

Peritoneal dialysis is less likely to cause rapid fluid and electrolyte shifts than hemodialysis, but it is less efficient in removing waste products. It does not require vascular access, but it places the client at risk for developing peritonitis. The indwelling peritoneal catheter also may cause a body image disturbance.

Kidney Transplant

Kidney transplant, implanting a functioning kidney, is the treatment of choice for many clients with end-stage renal disease. The client is no longer tied to a dialysis catheter, machine, or center. Dietary and fluid restrictions are reduced, and the body image is one of increased "wholeness."

About 30% of transplanted kidneys in the United States are from living related donors. The rest are from cadavers. Living relatives with normal kidneys who are in good physical health and have the same ABO blood group as the recipient may serve as donors. Predonation counseling is essential because of the risks involved. Cadaver kidneys are obtained from people who meet the criteria for brain death, are less than 65 years old, and are free of systemic disease, malignancy, or infection, including HIV and hepatitis B or C. Kidneys are removed before or immediately after cardiac arrest and are preserved by hypothermia or continuous perfusion until they are implanted.

The donor kidney is usually placed in the lower abdominal cavity of the recipient (Figure 21-20 ◆). It is connected to arterial and venous blood supplies, and its ureter is connected to one of the recipient's ureters or directly to the bladder, using a

BOX 21-21
NURSING CARE CHECKLIST

PERITONEAL DIALYSIS

Before Dialysis

☑ Use standard precautions at all times.

☑ Document vital signs including temperature, orthostatic blood pressures (lying and standing), apical pulse, respirations, and lung sounds.

☑ Weigh daily or between dialysis runs as indicated.

☑ Measure and record abdominal girth.

☑ Ask the client to urinate prior to peritoneal catheter insertion.

☑ Warm prescribed dialysate solution to body temperature (98.6° F or 37° C) using a warm water bath or heating pad on low setting.

☑ Explain all procedures and expected sensations.

During Dialysis

☑ Use aseptic technique during dialysis and when caring for the peritoneal catheter.

☑ Prime dialysis tubing with solution and connect it to the peritoneal catheter, avoiding kinks. Clamp drainage tubing.

☑ With the client sitting or in Fowler's position, instill dialysate into peritoneal cavity over approximately 10 minutes. Clamp tubing and allow the solution to remain in the abdomen for the prescribed dwell period.

☑ During instillation and the dwell time, observe for dyspnea, tachypnea, or other signs of respiratory distress.

☑ After the prescribed dwell time, open drainage tubing clamps and allow dialysate to drain by gravity into a sterile container. Observe solution for clarity and any evidence of blood, feces, odor, or cloudiness. Promptly report abnormal findings to the charge nurse or physician.

☑ Accurately record amount and type of solution instilled, including any added medications, the dwell time, and amount and character of the drainage.

☑ Monitor laboratory values, including BUN, serum creatinine, and serum electrolytes.

☑ Trouble-shoot for possible problems during dialysis:

   a. Slow instillation of dialysate: Raise the container and reposition the client. Check tubing and catheter for kinks. Check abdominal dressing for wetness, indicating leakage around the catheter.

   b. Excess dwell time.

   c. Poor dialysate drainage. Lower the bag; reposition the client, and check tubing for kinks.

After Dialysis

☑ Record vital signs, including temperature. Report significant changes from baseline.

☑ Time meals to correspond with solution drainage.

☑ Maintain fluid and dietary restrictions as ordered.

☑ Teach peritoneal dialysis procedure as indicated.

---

tunnel technique to prevent reflux. Review Box 21-19 for nursing care for a living kidney donor. Box 21-22 provides nursing care for the kidney recipient.

Figure 21-20. ◆ Placement of a transplanted kidney.

Unless the donor and recipient are identical twins, the transplanted organ stimulates a normal immune response to reject it. Drugs are given to suppress the immune system and the inflammatory response. Clients receiving immunosuppressive drugs have an increased risk of infections. Tumors may develop. Infants born to mothers undergoing immunosuppressive therapy have a higher risk of congenital defects. Corticosteroid use may lead to bone problems, peptic ulcer disease, and cataracts. (See nursing care of clients with altered immunity in Chapter 13.)

Even with immunosuppressive drugs, the transplanted kidney can be rejected at any time (Table 21-9 ◆).

NURSING CARE

ASSESSING

Nurses caring for clients at risk for developing renal failure collect data related to the cardiovascular system and kidney perfusion, as well as data related to urinary function.

Collect subjective data related to the client's current symptoms. Ask about urine output, including its color, quan-

---

BOX 21-22
NURSING CARE CHECKLIST

KIDNEY TRANSPLANT

Before Surgery

☑ Assess knowledge and reinforce teaching. Discuss concerns about surgery, the organ donor, and possible complications.

☑ Provide routine preoperative care as outlined in Chapter 7.

After Surgery

☑ Provide routine postoperative care as outlined in Chapter 7.

☑ Record urine output every 30 to 60 minutes initially. Maintain closed urinary drainage system.

☑ Closely monitor vital signs, arterial pressure, and hemodynamic pressures as ordered.

☑ Maintain intravenous fluids as ordered.

☑ Administer diuretics as ordered.

☑ Remove urinary catheter within 2 to 3 days or as ordered. Encourage voiding every 1 to 2 hours and assess frequently for urinary retention following catheter removal.

☑ Monitor serum electrolytes and renal function tests.

☑ Monitor for possible complications:
   a. Hemorrhage, as indicated by swelling at the operative site, increased abdominal girth, and changes in vital signs and level of consciousness.
   b. Urine leakage into the peritoneal cavity, as indicated by abdominal swelling and tenderness, and decreased urine output.
   c. Renal artery thrombosis, indicated by the abrupt onset of hypertension and a fall in GFR.
   d. Infection, indicated by possible fever, change in level of consciousness, cloudy or malodorous urine, or purulent drainage from the incision.
   e. Rejection, as indicated by fever, swelling and tenderness over the graft site, decreased urine output, and declining renal function.

☑ Reinforce teaching, including medications and potential side effects, vital sign and weight monitoring, signs of organ rejection, and any prescribed diet changes.

☑ Provide psychological support; address concerns and provide information as needed.

---

tity, and any difficulty initiating urine flow or emptying the bladder completely. Inquire about recent weight changes and any noticeable swelling of the face, hands, legs, or ankles. Ask about other symptoms such as nausea or vomiting. Obtain the client's medical history, including current or previous kidney problems, chronic diseases such as diabetes or lupus, recent surgery or diagnostic tests, and current or recent medications.

Objective data to obtain includes vital signs, current weight, and intake and output (if known). Note level of consciousness and mental status. Observe skin color, temperature, and moisture, and note presence of any edema. Auscultate heart, lung, and bowel sounds. Obtain a urine specimen for analysis, noting the color, clarity, character of the urine, and its specific gravity.

DIAGNOSING, PLANNING, AND IMPLEMENTING

EXCESS FLUID VOLUME

■ Maintain accurate I&O records. *Accurate I&O records help determine treatment, especially fluid restriction. Hourly urine output measurements may be done in acute renal failure.*

■ Weigh daily or as ordered. Use consistent technique and timing to ensure accuracy. *Weight often provides a more accurate assessment of fluid volume than intake and output records, particularly in oliguric clients.*

■ Document vital signs at least every 4 hours. *Changes in vital signs may indicate either fluid volume excess or deficit. Hypertension can further damage the kidneys.*

TABLE 21-9   **TYPES OF KIDNEY TRANSPLANT REJECTION**

TYPE OF REJECTION	MANIFESTATIONS	TREATMENT/OUTCOME
Hyperacute: Within hours of transplant *Accelerated:* Within 2–4 days	Urine output ceases; kidney appears blue and flaccid	Prevent by crossmatching before surgery. Transplant cannot be saved. Rarely occurs.
Acute: Days to months after transplant	Fall in kidney function; possible fever, graft tenderness and/or swelling	Increase immunosuppression with additional drugs or increased doses. Most common and treatable.
Chronic: Months to years after transplant	Gradual decline in kidney function	No treatment. Transplant cannot be saved.

■ Frequently assess heart and breath sounds. Assess the degree of peripheral edema and neck vein distention. *Excess fluid volume increases the risk for heart failure and pulmonary edema. An S_3 or S_4 gallop rhythm or crackles in the lungs may indicate heart failure and should be reported to the charge nurse or physician.*

■ Unless contraindicated, place in Fowler's position. *Fowler's position facilitates breathing and lung expansion and reduces the workload of the heart.*

■ Restrict fluids as ordered. Provide frequent mouth care and encourage using hard candies to decrease the thirst response. If ice chips are used to relieve thirst, include as intake (generally calculated as half of an equivalent volume of fluid; an 8 oz. or 240 mL container of ice chips yields 120 mL of water). *Fluid restriction helps minimize fluid retention and the complications of fluid volume excess, especially in the client being managed without dialysis.*

■ Administer medications with meals. *This reduces total liquid consumed.*

■ Turn frequently and provide good skin care. *Edema can lead to skin breakdown, especially in the older or debilitated client.*

■ Administer diuretics as ordered and monitor response. *Diuretics may promote urination.*

■ Monitor serum electrolytes and for manifestations of imbalances. Report abnormal results. *Electrolyte imbalances may develop because of water retention and impaired renal function.*

IMBALANCED NUTRITION: LESS THAN BODY REQUIREMENTS

The manifestations of uremia and dietary restrictions often affect food intake. The client may not eat enough to meet metabolic needs. *Catabolism* (breakdown of body proteins to meet energy needs) worsens azotemia and uremia.

■ Monitor and document food intake, including the amount and type of food consumed. *Food intake records help determine the adequacy of nutritional intake and identify the need for nutritional supplements.*

■ Administer antiemetic drugs 30 to 60 minutes before eating. *Anorexia, nausea, and vomiting are common. Antiemetics reduce nausea and the risk of vomiting with food intake.*

■ Provide mouth care just prior to meals. *The client may have a metallic taste and bad breath. Mouth care improves taste and stimulates the appetite.*

■ Provide frequent, small meals or between-meal snacks. *These measures promote food intake in the fatigued or anorectic client.*

■ Arrange for a dietary consultation. Provide preferred foods to the extent possible, and involve the client in planning menus. Allow family to prepare meals within dietary restrictions and encourage family members to eat with the client. *The client is more likely to eat favorite foods. Involving the client in planning promotes a sense of control and learning about dietary restrictions. Familiar foods and social interaction encourage eating and heighten the client's enjoyment of meals.*

■ Monitor serum electrolytes and albumin. *Changes in values may indicate either improving or declining nutritional status.*

■ Administer and monitor parenteral nutrition as ordered. *Parenteral nutrition may be necessary to prevent catabolism and increasing azotemia in the client with renal failure. Remember that intravenous lines and parenteral nutrition increase the risk for infection. Monitor sites carefully for signs of infection or inflammation.*

RISK FOR INFECTION

Renal failure affects immune function, increasing the risk for infection. Invasive treatments and catheters further increase this risk.

■ Use standard precautions and good handwashing at all times. *Handwashing and standard precautions help prevent spread of infection to and from the client. Clients on hemodialysis have an increased risk of hepatitis B, hepatitis C, and HIV infection.*

■ Use strict aseptic technique when handling ports, catheters, and incisions. *Aseptic technique is vital to reduce the risk of introducing an infectious organism.*

■ Monitor temperature and vital signs at least every 4 hours. *An elevated temperature or increased pulse rate may indicate infection.*

■ Monitor WBC count and differential. *High or low WBC counts may indicate an infection. Increasing numbers of immature WBCs in circulation also may indicate infection.*

■ Culture urine, peritoneal dialysis fluid, and other drainage as indicated. *Culture is used to determine the presence of pathogens.*

■ Turn or ambulate frequently; encourage coughing and deep breathing. *These measures decrease the risk of respiratory infection.*

■ Restrict visits from obviously ill family members. Teach the client and family how to reduce the spread of infection. *The client and family need to know and understand how to reduce the risk of infection at home and in the community.*

DISTURBED BODY IMAGE

■ Involve the client in decision making and encourage self-care. *Client involvement increases autonomy, improves acceptance, and promotes independence.*

■ Encourage expression of feelings and concerns. Accept perceptions and feelings without criticism. *Self-expression enhances the client's self-worth and acceptance.*

■ Work with the client to develop and achieve realistic goals. Provide positive reinforcement and feedback. Support positive gains. *Adapting to a change in body image and self-concept requires time and often occurs in a series of small steps. Realistic goals allow the client to see progress. Reinforcement helps develop positive coping strategies.*

■ Encourage contact with a support group. Refer for counseling or social services as indicated. *Peer support and counseling can help the client and family develop effective coping and adaptation strategies.*

EVALUATING

When evaluating the effectiveness of nursing interventions for the client with renal failure, collect data related to fluid volume status, such as weight, intake and output, degree of edema, and cardiovascular status. Assess skin and mucous membrane integrity as well. Evaluate food and nutrient intake, and compliance with prescribed diet. Assess for freedom from infection. Look at coping strategies employed by the client, as well as active participation in care.

Discharge Considerations

Renal failure may be an acute disorder or a chronic disease. Even when manifestations of acute renal failure resolve before discharge, the healing process lasts for up to 1 year. Both acute and chronic renal failure can require long-term, day-to-day management. Box 21-23 outlines assessment data to be collected before discharge.

Early teaching focuses on the nature of the renal failure. Teach clients with acute renal failure about the extended recovery period and the importance of avoiding exposure to nephrotoxins.

Educate all clients about prescribed dietary and fluid restrictions. Involve the client, a dietitian, and the family member usually responsible for cooking in teaching. Include strategies to improve flavor and to relieve thirst when fluid is restricted.

Teach the client on hemodialysis how to assess and protect the fistula or shunt. Refer home dialysis helpers for formal training. Teach and demonstrate catheter care and the dialysis procedure to the client who will perform CAPD and a family member or significant other. When a kidney transplant has been done, teach about the prescribed medications, their adverse effects and management, infection prevention, and signs and symptoms of organ rejection.

Refer clients to local or state chapters of the National Kidney Foundation or the American Association of Kidney Patients.

RESOURCES FOR HOME CARE

The following resources may be useful for clients with kidney disease:

American Association of Kidney Patients
800-749-2257
www.aakp.org

National Kidney Foundation
800-622-9010
www.kidney.org

BOX 21-23
ASSESSING FOR DISCHARGE

RENAL FAILURE
Client

- Self-care: Ability to independently perform ADLs; to prepare and eat prescribed diet; to manage peritoneal dialysis (CAPD or CCPD) or home hemodialysis
- Knowledge: Disease process; fluid and diet restrictions; treatment options; strategies to preserve kidney function; prevention and recognition of infection; complications to report to physician; follow-up care and/or scheduled treatments
- Psychosocial: Coping with diagnosis and treatments; support network and significant others; economic effects of treatments; acceptance of altered body image and roles
- Home environment: Clean running water, handwashing and toilet facilities; clean area for home dialysis; transportation options

Family and Caregivers

- Ability and willingness to assist with ADLs, to provide or assist with meal preparation and dialysis
- Financial and transportation resources; stability of family unit, effect of chronic illness on roles and relationships

Community

- Water and sanitation services; mass transit options; availability of dialysis center(s), home health and social support services; financial support options

Kidney Foundation of Canada
514-938-4515
www.kidney.ca

Nursing Process Case Study
■ CLIENT WITH CHRONIC RENAL FAILURE

Walter Cohen, 45 years old, has been a type 1 diabetic since the age of 20. He was diagnosed with diabetic nephropathy 10 years ago, and has now progressed to end-stage renal disease. He enters the nephrology unit for temporary hemodialysis to treat uremia and to prepare for CAPD.

Assessment During the nursing assessment, Mr. Cohen states that he thought his lack of appetite, nausea, vomiting, and fatigue over the past month was "a touch of the flu." His weight remained stable, so he didn't worry about not eating much.

Objective data includes BP 178/100; P 96; R 20; T 97.8° F (36.5° C) PO. His skin is cool and dry, with minor excoriations on his forearms and lower legs. Mr. Cohen has a fetid breath odor. A few fine crackles are noted in lung bases bilaterally. Both lower extremities have 3+ pitting edema to just below the knees; his hands also appear edematous. Bowel sounds are hypoactive. Urinalysis shows a specific gravity of 1.011 and gross proteinuria. CBC shows RBC 2.9 mill/mm^3; hemoglobin 9.4 g/dL; hematocrit 28%. His BUN is 198 mg/dL; creatinine 18.5 mg/dL; sodium 125 mEq/L; potassium 5.7 mEq/L; calcium 7.1 mg/dL; and phosphate 6.8 mg/dL.

Diagnosis The following nursing diagnoses are identified for Mr. Cohen:

- Excess Fluid Volume related to impaired kidney function
- Imbalanced Nutrition: Less Than Body Requirements related to effects of uremia
- Impaired Skin Integrity of extremities related to dry skin and itching
- Risk for Infection related to invasive catheters and impaired immune function

Expected Outcomes The expected outcomes for Mr. Cohen's plan of care are that he will:

- Adhere to the ordered fluid restriction of 750 mL per day.
- Demonstrate reduced fluid volume by weight loss, decreased peripheral edema, and clear lung sounds.
- Eat and retain 100% of prescribed diet, including snacks.
- Demonstrate healing of lesions on extremities.
- Remain free of infection.
- Demonstrate appropriate technique in performing catheter care and CAPD.

Planning and Implementation The following nursing interventions are planned and implemented for Mr. Cohen:

- Allocate fluids: 350 mL day shift, 250 mL evening shift, 100 mL at night.
- Provide mouth care every 4 hours and before every meal.
- Keep hard candy and ice chips at the bedside; include ice as fluid intake.
- Weigh daily; vital signs, including heart and lung sounds, every 4 hours.
- Intake and output every 4 hours.
- Arrange dietary consultation.
- Administer prescribed antiemetic 1 hour before meals.
- Monitor food intake.
- Clean lesions on lower extremities every 8 hours and assess healing.
- Teach CAPD procedure and peritoneal catheter care.

Evaluation Mr. Cohen underwent four hemodialysis sessions to treat his uremia. An arteriovenous fistula was created in his left arm for possible future hemodialysis. He began peritoneal dialysis, and by discharge was managing the catheter and dialysis runs with the help of his wife. His lungs are clear and his edema has resolved. The excoriations on his extremities have healed. His temperature is normal, and no evidence of infection is noted. Mr. Cohen remains anorectic and slightly nauseated but is eating most of his diet and snacks. After losing 10 pounds, his weight is now stable. Mr. Cohen and his wife have met another client who has been on CAPD for several years and who will help them with problem solving.

 Critical Thinking in the Nursing Process

1. How does diabetes mellitus damage the kidneys and lead to end-stage renal disease? Why is this seen more frequently in Type 1 diabetics than in Type 2?
2. How would discharge planning for Mr. Cohen differ if he planned to have hemodialysis at a dialysis center instead of CAPD?

Nursing Interventions Classification

Nursing interventions (McCloskey & Bulechek, 2000) that may be helpful in planning and implementing care for clients with renal and urinary tract disorders include the following:

- Fluid/Electrolyte Management
- Hemodialysis Therapy
- Infection Protection
- Nutritional Monitoring
- Ostomy Care
- Pelvic Floor Exercise
- Peritoneal Dialysis Therapy
- Teaching: Disease Process
- Tube Care: Urinary
- Urinary Catheterization: Intermittent
- Urinary Incontinence Care
- Urinary Retention Care

(*Note:* The bibliography listings for this and all chapters have been compiled at the back of the book.)

Chapter Review

key terms by topic

Use the CD-ROM disk enclosed with your textbook to hear the pronunciation of the key terms in the chapter.

Structure and function of the urinary system
glomeruli, nephrons, glomerular filtration rate (GFR)

Voiding disorders
urinary incontinence

Infectious and inflammatory disorders
cystitis, pyelonephritis, glomerulonephritis, proteinuria, azotemia, dysuria, nocturia, hematuria

Obstructive disorders
urolithiasis, hydronephrosis, renal colic

Kidney trauma
anuria

Tumors
cystectomy

Renal failure
renal failure, nephrotoxins, uremia, dialysis

key points

- Urinary incontinence, while often accepted as a normal part of aging in women, is not normal and can be treated.

- Lower urinary tract infections are common in women due to a short urethra and the proximity of the urethral meatus to the vagina and anus. Urinary tract infection in men, however, may indicate a structural, obstructive, or other problem of the urinary tract.

- Single-dose or a 3-day course of antibiotic therapy often is effective for treating uncomplicated UTIs. Added advantages are improved compliance and reduced adverse effects.

- Acute glomerulonephritis usually is due to an abnormal inflammatory response to beta-hemolytic streptococcal infection (strep throat). It usually resolves uneventfully in children and adults, but may lead to chronic glomerulonephritis and eventual kidney failure.

- Clients with a history of kidney or other urinary stones have a high risk of developing stones in the future. Emphasize the importance of maintaining a generous fluid intake, avoiding dehydration, and, for calcium stones, staying physically active and reducing calcium intake.

- Painless hematuria is a frequent initial manifestation of urinary tract cancer. Advise all clients with hematuria to see their physician for evaluation.

- Renal failure may be either acute or chronic.

  - Acute renal failure usually affects seriously ill older adults who experience hypovolemia or shock or who are exposed to a nephrotoxic drug or substance. Acute renal failure often resolves with treatment and kidney function is restored.

  - Chronic renal failure is the final stage of a long-term process of kidney destruction (due to diabetes, hypertension, lupus, or a primary kidney disease). Clients with chronic renal failure often require treatment to replace lost kidney function, such as dialysis or a kidney transplant.

Medialink

Additional interactive resources for this chapter can be found on the Companion Website at www.prenhall.com/burke. Click on Chapter 21 and "Begin" to select the activities for this chapter.

For NCLEX review questions and an audio glossary, access the accompanying CD-ROM in this book.

for further study

For more information on antidiuretic hormones, and the renin–angiotensin–aldosterone system, see Chapter 5.

For more about chemotherapy or radiation therapy, see Chapter 8.

For discussion of prostatectomy, see Chapter 32.

For further study about immunity, see Chapter 13.

For more information on calcium stones, see Chapter 16.

For more information about nursing implications for a kidney biopsy, see Box 21-13.

Critical Thinking Care Map

Caring for a Client with Urinary Incontinence
NCLEX-PN Focus Area: Health Promotion and Maintenance

Case Study: Anna Giovanni, a 76-year-old widow, lives alone. Her eldest daughter is concerned that her mother seems increasingly reluctant to leave the apartment to visit friends and family. She reports a strong odor of urine throughout her mother's apartment and that her mother's bed is often wet.

Nursing Diagnosis: Urinary Incontinence

COLLECT DATA

Subjective

_____

_____

_____

_____

_____

_____

Objective

_____

_____

_____

_____

_____

Would you report this data? Yes/No

If yes, to: _____

Nursing Care

_____

_____

_____

_____

_____

_____

_____

_____

How would you document this? _____

_____

_____

Data Collected
(use those that apply)

- Relates urine leakage when laughing, coughing, and on hearing the sound of running water
- Often unable to reach bathroom in time at night
- Hysterectomy at age 52
- Estrogen-replacement therapy for approximately 10 years after hysterectomy
- Takes digoxin 0.125 mg qd, furosemide 40 mg bid, and KCl 20 mEq tid
- Moderate cystourethrocele
- Atrophy of vaginal tissues
- Pelvic floor strength weak
- Urinalysis within normal limits
- Postvoiding residual urine 5 mL
- Average of nine daytime voidings and four at night
- Urine leakage usually occurs in late afternoon and at night

Nursing Interventions
(use those that apply)

- Teach how to identify pelvic floor muscles and perform Kegel exercises.
- Suggest decaffeinated tea and noncitrus fruit juices (grape, apple, and cranberry).
- Encourage minimizing fluid intake after evening meal.
- Change afternoon dose of furosemide from 9:00 P.M. to 4:00 P.M.
- Encourage voiding by the clock, gradually increasing intervals from every 45 to 60 minutes to every 2 to 2½ hours. Advise shorter intervals for 2 to 3 hours after furosemide doses.
- Suggest commercial products for protecting clothing and furniture.
- Provide bedside commode for nighttime use.
- Schedule follow-up visits and evaluations to reinforce teaching.

NCLEX-PN Exam Preparation

TEST-TAKING TIP

The LPN/LVN provides information to clients to prevent complications of disease or treatment. Be sure to study alterations in body systems and ways of teaching the client to manage his or her health after discharge from the health care facility.

1. A 79-year-old client with benign prostatic hypertrophy has not voided in the past 8 hours. The FIRST action by the LPN/LVN would be to:
   a. provide 500 mL fluids orally
   b. perform a catheterization with a 14 Fr. straight catheter
   c. palpate the lower abdomen
   d. notify the physician

2. A 50-year-old woman experiences stress incontinence. Which of the following assessment findings indicates a risk factor for this condition?
   a. total abdominal hysterectomy 9 years ago
   b. smokes one pack of cigarettes per day
   c. exercises four times a week
   d. history of two pregnancies

3. An LVN performs a residual urine on a client; 30 mL of clear yellow urine is returned. The appropriate action by the nurse would be to:
   a. notify the physician
   b. document the finding in the medical record
   c. implement measures to assist the client to void
   d. increase client's fluid intake

4. The nurse establishes a nursing diagnosis of Urinary Incontinence related to weak pelvic floor muscles for a 69-year-old client. Which of the following would be an appropriate nursing intervention?
   a. Encourage client to drink orange juice and tea at each meal.
   b. Schedule furosemide (Lasix) 40 mg at 8 P.M. daily.
   c. Teach to perform Kegel exercises every 2 hours while awake.
   d. Restrict fluid intake to 500 mL/day.

5. The nurse teaches a client to help prevent urinary tract infections by maintaining acidic urine. A means to accomplish this is to drink two glasses of _____ daily.
   a. skim milk
   b. cranberry juice
   c. water
   d. apple juice

6. A 9-year-old is admitted with acute glomerulonephritis. The nurse expects to obtain which of the following assessment findings?
   a. "strep throat" 2 weeks ago
   b. pneumonia 1 week ago
   c. gastroenteritis
   d. influenza 3 weeks ago

7. For a client with a ureteral calculus, a priority nursing action is to
   a. wash hands
   b. restrict fluids
   c. strain all urine
   d. collect a sterile urine specimen

8. A female client is discharged following a right nephrotomy to remove a urinary calculus. Discharge teaching should include:
   a. maintaining oral fluid intake of 1,500 mL daily
   b. avoiding all sources of calcium
   c. signs and symptoms of urinary tract infection
   d. maintaining alkaline urine

9. A client is diagnosed with chronic renal failure. The nurse explains that dietary management of a client with chronic renal failure includes:
   a. high protein, low carbohydrate
   b. low protein, high carbohydrate
   c. high fat, moderate sodium
   d. low fat, high sodium

10. A client has an arteriovenous (AV) fistula in his left arm for hemodialysis access. The nurse recognizes the need for further teaching if the client states:
    a. "My wife gets the best blood pressure in my left arm."
    b. "I check my fistula for pulsations."
    c. "I remind the lab personnel to take blood from my right arm."
    d. "I sleep on my left side with my left arm extended."

Answers for Review Questions, as well as discussion of Case Study Critical Thinking questions, appear in Appendix V.

Cultural Care STRATEGIES

Considering Cultural Variations Related to Time

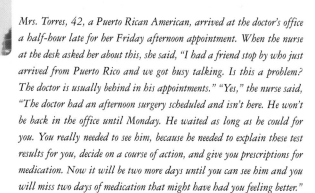

Mrs. Torres, 42, a Puerto Rican American, arrived at the doctor's office a half-hour late for her Friday afternoon appointment. When the nurse at the desk asked her about this, she said, "I had a friend stop by who just arrived from Puerto Rico and we got busy talking. Is this a problem? The doctor is usually behind in his appointments." "Yes," the nurse said, "The doctor had an afternoon surgery scheduled and isn't here. He won't be back in the office until Monday. He waited as long as he could for you. You really needed to see him, because he needed to explain these test results for you, decide on a course of action, and give you prescriptions for medication. Now it will be two more days until you can see him and you will miss two days of medication that might have had you feeling better."

Time is an important but seldom recognized aspect of interpersonal communication. While the phenomenon of time varies among individuals, a person's concept of time is largely the result of experiences within his or her culture of origin (Giger & Davidhizar, 1999). Individuals learn the concept of time from persons and events in their environment, and it becomes integrated into every segment of their behavior and thought. Thus, it is essential for nurses to understand how perceptions of time vary, so culturally competent and sensitive care can be delivered. In the case of Mrs. Torres, the failure to arrive at her appointment on time will delay her recovery. If the nurse had emphasized the need to keep this appointment exactly as scheduled, Mrs. Torres might have made this a higher priority than visiting with her friend.

Temporal Orientation

Temporal orientation refers to the ordering of past, present, and future events. People who focus on the past have little motivation for formulating future goals that include primary prevention and health promotion activities. For example, Native Americans or the Old Order Amish may be viewed as past-oriented individuals. They hold strongly to traditions and values passed from generation to generation. This belief pattern directly reflects their social order and health care practices (Buccalo, 1997).

For people whose culture is present-oriented, the present task is viewed as most important, such as visiting with a friend who has dropped by. These people are unlikely to adhere to rigid time schedules; instead, they focus on the current activity. Present time orientation may also result in nonadherence to medication regimens, visiting hours at the hospital, and follow up appointments. For example, a teenager may get caught up in an activity and miss an appointment that required arriving at a precise time (Davidhizar, Bechtel, & Giger, 1999).

People who have future time orientation organize and plan their activities to achieve future goals. Many middle-class Americans, regardless of ethnic or cultural origin, tend to be future oriented. They may delay starting a family, purchasing a house, or purchasing an expensive car until education is successfully completed and financial success has been attained. Future-oriented individuals may seem cold and detached and may focus more on tasks to accomplish future goals than on relationships.

Clock vs. Social Time

Most people in North America organize their activities around the clock, arriving at places or starting behaviors at a very specified time determined by hours and minutes. Some groups, however, initiate activities and behaviors on the basis of social time. For them, events such as weddings or church services may start when everyone arrives and stop when the event is completed. For these individuals, time is qualitative rather than quantitative (Giger & Davidhizar, 1999).

Nursing Implications

- **Assess individuals for time orientation.** The nurse needs to relate health care teaching to the client's perspective of time. For example, when a client is present rather than future oriented, the nurse needs to relate present actions to current health status, not to the future.
- **Care planning should be based on cultural orientation.** By acknowledging other time perceptions, the nurse can plan interventions to assist the client to adapt behavior to meet health needs. For example, stressing the importance of keeping appointments on time, of taking medication as ordered, and of complying with care regimens can increase the client's compliance.
- **Differences in behavior by health team members may be related to time perception.** Some team members who are social-time rather than clock-time oriented may have difficulty with punctuality and strict adherence to the time frames for treatments and medication administration.

Self-Reflection Questions

1. What is your predominant time orientation: past, present, or future?
2. Are you predominantly clock-time oriented or social-time oriented?
3. If your client or co-workers do not share your time orientation, what problems can occur?

chapter

22

Caring for Clients with Cardiac Disorders

CARING tip

❝Get involved at your facility. Volunteer for committees, quality management, risk management, etc.❞

Hilary H. Hamilton, BSN, MEd • Director, Practical Nursing Program •
Southeastern Technical Institute • South Easton, Massachusetts

LEARNING outcomes

After completing this chapter, you will be able to:
- Describe the structure and function of the heart.
- Discuss the mechanical and electrical properties of the heart.
- Compare and contrast the causes, pathophysiology, effects, and manifestations of common cardiac disorders.
- Identify nursing responsibilities for common diagnostic tests and monitors for clients with heart disease.
- Discuss nursing implications for drugs commonly prescribed for clients with heart disease.
- Describe nursing care for clients undergoing invasive procedures or surgery of the heart.
- Use the nursing process to collect assessment data, contribute to care planning, and provide individualized nursing care for clients with disorders of the heart.
- Provide and reinforce appropriate teaching for clients with heart disorders and their families.

MediaLink

 www.prenhall.com/burke

Use the above address to access the free, interactive Companion Website created for this textbook. Get hints, instant feedback, and textbook references to chapter-related multiple choice questions. Link to other interesting sites.

Cardiovascular disease (CVD) is the leading cause of death and disability in the United States. Approximately 21 million people are affected by heart disease and more than 700,000 people die from it each year. Public education efforts aimed at reducing fat intake, increasing exercise, and lowering stress levels have made people more aware of risk factors for heart disease, and the incidence of new cases has fallen.

Alterations in the electrical system of the heart, impaired blood flow to the heart muscle, and structural changes in the heart affect its ability to fulfill its major purpose: to pump enough blood to meet the body's demand for oxygen and nutrients. When the heart is unable to function effectively, other organ systems may fail because their fuel supply is impaired.

Nurses need to know about heart disease and its causes to teach and care for clients appropriately. This chapter provides the beginning nurse with the tools necessary to assess, plan, implement, and evaluate care for the client with cardiac disease.

Structure and Function of the Heart

The heart, a hollow, cone-shaped organ approximately the size of an adult's fist, weighs less than 1 lb. It is located behind the sternum and between the lungs in the thoracic cavity, slightly to the left of midline (Figure 22-1 ◆). The heart is a double pump: The right side receives blood from the body and pumps it to the lungs; the left side receives blood from the lungs and pumps it to the body.

STRUCTURE OF THE HEART

The heart is covered by the **pericardium.** The pericardium encases the heart and anchors it to surrounding structures. It has two layers: The *parietal pericardium* is the outermost layer, and the *visceral pericardium* (also called the *epicardium*) adheres to the heart surface. The small space between these layers contains serous lubricating fluid that cushions the heart as it beats. The epicardium is the outermost layer of the heart wall.

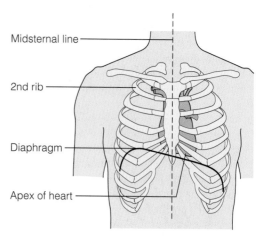

Figure 22-1. ◆ Location of the heart within the chest cavity.

The middle layer is the **myocardium,** or heart muscle, and the innermost layer, the **endocardium,** lines the inside of the heart's chambers and great vessels (Figure 22-2 ◆).

The heart has four hollow chambers: two upper *atria* and two lower *ventricles.* A septum (or wall) separates the two sides of the heart; *atrioventricular (AV) valves* separate the atria from the ventricles. The flaps of these valves are anchored to the muscles of the ventricles by the chordae tendineae. These structures prevent the backflow of blood during contraction of the higher-pressure ventricles.

The *right atrium* receives deoxygenated blood from the veins of the body via the *superior* and *inferior vena cavae.* The right atrium is separated from the right ventricle by the *tricuspid valve.* When open, deoxygenated blood flows through this valve into the *right ventricle,* which then pumps it through the *pulmonary artery* to the lungs (Figure 22-3 ◆).

The *left atrium* receives freshly oxygenated blood from the lungs through the *pulmonary veins.* The *left ventricle,* separated from the left atria by the *bicuspid* or *mitral valve,* pumps this freshly oxygenated blood out the *aorta* to the systemic circulation.

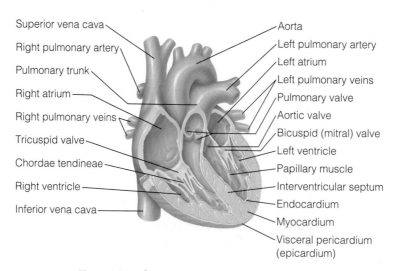

Figure 22-2. ◆ The internal anatomy of the heart.

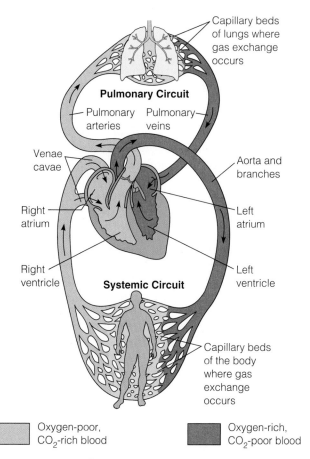

Figure 22-3. ◈ Pulmonary and systemic circulation.

Oxygen-poor,
CO_2-rich blood

Oxygen-rich,
CO_2-poor blood

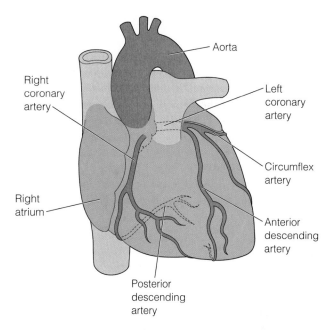

Figure 22-4. ◈ The coronary arteries.

The ventricles are connected to their great vessels by the *semilunar valves.* On the right, the *pulmonary valve* joins the right ventricle with the pulmonary artery. On the left, the *aortic valve* joins the left ventricle to the aorta.

The AV valves close as the ventricles start to contract, producing the first heart sound, or S_1 ("lub"). As the ventricles start to relax after contraction, the semilunar valves close, producing the second heart sound, or S_2 ("dup").

The *coronary circulation* supplies blood to the heart muscle. The *left* and *right coronary arteries* originate at the base of the aorta and branch out to encircle the myocardium (Figure 22-4 ◈). The coronary arteries fill with oxygen-rich blood during ventricular relaxation. Then, after the blood perfuses the heart muscle, the *cardiac veins* drain the blood into the coronary sinus, which empties into the right atrium of the heart.

CONDUCTION SYSTEM

Cardiac muscle is unique. Unlike skeletal muscle tissue, cardiac muscle can generate an electrical impulse and contraction independent of the nervous system. The heartbeat is controlled by specialized cells within the myocardium known as the *conduction system.* The structures of the cardiac conduction system include the sinoatrial node, internodal pathways, atrioventricular node, bundle of His, right and left bundle branches, and Purkinje fibers (Figure 22-5 ◈).

The *sinoatrial (SA) node,* located in the wall of the right atrium, acts as the "pacemaker" of the heart, usually generating an impulse 60 to 100 times per minute. This impulse travels through the *internodal pathways* to the *atrioventricular (AV) node* at the junction between the atria and ventricles. The impulse is slowed as it moves through the AV node, slightly delaying its transmission to the ventricles. It then passes through the *bundle of His* and continues down the interventricular septum through the *right* and *left bundle branches* and out to the *Purkinje fibers* in the ventricular muscle walls.

The electrical impulse, or *action potential,* generated by pacemaker cells is caused by the movement of ions across cell membranes. At rest, myocardial cells are *polarized,* or have a negative charge. The action potential causes the cell membrane to become more positive. This is known as *depolarization.* The action potential and depolarization cause the muscle

Sinoatrial (SA) node
(pacemaker)

Internodal
pathways

Atrioventricular (AV)
node

Bundle of His

Right bundle branch

Left bundle branch

Purkinje fibers

Figure 22-5. ◈ The cardiac conduction system.

to contract. With each beat, the heart muscle contracts to its fullest potential (the *all-or-nothing response*). *Repolarization* begins immediately after depolarization, returning the cell to its resting state. For a brief period during and after repolarization, the cell resists stimulation. This is known as the *refractory period*. It protects the heart muscle from going into spasm or tetany (continuous contraction). This electrical activity produces the waveforms represented on ECG strips.

Electrocardiography

The *electrocardiogram (ECG)* is a record of the heart's electrical activity detected by electrodes placed on the skin (Box 22-1).

ECG waveforms and patterns are used to detect dysrhythmias, myocardial damage or enlargement, and the effects of drugs.

Electrocardiography may be used on a continual or intermittent basis, depending on the client's needs.

CARDIAC CYCLE

The contraction and relaxation of the heart constitutes one heartbeat and is called the cardiac cycle (Figure 22-6 ◆). Ventricular filling occurs during *diastole*, when the ventricles are relaxed. Toward the end of diastole, the atria contract, pumping additional blood into the ventricles. During *ventricular systole*,

---

BOX 22-1   ELECTROCARDIOGRAM

An electrocardiogram (ECG) is a "picture" of the heart's electrical activity. Electrodes placed on different parts of the body allow different views of the heart's electrical activity, much like turning while holding a camera provides different views of the scenery.

A standard 12-lead ECG includes recordings of 6 limb leads and 6 precordial leads. The *limb leads* provide a view of the inferior and lateral walls of the heart. The *precordial leads* (chest or V leads) provide a view of the anterior, septal, lateral, and posterior walls of the heart.

ECG waveforms show the direction of electrical flow. Current moving toward the positive electrode causes an upward (positive) waveform; current moving away from it produces a downward (negative) waveform. When no electrical activity is occurring, a straight line, called the *isoelectric line*, is seen.

ECG waveforms are recorded on paper marked at intervals that represent time and voltage or amplitude (see first figure). Each small box represents 0.04 seconds. Five small boxes make one large box, equivalent to 0.20 seconds. Five large boxes represent 1 full second.

1 large box or 5 mm = 0.5 mV

1 large box or 5 mm = 0.20 second

1 small box or 1 mm = 0.04 second

1 mm = 0.1 mV

The P, Q, R, S, and T waves represent the cardiac cycle (see second figure). The P *wave* shows the SA node impulse and atrial depolarization. It precedes the QRS complex and is normally smooth, round, and upright. The PR *interval* is the time required for the impulse to travel to the AV node and the bundle branches. It is measured from beginning of P wave to beginning of QRS complex. The PR interval is normally 0.12 to 0.20 seconds.

The *QRS complex* indicates ventricular depolarization. It occurs rapidly, lasting from 0.06 to 0.10 seconds. The *ST segment*, the period from the end of the QRS complex to the beginning of the T wave, is normally isoelectric. The T wave represents ventricular repolarization. It is smooth and rounded, and points in the same direction as the QRS complex. The *QT interval*, measured from the beginning of the QRS to the end of the T wave, indicates the total time for ventricular depolarization and repolarization. Its duration varies with gender, age, and heart rate; usually, it is 0.32 to 0.44 seconds long. The *U wave* is not normally seen but may show repolarization of the terminal Purkinje fibers.

Left atrium
Right atrium
Left ventricle
Right ventricle

| Passive filling | Atrial contraction | AV valves close | Semilunar valves open; ventricles eject blood |

1

Ventricular diastole
(Ventricular filling)

2

Ventricular systole

Figure 22-6. ◆ The cardiac cycle. Ventricular filling occurs during diastole (1); blood is pumped out of the heart to the pulmonary and systemic circulation during ventricular systole (2).

the ventricles contract, ejecting blood into the pulmonary and systemic circuits. Normally, the complete cardiac cycle occurs about 70 to 80 times per minute (the *heart rate*).

CARDIAC OUTPUT

With each contraction, a certain volume of blood (approximately 70 mL in an adult), called the *stroke volume (SV),* is ejected from the heart. The *cardiac output (CO)* is the amount of blood pumped by the ventricles in 1 minute. Cardiac output indicates how well the heart is functioning as a pump. It is calculated by multiplying the stroke volume by the heart rate (HR):

$$CO = HR \times SV$$

The average adult cardiac output ranges from 4 to 8 liters per minute (L/min).

The heart regulates cardiac output to meet the body's needs. As oxygen demand increases, oxygen supply must also increase. *Cardiac reserve* is the ability of the heart to increase CO and blood pressure to meet the demand. Cardiac output is determined by four major factors: heart rate, preload, afterload, and contractility.

Heart rate is affected by activity level, the autonomic nervous system, and hormones. Increased heart rates increase cardiac output; however, very rapid heart rates allow less time for

ventricular filling and may reduce stroke volume and cardiac output. If the heart rate is too slow, cardiac output falls simply because the heart contracts less often.

Preload is the amount of blood in the ventricles prior to contraction. The blood in the ventricles stretches the muscle fibers, causing them to contract more forcefully. Preload is affected by venous return. If blood volume is low (e.g., due to hemorrhage or dehydration), it falls. To a certain point, the greater the blood volume, the greater force with which the ventricle contracts. Beyond a certain volume, however, the heart contracts less effectively. This is called *Starling's law of the heart.*

Afterload is the force the ventricles must develop to push blood into the circulation. The right ventricle pushes blood into the low-pressure pulmonary system. The left ventricle ejects its blood into the systemic circulation. Systemic arterial pressures are much higher than pulmonary pressures; therefore the left ventricle has to work much harder than the right ventricle.

Contractility is the natural ability of the cardiac muscle fibers to shorten during systole. Contractility is necessary to move blood into the circulation. Poor contractility reduces the ability of the ventricle to eject blood, decreasing stroke volume. The *ejection fraction,* or percentage of blood in the ventricle that is ejected with each contraction, is affected by the interaction of preload, afterload, and contractility.

Cardiac Rhythm Disorders

Cardiac Dysrhythmias

The heart contracts in response to electrical stimulation of its cells. In the normal heart, this produces a coordinated, rhythmic contraction that pushes blood into circulation. The normal heart rhythm is *normal sinus rhythm (NSR)*. Impulses originate in the SA node and travel through normal conduction pathways without delay. The rate is between 60 and 100 bpm. Changes from this rhythm can affect the heart's ability to pump blood effectively to body tissues.

A **cardiac dysrhythmia** is a disturbance or irregularity in the electrical system of the heart. Cardiac dysrhythmias may be benign or life threatening. Changes in heart rhythm occur due to "normal" events such as exercise or fear, as well as to pathologic changes. Any dysrhythmia can affect cardiac output. The effect of the dysrhythmia determines the need for treatment. Box 22-2 lists steps for heart rhythm analysis.

PATHOPHYSIOLOGY

Dysrhythmias develop when normal impulse formation is disrupted or conduction of the impulse through the heart is altered.

Abnormalities of impulse formation are caused by changes in automaticity. Impulses may develop more rapidly or more slowly than normal, or may originate outside the SA node. These are called *ectopic beats*.

An impulse may be blocked or delayed as it moves through the conduction pathways of the heart. This is known as *heart block*. In some cases, an impulse is delayed in one area of the heart but conducted normally through the rest. This pattern of normal and slow conduction, known as *reentry phenomenon*, may cause many dysrhythmias.

Cardiac rhythms are classified according to the site of impulse formation or the site and degree of conduction block (Table 22-1 ◆). In *supraventricular rhythms,* impulses form above the ventricles. *Ventricular rhythms* originate in the ventricles and may be fatal. *AV conduction blocks* result from impaired impulse transmission from the atria to the ventricles. See Box 22-3 for a discussion of dysrhythmias in older adults.

Supraventricular Rhythms

SINUS TACHYCARDIA. In *sinus tachycardia,* the heart rate is greater than 100 bpm. Tachycardia is a normal response to conditions that increase the body's demand for oxygen and nutrients, such as exercise. Other causes of sinus tachycardia include anxiety, pain, fever, hypoxia, hyperthyroidism, caffeine intake, and some drugs. Sinus tachycardia may be an early warning sign of cardiac problems such as heart failure.

The client with sinus tachycardia has a rapid pulse rate and may complain of a "racing" heart or shortness of breath. Clients with heart disease may experience chest pain.

SINUS BRADYCARDIA. *Sinus bradycardia* is a heart rate less than 60 bpm. It may be normal in some clients (e.g., clients with athletic heart syndrome) and during sleep. Bradycardia

---

BOX 22-2

ECG RHYTHM ANALYSIS

Interpreting an ECG strip is a skill that takes practice. Use a consistent, systematic method to determine the heart rhythm. A suggested sequence of steps follows.

1. *Determine rate.* Assess the heart rate using one of the following to determine number of beats per minute (bpm):
   • Count the number of R waves in a 6-second strip and multiply by 10.
   • Count the number of large boxes between two consecutive R waves, and divide 300 (the number of large boxes in 1 minute) by this number. For example, there are 6 large boxes between two R waves; 300 ÷ 6 = 50 BPM.
   • Memorize the following sequence: 300, 150, 100, 75, 60, 50. One large box between complexes equals a rate of 300; two = 150; three = 100, and so on.
2. *Determine regularity.* Measure the interval from one R wave to the next R wave, then evaluate successive R to R intervals for their regularity. Irregular rhythms may be *irregularly irregular* (if there is no pattern to the irregularity) or *regularly irregular* (if a consistent pattern can be identified).
3. *Assess P waves.* All the P waves should look alike in size and shape.
4. *Assess P to QRS relationship.* There should be one P wave before every QRS complex and one QRS complex following every P wave.
5. *Measure PR interval and QRS complex.* To determine the duration of any interval, count the number of small boxes from the beginning of the interval to the end, and multiply by 0.04 seconds. The normal PR interval is 0.12 to 0.20 seconds; the normal QRS complex lasts 0.06 to 0.10 seconds.
6. *Identify abnormalities.* Note any ectopic (abnormal) beats, deviation of the ST segment above or below the baseline, and abnormalities in waveform shape and duration.

TABLE 22-1

CHARACTERISTICS, CAUSES, AND MANAGEMENT OF SELECTED CARDIAC RHYTHMS

RHYTHM/ECG APPEARANCE	CHARACTERISTICS AND MANIFESTATIONS	MANAGEMENT
Supraventricular Rhythms Normal sinus rhythm (NSR)	Regular; rate 60–100 bpm. All waveforms and intervals are normal.	None; normal heart rhythm
Sinus tachycardia	Regular; rate > 100 bpm. Other characteristics as for NSR	Treated only if symptomatic or if client at risk for myocardial infarction (MI)
Sinus bradycardia	Regular; rate < 60 bpm. Other characteristics as for NSR	Treated only if symptomatic; may give atropine or require pacemaker
Premature atrial contractions (PACs)	Irregular, an ectopic atrial beat occurring earlier than expected	Usually require no treatment
Atrial flutter	Usually regular with sawtooth appearance of P waves. Atrial rate 240+ bpm; ventricular rate < 150 bpm	Synchronized cardioversion; medication to slow ventricular response

(continues)

TABLE 22-1 CHARACTERISTICS, CAUSES, AND MANAGEMENT OF SELECTED CARDIAC RHYTHMS (CONTINUED)

RHYTHM/ECG APPEARANCE	CHARACTERISTICS AND MANIFESTATIONS	MANAGEMENT
Atrial fibrillation 	Irregularly irregular; no identifiable P waves; variable ventricular rate	Synchronized cardioversion; medication to slow ventricular rate; anticoagulants to reduce risk of stroke
Ventricular Rhythms Premature ventricular contractions (PVCs) 	Irregular; ectopic ventricular beat interrupts normal rhythm; ectopic QRS wide and bizarre	Abstain from nicotine, caffeine; medication if symptomatic or if result of recent MI
Ventricular tachycardia (VT or V-tach) 	Regular; rate 100–250 bpm; no identifiable P waves, QRS wide and bizarre	Treated if symptomatic; intravenous drugs; cardioversion or defibrillation if unconscious or unstable
Ventricular fibrillation (V-fib) 	Grossly irregular; rate too rapid to count; no P waves, QRS bizarre and variable	Immediate defibrillation necessary to preserve life
AV Conduction Blocks First-degree AV block 	Regular; rate usually 60–100 bpm; PR interval > 0.21 sec	No treatment necessary

TABLE 22-1   CHARACTERISTICS, CAUSES, AND MANAGEMENT OF SELECTED CARDIAC RHYTHMS (CONTINUED)

RHYTHM/ECG APPEARANCE	CHARACTERISTICS AND MANIFESTATIONS	MANAGEMENT
Second-degree AV block	Atrial rate regular, ventricular rate irregular; some P waves not followed by QRS, PR interval may vary	Monitoring and observation; drug or pacemaker therapy may be required
Third-degree AV block (complete heart block)	Atrial rate regular (60–100 bpm), ventricular rate regular (30–40 bpm); no relationship between P waves and QRS complexes	Immediate pacemaker therapy

BOX 22-3   population FOCUS

Dysrhythmias in Older Adults

Aging affects the heart and the cardiac conduction system, increasing the risk for dysrhythmias, even when no other evidence of heart disease is found. Older adults are more likely to experience ectopic beats during exercise. AV blocks also are more common in people over the age of 65.

Assessing dysrhythmias in older adults focuses on the effect on function.

- Inquire about episodes of dizziness, light-headedness, fainting, palpitations, chest pain, or shortness of breath.
- Ask about the relationship of symptoms to food intake and caffeine-containing beverages.
- Evaluate other contributing factors such as heart disease, medications, smoking, or alcohol intake.
- Inquire about falls, particularly those occurring without apparent reason.

Teach older adults to reduce their risk for dysrhythmias and their consequences by:

- Taking medications (including over-the-counter drugs) as ordered.
- Eliminating caffeine intake.
- Stopping smoking and eliminate alcohol intake if appropriate.
- Engaging in regular exercise.
- Contacting their primary care provider for symptoms such as dizziness, fainting, frequent palpitations, shortness of breath, unexplained falls, or chest pain.

also may be caused by pain, increased intracranial pressure, hypothermia, heart disease, and certain drugs.

Clients with sinus bradycardia may be asymptomatic or may have manifestations of decreased cardiac output, such as decreased level of consciousness, syncope (faintness), or hypotension.

PREMATURE ATRIAL CONTRACTIONS. A *premature atrial contraction (PAC)* is an ectopic atrial beat that occurs earlier than the next expected sinus beat. PACs are usually asymptomatic and benign, but they may initiate supraventricular tachycardia in some people. PACs are common in older adults, and may occur without an obvious cause. Frequent PACs may cause heart palpitations or a fluttering sensation in the chest.

Supraventricular tachycardia (SVT) is usually characterized by a sudden onset and abrupt cessation. It may be caused by sympathetic nervous system stimulation and stressors such as fever, sepsis, and hyperthyroidism. Manifestations of SVT include complaints of palpitations and a "racing" heart, anxiety, dizziness, dyspnea, chest pain, diaphoresis, and fatigue.

ATRIAL FLUTTER. *Atrial flutter* is a very rapid and regular atrial rhythm. Causes include sympathetic nervous system stimulation due to anxiety, caffeine, and alcohol intake; thyrotoxicosis; and heart disease.

Clients with atrial flutter may complain of palpitations or a fluttering sensation in the chest or throat. If the ventricular rate is rapid, cardiac output falls, causing decreased level of consciousness, hypotension, decreased urinary output, and cool, clammy skin.

ATRIAL FIBRILLATION. *Atrial fibrillation* is a common dysrhythmia characterized by disorganized atrial activity without discrete atrial contractions. Extremely rapid impulses bombard the AV node, causing an irregularly irregular ventricular response. Atrial fibrillation may occur suddenly and recur, or it may become chronic. It is common in clients with heart failure.

Manifestations of atrial fibrillation include irregular pulses of variable strength. The client may have hypotension, shortness of breath, fatigue, and angina. Clients with extensive heart disease may develop syncope or heart failure.

Atrial fibrillation increases the risk of forming thromboemboli (blood clots). Stroke (brain attack) is a risk because these clots may travel to the brain.

Ventricular Dysrhythmias

Ventricular dysrhythmias originate in the ventricles. Because the ventricles pump blood into the pulmonary and systemic vasculature, any disturbance in their rhythm can affect cardiac output and tissue perfusion. A wide and bizarre QRS complex (greater than 0.12 sec) is a characteristic feature of ventricular dysrhythmias.

PREMATURE VENTRICULAR CONTRACTIONS. *Premature ventricular contractions (PVCs)* are ectopic ventricular beats that occur before the next expected beat of the normal rhythm. PVCs may be isolated or occur in patterns such as every other beat, in pairs, or in triplets (three in a row). Isolated PVCs often are benign. They may be triggered by anxiety or stress, tobacco, alcohol, or caffeine. Benign PVCs are common in older adults. In people with heart disease, PVCs are common. Frequent PVCs may signal an increased risk for lethal dysrhythmias.

Clients experiencing PVCs may complain of feeling their hearts "skip a beat" or of palpitations. The early beat may be heard on auscultation; it is felt as a "missed" beat on palpation of peripheral pulses.

VENTRICULAR TACHYCARDIA. *Ventricular tachycardia (VT; V-tach)* is three or more consecutive PVCs. VT may occur in short bursts, or "runs," or it may persist for longer periods. The rate is greater than 100 bpm, and the rhythm is usually regular. Myocardial ischemia and infarction are the most common causes of VT, although it also may occur with other heart diseases or in the absence of heart disease. It may be associated with anorexia nervosa, metabolic disorders, and drug toxicity.

Short bursts of VT may cause a sensation of fluttering in the chest, palpitations, and brief shortness of breath. Cardiac ouput drops with sustained VT, causing severe hypotension, a weak or nonpalpable pulse, and loss of consciousness. Allowed to continue, VT can deteriorate into ventricular fibrillation at any time. Sustained VT is a medical emergency that requires immediate intervention to preserve life.

VENTRICULAR FIBRILLATION. *Ventricular fibrillation (V-fib)* is defined as extremely rapid, chaotic ventricular depolarization that causes the ventricles to quiver and stop contracting; the heart does not pump. This is known as **cardiac arrest,** a medical emergency requiring immediate intervention with cardiopulmonary resuscitation (CPR) measures. Death will follow the onset of V-fib within 4 minutes if the rhythm is not recognized and terminated, with a return to a perfusing rhythm.

V-fib is usually triggered by severe myocardial ischemia or infarction. It occurs without warning 50% of the time. It is the terminal event in many disease processes or traumatic conditions. V-fib also may be caused by digitalis toxicity, electrolyte and acid base imbalances, certain drugs, mechanical stimulation (as with the insertion of cardiac catheters or pacing wires), and electric shock.

Clinically, loss of ventricular contraction causes the pulse to cease. The client loses consciousness and stops breathing *(cardiopulmonary arrest).*

Atrioventricular Conduction Blocks

Conduction defects that cause delayed or blocked transmission of sinus impulse through the AV node are called *atrioventricular (AV) conduction blocks.* AV blocks vary from benign to severe.

FIRST-DEGREE AV BLOCK. *First-degree AV block* is a benign conduction delay that poses no immediate threat and requires no treatment. There are no clinical manifestations except a prolonged PR interval. Causes of first degree block include myocardial infarction, digitalis therapy or toxicity, complications from cardiac surgery, chronic heart disease, or drug effects.

SECOND-DEGREE AV BLOCK. In *second-degree AV block,* some atrial impulses are totally blocked at the AV node, prevented from reaching the ventricles. Two types of second-degree block are recognized. *Type I,* also known as Mobitz I or Wenckebach, is characterized by a repeating pattern in which PR intervals become progressively longer until one QRS complex is not conducted, or dropped. It is usually asymptomatic, unless the heart rate slows and cardiac output falls.

Type II, also called Mobitz II, is characterized by a regular pattern of nonconducted impulses; usually, two atrial impulses occur for every one that is transmitted to the ventricles. Type II heart block is usually associated with acute myocardial infarction. Its manifestations depend on the ventricular rate and cardiac output.

THIRD-DEGREE AV BLOCK. *Third-degree AV block (complete heart block)* occurs when atrial impulses are completely blocked at the AV node and not conducted to the ventricles. Atrial and ventricular rhythms are completely independent of one another. The ventricular impulse is slow at a rate of 30 to 40 bpm, while the normal atrial rate of 60 to 100 bpm continues.

Third-degree block is frequently caused by an acute myocardial infarction. Other heart diseases, drugs, and electrolyte imbalances also can precipitate it. Cardiac output falls, leading to light-headedness, confusion, and syncope (fainting). Third-degree AV block is life threatening and requires immediate treatment to restore the cardiac output.

COLLABORATIVE CARE

While many dysrhythmias pose little risk, others, such as ventricular fibrillation, are life-threatening and require immediate intervention. Early recognition is vital. Clients at risk for dysrhythmias often are cared for in cardiac intensive care or other specialty units that allow constant monitoring of the ECG and client's status.

Cardiac Monitoring

Cardiac monitoring allows continuous observation of the client's cardiac rhythm. Different types of ECG monitoring are employed for different situations.

CONTINUOUS CARDIAC MONITORING. Electrodes placed on the client's chest are connected to monitoring system. The heart rate and rhythm are visually displayed on a bedside monitor and a central monitoring station. Alarms on the monitors warn of potential problems such as very rapid or very slow heart rates. Procedure 22-1 describes how to initiate cardiac monitoring.

PORTABLE CARDIAC MONITORING. Distance ECG monitoring (telemetry) is a type of continuous monitoring frequently used on medical-surgical or cardiac units. Chest electrodes are connected to portable transmitters worn around the neck or waist; the cardiac rhythm is transmitted electronically to a central monitoring station. Telemetry allows the client to get out of bed and walk around while being monitored.

Ambulatory or Holter monitoring may be used in community settings. Electrodes are applied and the leads attached to a portable unit that records and stores electrical activity. Some ambulatory monitors record continuously for a 24- to 72-hour period. Others allow the client to record cardiac activity intermittently when symptoms are experienced (such as chest pain or palpitations).

PROCEDURE 22-1   Initiating Cardiac Monitoring Checklist

- Gather supplies.
- Provide for privacy.
- Explain the reason for ECG monitoring, reassuring the client that it allows immediate treatment of abnormal rhythms if necessary. Explain alarms, their purpose, and possible causes such as loose or disconnected lead wires and other mechanical problems. Activity is permitted within ordered restrictions while on the monitor.
- Follow standard precautions.
- Check equipment for damage (i.e., fraying, bent, or broken wires). Connect lead wires to cable, and secure the connections.
- Select electrode sites on the chest wall, considering lead to be monitored, skin condition, and any incisions or catheters.
- Clean sites with soap and water, and dry thoroughly. Alcohol may be used to remove skin oils; allow the skin to dry for 60 seconds after use.
- Peel backing from a fresh electrode; check to ensure that the pad is moist with conductive gel.
- Apply electrode pads, pressing firmly to ensure contact.
- Attach leads and position cable with sufficient slack for comfort. Place telemetry unit (if used) in gown pouch or pocket.

- Assess ECG tracing on the monitor, adjusting settings as needed.
- Set ECG monitor alarm limits as indicated, typically at 20 bpm higher and lower than the baseline rate. Turn alarms on, and leave on at all times. Assess immediately if an alarm is triggered.
- Remove and apply new pads every 24 to 48 hours and as needed. Clean gel residue from previous site, and document skin condition. Use a different site if skin appears irritated or blistered. Time and date pads with every change.
- Save ECG strips according to unit policy, and when the rhythm or the client's condition changes. Note date, time, client, and monitor lead on each strip. Notify the charge nurse or physician of significant changes in heart rhythm.

■ SAMPLE DOCUMENTATION

| 12/8/03 | 1430 | Placed on cardiac monitor, lead 2. Monitor shows NSR at 75/min with no ectopy noted. Resting comfortably. |
| | | _____ S. Craven, LPN. |

Pharmacology

Antidysrhythmic drugs may be used to treat acute dysrhythmias or to manage chronic conditions. The overall goal of therapy is to maintain an effective cardiac output by stabilizing cardiac rhythm.

Many different classes of drugs are used to treat cardiac dysrhythmias. Table 22-2 ◆ identifies common antidysrhythmic drugs, their class, and the nursing implications in caring for the client receiving an antidysrhythmic drug.

CLINICAL alert

All antidysrhythmic drugs can also *cause* dysrhythmias. Closely monitor all clients receiving cardiac drugs for dysrhythmias.

Cardioversion/Defibrillation

Cardioversion (or defibrillation) is used to treat rhythms that affect cardiac output and the client's welfare. An electrical shock is administered to depolarize all cells of the heart at the same time. This often stops the abnormal rhythm and allows the sinus node to resume control of the rhythm.

Synchronized cardioversion delivers an electrical current synchronized with the client's rhythm to prevent ventricular fibrillation. It is used to treat rhythms that are not life threatening, such as supraventricular tachycardia and atrial fibrillation. It is usually an elective procedure, and the client is sedated prior to cardioversion. Anticoagulants may be given before cardioversion to reduce the risk of thromboembolism.

Defibrillation is an emergency treatment that delivers an electrical charge without regard to the cardiac cycle. Early defibrillation improves survival of clients experiencing V-fib. External defibrillation may be performed by any health care provider who has been trained in the procedure. Initiate CPR and the cardiac arrest (code) procedure when V-fib is recognized. Remove nitroglycerine patches from the

TABLE 22-2   NURSING IMPLICATIONS FOR PHARMACOLOGY: CLIENTS RECEIVING ANTIDYSRHYTHMIC DRUGS

CLASS/DRUGS	PURPOSE	NURSING RESPONSIBILITIES	CLIENT TEACHING
Class IA ■ Quinidine ■ Procainamide (Procan, Pronestyl) ■ Disopyramide (Norpace)	Used to treat symptomatic or frequent PVCs, supraventricular or ventricular tachycardias, and to prevent ventricular fibrillation	Obtain baseline vital signs, cardiac rhythm, and physical assessment. Monitor ECG. Notify the physician of new dysrhythmias. Notify the physician immediately if manifestations of toxicity develop: 　■ Signs of heart failure and 　■ Changes in ECG complex 　■ Skin rash or flulike symptoms 　■ Urinary retention 　■ Neurologic effects such as confusion, dizziness, agitation 　■ Shortness of breath 　■ Altered liver function tests Use an infusion pump to administer intravenous infusions. Monitor dose and its effectiveness.	Take the drug exactly as ordered. Do not skip or double doses. Check with your doctor if you miss a dose. Take and record your pulse rate daily before rising. Count pulse for 1 full minute. Bring the record to each office or clinic appointment. Report the following to your doctor: Irregular pulse rate or rhythm, dizziness, eye pain, vision changes, skin rashes, wheezing or other respiratory problems, behavior changes.
Class IB ■ Lidocaine ■ Tocainide (Tonocard) ■ Phenytoin (Dilantin)	Primarily used to treat ventricular dysrhythmias, including PVCs and ventricular tachycardia		
Class II: Beta Blockers ■ Esmolol (Brevibloc) ■ Propranolol (Inderal, others) ■ Acebutolol (Sectral)	Used to prevent SVT and possibly V-fib. May cause bronchospasm, so are contraindicated for clients with asthma or COPD		
Class III ■ Sotalol (Betapace) ■ Amiodarone (Cordarone) ■ Bretylium (Bretylol)	Primarily used to treat V-tach and V-fib		
Class IV: Calcium Channel Blockers ■ Verapamil (Calan, Isoptan) ■ Diltiazem (Cardizem, Dilacor)	Used to manage supraventricular tachycardias		

client's chest in preparation for defibrillation, but leave monitor pads in place. Conductive gel pads are applied to the chest wall at the apex and base of the heart (Figure 22-7 ◆), and an electrical shock is delivered by *automated external defibrillator (AED)* or manually. The cardiac rhythm is evaluated after each shock is delivered. After successful defibrillation, the client is transferred to the critical care unit for monitoring and therapy to prevent further episodes of V-fib.

AUTOMATIC IMPLANTABLE CARDIOVERTER–DEFIBRILLATOR.

The *automatic implantable cardioverter–defibrillator (AICD)* recognizes life-threatening changes in heart rhythm and automatically delivers an electric shock to convert the rhythm back into a normal rhythm. Electrodes surgically placed on the heart are attached to an implanted cardioverter–defibrillator device. The AICD is used for clients with recurrent ventricular tachycardia and people who have survived sudden cardiac death not associated with an acute myocardial infarction. When V-tach or V-fib occur, the AICD delivers a shock to convert the rhythm.

Pacemakers

Pacemakers may be used to treat AV blocks. *Temporary pacemakers* have an external generator attached to an electrode threaded intravenously into the right ventricle or to temporary pacing wires implanted during cardiac surgery. *Permanent pacemakers* have an implanted pulse generator attached to electrodes that are sewn directly onto the heart or passed into the heart via the subclavian or jugular vein (Figure 22-8 ◆).

Pacemakers have both sensing and pacing functions. *Sensing* detects the heart's own beats. When the pacemaker

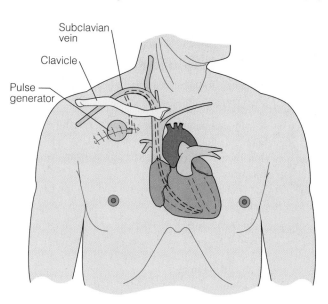

Figure 22-8. ◆ A permanent pacemaker with a transvenous electrode into the right ventricle.

senses a heart rate within preset limits, it provides no electrical stimuli. *Pacing,* or the delivery of an electical pulse to stimulate the heart to contract, occurs when the client's heart rate falls outside the programmed limits. Pacing is detected on the ECG strip (Figure 22-9 ◆) by the presence of pacing spike before the P wave (atrial pacing) or QRS complex (ventricular pacing). Box 22-4 outlines nursing care for the client having a permanent pacemaker implant.

Surgery

Surgical *ablation* (removal of a part or pathway) may be used when the site of an ectopic focus can be identified. The affected tissue may be excised or destroyed by freezing with liquid nitrogen, laser, or an electric current.

NURSING CARE

ASSESSING

It is vital to assess the client before treating any suspected dysrhythmia. What appears to be ventricular tachycardia on the monitor may be a client tapping the electrode pad or brushing

Figure 22-7. ◆ Placement of paddles for defibrillation.

Figure 22-9. ◆ Ventricular pacing. Note the presence of pacer spikes prior to the wide, ventricular QRS complexes, and the absence of spikes when the client's natural rhythm resumes.

BOX 22-4
NURSING CARE CHECKLIST

PERMANENT PACEMAKER IMPLANT

Before Surgery

☑ Assess knowledge and understanding; reinforce and clarify teaching as needed.

☑ Position ECG monitor electrodes away from potential incision sites.

☑ Provide routine preoperative care and teaching (see Chapter 7).

After Surgery

☑ Provide routine postoperative care, including monitoring and incision care.

☑ Obtain a chest x-ray as ordered.

☑ Administer analgesia and position for comfort. Restrict movement of affected arm and shoulder for 24 hours.

☑ After 24 hours, assist with gentle ROM exercises at least tid.

☑ Monitor pacemaker function and cardiac rhythm. Report pacemaker problems such as failure to pace or hiccups to the physician.

☑ Report dysrhythmias to the charge nurse or physician.

☑ Document date of insertion, pacemaker model and type, and settings.

☑ Provide a pacemaker identification card including manufacturer's name, model number, mode of operation, rate parameters, and expected battery life. Instruct to carry the card at all times, and to wear a Medic-Alert bracelet or tag.

☑ Teach about the pacemaker, its function, how to take and record the pulse rate, and usual battery replacement procedure.

☑ Instruct to report the following to the physician: pulse rate 5 or more bpm slower than preset pacemaker rate; fever; signs of pacemaker malfunction, such as dizziness, fainting, fatigue, weakness, chest pain, or palpitations.

☑ Notify all care providers of the pacemaker.

the teeth. Apparent asystole on the monitor may be a sleeping client whose electrode patch has come loose. Similarly, a heart rate of 52 bpm may be normal for some clients and not affect their functioning at all.

Ask about the presence of chest pain, shortness of breath, or palpitations. Inquire about dizziness or feeling light-headed, faint, or nauseated. Obtain vital signs and an ECG monitor strip. Assess skin color, temperature, and moisture; level of consciousness and mental status; heart sounds and peripheral pulses; respiratory status; and anxiety level. Check electrode placement, leads, the monitor cable, and connections.

CLINICAL alert

Remember: Treat the client, not the monitor!

DIAGNOSING, PLANNING, AND IMPLEMENTING

DECREASED CARDIAC OUTPUT

■ Assess for manifestations of decreased cardiac output: decreased level of consciousness; tachycardia; tachypnea; hypotension; diaphoresis; decreased urine output; cool, clammy, mottled skin; pallor or cyanosis; decreased peripheral pulses. *Manifestations of decreased cardiac output may indicate the client is not tolerating the dysrhythmia and needs immediate treatment.*

■ Monitor ECG rhythm and post ECG strip every shift and when rhythm changes occur. *Documenting ECG rhythms helps evaluate status and the effect of treatment.*

■ Frequently monitor vital signs during acute dysrhythmias and treatment. *Vital signs are an indicator of the effect of the dysrhythmia and treatment on cardiovascular status.*

■ Monitor lab values, especially serum electrolytes and drug levels as ordered. Report abnormal values to the charge nurse and physician. *Electrolyte imbalances can cause dysrhythmias. Serum drug levels need to be within the therapeutic range for optimal effectiveness.*

■ Maintain intravenous access with an intravenous infusion or saline lock. *Many drugs used to treat dysrhythmias are administered intravenously. In an emergency, an existing intravenous site facilitates rapid treatment of the dysrhythmia.*

■ On recognizing ventricular fibrillation, begin emergency procedures. Call for help. Begin CPR until a defibrillator is available. Initiate advanced cardiac life support (ACLS) protocols. Defibrillate as soon as possible. Assist the code team as needed. *V-fib is a medical emergency requiring immediate treatment to preserve life.*

■ After a cardiac arrest, transfer to critical care. *The period immediately following resuscitation is critical, and the client needs careful monitoring.*

ANXIETY

■ Notify family of significant changes in the client's condition or cardiac arrest, providing up-to-date information. Prepare family members for visits by explaining interventions such as invasive tubes, a ventilator, or additional equipment. *Concern for the family and significant others is part of holistic nursing. Family members need information, honest communication, and compassionate care. Preparing the family for changes in the client's condition and plan of care helps them to cope with a difficult situation.*

EVALUATING

To evaluate the effectiveness of nursing care for a client with a dysrhythmia, collect data related to cardiac output. For example, evaluate level of consciousness and mental status, skin color and temperature, vital signs, and urinary output.

Discharge Considerations

Dysrhythmias can have a significant physical and psychologic impact. The client and family may fear sudden cardiac death. Teaching focuses on coping strategies and specific treatments. Involve both the client and the family in teaching. Teach about prescribed drugs, including their desired and potential adverse or toxic effects. Stress the importance of follow-up visits with the cardiologist, and schedule them, if possible.

Teach clients with a pacemaker or an AICD about the device and how it works, how to take their pulse, signs of infection or other complications, resumption of and any limitations to activities, and safety issues. Stress the importance of promptly reporting problems to the physician, and attending follow-up appointments. In some states driving is prohibited for clients with AICDs; address the impact of this on lifestyle. Inform the client that magnetic interference can damage the AICD or cause it to discharge. Procedures such as magnetic resonance imaging (MRI) and equipment such as arc welders, radar, and theft prevention equipment can damage the AICD and should be avoided.

Encourage the client and family to learn and maintain current training in CPR. Refer to the American Heart Association or the American Red Cross for training.

Sudden Cardiac Death

Sudden cardiac death is defined as death occurring within 1 hour of the onset of cardiac symptoms. It usually is caused by ventricular fibrillation and cardiac arrest. Cardiac arrest occurs when effective circulation ceases. Nearly half of cardiac arrest victims die before reaching the hospital.

Coronary heart disease (CHD) is the most common cause of sudden cardiac deaths in the United States. Other causes include electrocution, pulmonary embolism, and rapid blood loss from a ruptured aortic aneurysm. Ventricular fibrillation is the most common dysrhythmia causing sudden cardiac death; asystole or cardiac standstill also leads to sudden death. The risk of sudden cardiac death is highest in the first 6 to 18 months following an acute myocardial infarction (MI) or other major cardiac event.

Effective CPR must be instituted within 2 to 4 minutes of cardiac arrest to prevent permanent brain damage. CPR is a mechanical means of maintaining tissue perfusion and oxy-genation using ventilation and external cardiac compressions. All health care providers need to be proficient in CPR or basic cardiac life support (BCLS). A review of CPR procedures is provided in Procedure 22-2. ACLS incorporates electrical and drug treatment in addition to mechanical compressions.

CPR can be traumatic, causing injuries to the skin, thorax, upper airway, abdomen, lungs, heart, and great vessels. These complications can be minimized by using appropriate CPR techniques.

Because most instances of sudden cardiac death result from ventricular fibrillation, the American Heart Association recommends early defibrillation when appropriate. Automated external defibrillators (AEDs) are easy to use. The device senses the heart rhythm through two electrodes placed on the chest, and delivers a shock when necessary. A shock can be delivered simply by pressing the "shock" button on the device.

The client who survives sudden cardiac death and family members have significant teaching needs to recognize and reduce the risk of subsequent events.

If the cause of cardiac arrest is identified, teach risk factor reduction. For example, if a myocardial infarction precipitated the cardiac arrest, teach the risk factors for MI and ways to reduce them. If the cause of cardiac arrest is unknown, explain diagnostic studies and discuss possible interventions such as the AICD. Stress the importance of carrying a card at all times listing all medications and the client's health care provider. In all cases, teach recognition of early manifestations or warning signs of cardiac arrest. All family members should become proficient in performing CPR.

To reduce death rates from cardiac arrest, teach community members how to perform effective CPR and the importance of early intervention. Work with community and emergency services agencies to provide and train community members to use the AED as well.

ADVANCE DIRECTIVES

Unless otherwise stipulated by the client, family, or an advance directive, all resuscitative measures necessary (CPR, respiratory and pharmacologic support) are used to treat cardiac arrest. *Advance directives* allow clients to make treatment decisions regarding care before a medical emergency occurs. The living will and the durable power of attorney for health care are two forms of advance directives.

Through an advance directive, a client may request that no or limited resuscitation procedures be used if cardiac arrest occurs. Without an advance directive, this decision falls to family members. A *"No code"* or *do-not-resuscitate (DNR)* order limits the use of resuscitative measures. Caring for clients with DNR orders does not mean withdrawing care. Nurses continue to provide optimal care for the clients and family.

PROCEDURE 22-2   Cardiopulmonary Resuscitation (CPR) Checklist

- Assess for responsiveness; shake and ask "Are you okay?"
- Call for help. Dial 911 (if outside the health care facility) or initiate the institutional cardiac arrest procedure.
- Open the airway using the head tilt–chin lift maneuver: Simultaneously press down on the client's forehead with one hand to tilt the head back. Lift the chin forward using the fingers of the other hand under the bony part of the chin (part A of the accompanying figure).

A

- Check for breathing. With the ear next to the client's mouth and nose, *look* for the chest to rise and fall with respirations, *listen* for exhalation, and *feel* for the flow of air.
- If not breathing, give two full breaths using a pocket mask, mouth shield, or bag-valve mask (see part B of the figure). Observe for chest rise and fall during ventilation.

B

- Check for a carotid pulse (take approximately 3 to 5 seconds to check the pulse).
- If pulse is present, continue rescue breathing at 10 to 12 breaths per minute. Recheck the carotid pulse every 12 breaths.

- If pulse is absent, begin chest compressions. Place the client on a firm surface. Place the heel of one hand on the lower half of the sternum so that the long axis of the heel of the hand is on the long axis of the sternum (see Part C of the figure). Place the other hand on top of the hand on the sternum with the fingers either extended or interlocked.

C

- With the arms straight and elbows locked, press straight down to depress the sternum 1½ to 2 inches (part D of the figure). Release pressure completely between compressions but do not lift the hands from the chest.

D

- Compress the chest 80 to 100 times per minute (one-and-two-and . . .).
  a. With one-rescuer CPR, provide 2 breaths after each 15 compressions. Assess the pulse after 4 complete cycles of 15 compressions and 2 breaths; continue CPR until help arrives.
  b. With two-rescuer CPR, provide 1 breath after every 5 compressions. Assess pulse every minute for 3 to 5 seconds. If no pulse is present, continue CPR until help arrives.

Coronary Heart Disease

Coronary heart disease (CHD), or coronary artery disease (CAD), causes about 500,000 deaths annually in the United States. CHD is caused by *atherosclerosis* in the coronary arteries that obstructs blood flow to the myocardium. Clients with CHD may have no symptoms, may experience episodic chest pain *(angina pectoris),* or may have a *myocardial infarction* resulting from complete obstruction of blood flow to part of the heart muscle (Figure 22-10 ◆).

Both men and women are affected by CHD. In women, however, it is seen about 10 years later because of the effects of estrogen. After menopause, women's risk is equal to that of men.

Atherosclerosis

Atherosclerosis is a disease in which the lining of medium and large arteries is affected by lesions called *atheromas* (or *plaque*). These lesions protrude into the artery and may affect blood flow through the artery. The cause of atherosclerosis is unknown. The process of lipid and cholesterol accumulation is thought to start with inflammation. Smooth muscle cells and connective tissue proliferate within the wall of the blood vessel, contributing to plaque growth. As the plaque develops, it gradually occludes the vessel lumen and impairs the vessel's ability to dilate in response to increased oxygen demands. Atheromas often develop where arteries divide, curve, or become narrow.

RISK FACTORS

While the cause of atherosclerosis is unknown, *risk factors* for its development and resulting CHD have been identified. Some risk factors for CHD (age, gender, and heredity) cannot be changed. Over 50% of heart attack victims are 65 or older. *Men* are affected at an earlier age than women. A *family history* of CHD is a risk factor for both men and women. Educating women about CHD is important, as many do not realize that their risk after menopause is just as high as men's risk.

Controllable risk factors can be controlled or completely eliminated. *Cigarette smoking* is a major risk factor, increasing the risk of heart disease by three to four times that of a nonsmoker. People who quit smoking reduce their risk almost immediately, no matter how long they have smoked. *Obesity* (body weight more 30% over ideal) and fat distribution affect the risk for CHD. Central or abdominal obesity is associated with abnormal blood lipids and a higher risk of CHD.

Physical inactivity, or a sedentary lifestyle, is associated with higher risk. People who maintain a regular program of physical activity are less likely to develop CHD than sedentary people.

Risk factors such as high blood pressure (hypertension), diabetes, and elevated blood lipid and cholesterol levels can usually be controlled through medication, weight control, and diet.

Hypertension, which affects more than 50 million people in the United States, is a systolic blood pressure greater than 140 mm Hg or a diastolic blood pressure greater than 90 mm Hg. Controlling blood pressure decreases the risk of heart disease, stroke, and renal failure. *Diabetes* affects both small and large blood vessels. It also is associated with a higher incidence of high blood lipids, high blood pressure, and obesity—all risk factors in their own right.

High blood lipids increase the risk for CHD. Lipoproteins carry cholesterol in the blood. LDL (low-density lipoprotein) is the primary carrier of cholesterol. High levels of LDL (remember **LDL** = *Less* healthy) promote atherosclerosis because LDL deposits cholesterol on the artery walls. In contrast, high-density lipoprotein, HDL (remember **HDL** = *Highly* healthy), helps clear cholesterol from the arteries, transporting it to the liver for excretion. HDL levels above 35 mg/dL reduce the risk of CHD. Table 22-3 ◆ lists desired levels of total cholesterol and LDL as identified by the National Heart, Lung, and Blood Institute. Triglycerides, used for fat storage by the body, also contribute to the development of CHD when elevated. *Stress* is a risk factor for CHD, although it is unclear how it contributes to developing CHD.

Risk Factor Management

DIET. A low-fat, low-cholesterol diet is suggested to help control blood lipid levels and promote weight loss. The American Heart Association recommends reducing total and saturated fat to less than 30% of the total daily calories. Much saturated fat is found in whole-milk products and in red meats. Eating nonfat dairy products, fish, and poultry as primary protein sources can lower cholesterol levels. Monounsaturated fats, found in olive, canola, and peanut oils, and omega-3 fatty acids found in certain cold-water fish, such as tuna, salmon, and mackerel, help reduce total serum cholesterol, LDL, and triglyceride levels. Several programs that combine diet, exercise, and other therapies have been proven to reduce atherosclerotic deposits. These programs are quite restrictive, however, and require significant commitment to follow (Box 22-5).

PHARMACOLOGY. Drug therapy may be used in addition to diet to lower serum cholesterol levels. Niacin or nicotinic acid

Figure 22-10. ◆ **Coronary heart disease.** Most cases of coronary heart disease are due to atherosclerosis, occlusion of the coronary arteries by fibrous, fatty plaque. Clients with coronary heart disease may experience *angina pectoris* or *myocardial infarction*. Risk factors for coronary heart disease include age, heredity, smoking, obesity, high serum cholesterol levels, hypertension, and diabetes mellitus. Other factors, such as stress and lack of exercise, also contribute to the risk of CHD.

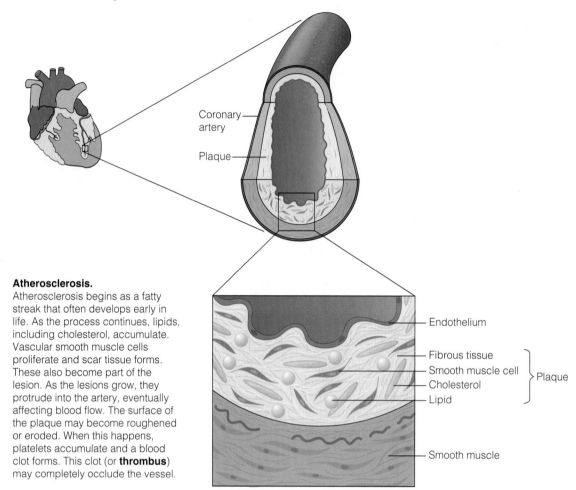

Coronary artery

Plaque

Endothelium

Fibrous tissue
Smooth muscle cell
Cholesterol   } Plaque
Lipid

Smooth muscle

Atherosclerosis.
Atherosclerosis begins as a fatty streak that often develops early in life. As the process continues, lipids, including cholesterol, accumulate. Vascular smooth muscle cells proliferate and scar tissue forms. These also become part of the lesion. As the lesions grow, they protrude into the artery, eventually affecting blood flow. The surface of the plaque may become roughened or eroded. When this happens, platelets accumulate and a blood clot forms. This clot (or **thrombus**) may completely occlude the vessel.

Angina pectoris.
Angina is characterized by episodes of chest pain. When the heart muscle needs more oxygen than partially occluded vessels can supply, the cells become ischemic. Lactic acid produced by ischemic cells stimulates nerve endings, causing pain. The pain subsides when cells again receive enough oxygen to meet their needs.

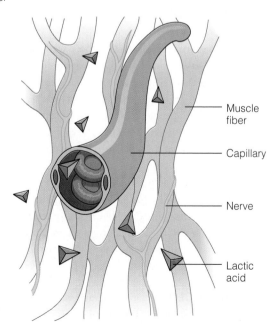

Muscle fiber

Capillary

Nerve

Lactic acid

Ischemia
Injury
Infarction

Myocardial infarction.
Myocardial infarction occurs when complete obstruction of a coronary artery interrupts blood supply to an area of heart muscle. Affected tissue becomes ischemic and eventually dies (*infarcts*) if the blood supply is not restored. Surrounding the area of infarction, there is an area of tissue injury. Surrounding the injured tissue is an area of ischemic but undamaged tissue.

TABLE 22-3 DESIRABLE CHOLESTEROL AND LDL LEVELS	TOTAL CHOLESTEROL (MG/DL)	LDL CHOLESTEROL (MG/DL)
DESIRABLE	< 200	< 130
BORDERLINE HIGH	200–239	120–159
HIGH	≥ 240	≥ 160

(Niacor, Nicobid, Nicolar) lowers LDL levels and raises HDL levels. Flushing, or "hot flashes," and pruritus are common side effects of niacin therapy. Cholestyramine (Questran) and colestipol (Colestid) bind with bile acids and cholesterol in the intestine, promoting their excretion in the feces. These drugs may have gastrointestinal (GI) side effects, such as constipation, gas, and abdominal cramping.

The statins, such as lovastatin (Mevacor), pravastatin (Pravachol), and simvastatin (Zocor) inhibit cholesterol synthesis in the liver. They are very effective in lowering LDL levels and also cause some increase in HDL levels. Headache and GI effects are the most common side effects of these drugs. Myalgias (muscle aches) or skin rashes may also develop. Liver function tests and muscle enzymes are monitored during therapy to assess for possible toxic effects.

NURSING CARE

Strongly encourage all clients to stop all forms of tobacco use. Discuss the effects of smoking on the body and the benefits of quitting. Resource materials to help clients stop smoking are available from the American Heart Association, the American Lung Association, and the American Cancer Society. Refer to a smoking cessation program to increase the likelihood of success in quitting.

Discuss the role of diet in CHD and obesity. Help assess food intake and patterns of eating to identify areas that can be improved. Refer to a dietitian for diet planning and further teaching. Encourage to make dietary changes gradually but progressively, maintaining a well-balanced low-fat diet. Advise to avoid fad diets for weight loss. Suggest American Heart Association and other cookbooks that offer low-fat recipes to encourage healthier eating.

Discuss the physical and psychosocial benefits of regular exercise. Help the client identify favorite forms of exercise and schedule exercise periods of 20 to 30 minutes of continuous aerobic activity (i.e., walking, running, bicycling, swimming) three to five times a week. Walking provides many benefits and is an easily accessible and low-cost form of exercise. Encourage identification of an "exercise buddy" to help maintain motivation.

Discuss the importance of controlling high blood pressure, diabetes, and elevated blood lipid levels. Refer clients to their primary care provider for treatment as needed, and provide teaching about specific diseases and/or prescribed treatments.

Stress is a normal part of every person's life. Assist the client to identify and develop stress-management techniques such as physical exercise or meditation. It is important to emphasize that relaxation techniques require practice.

Angina Pectoris

Angina pectoris is chest pain that occurs when there is a temporary imbalance between myocardial blood supply and demand. Angina often occurs in a pattern: Exercise brings on the pain; rest relieves the pain.

PATHOPHYSIOLOGY

Atherosclerosis and coronary heart disease often lead to angina. Obstruction of a coronary artery reduces blood flow to the part of the heart normally supplied by that vessel. Although the heart muscle may still receive enough blood and oxygen to meet its needs at rest, anything that further reduces blood flow or increases the oxygen demand of the heart muscle can cause angina. Exercise increases myocardial oxygen demand. The obstructed vessel is unable to provide an adequate supply, and cells are deprived of oxygen. Inadequate oxygen causes cells to switch from aerobic metabolism (a very efficient process that requires oxygen) to anaerobic metabolism (a very inefficient process that occurs in the absence of oxygen). Lactic acid and other substances that stimulate nerve fibers are released, causing pain.

Three types of angina have been identified:

1. *Stable angina* is the most common and predictable form of angina. It occurs with a known amount of activity or stress. Stable angina is relieved by rest and nitrates.

2. *Unstable angina* occurs with increasing frequency, severity, and duration. Pain is unpredictable and may occur at rest. Clients with unstable angina are at risk for myocardial infarction.

3. *Prinzmetal's angina* is atypical angina that occurs without an identified precipitating cause, usually at the same time each day, often waking the client from sleep. It is caused by coronary artery spasm.

Progression of the disease is marked by a change from stable angina to unstable angina. This change may herald an impending myocardial infarction.

The cardinal manifestation of angina is chest pain. The pain typically is precipitated by an identifiable event, such as physical activity, strong emotion, stress, eating a heavy meal, or exposure to cold. The classic sequence of angina is activity–pain, rest–relief. Anginal pain usually lasts less than 15 minutes and is relieved by rest. The manifestations of angina are summarized in Box 22-6.

COLLABORATIVE CARE

Angina is diagnosed by the client's symptoms, past medical history and family history, and physical assessment. Laboratory tests may confirm the presence of risk factors, such as abnormal blood lipids or the presence of diabetes mellitus.

Diagnostic Tests

Common diagnostic tests to determine the extent of coronary heart disease and angina include electrocardiography, stress testing, nuclear medicine studies, and coronary angiography.

ELECTROCARDIOGRAPHY. A resting ECG may be normal in clients with angina. However, characteristic changes are seen during anginal episodes. During periods of myocardial ischemia, the ST segment is depressed, and the T wave may flatten or invert (Figure 22-11 ◆). These changes reverse when adequate blood flow is restored.

STRESS ELECTROCARDIOGRAPHY (EXERCISE STRESS TESTS). *Stress electrocardiography* (also called treadmill testing) monitors the ECG during exercise on a treadmill or stationary bicycle. It is used to help diagnose angina and to identify clients at risk. During exercise, the workload of the heart increases. In

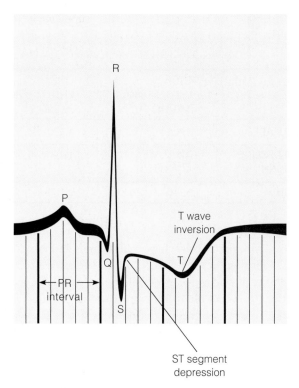

Figure 22-11. ◆ ECG changes during an episode of angina. Note the ST segment depression and T-wave inversion characteristic of myocardial ischemia.

coronary heart disease, the increased workload may cause myocardial ischemia and angina. *Pharmacologic stress testing* is used when physical exercise is not possible, such as for clients with orthopedic problems. A vasodilator drug may cause ischemia in areas of the heart affected by coronary heart disease, much like exercise does. The client's ECG, heart rate, and blood pressure are monitored continuously during testing.

CARDIAC RADIONUCLEAR SCAN. *Radionuclear scanning* is used to evaluate blood flow to the heart muscle. A radioactive substance such as thallium-201 is injected intravenously, and the heart is scanned with a radiation detector. Ischemic or infarcted cells of the myocardium do not take up the substance normally, appearing as a "cold spot" on the scan. The amount of radioisotope injected is very small; no special radiation precautions are required during or after the scan. Increased fluid intake is encouraged after the scan to speed elimination of the substance from the body.

CORONARY ANGIOGRAPHY. *Coronary angiography* is the "gold standard" for evaluating the coronary arteries. A catheter inserted into the femoral or brachial artery is threaded into the coronary artery, guided by a fluoroscope. Dye is injected to visualize the vessels and any abnormalities, such as stenosis or obstruction. Narrowing of a vessel by more than 50% is considered significant; most lesions that produce symptoms are more than 70% narrowed. Nursing care of the client undergoing a coronary angiogram is summarized in Box 22-7.

BOX 22-6
MANIFESTATIONS OF ANGINA

- Chest pain
  - Substernal or precordial (across the chest)
  - May radiate to neck, arms, shoulders, or jaw
  - Tight, squeezing, constricting, or heavy
  - Precipitated by exercise or activity, strong emotion, stress, cold, heavy meal
  - Relieved by rest, nitroglycerin
- Shortness of breath, pallor, anxiety, and fear

BOX 22-7
NURSING CARE CHECKLIST

CORONARY ANGIOGRAPHY AND PTCA

Before the Procedure

- ☑ Assess knowledge and understanding of the procedure. Reinforce teaching and provide additional information as needed.
- ☑ Provide routine preoperative care as ordered (see Chapter 7).
- ☑ Administer ordered cardiac medications with a small sip of water prior to the procedure unless contraindicated.
- ☑ Document and report any allergies to iodine, radiographic dyes, or seafood.
- ☑ Record height, weight, and vital signs. Record equality and amplitude of peripheral pulses; mark their locations.
- ☑ Explain that client will remain awake during the procedure, which lasts 1 to 2 hours. A sensation of warmth (a "hot flash") and a metallic taste may be experienced as the dye is injected. A rapid pulse or a few "skipped beats" also are common during the procedure.

After the Procedure

- ☑ Provide routine postoperative care (see Chapter 7).
- ☑ Monitor vital signs, distal pulses, color, movement, sensation, temperature, and capillary refill of affected extremity as ordered, usually every 15 minutes for the first hour, every 30 minutes the next hour, hourly for 8 hours, and then every 4 hours.
- ☑ Monitor cardiac rhythm continuously. Report dysrhythmias, ECG changes, or chest pain to the charge nurse or physician.
- ☑ Maintain bed rest with the affected extremity extended and the head of the bed elevated no more than 30 degrees.
- ☑ Keep a pressure dressing in place over arterial access sites. Place a 5-lb. sandbag over the access site for 6 hours or as ordered. Check frequently for bleeding (if the access site is in the groin, check for bleeding under the buttocks).
- ☑ Unless contraindicated, encourage liberal fluid consumption.
- ☑ Administer medications as ordered.
- ☑ Monitor intake, output, and laboratory values. Report abnormal values to the physician.

Pharmacology

Sublingual nitroglycerin (NTG) is the drug of choice to treat acute anginal attacks, acting within 1 to 2 minutes. Rapid-acting NTG is also available as a buccal spray in a metered-dose system. *Longer-acting nitroglycerin preparations* include oral tablets, ointment, and transdermal patches. In these forms,

NTG is used to prevent attacks of angina, not to treat an acute attack. Headache, nausea, dizziness, and hypotension are common adverse effects of NTG preparations.

Beta blockers (e.g., propranolol and atenolol) and *calcium channel blockers* (e.g., diltiazem and nifedipine) are used to prevent angina (Table 22-4 ◆). These drugs act too slowly to treat

---

TABLE 22-4

NURSING IMPLICATIONS FOR PHARMACOLOGY: CLIENTS RECEIVING ANTIANGINAL DRUGS

CLASS/DRUGS	PURPOSE	NURSING RESPONSIBILITIES	CLIENT TEACHING
Nitrates ▪ Nitroglycerin (Nitropaste, Nitro-Dur, Nitro-Bid, Nitrol, Transderm-Nitro, Nitrogard, Nitrodisc, Tridil) ▪ Isosorbide dinitrate (Isordil) ▪ Isosorbide mononitrate (Ismo)	Nitrates dilate blood vessels, increasing blood flow to the myocardium and reducing the workload of the heart. Sublingual nitroglycerin (NTG) tablets and buccal spray are used to prevent and	Administer sublingual NTG at the onset of chest pain. In some cases, tablets may be left at the bedside for prompt treatment of angina. Wear gloves when applying nitroglycerin ointment to prevent absorbing the drug through your skin. Measure dose carefully and spread evenly in a 2-by-3 inch area.	Use only the sublingual, buccal, and spray forms to treat acute anginal attacks. Carry your nitroglycerin with you. Use rapid-acting NTG at the onset of chest pain. Dissolve tablets under the tongue; do not swallow the tablet. If chest pain is not relieved within 5 minutes, take a second dose. After 5 minutes more, a third dose may be taken. If pain continues, seek medical help immediately.

(continues)

CLASS/DRUGS	PURPOSE	NURSING RESPONSIBILITIES	CLIENT TEACHING
Nitrates (continued)	treat acute angina. Oral and transdermal forms are used to reduce the frequency and severity of anginal attacks.	Remove nitroglycerin patches or ointment at night to help prevent the client from developing tolerance to the drug. Help the client identify events that precipitate anginal attacks.	Keep sublingual tablets in original amber glass bottle to protect them from heat, light, and moisture. Refill your prescription every 6 months and throw away any unused tablets. Apply ointment or transdermal patches to a hairless area; spread ointment evenly without rubbing or massaging. Remove the old patch or residual ointment before applying a fresh dose. Rotate sites. If you are using long-acting NTG, keep a supply of rapid-acting tablets to treat acute angina.
Beta Blockers ■ Atenolol (Tenormin) ■ Metoprolol (Lopressor) ■ Propranolol (Inderal) ■ Nadolol (Corgard)	Beta blockers decrease cardiac workload by blocking sympathetic nervous system stimulation. They are frequently ordered to prevent angina and treat hypertension.	Record heart rate and BP before giving. Withhold the drug if the heart rate is below 50 bpm or the BP is below identified levels. Notify the charge nurse or physician. Assess for possible contraindications to beta blockers, such as asthma, or COPD. These drugs should not be abruptly discontinued but gradually withdrawn when necessary.	Beta blockers do not work immediately; keep a supply of fast-acting NTG for acute chest pain. Do not abruptly stop taking this drug. Talk to your doctor about discontinuing its use. Take and record your pulse daily. Do not take the drug and notify your doctor if your heart rate is below 50 bpm. Have your BP checked frequently. Report to your doctor a slow or irregular pulse, swelling or weight gain, or difficulty breathing.
Calcium Channel Blockers ■ Nifedipine (Procardia) ■ Diltiazem (Cardizem) ■ Verapamil (Calan) ■ Bepridil (Vascor) ■ Felodipine (Plendil) ■ Isradipine (DynaCirc) ■ Nicardipine (Cardene) ■ Nimodipine (Nimotop)	Calcium channel blockers are used to control angina, hypertension, and dysrhythmias. They reduce cardiac workload and increase blood flow to the myocardium. They are often ordered for clients with coronary artery spasm (Prinzmetal's angina).	Record BP and heart rate before giving the drug. Withhold drug if the heart rate is below 50 bpm. Notify the charge nurse or physician if withheld. Nifedipine may be given by extracting the liquid from the capsule with a syringe and squirting the dose under the tongue (discard the needle first!). Immediately report manifestations of toxicity (nausea, generalized weakness, decreased cardiac output, hypotension, dysrhythmias).	Take your pulse before taking the drug. Do not take the drug and notify physician if your heart rate drops below 50 bpm. For acute angina, keep a fresh supply of rapid-acting NTG available (e.g., sublingual tablets). Calcium channel blockers will not work fast enough to relieve an acute attack.

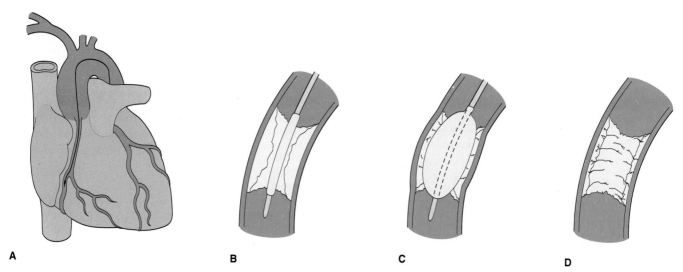

Figure 22-12. ◆ PTCA. (A) The balloon catheter is threaded into the affected coronary artery. (B) The balloon is positioned across the area of obstruction. (C) The balloon is then inflated, flattening the plaque against the arterial wall (D).

acute attacks of angina; they are used for long-term prophylaxis. Beta blockers may significantly slow the heart rate, and are contraindicated for clients with asthma or severe chronic obstructive pulmonary disease (COPD) (see Chapter 26) because they may cause severe bronchospasm in these clients.

The client with angina, particularly unstable angina, is at risk for myocardial infarction because of significant narrowing of the coronary arteries. Low-dose aspirin (75 mg/day) is often prescribed to reduce the risk that clots will form in narrowed arteries, causing a myocardial infarction.

Surgery and Revascularization Procedures

Clients with severe or unstable angina may undergo surgery or a nonsurgical procedure to restore blood flow to the myocardium.

Percutaneous transluminal coronary angioplasty (PTCA) is an invasive procedure used to increase blood flow to heart muscle. PTCA is performed in the cardiac catheterization laboratory under local anesthesia. Using the femoral artery, a small bal-

loon-tipped catheter is threaded into the obstructed coronary artery. The balloon is positioned across the area of narrowing (Figure 22-12 ◆). The balloon is inflated to reduce the narrowing and increase blood flow through the obstructed area. An intracoronary stent may be inserted at the same time. The stent remains in the artery as a prop after the balloon is deflated (Figure 22-13 ◆). Nursing care for the client having a PTCA is similar to care for clients undergoing coronary angiogram (see Box 22-7).

In a *coronary artery bypass graft (CABG)*, a vein or arterial graft is used to "bypass," or bridge, the coronary artery obstruction and provide blood to the ischemic portion of the heart. The internal mammary artery (IMA) in the chest and the saphenous vein from the leg are the most popular vessels used for cardiac bypass grafts. The distal end of the IMA is sutured to the coronary artery distal to the obstruction (Figure 22-14 ◆). When the saphenous vein is used, it is removed from the leg, reversed so that its valves do not interfere with blood flow, then grafted to the aorta and the coronary artery, distal to

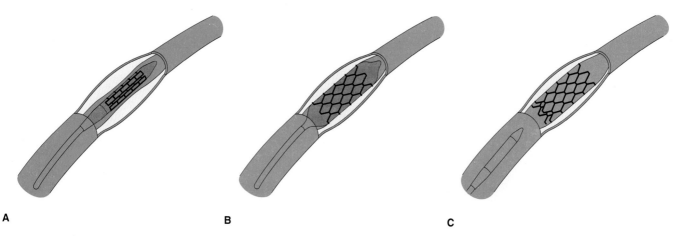

Figure 22-13. ◆ Placement of an intracoronary stent. (A) The stent is fitted over the balloon-tipped catheter. (B) The stent is positioned in the area of narrowing and expanded with balloon inflation. (C) The balloon is deflated and removed, leaving the stent in place.

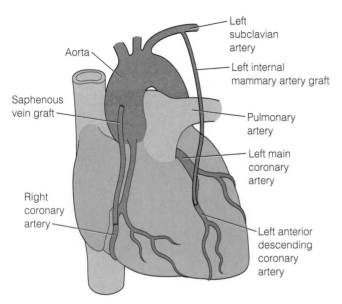

Figure 22-14. ◆ CABG using the internal mammary artery and a saphenous vein graft.

the occlusion. This provides a bridge for blood flow past the obstruction.

While CABG is a relatively safe procedure, the heart is usually stopped during surgery to make it easier to work on. The *cardiopulmonary bypass pump,* or *heart–lung machine,* is used to maintain blood flow to the rest of the organs during surgery

(Figure 22-15 ◆). The body temperature is lowered during surgery. Once the procedure has been completed, cardiopulmonary bypass is discontinued and the client is rewarmed. Nursing care for the client having cardiac surgery is outlined in Box 22-8.

Minimally invasive coronary artery surgery uses several small incisions to access the affected coronary arteries. Another revascularization procedure, *transmyocardial laser revascularization,* uses a laser to drill tiny holes into the myocardial muscle itself to provide blood to ischemic muscle.

NURSING CARE

Clients with angina are frequently treated in community-based settings; the primary nursing care focus is education. In an acute or long-term care setting, nursing care focuses on reducing the workload of the heart and improving its blood and oxygen supply.

ASSESSING

Assessment of the client with angina focuses on collecting data related to risk factors, the nature of the client's pain and associated manifestations, and measures the client is currently using to manage this condition. See Box 22-9 for focused assessment data to collect.

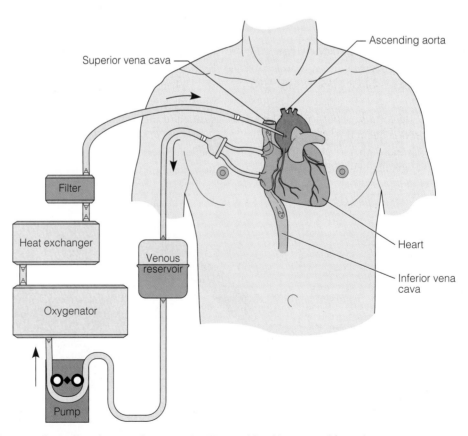

Figure 22-15. ◆ A diagram of a cardiopulmonary bypass pump. Venous blood is removed from the vena cavae, pumped through the oxygenator, and returned to the body via the ascending aorta.

BOX 22-8
NURSING CARE CHECKLIST

CARDIAC SURGERY

Before Surgery

☑ Provide routine preoperative care as outlined in Chapter 7.

☑ Teach the client and family what to expect after surgery, including:

  ☑ Returning to the cardiac recovery unit

  ☑ Tubes, drains, and general appearance

  ☑ Monitoring equipment (cardiac monitor, hemodynamic monitoring) and alarms

  ☑ Respiratory support (ventilator, endotracheal tube, suctioning, communication while intubated) and exercises

  ☑ Incisions and dressings

  ☑ Activity and diet progression

After Surgery

☑ Provide routine postoperative care as ordered (Chapter 7).

☑ Monitor vital signs including temperature, oxygen saturation, and hemodynamic measurements every 15 minutes until stable, then hourly. Report significant changes to the physician.

☑ Assess heart sounds and respiratory status at least every 4 hours. Monitor arterial blood gas (ABG) results. Report changes.

☑ Assess skin color and temperature, peripheral pulses, and level of consciousness with vital signs. Report changes.

☑ Monitor cardiac rhythm continuously; document rhythm every shift. Document and report any changes as they occur.

☑ Record intake and output hourly. Report urine output of under 30 mL/hr for 2 consecutive hours.

☑ Record chest tube output hourly. Monitor hemoglobin and hematocrit values. Report excessive blood loss or falling values to the surgeon immediately.

☑ Institute rewarming as needed (per orders or if temperature is below 96.8° F or 36° C), using warmed intravenous fluids or transfusions, warmed blankets, and other prescribed measures.

☑ Manage analgesia (PCA or by schedule) as ordered. Document effectiveness. Report anginal pain immediately to the physician.

☑ Note endotracheal tube (ETT) placement on chest x-ray; secure it in place. Insert an oral airway as needed to prevent biting and obstruction of the ETT.

☑ Maintain ventilator settings as ordered. Suction as needed. Hyperoxygenate before and after suctioning.

☑ After extubation, teach and assist with use of the incentive spirometer. Assist the client to splint the chest incision when coughing.

☑ Maintain a sterile dressing for the first 48 hours, then leave the incision open to the air. Use Steri-Strips as needed to maintain wound approximation.

☑ Monitor serum electrolytes and other lab values; report significant changes.

☑ Encourage the client and family to participate in care and decision making.

BOX 22-9
ASSESSING CLIENTS WITH ANGINA PECTORIS

SUBJECTIVE DATA

• Pain: Location, character (heavy, burning, tight, squeezing), intensity, radiation; timing (relationship to activity, meals, or other factors), duration; aggravating and relieving factors; associated manifestations

• History of angina or other heart disease, previous or current treatment measures

• Risk factors: Family history of CHD; history of hypertension, diabetes, high blood cholesterol levels; smoking and alcohol intake, use of other recreational drugs; perceived stress levels and techniques used to manage stress; for women, age of menopause, use of hormone replacement therapy or oral contraceptives

OBJECTIVE DATA

• Frequency and duration of angina; effectiveness of relief measures (oxygen, NTG, rest)

• Vital signs and ECG tracing during anginal episode

• Laboratory data: Hemoglobin and hematocrit; cardiac enzyme levels

DIAGNOSING, PLANNING, AND IMPLEMENTING

INEFFECTIVE TISSUE PERFUSION: CARDIOPULMONARY

- If short-acting NTG is ordered, keep it at the bedside so it can be taken at the onset of pain. *Immediate treatment can restore blood flow to the heart muscle and reduce the intensity and duration of anginal pain.*
- Start oxygen at 4 to 6 L/min per nasal cannula unless contraindicated. *Supplemental oxygen reduces myocardial hypoxia.*
- Space activities to allow rest between them. *Activity increases cardiac work and may precipitate angina. Spacing of activities allows the heart to recover.*
- Instruct the client to take a sublingual NTG tablet before engaging in activities that precipitate angina (e.g., climbing stairs, sexual intercourse). *This prophylactic dose of NTG helps maintain cardiac perfusion when increased work is anticipated, preventing ischemia and chest pain.*
- Encourage risk factor management, e.g., losing weight, making dietary changes (reducing fat, cholesterol, and kcal intake), reducing stress, and others as indicated. *Managing risk factors can slow the process of atherosclerosis and preserve myocardial perfusion.*
- Encourage the client to implement and maintain a progressive exercise program under the supervision of his or her primary care provider. *Exercise slows the atherosclerotic process and helps develop collateral circulation to the heart muscle.*
- Refer the client who smokes to a smoking cessation program. *Nicotine causes vasoconstriction and increases the heart rate, decreasing myocardial perfusion and increasing cardiac workload.*

RISK FOR INEFFECTIVE THERAPEUTIC REGIMEN MANAGEMENT

- Assess knowledge and understanding of angina. *Assessment allows teaching and interventions to be tailored to the needs of the client.*
- Teach about angina and atherosclerosis as needed. *Denial or exaggerated fear may be strong in clients with angina pectoris. Teaching helps the client understand that angina can be managed, pain controlled, and the disease progress slowed.*
- Provide written and verbal instructions about prescribed medications and their use. *Written instructions reinforce teaching and are available to the client for future reference.*
- Stress the importance of taking chest pains seriously while maintaining a positive attitude. *Chest pain is a warning and necessitates appropriate response.*
- Refer to a cardiac rehabilitation program or other organized activities and support groups for clients with coronary artery disease. *Programs such as these help the client develop strategies for risk factor management, maintain a program of supervised activity, and gain coping skills.*

EVALUATING

When evaluating the effectiveness of nursing care for the client with angina, collect data regarding the onset, duration, and management of anginal episodes. Use subjective and objective data to evaluate knowledge, understanding, and willingness to follow physician's orders and manage risk factors.

Discharge Considerations

Clients with stable angina often manage their pain effectively, continuing to live active and productive lives. Discuss the relationship between modifiable risk factors and angina. Provide information about risk factor management, as well as the disease process. Emphasize the relationship between reduced blood flow to the heart muscle and pain. Discuss the use of prescribed medications. Instruct to take NTG prophylactically, before activities that tend to cause chest pain. Advise taking NTG at the first indication of pain rather than waiting to see whether the pain develops. Emphasize the importance of seeking immediate medical assistance if three NTG tablets over 15 to 20 minutes do not relieve the pain. Instruct to call 911 or go to the emergency department immediately rather than contacting the physician.

Teach safe medication storage, especially for NTG. Because this is an unstable compound, instruct to store it in a cool, dry, dark place and to keep no more than a 6-month supply on hand. Advise to always carry a few tablets but not the whole supply, because body warmth (transmitted through a shirt or pants pocket) causes tablets to deteriorate more rapidly. If an NTG patch or ointment is prescribed, teach how to apply it. Explain the rationale for removing the patch or ointment at night.

Stress the importance of not discontinuing medications abruptly, particularly beta blockers. Review their adverse effects, and instruct when to notify the physician.

When cardiac surgery is anticipated, provide general preoperative teaching (see Chapter 7), as well as specifics related to the planned surgery. Reinforce instructions about respiratory care, activity, and pain management. Reinforce the importance of being an active participant in rehabilitation. Before discharge, teach about ordered medications, the manifestations of an infection, pain management, diet, and activity. Discuss posthospital cardiac rehabilitation.

See the Critical Thinking Care Map at the end of this chapter for an opportunity to apply what you have learned about angina.

Acute Myocardial Infarction

In an **acute myocardial infarction (MI),** cells in an area of cardiac muscle necrose (die) due to lack of blood and oxygen. It is a life-threatening event: If circulation to the affected cardiac muscle is not rapidly restored, functional muscle is lost and the heart may be unable to maintain an effective cardiac output. This can lead to cardiogenic shock and death. Most deaths from MI occur within the first hour following the onset of manifestations, often before the client reaches the hospital.

MI rarely occurs in clients without preexisting coronary artery disease. While no specific cause has been identified, the risk factors for MI are those for coronary heart disease: age, gender, heredity; smoking, obesity, hyperlipidemia, hypertension, diabetes, stress, and sedentary lifestyle.

PATHOPHYSIOLOGY

MI occurs when a coronary artery becomes occluded, blocking blood flow to a portion of cardiac muscle for a prolonged period of time. Occlusion is usually caused by development of a thrombus (clot) in an area of atherosclerotic narrowing. The occlusion blocks blood flow to myocardium distal to the obstruction.

When the cells are deprived of oxygen and nutrients for more than 20 to 45 minutes, they are irreversibly damaged, leading to cellular death and tissue necrosis. Intracellular enzymes are released as cells die. This necrotic tissue (*infarct*) is surrounded by an area of injured and ischemic tissues. If blood flow is restored, the injured and ishemic tissue recovers and heals. The infarcted tissue, however, no longer conducts electrical energy and ceases to contract. Because of this, cardiac output falls.

Collateral vessels connected to the smaller arteries in the coronary system dilate to maintain blood flow to the cardiac muscle when a larger coronary artery is occluded. In clients who remain active, collateral vessels develop and enlarge to meet the demand for blood flow as larger coronary arteries progressively narrow. Good collateral circulation can reduce the size of an infarction.

MI usually affects the left ventricle because it is the major "workhorse" of the heart; its muscle mass is greater, as are its oxygen demands.

MIs are described according to the area of the heart that is damaged. Occlusion of the left anterior descending (LAD) artery damages the *anterior* portion of the left ventricle; occlusion of the left circumflex artery (LCA) causes *lateral* damage. *Right ventricular, inferior,* and *posterior* MIs involve occlusions of the right coronary artery (RCA) and posterior descending artery (PDA). (See Figure 22-4.)

MIs may also be classified as either transmural or subendocardial. A *transmural* infarction involves all layers of the heart. A *subendocardial* infarction involves only the inner layer of the heart, and does not extend through the myocardium and epicardium.

Pain is a classic manifestation of MI. Chest pain is often described as crushing and severe; the client may call it a pressure, heavy, or squeezing sensation, or complain of chest tightness or burning. The pain begins in the center of the chest (in the substernal region), and may radiate to the shoulders, neck, jaw, or arms. It lasts more than 15 to 20 minutes and is not relieved by rest or NTG. The client often experiences a sense

---

BOX 22-10
MANIFESTATIONS OF MYOCARDIAL INFARCTION

- Chest pain
- Tachycardia
- Shortness of breath, dyspnea
- Cool, clammy skin
- Diaphoresis
- Anxiety
- Feeling of impending doom
- Nausea and vomiting
- Possible dysrhythmias

---

of impending doom and death. Typical signs and symptoms of MI are listed in Box 22-10.

Women and older adults may not have the "typical" manifestations of MI, increasing the risk that they will not seek treatment. Box 22-11 focuses on MI in women and older adults.

Cocaine-Induced MI

In recent years, acute MI associated with cocaine intoxication has been reported. Cocaine stimulates the heart rate, increases

---

BOX 22-11

population
FOCUS

Heart Disease in Women and Older Adults

Heart disease—myocardial infarction in particular—is the leading cause of death for women and older adults. In fact, more women than men die of heart disease every year. Women with symptoms of a myocardial infarction are likely to delay seeking treatment for several hours—an average of an hour longer than men. After an MI, the death rate for women is three times that of men, both in the hospital and within the first year.

Women and older adults are more likely than men to have a "silent" or unrecognized heart attack. Many women having an MI experience epigastric pain and nausea, causing them to believe their pain is due to heartburn. Chest pain in women often occurs during mental stress or while resting. Shortness of breath is common, as is fatigue and weakness of the shoulders and upper arms.

Older people may seek treatment for vague complaints of difficulty breathing, confusion, fainting, dizziness, abdominal pain, or cough. Many older adults who experience an MI do not complain of chest pain. When these clients seek care with vague symptoms and a history of cardiovascular problems, an MI should be suspected.

When teaching women and older adults about heart disease, emphasize the importance of seeking immediate medical care for manifestations of an acute MI. With prompt treatment, survival in both groups is improved.

its contractility, and causes vasoconstriction and hypertension. As a result, the workload of the heart increases. Cocaine also increases the risk of dysrhythmias. The client with cocaine-induced MI may have an altered level of consciousness, confusion and restlessness, seizure activity, tachycardia, hypotension, increased respiratory rate, and respiratory crackles.

Complications

The risk of complications associated with MI is related to the size and location of infarcted tissue.

DYSRHYTHMIAS. Dysrhythmias are the most frequent complication. Sinus tachycardia is common. Clients may develop symptomatic bradycardia or heart blocks. Premature atrial contractions (PACs) and atrial fibrillation may occur. Premature ventricular contractions (PVCs) are common, particularly in the first few hours following an MI. Frequent PVCs (more than 6 per minute), couplets, short bursts of ventricular tachycardia, and early PVCs (R on T wave) are treated with drugs to reduce the risk of ventricular fibrillation. The risk of V-fib is greatest the first hour after MI; it is a frequent cause of sudden cardiac death associated with acute MI. (See Table 22-1.)

PUMP FAILURE. MI reduces myocardial contractility and ventricular filling. Heart failure may develop, particularly when large portions of the left ventricle are affected. With loss of 20% to 30% of the left ventricular muscle, the client may develop manifestations of left-sided heart failure, including dyspnea, fatigue, weakness, and respiratory crackles on auscultation. Heart failure and its manifestations are discussed in greater depth later in this chapter.

If more than 40% of the left ventricle is infarcted, **cardiogenic shock,** impaired tissue perfusion due to pump failure, results. The client is hypotensive and has signs of impaired tissue perfusion, such as low urinary output, decreased level of consciousness, and cool, clammy skin. Perfusion of the heart itself also is affected, further increasing tissue damage. See Chapter 10 for a more extensive discussion of shock.

OTHER COMPLICATIONS. Pericarditis (inflammation of the pericardium) may develop after an MI, usually within 2 to 3 days. Chest pain associated with pericarditis is sharp and stabbing, aggravated by movement or deep breathing. A pericardial friction rub may be noted on auscultation of heart sounds.

Approximately 10% of clients experience *extension* or *expansion* of MI within 10 to 14 days. The client may have continuing chest pain, unstable vital signs, or worsening heart failure. Because the scar tissue that replaces necrotic muscle is thinner than the ventricular muscle mass, a *ventricular aneurysm* may develop or rupture may occur. A ventricular aneurysm is an outpouching of the ventricular wall. *Myocardial rupture* is often fatal, and may occur between days 4 and 7 after MI, when the injured tissue is soft and weak.

COLLABORATIVE CARE

Rapid assessment and early diagnosis are vital in an MI. "Time is muscle"—the quicker the artery is reopened (medically or surgically), the more myocardium can be saved and fewer complications develop. The American Heart Association (AHA) recommends definitive treatment be initiated within 1 hour of arrival at the emergency center.

The major problem is delay in seeking medical care after the onset of chest pain or other cardiac symptoms. Up to 44% of clients with symptoms of MI wait more than 4 hours before seeking treatment.

Laboratory Tests

The principal laboratory tests ordered when an MI is suspected MI are *serum cardiac markers.* As cardiac cells die, their contents are released into the bloodstream. Serum levels of these proteins can then be measured. The serum creatine kinase (CK; also called creatinine phosphokinase, or CPK) and cardiac-specific troponins are most specific for diagnosis of MI. *Creatine kinase* is an enzyme found in cardiac muscle. CK levels rise rapidly following MI; it is detectable in the serum within 3 to 6 hours, peaks within 12 to 24 hours, and then declines over the next 48 to 72 hours. The greater the amount of infarcted tissue, the higher its level. A CK *isoenzyme* specific to cardiac muscle, CK-MB (also called MB-bands), is the most sensitive indicator of MI (Table 22-5 ◆).

Cardiac muscle troponins, *cardiac-specific troponin T (cT_nT) and cardiac-specific troponin I (cT_nI),* are proteins that normally cannot be detected in the blood. With cardiac muscle necrosis, troponins are released and blood levels rise. Because they remain in the blood for 10 to 14 days, they can help diagnose an MI when treatment is delayed by several days.

Lactic dehydrogenase (LDH) is an enzyme found in many body tissues, and is a less specific indicator of myocardial damage.

Serum levels of cardiac markers are ordered on admission and for 3 succeeding days. Serial blood levels are used to establish the diagnosis and to evaluate the extent of myocardial damage.

Diagnostic Tests

Electrocardiography, echocardiography, and myocardial nuclear scans are the most common diagnostic tests performed for a suspected MI. Ischemic or necrotic cardiac cells do not respond normally to electrical stimulation. This causes a change in ECG waveforms. The location of myocardial damage can be identified on the 12-lead ECG. Characteristic changes in the ECG with an acute MI include:

- Inversion of the T wave
- Depression or elevation of the ST segment
- Formation of a Q wave

Echocardiography uses ultrasound to evaluate cardiac structures and left ventricular function. Images are produced

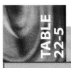

TABLE 22-5   CARDIAC MARKERS

MARKER	NORMAL LEVEL	PRIMARY TISSUE LOCATION	SIGNIFICANCE OF ELEVATION	CHANGES OCCURRING IN AN MI		
				Appears	*Peaks*	*Duration*
Creatine kinase (CK or CPK)	Male: 12–80 U/L Female: 10–70 U/L	Cardiac and skeletal muscle, brain	Injury to muscle cells	3–6 hours	12–24 hours	24–48 hours
Creatine kindase M-bands (CK-MB)	0–3% of total CK	Cardiac muscle	MI, myocarditis, cardiac contusion, defibrillation	4–8 hours	18–24 hours	72 hours
Cardiac-specific troponin T (cT$_n$T)	< 0.2 µg/L	Cardiac muscle	Acute MI, unstable angina	2–4 hours	24–36 hours	10–14 days
Cardiac-specific troponin I (cT$_n$I)	< 3.1 µg/L	Cardiac muscle	Acute MI, unstable angina	2–4 hours	24–36 hours	7–10 days
Lactic dehydrogenase (LDH)	45–90 U/L	Heart, liver, kidneys, skeletal muscle, brain, RBCs, lungs	MI; disease of other organs or tissues containing LDH	24–72 hours	3–4 days	10–14 days

as ultrasound waves strike cardiac structures and are reflected back through a transducer. Echocardiography can be performed at the bedside and is used to diagnose MI and complications such as ventricular aneurysm.

Myocardial perfusion imaging scans are nuclear scans used to detect changes in coronary blood flow and myocardial tissue.

Medical Management

The client with a suspected or confirmed MI is monitored continuously from entry into the medical system. Care is provided in the intensive coronary care unit for the first 24 to 48 hours, after which less intensive monitoring (e.g., telemetry) may be required. An intravenous line is established to allow rapid administration of emergency drugs.

Bed rest with bedside commode is ordered initially to reduce the cardiac workload. After 12 to 24 hours, activities are gradually increased. A quiet, calm environment with limited outside stimuli, such as television and telephone, is preferred. Visitors are limited to close family members for short periods of time. Oxygen is administered by nasal cannula at 2 to 6 L/min to improve oxygenation of the myocardium and other tissues.

A low-fat, low-cholesterol, reduced-sodium diet is allowed. Small, frequent feedings are often recommended. Drinks containing caffeine and very hot and cold foods may be limited.

Pharmacology

Pain relief is vital in treating the client with an acute MI. Pain stimulates the sympathetic nervous system, increasing the heart rate and blood pressure and, in turn, myocardial workload. *Morphine sulfate* is the drug of choice for pain and sedation. It is given intravenously in small doses until pain is relieved. *Sublingual NTG* may be ordered to relieve pain and improve blood flow to the myocardium. It is important to assess frequently for pain relief and possible adverse effects of analgesia, such as excessive sedation. Antianxiety agents, such as diazepam (Valium) may also be given to promote rest.

Thrombolytic agents, drugs that dissolve or break up blood clots, are used to treat acute MI. These drugs activate the fibrinolytic system to destroy the clot, restoring blood flow to the obstructed artery. When given within the first 6 hours of MI symptoms, thrombolytics limit infarct size, reduce heart damage, and improve the chances of survival. These drugs also can cause multiple complications; up to 5% of clients receiv-

ity of the ventricles. The heart rate increases when cardiac output falls, increasing the workload of the heart.

- Report changes in level of consciousness; decreased urine output; moist, cool, pale, mottled or cyanotic skin; dusky or cyanotic mucous membranes and nail beds; diminished to absent peripheral pulses; delayed capillary refill. *These are manifestations of decreased tissue perfusion. A change in level of consciousness is often the first manifestation of altered perfusion because brain tissue and cerebral function depend on a continuous supply of oxygen.*
- Auscultate heart and breath sounds. Note abnormal heart sounds (e.g., an S_3 or S_4 gallop or murmur) or adventitious lung sounds. *Abnormal heart or lung sounds may indicate impaired cardiac function.*
- Monitor ECG rhythm continuously. Report dysrhythmias. *Dysrhythmias can further impair cardiac output and tissue perfusion.*
- Administer antidysrhythmic medications as needed. *Dysrhythmias affect tissue perfusion by altering cardiac output.*

INEFFECTIVE COPING

- Establish an environment of caring and trust. Encourage the client to express feelings. *A trusting nurse–client relationship provides a safe environment for the client to discuss feelings of helplessness, powerlessness, anxiety, and hopelessness.*
- Accept denial as a coping mechanism, but do not reinforce it. *Denial may initially help decrease anxiety by diminishing the perceived threat to health. Prolonged denial can interfere with acceptance of reality and cooperation, possibly delaying treatment and hindering recovery.*
- Note aggressive behaviors, hostility, or anger. Document any failure to comply with treatments. *These behaviors may indicate anxiety and denial.*
- Help identify positive coping skills used in the past (e.g., problem-solving skills, verbalization of feelings, asking for help, prayer). Reinforce positive coping behaviors. *Previously successful coping behaviors can help the client deal with the current situation. These familiar methods can decrease feelings of powerlessness.*
- Allow the client to make decisions about care, as possible. *Participating in care planning gives a sense of control and the opportunity to use positive coping skills.*
- Provide privacy for the client and significant other to share their questions and concerns. *Privacy allows the client and partner the opportunity to share their feelings and fears, offer support and encouragement to one another, relieve anxiety, and establish effective coping methods.*

FEAR

- Acknowledge the client's perception of the situation. Allow to verbalize concerns. *The sudden change in health status brings on anxiety and fear of the unknown. Verbalizing these fears may help the client cope with the changes and allow the health care team to provide information and correct misconceptions.*

- Encourage questions, and provide consistent, factual answers. Repeat information as needed. *Accurate and consistent information can reduce fear and help develop realistic expectations. Anxiety and fear decrease the ability to concentrate and retain information; information may need to be repeated.*
- Administer antianxiety medications as ordered. *These medications promote rest and relaxation and decrease feelings of anxiety, which may act as barriers to restoration of health.*
- Teach nonpharmacologic methods of stress reduction (e.g., relaxation methods, mental imagery, music therapy, breathing exercises, meditation, massage). *Stress management techniques may help reduce tension and anxiety, provide the client with a sense of control, and enhance coping skills.*

EVALUATING

To evaluate the effectiveness of nursing care for the client with an MI, collect data such as the following:

- Pain level and relief with prescribed analgesic
- Evidence of adequate tissue perfusion: Level of consciousness, urine output, heart and lung sounds, skin color and temperature, peripheral pulses, ECG rhythm
- Acceptance of diagnosis, involvement in care, and participation in care planning
- Expressions or nonverbal evidence of fear and anxiety

Discharge Considerations

Teaching and planning for home care begins with admission to the coronary care unit and continues through the hospital stay and after discharge into the rehabilitation period. The emphasis is on restoring optimal health and reducing the risk of future cardiac events.

Assessing readiness to learn is an important first step. The client in strong denial may not believe that the information being taught has any relevance. Evaluate ability to learn, assessing knowledge base, physiologic and psychologic health, health beliefs, and expectations of the health care system.

Teach about CHD and myocardial infarction. Explain the purpose of prescribed dietary changes and activity restrictions. Discuss prescribed medications, including their purposes and side effects. Encourage the client to ask questions. Reinforce teaching with written materials.

Provide referral to a cardiac rehabilitation program. Emphasize the importance of complying with the medical regimen and cardiac rehabilitation program and of keeping follow-up appointments. Provide telephone numbers of resource personnel who are available to respond to questions and concerns after the client's discharge.

Provide information about community resources, such as the local chapter of the AHA. Encourage family members to learn CPR in the event of an emergency, and provide information about other community agencies that offer CPR classes.

Nursing Process Case Study
■ CLIENT WITH ACUTE MYOCARDIAL INFARCTION

Betty Williams, a 62-year-old psychologist, is admitted to the emergency department complaining of severe substernal chest pain. She thought the pain, which started after lunch, was indigestion. She describes the pain as "like someone sitting on my chest." The pain radiates to her jaw and left arm, and is accompanied by a "choking feeling," severe shortness of breath, and diaphoresis. The pain is unrelieved by rest, antacids, or three sublingual NTG tablets (gr 1/150).

After inserting an intravenous catheter and beginning oxygen at 6 L/min per nasal cannula, a 12-lead ECG and cardiac enzymes are obtained. Mrs. Williams's pain is relieved by intravenous morphine sulfate. Based on her history, assessment, and ECG, an acute anterior wall MI is diagnosed. Intravenous alteplase (t-PA) is administered followed by intravenous infusions of heparin. Mrs. Williams is transferred to the coronary care unit (CCU).

Assessment Mrs. Williams's medical history includes Type 2 diabetes, angina, and hypertension. She has smoked cigarettes for 45 years, averaging 1½ to 2 packs per day. Her father died at age 42 of MI, and her paternal grandfather died at age 65 of MI. Mrs. Williams is currently taking tolbutamide (Orinase) and metoprolol (Lopressor).

On admission to the CCU, Mrs. Williams is alert and oriented to time, place, and person; P 118; BP 172/92; R 24; T 99.6° F (37.5° C). Auscultation reveals an S_4 and fine crackles in the bases of both lungs. The ECG shows sinus tachycardia with occasional PVCs. Her skin is cool and slightly diaphoretic. Capillary refill is less than 3 seconds, and peripheral pulses are strong and equal. Her nail beds are pink.

A triple-lumen central line is in place, with nitroglycerine, t-PA, and heparin infusions controlled by infusion pumps. A solution of 5% dextrose in ¼ normal saline solution is infusing in a peripheral intravenous line. Mrs. Williams states, "The pain is better since the nurse in the ER gave me a shot. But it has been coming and going. I would rate it a 4 right now, but it was terrible before. The doctor told me that this drug I'm getting will quickly open up the artery that is blocked. I hope it works! Do many people get this drug?"

Diagnosis The CCU nurses formulate the following nursing diagnoses for Mrs. Williams:

■ Pain related to cardiac muscle ischemia and infarct
■ Anxiety related to change in health status
■ Ineffective Protection related to the risk of bleeding secondary to thrombolytic therapy
■ Risk for Injury related to altered cardiac rate and rhythm

Expected Outcomes The expected outcomes of the plan of care specify that Mrs. Williams will:

■ Verbalize relief of chest pain.
■ Verbalize a reduced anxiety and fear.
■ Exhibit no signs of internal or external bleeding.
■ Maintain an adequate cardiac output.

Planning and Implementation The following interventions are planned and implemented:

■ Instruct to report any chest pain. Titrate NTG infusion for chest pain; stop infusion if systolic BP drops below 100 mm Hg. Administer 2 to 4 mg morphine intravenously for chest pain unrelieved by nitroglycerin infusion.
■ Encourage verbalization of fears and concerns. Answer questions honestly, and correct any misconceptions about disease process, therapeutic interventions, or prognosis.
■ Explain that the tPA will dissolve the clot obstructing blood flow to the heart muscle, thus limiting heart damage.
■ Explain the need for frequent assessment.
■ Assess for evidence of internal or intracranial bleeding: Back or abdominal pain, headache, decreased level of consciousness, dizziness, bloody secretions or excretions, or pallor. Test all stools, urine, and vomitus for occult blood. Notify physician immediately of any abnormal findings.
■ Continuously monitor ECG.
■ Immediately treat dysrhythmias or other cardiac emergencies per unit protocol.

Evaluation Mrs. Williams's chest pain is relieved with the morphine, NTG infusion, and thrombolytic therapy. She states that she feels "much better now that the pain is gone. I was afraid it would just get worse." No indication of bleeding problems are noted, and while her PVCs increase with reperfusion therapy, she experiences no significant dysrhythmias. Mrs. Williams remains in CCU for 2 days and is transferred to the floor.

Critical Thinking in the Nursing Process

1. You are admitting Mrs. Williams to the medical unit from CCU. What assessment data will you obtain? What nursing diagnoses and interventions will you anticipate as part of Mrs. Williams's care at this point in her recovery?

2. Two days after her initial therapy, Mrs. Williams complains of palpitations. You notice frequent PVCs on the ECG monitor. What do you do?

3. Mrs. Williams states, "I have been smoking for over 45 years, and I am not going to stop now! Besides, it calms me down when I am feeling anxious." How would you respond to this statement?

Disorders of Cardiac Function

Heart Failure

Heart failure is defined as the inability of the heart to function as a pump to meet the needs of the body. Heart failure may result from any condition that (a) increases the workload of the heart beyond its limits, (b) affects the ability of the heart muscle to contract effectively, or (c) affects blood flow through or within the heart (Table 22-6 ◆). Hypertension and coronary heart disease with myocardial ischemia and infarction are the leading causes of heart failure in the United States.

The incidence of heart failure increases significantly with age; 10% or more of people aged 75 or older are affected (Box 22-14). African-Americans, who have a high incidence of hypertension, also have a significant risk of developing heart failure. Heart failure generally is a progressive disease, with the client experiencing declining heart function and more frequent episodes of failure. Box 22-15 shows the American Heart Association classification for heart failure.

PATHOPHYSIOLOGY

When the cardiac output falls, *compensatory mechanisms* are activated to maintain tissue perfusion. The sympathetic nervous system (SNS) is stimulated. As a result, the heart rate and stroke volume increase. SNS stimulation also causes arterial and venous vasoconstriction, increasing venous return to the heart. Increased venous return increases ventricular filling and myocardial stretch (preload), increasing the force of contraction. Blood flow is redistributed to the brain and the heart to maintain perfusion of these vital organs.

A fall in cardiac output also activates the renin–angiotensin–aldosterone system, which produces additional vasoconstriction and salt and water retention. Salt and water retention increase the blood volume to help restore cardiac output.

The chambers of the heart dilate to accommodate the additional fluid volume. Initially, this leads to more effective contractions. Cardiac muscle cells enlarge, leading to *ventricular hypertrophy.*

Although all of these responses may initially help maintain cardiac output, their long-term effects hasten the deterioration of cardiac function. Heart failure occurs when these mechanisms no longer maintain a cardiac output that meets the metabolic needs of the body.

The rapid heart rate, salt and water retention, increased preload, and arterial vasoconstriction increase the workload of the heart. The ventricles continue to dilate to accommodate the excess fluid, but the heart loses its ability to contract forcefully. The heart muscle may eventually become so large that the coronary blood supply is inadequate, causing ischemia.

In normal hearts, the cardiac reserve allows the heart to adjust its output to meet metabolic needs of the body. Clients with heart failure have very little cardiac reserve. At rest, they

TABLE 22-6	SELECTED CAUSES OF HEART FAILURE	
INCREASED WORKLOAD	**ALTERED FUNCTION**	**ALTERED FILLING AND FLOW**
Hypertension	Myocardial infarction	Valve stenosis
Fluid overload	Cardiomyopathy	Cardiac tamponade
Anemia	Rheumatic fever	Restrictive pericarditis
Pregnancy	Dysrhythmias	Congenital heart defects

BOX 22-14

population
FOCUS

Older Adults and Cardiac Function

Aging affects cardiac function. Ventricular walls become stiffer, affecting filling. The response to exercise and sympathetic stimulation is slowed, and cardiac reserve is reduced. Other health problems (e.g., arthritis) often contribute to a more sedentary lifestyle, further decreasing the heart's ability to respond to stress. Salt intake often increases with aging as taste decreases. Limited mobility or visual acuity may cause the older adult to rely on high-sodium foods like canned soups and frozen meals. Teach older adults how to adapt to changes in cardiovascular function:

- Allow longer warm-up and cool-down periods during exercise.
- Engage in regular exercise such as walking 3 to 4 times a week.
- Rest with feet elevated (e.g., in a recliner) when fatigued.
- Maintain adequate fluid intake.
- Reduce sodium intake by using herbs and other flavorings; read food labels for sodium content.

may be unaffected; however, any stressor (e.g., exercise, illness) taxes their ability to meet the demand for oxygen and nutrients.

Heart failure is often classified by the primary pumping chamber affected and by its effects. Clients may have manifestations of *left-sided* and/or *right-sided failure.* The effects of heart failure on cardiac output and venous congestion are referred to as *forward* and *backward effects.*

Left-Sided Heart Failure

Although either side of the heart can fail, the left ventricle is affected more often than the right because of its high workload and oxygen demand. Left-sided heart failure results from ventricular muscle damage or overloading. As left ventricular function deteriorates, cardiac output falls *(forward effect).* Impaired emptying of the left ventricle leads to increased pressures on the left side of the heart and in the pulmonary vascular system *(backward effects).* Increased pressures in this normally low-pressure system push fluid from the blood vessels into interstitial tissues and the alveoli (Figure 22-17 ◆).

The manifestations of left-sided heart failure result from pulmonary congestion and decreased cardiac output (Box 22-16). Fatigue, activity intolerance, and dyspnea on exertion (DOE) are common early manifestations. **Orthopnea** (breathing difficulty while lying down), may prompt the client to sleep propped up on two or three pillows or in a recliner. Inspiratory crackles (rales) and wheezes may be heard in lung bases.

ACUTE PULMONARY EDEMA. *Acute pulmonary edema,* accumulation of fluid in the interstitial spaces and alveoli of the lungs, may occur with severe left-ventricular failure. The client in pulmonary edema has acute and severe dyspnea, shortness of breath, and anxiety. The skin is cool, clammy, and cyanotic. A productive cough with pink, frothy sputum is also present. If cerebral hypoxia occurs, the client may be confused or lethargic. Crackles are heard throughout the lung fields. As the condition worsens, breathing becomes more labored and lung sounds harsher. Pulmonary edema is a medical emergency: The client is "drowning" as a result of fluid in the alveolar and pulmonary spaces and must be treated immediately.

Right-Sided Heart Failure

The most common cause of right ventricular failure is left ventricular failure. Increased pressures in the pulmonary system

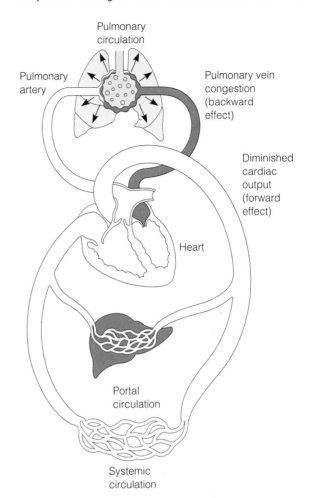

Figure 22-17. ◆ The forward and backward effects of left-sided heart failure.

or damage to the right ventricle impair blood flow into the pulmonary circulation. The right ventricle and atrium become distended, and blood accumulates in the systemic venous system. Increased venous pressures lead to abdominal organ congestion and peripheral tissue edema (Figure 22-18 ◆).

Fluid collects in dependent tissues because of the effects of gravity. Edema develops in the feet and legs of an upright client and in the sacrum of one who is reclining. Congestion of vessels in the abdomen can lead to right upper quadrant pain, anorexia and nausea. Distended jugular veins may be visible even when the client is standing (see Box 22-16).

Biventricular Failure

When both ventricles fail to function adequately, the client has manifestations of both right- and left-sided or *biventricular* heart failure. *Paroxysmal nocturnal dyspnea (PND),* a frightening condition in which the client awakens at night acutely short of breath, may occur. PND occurs when edema fluid that has accumulated during the day is reabsorbed into the circulation at night, causing fluid overload and pulmonary congestion. The client in severe heart failure may be dyspneic at rest as well as with activity, signifying little or no cardiac reserve.

BOX 22-16
MANIFESTATIONS OF HEART FAILURE

LEFT-SIDED
Forward Effects

Activity intolerance
Fatigue
Weakness
Dizziness and syncope

Backward Effects

Shortness of breath
Dyspnea, orthopnea
Cough
Tachycardia
Crackles in lung bases

RIGHT-SIDED
Forward Effects

Fatigue
Activity intolerance

Backward Effects

Jugular vein distention
Peripheral edema
Anorexia, nausea
Abdominal distention, ascites
Liver, spleen enlargement, tenderness

COLLABORATIVE CARE

The main goals for the client with heart failure are to reduce cardiac workload, improve cardiac pumping ability, and control fluid retention. The focus is on improving activity tolerance and decreasing mortality and morbidity.

Diagnostic tests are used to evaluate the effects of heart failure. *Serum electrolytes* are measured to evaluate fluid and electrolyte status, as well as the effects of treatment. The *chest x-ray* may show pulmonary vascular congestion and cardiomegaly if the heart has hypertrophied or dilated. An *echocardiogram* is done to evaluate left ventricular function and assess for ventricular dilation and hypertrophy. The *ECG* shows changes associated with ventricular enlargement, and may show dysrhythmias, myocardial ischemia, or infarction.

Hemodynamic Monitoring

Hemodynamic monitoring may be used to assess cardiovascular function and the response to treatment. A multilumen catheter inserted through a central vein into the right side of the heart and pulmonary artery is used to measure central venous pressure, pulmonary artery pressures, and cardiac output. These pressures and the cardiac output are used to evaluate fluid balance, ventricular function, and the effects of interventions (e.g., drug therapy). The arterial blood pressure can be measured using a peripheral arterial line.

The pressure within a vessel is converted into an electrical signal. The electrical signal is then recorded on graph paper and displayed on a monitor (Figure 22-19 ◆). While hemodynamic monitoring provides valuable information to help manage heart failure, it has some risks. The presence of an invasive catheter increases the risk of infection, bleeding, and thrombus formation. The lung may be punctured during insertion of the catheter into the subclavian vein, causing a pneumothorax. Dysrhythmias may develop as the catheter passes through the right ventricle.

Pharmacology

Clients with heart failure typically receive multiple medications to reduce cardiac work and improve cardiac function.

Pulmonary circulation

Pulmonary artery

Pulmonary veins

Heart

Congested portal circulation

Congested systemic circulation

Figure 22-18. ◆ The effects of right-sided heart failure.

Figure 22-19. ◆ A hemodynamic monitoring setup.

The main drug classes used to treat heart failure are the angiotensin-converting enzyme (ACE) inhibitors, diuretics, inotropic medications (such as digitalis and dopamine), and direct vasodilators (Table 22-7 ◆). Complementary treatment with hawthorn is discussed in Box 22-17.

Morphine sulfate is a drug of choice for treating acute pulmonary edema. Morphine relieves anxiety, improves breathing, and also is a venous vasodilator. It reduces venous return and lowers left atrial pressure. Potent loop diuretics such as furosemide or bumetanide are administered intravenously to promote rapid diuresis.

DIGITALIS. Digitalis has a positive inotropic effect on the heart, increasing the strength of myocardial contraction. Digitalis has a *narrow therapeutic index;* in other words, thera-

TABLE 22-7

NURSING IMPLICATIONS FOR PHARMACOLOGY: CLIENTS WITH HEART FAILURE

CLASS/DRUGS	PURPOSE	NURSING RESPONSIBILITIES	CLIENT TEACHING
Positive Inotropic Agents *Digitalis Glycosides* <ul><li>Digoxin (Lanoxin)</li><li>Digitoxin (Crystodigin)</li></ul>	Improve myocardial contractility, increasing stroke volume and cardiac output. Greater cardiac output improves renal perfusion, decreasing renin secretion and cardiac work. Slow heart rate and reduce oxygen consumption.	Assess apical pulse before giving digitalis. Hold the drug and notify the physician if HR < 60 bpm. Record HR on medication record. Assess serum electrolytes and digoxin levels. Hypokalemia increases the risk of digitalis toxicity. Report manifestations of digitalis toxicity: Anorexia, nausea, vomiting, abdominal pain, weakness, vision changes (diplopia, blurred vision, halos seen around objects), and dysrhythmias.	Take your pulse before each dose. Do not take the digitalis if your pulse is < 60. Notify your doctor immediately. Call your doctor if you develop palpitations, weakness, loss of appetite, nausea, vomiting, abdominal pain, blurred or colored vision, double vision. Avoid antacids and laxatives; they decrease the absorption of digoxin. Include high-potassium foods in your diet: Orange or tomato juice, bananas, raisins, dates, figs, prunes, apricots, spinach, cauliflower, and potatoes.
Sympathomimetic Agents <ul><li>Dopamine (Inotropin)</li><li>Dobutamine (Dobutrex)</li></ul> **Phosphodiesterase Inhibitors** <ul><li>Amrinone (Inocor)</li><li>Milrinone (Primacor)</li></ul>	These drugs improve the force of ventricular contraction. Sympathomimetic drugs are given intravenously, adjusting the dose to obtain maximal effect. Phosphodiesterase inhibitors also cause vasodilation, reducing cardiac workload.	Use an infusion pump to administer these drugs. Frequently monitor vital signs and hemodynamic measurements. Titrate the drug to maintain the BP and heart rate. Avoid discontinuing these agents abruptly. Change solutions and tubing every 24 hours.	Notify the nursing staff if you experience abdominal pain or notice a skin rash or bruising.

(continues)

TABLE 22-7   NURSING IMPLICATIONS FOR PHARMACOLOGY: CLIENTS WITH HEART FAILURE (CONTINUED)

CLASS/DRUGS	PURPOSE	NURSING RESPONSIBILITIES	CLIENT TEACHING
Angiotensin-Converting Enzyme (ACE) Inhibitors ▪ Enalapril maleate (Vasotec) ▪ Lisinopril (Prinivil, Zestril) ▪ Captopril (Capoten)	ACE inhibitors block the effect of the renin–angiotensin–aldosterone system, reducing vasoconstriction and sodium and water retention. The result is decreased cardiac workload and reduced edema.	Avoid discontinuing these agents abruptly. Give captopril 1 hour before meals. Maintain bed rest and monitor BP for 3 hours following the initial dose as significant hypotension can develop. Monitor serum potassium levels during treatment as hyperkalemia may develop.	Do not stop taking your drugs without talking to your doctor. Keep follow-up medical appointments. Avoid sudden position changes; for example, rise from bed slowly. Report easy bruising and bleeding, sore throat, or fever, weight gain of 2 lbs. or more per day, edema, dizziness, or skin rash. Immediately report swelling of the face, lips, or eyelids, itching, or breathing problems.
Diuretics ▪ Hydrochlorothiazide (Hydrodiuril) ▪ Chlorothiazide (Diuril) ▪ Furosemide (Lasix) ▪ Ethacrynic acid (Edecrin) ▪ Bumetanide (Bumex) ▪ Spironolactone (Aldactone) ▪ Triamterene (Dyrenium) ▪ Amiloride (Midamor) ▪ Acetazolamide (Diamox)	Diuretics act on different portions of the kidney tubule to promote sodium and water excretion. With the exception of the potassium-sparing diuretics—spironolactone, triamterene, and amiloride—diuretics also promote potassium excretion, increasing the risk of hypokalemia.	Monitor fluid volume status: BP, intake and output, weight, skin turgor, edema. Assess for volume depletion, particularly with loop diuretics (furosemide, ethacrynic acid, and bumetanide): Dizziness, orthostatic hypotension, tachycardia, muscle cramping. Notify the charge nurse or physician of abnormal serum electrolyte values. Administer intravenous furosemide slowly, no more than 20 mg/min. Notify the physician if the client is on an aminoglycoside antibiotic. When given concurrently with furosemide or ethacrynic acid, there is an increased risk of ototoxicity and hearing loss.	Report abdominal pain, jaundice, dark urine, abnormal bleeding or bruising, flulike symptoms, signs of electrolyte imbalance, or dehydration (Chapter 5) to your doctor. Monitor your blood pressure, pulse, and weight daily. Report changes in your weight of 2 lbs. or more per day. Avoid making sudden position changes. You may feel dizzy, light-headed, or faint. Drink at least 6 to 8 glasses of water per day. Take your diuretic when it will be the least disruptive to your lifestyle. Take with meals to decrease GI symptoms. Unless you are taking a potassium-sparing diuretic, increase intake of potassium-rich foods. Limit salt intake.

peutic levels are very close to toxic levels. Early manifestations of digitalis toxicity include anorexia, nausea and vomiting, headache, alterations in vision, and confusion. A number of dysrhythmias are also associated with digitalis toxicity. Low serum potassium levels increase the risk of digitalis toxicity, as do low magnesium and high calcium levels. Older adults are at particular risk for digitalis toxicity.

CLINICAL alert

Always take an apical pulse before administering any digitalis drug. If the pulse rate is less than 60 per minute or if the client has manifestations of digitalis toxicity, hold the drug and notify the charge nurse or physician.

Diet and Activity

Clients in heart failure are generally put on a restricted sodium diet to minimize sodium and water retention. An intake of 1.5 to 2 g of sodium per day, a moderate restriction, is recommended. Activity may be limited to bed rest during acute episodes of heart failure to reduce cardiac workload and allow the heart to recompensate. Activity is gradually increased as the condition improves, and is encouraged to tolerance to improve cardiovascular performance.

Surgery

In the end-stage of chronic heart failure, surgery may be done to improve quality of life. Two primary options are available at this time: dynamic cardiomyoplasty, to improve function in the existing heart, and cardiac transplantation. *Dynamic cardiomyoplasty* involves wrapping a skeletal muscle graft around the heart to lend support to the failing myocardium. The grafted skeletal muscle is stimulated to contract with the heart muscle, providing a more forceful contraction and increasing cardiac output. *Cardiac transplantation* provides another option for end-stage heart disease. There are two types of transplant techniques: The client's diseased heart is removed and replaced with a donor heart (Figure 22-20 ◆); in the "piggyback transplant," the client's heart is left in place and the

donor heart is sutured to it. The client then has two functioning hearts, although most of the work is performed by the donor heart. Although cardiac transplantation benefits many clients with end-stage heart disease, it is limited by the availability of donor hearts. Transplanted organs typically are obtained from young accident victims with no evidence of cardiac trauma. Ventricular assist devices are often used as a bridge to transplantation. Mechanical heart transplants are in development.

Nursing care of the heart transplant client is similar to the care of any cardiac surgery client. Infection and rejection are major postoperative concerns. Immunosuppressive drugs are given to prevent rejection of the transplanted organ (see Chapter 13). Although immunosuppressive drugs help prevent rejection, they also leave the client with impaired defenses against infection.

NURSING CARE

Heart failure impacts quality of life, interfering with such day-to-day activities as self-care and role performance. Reducing the oxygen demand of the heart is a major nursing care goal. This includes providing both physical and psychological rest, as well as administering and monitoring multiple drugs to reduce cardiac work, improve contractility, and manage symptoms.

ASSESSING

Clients with heart failure require frequent and careful nursing assessment. Box 22-18 outlines assessment data to be collected by the nurse.

DIAGNOSING, PLANNING, AND IMPLEMENTING

DECREASED CARDIAC OUTPUT

■ Auscultate heart and breath sounds regularly. *An S_3 or an S_4 may be heard in heart failure. Crackles are often heard in the*

Figure 22-20. ◆ Cardiac transplantation. (A) The heart is removed, leaving the posterior walls of the atria intact. The donor heart is sutured to the atria (B) and the great vessels (C).

BOX 22-18
ASSESSING CLIENTS WITH HEART FAILURE

SUBJECTIVE DATA

- Shortness of breath, level of activity, number of pillows used to sleep; swelling of legs and feet; weight changes; appetite, nausea, abdominal discomfort
- History of MI or other heart disease, recent stressors such as upper respiratory infection; previous or current treatment; current medications
- Risk factors: Family history of heart disease; history of hypertension, diabetes, high blood cholesterol levels; smoking and alcohol intake
- Understanding of disease and treatment, compliance with activity prescriptions; current diet and use of salt

OBJECTIVE DATA

- Vital signs at rest and changes with activity; cardiac rhythm, any dysrhythmias
- Dyspnea and its relationship to activity; oxygen saturation levels
- Skin color, temperature, and moisture; capillary refill; extent and degree of dependent edema; presence of neck vein distention
- Heart and lung sounds; presence of S_3 or S_4 heart sounds; presence and extent of crackles or wheezes on auscultation of lungs
- Intake and output; daily weight
- Level of consciousness; anxiety or fear
- Central venous pressure, pulmonary artery pressure, or cardiac output as ordered

lung bases; increasing crackles, dyspnea, and shortness of breath indicate worsening failure.

- Report manifestations of decreased cardiac output: changes in mental status; decreased urine output; cool, clammy skin; tachycardia, diminished pulses; pallor or cyanosis; dysrhythmias. These are manifestations of decreased tissue perfusion.
- Administer oxygen as needed. This improves oxygenation of the blood, decreasing the effects of hypoxia and ischemia.
- Administer medications as ordered. Drugs are used to decrease the cardiac workload and increase the effectiveness of contractions.
- Encourage rest, explaining its purpose. Keep the head of the bed elevated to reduce the work of breathing. Provide a bedside commode, and assist with personal needs. These measures reduce cardiac workload.
- Maintain a quiet environment, allow the client to express fears and feelings, and explain the reasons for medical and nursing care. These measures reduce anxiety and decrease oxygen consumption.

EXCESS FLUID VOLUME

- Immediately notify the physician if the client develops air hunger, an overwhelming sense of impending doom or panic, tachypnea, orthopnea, or a cough productive of pink, frothy sputum. Acute pulmonary edema, a medical emergency, can develop rapidly, requiring immediate intervention to preserve life.
- Monitor intake and output. Notify the physician if urine output drops to less than 30 mL/hr. Intake and output records help evaluate the effectiveness of treatment. A drop in urine output may indicate reduced cardiac output.
- Weigh daily. Weight is an accurate measure of fluid status; 1 liter of fluid is equal to 1 kg or 2.2 lbs. of weight.
- Place in Fowler's or high Fowler's position, with the head of bed elevated to 45 degrees. Elevating the head of the bed reduces venous return to the heart, decreasing its work. It also improves lung expansion.
- Report decreased urine output, vital sign changes, distended neck veins, peripheral edema, weight gain, increased dyspnea, or dysrhythmias to the charge nurse or physician. These may indicate progressive worsening of the client's condition.
- Administer diuretics and other medications as ordered. Diuretics increase sodium and water excretion.
- Restrict fluids as ordered. Encourage the client to help choose the time and type of fluid consumed. Schedule the majority of intake during the morning and afternoon. Offer ice chips and frequent mouth care; provide hard candies if allowed. Involving the client increases the sense of control. Ice chips, hard candies, and mouth care relieve dry mouth and thirst and promote comfort.

ACTIVITY INTOLERANCE

- Assess vital signs and heart rhythm before and after activity. Tachycardia, dysrhythmias, changes in blood pressure, diaphoresis, pallor, or complaints of increasing dyspnea, chest pain, excessive fatigue, or palpitations indicate activity intolerance. Instruct to rest if these manifestations are noted.
- Organize nursing care to allow for rest periods. Grouping care activities as much as possible allows adequate time to "recharge."
- Assist as needed with self-care. Encourage independent performance of activities of daily living (ADLs) within prescribed limits. Assisting with ADLs helps meet care needs while reducing the cardiac workload. Involving the client promotes a sense of control and reduces helplessness.
- Plan and implement progressive activity plan. Employ passive and active range-of-motion (ROM) exercises as appropriate. Consult with physical therapist on activity plan. Progressive activity slowly increases exercise capacity by strengthening and improving cardiac function without strain. Progressive activity also helps prevent skeletal muscle atrophy. ROM exercises prevent complications of immobility in bedridden or severely compromised clients.

- Encourage small, frequent meals rather than three heavy meals per day. *Small, frequent meals provide continuing energy resources and decrease the work required to digest a large meal.*

EVALUATING

Collect data such as the following to evaluate the effectiveness of nursing care:

- Vital signs, urine output, and degree of dyspnea at rest and during activity
- Presence or absence of abnormal heart or lung sounds and edema
- Ability to tolerate gradually increased activity levels

Discharge Considerations

The chronic and progressive nature of heart failure requires that the client and family actively participate in managing the disease. When planning for discharge care, carefully assess the client's and family's knowledge, abilities, and resources (Box 22-19).

BOX 22-19
ASSESSING FOR DISCHARGE

HEART FAILURE
Client
- Ability to independently perform ADLs; to participate in cardiac rehabilitation program; to prepare and eat prescribed diet; to manage medications
- Understanding of disease, medications, diet and activities, health maintenance measures, symptoms to report to physician, follow-up care
- Ability to cope with activity and employment restrictions and economic effects; acceptance of altered roles/relationships
- Home environment: Stairs, other factors that increase cardiac work (such as reliance on wood heat or lack of running water)

Family and Caregivers
- Ability and willingness to assist with ADLs and pre-scribed care measures (e.g., diet, exercise, and avoidance of smoking) as needed, acceptance of altered roles
- Income; effect of chronic progressive disease on financial and family stability

Community
- Availability of cardiac rehabilitation programs, home health and social support services; public transportation; access to medical services, pharmacies
- Safe environment/facilities for exercise

Explain heart failure and its effects on the client's life. This helps the client understand the reasons for ordered treatments. Discuss the warning signs of impending failure and when to contact the physician. Teach about prescribed drugs and their potential adverse effects. Stress the importance of the medications in managing heart failure. Provide verbal and written information regarding each specific medication to encourage compliance. Instruct to keep regular follow-up appointments to monitor disease progression and the effects of therapy.

Lifestyle changes are important, although they may be the most difficult to achieve. Teach the client and family about the prescribed diet. Give practical suggestions for reducing salt intake. The AHA has written materials and recipes that may make adjusting to a low-sodium diet easier to tolerate. Refer to a dietitian for further teaching and diet planning as needed.

Encourage exercise within prescribed limits to strengthen the heart muscle and improve aerobic capacity. Box 22-20 provides activity guidelines for clients with heart failure.

Provide referrals to a home health agency and community agencies, such as local cardiac rehabilitation programs, heart support groups, or the AHA, as needed for further nursing evaluation and care, education, and psychosocial support.

Nursing Process Case Study
■ CLIENT WITH HEART FAILURE

One year ago, Arthur Jackson, 67 years old, had an anterior MI followed by coronary artery bypass surgery. On discharge, he was started on digoxin, furosemide, coumadin, and a potassium chloride supplement. He has now been admitted to the medical intensive care unit (MICU) after developing severe shortness of breath, a productive cough, and no appetite for one week. He is diagnosed with heart failure.

Assessment On entering his room, Mr. Jackson's nurse, Myumi Takashi, notices that he is sitting in the bedside recliner in high Fowler's position. He says, "Lately, this is the only way I feel fairly comfortable." He states that he gets short of breath working in his garden and complains of his shoes and belt being too tight. On questioning, Mr. Jackson insists that he takes his medications regularly. He admits to a fondness for bacon and Chinese food and sheepishly says he snacks between meals "even though I need to lose weight."

Mr. Jackson's vital signs are BP 95/72 mm Hg; AP 124, irregular; R 28 and labored; and T 97.5° F (36.5° C). The ECG shows atrial fibrillation. An S_3 is heard on auscultation. He has crackles and diminished breath sounds in the bases of both lungs. Neck veins distended, 3+ pitting edema of ankles and feet, and abdominal distention are noted. Skin is cool and diaphoretic. Chest x-ray shows cardiomegaly and pulmonary infiltrates.

> **BOX 22-20**
> **TEACHING FOR DISCHARGE**
>
> ## ACTIVITY GUIDELINES FOR CLIENTS WITH HEART FAILURE
>
> - Perform as many activities as independently as you can.
> - Space meals and activities. Eat six small meals a day. Allow rest periods during the day.
> - Perform all activities at a comfortable pace; rest for 15 minutes if you get tired.
> - Stop any activity that causes chest pain, shortness of breath, dizziness, excessive weakness, or sweating. Rest. Notify your doctor if your activity tolerance changes and if symptoms continue after rest.
> - Avoid straining. Do not lift heavy objects. Eat a high-fiber diet and drink plenty of water to prevent constipation. Use bulk-forming laxatives or stool softeners, as allowed, to avoid constipation and straining.
> - Begin a graded exercise program. Walking is good exercise. Plan to walk twice a day at a comfortable, slow pace for the first couple of weeks, and then gradually increase the distance and pace. Below is a suggested schedule:
>
> | Week 1 | 200 to 400 yards (¼ mile) | Twice a day, slow leisurely pace |
> | Week 2 | ¼ mile | 15 min, minimum of 3 times per week |
> | Week 3 | ½ mile | 30 min, minimum of 3 times per week |
> | Week 4 | 1 mile | 30 min, minimum of 3 times per week |
> | Week 5 | 1½ mile | 30 min, minimum of 3 times per week |
> | Week 6 | 2 miles | 40 min, minimum of 3 times per week |

Diagnosis Ms. Takashi identifies the following nursing diagnoses for Mr. Jackson:

- Excess Fluid Volume related to impaired cardiac pump and salt and water retention
- Activity Intolerance related to imbalance between oxygen supply and demand
- Deficient Knowledge regarding diet and fluid restrictions

Expected Outcomes The expected outcomes specify that Mr. Jackson will:

- Demonstrate weight loss, and decreased edema, jugular venous distention, and abdominal distention.
- Achieve improved activity tolerance.
- Verbalize understanding of diet and fluid restrictions.

Planning and Implementation Ms. Takashi plans and implements the following interventions for Mr. Jackson:

- Hourly vital signs until stable.
- Weigh daily. Record intake and output (I&O).
- Restrict fluids to 1,500 mL/24 hr (as ordered by physician); 600 mL day shift, 600 mL evenings, 300 mL at night.
- Auscultate breath and heart sounds every 4 hours and as necessary.
- Monitor oxygen saturation levels. Notify physician if below 94%.
- High Fowler's position to maintain comfort.
- Teach about all medications and how to take and record his pulse daily.
- Design an activity plan that incorporates preferred activities and scheduled rest periods throughout the day.
- Instruct on a sodium-restricted diet. Allow choices for meals within allowed limits.

- Consult dietitian to assist Mr. and Mrs. Jackson in planning a low-sodium diet.

Evaluation Mr. Jackson is transferred to the medical unit after 2 days in MICU. He has lost 8 lbs. His respirations are unlabored at rest, and his edema is significantly reduced. He is able to sleep in low Fowler's with only one pillow. The dietitian is helping Mr. and Mrs. Jackson develop a realistic eating plan to limit sodium, sugar, and fats. Mr. Jackson is relieved to know that he can still enjoy Chinese food that is prepared without monosodium glutamate (MSG) or added salt. The physical therapist has designed a progressive activity plan with Mr. Jackson for both in-hospital and at-home activity. Mr. Jackson's knowledge about his medications is assessed and reinforced. Mr. Jackson is discharged 5 days after his admission.

Critical Thinking in the Nursing Process

1. Design an exercise plan for Mr. Jackson to follow after discharge.
2. Mr. Jackson tells you, "Talk to my wife about my medications—she's Tarzan and I'm Jane now." How would you respond?

Cardiomyopathy

Cardiomyopathy affects the structure or function of the heart muscle. Cardiomyopathies are a diverse group of disorders that often lead to heart failure. In many cases, the cause is unknown. Cardiomyopathy also may be related to another dis-

TABLE 22-8	CLASSIFICATIONS OF CARDIOMYOPATHY		
	DILATED	**HYPERTROPHIC**	**RESTRICTIVE**
DESCRIPTION	Ventricles dilate; ventricular contraction is impaired	Left ventricular hypertrophy interferes with filling and outflow	Rigidity of ventricular walls interferes with filling
MANIFESTATIONS	Heart failure Cardiomegaly Dysrhythmias S_3 and S_4 heard on auscultation	Dyspnea Anginal pain Syncope Dysrhythmias Possible sudden death	Dyspnea on exertion Fatigue Heart failure S_3 and S_4 on auscultation

ease or condition, such as chronic alcohol abuse, myocardial ischemia, or a viral infection.

Cardiomyopathies are categorized by their effects on the heart (Table 22-8 ◆).

Dilated cardiomyopathy is the most common type of cardiomyopathy. The heart chambers dilate, and ventricular contraction is impaired. Manifestations develop gradually. Heart failure may develop years after the onset of dilation and pump failure. Dysrhythmias are common, increasing the risk of sudden cardiac death. The prognosis of dilated cardiomyopathy is grim; most clients get progressively worse and die within 2 years of the onset of symptoms.

Hypertrophic cardiomyopathy is characterized by hypertrophy and decreased compliance of the left ventricle. The interventricular septum tends to hypertrophy to a greater extent than the free wall of the ventricle. This impairs left ventricular filling and outflow. This may be a hereditary disorder. Sudden cardiac death may be the first sign of the disorder; manifestations can occur suddenly during or after physical activity. Frequent manifestations include dyspnea, angina, and syncope.

Restrictive cardiomyopathy is the least common form of cardiomyopathy. Rigidity of the ventricular walls impairs filling, resulting in decreased ventricular size, and decreased cardiac output. The manifestations of restrictive cardiomyopathy are those of heart failure and decreased tissue perfusion. The prognosis is poor.

Unless a treatable cause can be identified, little can be done to treat cardiomyopathy. Management focuses on minimizing heart failure and treating dysrhythmias. Goals for the client with hypertrophic cardiomyopathy are aimed at reducing contractility and preventing sudden cardiac death. All clients should be restricted from strenuous physical exertion, which may precipitate dysrhythmias and/or sudden cardiac death. Dietary and sodium restrictions may help diminish the manifestations. Cardiac transplant is the definitive treatment for dilated cardiomyopathy; without transplant, survival time is limited. Obstructive hypertrophic cardiomyopathy may be surgically treated by resecting excess muscle away from the aortic valve outflow tract.

Nursing goals for clients with cardiomyopathies are to prevent complications, assist the client to conserve energy while encouraging self-care, and support coping skills. If surgery is done, nursing care is similar to that for any client undergoing open heart surgery or cardiac transplant (see Box 22-8).

Client and family teaching focuses on self-care measures such as activity restrictions, dietary changes, and drugs used to reduce symptoms and/or prevent complications. Educate about the disease process, its ultimate outcome, and treatment options. Teach clients who are undergoing invasive procedures for diagnosis or treatment about the procedure, including preparation and care following the procedure. If heart transplant is an option, provide information about the procedure and initiate preoperative teaching.

Inflammatory Cardiac Disorders

Any layer of the heart—the endocardium, myocardium, or pericardium—can become inflamed, damaging the heart valves, heart muscle, or pericardium. Manifestations of inflammation may range from very mild to life threatening. This section discusses rheumatic heart disease, endocarditis, myocarditis, and pericarditis.

Rheumatic Fever and Rheumatic Heart Disease

Rheumatic fever is a systemic inflammatory disease caused by an abnormal immune response to infection by group A beta-hemolytic streptococci (usually streptococcal pharyngitis or strep throat). While children between ages 5 and 15 have the highest incidence, rheumatic fever may affect people of any age. Rheumatic fever can damage the heart valves, and often leads to mitral and aortic valve disorders (discussed in the next section of this chapter).

PATHOPHYSIOLOGY

Rheumatic fever is thought to result from an abnormal immune response to the *Streptococcus* bacterium or its toxins. Antibodies produced to attack the invading bacteria (the antigen) appear to also attack connective tissues of the heart, blood vessels, joints, and subcutaneous tissues, initiating an inflammatory response.

Any layer of the heart may be affected in acute rheumatic fever; usually all three are involved. The valves become red and swollen, and small vegetative lesions develop on the leaflets. As the inflammation resolves, scarring occurs, causing deformity. Myocarditis and pericarditis associated with rheumatic fever are generally mild and have no long-term effects.

Rheumatic heart disease (RHD) is slowly progressive valve deformity following acute or repeated attacks of rheumatic fever. Valve leaflets become rigid and deformed, resulting in stenosis or regurgitation of the valve. In **stenosis,** the valve leaflets fuse, obstructing forward blood flow. In **regurgitation,** the valve fails to close properly, allowing blood to flow back through it. Valves on the left side of the heart, the mitral valve in particular, are most often affected.

Manifestations of rheumatic fever typically follow the initial streptococcal infection by about 2 to 3 weeks (Box 22-21). About 50% of clients with rheumatic fever develop some form of rheumatic heart disease.

COLLABORATIVE CARE

The diagnosis of rheumatic fever is based on the client's history and physical examination. Laboratory testing helps estab-lish the diagnosis. The *WBC count* is elevated, as is the *erythrocyte sedimentation rate (ESR),* a general indicator of inflammation. A positive *C-reactive protein (CRP)* indicates active inflammation. The *antistreptolysin-O (ASO)* titer is a streptococcal antibody test that rises within 2 months of the disease's onset and is found in most clients with rheumatic fever.

Management of rheumatic heart disease focuses on treating the primary infection, managing its manifestations, and preventing complications and recurrences of the disease. In clients with acute carditis, treatment focuses on decreasing myocardial work. Activity is limited during the acute phase, then gradually increased after about 4 to 5 weeks.

Antibiotics are prescribed to eliminate the streptococcal infection. Joint pain and fever are treated with salicylates (e.g., aspirin); corticosteroids may be used for severe pain.

NURSING CARE

Nurses have a significant role in identifying clients at risk for rheumatic heart disease and teaching for primary prevention. Identify risk factors for streptococcal infections. These include crowded living conditions, poor nutrition, immunodeficiency, and poor access to health care.

ASSESSING

Ask about recent sore throat or "strep throat" and treatment. Other subjective data includes complaints of chest pain, shortness of breath, fatigue, weakness, fever, or joint pain. Obtain objective data such as heart rate and heart sounds, respiratory rate, and ease of breathing. Observe for joint redness, swelling, or heat, and the presence of a rash on trunk or extremities. Note mental status and any abnormal muscle movements.

BOX 22-21
MANIFESTATIONS OF RHEUMATIC FEVER

- Fever
- Migratory joint pain and inflammation
- Rash on trunk and proximal extremities
- Chest pain or discomfort
- Tachycardia, shortness of breath
- Cardiac friction rub, S_3, S_4, possible murmur
- Involuntary muscle spasms, difficulty concentrating

DIAGNOSING, PLANNING, AND IMPLEMENTING

PAIN

■ Administer anti-inflammatory drugs as ordered. Give aspirin and other nonsteroidal anti-inflammatory drugs (NSAIDs) with food, milk, or antacids to minimize gastric irritation. Report tinnitus (a symptom of aspirin toxicity), vomiting, or GI bleeding. *Anti-inflammatory drugs are given to control inflammation. The dose of aspirin and NSAIDs may be high, and the drugs are given around the clock rather than as needed.*

■ Provide warm, moist compresses for local pain relief. *Direct application of moist heat may help relieve the pain associated with inflamed joints.*

■ Auscultate heart sounds every shift and as necessary. Notify the physician if a pericardial friction rub or a new murmur appears. *A friction rub may be produced by an inflamed pericardium. This also causes chest pain and discomfort.*

ACTIVITY INTOLERANCE

■ Explain the importance of activity limitations. Instruct to avoid or stop any activity that causes dyspnea or shortness of breath. *Activities are limited for 4 to 6 weeks to decrease the stress on the heart.*

■ Encourage visits from friends and family members and diversional activities, such as reading, playing games, watching television, listening to radio or favorite music cassettes, and so on. *Diversionary activities help reduce boredom when activity is limited.*

■ Monitor activity tolerance (vital signs, fatigue, shortness of breath) as activity is gradually increased. *The client may require bed rest or limited activity for a longer period of time to allow carditis to resolve and prevent permanent heart damage.*

EVALUATING

To evaluate the effectiveness of nursing care, collect data such as: The client's reports of pain and discomfort; vital signs at rest and with activity, and response to increasing activity levels.

Discharge Considerations

Rheumatic fever is preventable. Prompt treatment of streptococcal throat infections helps decrease the spread of this pathogen and the risk of rheumatic fever. Manifestations of strep throat include a red, fiery-looking throat, pain upon swallowing, enlarged and tender cervical lymph nodes, fever in the range of 101° to 104° F (38.3° to 40.0° C), and headache. Emphasize the importance of finishing the complete course of antibiotic to eradicate the pathogen.

To prevent recurrence of rheumatic fever, emphasize the importance of continuing antibiotic prophylaxis as ordered.

Teach the client with chronic RHD about the importance of antibiotic prophylaxis for any invasive procedure (e.g., dental care, endoscopy, or surgery) to prevent bacterial endocarditis. Preventive dental care and good oral hygiene help discourage gingival infections, and are important.

Instruct the client with rheumatic carditis to limit salt intake to reduce the workload of the heart. A high-carbohydrate, high-protein diet is usually recommended to promote healing and to combat weakness and fatigue. Teach the early manifestations of heart failure. Provide instructions about prescribed medications, including dosage, signs of adverse or allergic reactions, and possible drug interactions. Assess the need for home health care, and provide a referral as needed.

 # Infective Endocarditis

Endocarditis, inflammation of the endocardium, is an infectious process that usually affects clients with underlying heart disease. Lesions develop on deformed valves, on valve prostheses, or in areas of tissue damage within the heart. The disease also occurs in intravenous drug users. The left side of the heart, the mitral valve in particular, is the most common site of infection; in intravenous drug users, the right side (the tricuspid valve) is often involved. Bacteria may enter through intravenous drug use; through oral lesions or during dental work; as a result of invasive procedures, such as intravenous catheter insertion, surgery, or urinary catheterization; or as a result of urinary tract or upper respiratory infection.

Endocarditis is frequently classified by its onset and disease course (Table 22-9 ◆). *Acute endocarditis* has an abrupt onset and is a rapidly progressive, severe disease. *Staphylococcus aureus* is the usual infective organism in acute endocarditis. In contrast, *subacute endocarditis* has a more gradual onset. It is more likely to occur in clients with preexisting heart disease. *Streptococcus viridans* is the most common organism causing subacute endocarditis.

PATHOPHYSIOLOGY

Organisms in the bloodstream attach to the endocardial lining of the heart and become enmeshed in deposits of fibrin and platelets. This covering "protects" the bacteria from quick removal by the immune system. These vegetations develop on heart valve leaflets, varying in size and shape. *Friable* (easily broken, fragile) vegetations can break off, traveling through the bloodstream to other organs. When they lodge in small vessels, they may cause hemorrhages, infarcts, or abscesses. The vegetations prevent normal valve closure, causing regurgitation of blood through the valve and heart murmurs.

Infective endocarditis generally causes elevated temperature (above 101.5° F or 39.4° C) and flulike symptoms. The client may have a cough, shortness of breath, and complain of joint pain. Acute staphylococcal endocarditis presents with sudden and more severe manifestations, including a high fever. Heart murmurs are common.

Peripheral manifestations of endocarditis may include *petechiae* (small, purplish-red spots) on the trunk, conjunctiva,

TABLE 22-9 CLASSIFICATIONS OF INFECTIVE ENDOCARDITIS

	ACUTE INFECTIVE ENDOCARDITIS	SUBACUTE INFECTIVE ENDOCARDITIS
ONSET	Sudden	Gradual
USUAL ORGANISM	*Staphylococcus aureus*	*Streptococcus viridans;* others
RISK FACTORS	Intravenous drug use, sepsis	Previous heart or valve damage or deformity; dental work, invasive procedures
PATHOLOGIC PROCESSES	Rapid valve destruction	Valve destruction with regurgitation; embolization of friable vegetations
PRESENTATION	Abrupt onset with spiking fever and chills; manifestations of heart failure	Gradual onset of febrile illness with cough, dyspnea, arthralgias, abdominal pain

and mucous membranes; *splinter hemorrhages* (red streaks under the fingernails or toenails); small, painful growths on the fingers and toes; or small, purplish-red lesions on the palms of the hands and soles of the feet.

Complications of infective endocarditis include heart failure, and infarctions of other organs (lungs, brain, kidneys, or bowel) from embolization of vegetative fragments.

COLLABORATIVE CARE

Prevention is key; education of clients at high risk for the disease is essential. Teaching the public about the risks of intravenous drug use, including endocarditis, can also help reduce the incidence of this frightening disease. The management priorities for infective endocarditis are to eradicate the infecting organism and minimize valve damage and complications of the disease.

There are no definitive tests for infective endocarditis. A *CBC* and *blood cultures* are done. *Echocardiography* is performed to identify vegetations and evaluate valve function.

Pharmacology

To prevent infective endocarditis, antibiotics are commonly prescribed prior to high-risk procedures for clients with preexisting heart disease or damage. Table 22-10 ◆ lists conditions and procedures for which prophylactic antibiotic therapy is recommended.

Antibiotics are prescribed to eradicate the infecting organism from the blood and heart lesions. Because the fibrin covering that protects organisms from the immune system also protects them from the antibiotic, an extended course of multiple intravenous antibiotics is required. Intravenous drug therapy is continued for 2 to 4 weeks.

Some clients with infective endocarditis require surgery to repair or replace damaged valves. The most common indication for surgery is valvular regurgitation that causes heart failure. When the infection has not responded to antibiotic therapy within 7 to 10 days, the infected valve may be replaced to help eliminate the organism.

NURSING CARE

Nursing care of the client with infective endocarditis focuses on managing its manifestations, administering antibiotics, and educating the client and family members. Preventing and identifying complications promptly is also a nursing priority.

RISK FOR IMBALANCED BODY TEMPERATURE

- Record temperature every 2 to 4 hours. Notify physician if above 101.5° F (39.4° C). *Body temperature usually returns to normal within 1 week of antibiotic therapy. Continuing fever may indicate a need to modify the treatment regimen.*
- Obtain blood cultures as ordered, before giving the first dose of antibiotics. *Blood cultures can identify the causative organism and direct the choice of antibiotic. Initial blood cultures must be obtained before antibiotic therapy is started to obtain enough organisms for culture. Follow-up cultures are used to assess the effectiveness of therapy.*
- Administer anti-inflammatory or antipyretic agents as prescribed. *Fever may be treated with aspirin, ibuprofen, or acetaminophen.*

TABLE 22-10 INDICATIONS FOR ANTIBIOTIC PROPHYLAXIS TO PREVENT ENDOCARDITIS

CONDITIONS	PROCEDURES
Rheumatic heart disease Prosthetic heart valves Previous episodes of infective endocarditis Congenital heart conditions Mitral valve prolapse	Dental procedures, including cleaning Surgery Bronchoscopy or cystoscopy Urinary catheterization Incision and drainage of infected tissue

■ Administer antibiotics as ordered; obtain peak and trough drug levels as indicated. *Intravenous antibiotics are given for 2 to 6 weeks to eradicate the pathogen. Peak and trough levels evaluate the adequacy of the dose to maintain a therapeutic blood level.*

RISK FOR INEFFECTIVE TISSUE PERFUSION

■ Notify the charge nurse or physician of manifestations of altered organ perfusion:
  ■ Brain: Altered level of consciousness, numbness or tingling in extremities, hemiplegia, visual disturbances, or manifestations of stroke
  ■ Kidneys: Decreased urine output, hematuria, elevated blood urea nitrogen (BUN) or creatinine
  ■ Lungs: Dyspnea, hemoptysis, shortness of breath, diminished breath sounds, restlessness, sudden chest or shoulder pain
  ■ Heart: Chest pain radiating to jaw or arms, tachycardia, anxiety, tachypnea, hypotension
  ■ Bowel: Abdominal pain, tenderness, guarding; decreased or absent bowel sounds, nausea, vomiting
    Embolization of vegetative lesions can affect tissue perfusion. Vegetations from the left heart may lodge in vessels of the brain, kidneys, or peripheral tissues, causing infarction or abscess. Emboli from the right side of the heart can lead to manifestations of a pulmonary embolism.
■ Assess skin color and temperature, quality of peripheral pulses, and capillary refill. *Assessment of peripheral tissue perfusion is important to reduce the risk of tissue necrosis and possible extremity loss.*

 ## Discharge Considerations

The client with infective endocarditis needs education and support throughout the course of the disease, as well as teaching to prevent future recurrences. In basic terms, teach the client what is happening in the heart and the reasons for the symptoms. Emphasize that infective endocarditis, although serious and frightening, can usually be treated effectively with intravenous antibiotics. Stress the importance of promptly reporting any unusual manifestation, such as a change in vision, sudden pain, or weakness, so that treatment can be promptly implemented. Explain the rationale for all treatments and procedures, including activity restrictions, to reduce anxiety and enhance cooperation. Describe the manifestations of heart failure, and instruct the client to notify his or her care provider if these manifestations develop.

Client and family education is also extremely important to prevent recurrences of infective endocarditis. Box 22-22 outlines a teaching plan for clients at risk.

Clients who acquire infective endocarditis from intravenous drug use need additional teaching about the risks of intravenous drug injection. Refer the client and significant

BOX 22-22
TEACHING FOR DISCHARGE

PREVENTING ENDOCARDITIS

• Teach the function of the heart valves and the effects of endocarditis. Define endocarditis, and explain why the client is at risk.
• Stress the importance of notifying care providers of valve disease, heart murmur, or valve replacement before undergoing any invasive procedures.
• Encourage good oral and dental hygiene and regular dental checkups. Discuss the importance of preventing oral trauma (e.g., gentle toothbrushing, proper fitting dentures, and avoiding toothpicks, dental floss, and high-flow water devices).
• Encourage pneumococcal vaccine and annual influenza immunizations.

others as appropriate to a drug or substance abuse treatment program or facility.

Myocarditis

Myocarditis is an inflammatory disorder of the heart muscle that may be infectious (viral, bacterial, protozoal), an immunologic response, or result from radiation, chemical poisons, drugs, or burns. Myocarditis may occur at any age, and it is more common in men than women. Immunosuppressed clients, people with acquired immunodeficiency syndrome (AIDS) in particular, are at risk. Factors that alter immune response—such as malnutrition, alcohol use, immunosuppressive drugs, radiation, stress, and advanced age—increase the risk for myocarditis.

The client with myocarditis may be asymptomatic or have nonspecific symptoms such as fever, fatigue, general malaise, dyspnea, palpitations, and arthralgias. Often, there is a history of recent nonspecific illness or upper respiratory infection. Manifestations of heart failure, including tachycardia, dysrhythmias, and an S_3 and S_4 may be present. A heart murmur, pericardial friction rub, cardiomegaly, and ECG abnormalities may be noted. The long-term effects of the disease depend on the extent of damage to the heart muscle. While many clients recover fully, others may develop progressive heart failure and cardiomyopathy.

Care for the client with myocarditis is focuses on treating the inflammatory process to prevent further damage to the heart muscle. Bed rest and activity restrictions are ordered during the acute stage to reduce myocardial work. Oxygen is administered to clients with signs of cardiac dysfunction. If the cause is infectious, antimicrobial therapy is prescribed. Corticosteroids or other immunosuppressive agents (see

Chapter 13) may be given to reduce inflammation. Digoxin may be ordered to manage heart failure.

Nursing care is directed at decreasing myocardial work and increasing oxygen supply. Encourage strict bed rest to reduce physical activity. Emotional rest also is indicated, because anxiety increases myocardial oxygen demand. Closely monitor vital signs, heart rhythm, and pump effectiveness during the acute phase of the illness. Consider the following nursing diagnoses for the client with myocarditis:

- Decreased Cardiac Output related to impaired cardiac muscle function
- Fatigue related to the inflammatory process and inadequate cardiac output
- Anxiety related to possible long-term effects of the disorder
- Excess Fluid Volume related to compensatory mechanisms for decreased cardiac output

Explain all procedures, tests, and treatments to decrease anxiety and cardiac workload. Teach the early manifestations of heart failure to report to the physician. Stress the importance of following the treatment regimen, including activity restrictions, any dietary modifications (such as a low-salt diet if signs of heart failure are present), and medications. Emphasize that adhering to the treatment plan can reduce the risk of long-term consequences, such as cardiomyopathy.

Pericarditis

Pericarditis is inflammation of the pericardium, the outermost layer of the heart. Acute pericarditis is usually viral. Pericarditis is a frequent complication of uremia or end-stage renal disease. Pericarditis also may follow a myocardial infarction or open heart surgery.

PATHOPHYSIOLOGY
Damage to pericardial tissue triggers an inflammatory response. The inflammatory response causes fluid and exudate to collect in the pericardial space. If the volume of fluid and exudate is significant, cardiac filling may be impaired. The inflammatory process may resolve without long-term consequences, or scar tissue and adhesions may form between the pericardial layers. Fibrosis and scarring of the pericardium can restrict the heart's ability to function effectively.

Classic manifestations of acute pericarditis include chest pain, a pericardial friction rub, and fever. The onset of chest pain is often abrupt. It is usually sharp and may radiate to the back or neck. The pain may be steady or intermittent, and is aggravated by deep breathing, coughing, movement, or swallowing. The client often sits upright and leans forward to reduce the discomfort.

A **pericardial friction rub** is the characteristic sign of pericarditis. It is a leathery, grating sound produced by the inflamed pericardial layers rubbing against the chest wall or pleura. The rub is best heard at the left lower sternal border with the client sitting up or leaning forward. It may be constant, or it may disappear and then reappear hours later. A

low-grade fever (below 100° F [38.4° C]) is often present. Dyspnea and tachycardia are common.

A *pericardial effusion,* an abnormal collection of fluid between the pericardial layers, may develop in pericarditis. If the fluid collects gradually, the pericardial sac stretches to accommodate it. Heart function is not affected, although heart sounds may be muffled. In contrast, a rapid buildup of pericardial fluid (as little as 100 mL) does not allow the sac to stretch and can compress the heart, interfering with myocardial function. This is known as **cardiac tamponade.** It is a medical emergency that is fatal if it is not aggressively treated.

In cardiac tamponade, cardiac output is critically reduced. A hallmark sign of cardiac tamponade is a *paradoxical pulse,* in which the systolic blood pressure drops more than 10 mm Hg during inspiration. Peripheral pulses weaken or disappear as well during inspiration. The increased pressure in the chest cavity during inspiration further interferes with cardiac output, causing paradoxical pulse. Other manifestations of cardiac tamponade include muffled heart sounds, dyspnea and tachypnea, tachycardia, and a narrowed pulse pressure.

COLLABORATIVE CARE
Although it is uncomfortable, acute pericarditis is usually self-limiting, and will resolve with or without treatment. However, close observation is important to detect early manifestations of increasing effusion or cardiac tamponade.

In acute pericarditis, *cardiac enzymes* may be slightly elevated. Acute pericarditis produces characteristic changes on the *electrocardiogram. Echocardiography* is used to evaluate for pericardial effusion or restricted heart motion. *Computed tomography (CT scan)* or *magnetic resonance imaging (MRI)* may also be used to identify pericardial effusions.

Aspirin, acetaminophen, or NSAIDs are ordered to reduce fever and inflammation, and to promote comfort. If heart function is affected, activity may be restricted.

Pericardiocentesis
Pericardiocentesis may be done to remove fluid from the pericardial sac (Figure 22-21 ◆). The physician inserts a large (16- to 18-gauge) needle into the pericardial sac and withdraws excess fluid. Pericardiocentesis may be be done as an emergency procedure for cardiac tamponade. Nursing implications for the client undergoing pericardiocentesis are outlined in Box 22-23.

NURSING CARE

PAIN

- Assess chest pain on a standarized scale; note quality and radiation of the pain. Ask about factors that aggravate or relieve the pain. *Assessing the severity, quality, and characteristics of chest pain help differentiate the pain of pericarditis from angina.*
- Administer NSAIDs on a regular basis as prescribed with food. *NSAIDs are ordered to reduce fever, inflammation, and*

Figure 22-21. ◆ Pericardiocentesis.

pericardial pain. They are most effective when given on a regular schedule. Administering the drugs with food helps decrease GI distress.

■ Maintain a quiet, calm environment. Provide position changes, back rubs, heat/cold therapy, diversional activity,

and emotional support. Supportive interventions convey caring, enhance the effects of the medication, and decrease the perception of pain.

INEFFECTIVE BREATHING PATTERN

The pain of pericarditis increases with respiratory movement, leading the client to breathe shallowly.

■ Assess respiratory rate and effort, and auscultate breath sounds every 4 hours. Report adventitious or diminished breath sounds. Congestion or atelectasis may result from decreased ventilation of peripheral alveoli due to shallow respirations.

■ Assist to use the incentive spirometer at least every 2 hours. Provide pain medication before respiratory therapy treatments, as needed. Deep breathing and the incentive spirometer help ensure alveolar ventilation and prevent atelectasis. Analgesia prior to painful treatments promotes comfort and facilitates participation.

■ Administer oxygen as needed. Supplementary oxygen promotes optimal gas exchange and tissue oxygenation.

■ Place in Fowler's or high Fowler's position. Elevating the head of the bed reduces the work of breathing and decreases pericardial chest pain.

BOX 22-23
NURSING CARE CHECKLIST

PERICARDIOCENTESIS
Before the Procedure

☑ Gather all supplies.
☑ Reinforce teaching about the procedure, clarifying information and answering questions. Provide emotional support.
☑ Verify informed consent for the procedure.
☑ Provide for privacy.
☑ Obtain baseline vital signs.
☑ Initiate cardiac monitoring and obtain a baseline rhythm strip.
☑ Have emergency resuscitation equipment at the bedside.
☑ Administer oxygen as ordered.

During the Procedure

☑ Follow standard precautions.
☑ Position at a 45- to 60-degree angle. Position a dry towel to catch blood or fluid.
☑ Assist physician with the aspiration as directed.
☑ Notify physician of changes in cardiac rhythm, vital signs, level of consciousness, and urine output.

After the Procedure

☑ Monitor vital signs and cardiac rhythm every 15 minutes for first hour, every 30 minutes next hour, then hourly for 24 hours.
☑ Record fluid removed as output on the intake and output record.
☑ If indicated, send aspirated fluid for culture and sensitivity and laboratory analysis.
☑ Assess heart and breath sounds.
☑ Document the procedure and the client's response.

■ SAMPLE DOCUMENTATION

3/15/03	0915	Pericardiocentesis performed
		by Dr. Smith at bedside. 250 mL clear
		yellow fluid obtained; specimen to lab
		for analysis. Tolerated procedure well
		with stable vital signs and heart
		rhythm.
		___ M. May, LPN.

RISK FOR DECREASED CARDIAC OUTPUT

- Assess vital signs hourly during acute inflammatory processes. *Frequent assessment allows early identification of manifestations of decreased cardiac output, such as tachycardia, hypotension, or changes in pulse pressure.*
- Assess heart sounds and peripheral pulses, and observe for neck vein distention and pulsus paradoxus every hour. Notify the physician of distant, muffled heart sounds, new murmurs or extra heart sounds, decreasing quality of peripheral pulses, and distended neck veins. *Acute pericardial effusion interferes with cardiac filling and pumping, causing venous congestion and decreased cardiac output.*
- Promptly notify physician of altered level of consciousness; decreased urine output; cold, clammy, mottled skin; delayed capillary refill; and weak peripheral pulses. *These signs of decreased organ and tissue perfusion indicate a significant drop in cardiac output.*
- If emergency pericardiocentesis and/or surgery is needed to remove pericardial fluid, prepare the client for the procedure, providing appropriate explanations and reassurance. Observe for adverse effects during pericardiocentesis. *Emotional support and explanations reduce anxiety and promote a caring atmosphere.*

Discharge Considerations

Stress the importance of continuing anti-inflammatory medications as ordered. Teach about prescribed drugs, including dose, desired and possible adverse effects, and interactions with other drugs or food. Instruct to take anti-inflammatory medications with food, milk, or antacids to minimize gastric distress, and to contact the physician if unable to tolerate the drug. Tell clients taking NSAIDs to monitor their weight at least weekly, because these drugs may cause fluid retention. Encourage to maintain a fluid intake of at least 2,500 mL/day to minimize the risk of kidney damage. Advise to avoid aspirin while taking other NSAIDs because it may interfere with their activity. Instruct to avoid over-the-counter preparations containing aspirin, as well.

If an activity restriction is ordered, suggest measures to maintain this restriction. Emphasize that activity will be gradually increased once the inflammatory process has resolved.

The client may be at risk for recurrence of pericarditis. Teach manifestations that may indicate recurrent pericarditis, and stress the importance of promptly reporting these to the physician.

Disorders of Cardiac Structure

Valvular Heart Disease

Proper functioning of the heart valves is necessary to ensure one-way blood flow through the heart and vascular system. **Valvular heart disease** interferes with blood flow to and from the heart. Rheumatic heart disease is the most common cause of valvular disease, especially in older adults. Valve disorders also can result from endocarditis or after myocardial infarction, due to damaged papillary muscles. Congenital heart defects may affect heart valves, often with no symptoms until adulthood. Changes in the heart that occur with normal aging also may lead to valvular disease.

PATHOPHYSIOLOGY

There are two major types of heart valve disorders: stenosis and regurgitation. **Stenosis** occurs when valve leaflets fuse together and are unable to open or close fully. The valve opening narrows, impairing the forward flow of blood. *Regurgitant valves* (also called *insufficient* or *incompetent* valves) do not close completely. This allows **regurgitation,** or backflow of blood, through the incompletely closed valve into the area it just left.

With valvular disease, pressures and blood flow are affected both in front of and behind the affected valve. Stenosis increases the work of the chamber behind the affected valve as the heart attempts to move blood through the narrowed opening. Excess blood volume behind regurgitant valves causes the chamber to dilate. Blood volume and pressures are reduced in front of the diseased valve, because flow is impeded through a stenotic valve and backflow occurs through a regurgitant valve. These changes can lead to pulmonary complications or heart failure. The heart muscle hypertrophies as the heart attempts to maintain cardiac output.

The valves on the left side of the heart (mitral and aortic) are subjected to higher pressures, increasing their risk of damage. Blood flow through the heart becomes turbulent as blood moves or attempts to move through damaged valves; the result is a murmur, one of the characteristic manifestations of valvular disease (Table 22-11 ◆).

Mitral Stenosis

Mitral stenosis is a narrowing of the mitral valve that obstructs blood flow from the left atrium into the left ventricle during diastole. Mitral stenosis is usually caused by rheumatic heart disease.

TABLE 22-11 CHARACTERISTICS OF COMMON HEART MURMURS

MURMUR	TIMING IN CARDIAC CYCLE	LOCATION	CONFIGURATION	QUALITY
Mitral stenosis	Diastole	Apex—5th intercostal space (ICS), midclavicular line (MCL)	S₂ ～ S₁	Continuous rumble, increasing toward end of diastole
Mitral regurgitation	Systole	Apex	S₁ ～ S₂	Continuous throughout systole (holosystolic)
Aortic stenosis	Systole	Right sternal border, 2nd ICS	S₁ ～ S₂	Crescendo–decrescendo, continuous
Aortic regurgitation	Early diastole	3rd ICS, left sternal border	S₂ ～ S₁	Decrescendo, continuous

The narrowed mitral opening impairs left ventricular filling and cardiac output. It also causes the left atrium to dilate and hypertrophy. High atrial pressures are reflected back into the pulmonary system (Figure 22-22 ◆). Increased pressure in the pulmonary system increases the workload of the right ventricle, causing it also to dilate and hypertrophy. Eventually, right-sided heart failure occurs. Chronic atrial distention often leads to atrial dysrhythmias such as atrial fibrillation. Thrombi may form in the left atrium and become emboli to the brain, coronary arteries, kidney, spleen, and extremities—potentially devastating complications.

Dyspnea on exertion (DOE) is typically the earliest manifestation of mitral stenosis. Others include cough, hemoptysis, frequent respiratory infections such as bronchitis and pneumonia, paroxysmal nocturnal dyspnea, orthopnea, weakness, fatigue, and palpitations. As the stenosis increases, manifestations become more severe. Signs of right heart failure, such as distended neck veins and peripheral edema, may develop. The client with severe mitral stenosis may be cyanotic.

CLINICAL alert

Women with mitral stenosis may be asymptomatic until they become pregnant. The increased circulating volume (30% more in pregnancy) can precipitate sudden pulmonary edema and heart failure, threatening the lives of the mother and fetus.

On auscultation, a diastolic murmur characterized as low pitched and rumbling may be heard in the apical region. It is heard best with the bell of the stethoscope. The murmur may

➡ Blood flow

➡ Reduced blood flow

→ Backward pressure against flow

Figure 22-22. ◆ Mitral stenosis.

be accompanied by a palpable *thrill* (a palpable tremor or vibration). Crackles may be noted in the lungs.

Mitral Regurgitation

Mitral regurgitation or *insufficiency* allows blood to flow back into the left atrium during systole because the valve does not close completely. Rheumatic heart disease is a common cause of mitral regurgitation. Only a portion of the blood in the ventricle is ejected into the systemic circulation during systole; the rest returns to the left atrium through the deformed valve. This is added to the blood from the pulmonary system (Figure 22-23 ◆). The left atrium dilates to accommodate the extra volume; the left ventricle dilates to compensate for increased preload and low cardiac output.

Clients with mitral regurgitation may experience fatigue, weakness, exertional dyspnea, and orthopnea. In severe or acute mitral regurgitation, manifestations of left heart failure may develop, including pulmonary congestion and edema. With high pulmonary pressures, right-sided heart failure may develop as well.

The murmur of mitral regurgitation is usually loud, high pitched, and rumbling. It may be described as "cooing" or "sea gull-like" or have a musical quality. It is heard best at the apex of the heart and often is accompanied by a palpable thrill.

Mitral Valve Prolapse

Mitral valve prolapse (MVP) is a form of mitral insufficiency that occurs when the posterior cusp of the mitral valve flops back into the left atrium during systole. It is probably congenital and is commonly found in young women between ages 14 and 30. Its incidence declines with age. Most clients with MVP are asymptomatic. Chest pain, usually related to fatigue rather than exertion, is the most common symptom of MVP. Dysrhythmias can cause palpitations, light-headedness, and syncope. A high-pitched late systolic murmur, sometimes described as a "whoop" or "honk," may be present.

Aortic Stenosis

Aortic stenosis obstructs blood flow from the left ventricle into the aorta during systole. Aortic stenosis is more common in males (80%) than females. It may be *idiopathic* (unknown cause), congenital, or related to rheumatic heart disease. The older adult may develop aortic stenosis from changes associated with aging.

As aortic stenosis progresses, the left ventricle has to work harder to eject blood through the narrowed opening. The ventricle hypertrophies to maintain the cardiac output (Figure 22-24 ◆). Because of the extra work, myocardial oxygen needs increase. The increased oxygen consumption can lead

➡ Blood flow
➡ Reduced blood flow
→| Backward pressure against flow

Figure 22-23. ◆ Mitral regurgitation.

➡ Blood flow
➡ Reduced blood flow
→| Backward pressure against flow

Figure 22-24. ◆ Aortic stenosis.

to myocardial ischemia. Increased pressures in the left heart are reflected back to the pulmonary vascular system; congestion and pulmonary edema may result.

Manifestations of aortic stenosis usually develop after age 50. They include dyspnea on exertion, angina, and exertional syncope (light-headedness with activity). The pulse pressure narrows as stoke volume and cardiac output fall. Clients with aortic stenosis are at risk for sudden cardiac death.

A harsh systolic murmur can be heard in the second intercostal space to the right of the sternum. A palpable thrill is often noted. As the condition becomes more severe, S_3 and S_4 heart sounds may be heard.

Aortic Regurgitation

In *aortic regurgitation* or *insufficiency,* the aortic valve fails to close completely, allowing blood to flow back into the left ventricle from the aorta during diastole (Figure 22-25 ◆). Rheumatic heart disease is the most common cause of aortic regurgitation.

Blood from the aorta causes volume overload of the left ventricle. The ventricle dilates, and stroke volume increases. Over time, the left ventricle hypertrophies, and cardiac output falls. Eventually, pulmonary congestion and possibly right heart failure develop from increased pressures on the left side of the heart. Unlike many other valve disorders, exercise reduces regurgitation and improves heart function in this disorder.

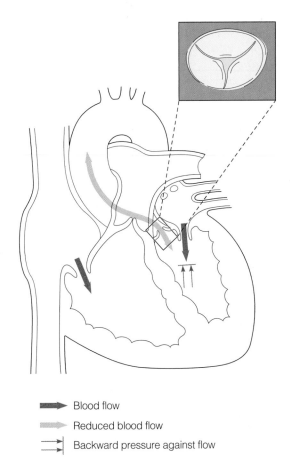

▬▶ Blood flow

▬▶ Reduced blood flow

→| Backward pressure against flow

Figure 22-25. ◆ Aortic regurgitation.

People with mild to moderate aortic regurgitation may complain of palpitations, especially when flat or in a left-lying position. The heartbeat is visible as a throbbing pulse in the arteries of the neck. Sometimes the force of contraction causes a head bob and shakes the whole body. Other manifestations include dizziness, exercise intolerance, fatigue, exertional dyspnea, and angina. Angina often occurs at night and may not respond to common treatments. The pulse pressure often is widened.

The murmur of aortic regurgitation is heard in diastole as blood flows back into the left ventricle from the aorta. It is described as a "blowing," high-pitched sound heard most clearly at the third left intercostal space. It may be associated with a thrill. An S_3 and S_4 may be heard. Because the heart is enlarged, the apical impulse is displaced to the left.

COLLABORATIVE CARE

Valvular disease may be asymptomatic for many years. The initial indication often is a heart murmur heard during a routine physical examination. *Echocardiography* is used to diagnose valvular disease. *Cardiac catheterization* is used to assess the effects of valve disease on heart function.

Asymptomatic clients and those with mild manifestations often require no treatment. They are closely observed for signs of disease progression. Valve damage increases the risk for infective endocarditis because altered blood flow through the heart and deformed valve allows bacterial colonization. Antibiotics are given prophylactically prior to any dental work, invasive procedures, or surgery (see Table 22-10). Manifestations of heart failure are treated with diet and medications (see the preceding section on heart failure). When medical treatment no longer controls the disease, surgery is considered.

Percutaneous Balloon Valvuloplasty

Stenotic valve disease may be treated with *percutaneous balloon valvuloplasty.* A balloon catheter is inserted into the femoral vein or artery, and advanced to the stenotic valve. The balloon is then inflated for approximately 90 seconds to divide the fused leaflets and enlarge the valve opening (Figure 22-26 ◆). Nursing care of the client with a balloon valvuloplasty is similar to that of the client following PTCA (see Box 22-7).

Surgery

Surgery to repair or replace the diseased valve may be required to restore valve function, relieve symptoms, and prevent complications. *Valvuloplasty* is a general term for reconstruction or repair of a heart valve. Methods include "patching" the perforated portion of the leaflet, resecting excess tissue, removing vegetations or calcification, and other techniques. A *commissurotomy* may be done to open stenotic valves.

Severely damaged valves may be replaced. Many different prosthetic heart valves are available, including mechanical and biologic tissue valves (Figure 22-27 ◆). Biologic tissue valves (from animal tissue or a human cadaver) allow more normal blood flow and are less likely to cause clots to form. Mechanical prosthetic valves are more durable, but require lifetime antico-

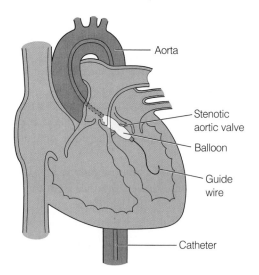

Figure 22-26. ◆ Balloon valvuloplasty. The balloon catheter is positioned across the stenosed valve. The balloon is then inflated to increase the size of the valve opening.

agulation to prevent clot formation on the valve. Both biologic and mechanical valves increase the risk of emboli and endocarditis, although the incidence of these complications is fairly low. Nursing care of the client having valve surgery is similar to that for other types of open heart surgery (see Box 22-8).

NURSING CARE

Nursing care focuses on maintaining the cardiac output, managing manifestations of the disorder, teaching about the disease and its treatment, and preventing complications.

DECREASED CARDIAC OUTPUT

■ Monitor vital signs and hemodynamic pressures, reporting changes. *A drop in systolic blood pressure and increasing pulse rate may indicate decreased cardiac output.*

■ Assess indicators of cardiac output every 8 hours, including level of consciousness, neck vein distention, respiratory effort and lung sounds, urine output, skin color and temperature, peripheral edema, and peripheral pulses and capillary refill. Notify the physician of significant changes. *Decreased cardiac output impairs tissue and organ perfusion, producing clinical manifestations.*

■ Monitor intake and output; weigh daily, reporting any gain of 3 to 5 lbs. (1 to 2 kg) within 24 hours. *Fluid retention may indicate decreased cardiac output; 2.2 lbs. (1 kg) of weight is equal to 1 liter of retained fluid.*

■ Maintain fluid restriction as ordered. *Fluid intake may be restricted to minimize cardiac workload.*

■ Elevate head of the bed, and administer oxygen as ordered. *These measures facilitate lung ventilation and improve oxygenation.*

■ Monitor pulse oximetry. *Pulse oximetry allows assessment of oxygenation.*

■ Promote physical, emotional, and mental rest. *Physical and psychological rest decreases the cardiac workload.*

■ Administer medications as ordered. *Diuretics, ACE inhibitors, and direct vasodilators are often ordered to reduce or redistribute excess fluid volume and reduce the cardiac workload.*

ACTIVITY INTOLERANCE

■ Obtain vital signs before and during activities. *An increased heart rate, change in BP, diaphoresis, or complaints of shortness of breath, fatigue, or chest pain may indicate poor tolerance of the level of activity.*

■ Encourage gradual increases in activity/self-care as tolerated. *Progressive activity prevents sudden stress on the heart and helps improve exercise tolerance.*

■ Provide assistance as needed. Suggest using a shower chair, sitting while brushing hair or teeth, and so on. *Energy-saving techniques reduce cardiac workload.*

Figure 22-27. ◆ Prosthetic heart valves. (A) Carpentier–Edwards porcine xenograft. (B) Medtronic Hall prosthetic valve.

INEFFECTIVE PROTECTION

Anticoagulant therapy may be ordered to reduce the risk of clotting with valve disorders or an artificial valve. This increases the risk for bleeding and hemorrhage.

- Test stools and emesis for occult blood. *Bleeding in the GI tract may not be visible.*
- Caution to avoid using aspirin or other NSAIDs. Instruct to read ingredient labels on over-the-counter drugs; many contain aspirin. *Aspirin and other NSAIDs interfere with clotting and may increase the risk of bleeding.*
- Instruct to use a soft-bristled toothbrush and an electric razor, and to clean fragile skin gently. *These measures reduce the risk of bleeding from skin nicks and cuts or the gums.*
- Monitor hemoglobin, hematocrit, and platelet counts. Notify the charge nurse of significant changes. *Low hemoglobin and hematocrit may indicate blood loss. Platelet counts below 50,000/mm^3 significantly increase the risk of bleeding.*

Discharge Considerations

Preventing rheumatic fever is important to prevent heart valve disorders. Early treatment of strep throat usually prevents rheumatic fever. Teach individual clients, families, and communities the importance of timely and effective treatment of strep throat. Emphasize the importance of completing the full prescription of antibiotics to prevent development of resistant bacteria.

Explain all tests and procedures, including corrective surgery, to increase understanding and decrease anxiety. Discuss symptom management, including activity restrictions or lifestyle changes related to the valve disease. Advise to schedule rest periods to prevent fatigue. Teach about diet restrictions to control heart failure; arrange a consultation with the dietitian for teaching and menu planning. Provide information about prescribed medications, including their purpose, desired and possible adverse effects, scheduling, and possible interactions with other drugs. Refer the client and family to community resources prior to discharge. Emphasize the importance of keeping follow-up appointments to monitor the disease and treatment. Emphasize the importance of notifying all health care providers about valve disease or surgery so that antibiotics can be given before any procedure that might cause infection.

Instruct the client and family to report increasing severity of symptoms, particularly of heart failure and pulmonary edema, to the doctor. The treatment regimen may need to be modified or surgery considered to repair or replace the diseased valve. Advise to report neurologic changes and other symptoms of emboli so anticoagulant therapy can be adjusted. Instruct to notify the physician of manifestations of bleeding, such as joint pain, easy bruising, black and tarry stools, bleeding gums, or blood in the urine or sputum.

Nursing Interventions Classification

Consider the following nursing interventions (McCloskey & Bulechek, 2000) when providing care for clients with cardiac disorders:

- Analgesic Administration
- Anxiety Reduction
- Cardiac Care
- Fluid/Electrolyte Management
- Invasive Hemodynamic Monitoring
- Oxygen Therapy
- Respiratory Monitoring
- Teaching: Procedure/Treatment
- Vital Signs Monitoring

(*Note:* The bibliography listings for this and all chapters have been compiled at the back of the book.)

Chapter Review

key terms by topic

Use the CD-ROM disk enclosed with your textbook to hear the pronunciation of the key terms in the chapter.

Cardiac structure and function
pericardium, myocardium, endocardium

Rhythm disorders
dysrhythmia

Coronary heart disease
atherosclerosis, angina pectoris, myocardial infarct (MI), cardiogenic shock, pericarditis

Disorders of cardiac function
heart failure, orthopnea, paroxysmal nocturnal dyspnea

Inflammatory cardiac disorders
rheumatic fever, stenosis, regurgitation, endocarditis, myocarditis, pericarditis, pericardial friction rub, cardiac tamponade

key points

- The heart is a simple pump: The right side receives blood from the veins and pumps it into the low-pressure pulmonary system; the left side receives blood from the lungs, and pumps it to the higher pressure systemic circulation.

- Electrical impulses, usually generated by the sinoatrial (SA) node, travel through conduction pathways in the heart, causing the muscle to contract. Heart disease and other factors (e.g., drugs, the autonomic nervous system) can affect generation and conduction of these electrical impulses. This can lead to dysrhythmias, disorders of heart rate and regularity. Cardiac output can be affected by very slow, very fast, or very irregular dysrhythmias.

- The coronary arteries provide the "fuel" for the myocardium. These arteries often are affected by atherosclerosis. Narrowing of the vessel affects myocardial blood supply and can lead to angina or myocardial infarction.

- Angina is caused by myocardial ischemia, a temporary imbalance between myocardial oxygen supply and demand.

- Myocardial infarction, on the other hand, results from total blockage of the blood supply to a part of the myocardium. Unless blood flow is restored within a few hours, the affected myocardium will infarct and die. This affects function of the heart muscle and cardiac output.

- Heart failure, inability of the heart to meet the body's needs for fuel and oxygen, is caused by impaired pumping of the heart. It usually is caused by extensive heart muscle damage from myocardial infarction, but also can result from inflammatory, congenital, or valve disorders.

- Any layer of heart tissue can be affected by infection or inflammation. Inflammatory disorders can lead to either structural damage or impaired cardiac function.

- Prophylactic antibiotic therapy is an important measure to prevent infective endocarditis in clients with previous heart damage or deformity.

- The aortic and mitral valves are more likely to be affected by valve disorders because of the high pressures on the left side of the heart. When these valves are affected by either stenosis or reguritation, heart failure is likely to develop.

Medialink

Additional interactive resources for this chapter can be found on the Companion Website at www.prenhall.com/burke. Click on Chapter 22 and "Begin" to select the activities for this chapter.

For NCLEX review questions and an audio glossary, access the accompanying CD-ROM in this book.

for further study

For nursing measures related to pain, see Chapter 6.
For further information about cardiogenic shock, see Chapter 10.
For information about diet and nutrition, see Chapter 18.
For more information about thrombolytic therapy, see Chapter 24.

Critical Thinking Care Map

Caring for a Client after Coronary Artery Bypass Surgery
NCLEX-PN Focus Area: Coping and Adaptation

Case Study: John Clements, 50 years old, had emergency triple bypass surgery 3 days ago. His initial recovery has been uneventful, and he has transferred from the cardiac recovery unit to the cardiac unit for the remainder of his hospital stay.

Nursing Diagnosis: Ineffective Role Performance

COLLECT DATA

Subjective	Objective
_____	_____
_____	_____
_____	_____
_____	_____
_____	_____
_____	_____

Would you report this data? Yes/No

If yes, to: _____

Nursing Care

_____
_____
_____
_____
_____
_____
_____
_____

How would you document this? _____
_____
_____

Data Collected
(use those that apply)

- History of progressive angina for 4 years
- Anterior wall myocardial infarction 2 years ago; treated with immediate thrombolytic therapy and percutaneous balloon angioplasty
- BP 138/72, P 86, regular, R 24, T 99.1° F PO
- Faint crackles left lung base
- Strong family history of CHD (father died age 51, brother died age 48 of myocardial infarctions)
- Does not smoke, uses alcohol occasionally
- Enjoys "good Southern-style cooking" and watching TV; rarely exercises other than dancing with wife and friends about once a month
- Incision clean and dry, healing well
- Color good; O_2 sats 95% on 4 L O_2 per cannula
- Bowel sounds active, taking regular diet in small amounts
- Usually works 50 to 60 hours per week at own contracting business
- States, "I have got to get back to work! You just can't sit around in my business—you have to make sure that the work is getting done on time."

Nursing Interventions
(use those that apply)

- Teach about: The heart and coronary heart disease; exercise and activities; lifestyle modifications, including diet and stress management.
- Discuss emotional reactions to CHD and sexual activity after discharge.
- Provide analgesics as needed for comfort.
- Ambulate at least four times per day for increasing distances.
- Encourage use of incentive spirometer every 1 to 2 hours.
- Encourage rest before and after activity/exercise.
- Provide information about community resources for emotional support.
- Help identify coping strategies for concerns about role in business.

NCLEX-PN Exam Preparation

Nursing responsibility includes caring for clients who are attempting to adapt to various alterations in physiological status. When answering NCLEX questions that require priority setting, use Maslow's Hierarchy of Needs to determine which client is most at risk for physiologic complications. Ask yourself which client has the most acute medical process, is most physiologically unstable, or is most at risk for developing medical complications. Intervene with physiologic problems before psychological conditions are addressed.

1. A client asks the nurse how he can distinguish between angina and chest pain associated with a myocardial infarction. An accurate response by the nurse would be:
   a. "Chest pain associated with myocardial infarction is relieved by nitroglycerin."
   b. "Chest pain associated with angina is unrelieved by nitroglycerin."
   c. "Chest pain associated with angina is relieved by rest."
   d. "Chest pain associated with myocardial infarction is relieved by rest."

2. A male client has experienced a myocardial infarction. The nurse assesses him for signs of complications. Which of the following would concern the nurse MOST?
   a. B/P 138/84, P 72
   b. B/P 90/50, urinary output 20 mL/hr
   c. P 92, urinary output 50 mL/hr
   d. B/P 150/70, P 100

3. Teaching for a client with a diagnosis of myocardial infarction should include which of the following?
   a. Take nitroglycerin sublingually every 5 minutes until chest pain disappears.
   b. Call 911 immediately if chest pain occurs.
   c. Avoid all stress.
   d. Adjust diet to low cholesterol, low fat, low sodium.

4. A client develops left-sided heart failure. An appropriate nursing diagnosis is:
   a. Activity Intolerance
   b. Ineffective Airway Clearance
   c. Deficient Fluid Volume
   d. Pain

5. A client develops right-sided heart failure. Which of the following symptoms would the nurse expect to find?
   a. pulmonary edema
   b. edematous legs and ankles
   c. decreased heart rate
   d. increased urinary output

6. The nurse is to administer digoxin (Lanoxin) 0.25 mg PO. The client's apical pulse is 48. The appropriate nursing action is to:
   a. check the digoxin level and administer the drug if the level is < 2 ng/mL.
   b. hold the drug and recheck the apical pulse in 1 hour
   c. hold the drug and notify the physician
   d. administer the drug and report the apical pulse when the physician makes rounds

7. A man who has been diagnosed with congestive heart failure is prescribed a low-fat, low-cholesterol, and low-sodium diet. Which of the following food items, if chosen by the client, indicates a need for further teaching?
   a. baked chicken, green beans, sliced carrots
   b. macaroni and cheese, smoked turkey leg, broccoli
   c. grilled fish, baked potato, tossed salad
   d. turkey bacon, egg white omelet, wheat toast, apple

8. A priority nursing goal for a client diagnosed with rheumatic heart disease includes:
   a. determining the etiology of the disease
   b. encouraging visits from friends and family
   c. enforcing prescribed activity limitations
   d. assessing for signs of recurring streptococcal infection

9. A female client is diagnosed with pericarditis. The nurse expects which of the following assessment findings?
   a. peripheral edema
   b. wheezing breath sounds
   c. absence of chest pain
   d. pericardial friction rub

10. A client is diagnosed with mitral stenosis. Discharge teaching should include all but which of the following?
    a. How to auscultate heart for murmurs twice per day.
    b. Signs and symptoms of heart failure.
    c. Notify physician of temperature elevation > 100° F for more than 2 days.
    d. Report signs and symptoms of activity intolerance to the physician.

chapter

23

Caring for Clients with Peripheral Vascular Disorders

CARING tip

❝Choose to learn something new every day. Realize you can learn from clients and co-workers and especially yourself.❞

Geneo A. Roberts, RN, C • PICU Staff Nurse, VN Supervisor • Medical Center Hospital • Odessa, Texas • Former Vocational Nursing Director • Odessa College–Monahans Extension • Monahans, Texas

LEARNING outcomes

After completing this chapter, you will be able to:

- Relate physiology of the peripheral vascular system to common disorders affecting the peripheral vascular system.
- Describe the pathophysiology of common peripheral vascular disorders.
- Identify subjective and objective assessment data to collect for clients with peripheral vascular disorders.
- Explain the nursing implications of drugs used to treat clients with peripheral vascular disorders.
- Describe pre- and postoperative care for clients having vascular surgery.
- Reinforce client and family teaching to promote and maintain health in clients with common peripheral vascular disorders.
- Use the nursing process to provide individualized care to clients with peripheral vascular disorders.

MediaLink

 www.prenhall.com/burke

Use the above address to access the free, interactive Companion Website created for this textbook. Get hints, instant feedback, and textbook references to chapter-related multiple choice questions. Link to other interesting sites.

Nursing care for clients with peripheral vascular disorders focuses on relieving pain, improving peripheral circulation, preventing tissue damage, and promoting healing. A holistic approach to caring is important to address the emotional, social, and economic effects of these often chronic and potentially disabling disorders.

Several processes can affect blood vessels and interfere with peripheral blood flow: constriction, obstruction, inflammation, and spasm. In conditions like aneurysms and varicose veins, the structure of the vessel itself is altered.

Structure and Function of the Peripheral Vascular System

The **peripheral vascular system** is a network of blood vessels that carry blood to peripheral tissues and then return it to the heart. This network includes arteries, veins, and capillaries.

ARTERIES AND VEINS

Arteries carry blood away from the heart. Oxygenated blood leaves the left ventricle via the *aorta.* Major arteries branch off the aorta and into successively smaller arteries. These eventually divide into *arterioles.* Arterioles feed into beds of hairlike *capillaries* within the organs and tissues.

In the capillary beds, oxygen and nutrients are exchanged for metabolic wastes, and deoxygenated blood begins its journey back to the heart through *venules.* Venules join onto veins, which in turn join larger and larger veins. **Veins** carry blood toward the heart. Peripheral veins empty into the *superior* and *inferior venae cavae,* and then into the right atrium.

Blood Vessel Structure

The structure of blood vessels reflects their different functions within the circulatory system. Except for the capillaries, blood vessel walls have three layers: the tunica intima, the tunica media, and the tunica adventitia (Figure 23-1 ◆). The innermost layer, the *tunica intima,* or *endothelium,* has a slick surface to assist blood flow. The middle layer, or *tunica media,* contains smooth muscle. This layer is thicker and more elastic in arteries than it is in veins. It allows arteries to expand and contract, maintaining blood flow to the capillaries between heart beats. *Constriction* (narrowing) and *dilation* (widening) of the arterioles is the major factor controlling blood pressure. The *tunica adventitia,* or outermost layer, is connective tissue that protects and anchors the vessel. Veins have a thicker tunica adventitia than arteries do.

The pressure in the veins is much lower than in the arteries. Veins have thinner walls, a larger lumen, and greater capacity than arteries. Many have valves that help move blood against gravity back to the heart. Skeletal muscle contraction helps: When skeletal muscles contract against veins, the valves open, and blood is propelled toward the heart. Changes in abdominal and thoracic pressure that occur with breathing also propel blood toward the heart.

The tiny capillaries, which connect the arterioles and venules, contain only one thin layer of tunica intima. This allows gases and nutrients to escape the blood vessels and reach tissue cells. Waste products from metabolism enter the capillaries for elimination. Capillaries are found in interwoven networks.

ARTERIAL CIRCULATION

Arterial circulation is maintained by a balance of blood flow, peripheral vascular resistance, and blood pressure. *Blood flow* is the amount of blood transported.

Peripheral vascular resistance (PVR) is the force opposing blood flow. PVR is determined by three factors:

1. *Blood viscosity* (thickness): The greater the viscosity of the blood, the greater its resistance to moving and flowing.
2. *Vessel length:* The longer the vessel, the greater the resistance to blood flow.

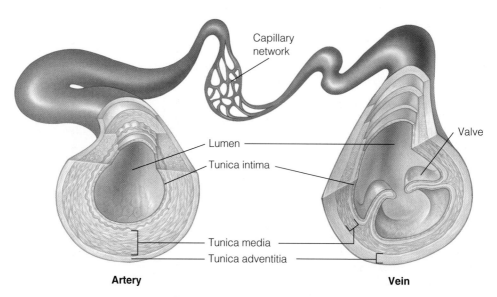

Artery   **Vein**

Figure 23-1. ◆ Structure of arteries, veins, and capillaries.

3. *Vessel diameter:* The smaller a vessel is, the more friction is produced, and the greater the resistance is to blood flow.

Blood pressure (BP) is the force exerted by blood against the walls of the arteries. The *systolic* pressure is the force exerted as the heart contracts (systole). The *diastolic* pressure reflects the force exerted when the heart is filling (diastole). The average adult BP is 120/80 mm Hg. The blood pressure is regulated mainly by cardiac output (CO) and peripheral vascular resistance (PVR). A number of factors affect CO and PVR:

- Sympathetic nervous system (SNS) stimulation increases cardiac output and constricts arterioles, increasing blood pressure. Pressure-sensitive receptors *(baroreceptors)* and *chemoreceptors* in the aortic arch, carotid sinus, and other large vessels stimulate the SNS.
- Parasympathetic stimulation causes dilation of arterioles, lowering the blood pressure.
- The kidneys help regulate BP. A fall in BP stimulates the renin–angiotensin–aldosterone mechanism, causing vasoconstriction and salt and water retention. Antidiuretic hormone (ADH) from the pituitary gland promotes water retention, increasing blood volume, cardiac output, and blood pressure.
- Temperatures affect peripheral resistance: Cold causes vasoconstriction; warmth produces vasodilation.
- Many chemicals, hormones, and drugs affect cardiac output or peripheral vascular resistance.

Other factors that affect cardiac output, peripheral vascular resistance, and BP include diet (e.g., sodium and calcium intake), race, gender, age, weight, time of day, position, exercise, and emotional state.

Hypertension

In adults, **hypertension** is defined as a blood pressure higher than 140 mm Hg systolic or 90 mm Hg diastolic on three separate readings several weeks apart. Hypertension is common, affecting about 50 million people in the United States. People between age 25 and 55 are primarily affected by this disorder. African Americans are more commonly affected than Caucasians. Hypertension is often called the "silent killer," because it has few symptoms. Its impact is significant because of the conditions that result from persistent high blood pressure: brain attack (stroke), coronary heart disease, and chronic renal failure. Only about 20% of people with hypertension have satisfactory blood pressure control.

PATHOPHYSIOLOGY
Peripheral vascular resistance is the primary factor in determining the blood pressure. In hypertension, the resistance to blood flow is increased, primarily in the arterioles. This increases the workload of the left ventricle. As a result, left ventricular muscle mass increases. More blood flow and oxy-

gen is required to meet the needs of the heart, increasing the risk for coronary heart disease.

Hypertension is classified both by its cause and its course. **Primary** (or *essential*) **hypertension** has no identified cause, although risk factors have been identified (Box 23-1). **Secondary hypertension** results from a known cause, such as kidney disease. When the systolic pressure is high but the diastolic pressure remains within normal limits, it is known as *isolated systolic hypertension.* Isolated systolic hypertension is common in older adults (Box 23-2).

BOX 23-1
RISK FACTORS FOR HYPERTENSION

RISK FACTORS THAT CAN BE CHANGED
- High sodium intake
- Obesity
- Excess alcohol consumption
- Low calcium and/or potassium intake
- Smoking

RISK FACTORS THAT CANNOT BE CHANGED
- Family history
- Age
- Race

BOX 23-2

population FOCUS

Hypertension in Older Adults

Until recently, a gradual increase in blood pressure was thought to be normal with aging. It is now recognized that blood pressure control is as important in older adults as in the rest of the population. Changes associated with aging that can affect older adults include the following:

- Isolated systolic hypertension is common. It increases the risk of stroke and death due to cardiovascular disease. It develops as blood vessels become more rigid. Their ability to expand and contract decreases, and PVR increases.
- An *auscultatory gap* (temporary disappearance of sounds when measuring the BP) is common. This gap can lead to inaccurate blood pressure readings if the cuff is not first inflated above the systolic pressure (see Box 23-4).
- The reflexes that maintain BP with position changes diminish. This can lead to a temporary fall in BP. When assessing for orthostatic hypotension, allow 2 to 5 minutes after position changes before measuring the blood pressure. Instruct older clients to change positions slowly, especially when rising from bed or a chair.

The stages of hypertension are:

Stage 1 (mild)	140–159/90–99
Stage 2 (moderate)	160–179/100–109
Stage 3 (severe)	180–209/110–119
Stage 4 (very severe)	> 210/120

People with stage 1 or stage 2 (mild or moderate) hypertension usually have no symptoms other than an increased blood pressure. They may complain of vague headaches or occasional dizziness. Hypertension is usually advanced when symptoms develop. These may include morning headache, blurred vision, unsteadiness, depression, and nocturia.

Without treatment, hypertension affects other organs and can lead to premature death (Table 23-1 ◆).

Hypertensive Crisis

Clients with hypertension may experience *hypertensive crisis,* a rapid increase in systolic pressure to greater than 240 mm Hg and/or diastolic pressure to greater than 120 mm Hg. *Malignant hypertension* is a diastolic pressure greater than 130 mm Hg. Hypertensive crisis requires immediate treatment (within 1 hour) to prevent irreversible damage to the brain, kidneys, and heart. Clients may have manifestations such as headache, confusion, blurred vision, restlessness, and motor and sensory deficits.

CLINICAL alert

Frequently monitor blood pressure (every 5 to 30 minutes) during a hypertensive emergency.

COLLABORATIVE CARE

Hypertension is diagnosed by blood pressure readings. The BP is measured after resting for at least 5 minutes and avoiding caffeine and smoking for at least 30 minutes.

No specific diagnostic tests are ordered to diagnose hypertension. Laboratory tests such as blood chemistries (including electrolytes, glucose, and cholesterol levels) are done to identify secondary hypertension and to provide baseline data before treatment is started.

Hypertension treatment focuses on lowering the blood pressure to less than 140 mm Hg systolic and 90 mm Hg diastolic. Treatment is directed at reducing the risk of damage to the cardiovascular system and other target organs. Developing a plan of care that the client can and will follow is vital to prevent long-term complications. While essential hypertension cannot be cured, it can be controlled with lifestyle management and medications (Table 23-2 ◆).

Lifestyle Modifications

Lifestyle modifications to reduce blood pressure include weight loss, dietary changes, restricted alcohol use and cigarette smoking, increased physical activity, and stress reduction.

TABLE 23-1 EFFECTS OF HYPERTENSION

ORGAN	EFFECT
Eyes	Retinopathy: Narrowed blood vessels, hemorrhages, fluid leakage, and swelling of the optic nerve
Heart	Coronary heart disease: Angina and myocardial infarction Left ventricular hypertrophy Heart failure Dysrhythmias
Vascular system	Peripheral vascular disease Aneurysms
Brain	Brain attack (stroke) Cerebral edema and changes in brain tissue
Kidneys	Renal insufficiency Renal failure

DIET. Dietary changes include limiting sodium and fat in the diet and promoting weight loss if overweight. Foods high in sodium, such as processed foods, canned fruits and vegetables, carbonated beverages, snack foods, and fast foods are avoided (see Box 5-5 in Chapter 5). These foods are often high in fats as well, contributing to weight gain. High-sodium, high-fat foods should be replaced with foods higher in potassium and lower in fat (such as fresh fruit and vegetables, freshly cooked meats, and whole grains).

ALCOHOL AND SMOKING. Alcohol intake is limited to no more than 1 ounce of ethanol per day. This translates to 24 ounces of beer, 10 ounces of wine, or 2 ounces of whiskey. Women and lighter-weight people should reduce this limit by half. Because both smoking and hypertension increase the risk of heart disease, clients are strongly urged to quit. Smoking reduces the benefits of some antihypertensive medications such as propranolol (Inderal).

PHYSICAL ACTIVITY. Regular exercise (such as walking, cycling, jogging, or swimming) decreases blood pressure and contributes to weight loss, stress reduction, and feelings of overall well-being. Exercises that oppose one muscle group to another (isometric), however, can raise blood pressure severely and should be avoided.

STRESS REDUCTION. Stress constricts blood vessels, raising the blood pressure. Regular, moderate exercise is the treatment of choice for reducing stress in the hypertensive client. Other stress reduction techniques may also benefit the client (Box 23-3).

Pharmacology

One or more of the following drug classes may be used to treat hypertension: diuretics, beta-adrenergic blockers, centrally

| TABLE 23-2 | RECOMMENDED FOLLOW-UP AND TREATMENT FOR HYPERTENSION |

STAGE	FOLLOW-UP RECOMMENDATION	TREATMENT RECOMMENDATION		
		Risk Group A[a]	*Risk Group B[b]*	*Risk Group C[c]*
Normal (< 130/< 85)	Recheck in 2 years	Lifestyle modification	Lifestyle modification	Lifestyle modification
High-normal (130–139/ 85–89)	Recheck in 1 year	Lifestyle modification	Lifestyle modification	Medication plus lifestyle modification
Stage 1 (140–159/ 90–99)	Confirm within 2 months	Lifestyle modification for up to 1 year, then medication	Lifestyle modification for up to 6 months, then medication	Medication plus lifestyle modification
Stage 2 (160–179/ 100–109)	Refer for evaluation within 1 month	Medication plus lifestyle modification	Medication plus lifestyle modification	Medication plus lifestyle modification
Stage 3 (> 180/110)	Refer for evaluation within 1 week			

[a]Risk Group A: No evidence of cardiovascular disease, target organ damage, or other risk factors
[b]Risk Group B: No evidence of cardiovascular disease or target organ damage; major risk factors (e.g., smoking, hyperlipidemia, older age, male gender, or family history of cardiovascular disease) are present
[c]Risk Group C: Evidence of cardiovascular or target organ damage; presence of diabetes
Source: Adapted from National Institutes of Health, National Heart, Lung, and Blood Institute. (1997, November). *The Sixth Report of the Joint National Committee on Prevention, Detection, Evaluation, and Treatment of High Blood Pressure.* NIH Publication No. 98-4080.

acting sympatholytics, vasodilators, angiotensin-converting enzyme (ACE) inhibitors, and calcium channel blockers.

BOX 23-3

COMPLEMENTARY THERAPIES

Hypertension

Stress management is an important part of the lifestyle changes recommended for clients with hypertension. All of the following may help reduce stress:

- Animal-assisted therapy
- Aromatherapy with ylang-ylang, clary sage, lavender, or marjoram
- Biofeedback
- Massage
- Meditation
- Qigong, a Chinese discipline of breathing and mental exercises that may be combined with arm movements (similar to T'ai Chi)
- T'ai Chi
- Yoga
- Herbal supplements such as garlic and hawthorn

Diuretics and ACE inhibitors reduce circulating blood volume. Beta blockers reduce cardiac output. Centrally acting sympatholytics and vasodilators reduce peripheral resistance. Calcium channel blockers produce vasodilation. There is no one primary antihypertensive drug used to treat hypertension. A combination of drugs or a trial with a different category of antihypertensives is often used. Nursing implications for administering antihypertensive drugs (other than diuretics) are outlined in Table 23-3 ◆. (See also Table 5-4 for the nursing implications of diuretics.)

Treatment of clients in risk group C is more aggressive to reduce the risk of an MI, heart failure, or stroke. When the client's average blood pressure is greater than 200/120, immediate treatment is vital. Parenteral medications are given to reduce the blood pressure rapidly and prevent long-term consequences of the emergency.

NURSING CARE

ASSESSING

Obtaining accurate blood pressure measurements is key when assessing clients with hypertension. Inaccurate readings often

TABLE 23-3   NURSING IMPLICATIONS FOR PHARMACOLOGY: CLIENTS WITH HYPERTENSION

CLASS/DRUGS	MECHANISM OF ACTION	NURSING IMPLICATIONS	CLIENT AND FAMILY TEACHING
Angiotensin-converting Enzyme (ACE) Inhibitors ▪ Benazepril (Lotensin) ▪ Captopril (Capoten) ▪ Enalapril (Vasotec) ▪ Lisinopril (Zestril) ▪ Moexipril (Univasc) ▪ Ramipril (Altace) ▪ Others	ACE inhibitors inhibit the renin–angiotensin system, stimulate vasodilation, and may reduce sympathetic nervous system activity. These drugs have relatively few side effects in clients with essential hypertension.	Give 1 hour before meals to increase absorption; tablets may be crushed. Report abnormal laboratory values to the primary care provider. Take blood pressure before each dose. If hypotension occurs, keep flat with legs elevated. Monitor for rash or hives. Report peripheral edema.	Report peripheral edema, infection, or difficulty breathing to your health care provider. Change position (lying to sitting and sitting to standing) slowly to prevent dizziness and possible falls. Do not skip doses or stop taking drugs, this could cause your blood pressure to rise significantly.
Beta-Adrenergic Blockers ▪ Atenolol (Tenormin) ▪ Labetalol (Normodyne) ▪ Metoprolol tartrate (Lopressor) ▪ Nadolol (Corgard) ▪ Penbutolol (Levatol) ▪ Propranolol (Inderal) ▪ Timolol (Blocadren) ▪ Others	Beta blockers block sympathetic input to the heart. This reduces heart rate and cardiac output. They also interfere with the renin–angiotensin system, blocking vasoconstriction. Beta blockers can have serious side effects and should not be taken by clients with asthma, COPD, or heart block.	Assess blood pressure and apical pulse before giving; notify the charge nurse if they are not within established limits. Monitor for hypotension if client is also taking a diuretic. Carefully monitor diabetic clients for hypoglycemia.	Take your pulse and blood pressure daily. Change positions slowly to prevent dizziness and possible falls. Report fatigue, lethargy, or impotence to your doctor. If diabetic, check blood glucose more frequently; this medication may block hypoglycemia symptoms. Do not stop taking the drug unless instructed to by your doctor.
Centrally Acting Sympatholytics ▪ Clonidine (Catapres) ▪ Guanabenz (Wytensin) ▪ Guanfacine (Tenex) ▪ Methyldopa (Aldomet)	These drugs slow the heart rate and reduce vasoconstriction, lowering the blood pressure. They may be given in combination with a diuretic.	Administer PO; tablets may be crushed. Methyldopa may be given IV over 30 to 60 minutes; do not give subq or IM. Apply transdermal forms to dry, hairless, intact skin on the chest or upper arm. Report rash to physician. Report abnormal laboratory values to the primary care provider. Record baseline BP, pulse, and weight; assess VS before giving drug. Report peripheral edema or other side effects to the physician.	Relieve dry mouth by sipping water or chewing sugarless gum. Use unsalted crackers, noncola beverages, or dry toast to relieve nausea. Change positions slowly to prevent dizziness and possible falls. Do not stop taking or skip doses of this drug. The drug may darken your urine. Report depression or difficulty thinking to your doctor. Side effects tend to diminish over time. Do not drive if the drug causes drowsiness.

TABLE 23-3 NURSING IMPLICATIONS FOR PHARMACOLOGY: CLIENTS WITH HYPERTENSION (CONTINUED)

CLASS/DRUGS	MECHANISM OF ACTION	NURSING IMPLICATIONS	CLIENT AND FAMILY TEACHING
Vasodilators ▪ Hydralazine (Apresoline) ▪ Minoxidil (Loniten)	Vasodilators reduce blood pressure by relaxing vascular smooth muscle and decreasing peripheral vascular resistance.	Administer PO with meals or food; tablets may be crushed. Assess BP and pulse before giving the drug. Monitor bowel movements. Monitor for heart failure, fluid retention, and angina.	Change positions slowly to prevent dizziness and possible falls. Eat dry toast or unsalted crackers to relieve nausea. Report muscle, joint aches, and fever to your doctor. Tearing and nasal congestion may occur. Headache, palpitations, and rapid pulse should stop in about 10 days. Do not stop this drug unless your doctor approves. Report black, tarry stools or red blood in stools to your doctor.
Alpha-Adrenergic Blockers ▪ Doxazosin (Cardura) ▪ Prazosin (Minipress) ▪ Terazosin (Hytrin)	Alpha-adrenergic blockers promote vasodilatation, lowering blood pressure. They also reduce LDL and VLDL levels. Doxazosin and terazosin may cause tachycardia and palpitations, and other unwanted side effects. For these reasons, they are primarily used in acute situations.	Maintain safety during position changes; severe hypotension may develop. Give first dose at bedtime to reduce risk of fainting ("first-dose syncope"). Assess apical pulse and BP immediately before each dose and every 15 to 30 minutes thereafter until stable.	Use sips of water or sugarless gum to relieve dry mouth. Eat dry toast or unsalted crackers to relieve nausea. You may experience nasal congestion. Do not expect full benefit for 3–4 weeks. Change positions slowly to prevent dizziness and possible falls. Do not stop the drug without contacting your doctor.
Calcium Channel Blockers ▪ Amlodipine (Norvasc) ▪ Diltiazem (Cardizem) ▪ Felodipine (Plendil) ▪ Isradipine (DynaCirc) ▪ Nicardipine (Cardene) ▪ Nifedipine (Procardia) ▪ Verapamil (Isoptin)	Calcium channel blockers relax arterial smooth muscle causing vasodilatation.	If given parenterally, monitor heart rhythm continuously. Assess apical pulse and BP before giving. Notify charge nurse if outside identified limits. Monitor frequency and consistency of stools. Assess lungs for crackles and wheezes. Monitor intake and output. Assess extremities for peripheral edema.	Take BP and pulse daily. Change positions slowly to prevent dizziness and possible falls. Drink 6 to 8 glasses of water daily, and increase fiber in diet. Do not abruptly stop taking medications. Report difficulty breathing or chest pain to your doctor.

BOX 23-4
NURSING CARE CHECKLIST

ACCURATE BLOOD PRESSURE MEASUREMENT

☑ Choose blood pressure cuff that is the correct size: The cuff width should be about 40% of the circumference of the arm (or thigh) (see figure).

Bladder of cuff

☑ Position the cuff on the extremity with the center of the bladder directly over the artery.

☑ While palpating the artery (brachial if using the upper arm, radial if using the forearm, and popliteal if using the thigh), inflate the cuff until the pulse is no longer felt. Note the pressure and rapidly deflate the cuff. Wait approximately 1 to 2 minutes.

☑ Position the stethoscope over the artery and inflate the cuff to 30 mm Hg above the level at which the pulse was no longer felt. Slowly deflate the cuff at a rate of 2 to 3 mm Hg per second.

☑ Note the systolic reading where the first clear tapping sound (Korotkoff sound) is heard. Note the diastolic reading when the sounds change from distinct, crisp sounds to muffled sounds. In some facilities, a third reading is noted at the point where the last sound is heard.

☑ If possible, measure the pressure on both arms. If there is a difference of more than 5 to 10 mm Hg in the pressures, use the arm with the higher pressure reading for subsequent measurements because it more accurately reflects the systemic blood pressure.

---

occur because of inappropriate cuff size or incorrect technique. Box 23-4 gives guidelines that help ensure accurate blood pressure readings.

DIAGNOSING, PLANNING, AND IMPLEMENTING

INEFFECTIVE HEALTH MAINTENANCE

■ Explain the physiology and significance of the blood pressure. *Many people do not understand the significance of the blood pressure and its effects on the body.*

■ Emphasize the importance of adhering to prescribed treatment. *Keeping the blood pressure within normal levels reduces the risk for target organ damage.*

■ Discuss lifestyle changes with all clients at risk for or with hypertension. *Lifestyle changes may help reduce the risk of hypertension and its consequences. These changes alone will not control stage 2 or stage 3 hypertension but may lower the amount of medication needed to maintain blood pressure within appropriate levels.*

■ Discuss the relationship between sodium intake and blood pressure. Refer to dietary services for teaching about a low-sodium diet. Provide opportunities to choose low-sodium foods from simulated menus. *Knowledge and practice help clients understand and take control of their disease.*

■ Discuss weight-loss strategies and a low-fat diet. If appropriate, refer the client to an approved weight-loss program (*Weight Watchers, Overeaters Anonymous, Diet Workshop*).

Many overweight clients "diet" frequently without a good understanding of nutrition. Teaching and the support of a weight-loss program help the client learn to make more appropriate food choices.

■ Help identify realistic and appropriate life-style changes such as increasing exercise, stopping smoking, reducing alcohol intake, and controlling stress. *A plan that fits with the client's lifestyle is more likely to succeed. Family support is vital for maintaining lifestyle changes.*

■ Help identify strengths and weaknesses in maintaining health. *Anticipating potential difficulties allows the client and family to plan strategies to overcome these hurdles.*

EVALUATING

When evaluating the effectiveness of nursing care related to hypertension, collect data to assess the client's knowledge and understanding of the disease and its treatment. Inquire about continued compliance with recommended diet, exercise, smoking cessation, and other lifestyle changes.

 Discharge Considerations

Hypertension is primarily managed in community settings with regular visits to the primary care provider or hypertension clinic to monitor treatment. Because the client is primarily responsible for managing this chronic disease, careful assessment of the resources for home care is important (Box 23-5).

Stress the importance of taking medications as ordered. Discuss common side effects and their management. Inform the client that initial drug side effects may be unpleasant, but these effects diminish within two to three weeks of starting the medication. Review symptoms that should be reported to the primary care provider.

Help clients develop a realistic, regular exercise program that can be continued for life. Aerobic exercise such as walking, swimming, or cycling increases stamina and endurance, reduces stress, and helps manage obesity. Isometric activities (such as weight lifting) should be avoided unless approved by the physician, because they increase blood pressure.

Discuss the impact of stress on blood pressure. Teach stress reduction techniques such as meditation, relaxation, or deep breathing. Discuss the vasoconstrictive effects of anger and hostility, and help identify ways to diffuse these emotions. Explore alternative coping mechanisms to use during stressful situations.

Emphasize the need for regular follow-up care, even if progress is slow or if they have been unable to adhere to the plan. Comparing hypertension to diabetes, another chronic disease that requires lifelong management, may help the client and family understand the importance of continued care and follow-up.

BOX 23-5
ASSESSING FOR DISCHARGE

HYPERTENSION
Client

- Self-care: Ability to prepare and eat low-sodium, low-fat, low-cholesterol diet; to engage in aerobic exercise; to manage medications
- Knowledge: Understanding of disease, prescribed drugs, diet and activity recommendations, lifestyle changes, recommendations for follow-up care
- Psychosocial: Support network and significant others; ability to cope with lifestyle changes (e.g., smoking cessation, limiting alcohol intake, and stress reduction)
- Home environment: Cooking and food storage to allow less reliance on prepared foods; exposure to secondhand smoke

Family and Caregivers

- Ability and willingness to support lifestyle changes and risk factor reduction
- Financial resources for dietary changes and prescribed medications

Community

- Availability of blood pressure clinics, smoking-cessation programs, alcohol treatment programs; safe environment for exercise

Nursing Process Case Study
■ CLIENT WITH HYPERTENSION

Margaret Spezia is a married, 49-year-old Italian American woman with eight children, currently ranging in age from 3 to 18 years. During her annual physical examination 2 months ago, her blood pressure was found to be 146/98. Mrs. Spezia was instructed to reduce her cholesterol intake, to avoid salty foods, and not to add any salt to her foods either at the table or during cooking. An exercise program of short, daily walks was suggested for exercise and to reduce stress. She returns for follow-up.

Assessment Lisa Christos, the clinic nurse, obtains a nursing history. Mrs. Spezia reveals that between raising their children and working part-time, she rarely gets enough rest. Although her husband has a steady job, money is tight. She admits to a steady weight gain over the past 18 years. There is no known family history of hypertension. Physical assessment data includes: height 5'3" (160 cm); weight 225 lbs. (102 kg); T 99° F (37.2° C); P 100, regular; R 16; BP 170/110 (sitting). Skin cool and dry; capillary refill 3 seconds in upper extremities. Total serum cholesterol 245 mg/dL (normal adult value < 200 mg/dL). All other blood and urine studies within normal limits.

Captopril (Capoten), 25 mg by mouth twice daily, and hydrochlorothiazide, 50 mg by mouth daily are ordered. She is placed on a low-cholesterol, no-added-salt diet.

Diagnosis The following nursing diagnoses are identified:

- Imbalanced Nutrition: More Than Body Requirements related to excess food intake
- Ineffective Health Maintenance related to lifestyle behaviors
- Deficient Knowledge related to lack of information about prescribed treatment

Expected Outcomes The expected outcomes for the plan of care specify that Mrs. Spezia will:

- Lower blood pressure to less than 150 systolic and 90 diastolic within one week.
- Incorporate in her diet low-sodium and low-fat foods from a list provided.
- Develop a plan for regular exercise.
- Verbalize how prescribed medications, dietary restrictions, exercise, and follow-up visits will help her control her hypertension.

Planning and Implementation The following nursing interventions are planned and implemented:

- Teach how and when to monitor her blood pressure.

■ Instruct to withhold medications and contact the clinic if BP is less than 90 mm Hg systolic or 60 mm Hg diastolic.

■ Provide written and verbal instructions including the name, dose, action, and side effects of antihypertensive medications.

■ Help develop an exercise plan that includes a daily 15 minute walk and possible swimming classes at local YWCA.

■ Discuss a realistic weight-loss goal and plan.

■ Refer for dietary consultation and teaching about fat and sodium restrictions and weight loss.

■ Teach stress-reducing techniques.

Evaluation When Mrs. Spezia returns to the clinic 1 week later, her blood pressure is 142/88. She has lost 1.5 lbs. and says her oldest daughter is encouraging her to join a weight-reduction program. Mrs. Spezia is walking about 20 minutes a day at a local mall. She has met with the dietitian to discuss

ways to replace salt with herbs and spices. She has a list of low-fat, low-sodium foods and recommended cookbooks. Mrs. Spezia verbalizes the importance of taking her medications as ordered and managing her stress. She tells Ms. Christos, "I just can't believe that I feel better already. I've actually lost some weight—and I want to keep going. I think I can stick with this plan, even though it's like learning to cook all over again."

 Critical Thinking in the Nursing Process

1. Identify factors that contributed to Mrs. Spezia's hypertension. Which were modifiable and which were not?

2. What are the reasons for reducing sodium and fat in Mrs. Spezia's diet?

Arterial Disorders

Arterial blood flow is essential to provide oxygen and nutrients to tissues and cells. This blood flow can be affected by arterial wall defects, compression of the blood vessel, or vasospasm. Arteriosclerosis is the most common chronic disorder affecting the arteries. Others include arterial embolism or thrombus, thromboangitis obliterans (Buerger's disease), Raynaud's phenomenon, and aneurysms.

 ## Peripheral Arteriosclerosis

Arteriosclerosis is a common arterial disorder characterized by thickening, loss of elasticity, and calcification of arterial walls. *Atherosclerosis* is a form of arteriosclerosis in which the arterial walls thicken and harden due to deposits of fat and fibrin (see Chapter 22). In the peripheral circulation, arteriosclerosis and atherosclerosis decrease the blood supply to tissues, leading to peripheral vascular disease (PVD). PVD usually affects the lower extremities.

Peripheral arterial disease is more common in people over the age of 50 and is seen in men more than in women. Risk factors include a high fat diet, hypertension, diabetes mellitus, smoking, obesity, and stress (see Chapter 22).

PATHOPHYSIOLOGY

As peripheral arteries thicken and harden because of plaque deposits, the vessel lumen narrows. Plaque tends to form at arterial *bifurcations* (where the artery divides into two smaller arteries). Blood flow and oxygen delivery to the distal tissues decreases. If the occlusion develops slowly, collateral circula-

tion often develops, but it is usually not adequate to supply tissue needs. Few symptoms are seen until 60% or more of the blood supply to the tissues is occluded.

Peripheral plaque deposits usually affect the femoral arteries, the common iliac arteries, and the abdominal aorta. Arteriosclerosis of the abdominal aorta weakens the vessel wall and may lead to an aneurysm.

Pain is the primary symptom of peripheral arterial disease. One type of pain, called **intermittent claudication,** is usually described as a cramping or aching sensation in the calves of the legs or the arch of the foot. It develops with exercise such as walking, and is relieved by rest.

Rest pain, in contrast, occurs during periods of inactivity. It is a gnawing, aching, or burning sensation in the lower legs, feet, or toes. Rest pain often occurs at night. It increases when the legs are elevated and decreases when the legs are dependent (e.g., hanging over the side of the bed). Clients often complain that the legs feel cold or numb as well as painful.

The skin is pale when the legs are elevated but often dark red *(dependent rubor)* when the legs are dependent. The skin is often thin and shiny, with areas of discoloration and hair loss. The toenails may be thickened. In addition, areas of skin breakdown may be present. These may lead to ulcerations or gangrene.

Peripheral pulses often are decreased or absent. A **bruit** (a harsh or musical sound caused by turbulent blood flow) may be heard over large affected arteries, such as the femoral artery and the abdominal aorta.

The complications of peripheral arteriosclerosis include gangrene and amputation of one or both lower extremities.

Arterial Thrombus or Embolism

An arterial thrombus or embolism may develop, often as a complication of another disease, occluding blood flow through the artery.

Atherosclerotic changes in blood vessels can cause a **thrombus,** or blood clot, to develop. If the blood clot breaks away from the vessel wall and moves, it becomes an **embolus.** Foreign matter such as fat, bacteria, amniotic fluid, and air bubbles also may become emboli. An embolus eventually lodges in a vessel that is too small to allow it to pass through. Both thrombi and emboli block blood flow through the affected vessel to distal tissues. When arterial flow is interrupted, tissue necrosis and gangrene may result. Manifestations of arterial occlusion by a thrombus or embolus are listed in Box 23-6. A clear line between normal and pale, cold skin may be noted with an embolus.

Buerger's Disease

Buerger's disease (thromboangiitis obliterans) is an occlusive disease of small and medium-sized peripheral arteries. Affected vessels become inflamed, spastic, and thrombotic. It usually affects a leg or foot, although either the upper or lower extremities can be affected.

Buerger's disease primarily (95%) affects men under the age of 40 who smoke. Cigarette smoking is the single most significant cause. There also may be a genetic link.

The course of the disease is intermittent, with episodes of pain and impaired blood flow, and periods of remission. It may be dormant for weeks, months, or years. As the disease progresses, arteries become more widely involved, and episodes are more intense and longer. The risk of tissue ulceration and gangrene increases.

Pain in the involved extremity is the major symptom of Buerger's disease. The client complains of cramping pain in the instep of the foot or the calves of the legs that is relieved

Figure 23-2. ◆ A Doppler (ultrasound) stethoscope.

by rest (intermittent claudication), or of rest pain in the fingers and toes. Smoking, cold, and emotional distress often trigger burning pain.

The involved digits and/or extremities are pale, and cool or cold to the touch. The skin may be shiny and thin, and the nails are often thick and malformed. Distal pulses often are either difficult to locate or absent, even when a Doppler device is used (Figure 23-2 ◆). *Rubor* (redness) is intense when the extremity is dependent.

Raynaud's Phenomenon

Raynaud's phenomenon is characterized by spasms of the small arteries and arterioles of the extremities. The arterial spasms limit blood flow to the fingers and, on occasion, to the toes, ears, or nose. Raynaud's phenomenon is often secondary to another disorder. When the cause is unknown *(idiopathic),* it is known as *Raynaud's disease.* In either case, it almost always affects women between the ages of 15 and 45. A genetic predisposition may have some part in this disease.

The signs and symptoms of Raynaud's occur intermittently, often following exposure to cold or work-related vibration. The attacks tend to become more frequent and prolonged. Raynaud's has been called the blue–white–red disease. Vasospasm causes the fingers to first turn blue, then white as blood flow is severely limited, and finally very red as the fingers are warmed and the spasm resolves. Numbness, stiffness, decreased sensation, and aching pain may accompany the color changes.

COLLABORATIVE CARE

Management of clients with peripheral vascular disease focuses on maintaining or improving the blood supply to tissues and relieving symptoms.

Diagnostic Tests

■ *Doppler ultrasound studies* are done to evaluate blood flow. Low-intensity sound waves directed at the affected vessel strike moving RBCs and bounce back to the transducer–receiver. Blood flow within the vessel can be evaluated by an audible sound or a graphic recording.

BOX 23-6
MANIFESTATIONS OF ARTERIAL THROMBOSIS OR EMBOLUS

- Pain in the affected area; may be sudden or insidious
- Numbness or tingling of affected extremity
- Coldness of the extremity
- Pallor or mottling of the skin
- Absent pulses distal to the blockage
- Muscle weakness or spasms
- Possible paralysis

■ *Angiography* may be performed. A contrast medium is injected into the vessels and x-rays are obtained to evaluate the extent of arteriosclerosis and occlusion.

Conservative Therapy

Smoking cessation is vital in managing peripheral vascular disorders. Nicotine causes vasoconstriction, further decreasing blood supply to the extremities. Continued smoking increases the risk for ulcerations, gangrene, and amputation.

Exercise (e.g., walking for 30 minutes twice a day) often is prescribed for clients with PVD. Exercise improves collateral circulation and is an effective stress management strategy.

Buerger–Allen exercises may be ordered when clients with Buerger's disease are unable to participate in other forms of exercise. The client is taught to slowly raise the extremities from a horizontal position to a 45-degree angle, then lower them to a dependent position sitting on the side of the bed. Each repetition takes about 2 minutes. A set of five exercises is done three to four times daily. The position changes dilate distal arterioles, improving oxygenation and nutrition of cells.

Weight reduction improves activity tolerance. A low-fat, low-cholesterol diet is prescribed for clients with atherosclerosis.

Other measures to prevent vasoconstriction and improve blood flow include keeping extremities warm and protecting them from injury, and managing stress. Stress management is particularly important for clients with Raynaud's phenomenon. Complementary therapies for PVD are outlined in Box 23-7.

Pharmacology

Medications used to manage peripheral vascular disease vary, depending on the disease process. Vasodilators and calcium channel blockers may be ordered to reduce vasoconstriction. Pentoxifylliune (Trental) decreases blood viscosity (thickness), increasing blood flow to the extremities. Low doses of aspirin are recommended to reduce the risk of inflammation and clotting.

Arterial thrombosis or embolism may be treated with a thrombolytic drug (see also Chapter 22). Thrombolytic therapy is avoided if the client is bleeding, has had recent surgery, has uncontrolled hypertension, or is pregnant.

Surgery

Surgery may be done to remove an obstruction, thrombus, or embolus. Acute arterial embolus requires emergency surgery to restore blood flow and prevent gangrene. Clients with severe intermittent claudication, rest pain, or gangrenous lesions may have a balloon angioplasty to dilate partially occluded blood vessels, or an arterial graft to bypass a blocked section of an artery. These procedures are explained in Chapter 22.

Amputation is necessary if blood flow cannot be restored and tissue necrosis has occurred. As much healthy tissue as possible is saved, so only part of a limb or digit may be amputated. A below-the-knee amputation is sometimes done for gangrene of the lower leg or for foot pain that cannot be relieved. Arterial thrombosis or embolism may be treated with a thrombolytic drug (see Chapter 22).

NURSING CARE

ASSESSING

Assessment of the peripheral vascular system may focus on the chief complaint (such as swelling or pain in the legs), or may be a part of a full cardiovascular assessment (Box 23-8).

DIAGNOSING, PLANNING, AND IMPLEMENTING

Peripheral vascular disease impairs peripheral blood flow. Managing the effects of chronic diseases such as arteriosclerosis may mean lifetime changes in activities and diet. Acute conditions such as emboli require immediate care to preserve life. In all cases, nurses intervene to help promote blood flow and protect tissues from damage.

INEFFECTIVE TISSUE PERFUSION: PERIPHERAL

■ Assess peripheral pulses, color, temperature, and capillary refill every 4 hours and as needed. If pulses cannot be felt, use a Doppler device to assess pulses. *Continuing assessment is important to detect changes in blood flow that could affect tissue integrity.*

BOX 23-7

COMPLEMENTARY THERAPIES

Peripheral Vascular Disease

To Improve Circulation
- Aromatherapy with rosemary or vetiver
- Biofeedback
- Healing touch
- Herbs: Ginkgo, garlic, cayenne, hawthorn, bilberry
- Imagery
- Magnets
- Massage
- Therapeutic touch
- Yoga

To Reduce Stress
- Aromatherapy with juniper, lavender, vetiver, ylang-ylang, or jasmine
- Breathing exercises
- Counseling
- Meditation
- Yoga

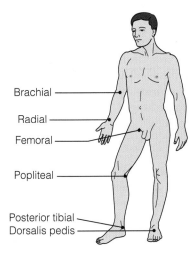

BOX 23-8
ASSESSING CLIENTS WITH PERIPHERAL VASCULAR DISEASE

SUBJECTIVE DATA

- Pain: Onset, relationship to activities, characteristics, severity, precipitating and relieving factors
- Other manifestations: Burning, numbness, or tingling in limbs or digits; leg fatigue or cramps; ankle swelling and when it occurs; effect of temperature or position on symptoms
- Medical and family history of cardiovascular disorders, peripheral vascular disease, stroke, hypertension, hyperlipidemia, blood clots, or other chronic illnesses (e.g., diabetes); previous surgery or evaluation of blood vessels; current medications
- Usual diet, including caffeine and alcohol consumption; smoking history (in pack years) or other tobacco use; activity level, exercise habits and exercise tolerance.

OBJECTIVE DATA

- Vital signs
- Capillary refill on upper and lower extremities; strength and equality of peripheral pulses (brachial, radial on upper extremities; femoral, popliteal, posterior tibial, and dorsalis pedis pulses on lower extemities—see figure below)

Brachial

Radial

Femoral

Popliteal

Posterior tibial

Dorsalis pedis

- Presence and degree of edema
- Skin color, temperature, texture and hair distribution on trunk, upper and lower extremities; any skin lesions or ulcers

---

- Instruct client to keep extremities in a dependent position. *Gravity helps maintain arterial blood flow to distal tissues.*
- Keep extremities warm using lightweight blankets, socks, and slippers. Do not use electric heating pads or hot water bottles. *Warmth helps prevent vasospasm and promotes arterial flow. Sensation of affected extremities may be decreased; avoid electric heating pads and hot water bottles to reduce the risk of burns.*

- Avoid raising the knee gatch, placing pillows under the knees, or positioning with 90-degree hip flexion. *These positions may further impair peripheral blood flow.*
- Encourage frequent position changes and remind the client to avoid crossing legs. *Changing position promotes blood flow. Leg crossing may compress arteries, leading to further compromise of circulation.*

PAIN

- Assess pain level using a pain scale at least every 4 hours and more often if needed. Immediately report acute or very severe pain accompanied by a pale, cold extremity. *The pain scale helps evaluate the severity of pain and the effectiveness of relief measures. Very severe acute pain and a pale, cold extremity may indicate an arterial embolism. Immediate treatment is vital to save the extremity.*
- Keep extremities warm, using socks, slippers, or light blankets. *Cooling causes vasoconstriction and increases pain.*
- Explain the relationship between smoking and pain, and assist develop a plan for smoking cessation. *Smoking causes vessel constriction and spasm, increasing the pain of PVD.*
- Provide time to discuss issues related to pain. Assist to refocus on positive aspects of life rather than on the pain. *Expressing concerns about pain reduces anxiety and may help relieve pain.*
- Teach stress reduction and pain relief measures such as relaxation, meditation, and guided imagery. *Stress increases vasoconstriction and pain. Many nonpharmacologic techniques may be used to relieve stress and minimize pain.*

IMPAIRED SKIN INTEGRITY

- Assess skin of extremities at least every 8 hours and more often if needed. Report changes to the charge nurse or physician. *Clients may be unaware of accidental injury or skin damage. Early identification helps prevent complications.*
- Provide meticulous leg and foot care daily, using mild soaps and moisturizing lotions. *Proper skin care helps prevent drying and cracking, reducing the risk of skin breakdown and infection. Once the skin is broken, the warm, moist, dark tissues of the injured extremity provide an excellent medium for bacterial growth.*
- Use a foot or bed cradle to prevent linens from rubbing against or putting pressure on extremities. *A cradle provides warmth while avoiding pressure on injured or damaged tissues.*

INEFFECTIVE PROTECTION

Thrombolytic drugs or anticoagulants may be given to dissolve or prevent clots. These drugs interfere with normal clotting, increasing the risk for bleeding.

- Report evidence of bleeding, such as excessive bleeding from incisions or injection sites, bleeding from gums or nose, hematuria, or mutiple bruises, petechiae, purpura, or ecchymoses. *Rapid identification and treatment of bleeding can prevent significant blood loss.*

■ Report abnormal hemoglobin and hematocrit levels, and activated partial thromboplastin time (APTT) and pro-thrombin time (PT) values greater than the target therapeutic range. *Low hemoglobin and hematocrit levels may indicate undetected bleeding. APTT and PT times are prolonged by anticoagulant therapy. The therapeutic range is from 1.5 to 2 times normal.*

EVALUATING

To evaluate the effectiveness of nursing care for a client with peripheral vascular disease, collect data such as: strength and equality of peripheral pulses and capillary refill; skin color, temperature, and condition of extremities; reports of pain and its relief; and evidence of bleeding.

Discharge Considerations

Teach measures such as exercise to help manage peripheral vascular disease. Stress the importance of smoking cessation. Provide a referral to smoking-cessation classes and encourage the client to discuss alternative methods of nicotine withdrawal with physicians. Teach care of the legs and feet, as described in Box 23-9.

Provide information about progressive exercise and its benefits for peripheral circulation. Discuss stress reduction, medications, and ways to keep the extremities warm. Teach Buerger–Allen exercises (discussed above) as indicated, and help develop a schedule to incorporate these exercises into daily routines. Provide a list of resources such as support groups, public health services, and other community agencies.

If surgery is planned, provide preoperative teaching as outlined in Chapter 7. Discuss expected postoperative measures such as anticoagulant drugs, diet and activity restrictions, and risk factor reduction strategies. Prior to discharge, teach the signs and symptoms of postoperative wound infection and other manifestations that should be reported to their physician. Stress the importance of regular follow-up care.

 Older Adults and PVD

Blood vessels thicken and become less compliant with age. These changes reduce oxygen delivery to tissues, and impair the removal of carbon dioxide and waste products. Impaired vision may make it more difficult for an older adult to provide careful and safe foot care. Long-standing smoking addiction is difficult to break. The client who lives alone may resist walking. Home and community safety is an additional concern. It is often helpful to arrange periodic visits by a community health or home health nurse. Encourage the client to join a support group for stopping smoking, changing eating habits, and taking part in regular activity.

BOX 23-9
TEACHING FOR DISCHARGE

LEG AND FOOT CARE FOR CLIENTS WITH PERIPHERAL VASCULAR DISEASE

- Keep legs and feet clean, dry, and comfortable.
  - Wash legs and feet daily using a mild soap and warm water.
  - Pat dry with a soft towel; do not rub, and be sure to dry between toes.
  - Apply lotion that does not contain alcohol to dry, scaly skin.
  - Use powder on feet and between toes.
  - Buy shoes in the afternoon (when feet are largest). Never buy shoes that are uncomfortable. Be sure the toes have adequate room.
  - Wear a clean pair of cotton socks each day.
- Prevent accidents and injuries to the feet.
  - Always wear shoes or slippers when getting out of bed.
  - Walk on level ground and avoid crowds, if possible.
  - Do not go barefoot.
  - Inspect legs and feet daily. Use a mirror to examine the backs of your legs and the bottoms of your feet.
  - Have a professional foot care provider trim toenails and care for corns, calluses, ingrown toenails, or athlete's foot.
  - Always check the temperature of bath water before stepping into the tub.
  - Use sunblock on your legs and the tops of your feet.
  - Report increased pain, cuts, bruises, blistering, redness, or open areas of your legs or feet to your health care provider.
- Improve blood supply to the legs and feet.
  - Do not cross your legs when sitting or in bed.
  - Do not wear garters or knee stockings.
  - Do not go swimming in cold water.
  - Do not smoke cigarettes or inhale passive smoke.
  - Walk until you develop pain, stop for 3 minutes, then resume walking until fatigued. Do this eight times a day.
  - Take medications as prescribed.

 Aneurysm

An **aneurysm** is weakness and localized dilation of a blood vessel wall. Aneurysms usually affect the aorta and arteries, because of the high pressure within these vessels. Most aneurysms are caused by arteriosclerosis or atherosclerosis. Trauma and congenital weakness of a vessel also may cause an aneurysm to form.

PATHOPHYSIOLOGY

Aneurysms are commonly classified by their shape and location (Figure 23-3 ◆). *Fusiform aneurysms* involve the entire circumference of the vessel. They generally grow slowly but progressively. Their length and diameter vary considerably from client to client. *Saccular aneurysms* involve only a portion of the vessel. They are more often associated with congenital malformations or syphilis than with arteriosclerosis. *Berry aneurysms* are a common type of congenital saccular aneurysm found in a section of cerebral arteries (the circle of Willis) in the brain. *Aortic dissection* (also called a *dissecting aneurysm*) develops due to weakening of the medial layer of the aorta. Blood leaks into the vessel wall, separating the intimal (innermost) layer of the artery from the adventia (outermost layer). Aortic dissection usually occurs in the ascending aorta.

Aneurysms often have no symptoms and are discovered during a routine physical examination. When manifestations occur, they are due to the pressure of the aneurysm on adjacent tissues and organs (Table 23-4 ◆).

Thoracic Aortic Aneurysms

Thoracic aortic aneurysms frequently cause no symptoms. Substernal (anginal), neck, or back pain may occur. Pressure on the trachea, esophagus, laryngeal nerve, or superior vena cava may cause difficulty breathing, stridor, cough, difficult or painful swallowing, hoarseness, edema of the face and neck, and distended neck veins. Aneurysms of the thoracic aorta tend to enlarge progressively and may rupture, causing death.

Abdominal Aortic Aneurysms

Abdominal aortic aneurysms are associated with arteriosclerosis, hypertension, smoking, and increasing age. Most abdominal aortic aneurysms are found in adults over age 70.

Most clients with abdominal aneurysms are asymptomatic, but on examination have a pulsating mass in the mid and upper abdomen and a bruit over the mass. The client may complain of mild to severe midabdominal or lower back pain. The degree of pain commonly indicates the severity (and

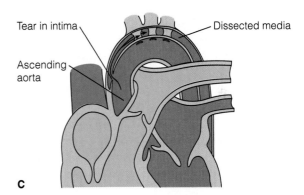

Figure 23-3. ◆ Aortic aneurysms. (A) Fusiform aneurysm of the abdominal aorta. (B) Saccular aneurysm of the descending thoracic aorta. (C) Dissecting aneurysm of the ascending thoracic aorta.

TABLE 23-4	MANIFESTATIONS AND COMPLICATIONS OF AORTIC ANEURYSMS		
TYPE OR LOCATION	**THORACIC**	**ABDOMINAL**	**DISSECTING**
Manifestations	Chest, back, or neck pain Dyspnea, cough Hoarseness, dysphagia Distended neck veins, edema of face and neck	Pulsating abdominal mass Abdominal or lower back pain Cool, pale, or cyanotic lower extremities	Sudden, severe chest pain Decreased blood pressure in upper extremities Absent radial pulses
Complications	Rupture and hemorrhage	Emboli to lower extremities Rupture and hemorrhage	Hemorrhage Renal failure, cardiac tamponade, sepsis

urgency) of the problem. Pain may be an indication of an impending rupture.

Emboli may form due to sluggish blood flow within the aneurysm and travel to the lower extremities. The aneurysm may also rupture and lead to death due to hemorrhage and hypovolemic shock.

Aortic Dissections

Dissection is a life-threatening emergency caused by a tear in the inner layer of the aorta and bleeding into the middle layer. This *dissects* or splits the vessel wall, forming a blood-filled channel between its layers. Dissection can occur anywhere along the aorta, but is most common in the ascending aorta where pressures are high.

Hypertension is a major risk factor for aortic dissection. Clients with a genetic disorder called Marfan syndrome are at risk for aortic dissection (Box 23-10).

The primary symptom of aortic dissection is sudden, excruciating pain. Pain often is described as a ripping or tearing sensation. It is usually located in the area of dissection (e.g., anterior chest if thoracic, back if abdominal). Blood pressure may initially rise, but it falls rapidly and is often inaudible as the dissection occludes blood flow. Peripheral pulses are also are absent.

COLLABORATIVE CARE

Aneurysms often are detected by a *chest* or *abdominal x-ray*. An *abdominal ultrasound* is done when an abdominal aneurysm is suspected. A *CT scan* or *MRI* may be ordered to measure the aneurysm size.

Pharmacology

Clients with aortic aneurysms often are treated with antihypertensive medications to lower blood pressure. Anticoagulant therapy (discussed in the following section) may be started to

BOX 23-10

population
FOCUS

Clients with Marfan Syndrome

Marfan syndrome is a connective tissue disorder with three distinctive features: (1) long, thin extremities, hyperextensible joints, and other skeletal deformities; (2) impaired vision; and (3) cardiovascular defects, including mitral valve prolapse and weakness of the aorta with frequent aortic dissection and rupture. Marfan syndrome affects about 1 in 10,000 people. It is inherited as an autosomal dominant trait.

There is no cure for Marfan syndrome, so teaching is vital. Severe physical and emotional stress and pregnancy increase the risk of aortic dissection and cardiac complications. Encourage to avoid vigorous physical exertion and the physical stress of pregnancy. Teach measures to reduce the risk of endocarditis (see Chapter 22). Scoliosis and kyphosis are common; refer for physical therapy and bracing as needed. Stress the importance of regular eye examinations and immediate care if symptoms of retinal detachment develop (see Chapter 31). Discuss the genetic nature of Marfan syndrome: Each child has a 50% risk of being affected. Encourage consideration of alternatives such as adoption. Make referrals as appropriate.

prevent emboli from forming or after surgical repair of an aneurysm.

Surgery

Surgery is done to repair aneurysms that are tender or enlarging. The client's general health and surgical risk are considered, unless immediate surgery is necessary to preserve life. In most cases, the aneurysm is excised and replaced with a synthetic fabric graft (Figure 23-4 ◆). Nursing care of the client having surgery on the aorta is outlined in Box 23-11.

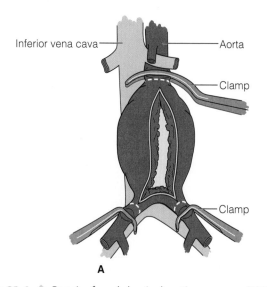

Inferior vena cava — Aorta
— Clamp
— Clamp

A

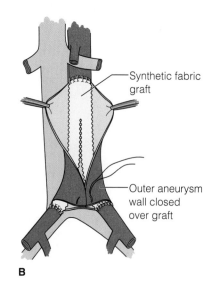

— Synthetic fabric graft
— Outer aneurysm wall closed over graft

B

Figure 23-4. ◆ Repair of an abdominal aortic aneurysm. (A) The aneurysm is exposed and clamped above and below the vessel dilation. (B) A synthetic graft is used to replace the aneurysm. The arterial wall is then sutured around the graft.

BOX 23-11
NURSING CARE CHECKLIST

SURGERY OF THE AORTA

Before Surgery

☑ Provide routine preoperative care and teaching as time permits (see Chapter 7).

☑ Orient to intensive care unit. Describe anticipated equipment, tubes, sights and sounds, and postoperative communication. Allow time for questions and to clarify information.

☑ Immediately report changes in blood pressure in upper and lower extremities, peripheral pulses, pain, abdominal girth, and sensation and movement of lower extremities.

☑ Maintain bed rest with legs flat. Instruct to avoid holding breath while moving or defecating.

☑ Report absent peripheral pulses; pale, cyanotic, or cool extremities; diffuse abdominal pain; or an increase in groin, lumbar, or lower extremity pain.

After Surgery

☑ Provide general postoperative care (see Chapter 7).

☑ Monitor chest tube drainage and status as needed (see Chapter 26).

☑ Frequently assess for bleeding. Immediately report signs of graft leakage such as:
  a. Bruising of scrotum, perineum, or penis; hematoma at incision
  b. Increased abdominal girth
  c. Weak or absent peripheral pulses; impaired movement or sensation of extremities
  d. Decreased blood pressure, increased pulse; low urine output (< 30 mL/hr)
  e. Increased abdominal, back, or groin pain
  f. Drop in hematocrit, hemoglobin, and red blood cell levels

☑ Maintain intravenous fluids and administer blood as ordered.

☑ Report evidence of complications:
  a. Lower extremity embolism: Pain and numbness, diminished pulses, and pale, cool, or cyanotic skin
  b. Bowel ischemia: Blood in stools, diarrhea, severe abdominal pain, and abdominal distention
  c. Impaired renal function: Output less than 30 mL/hour, fixed specific gravity, increasing BUN and serum creatinine levels
  d. Spinal cord ischemia: Lower extremity weakness and paraplegia

NURSING CARE

Nurses most often care for clients with an aneurysm before and after surgical repair or treatment of an expanding or ruptured aneurysm. Clients are often highly anxious because of the urgent nature of their disorder. Managing anxiety levels is an important component of nursing care. Establish trust through active listening. Acknowledge the fears and concerns of the client and family. Use a calm demeanor, appropriate and reassuring manner, and factual explanations to keep clients calm and prevent any additional stress, which might worsen hypertension.

The nursing diagnoses and interventions described for clients with peripheral vascular disease are also appropriate for the client with an aortic aneurysm: Anxiety, Pain, Ineffective Tissue Perfusion, and Ineffective Protection.

Discharge Considerations

Small or asymptomatic aneurysms often are treated conservatively. Teach measures to control hypertension, discussing diet, stress reduction, alcohol, smoking, and medications. Stress the importance of keeping blood pressure within normal limits to slow growth of the aneurysm. Emphasize the necessity of following the prescribed treatment to prevent complications.

After surgery, provide verbal and written instructions about preventing and recognizing infection, caring for the incision, taking medications to control blood pressure and prevent blood clotting, and recognizing complications. Discuss the importance of regular rest. Suggest ways to prevent constipation and straining at stool (such as increasing fluid and fiber in the diet). Instruct to avoid prolonged sitting, lifting heavy objects, exercising strenuously, and having sexual intercourse until approved by the physician (usually 6 to 12 weeks). Provide information about return appointments. Refer to a home health agency or community health service as necessary for continuing care after discharge.

Venous Disorders

Because the pressure is lower and blood flow is slower in the veins than in the arteries, blood can stagnate or pool. As a result, clots may form, the veins may become inflamed, or chronic venous insufficiency may develop. Three of the most common disorders of venous circulation are thrombosis, chronic venous insufficiency, and varicose veins.

Venous Thrombosis

Venous thrombosis occurs when a blood clot *(thrombus)* forms on the wall of a vein and partially or completely blocks blood flow back to the heart. Because inflammation often accompanies the clot, the term *thrombophlebitis* often is used *(thrombo* = clot; *phlebo* = vein; *-itis* = inflammation).

A number of risk factors have been identified for venous thrombosis (Box 23-12). There is an increased risk in people with impaired heart function, older clients, and people with certain cancers. The major complications of thrombophlebitis are chronic venous insufficiency and pulmonary embolism.

PATHOPHYSIOLOGY

Small, localized clots may develop in small veins. In larger veins, extensive thrombi may form. Three pathologic factors, called *Virchow's triad,* are associated with thrombosis: venous stasis, increased blood coagulability, and vessel wall injury.

Damage to the lining of a vein attracts platelets to the area, especially if venous stasis is present. So a clot or thrombus develops. The thrombus may partially or totally block blood flow through the vein. Either deep or superficial veins may be affected. Venous blood returns to the heart through collateral vessels. The thrombus may break loose or fragment, becoming an embolus. Emboli from venous clots tend to lodge in the vessels of the pulmonary vascular system.

Deep Vein Thrombosis

The deep veins of the legs, especially in the calf, provide the best environment for thrombus formation in the lower extremities (Figure 23-5 ◆). Most thrombi originate in the vessels of the calf.

Deep vein thrombosis (DVT) may cause calf pain and muscle tenderness. The client may experience dull, aching pain in the leg, particularly when walking. The calf is enlarged and the affected leg may be slightly cyanotic. An elevated temperature and general malaise may be present. A *positive Homan's sign* (pain in the calf when the foot is dorsiflexed) may be noted, but it is not specific to DVT.

Pulmonary embolism is a serious, potentially fatal complication of DVT. Most pulmonary emboli arise in the proxi-

---

> **BOX 23-12**
> **RISK FACTORS FOR VENOUS THROMBOSIS**
>
> - Previous venous thrombosis
> - Prolonged immobility, leg paralysis
> - Major general surgery or trauma
> - Myocardial infarction, heart failure
> - Cancer of the breast, pancreas, prostate, or ovary
> - Pregnancy or childbirth
> - Estrogen therapy, oral contraceptives, especially in women who smoke
> - Obesity

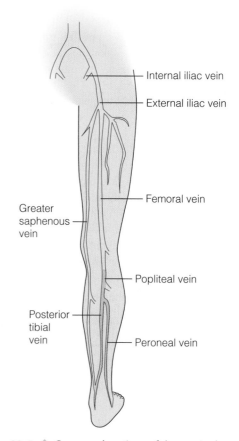

Figure 23-5. ◆ Common locations of deep vein thrombosis.

mal leg veins (above the knee). Pulmonary embolism is discussed in Chapter 26.

Superficial Vein Thrombophlebitis

Thrombophlebitis of the arm veins is a common complication of trauma to the vein wall caused by venous catheters, repeated venous punctures, or intravenous solutions that irritate and inflame the vein. Superficial venous thrombi are also found in pregnant or postpartum women, but the cause is unknown.

The clinical manifestations of superficial and deep vein thrombosis are listed in Box 23-13.

Venous Insufficiency

Chronic **venous insufficiency** is *stasis* (stagnation) of venous blood flow in the lower extremities. Chronic venous insufficiency often results from venous thrombosis and incompetent venous valves.

PATHOPHYSIOLOGY

When valves in the veins of the legs are *incompetent* and fail to close, the muscle-pumping action on veins during activity is unable to move blood back to the heart. The blood collects and stagnates in the lower leg. This increases pressure in the veins, leading to congestion and edema of leg tissue. Edema develops in the lower leg, and the leg and foot become darkly colored. Subcutaneous tissue changes make the leg and foot feel hard or firm to palpation.

As the congestion worsens, the body is unable to provide adequate oxygen and nutrients to the cells. Eventually, cells begin to die, forming venous stasis ulcers (Figure 23-6 ◆). As the condition worsens, the ulcers enlarge. The impaired circulation also increases the risk of wound infection.

Skin around stasis ulcers appears shiny, atrophic, and cyanotic. The color of the skin is brownish. Scar tissue com-

Figure 23-6. ◆ Chronic venous insufficiency. Note the discoloration of the ankle and the stasis ulcer.

monly forms, causing the affected area of the leg to feel hard and somewhat leathery to the touch, but even the slightest trauma to the area can lead to serious tissue breakdown.

COLLABORATIVE CARE

Prevention is important to reduce the complications of venous thrombosis (see below). When thrombosis develops, treatment is started to prevent further clots from forming, treat inflammation, and, in some cases, to dissolve existing clots.

Diagnostic Tests

- *Ascending phlebography* (or ascending *venous venography*) uses a contrast medium injected into the veins of the leg to identify the location and extent of thrombophlebitis.
- *Doppler ultrasound* is used to identify obstruction of the larger veins of the legs. It is a noninvasive test that uses sound waves reflected off blood cells to assess flow.
- *Plethysmography* is often used in conjunction with Doppler ultrasonography. Plethysmography measures changes in the volume of fluid passing through the veins.

Conservative Therapy

Whenever possible, prevention is key. Elastic stockings and pneumatic compression devices are ordered for postoperative clients, people who are immobile for long periods, and for clients who cannot tolerate anticoagulants. Leg exercises and early ambulation are ordered after surgery to minimize venous stasis. Teach clients not to cross their legs, to wear loose-fitting garments, and to incorporate exercise into their daily schedule.

Warm, moist compresses are applied over superficial venous thrombosis to relieve symptoms. Clients with deep vein thrombosis are placed on strict bed rest until the symptoms of tenderness and edema resolve.

BOX 23-13
MANIFESTATIONS OF DEEP AND SUPERFICIAL VEIN THROMBOSIS

DEEP VEIN THROMBOSIS (DVT)
- Dull, aching pain, tenderness in affected extremity
- Pain aggravated by walking
- Increased calf size
- Cyanosis
- Positive Homan's sign
- Slightly elevated temperature; general malaise

SUPERFICIAL VEIN THROMBOSIS (SVT)
- Dull, aching pain over affected vein
- Redness and warmth along affected vein
- Palpable cordlike structure

The legs are elevated, with the knees slightly flexed, above the level of the heart to promote venous return and discourage venous pooling. Elastic antiembolism stockings (compression stockings or TED hose) or pneumatic compression devices are often ordered to simulate the muscle-pumping mechanism that promotes blood return to the heart. When permitted, ambulation is encouraged with the caution to avoid prolonged standing or sitting that may contribute to venous stasis.

Stasis Dermatitis and Stasis Ulcer Care

Stasis dermatitis may be treated with wet compresses with boric acid, Burow's solution, or isotonic saline four times daily, for 1-hour intervals. Following the wet compress, topical ointments (such as 0.5% hydrocortisone cream) are applied. Other topical agents such as zinc oxide ointment or broad-spectrum antifungal agents may also be ordered.

Stasis ulcers may be treated with saline compresses or a semirigid boot applied to the foot and lower leg. This device may be made of Unna's paste or Gauzetex bandage. Bony prominences must be well padded. The boot is changed every 1 to 2 weeks, depending on the amount of drainage from the ulcer. This device often allows ambulatory treatment. Once the ulcer is healed, a heavy elastic stocking is worn to promote adequate venous return and to prevent ulcer recurrence.

Pharmacology

Nonsteroidal anti-inflammatory agents (NSAIDs) such as indomethacin (Indocin) or naproxen (Naprosyn) are used to reduce inflammation in clients with thrombophlebitis.

ANTICOAGULANTS. Anticoagulants are ordered for clients with deep vein thromboses to prevent expansion of the clot and possible pulmonary embolism. Anticoagulation is started with intravenous or subcutaneous heparin. If a heparin infusion is ordered, an infusion pump should be used, and the dose should be checked every hour. Anticoagulation is monitored using a blood test, the *activated partial thromboplastin time (APTT)*. The heparin dosage is adjusted so that the APTT is 1.5 to 2 times the normal value.

Oral warfarin is initiated while the client continues to receive heparin. This overlap of therapy is important because the full anticoagulant effect of warfarin is delayed. The *prothrombin time (PT)* or *International Normalized Ratio (INR)* are used to assess the effect of warfarin on clotting. The dosage is adjusted to achieve a PT that is 1.5 to 2.5 times greater than the normal value or an INR of 2.0 to 3.0.

Once this level is achieved, a maintenance dose of warfarin is continued for 2 to 4 months. Anticoagulant treatment (Table 23-5 ◆) may be extended if a complication such as pulmonary embolus has occurred. Regular follow-up is important to monitor coagulation.

THROMBOLYTICS. Thrombolytic drugs dissolve blood clots in the body. They may be used to destroy venous thrombi and prevent additional damage to venous valves. Thrombolytic therapy, however, increases the risk of bleeding and hemorrhage. Box 22-12 reviews nursing care related to thrombolytic drugs.

Surgery

Surgery may be done to remove a venous thrombus or to prevent complications such as pulmonary embolism. A venous thrombectomy may be done to remove the clot. A filtering device may be inserted into the inferior vena cava via the femoral or jugular vein. This umbrella-like device captures venous thrombi, preventing pulmonary emboli.

NURSING CARE

Nurses play a vital role in identifying clients at risk for venous thrombosis, preventing it from occurring, and collecting data to evaluate the effectiveness of treatment.

ASSESSING

Assessment for problems of venous circulation is not limited to clients with diagnosed venous thrombosis, but also includes all clients who are at risk. Box 23-14 outlines subjective and objective assessment data related to venous circulation. (See Table 23-6 ◆ for assessment of peripheral edema.)

DIAGNOSING, PLANNING, AND IMPLEMENTING

PAIN

■ Regularly assess pain. Immediately report increased pain. *Venous thrombosis causes pain that is not affected by exercise or relieved by elevating the leg. Increased pain may indicate extension of the inflammation and clot.*

■ Apply warm, moist heat to affected extremity at least four times daily, using warm, moist compresses or an aqua-K pad. *Heat dilates the vessels and promotes the reabsorption of edema fluid, thus improving circulation and reducing pain.*

■ Maintain bed rest; explain the reason. *Using leg muscles during ambulation increases inflammation and pain.*

INEFFECTIVE TISSUE PERFUSION: PERIPHERAL

■ Assess peripheral pulses, skin integrity, capillary refill, and color of the extremities at least every 8 hours. Report changes promptly. *Swelling from obstructed venous blood flow can impair arterial circulation to the tissues, increasing the risk for ischemia and necrosis.*

■ Measure calf and thigh diameter on the affected extremity on admission and daily thereafter. Report increases. *As venous thrombosis resolves, the diameter will decrease. Increased diameters may indicate further inflammation.*

TABLE 23-5	NURSING IMPLICATIONS FOR PHARMACOLOGY: CLIENTS WITH ANTICOAGULATION		
DRUGS	**MECHANISM OF ACTION**	**NURSING IMPLICATIONS**	**CLIENT AND FAMILY TEACHING**
Heparin sodium	Heparin interferes with normal clotting, preventing the formation of new clots and the extension of existing clots.	May be given by intravenous or subcutaneous routes. Check dose with a second licensed person before giving. SC: Administer deep into SC tissue, rotating sites in the lower abdomen. Do not aspirate or massage. IV: Use an infusion pump for continuous infusions; do not mix with other drugs. Report signs of bleeding: Bleeding gums, nosebleed, bruising; black, tarry stools; hematuria. Test stools for occult blood. Monitor APTT, platelet count, hemoglobin, and hematocrit. Report results outside the expected range.	Report any unusual bleeding or bruising to your health care provider. Do not take any drugs containing aspirin or NSAIDs while on heparin therapy. Avoid activities that increase your risk of injury. Use a soft toothbrush and electric razor while you are receiving heparin. Tell all health care providers that you are on heparin therapy, and carry an identification card with you at all times.
Warfarin (Coumadin)	Interferes with synthesis of clotting factors, preventing clot formation. Requires 3–5 days to reach effective levels.	Give at the same time each day. Report signs of bleeding: Bleeding gums, nosebleed, bruising; black, tarry stools; hematuria. Test stools for occult blood. Monitor PT or INR, CBC, and liver function studies. Report results outside the expected range. Drug interactions are common; monitor carefully when new drugs are added to medication regimen or other drugs are discontinued.	Take the drug as ordered. If you miss a dose, take it as soon as you remember that day. Do not double your dose. Limit your intake of foods rich in vitamin K (asparagus, beans, broccoli, brussel sprouts, cabbage, cauliflower, cheeses, fish, greens, milk, pork, rice, spinach, turnips, yogurt). Report any unusual bleeding or bruising to your doctor. Do not drink alcohol or take drugs containing aspirin or NSAIDs. Use a soft toothbrush and electric razor. Tell all health care providers that you are taking an anticoagulant, and carry an identification card with this information with you at all times. Keep all follow-up appointments for lab work and with your doctor.

■ Elevate legs, keeping knees slightly flexed. Avoid flexing hips more than 60 degrees. *Elevation promotes venous return and reduces peripheral edema. Knee flexion promotes comfort.*

■ Apply antiembolic stockings or pneumatic compression devices as ordered, removing them for short periods (30 to 60 minutes) during daily hygiene. *Antiembolic stockings and*

BOX 23-14
ASSESSING CLIENTS WITH VENOUS THROMBOSIS

SUBJECTIVE DATA

- Describe any leg pain, including characteristics, intensity, timing (with activity, when standing or sitting for prolonged periods, at rest), aggravating and relieving factors, and any associated manifestations
- Inquire about ankle swelling, its timing (end of day, after sitting or standing for prolonged periods), extent, effect of temperature; use of support stockings
- Past history of cardiovascular disorders, peripheral vascular disease, blood clots, or chronic conditions; heart or vascular surgery; cancer
- Diet, exercise, and smoking history; occupational factors such as prolonged standing or sitting

OBJECTIVE DATA

- Skin of extremities, particularly legs and feet: Color, texture, and hair distribution; presence of ulcers (particularly over the medial malleolus) or irritation; healing
- Venous pattern on hands, arms, and legs
- Note edema; grade as 1+ to 4+ (see Table 23-7) if present.
- Palpate calves for tenderness, warmth, swelling; presence of cords.
- If indicated, check Homan's sign: Dorsiflex the foot while holding knee flat or slightly flexed (see figure). Calf pain with dorsiflexion of the foot (positive Homan's sign) may indicate venous thrombosis.

- Measure leg circumference at forefoot, above ankle, calf, and midthigh.

pneumatic compression devices promote venous return to the heart by gently compressing the extremity.

- Encourage frequent position changes. *Position changes help prevent further venous stasis and other complications of immobility.*
- Administer and monitor the effectiveness of anticoagulants or thrombolytic drugs as ordered. Monitor laboratory values (APTT, INR, and PT) before giving prescribed anticoagulants. Promptly report values outside the expected range. *Monitoring is vital to evaluate the effectiveness of therapy and prevent complications of treatment.*

IMPAIRED SKIN INTEGRITY

- Assess skin of the affected leg and foot at least every 8 hours and more often as needed. *Careful, frequent assessment allows early detection of signs of potential skin breakdown and early intervention to prevent further problems.*
- Use mild soaps, solutions, and lotions to clean the affected leg and foot daily. Avoid harsh soaps or alcohol-based solutions. Pat dry. *Gentle cleansing with mild agents helps maintain skin integrity, prevent excessive drying and itching, and prevent infection.*
- Use egg crate mattresses or sheepskin as needed. *Egg crate mattresses and sheepskin distribute the weight more equally and prevent skin breakdown and discomfort.*
- Encourage active or perform passive range-of-motion (ROM) exercises at least every 8 hours. *ROM exercises help preserve joint function, promote circulation, and prevent skin breakdown.*
- Assist with progressive ambulation as ordered. *Daily increases in activity improve circulation and increase stamina and endurance.*

EVALUATING

In order to evaluate the effectiveness of nursing care for venous thrombosis or venous insufficiency, assess the client's comfort, peripheral circulation (especially of the legs), and skin condition.

Discharge Considerations

Clients who have experienced an episode of venous thrombosis or who have venous insufficiency often will manage their treatment after discharge. Explain the disease process and course of treatment, including:

- Ordered laboratory tests, their purposes and frequency
- Prescribed medications, including dosage, time of day to take the drug, and side effects that should be reported
- Any continuing order for heat application or wound care, including precautions to avoid burns and infection, and symptoms to report to the health care provider
- Activity restrictions and their duration
- Measures to prevent future episodes of venous thrombosis
- The importance of follow-up visits

Reinforce teaching with written instructions, and have the client demonstrate wound care before discharge.

Teach the following measures to reduce the risk of complications:

- Elevate legs while resting and during sleep.

TABLE 23-6	**EVALUATING EDEMA**	

2 mm / 1+		1+ No visible change in the leg, slight pitting
4 mm / 2+		2+ No marked change in the shape of the leg; pitting slightly deeper
6 mm / 3+		3+ Leg visibly swollen; deep pitting
8 mm / 4+		4+ Leg very swollen; very deep pitting

- Walk as much as possible, and avoid sitting or standing for long periods of time.
- When sitting, do not cross your legs or put pressure on the back of the knees (such as when sitting on the side of the bed).
- Do not wear anything that constricts your legs (knee-high hose, garters, or girdles).
- Wear elastic hose as prescribed. Put on the hose after the legs have been elevated. The elastic hose should be tighter over the feet than at the top of the leg, and the tops should not cut into the legs.
- Keep skin on feet and legs clean, soft, and dry. Follow guidelines for care of the legs and feet (see Box 23-9).

Nursing Process Case Study
■ CLIENT WITH DEEP VEIN THROMBOSIS

Mrs. Opal Hipps is a 75-year-old widow who lives alone with her dog Chester. She retired from her job as a postal clerk 10 years ago and now spends a lot of time reading and watching television. Over the past week she developed a vague aching pain in her right leg. Last night it became more severe, especially in her right calf. She noticed that her right lower leg seemed larger than the left, and it was very tender to the touch. Mrs. Hipps is admitted to the hospital with deep vein thrombosis in the right leg. She is placed on bed rest and intravenous heparin. Michael Cookson is her admitting nurse.

Assessment Mrs. Hipps tells Mr. Cookson, "This business about a blood clot really has me worried." She also says she is worried about who will care for her dog while she is in the hospital. Objective data includes: height 5′2″ (157 cm); weight 149 lbs. (68 kg); T 99.2° F (37.3° C); vital signs within normal limits. Her left leg is warm, pink, and supple with good skin turgor. Her right calf is warm, red, dry, and

tender to touch. Femoral and popliteal pulses are strong bilaterally. Right pedal and posterior tibial pulses are difficult to locate, and the diameter of the right calf is 0.5 inch (1.27 cm) larger than that of the left.

Diagnosis Mr. Cookson makes the following nursing diagnosis for Mrs. Hipps:

- Pain related to venous inflammation in the right leg
- Anxiety related to unexpected hospitalization
- Ineffective Tissue Perfusion: Peripheral related to decreased venous circulation in the right leg
- Risk for Impaired Skin Integrity related to bed rest and altered tissue perfusion

Expected Outcomes The expected outcomes of the plan of care are that Mrs. Hipps will:

- State that her leg pain is relieved by the day of discharge.
- Verbalize reduced anxiety by the second day of her hospitalization.
- Have a reduced right leg diameter by 0.25 inch (0.64 cm) by the fifth day of hospitalization.
- Maintain intact skin throughout the hospital stay.

Planning and Implementation The following interventions are planned and implemented for Mrs. Hipps:

- Elevate legs, with knees slightly flexed, throughout hospital stay.
- Apply warm, moist compresses to right leg using 2-hour-on, 2-hour-off schedule around the clock.
- Provide analgesics as ordered and needed; evaluate effectiveness.
- Provide time to discuss fears and concerns.
- Arrange for a friend or neighbor to care for dog.
- Apply antiembolism stockings; remove for 30 minutes each shift.
- Administer anticoagulants as ordered; monitor laboratory values.
- Assist with progressive ambulation as ordered.
- Document skin condition each shift.

Evaluation Ten days after admission, Mrs. Hipps's pain has subsided and her right calf diameter is equal to the left. After talking about her condition and how she can prevent recurrence, Mrs. Hipps is much less anxious. Before discharge, Mr. Cookson reviews instructions for antiembolism stockings, activity, daily warfarin, and scheduled follow-up. Her neighbor, Kate, came to pick her up, handing Mrs. Hipps a small brown dog. Kate said, "Chester missed you." Mrs. Hipps promised to call the number Mr. Cookson had given her if she had any questions.

 Critical Thinking in the Nursing Process

1. Describe the cause of the pain in Mrs. Hipps's right leg.
2. How would you respond if Mrs. Hipps tells you she does not have the money to buy the prescribed anticoagulant when she goes home?
3. Design teaching plan for Mrs. Hipps to prevent future episodes of venous thrombosis.

 # Varicose Veins

Varicose veins are irregular, tortuous veins with poorly functioning (incompetent) valves. *Varicosities* may develop in veins anywhere in the body. In the rectum they are called hemorrhoids; when they develop in the esophagus, they are known as varices. They commonly affect the lower extremities. The long saphenous vein of the leg is most often affected by varicosities (Figure 23-7 ◆). Varicose veins affect about one in five people in the world. They are more common in women over the age of 35, perhaps because of venous stasis that occurs during pregnancy. People who stand for long periods at work (waiters, beauticians, nurses) are also prone to develop varicose veins.

PATHOPHYSIOLOGY

Increased pressure that stretches the vessel wall is the major factor leading to varicose veins. Standing increases pressure in the leg veins and decreases venous return to the heart. Blood collects in the leg veins, stretching the vessel wall. As the vessels stretch, their valves cannot close properly and become incompetent. Prolonged standing, obesity, venous thrombosis, and increased pressure on the veins of the abdomen (from pregnancy or an abdominal tumor) contribute to varicose vein development.

Some clients are asymptomatic, but most complain of one or more of the manifestations listed in Box 23-15. The menstrual cycle tends to increase symptoms in women.

Varicose veins can lead to venous insufficiency, stasis dermatitis, and stasis ulcers. The skin above the ankles may be thin and discolored. Venous thrombosis may develop in varicose veins, especially in pregnant or postpartal clients, postoperative clients, or clients taking oral contraceptives.

COLLABORATIVE CARE

Doppler ultrasonic flow tests and *angiographic studies* with contrast media may be done to evaluate the extent of varicose veins. Surgery may relieve major symptoms of the disease, but there is no real cure for varicose veins.

Conservative Therapy

Most clients are managed conservatively with measures to improve venous circulation and relieve the pressure on vein

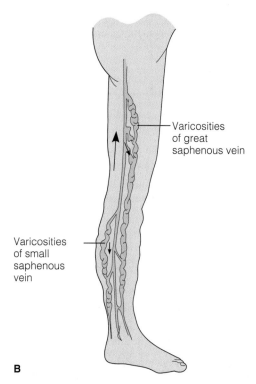

A   **B**

Figure 23-7. ◆ (A) Normal leg veins. (B) Varicose veins.

> ### BOX 23-15
> ### MANIFESTATIONS OF VARICOSE VEINS
>
> • Severe, aching leg pain
> • Leg fatigue or heaviness
> • Itching of the affected leg
> • Heat in the affected leg after prolonged standing
> • Visibly dilated veins in the leg

walls and valves. Properly fitted antiembolism (elastic) stockings compress veins, helping move blood back to the heart. Regular, daily walking is an important part of treatment. Prolonged sitting and standing are avoided. The legs are elevated for specified periods of time throughout the day.

Surgery

Two surgical techniques are generally used to treat varicose veins: compression sclerotherapy and vein stripping. In *compression sclerotherapy,* a sclerosing (hardening) agent is injected into the varicosed vein. A compression dressing is then applied to compress and obliterate the vein. Venous blood is rerouted through healthy vessels. In *vein stripping,* the varicose veins are surgically removed. Pressure bandages are applied and the legs are elevated to reduce edema. Ambulation is gradually increased, but sitting and standing are forbidden during the recovery period.

NURSING CARE

Nurses rarely interact with clients whose primary diagnosis is varicose veins, except when surgery is planned. Through teaching and referral, however, nurses can be instrumental in helping clients slow their development and minimize the symptoms of varicose veins.

INEFFECTIVE TISSUE PERFUSION: PERIPHERAL

■ Assess peripheral pulses, capillary refill, skin temperature, and degree of edema. *Assessment helps determine the effects of impaired venous return on blood flow to and perfusion of the extremities.*

■ Apply properly fitted support or antiembolic stockings. Remove stockings daily for 30 to 60 minutes. Inspect and clean the skin while stockings are off. *Antiembolic stockings exert pressure on the veins of the lower extremities, promoting venous return to the heart. During ambulation, they assist the blood-pumping action of the muscles. Because elastic stockings can impair blood flow through small superficial vessels, they should be removed at least once daily for 30 minutes or more.*

■ Wrap the leg(s) with ace bandages as directed if sclerotherapy or vein stripping has been done. Assess pulses, color,

temperature, and capillary refill distal to wrappings. Frequently inspect the wrappings, and rewrap as needed to prevent skin irritation or obstruction of blood flow to or from the extremity. *Ace bandages compress the leg from ankle to thigh, obliterating the sclerosed veins, and minimizing the risk of bleeding or edema following surgery. Wrinkled or excessively tight bandages can impair skin integrity or interfere with arterial blood flow.*

■ Assist with or instruct to exercise legs at regular intervals. *Exercise (e.g., ROM and Buerger–Allen exercises) promotes normal blood flow and venous return. Walking is excellent exercise and is encouraged.*

■ Position with legs elevated when supine. When sitting, use a recliner chair to elevate the legs and reduce the angle of hip flexion. Change position frequently. *Leg elevation and limited hip flexion promote venous return and minimize pressure on lower extremity veins.*

Discharge Considerations

Most clients with varicose veins provide self-care at home. Emphasize the importance of daily walks. Teach technique for applying antiembolism stockings. Instruct to elevate legs for specified periods of time throughout the day. Help identify strategies to avoid prolonged periods of standing or sitting. If the client's job requires prolonged standing, encourage to wear elastic stockings. Teach calf and thigh muscle tightening and relaxation exercises to perform while standing. Encourage clients whose job requires extensive sitting to work on incorporating frequent activity into the job.

Provide referrals for home health services as needed for clients recovering from surgery. In some instances, temporary placement in an extended care facility may be necessary before returning home.

Nursing Interventions Classification

The following Nursing Interventions (McCloskey & Bulechek, 2000) may be helpful when planning care for clients with peripheral vascular disorders:

■ Circulatory Care: Arterial/Venous Insufficiency
■ Embolus Care: Peripheral
■ Exercise Promotion
■ Foot Care
■ Pressure Ulcer Prevention
■ Skin Surveillance
■ Smoking Cessation Assistance
■ Teaching: Disease Process
■ Teaching: Prescribed Diet/Medication

(*Note:* The bibliography listings for this and all chapters have been compiled at the back of the book.)

Chapter Review

key terms by topic

Use the CD-ROM disk enclosed with your textbook to hear the pronunciation of the key terms in the chapter.

Structure and function
peripheral vascular system, arteries, veins, peripheral vascular resistance (PVR), blood pressure (BP)

Hypertension
primary hypertension, secondary hypertension

Arterial disorders
arteriosclerosis, intermittent claudication, bruit, thrombus, embolus, aneurysm

Venous disorders
venous thrombosis, venous insufficiency, varicose veins

key points

■ Hypertension is a leading, often undiagnosed, cause of cardiovascular disability and mortality. Few people with hypertension have symptoms of the disorder, yet it can lead to heart failure, stroke, and chronic renal failure.

■ Encourage all clients to regularly monitor their blood pressure, reduce their salt intake, stop smoking, limit alcohol intake, exercise regularly, and reduce stress.

■ Stress the importance of continuing hypertension treatment: this disease can be managed but cannot, at this time, be cured.

■ Both arterial and venous disorders can affect circulation to the extremities.

■ Arterial disorders are characterized by cool, pale, hairless skin, diminished peripheral pulses, and often by pain from ischemic tissues.

■ Venous disorders are more often characterized by rubor, brown, leathery skin, and edema.

■ Peripheral vascular disorders increase the risk of skin trauma and breakdown. Provide meticulous foot and skin care for clients with peripheral vascular disorders, and protect from injury.

■ Encourage all clients with peripheral vascular disease to engage in regular activity as approved by their primary care provider.

Medialink

Additional interactive resources for this chapter can be found on the Companion Website at www.prenhall.com/burke. Click on Chapter 23 and "Begin" to select the activities for this chapter.

For NCLEX review questions and an audio glossary, access the accompanying CD-ROM in this book.

for further study

For more information about foods high in sodium, see Box 5-5. For nursing implications for diuretics, see Table 5-4 in Chapter 5.

For more discussion about atherosclerosis, its causes, and treatment, see Chapter 22.

For in-depth review about surgery, see Chapter 7.

For more information about pulmonary embolism, see Chapter 26.

Critical Thinking Care Map

Caring for a Client with Buerger's Disease
NCLEX-PN Focus Area: Reduction of Risk Potential

Case Study: John Kirvis, a 34-year-old computer programmer, has developed leg cramps when he climbs the two flights of stairs to his office each day. The cramps began about 2 months ago, and have become so painful over the last week that he cannot walk more than about 50 feet without resting and he is now taking the elevator to his office. Mr. Kirvis makes an appointment with his primary care provider.

Nursing Diagnosis: Ineffective Tissue Perfusion: Peripheral

COLLECT DATA

Subjective   Objective

_____   _____
_____   _____
_____   _____
_____   _____
_____   _____
_____   _____

Would you report this data? Yes/No

If yes, to: _____

Nursing Care

_____
_____
_____
_____
_____
_____
_____
_____

How would you document this? _____
_____
_____

Data Collected
(use those that apply)

- Has smoked over two packs of cigarettes a day for 20 years
- Calf pain with activity progressing over past 2 months
- Must rest frequently when walking
- Anxious about seriousness of symptoms
- Weak peripheral pulses in right leg
- Absent pedal and posterior tibial pulses in left foot
- Third, fourth, and fifth toes of left foot pale
- Relates numbness and tingling of toes of left food
- Right foot pink and warm; left foot cool to touch
- Skin on left leg shiny and thin; hairless below knee
- Moderate amount evenly distributed hair right leg

Nursing Interventions
(use those that apply)

- Assess pain at rest and during activity using a scale of 0 to 10.
- Mutually determine most effective methods of managing pain.
- Teach Buerger–Allen exercises; instruct to perform exercises three times per day.
- Teach the importance of smoking cessation.
- Teach foot care measures.
- Provide time to discuss issues that contribute to anxiety.
- Encourage questions about the disease and its management.

NCLEX-PN Exam Preparation

TEST-TAKING TIP

Be familiar with the anticoagulant drugs used for various vascular disorders. You will need to know this information in order to answer questions related to the care of clients with vascular disorders.

1. When assessing a bedridden client with a total arterial occlusion, the nurse can expect to find:
   a. palpable pulses in the area below the occlusion
   b. cyanosis or mottling of the area above the occlusion
   c. cyanosis or mottling of the area below the occlusion
   d. extreme pallor, cold and pain in the area below the occlusion

2. When the client's extremity is affected by peripheral arteriosclerosis, blood flow to the extremity can be enhanced by:
   a. placing the affected extremity in a dependent position
   b. elevating the affected extremity
   c. wrapping the affected extremity with an elastic bandage
   d. range of motion exercises to the affected extremity

3. You are admitting a client diagnosed with thrombophlebitis. Which of the following medications should you prepare to administer?
   a. heparin
   b. coumadin
   c. aspirin
   d. nonsteroidal anti-inflammatory drug

4. The nurse can educate the client with Raynaud's disease by offering the following information:
   a. Elevate the extremities above the heart during an episode.
   b. Wear support hose during cold weather.
   c. Practice relaxation techniques to reduce stress.
   d. Avoid any activities that involve repetitive movement.

5. You are caring for a client with Raynaud's disease. Signs and symptoms characteristic of Raynaud's include:
   a. persistent mottling of the hands and feet
   b. consistent pain and numbness in the feet
   c. periodic cyanosis and pallor of the hands and feet
   d. alternating periods of vasodilation and vasoconstriction

6. The nurse is caring for a client who has recently been diagnosed with stage 2 hypertension. When educating the client about hypertension it is important to emphasize that they commonly:
   a. experience severe headaches
   b. have no symptoms other than an increased blood pressure
   c. experience symptoms of kidney failure
   d. experience visual disturbances

7. When educating a client with stage 2 hypertension about how to manage their hypertension, the nurse should stress:
   a. adhering to medication schedules
   b. the short-term aspect of managing hypertension
   c. making all recommended life style changes
   d. engaging in range of motion exercises

8. A 70-year-old male comes to the clinic complaining of severe headaches and dizziness and also states that he recently fell and bumped his head. When reviewing the client's medication history, the nurse should note that the client is taking:
   a. cardizem
   b. inderal
   c. digoxin
   d. coumadin

9. Your 54-year-old female client has recently been diagnosed with stage 2 hypertension. She states that she cannot understand why smoking is bad for her as it usually helps her to relax. The nurse responds by stating that smoking affects blood pressure because nicotine:
   a. stimulates blood vessels
   b. increases the pulse rate
   c. constricts blood vessels
   d. dilates blood vessels

10. Which of the following is a symptom of a dissecting aneurysm of the ascending aorta?
    a. sudden, excruciating pain
    b. paralysis of the lower extremities
    c. diminished or absent peripheral pulses
    d. cyanosis

Caring for Clients with Hematologic and Lymphatic Disorders

chapter 24

CARING tip

"Remember these 3-H's (Hands, Heart, Head)

Hands—Competence and safety on the job skills

Heart—Commitment and dedication

Head—Wide theory base and knowledge of nursing"

Eva Talastas, RN, MSN • Nursing Professor • Long Beach City College • Long Beach, California

LEARNING outcomes

After completing this chapter, you will be able to:

- Describe the physiology of the hematologic system.
- Identify and describe the structures and functions of the lymphatic system.
- Describe the pathophysiology and manifestations of common hematologic and lymphatic disorders.
- Discuss the collaborative care of clients with hematologic or lymphatic disorders, including diagnostic tests and commonly prescribed medications.
- Discuss the nursing implications for selected treatment measures for clients with hematologic or lymphatic disorders.
- Provide individualized nursing care for clients with hematologic or lymphatic disorders.
- Identify discharge considerations for clients with hematologic or lymphatic disorders.

Blood transports oxygen and nutrients to cells, essential substances (such as hormones and other chemical messengers) to cells and tissues, and waste products away from tissues for removal from the body. Blood is made up of **plasma,** a clear yellow, protein-rich fluid, and the cells suspended in it: *red blood cells* (RBCs or **erythrocytes**), *white blood cells* (WBCs or **leukocytes**), and **platelets** (or *thrombocytes*).

A number of body systems are involved in forming blood. Many of the plasma proteins are formed in the liver.

Blood cells are formed in bone marrow. All blood cells begin as *stem cells,* or *hemocytoblasts.* Stem cells then differentiate (mature) into the different types of blood cells (red blood cells, platelets, and several kinds of white cells) (Figure 24-1 ◆).

This chapter provides an overview of each type of blood cell and its function prior to discussion of disorders that affect that cell and its functions.

Red Blood Cell Disorders

Red blood cells (RBCs) and the hemoglobin they contain are vital for transporting oxygen to body tissues. They also help carry carbon dioxide from the tissues to the lungs for excretion.

Red blood cells (erythrocytes) are shaped like *biconcave disks* (Figure 24-2 ◆). The shape of the RBC increases its surface area for gas exchange and allows it to change shape as it moves through very small capillaries. RBCs are formed in bone marrow through a process known as *erythropoiesis.* Tissue hypoxia stimulates the kidneys to release a hormone, *erythropoietin,* that stimulates the bone marrow to produce RBCs. The complete sequence from stem cell to RBC (see Figure 24-1) takes from 3 to 5 days.

RBCs contain **hemoglobin,** an oxygen-carrying protein. Hemoglobin consists of *heme* molecules within a protein structure. Heme contains iron, which binds with oxygen. Hemoglobin molecules are synthesized within the RBC.

RBCs have a life span of about 120 days. Old or damaged RBCs are destroyed by phagocytes in the spleen, liver, bone marrow, and lymph nodes. The process of RBC destruction is called **hemolysis.** The amino acids and iron from destroyed RBCs are saved and reused by the body. Most of the heme unit is converted to *bilirubin,* an orange-yellow pigment that is removed from the blood by the liver and excreted in the bile.

Normal RBC laboratory values often differ by gender (Table 24-1 ◆). Other terms are used to describe RBCs include: *normocytic* (normal size), *microcytic* (smaller than normal), or *macrocytic* (larger than normal); and *normochromic* (normal color) or *hypochromic* (decreased color).

 Anemia

Anemia is a condition in which the hemoglobin concentration or the number of circulating RBCs is decreased. Anemia typically is caused by either impaired RBC formation or excessive loss or destruction of RBCs (Table 24-2 ◆). Hemorrhage

or chronic bleeding (e.g., from a bleeding ulcer) can lead to anemia, as can nutritional problems that interfere with the body's ability to form red blood cells.

PATHOPHYSIOLOGY
Anemia reduces the oxygen-carrying capacity of the blood, leading to tissue hypoxia. As tissue oxygenation decreases, the heart rate and the respiratory rate rise. Tissue hypoxia may cause angina, fatigue, dyspnea on exertion, and night cramps. The skin, mucous membranes, nail beds, and conjunctiva appear pale. The severity of the manifestations of anemia (Figure 24-3 ◆) depends on the cause and severity of the disorder. For example, rapid blood loss causes immediate symptoms, whereas the person with slowly developing anemia may have no symptoms until the condition is advanced.

Blood Loss Anemia
Red blood cells and hemoglobin are lost from the body with acute or chronic bleeding. With acute bleeding, the risk of hypovolemia and shock is greater than the risk of anemia. Chronic bleeding, however, often leads to anemia. The symptoms of the anemia may actually alert the client and care provider to the bleeding problem. In blood loss anemia, RBCs are normal in size, shape, and color, but their numbers are reduced. The RBC, hemoglobin, and hematocrit fall.

Nutritional Anemias
Nutritional anemias result when RBC development or hemoglobin synthesis are disrupted by a lack of one or more necessary components. The nutrient deficiency may be due to a poor diet, impaired absorption of the nutrient, or an increased need for the nutrient. The most common nutritional anemias are iron deficiency anemia, vitamin B_{12} deficiency (pernicious) anemia, and folic acid deficiency anemia.

IRON DEFICIENCY ANEMIA. Iron deficiency anemia is caused by an inadequate supply of iron for RBC formation. It is the most common type of anemia. The body cannot make hemo-

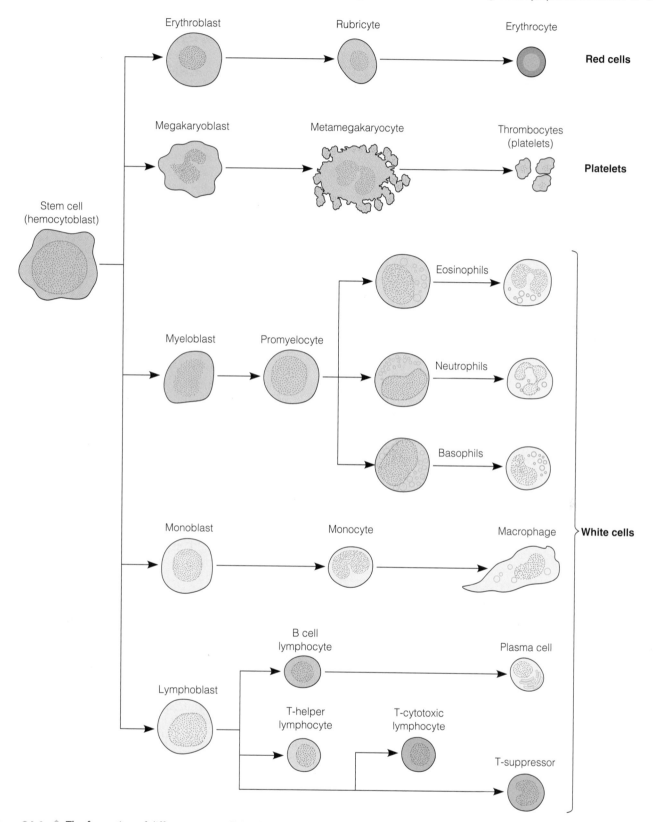

Figure 24-1. ◆ The formation of different types of blood cells from the stem cell. The stem cell differentiates into one of five types of blast cells, which then mature into red blood cells (erythrocytes), platelets (thrombocytes), or white blood cells (leukocytes).

globin without iron. Iron deficiency leads to fewer RBCs, microcytic (small) RBCs, and hypochromic (pale) RBCs. The RBCs also may be malformed.

In adults, iron loss due to bleeding is the usual cause of iron deficiency anemia. Menstrual blood loss is the common cause in adult females. Chronic, occult (hidden) blood loss

Top view

Side view

Figure 24-2. ◆ Top and side view of a red blood cell. Note the distinctive concave shape.

may occur from disorders such as bleeding ulcers, gastrointestinal inflammation, hemorrhoids, and cancer.

Inadequate iron intake (< 1 mg/day) or impaired iron absorption also can lead to iron deficiency anemia. This is common in older adults. Women may develop anemia during pregnancy and lactation because the need for iron is higher.

In addition to the manifestations shown in Figure 24-3, chronic iron deficiency can cause brittle, spoon-shaped nails; *cheilosis* (cracks at the corners of the mouth); a smooth, sore tongue; and *pica* (a craving to eat unusual substances, such as clay or starch).

VITAMIN B$_{12}$ DEFICIENCY (PERNICIOUS) ANEMIA. Vitamin B$_{12}$ is required for RBC formation and maturation. The usual cause of vitamin B$_{12}$ deficiency is impaired absorption of the nutrient from the GI tract. This is known as *pernicious anemia. Intrinsic factor,* a substance secreted by the gastric mucosa, binds with dietary vitamin B$_{12}$ so it can be absorbed by the body.

Vitamin B$_{12}$ deficit interferes with maturation of red blood cells. Great numbers of large, immature RBCs move into the circulation. These cells are fragile and incapable of carrying oxygen in adequate amounts.

Clients with pernicious anemia may develop a smooth, sore, beefy red tongue and diarrhea. Because vitamin B$_{12}$ is important for neurologic function, *paresthesias* (altered sensations, such as numbness or tingling) in the extremities and problems with *proprioception* (the sense of one's position in space) also may develop.

FOLIC ACID DEFICIENCY ANEMIA. Like vitamin B$_{12}$, folic acid is required for normal production and maturation of red blood cells. Folic acid is absorbed from the intestines and is found in green, leafy vegetables; fruits; cereals; and meats. Folic acid deficiency produces an anemia characterized by fragile, megaloblastic (big and immature) cells.

Folic acid deficiency anemia is more common among people who are chronically undernourished (e.g., older adults, alcoholics, and drug users). People receiving total parenteral nutrition (TPN) may develop folate deficiency. Pregnant women, who have increased metabolic requirements for folic acid, and clients with certain malabsorption disorders also are at risk.

The manifestations of folic acid deficiency anemia develop gradually. In addition to the symptoms common to anemia, gastrointestinal manifestations such as glossitis, cheilosis, and diarrhea often develop.

TABLE 24-1	LABORATORY VALUES RELATED TO RED BLOOD CELLS	
LABORATORY TEST	**NORMAL VALUE**	**MEASURES**
Red blood cell (RBC) count ■ Men ■ Women	4.2–5.4 million/mm³ 3.6–5.0 million/mm³	Number of circulating RBCs in one cubic millimeter (mm³) of blood
Reticulocyte count	1%–1.5% of total RBC	Number of immature RBCs in 1 mm³ of blood
Hemoglobin (Hgb) ■ Men ■ Women	14–16.5 g/dL 12–15 g/dL	Amount of hemoglobin in 100 mL (1 dL) of blood
Hematocrit (Hct) ■ Men ■ Women	40%–50% 37%–47%	Packed volume of RBCs in 100 mL of blood; reported as a percentage
Mean corpuscular volume (MCV)	85–100 µm³/cell	Average volume of individual RBCs
Mean corpuscular hemoglobin (MCH)	31–35 g/dL	Weight of the hemoglobin in an average RBC
Mean corpuscular hemoglobin concentration (MCHC)	33.4%–35.5%	Average concentration (percent) of hemoglobin within RBC

TABLE 24-2   SELECTED CLASSIFICATIONS AND CAUSES OF ANEMIA

CLASSIFICATION	CAUSE	EXAMPLES
Blood loss	Acute or chronic bleeding	Trauma Internal bleeding Complications of pregnancy
Nutritional	Decreased RBC or hemoglobin production	Iron deficiency anemia Pernicious or vitamin B$_{12}$ anemia Folic acid deficiency anemia
Hemolytic	Defective hemoglobin synthesis	Sickle cell disease Thalassemia
	Increased hemolysis	Immune reactions Chemical or physical agents
Aplastic (bone marrow failure)	Suppression of bone marrow function	Leukemias Chemical or physical agents

Hemolytic Anemias

Hemolytic anemias are characterized by the premature destruction of RBCs. RBCs may be destroyed because the cell itself is improperly formed *(intrinsic)* or because it has been damaged by an outside source *(acquired)*. Intrinsic causes include defects in the cell membrane or hemoglobin structure and function, and inherited enzyme deficiencies. External causes of hemolytic anemia include drugs, bacterial and other toxins, and trauma.

SICKLE CELL DISORDERS. Sickle cell disorders are inherited as an autosomal recessive trait (Figure 24-4 ◆). They are characterized by abnormal hemoglobin, hemoglobin S (HbS), in the RBCs. This abnormal hemoglobin affects how RBCs respond to stress. At low blood oxygen levels, the cells become sickle-shaped and obstruct small blood vessels (Figure 24-5 ◆). Although the shape returns to normal when normal oxygen levels are restored, repeated episodes of sickling damage RBC membranes. The damaged RBCs break down (hemolysis), leading to anemia. Events likely to trigger a sickling event include hypoxia, low temperatures, excessive exercise, anesthesia, dehy-

Neurologic
• Headache
• Fatigue
• Difficulty concentrating
• Dizziness

Respiratory
• Tachypnea
• Dyspnea on exertion

Urinary
• Hemoglobinuria

Gastrointestinal
• Constipation
• Decreased bowel sounds

Cardiovascular
• Tachycardia
• Palpitations
• Heart murmur
• Angina
Potential Complication
• Heart failure

Musculoskeletal
• Night cramps
• Bone pain
• Muscle weakness

Integumentary
• Pallor
  – Skin
  – Mucous membranes
  – Conjunctiva
  – Nail beds

Figure 24-3. ◆ The multisystem effects of anemia.

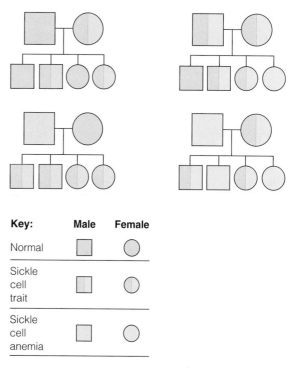

Key:

	Male	Female
Normal		
Sickle cell trait		
Sickle cell anemia		

Figure 24-4. ◆ The inheritance pattern for sickle cell anemia.

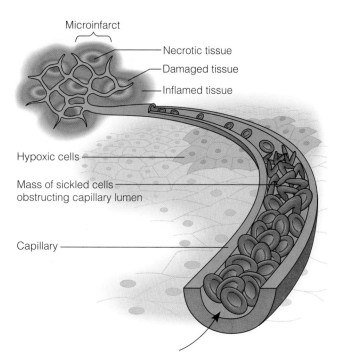

Figure 24-5. ◆ Pathophysiology Illustrated: Sickle cell anemia. **Hemoglobin S and Red Blood Cell Sickling.** Sickle cell anemia is caused by an inherited defect in hemoglobin (Hb) synthesis. When sickle cell hemoglobin (Hb S) is oxygenated, it has the same globular shape as normal hemoglobin. However, when Hb S is not bound with oxygen, it becomes insoluble and crystallizes into rod-like structures. Clusters of these rods form long chains that bend the erythrocyte into the characteristic crescent shape of the sickle cell.

The Sickle Cell Disease Process. Sickle cell disease is characterized by episodes of acute painful crises. Sickling crises are triggered by conditions that affect the oxygen supply, increase the oxygen demand, or change the pH. As a sickle cell crisis begins, sickled RBCs cling to capillary walls and each other, obstructing blood flow and causing cellular hypoxia. The crisis accelerates as hypoxia and acidic waste products cause further sickling and cell damage. Sickle cell crises cause small infarctions in joints and organs. Repeated crises slowly destroy organs and tissues. The spleen and kidneys are especially prone to sickling damage.

dration, infections, or acidosis. Box 24-1 provides more information about sickle cell disorders.

Sickling is usually marked by an abrupt onset of intense pain, often in the abdomen. The acute pain also may occur in the chest, back, or joints. The client also has manifestations of anemia and may become jaundiced as bilirubin is released from the red blood cells.

THALASSEMIA. *Thalassemia* is an inherited disorder also caused by abnormal hemoglobin synthesis. It commonly affects people of Mediterranean, Asian, or African descent. Depending on the form of the disorder and whether the person has inherited one or both defective genes, the client may have few symptoms or severe disease.

Manifestations of thalassemia include liver and spleen enlargement from increased red cell destruction. Stress on the bone marrow to produce RBCs can lead to thinning of bones and fractures. People with severe thalassemia may require blood transfusions to sustain life.

ACQUIRED HEMOLYTIC ANEMIA. *Acquired hemolytic anemia* results when RBCs are damaged by outside factors, such as:

- Mechanical trauma (prosthetic heart valves, severe burns, hemodialysis, or radiation)

- Antibody reactions following infection
- Immune responses (transfusion reactions)
- Drugs, toxins, chemical agents, or venoms

The manifestations of acquired hemolytic anemia depend on the extent of hemolysis. The spleen enlarges as it removes large numbers of damaged or destroyed RBCs. Bilirubin released from the hemoglobin of damaged RBCs can cause jaundice. In severe cases, bones may become deformed or develop pathologic fractures.

Aplastic Anemia

In *aplastic anemia,* the bone marrow fails to produce RBCs. The cause is usually unknown. Aplastic anemia may follow injury to stem cells in bone marrow caused by radiation or certain chemicals. Benzene, arsenic, nitrogen mustard, certain antibiotics (especially chloramphenicol), and chemotherapeutic drugs can cause aplastic anemia. Aplastic anemia also is associated with some viral infections such as mononucleosis, hepatitis C, and HIV.

People with aplastic anemia usually have *pancytopenia;* that is, they have decreased numbers of red blood cells, white cells, and platelets. Signs and symptoms of aplastic anemia may develop gradually or suddenly. These include fatigue, pallor, progressive weakness, exertional dyspnea, headache, tachy-

BOX 24-1 population FOCUS

Sickle Cell Disorders

Inherited sickle cell disorders include sickle cell anemia, sickle cell trait, and related disorders. In *sickle cell anemia*, abnormal hemoglobin (hemoglobin S) is formed within red blood cells.

Sickle cell anemia usually affects people of African descent. About 8% of African Americans have inherited the Hb S gene from a parent. They have *sickle cell trait*. They have few symptoms. Each child of a person with sickle cell trait has a 50% risk of inheriting the Hb S gene (Figure 24-4). If both parents have sickle cell trait, each child has a 25% risk of inheriting the Hb S gene from both parents. These children are likely to develop sickle cell anemia. Hispanics from the Caribbean and Central and South America also may have the Hb S gene.

Sickled cells obstruct blood vessels, causing tissue ischemia (Figure 24-5). Every organ of the body can be damaged, especially the spleen, bone marrow, lung, eye, and head of the femur and humerus. Good general health maintenance through nutrition, exercise, and avoiding smoking and excess alcohol intake are important to prevent sickling crises.

Sickle cell anemia is chronic, unpredictable, and recurrent, leading to psychosocial stress. The risk of passing the disease to offspring compounds this stress. Genetic counseling is recommended.

BOX 24-2 NURSING CARE CHECKLIST

BONE MARROW ASPIRATION

Bone marrow studies are used to diagnose aplastic anemia, leukemias, and other cancers. A sample of bone marrow is obtained by inserting a needle or biopsy instrument into a bone (usually the posterior iliac crest or sternum).

Before the Procedure

☑ Verify a signed consent for the procedure.
☑ Explain the purpose and procedure of the test.
☑ Record vital signs. Have the client void.
☑ Place in supine position if sternum or anterior iliac crest will be used, in prone position if posterior iliac crest is to be used.

After the Procedure

☑ Apply pressure to the puncture site for 5 to 10 minutes.
☑ Assess vital signs; report changes from baseline.
☑ Apply dressing to puncture site. Monitor for bleeding and infection.

Client and Family Teaching

☑ The procedure takes about 20 minutes.
☑ A local anesthetic will be used; you will feel some pain during insertion. Take deep breaths to help relieve pain during this time.
☑ It is important to remain very still during the procedure.
☑ The site of the aspiration may ache for a day or two.
☑ Report any unusual bleeding immediately.

---

cardia, and ultimately heart failure. Platelet deficiency may cause bleeding problems. A deficiency of white blood cells increases the risk of infection.

COLLABORATIVE CARE
Diagnostic Tests

When anemia is suspected, the following diagnostic tests may be ordered:

- A *complete blood count (CBC)* to determine the RBC count, hemoglobin, and hematocrit.
- *Iron levels* and *total iron-binding capacity tests* to identify iron deficiency. If iron deficiency anemia is present, the serum iron concentration will be low, and the total iron-binding capacity will be high.
- *Serum ferritin* is low in iron deficiency anemia. Ferritin is an iron-storage protein produced by the liver, spleen, and bone marrow.
- *Sickle-cell screening test* is ordered to identify hemoglobin S if sickle cell anemia is suspected.
- *Schilling's test,* which includes consuming radioactive vitamin B_{12} and a 24-hour urine sample, is ordered to diagnose pernicious anemia.
- *Bone marrow examination* may be done to diagnose aplastic anemia. Nursing care for a client having a bone marrow study is described in Box 24-2.

Pharmacology

Drugs used to treat anemia depend on the type of anemia. Iron replacement is prescribed for clients with iron deficiency ane-

mia. Supplemental iron may be given orally or intramuscularly. Vitamin B_{12} is given by injection to clients with pernicious anemia. Folic acid supplements are ordered for clients with a folic acid deficiency or sickle cell anemia to meet the increased demands of the bone marrow. Hydroxyurea may be prescribed for clients with severe sickle cell disease. This drug promotes fetal hemoglobin production. Fetal hemoglobin reduces sickling and painful crises. Nursing implications for iron, vitamin B_{12}, and folic acid are found in Table 24-3 ◆. Procedure 24-1 reviews Z-track technique to administer iron dextran solution.

Dietary Modifications

Dietary modifications may be ordered for nutritional deficiency anemias, such as iron deficiency anemia or folic acid deficiency anemia. Meats, poultry, and fish provide iron that is readily absorbed. The iron contained in vegetables and grains is less readily absorbed, but accounts for most of the daily iron

TABLE 24-3 NURSING IMPLICATIONS FOR PHARMACOLOGY: CLIENTS WITH ANEMIA

DRUG/CLASS	ACTION	NURSING IMPLICATIONS	CLIENT AND FAMILY TEACHING
Iron Sources ▪ Ferrous sulfate (Feosol, Fer-in-sol) ▪ Ferrous gluconate (Fergon, Ferralet, Fertinic) ▪ Iron dextran injection (Imferon) ▪ Iron polysaccharide	Iron preparations are used to treat iron deficiency anemias. They are usually taken by mouth and are absorbed from the gastrointestinal tract.	Assess for drug interactions and GI bleeding. Give with orange juice to improve absorption. Administer elixirs through a straw to prevent staining of teeth. Use Z-technique when administering parenteral iron (see Procedure 24-1). Report manifestations of iron toxicity: Nausea, diarrhea, or constipation. Monitor hemoglobin and RBC counts.	Take with food (not milk) to reduce gastric distress. Stools may be dark green or black; this is harmless. Increase fluid and fiber intake to decrease constipation. A delayed reaction to iron dextran injection can occur. Report fever, chills, malaise, muscle and joint aches, nausea or vomiting, dizziness, or backache to your primary care provider.
Vitamin B$_{12}$ Sources ▪ Cyanocobalamin (Kaybovite [oral], Anacobin [parenteral], Bedoz)	Cyanocobalamin is used to treat vitamin B$_{12}$ deficiencies and pernicious anemia. It is rapidly absorbed and is stored in the liver. Intrinsic factor is required for absorption from the GI tract.	Do not expose injection to light. Do not mix in a syringe with other medications. Administer injections IM or deep SC to decrease local irritation. Monitor hemoglobin, RBC, reticulocyte counts, and potassium levels.	The burning sensation that may occur with injection is temporary. Avoid alcohol, which interferes with absorption. If used to treat pernicious anemia, the medication must be taken for life.
Folic Acid Sources ▪ Folic acid (Folvite, novofolacid)	Folic acid is used to treat folic acid deficiency and resulting anemia. Synthetic folic acid is absorbed from the GI tract and stored in the liver.	Do not mix folic acid with other medications in the same syringe. Report hypersensitivity response of skin rash.	Large doses may darken the urine. Excess alcohol intake increases folic acid requirements.

intake. Selected dietary sources of iron, vitamin B$_{12}$, and folic acid are outlined in Box 24-3.

Blood Transfusion

When anemia is due to a major blood loss, such as from trauma or major surgery, blood transfusions may be given to replace red blood cells. If the bleeding is acute (hemorrhage), whole blood may be given. If the blood loss is chronic, packed red cells may be given. Clients with severe anemia from other causes (such sickle cell anemia or aplastic anemia) also may

require blood transfusions. See Chapter 10 for more information about blood transfusions.

CLINICAL alert

Members of the Jehovah's Witness faith do not accept blood and blood products. Alternatives to blood transfusion include intravenous solutions to increase blood volume and colony-stimulating factors to increase RBC production. Oxygen-carrying blood substitutes are in the process of being developed.

PROCEDURE 24-1   Z-Track Technique Checklist

■ PURPOSE

Z-track technique is used to seal medication within a muscle and prevent staining or irritation of subcutaneous tissues.

■ BEFORE THE PROCEDURE

- Verify medication order, including drug, dose, route, and time.
- Gather all supplies. After drawing the correct dosage into the syringe, draw an additional 0.2 mL of air into the syringe and change the needle.
- Identify client and provide for privacy.
- Position appropriately for the site to be used (prone or side-lying).

■ PROCEDURE

- Follow standard precautions.
- Identify and cleanse the site.
- Using nondominant hand, pull skin laterally approximately 1″ (2.5 cm).
- Holding the skin taut, administer the medication and withdraw the needle. Release the skin and apply direct pressure to the injection site.
- Document the medication administration, site, and client response.

Z-Track Injection

Medication

■ SAMPLE DOCUMENTATION

12/20/03	0900	1 mL Imferon given R
		ventral gluteal site using Z-technique.
		Tolerated well.
		S. Meyer, LPN.

NURSING CARE

Unless anemia is related to acute blood loss, care is usually provided in community-based settings. Nurses in these settings play an important role in identifying clients with anemia, monitoring their status and treatment, and providing appropriate teaching.

ASSESSING

Assessment data can reveal manifestations of anemia, as well as provide clues about potential causes of anemia. Assessment data related to anemia is outlined in Box 24-4.

DIAGNOSING, PLANNING, AND IMPLEMENTING

ACTIVITY INTOLERANCE

Inadequate oxygen delivery to the tissues can lead to weakness, fatigue, and shortness of breath with activity.

- Monitor vital signs, especially heart and respiratory rates, before and after activity. *Vital signs are an objective measure of activity tolerance. Heart and respiratory rates should remain within normal limits during and after normal activities.*
- Discontinue activity and allow rest for complaints of chest pain, shortness of breath, palpitations, or dizziness; tachycardia that does not return to normal within four minutes of resting; rapid or labored respirations. *These signs and symptoms indicate intolerance of the activity.*

DIETARY SOURCES OF IRON, FOLIC ACID, AND VITAMIN B12

BOX 24-3

Iron
- Beef, beef liver, pork, ham, chicken, turkey, tuna, shrimp, clams, tofu
- Dried beans, green beans, green peas, spinach, broccoli
- Potatoes, whole grains, brown rice

Folic Acid (Folate)
- Asparagus, okra, spinach and other greens, broccoli
- Green beans and other legumes, dried beans
- Fortified grain products (corn flakes, oatmeal, pasta)

Vitamin B12 (Cobalamin)
- Meat, poultry, eggs
- Fish and shellfish
- Milk and cheese

■ Help identify ways to conserve energy during activities of daily living (ADLs), e.g., sitting to shower, spacing activities throughout the day. *Reducing energy use allows greater independence while avoiding excess fatigue or shortness of breath.*

BOX 24-4 ASSESSING CLIENTS WITH ANEMIA

SUBJECTIVE DATA
- Complaints of fatigue, headache, difficulty concentrating, shortness of breath, palpitations, or dizziness; chest pain, muscle cramps or aching bone pain; sore mouth or tongue, cracking at corners of lips
- Reports of obvious bleeding (excessive menstrual flow, rectal bleeding, or vomiting blood) or black or tarry stools

OBJECTIVE DATA
- Vital signs, including orthostatic blood pressure if bleeding is suspected
- Inspect skin, mucous membranes, nail beds, and conjunctiva for color, condition, presence of petechiae or ulcers; mouth and lips for *glossitis* (inflammation of the tongue), a beefy, red tongue, and *cheilosis* (cracking at the corners); incisions and dressings for acute bleeding
- Observe for dyspnea or shortness of breath.
- Auscultate heart, breath, and bowel sounds.
- Check stool and vomitus for occult blood.
- Laboratory reports for RBC, hemoglobin, and hematocrit levels.

■ Help prioritize activities and distribute tasks among family members. *This allows the client to conserve energy while relieving concerns that necessary tasks are being performed.*

■ Help plan a schedule of balanced rest and activity during the day and 8 to 10 hours of sleep at night. *Rest decreases oxygen demand and reduces fatigue.*

■ Instruct not to smoke. *Smoking is a vasoconstrictor that further increases the workload of the heart and impairs tissue oxygenation.*

IMPAIRED ORAL MUCOUS MEMBRANE

■ Assess condition of lips and tongue daily. *Glossitis and cheilosis increase the risk for bleeding and infection. These conditions also may cause pain and discomfort with eating, interfering with oral intake.*

■ Use a mouthwash of saline, salt water, or half-strength peroxide and water to rinse mouth every 2 to 4 hours. *This cleans and soothes oral mucous membranes.*

■ Provide frequent oral hygiene (after meals and at bedtime) with a soft bristle toothbrush or sponge. *Removing food debris promotes comfort and reduces the risk of infection. A soft toothbrush is less likely to cause irritation or bleeding of the oral mucosa.*

■ Instruct to avoid alcohol-based mouthwashes. *Alcohol is drying and will aggravate cracking of the mucous membranes.*

■ Apply a petroleum-based lubricating jelly or ointment to lips after oral care. *A lubricating ointment helps to retain moisture, facilitate healing, and protect the lips from other drying agents.*

■ Instruct to avoid hot, spicy, or acidic foods. *These foods may irritate and dry damaged mucous membranes.*

■ Encourage soft, cool, bland foods. *Foods that are soothing to the mucous membranes promote comfort and help maintain adequate intake.*

■ Encourage four to six small, high-protein, nutritionally balanced meals daily. *Small, frequent meals reduce fatigue. High-protein, well-balanced meals promote healing.*

SELF-CARE DEFICIT

■ Assist with ADLs, such as bathing, grooming, and eating. *Assistance decreases energy expenditures and tissue requirements for oxygen.*

■ Instruct to rest between activities such as bathing and dressing. *Rest reduces oxygen demand and cardiac workload, promoting independence and self-esteem.*

■ Listen to and acknowledge concerns about inability to maintain self-care. *Dependence on others for ADLs may signify a loss of control and lead to a loss of self-esteem.*

EVALUATING

To evaluate the effectiveness of nursing care, assess the client's ability to independently perform ADLs, and gradually increase level of activity. Assess skin and oral mucous membrane condition, and ability to consume the recommended diet.

Discharge Considerations

Clients with anemia are primarily managed in the home and community-based health care settings. Assessing for home care, planning, and teaching are vital nursing responsibilities. See Box 24-5 for assessment data to consider when planning for discharge.

Teach about the type of anemia, its causes, effects, and treatment. Provide a list of foods that should be included in the diet. Refer to a dietitian or nutritionist for further teaching as indicated. Discuss ordered medications, including dose, how and when to take the drug, and anticipated side effects and their management. Stress the importance of keeping scheduled appointments with the health care provider for follow-up.

Refer the client with an inherited form of anemia for genetic counseling, and discuss the risks of transmitting the condition to offspring. With clients who have sickle cell dis-

ease, discuss measures to prevent and treat sickling crises. Provide information about when to contact the primary care provider or seek treatment in the emergency department. Provide contacts for local support groups and national organizations, including:

American Sickle Cell Anemia Association
10300 Carnegie Avenue
Cleveland Clinic/East Office Building (Eeb 18)
Cleveland, OH 44106
1-216-229-8600
www.ccf.org

Have a Heart for Sickle Cell Foundation
47 West Polk, #100-130
Chicago, IL 60605
1-312-828-1106
www.4sicklecellanemia.org

Nursing Process Case Study
■ CLIENT WITH FOLIC ACID DEFICIENCY ANEMIA

Sheri Matthews is a 76-year-old widow who lives alone. She tells the clinic nurse, Lisa Apana, that she liked to cook when her husband was alive but that preparing an entire meal just for herself seems senseless. She relates she typically has nothing for breakfast, a bologna sandwich and cup of coffee for lunch, and a hot dog or two, a few cookies, and a glass of milk for dinner.

Assessment   Mrs. Matthews has lost 20 lbs. (9 kg) since her husband died 8 months ago. She says she feels weak and sometimes has heart palpitations. Physical assessment data include: T 98.8° F (37.1° C); BP 90/52; P 110; R 22. Skin is warm, pale, and dry. Diagnostic tests indicate folic acid deficiency anemia. Mrs. Matthews is started on an oral folic acid supplement and is instructed to increase her intake of foods containing folic acid.

Diagnosis   The following nursing diagnoses are identified:

■ Activity Intolerance related to weakness
■ Imbalanced Nutrition: Less Than Body Requirements related to lack of motivation to cook and understanding of nutritional needs

Expected Outcomes   The expected outcomes for the plan of care specify that Mrs. Matthews will:

■ Gain at least 1 lb. (0.45 kg) per week.
■ Regain previous energy level.
■ Eat a balanced diet, including foods containing folic acid.
■ Verbalize the importance of taking folic acid supplements.

Planning and Implementation   The following interventions are planned and implemented for Mrs. Matthews:

BOX 24-5
ASSESSING FOR DISCHARGE

ANEMIA
Client

• Self-care: Ability to independently perform ADLs, prepare and eat ordered diet, manage medications
• Knowledge: Understanding of anemia and its effects, prescribed medications, diet, and activity progression; recommendations for follow-up care
• Psychosocial: Support network; coping with activity and role limitations and effects; willingness to seek genetic counseling if indicated
• Home environment: Stairs, other environmental features that increase oxygen consumption (e.g., reliance on wood heat or lack of running water)

Family and Caregivers

• Members of household: Ability to assist with ADLs; willingness to participate in genetic counseling if indicated
• Resources: Financial; for prescribed diet and medications

Community

• Availability of home health, social support services, and support groups
• Access to public transportation, medical services, pharmacies

■ Discuss foods in a well-balanced diet. Provide a list of food sources of folic acid. Help plan balanced meals that include foods that are easy and quick to prepare.

■ Discuss the importance of taking folic acid supplement. Advise to continue taking it even after she begins to feel better.

■ Help develop a schedule of activities to ensure adequate energy to prepare meals.

Evaluation Mrs. Matthews gained 1 lb. (0.45 kg) during the first week of treatment. She rests before and after preparing her meals and is beginning to enjoy cooking again now that she has a reason to cook. She verbalizes an understanding of the need to keep taking her folic acid supplement. Ms. Apana refers her to a home health agency to determine whether Mrs. Matthews is able to participate in the local "Meals-on-Wheels" program.

 Critical Thinking in the Nursing Process

1. Design a week's menu that includes foods high in folic acid.
2. Why was Mrs. Matthews placed on a folic acid supplement in addition to dietary modifications?
3. Why is the older adult at increased risk for developing folic acid deficiency anemia? Consider physiologic, economic, and social factors.

 Polycythemia

Polycythemia (also called *erythrocytosis*) is an abnormally high red blood cell count with high hematocrit. When the hematocrit is greater than 50%, the blood becomes more viscous or "sticky."

PATHOPHYSIOLOGY

Polycythemia usually develops secondarily to chronic hypoxemia or excess production of erythropoietin. Decreased tissue oxygenation stimulates erythropoietin production, which in turn stimulates the bone marrow to produce more RBCs. People who live at high altitudes, where the atmospheric oxygen level is low, have a gradual increase in RBCs to adapt to the lower oxygen levels. People who have chronic lung disease or are heavy smokers also often develop polycythemia. Excess erythropoietin production may be due to kidney disease or malignancy.

Polycythemia vera is a primary condition in which the production of all blood cells (red, white, and platelets) is increased. Its cause is unknown. Polycythemia vera is relatively rare, and usually affects people over the age of 50. In polycythemia vera, RBC, WBC, and platelet counts increase, as does the hematocrit and blood volume. The liver and spleen become congested with RBCs. The client is at risk for thrombosis and infarction.

The onset of polycythemia vera is insidious. Its symptoms are related to excess blood volume, increased blood viscosity, and changes in cerebral blood flow. The client may complain of headaches, dizziness, tinnitus, and blurred vision. Hypertension often develops. Ruddy or dusky cyanosis of the face is common, as is pruritus. The client may develop heart failure, thrombophlebitis, and thrombosis in distal arteries. Gangrene of fingers or toes is a potential complication.

COLLABORATIVE CARE

The *RBC count* and *hematocrit* are elevated in polycythemia. In polycythemia vera, *WBC* and *platelet counts* also are increased. *Erythropoietin levels* are high in secondary polycythmia, but low in polycythemia vera.

Treatment of polycythemia focuses on reducing blood viscosity and volume and relieving symptoms. Phlebotomy, removal of 300 to 500 mL of blood through a vein, can be done repeatedly to keep blood volume and viscosity within normal levels. In some cases, chemotherapy drugs may be used to suppress the bone marrow in clients with polycythemia vera.

 NURSING CARE

Nursing care focuses on teaching the importance of maintaining adequate hydration and preventing blood stasis: elevating the legs when sitting, using support stockings, and complying with treatment measures. To smokers, emphasize the importance of smoking cessation. Instruct to immediately report symptoms of thrombosis such as pallor or pain in an extremity, chest or abdominal pain, and any abnormal bleeding.

Platelet and Coagulation Disorders

Platelets are an essential part of the body's clotting mechanism. They are small fragments of cytoplasm without nuclei that contain many granules. Most platelets are stored in the spleen before being released into the circulation. There are about 250,000 to 400,000 platelets in each milliliter of blood. An excess of platelets is *thrombocytosis.* A deficit of platelets is **thrombocytopenia.** Platelets live approximately 10 days in circulating blood.

Hemostasis

Hemostasis, or blood clotting, is a complex process the body uses to stop bleeding. There are five stages in hemostasis:

1. *Vessel spasm:* Damage to a blood vessel causes it to spasm. This spasm, which lasts more than a minute, constricts the vessel and reduces blood flow.
2. *Formation of the platelet plug:* Platelets adhere to the damaged vessel wall and to one another, forming a platelet plug. Von Willebrand's factor is necessary for platelets to adhere to one another. The platelet plug is stabilized by fibrin.
3. *Clot formation.* Coagulation occurs as fibrin forms a meshwork that cements blood components together into an insoluble clot. The process involves two different clotting pathways. The *intrinsic pathway* is activated by vessel injury; the *extrinsic pathway* is activated by blood leaking out of the vessel into the tissues. The final outcome is fibrin clot formation. Each clotting factor is activated in sequence; activation of one clotting factor activates another in turn. A deficiency of one or more factors interrupts blood clotting.
4. *Clot retraction:* After about 30 minutes, platelets trapped within the clot begin to contract. This pulls the broken portions of the ruptured blood vessel closer together. At the same time, platelets release growth factors that stimulate cell division and tissue repair in the damaged vessel.
5. *Clot dissolution:* A process called *fibrinolysis* removes the clot after tissue has been repaired. Fibrinolysis begins within a few days of clot formation and continues until the clot is dissolved.

Thrombocytopenia

Thrombocytopenia is a platelet count of less than 100,000 platelets per milliliter of blood. It is the most common cause of abnormal bleeding. If the number of circulating platelets continues to decrease, falling below 20,000/mL, spontaneous bleeding (internal and external) is likely. *Primary idiopathic*

thrombocytopenia purpura is the most common form of thrombocytopenia. Its cause is unknown.

PATHOPHYSIOLOGY

In idiopathic thrombocytopenia purpura (ITP), platelets are destroyed much more rapidly than normal. It appears that the platelets are destroyed by the body's immune system (an autoimmune disorder). Idiopathic thrombocytopenia may be an acute or a chronic condition. Acute ITP is seen in children and is often preceded by a viral infection. Chronic ITP affects adults and has no known precipitating factors.

The manifestations of ITP are caused by abnormal bleeding, particularly into the skin and mucous membranes. *Purpura* (hemorrhage into the tissues), *ecchymoses* (buises), and **petechiae** (small, flat, purple, or red spots on the skin or mucous membranes) develop on the anterior chest, arms, and neck. Other bleeding may occur as well: *epistaxis* (nosebleed), *menorrhagia* (prolonged and heavy menstrual periods), hematuria, and gastrointestinal bleeding. Spontaneous bleeding into the brain can be fatal.

COLLABORATIVE CARE

Thrombocytopenia is diagnosed by its manifestations and diagnostic test results. A *CBC with platelet count* is ordered; the platelet count is decreased to less than 100,000/mL. A *bone marrow examination* may be ordered.

Pharmacology

Corticosteroids such as prednisone are given to suppress the immune response and the antibodies targeted for the platelets. See Chapter 13 for more information about corticosteroids. Although the exact mechanism of action is not well understood, corticosteriods also reduce bleeding time.

Platelet Transfusion

Platelet transfusions may be needed to restore the platelet count and prevent bleeding. Platelets are prepared from fresh whole blood; one unit contains 30 to 60 mL of platelet concentrate.

CLINICAL alert

Platelets must be administered as soon as they are obtained from the blood bank. As with whole blood, platelets are typed and cross-matched to the individual.

Surgery

A *splenectomy* (surgical removal of the spleen) may be necessary. The spleen is the site of platelet destruction and antibody production. This surgery often leads to remission or even cure of the disorder.

NURSING CARE

Nursing care for the client with thrombocytopenia focuses on the risk for injury resulting from bleeding. This diagnosis, with related nursing interventions and rationale, is discussed in the section on leukemia that follows.

Discuss the need to continue treatment to maintain remission of this chronic disease, and the risks and benefits of long-term corticosteroid therapy. Respond to questions about splenectomy. While surgery is an invasive treatment, most people experience partial or complete remission of the disease following surgery. Teach measures to avoid injury and bleeding.

Disseminated Intravascular Coagulopathy

Disseminated intravascular coagulopathy (DIC) is a complex coagulation disorder characterized by simultaneous blood clotting and hemorrhage. It is a complication of other disorders, such as shock, sepsis, or other conditions listed in Box 24-6. This critical condition has a mortality rate of 50% to 80%.

PATHOPHYSIOLOGY

DIC is a complex process in which the intrinsic and/or extrinsic clotting cascades are activated. Widespread clotting occurs within small blood vessels. Clotting obstructs small blood vessels in the organs, leading to tissue ischemia, infarction, and necrosis. The widespread clotting activates the fibrinolytic pathway that normally breaks down existing clots. Fibrinolytic products interfere with platelet function. Clotting factors are depleted by the abnormal coagulation process, leading to bleeding. Thus, in the client with DIC,

---

> ### BOX 24-6
> ### RISK FACTORS FOR DISSEMINATED INTRAVASCULAR COAGULOPATHY
>
> - Hypovolemic or septic shock
> - Infection and sepsis
> - Malignancy
> - Obstetric complications
> - Trauma
> - Liver disease
> - Hematologic or immune disorders
> - Acute respiratory distress syndrome
> - Venomous snakebite

> ### BOX 24-7
> ### MANIFESTATIONS OF DISSEMINATED INTRAVASCULAR COAGULOPATHY
>
> - Petechiae, purpura, ecchymoses
> - Bleeding from wounds
> - Tachycardia, hypotension
> - Cold, mottled fingers and toes
> - Tachypnea
> - Obvious or occult blood in vomitus and/or stool
> - Abdominal distention
> - Hematuria
> - Oliguria, renal failure
> - Anxiety, confusion
> - Decreased level of consciousness

---

both intravascular clotting and hemorrhage are occurring at the same time.

Bleeding is the most obvious manifestation of DIC. The bleeding ranges from oozing blood following an injection to frank hemorrhage from every body orifice. Clotting leads to symptoms of tissue ischemia. The manifestations of DIC are listed in Box 24-7.

> ### CLINICAL alert
>
> Promptly report abnormal bleeding (e.g., oozing from injection sites, nosebleed) in critically ill clients as it may be an early sign of DIC.

COLLABORATIVE CARE

Clotting studies are ordered to establish the diagnosis of DIC. Treatment focuses on treating the underlying disease and interrupting the clotting/bleeding process. If liver function is intact, it can restore depleted clotting factors in 24 to 48 hours.

Fresh frozen plasma and platelet concentrates are given to control bleeding. Heparin also may be ordered. Heparin interferes with the clotting cascade and may prevent depletion of clotting factors due to uncontrolled clotting. It is used when bleeding is not controlled by plasma and platelets, and when the client is at risk for tissue necrosis and gangrene.

NURSING CARE

INEFFECTIVE TISSUE PERFUSION

Tiny blood clots forming within blood vessels impair perfusion of body tissues.

- Assess peripheral pulses and warmth and capillary refill of extremities. Monitor level of consciousness and mental status. Assess bowel sounds and monitor urine output. Promptly report changes to the charge nurse or physician. *Early treatment of impaired circulation is important to preserve organ function.*

■ Carefully turn from side to side at least every 2 hours. *Frequent position changes help relieve pressure, maintain tissue perfusion, and preserve skin integrity. Position changes also provide an opportunity to assess tissue integrity and check for bleeding.*

■ Discourage from crossing the legs; do not use the knee gatch on the bed. *These positions can impair blood flow and tissue perfusion of the legs.*

■ Minimize tape use. *Tape can damage the skin, causing bleeding.*

IMPAIRED GAS EXCHANGE

Microclots in the pulmonary vascular system can interfere with gas exchange.

■ Report oxygen saturation levels and ABGs outside established limits to the physician. *Oxygen saturation levels and ABGs are objective measures of gas exchange.*

■ Administer oxygen as ordered. *Supplemental oxygen helps maintain adequate gas exchange and relieve dyspnea.*

■ Place in semi-Fowler's or Fowler's position. *Elevating the head of the bed improves lung ventilation and gas exchange.*

■ Maintain bed rest. *Bed rest reduces oxygen demands and improves pulmonary circulation for better gas exchange.*

■ Encourage deep breathing and coughing. *Coughing and deep breathing help maintain airway patency, facilitating alveolar ventilation.*

PAIN

■ Assess pain using a pain scale. Document location, severity, and character of all reported pain. Promptly notify the charge nurse or physician of new or different pain, or if its intensity changes. *The pain scale provides an objective assessment of pain. Changes in the location or severity of pain may indicate tissue ischemia or bleeding into tissues.*

■ Handle extremities gently. *Gentle handling minimizes trauma and pain.*

■ Apply cool compresses to painful joints. *Application of cold decreases pain perception and may reduce bleeding into joint tissues.*

FEAR

DIC is a frightening complication of critical illness.

■ Allow client and family to verbalize concerns. *This helps identify concerns and questions.*

■ Answer questions truthfully. *Providing truthful answers establishes trust and helps the client and family understand what is happening.*

■ Help identify coping strategies. *Past effective coping methods may provide skills to manage the current crisis.*

■ Provide emotional support. *The presence of a caring nurse may help reduce the fear and anxiety associated with the crisis.*

■ Maintain a calm environment. *A calm, quiet environment and evidence that the staff is in control of the situation help relieve fears and promote rest.*

■ Respond promptly to calls for help. *Prompt responses help develop a trusting relationship and reduce anxiety.*

■ Teach relaxation techniques. *Relaxation techniques can reduce muscle tension and help the client gain a sense of control.*

Hemophilia

Hemophilia is not a single disease but a group of hereditary clotting factor deficiencies. Lack of a clotting factor disrupts blood coagulation, leading to persistent and sometimes severe bleeding. Although it usually is considered a disease of children, hemophilia may be diagnosed in adults.

PATHOPHYSIOLOGY

In hemophilia, the first steps of hemostasis, vasoconstriction and the platelet plug, occur normally. The third step, blood clotting, is disrupted by lack of a specific factor required in the clotting cascade. *Hemophilia A* is the most common type of hemophilia. It is caused by a deficiency in factor VIII. *Hemophilia B* (also called Christmas disease) is less common. It is caused by a deficiency in factor IX. The clinical manifestations of hemophilia A and B are the same. Both are transmitted from mother to son as sex-linked recessive disorders on the X chromosome (Figure 24-6 ◆).

People with hemophilia A or B experience hemorrhages into body tissues. Severe clotting factor deficiencies can lead to spontaneous bleeding episodes. Bleeding of the mouth, gums, lips, and tongue are common, as is hematuria. Bleeding into joints *(hemarthrosis)* causes severe pain and can affect joint structure and function.

Von Willebrand's disease is a common hereditary bleeding disorder that is usually seen in adults. It is caused by a deficiency of von Willebrand (vW) factor; factor VIII is often lacking as well. This clotting disorder affects both men and women. Von Willebrand's disease causes less severe bleeding than hemophilia A or B. It is often diagnosed when surgery or a dental extraction causes prolonged bleeding. A comparison of the types of hemophilia is found in Table 24-4 ◆.

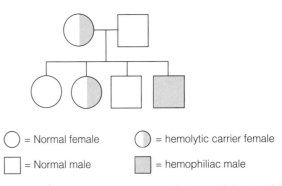

Figure 24-6. ◆ The inheritance pattern for hemophilia A and B. Both are X-linked recessive disorders; females may carry the trait, but only males develop the disorder.

TABLE 24-4 COMPARISON OF TYPES OF HEMOPHILIA			
TYPE	**DEFICIENCY**	**CHARACTERISTICS**	**TREATMENT**
Hemophilia A (classic hemophilia)	Factor VIII	Most common form of hemophilia; transmitted from mother with defective gene to sons	Factor VIII concentrate or cryoprecipitate
Hemophilia B (Christmas disease)	Factor IX	Less common; transmitted from mother with defective gene to sons	Factor IX concentrate
von Willebrand's disease	vW factor	Most common hereditary bleeding disorder; affects both males and females	Cryoprecipitate, factor VIII products, or DDAVP

COLLABORATIVE CARE

Treatment of hemophilia focuses on preventing and/or treating bleeding, primarily by replacing deficient clotting factors. Treatment varies, depending on the clotting defect and the severity of the illness.

The *platelet count* is measured and coagulation studies, including the *APTT, bleeding time,* and *prothrombin time* are done as screening tests for hemophilia. *Clotting factor assays* are done to identify specific clotting factor deficiencies.

Pharmacology

Replacement of clotting factors is treatment for hemophilia. They may be given on a regular basis, as a prophylactic measure before surgery and dental procedures, and to control bleeding. Clotting factors may be given in the form of fresh frozen plasma, cryoprecipitates, or concentrates. They may be given intravenously, and may be self-administered. Fresh frozen plasma replaces all clotting factors (including both factor VIII and factor IX) except platelets. People who were treated for hemophilia between 1978 and 1985 have a high incidence of HIV disease, because donated blood was not routinely tested. Rigorous screening of donors, testing of donated blood, and heat treating of blood products have significantly reduced this risk. Factor VIII prepared by recombinant DNA does not contain human plasma, so it carries no risk of infectious disease. It is, however, very expensive.

Desmopressin acetate (DDAVP) also may be used to treat mild hemophilia and von Willebrand's disease. This drug stimulates the body to release vW factor, helping promote clotting.

 NURSING CARE

RISK FOR INJURY

Because hemophilia increases the risk for bleeding, preventing injury is a major nursing concern.

- Monitor for signs of bleeding, including hematomas, ecchymoses, purpura, and obvious oozing or bleeding. *Careful assessment is necessary to identify hidden or occult bleeding.*
- Notify the charge nurse or physician at the first sign of bleeding. *Prompt intervention decreases the risk of hemorrhage.*

- If bleeding occurs, apply gentle pressure until bleeding stops; apply ice; or apply a topical agent to stop bleeding as ordered. *These measures reduce bleeding until definitive treatment can be given.*
- Avoid intramuscular injections, rectal temperatures, and enemas. *These can cause tissue trauma, leading to bleeding.*
- Use safety measures such as a soft toothbrush and electric razor in personal care. *Use of a soft toothbrush and electric razor minimize the risk of skin and mucous membrane trauma that may result in bleeding.*
- Protect from injury as needed:
  - Pad side rails of the bed if restless or confused.
  - Assist with ambulation and activities as needed to prevent falling.
  - Provide adequate lighting, especially at night.
  - Keep halls and pathways free of obstruction; make no unnecessary changes in furniture arrangements.
  - Encourage to wear shoes with nonskid soles when ambulating.
  These measures help prevent accidental falls or tissue trauma from bumping into objects.

RISK FOR INEFFECTIVE THERAPEUTIC REGIMEN MANAGEMENT

- Assess knowledge and reinforce teaching about disorder and its treatments. *Teaching based on current level of knowledge and understanding is more effective.*
- Provide emotional support, and express confidence in self-care abilities. *Support and confidence are necessary to incorporate a care regimen into the client's lifestyle.*
- Provide opportunities to learn and practice administering clotting factors and topical hemostatic preparations under supervision. *Practice helps with mastery of psychomotor skills and confidence in the ability to perform self-care.*

 Discharge Considerations

Clients with bleeding disorders need to know how to prevent bleeding, how to treat it at home, and how to administer prescribed drugs. Teach to:

- Recognize and immediately report manifestations of internal bleeding: pallor, weakness, restlessness, headache, disorientation, pain, swelling.
- Apply cold packs and immobilize the joint for up to 24 to 48 hours if hemarthrosis occurs.
- Request a prescription for analgesia if pain is severe. Avoid aspirin, which increases the risk of continued bleeding.
- Ensure a safe home environment. For example, pad sharp furniture edges, leave on a light at night, do not use scatter rugs, and wear gloves when working in the house or yard.
- Use only electric razors.
- Wear a Medic-Alert bracelet in case of accident.

- Practice good dental hygiene to maintain dental health. If dental procedures are necessary, discuss the need for prophylactic clotting factor with dentist and physician.
- Avoid activities that increase the risk of injury, such as contact sports or racquetball.
- Consider physical demands of the job and risk for injury when planning a career or seeking employment.
- Follow safer-sex practices.
- Prepare and administer intravenous medications.

Refer clients with hemophilia or a family history of hemophilia who wish to have a family for genetic counseling.

White Blood Cell Disorders

White blood cells (WBCs), also called **leukocytes,** are part of the body's defense against infection and disease. On average, there are 5,000 to 10,000 WBCs per cubic millimeter of blood. WBCs make up about 1% of total blood volume. *Leukocytosis* is higher than normal WBC count; in *leukopenia,* the WBC count is lower than normal.

WBCs originate from stem cells in the bone marrow (see Figure 24-1). Unlike RBCs, which remain within blood vessels, WBCs use the circulation to move to where they are needed, and can migrate into other tissues. There are three major types of WBCs: granulocytes, monocytes, and lymphocytes.

Granulocytes are the most plentiful WBCs, accounting for 60% to 80% of the total leukocytes. Their cytoplasm looks granular and their nuclei have multiple lobes, giving them a distinctive appearance. Granulocytes play a key role in protecting the body from harmful microorganisms during acute inflammation and infection. There are three types of granulocytes:

1. *Neutrophils* make up 60% to 70% of circulating WBCs. They are also called *polymorphonuclear leukocytes (PMNs* or polys). Neutrophils are *phagocytic,* responsible for engulfing and destroying foreign matter. They are the first cells to arrive at a site of invasion. Neutrophils have a life span of about 10 hours and must constantly be replaced. *Segmented neutrophils* are mature cells, *bands* are immature neutrophils.
2. *Eosinophils* make up 1% to 3% of WBCs. Their numbers increase during allergic reactions and during infestations with parasites.
3. *Basophils* make up 0.3% to 0.5% of total WBCs and are believed to be a part of the hypersensitivity and stress responses.

Monocytes are the largest of the WBCs and make up approximately 3% to 8% of the total WBC count. Monocytes migrate into body tissues such as the skin, subcutaneous tissue, lungs, and liver. There they mature into *macrophages.* Both monocytes and macrophages are phagocytic cells.

Lymphocytes account for 20% to 30% of WBCs. Although they are small and nondescript, lymphocytes are the primary effectors and regulators of specific immune responses. *B lymphocytes (B cells)* are involved in forming antibodies, whereas *T lymphocytes (T cells)* take part in cell-mediated immunity. A third type of lymphocyte, *natural killer cells (NK cells)* also provide immune surveillance and resistance to infection. Normal laboratory values for WBCs are outlined in Table 24-5 ◆.

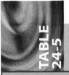

Agranulocytosis

Agranulocytosis (also called *neutropenia*) is a decrease in granulocytes. In agranulocytosis, both the total granulocyte count

TABLE 24-5	NORMAL WHITE BLOOD CELL COUNT AND DIFFERENTIAL	

LABORATORY TEST	NORMAL VALUES
WBC count	5,000–10,000/mm^3
Differential WBC count	
Neutrophils	60%–70% (3,000–7,000/mm^3)
Eosinophils	1%–3% (50–400/mm^3)
Basophils	0.3%–0.5% (25–200/mm^3)
Lymphocytes	20%–30% (1,000–4,000/mm^3)
Monocytes	3%–8% (100–600/mm^3)

and the number of neutrophils are significantly reduced. Impaired WBC formation in the bone marrow is the usual cause of agranulocytosis. Chemotherapy used in cancer treatment and other drugs can suppress bone marrow function. Increased cell destruction also can lead to low WBC levels.

CLINICAL alert

Decreased neutrophil counts greatly increase the risk of infection. Protect the client by providing a private room, using excellent handwashing, and limiting visitors.

Fatigue, weakness, sore throat, and stomatitis, *dysphagia* (difficult or painful swallowing), and fever and chills are the usual symptoms of agranulocytosis. It is diagnosed by the WBC count. The neutrophil count is less than 1,500 cells/mm^3; it may be less than 500/mm^3 when the condition is severe.

Any drug suspected of causing agranulocytosis is discontinued and infections are treated. Filgrastin (Neupogen), a drug that stimulates the growth and development of WBCs in bone marrow, may be given, particularly when neutropenia is associated with chemotherapy. This drug, which is given parenterally, is generally safe. Many clients develop bone pain while taking this drug. (See Table 24-7 later in the chapter for more information about filgrastin.)

Leukemia

Leukemia (literally, "white blood") is a malignant production of WBCs. Bone marrow is gradually replaced by immature, abnormal cells. Eventually, these abnormal cells spill into the circulation and invade other organs such as the liver, spleen, and lymph nodes. If the disease is not treated, leukemic cells replace all normal blood cells, leading to death.

Although leukemia is often considered a childhood disease, it affects many more adults than children each year. It is more common in people over age 50.

The cause of leukemia is unknown. Identified risk factors include exposure to chemicals such as benzene, genetic factors, viruses, immune disorders, certain cancer drugs, and exposure to large doses of radiation. Its incidence is higher in people who have been treated with radiation or chemotherapy, people living near sites of radiation testing, survivors of atomic bombing sites, radiologists, and people with Down syndrome or other genetic abnormalities.

PATHOPHYSIOLOGY

In leukemia, the bone marrow becomes almost totally filled with leukemic cells. These cells proliferate rapidly but are unable to function as normal WBCs. They cannot combat infection or maintain immune function. Because cells that produce RBCs and platelets are crowded out, severe anemia and bleeding results.

Leukemic cells leave the bone marrow and infiltrate other tissues such as the central nervous system, testes, skin,

GI tract, and the lymph nodes, liver, and spleen. Death usually results from internal hemorrhage and infections.

The manifestations of leukemia result from anemia, infection, and bleeding. Anemia causes pallor, fatigue, tachycardia, malaise, lethargy, and dyspnea. Infection, due to impaired WBC function, causes fever, night sweats, ulcers of the mouth and pharynx, respiratory, urinary tract, and skin infections. Septicemia may develop. Thrombocytopenia increases the risk of bleeding, leading to bruising, petechiae, and hematomas, as well as overt and hidden bleeding into organs. As leukemic cells infiltrate other organs, pain and other symptoms may occur. The manifestations of leukemia are summarized in Box 24-8.

Leukemia is classified by its onset and duration (acute or chronic) and by the type of abnormal cells (myelogenous or lymphocytic). *Acute leukemia* has an abrupt onset and progresses rapidly. The onset and progression of *chronic leukemia* is more gradual. *Myelocytic* (also known as *myelogenous*) *leukemias* involve myeloid stem cells in the bone marrow. These are the cells that normally become granulocytes (see Figure 24-1). Myelocytic leukemias interfere with the maturation of all blood cells, including RBCs and platelets. *Lymphocytic leukemias* involve immature lymphocytes in the bone marrow, spleen, lymph nodes, CNS, and other tissues. Table 24-6 ◆ compares the four major types of leukemia.

BOX 24-8
MANIFESTATIONS OF LEUKEMIA

SKIN AND MUCOUS MEMBRANES

- Pale lips and conjunctiva
- Petechiae, ecchymoses
- Skin and oral lesions
- Bleeding gums

NEUROLOGIC

- Headache
- Altered LOC

CARDIOVASCULAR

- Tachycardia, palpitations, murmurs
- Orthostatic hypotension
- Hemorrhage

RESPIRATORY

- Dyspnea

GASTROINTESTINAL

- Anorexia, nausea
- Abdominal pain
- Constipation, diarrhea
- Occult blood in stools
- Weight loss

TABLE 24-6 MAJOR CLASSIFICATIONS OF LEUKEMIA

CLASSIFICATION	CHARACTERISTICS	MANIFESTATIONS	TREATMENT
Acute myelocytic leukemia (AML)	Common in older adults; may affect children and young adults. Strongly associated with toxins, genetic disorders, and treatment of other cancers	Fatigue, weakness; fever; anemia; headache, bone and joint pain; abnormal bleeding and bruising; recurrent infection; lymph node, liver, and spleen enlargement	Chemotherapy; bone marrow transplant (BMT)
Chronic myelocytic leukemia (CML)	Primarily affects adults; early course is slow and stable, progressing to aggressive phase in 3–4 years.	Early: Weakness, fatigue, dyspnea on exertion; possible spleen enlargement Later: Fever, weight loss, night sweats	Interferon-alpha; chemotherapy, BMT
Acute lymphocytic leukemia (ALL)	Primarily affects children and young adults; leukemic cells may infiltrate CNS; 70% cure rate in children with aggressive treatment	Recurrent infections; bleeding; pallor, bone pain, weight loss, sore throat, fatigue, night sweats, weakness	Chemotherapy; BMT or stem cell transplant
Chronic lymphocytic leukemia (CLL)	Primarily affects older adults; insidious onset and slow, chronic course	Fatigue; exercise intolerance; enlarged lymph nodes and spleen; recurrent infections, pallor, edema, thrombophlebitis	Often requires no treatment; chemotherapy

COLLABORATIVE CARE

Treatment for leukemia focuses on achieving remission or cure and relieving symptoms. Cure is more likely in children than adults. The prognosis for each type of leukemia differs.

Laboratory tests that may be ordered include a *CBC with WBC differential* and *platelet count.* In all types of leukemia, the RBC is low, as are the hemoglobin and hematocrit. The platelet count also is low in most cases, while the WBC tends to be high. The *bone marrow* is examined to look for abnormal cells.

Chemotherapy

Systemic chemotherapy is used to destroy leukemic cells and produce remission. Chemotherapy interferes with the proliferation of rapidly dividing cells in the bone marrow. A combination of chemotherapy drugs is usually used to treat leukemia. Combining drugs reduces drug resistance, reduces toxicity from high doses of single agents, and interrupts cell growth at various stages of the cell cycle. Cancer treatment with chemotherapy is discussed in greater detail in Chapter 8.

Radiation Therapy

Radiation therapy may be used to shrink enlarged lymph nodes and destroy leukemic cells in the central nervous system (CNS). Radiation damages the cell DNA so that it is unable to reproduce and multiply. Although normal cells are affected, they are better able to recover from the damage caused by the radiation than are cancer cells. Radiation therapy is discussed in greater detail in Chapter 8.

Bone Marrow Transplantation

Bone marrow transplantation (BMT) may be used along with chemotherapy or radiation to treat some types of leukemia. There are two major categories of BMT. In *allogenic BMT,* the bone marrow of a healthy donor is infused into the client with the illness; in *autologous BMT,* the client is infused with his or her own bone marrow.

ALLOGENIC BMT. Prior to an allogenic BMT, high doses of chemotherapy and/or total body irradiation are given to eliminate leukemic cells. Then new marrow from a donor (often a sibling with a closely matched tissue type) is infused through a central venous line.

Following allogenic BMT, the client is at risk for *graft-versus-host disease.* In this disorder, immune cells in the donated bone marrow see the recipient's body tissue as foreign. Consequently, T lymphocytes in the donated marrow attack the liver, skin, and gastrointestinal tract, causing skin rashes and sloughing, diarrhea, gastrointestinal bleeding, and liver damage. The disorder is treated with antibiotics, steroids, and, if necessary, other drugs to suppress the immune response.

AUTOLOGOUS BMT. In an autologous bone marrow transplant, about 1 liter of the client's own bone marrow is withdrawn, treated to kill any tumor cells, and then frozen for storage.

Massive doses of chemotherapy and/or radiation are then given to destroy tumor cells in the client's body. These high doses destroy any remaining bone marrow and the client's immune system. The stored bone marrow then is thawed and infused through a central venous catheter. The infused bone marrow gradually restores bone marrow and immune function. In an alternative to autologous BMT, stem cells may be harvested from peripheral blood and then reinfused.

During autologous BMT, the client is hospitalized in a private room for at least 6 to 8 weeks. The risk of death due to immunosuppression is a major stressor. Complications that may occur are malnutrition, infection, and bleeding.

Biologic Therapy

Biologic agents such as interferons and interleukins may be used to treat some leukemias. These agents have multiple effects, including moderating immune function and slowing abnormal cell proliferation and growth. Side effects of interferon therapy include flulike symptoms, persistent fatigue and lethargy, weight loss, and muscle and joint pain.

Colony-stimulating factors (CSFs) regulate the growth and differentiation of blood cells. They often are given to clients whose bone marrow function is suppressed due to chemotherapy or leukemic changes. They also are given to stimulate stem cell development prior to harvesting bone marrow for autologous transplant. Bone pain is a common side effect of these agents. Clients also may experience fevers, chills, anorexia, muscle aches, and lethargy. See Table 24-7 ◆ for the nursing implications for colony stimulating factors.

NURSING CARE

ASSESSING

In all settings, it is important to recognize the manifestations of leukemia. This is particularly important when working with groups at higher risk (e.g., older adults and children). Assessment data related to manifestations of the disease or the current status of the client with leukemia is outlined in Box 24-9.

DIAGNOSING, PLANNING, AND IMPLEMENTING

Leukemia can be both a chronic and a life-threatening disease. Treatment may require toxic chemotherapy drugs, radiation, or bone marrow transplant. All these therapies have undesirable side effects. Nursing care focuses on the physical and psychosocial effects of the disease and its treatment.

RISK FOR INFECTION

- Institute infection precautions, including the following:
  - If prescribed, maintain protective isolation.
  - Use good handwashing, and remind all care providers and visitors to do the same.
- Assist to maintain good daily hygiene.
- Restrict visitors with colds, flu, or infections.
- Provide oral hygiene after every meal.
- As much as possible, avoid invasive procedures such as injections, intravenous catheters, catheterizations, and rectal and vaginal procedures. When necessary to perform these procedures, use strict aseptic technique. *These precautions minimize the client's exposure to bacterial, viral, and fungal pathogens.*
- Promptly report evidence of infection: fever, chills, sore throat, cough, chest pain, burning on urination, purulent drainage, and itching and burning in vaginal or rectal areas. *Early detection of infection allows prompt treatment and is vital when the immune system is suppressed.*
- Monitor vital signs and oxygen saturation at least every 4 hours. Promptly report increased pulse or respiratory rate, restlessness, hypotension, or changes in oxygen saturation. *The client with leukemia may not show typical manifestations of infection such as fever. It is important to be alert for other manifestations of infection or sepsis.*
- Report decreasing WBC levels to the charge nurse or physician. *The risk for infection increases as the WBC count declines.*
- Explain the precautions and restrictions to the client and family. Advise that strict precautions are usually temporary. *Understanding increases compliance and thereby lowers the risk of infection.*

IMBALANCED NUTRITION: LESS THAN BODY REQUIREMENTS

- Regularly monitor weight. *Continued weight loss or a weight below the normal range for height and age may indicate malnutrition. Maintaining adequate nutrition is vital during cancer treatment.*
- Implement measures to promote food and fluid intake, such as:
  - Provide oral hygiene before and after meals; use a soft toothbrush or sponges as necessary.
  - Experiment with food and liquids that have different textures and tastes to identify those best tolerated.
  - Increase liquid intake with meals.
  - Minimize intake of milk and milk products, which makes mucus more tenacious.
  - Encourage to sit upright when eating.
  - Ensure a clean and odor-free environment.
  - Provide medications for pain or nausea 30 minutes before meals, as needed.
  - Provide rest periods before meals.
  - Offer small, frequent meals six times a day. Encourage to avoid very sweet, rich, or greasy foods.
  - Use commercial supplements, such as Ensure.
  - Avoid painful or unpleasant procedures immediately before or after meals.
  Measures to reduce mouth inflammation, sore throat, nausea, and other effects of the disease and its treatment help promote

DRUG/CLASS	ACTION	NURSING IMPLICATIONS	CLIENT AND FAMILY TEACHING
Erythropoietin ▪ Epoetin alfa (Epogen, Procrit)	Epoetin alfa mimics the action of the hormone erythropoietin in stimulating RBC production. It is used to restore and maintain RBC counts during chemotherapy, renal failure, or zidovudine therapy for HIV disease.	Administer parenterally (IV or SC). Do not shake and do not mix with other drugs. Use only one dose per vial. Monitor BP during treatment; report elevations. Monitor hemoglobin and hematocrit levels.	This drug will be given 3 times per week by injection. Keep all scheduled appointments and BP checks. If you have high blood pressure, take your medication and follow your diet closely. This drug can increase your blood pressure. Headache is common while taking this drug. If it becomes severe, contact your doctor.
Granulocyte colony-stimulating factor ▪ Filgrastim (Neupogen)	Filgrastim acts on cells in the bone marrow to increase neutrophil (granulocyte) production. It also enhances the immune function of mature neutrophils. It is used to improve neutrophil counts during chemotherapy, after BMT, and in chronic neutrophilia.	Administer parenterally (IV or SC). Use only one dose per vial. Store refrigerated. Can be allowed to reach room temperature for up to 6 hours before giving. Report elevated WBC and neutrophil counts. Monitor temperature every 4 hours.	This drug is given by injection; you may be taught how to give it to yourself. Bone pain is a common side effect of this drug. Report it to your doctor if you need analgesics for pain relief. Keep all scheduled appointments.
Granulocyte–macrophage colony-stimulating factor ▪ Sargramostim (Leukine)	Sargramostim stimulates bone marrow production of granulocytes and monocytes/macrophages. It also increases the function of mature WBCs. It is given after BMT to stimulate WBC production.	Administer parenterally by IV infusion or SC injection. Give within 6 hours of reconstitution. Slow IV infusion to half rate if dyspnea develops. Notify physician if dyspnea worsens.	Immediately contact the nurse if you develop difficulty breathing or palpitations during the infusion. Keep all scheduled appointments.
Thrombopoietic growth factor ▪ Oprelvekin (Neumega)	Oprelvekin (interleukin-11) increases platelet production. It may be given during chemotherapy to treat resulting thrombocytopenia.	Administer by SC injection. Use reconstituted solution within 3 hours. Causes sodium and water retention; immediately report manifestations of fluid overload. Report hypokalemia and cardiac dysrhythmias.	You may be taught how to give this drug to yourself. Keep all scheduled appointments. Report any of the following to your doctor: Shortness of breath, swelling of arms or legs, chest pain, fatigue or weakness, irregular heartbeat, blurred vision.

food and fluid intake. Small, frequent meals are often better tolerated, especially high-protein, high-kcal foods.

IMPAIRED ORAL MUCOUS MEMBRANE

- Frequently assess mouth for swelling, lesions, or bleeding. Report complaints of mouth pain or difficulty swallowing to the charge nurse or physician. Culture oral lesions as ordered. *The client with leukemia is at risk for bacterial, viral (especially herpes simplex), and fungal (especially* Candida*) infections of the oral mucosa.*
- Provide a 1:1 solution of hydrogen peroxide and water or warm saline as a mouth rinse for use every 2 to 4 hours. Apply petroleum jelly to the lips as needed to prevent dryness and cracking. *These measures promote healing and comfort and help prevent infection.*
- Encourage use of soft-bristle toothbrush or sponge to clean the teeth and gums. *Soft-bristle brushes reduce trauma to the gums and mucous membranes of the mouth.*
- Administer drugs as ordered to treat infections or relieve pain. *Topical antifungal agents such as nystatin may be ordered for* Candida *infections. Topical anesthetics such as lidocaine may be prescribed to promote comfort.*

- Instruct to avoid alcohol-based mouthwashes, citrus fruit juices, spicy foods, foods that are either very hot or very cold, alcohol, and crusty foods. Encourage bland, cool foods and cool liquids. *Avoiding food and liquids that irritate the mucosa increases comfort and oral intake.*

INEFFECTIVE PROTECTION

Bleeding due to decreased platelets is a common cause of death in leukemia.

- Monitor level of consciousness (LOC) and vital signs every 4 hours and report changes such as hypotension or tachycardia to the charge nurse or physician. *A change in LOC or tachycardia can be early signs of bleeding; hypotension is a later sign.*
- Promptly report manifestations of bleeding:
  - Increased petechiae, bruising, or hematoma formation
  - Obvious bleeding from gums, nose, prolonged bleeding from puncture sites
  - Bright red or coffee-ground emesis; rectal bleeding or tarry stools
  - Hematuria (blood in the urine)
  - Vaginal bleeding
  - Changes in neurologic status: headache, visual changes, altered mental status, decreasing LOC, seizures
  - Complaints of epigastric pain, absent bowel sounds, increasing abdominal girth, abdominal rigidity
  Prompt reporting allows early treatment of bleeding or hemorrhage. Bleeding into the abdomen or intracranial bleeding may not be readily apparent, and identified only by changes in neurologic status or abdominal assessment data.
- Avoid invasive rectal, vaginal, or urinary tract procedures, and parenteral injections if possible. *Invasive procedures can damage mucous membranes and tissues, increasing the risk of bleeding.*
- Apply pressure to puncture sites for 3 to 5 minutes; apply pressure to arterial blood gas sites for 15 to 20 minutes. *Pressure prevents prolonged bleeding by prompting hemostasis and clot formation.*
- Instruct to avoid straining to have a bowel movement and forceful coughing, sneezing, and blowing the nose. *Avoiding these activities reduces the risk of external or internal bleeding.*

ANTICIPATORY GRIEVING

Grieving is an emotional response to the losses associated with a life-threatening illness such as leukemia. See Chapter 9 for more information about loss and grieving.

- Use therapeutic communication skills to allow open discussion of losses as well as permission to grieve. *Encouraging discussion about the meaning of the loss helps to decrease some of the anxiety associated with loss.*
- Accept the client's and family's responses to the diagnosis without making judgments. *People respond to stress and griev-*

ing in many different ways. *Denial, anger, bargaining, and depression are common. Demonstrating acceptance of responses and behaviors promotes trust.*

■ Assist to identify ways of managing past stressful situations. In addition, help identify effective coping strategies; sources of strength; reactions to changing family roles; and spiritual or cultural influences on grief reactions. *Grieving is a normal response to a real or potential loss that begins at the time of diagnosis. Identifying resources and strategies that have been successfully used in the past helps the client and family members use these resources during the early crisis of dealing with the diagnosis.*

■ Identify agencies, groups, and organizations that may help with the grieving process, and make referrals as indicated. Consider self-help groups, cancer support groups, single-parent groups, and bereavement groups. *A support group that includes others who are anticipating or have experienced a similar loss can decrease the client's feelings of isolation.*

EVALUATING

When evaluating the effectiveness of nursing care for the client with leukemia, look at data that demonstrates freedom from infection (e.g., no fever, vital signs within normal limits, etc.). Evaluate weight, food intake, and the integrity of oral mucous membranes. Assess for evidence of bleeding. Finally, look at data that demonstrates coping with the diagnosis, such as talking about the disease and its potential effect on lifestyle and family relationships.

Discharge Considerations

Because leukemia is a chronic disease requiring long-term management, most required care is provided by the client and family members. Teaching is vital to prepare for discharge.

Reinforce teaching about leukemia and its effects, the function of bone marrow, and potential complications. Discuss cancer as a chronic illness that often can be cured or controlled. Provide information about planned treatment, including chemotherapy, radiation, and/or bone marrow transplantation. Discuss the rationale for each type of treatment and techniques to manage undesirable side effects of the treatment.

Encourage a balance of activity with rest to reduce fatigue. Discuss measures to maintain weight and nutrition: eat several small, bland meals each day; maintain an ample fluid intake by drinking 4 to 6 glasses of water daily. Instruct to report any continued weight loss, loss of appetite, or an inability to eat for 24 hours. Refer to a dietitian for further teaching and diet planning.

Discuss the importance of measures to prevent infection: wash hands frequently, especially after using the toilet and before preparing foods or eating; bathe daily; avoid using per-

ineal powders or sprays that could dry mucous membranes; brush teeth using a soft-bristle toothbrush after meals and see a dentist regularly; avoid crowds and contact with people who are ill. Instruct to regularly inspect skin and mucous membranes for signs of bleeding or infection. Instruct to report signs of infection such as fever, chills, burning on urination, foul-smelling urine, vaginal or rectal discharge, or skin lesions to the health care provider. Advise to avoid immunizations unless specifically ordered by the oncologist.

Discuss measures to reduce the risk of bleeding or injury: Avoid contact sports or strenuous exercise if platelet count is low; use an electric razor for shaving; avoid using rectal or vaginal suppositories, vaginal tampons, or enemas to minimize trauma to mucous membranes; increase fiber in the diet, and drink ample water to maintain soft stool and prevent straining. Advise to avoid over-the-counter drugs that increase the risk of bleeding, such as aspirin and preparations containing aspirin, and NSAIDs. Instruct to report any bleeding (nosebleeds, rectal bleeding, vomiting blood, excessive menstrual periods, blood in the urine, bleeding gums, bruises, or collections of blood under the skin) or changes in behavior to the health care provider.

The client and family may need help with physical care, finances, and transportation after discharge. Provide referrals to social services, support groups, home care services if needed, and other agencies that can provide needed services (such as local chapters of the American Cancer Society, which can provide hospital beds and transportation for outpatient cancer treatment).

See the Critical Thinking Care Map at the end of this chapter for an opportunity to use the nursing process to plan care for a client with acute myelocytic leukemia.

Multiple Myeloma

Multiple myeloma is a malignancy in which plasma cells multiply uncontrollably and infiltrate bone marrow, lymph nodes, and other tissues. *Plasma cells* are B-cell lymphocytes that develop to produce antibodies (*immunoglobins*).

The incidence of multiple myeloma is higher in African Americans than Caucasians. It affects men more often than women, and its incidence increases with age. Multiple myeloma rarely occurs before age 40.

PATHOPHYSIOLOGY

As myeloma cells proliferate, they replace the bone marrow and infiltrate the bone itself. The bone is weakened by these abnormal cells, and may break without trauma (a *pathologic fracture*). Myeloma cells also secrete abnormal immunoglobins. These abnormal proteins are ineffective as antibodies to maintain B-cell or humoral immunity (see Chapter 13). They also increase the viscosity of the blood and damage kidney tubules.

The disease develops slowly. Bone or back pain is the most common symptom. As the disease progresses, the pain becomes more severe. Pathologic fractures occur, particularly in weight-bearing bones such as the vertebrae, pelvis, and femur. Vertebral fractures may compress the spinal cord, causing neurologic symptoms. The client becomes more susceptible to infections and develops signs of anemia and bleeding tendencies. Kidney damage may cause manifestations of renal failure (see Chapter 21).

COLLABORATIVE CARE

Laboratory and diagnostic tests are ordered to confirm the diagnosis of multiple myeloma. Urine samples usually are positive for *Bence Jones proteins,* abnormal proteins produced by plasma cells in some forms of multiple myeloma. The *CBC* reveals moderate to severe anemia. *Bone marrow studies* show excessive immature plasma cells. *Bone x-rays* reveal punched-out holes in the bone, particularly in the vertebrae, ribs, skull, pelvis, femurs, clavicles, and scapulae.

There is no cure for multiple myeloma. Treatment focuses on symptom relief *(palliative).* The disease course typically is chronic and progressive; death usually occurs within 2 to 5 years of the diagnosis.

Chemotherapy, radiation therapy, and pharmacology are used to decrease the tumor size and reduce bone pain. Pain is controlled with analgesics. Blood transfusions are used to treat anemia, and infections are controlled with antibiotics. Braces or splints may be ordered as needed to maintain mobility.

NURSING CARE

Clients with multiple myeloma require nursing care similar to that required by clients with leukemia. Pain and the risk for pathologic fractures are additional nursing care considerations discussed in this section.

CHRONIC PAIN

- Assess pain, including location, onset, duration, precipitating factors, and effective relief measures. *Assessment provides baseline data for evaluating the effectiveness of pain relief measures.*
- Assist into the position of greatest comfort. *A client who is weak and uncomfortable may need assistance with repositioning.*
- Support position with pillows. *The client may have painful bony prominences and require the support of many pillows for comfort.*
- Teach effective use of prescribed analgesics. Involve the family as needed to help ensure that pain is relieved. *Taking analgesics on a regular schedule and before pain becomes severe increases their effectiveness.*
- Teach use of nonpharmacologic methods of pain control, including relaxation or guided imagery. *Nonpharmacologic pain management strategies augment the effectiveness of analgesics.*
- Provide for uninterrupted rest periods. *Rest promotes muscle relaxation and emotional equilibrium, increasing the ability to manage pain.*
- Report unrelieved pain to the physician. *Because of the chronic and increasing nature of cancer pain, different or additional medications may be necessary. See Chapter 8 for more information about cancer pain management.*

IMPAIRED PHYSICAL MOBILITY

- Reposition carefully and gently. *Fractures may occur during common activities such as turning or repositioning. Gentle handling reduces the risk of pathologic fracture.*
- Change position at least every 2 hours; more frequently as needed. *Repositioning promotes comfort and minimizes the risk of skin breakdown.*
- Provide a trapeze to assist in repositioning. *A trapeze enables the client to assist with repositioning and promotes self-care.*
- Place needed items close at hand. *This reduces the need to reach for objects and the risk of falling.*
- Place bed in low position, use side rails as indicated, and place the call bell within reach. Keep halls and pathways free of clutter, remove scatter rugs, and provide adequate lighting, a nonslippery floor, and nonskid soles on shoes. *These safety measures reduce the risk for falling and injury.*

Discharge Considerations

As with leukemia, clients with multiple myeloma must be actively involved in their disease management. Teach signs and symptoms that indicate complications and the need to seek medical help. These complications include infection, pathologic fractures, bleeding, and severe anemia. Infection is the leading cause of death for clients with multiple myeloma. Discuss hospice services with the client and family. Although clients qualify for hospice services during the last 6 months of life, many do not seek services until death is imminent. Hospice services provide pain management, emotional support, and respite services for caregivers.

Lymphatic System Disorders

Lymphoid tissues are connective tissues that contain many lymphocytes, the WBCs primarily responsible for specific immune responses. Lymphoid tissue can be found throughout the body. The tonsils are examples of lymphoid tissue.

The **lymphatic system** of the body is made up of lymphoid organs, including the lymph vessels, the lymph nodes, the spleen, and the thymus. *Lymph* resembles plasma, but contains fewer proteins. *Lymph vessels* collect lymph from body tissues and return it to the circulation. *Lymph nodes* located along lymphatic vessels filter bacteria and other debris from the lymph before it is returned to the bloodstream. **Lymphadenopathy** is swelling and enlargement of the lymph nodes. It may occur in response to infections, inflammation, or cancers. T cells mature in the *thymus,* an important organ in the developing immune system of infants. The *spleen* filters bacteria and aged blood cells from the blood and also is involved in the immune response.

Lymphangitis and Lymphedema

Lymphangitis is inflammation of the lymph vessels. It is usually caused by a bacterial infection. Clients with lymphangitis develop painful red streaks following the lymph vessels and extending up an arm or leg. If lymph nodes also become inflamed, it is called *lymphadenitis.* The lymph nodes are swollen and may be tender. Fever, malaise, and chills also accompany lymphangitis or lymphadenitis.

Lymphedema is edema caused by obstruction of lymph vessels. Obstruction of the lymph vessels from surgical removal of lymph nodes (as is done in a radical mastectomy), scarring of lymph nodes following radiation, or invasion of lymph nodes by tumor may cause lymphedema. Clients who live in the tropics may develop *elephantiasis,* a type of lymphedema caused by filaria, a nematode worm.

The affected extremity is swollen and edematous (Figure 24-7 ◆). Early in the course of the disorder, the edema is soft and pitting. With time, the edematous tissue becomes hard to the touch *(brawny edema)*. The skin appears thick and hardened and may resemble an orange peel. The edema may worsen in warm weather and (if the legs are affected) after standing for long periods.

COLLABORATIVE CARE

Collaborative care for clients with lymphatic system disorders focuses on relieving edema, maintaining skin integrity in the affected extremity, and preventing or treating infection.

For lymphangitis, moist heat is applied and the affected extremity is elevated and immobilized. Meticulous skin and wound care is vital. Antibiotics are prescribed to treat the infection. Penicillin G is often used because streptococcal bacteria are common causative organisms.

Lymphedema is often chronic and requires longer-term treatment. Measures such as the following are ordered:

- Elevate the extremity, especially during sleep.
- Use elastic stockings, elastic bandages, or pneumatic pressure devices.
- Provide meticulous skin hygiene.
- Remain on bed rest.
- Restrict dietary sodium.

Occasionally, surgery may be performed to relieve pain, remove cancerous tissue, or treat repeated episodes of lymphangitis in the affected extremity.

Figure 24-7. ◆ Severe lymphedema of the lower extremity.

NURSING CARE

The nursing care focus for clients with lymphatic system disorders is the same as the collaborative care focus: relieving edema, maintaining skin integrity, and preventing infection.

Measure the circumference of the affected extremity daily or as ordered. Maintain intake and output records, and weigh daily. Report changes to the charge nurse or physician. Restrict sodium intake and help choose low-sodium foods.

Apply antiembolic stockings and intermittent pressure devices as ordered. Remove stockings and pressure devices at least once each shift to inspect the underlying skin for redness, irritation, dryness, or breakdown. Document findings. Elevate extremities while seated or in bed. Keep skin clean and dry, especially between toes. Use protective devices such as egg crate foam, sheepskin, pillows, or padding to reduce the risk of skin breakdown.

Discharge Considerations

Teach how to apply and use intermittent pressure devices and/or elastic stockings. Instruct to wear elastic stockings during waking hours and to remove them while sleeping. Emphasize the importance of inspecting the skin at least daily for signs of breakdown or cracking.

Teach skin care to promote its integrity, prevent breakdown, and reduce the risk for infection. Help develop a schedule and plan for elevating the affected extremity that interferes as little as possible with daily schedules. Discuss other prescribed measures such as any activity restriction, dietary sodium restriction, and diuretic therapy. Provide a list of high-sodium foods to avoid, and refer to a dietitian for further teaching about salt-restricted diets. If the client is taking a potassium-wasting diuretic, provide a list of foods that are high in potassium (see Box 5-9 in Chapter 5).

Provide information about contacts for questions, and make referrals as needed. The client may face long years of self-management and may need assistance with health care management, meals, and housework.

> **BOX 24-10**
> **MANIFESTATIONS**
> **OF HODGKIN'S DISEASE**
>
> - One or more painless, enlarged lymph nodes
> - Fever
> - Night sweats
> - Pruritus
> - Weight loss
> - Fatigue
> - Malaise

Infectious Mononucleosis

Infectious mononucleosis is an acute infectious disease caused by the Epstein–Barr virus (EBV). This disease, which primarily affects young adults, is usually benign and self-limiting. It appears to be transmitted by saliva; hence, it is often called the "kissing disease."

When the virus enters the body, it invades B cells in the lymphoid tissues of the oropharynx. The infection causes increased lymphocyte production and swelling of lymph glands. The manifestations begin with headache, malaise, and fatigue. Most clients with infectious mononucleosis have fever, sore throat, and enlargement and pain in the cervical lymph nodes. Enlargement of the spleen occurs in about half of all people with the illness.

Laboratory findings include increased lymphocytes and monocytes; about one fifth of the cells are atypical in form. The WBC count increases and remains high for 4 to 8 weeks. Platelet counts are often low during the illness.

Recovery occurs in 2 to 3 weeks. However, weakness and lethargy may last for up to 3 months. Treatment includes bed rest and analgesics to relieve the symptoms.

Malignant Lymphoma

Malignant lymphomas are cancerous tumors of lymphoid tissue. They are characterized by lymphocyte proliferation and progressive, painless enlargement of the lymph nodes.

PATHOPHYSIOLOGY

Lymphomas are classified as Hodgkin's disease (or Hodgkin's lymphoma) and non-Hodgkin's lymphomas.

Hodgkin's Disease

Hodgkin's disease is one of the most curable of all cancers. It is characterized by painless, progressive enlargement of one or more lymph nodes and the presence of *Reed–Sternberg* cells in the affected node. It usually affects people between the ages of 15 and 35 or over age 50. It is more common in men than women. The cause of Hodgkin's disease is unknown, but it may be linked to viral infection (Epstein–Barr virus). The lymph nodes of the neck or above the clavicle often are the first affected. If untreated, it spreads via the lymphatic system to nodes throughout the body.

The most common manifestation of Hodgkin's disease is an enlarged lymph node that is not painful or tender. The node or nodes are firm but movable. Other common symptoms are listed in Box 24-10.

Non-Hodgkin's Lymphoma

Non-Hodgkin's lymphomas are more common than Hodgkin's disease. Unlike Hodgkin's disease, multiple lymph nodes and lymphoid tissue in other body tissues are involved. Non-Hodgkin's lymphomas tend to occur in older adults. They also are more common in people whose immune system has been suppressed by HIV disease or immunosuppressive drugs (e.g., people who have had an organ transplant).

The first symptom of non-Hodgkin's lymphoma often is an enlarged lymph node. The client may, however, have symptoms such as abdominal pain, nausea, vomiting, or bloody diarrhea. Involvement of other organs can lead to symptoms of urinary tract obstruction or infection, neurologic symptoms, shortness of breath, cough, or chest pain. Systemic manifestations such as weight loss, fatigue, and night sweats also may be present. The prognosis for non-Hodgkin's lymphoma is not as good as it is for Hodgkin's disease.

COLLABORATIVE CARE

The diagnosis of lymphoma is made based on *biopsy* of tissue from the enlarged node or tissue mass. If Reed–Sternberg cells are present, the diagnosis of Hodgkin's disease is confirmed. For both Hodgkin's disease and non-Hodgkin's lymphoma, the *Ann Arbor staging system* is used to determine the extent and severity of the disease and to estimate the prognosis. This system uses the number and location of involved lymph nodes, as well as the presence of systemic symptoms to stage the disease.

Radiation Therapy

Radiation therapy is used to treat both Hodgkin's disease and non-Hodgkin's lymphoma. Therapy usually involves external radiation of the involved lymph node region. If the disease is advanced, total nodal irradiation may be done (Figure 24-8 ◆). This may cause permanent sterility. In many cases, radiation therapy is used in conjunction with chemotherapy.

Chemotherapy

Single-agent or combination chemotherapy is also used to treat both Hodgkin's disease and non-Hodgkin's lymphoma. The choice of drug combination depends on the stage of the disease as well as the client's age and general condition.

NURSING CARE

Nursing care of the client with malignant lymphoma involves providing physical and emotional support throughout the course of treatment. The client is at risk for infection because cancerous lymphocytes are less effective in mounting an immune response. Nutritional status also must be considered due to the effects of the disease and treatment on appetite and food tolerance. See *Risk for Infection* and *Imbalanced Nutrition: Less Than Body Requirements* in the nursing care section for leukemia for nursing activities to address these problems.

RISK FOR IMPAIRED SKIN INTEGRITY

Pruritus and night sweats (symptoms of lymphoma) increase the risk for skin lesions. Radiation therapy also can damage the skin.

■ Discuss measures to relieve itching:

Figure 24-8. ◆ Areas of radiation for total nodal radiation therapy.

■ Use cool water and a mild soap to bathe.
■ Blot (rather than rub) dry skin; apply plain cornstarch or nonperfumed lotion or powder to the skin unless contraindicated (lotions and powders may not be allowed if undergoing radiation therapy).
■ Use lightweight cotton blankets and clothing.
■ Maintain adequate humidity and a cool room temperature.
■ Wash bedding and clothes in mild detergent, and put them through second rinse cycle.
   Pruritus is aggravated by excessive warmth, excessive dryness, rough fabrics, fatigue, and stress. These interventions reduce mechanical or chemical irritation of the skin.

NAUSEA

■ Administer ordered antiemetics before chemotherapy is started. *Premedication with an antiemetic can prevent nausea and reduce the psychological association between chemotherapy and nausea.*
■ Teach measures to prevent or relieve nausea and vomiting:
   ■ Eat soda crackers and suck on hard candy.
   ■ Eat soft, bland foods that are cold or at room temperature.
   ■ Avoid unpleasant odors, and get fresh air.
   ■ Do not eat immediately before chemotherapy.

- Use distraction or progressive muscle relaxation when nauseated.
  Crackers and hard candy often relieve queasiness. Foods that are hot, warm, salty, sweet, or have strong odors often increase nausea. Alternative methods of relieving nausea may be effective.

FATIGUE

- Assess complaints of malaise (a vague feeling of body weakness or discomfort) and fatigue (a pervasive, drained feeling that cannot be eliminated). *Malaise and fatigue are subjective experiences.*
- Encourage expression of feelings about the disease and its impact on lifestyle and roles. *Discussion may help the client identify lifestyle priorities.*
- Encourage enjoyable but quiet activities, such as reading, listening to music, or doing puzzles. *Enjoyable activities such as these help conserve energy and decrease fatigue.*
- Help establish priorities, and include rest periods or naps when scheduling daily activities. *This helps the client maintain control and self-esteem while conserving energy.*
- Encourage to delegate some responsibilities to others. *Delegating responsibilities helps conserve energy while allowing others to be more involved in care and decision making.*
- Encourage a diet high in carbohydrates and fluids. *A high-carbohydrate diet helps maintain energy stores, while increased fluid intake promotes excretion of waste products that may cause malaise and fatigue.*

DISTURBED BODY IMAGE

- Collect subjective data related to body image by asking questions such as:
  - What do you like the most/least about your body?
  - What do you understand about your disease?
  - How do you feel about this illness?
  - How do you think your illness or treatment will affect you?
  - Has the illness changed the way you believe others will respond to you?
    A person's image of his or her body is based on past and present experiences. It includes both the physical body and emotional responses to that body. Body image changes constantly.
- Assess for objective signs of altered body image, such as refusal to touch or look at a body part or to look in a mirror; refusal to discuss body changes; refusal to participate in self-care or rehabilitation; increasing dependence on others; signs of grieving (weeping, despair, anger); hostility toward healthy people; or withdrawal from social contacts.
  Although there is no one response to an altered body image, clients may demonstrate any of the above signs.
- Teach ways to cope with *alopecia* (hair loss). Discuss using wigs, scarves, hats, and caps during hair loss and regrowth. Teach scalp care using baby shampoo or mild soap, a soft brush, and mineral oil to reduce itching. Emphasize the importance of using sunscreen and covering the head to prevent sunburn. If eyelashes and eyebrows are lost, teach methods of protecting the eyes, such as eyeglasses and caps with wide brims. Discuss and refer to resources (such as the American Cancer Society or insurance) for financial assistance to buy wigs. *Alopecia may range from thinning of hair to total hair loss. Regrowth usually begins 2 to 3 months after treatment ends. New hair may be softer, more curly, and slightly different in color.*
- Assess knowledge of the effects of illness and treatment on sexuality and reproduction. Provide information and clarify misconceptions as needed. Encourage the client and significant other to verbalize concerns. Discuss options such as storing sperm in a sperm bank prior to undergoing radiation therapy. Refer for counseling as indicated. *Sexual function often is altered by the disease and the effects of treatment. This may include temporary or permanent sterility, changes in menstruation, and changes in libido (sexual desire).*
- Encourage participation in support groups. *Support groups are often effective in helping the client and family deal with loss and altered body image.*

Discharge Considerations

Teach about lymphoma, its treatment, and the side effects of treatments. Topics that are appropriate for the client with leukemia are also appropriate for the client with a malignant lymphoma. In addition, teach the client and family to:

- Care for the skin and avoid scratching to reduce the risk of infection.
- Report new or different symptoms that may indicate extension of the disease.
- Use complementary pain management strategies as well as prescribed drugs to promote comfort. See Chapter 8 for more information about cancer pain management.
- Plan activities of daily living to ensure adequate rest and exercise.
- Eat a well-balanced diet.

Refer to the local chapter of the American Cancer Society for information, financial assistance, and counseling. Clients with malignant lymphomas may obtain a list of state and local agencies that offer information about the disease and financial assistance from the Leukemia Society of America.

Nursing Process Case Study
■ CLIENT WITH HODGKIN'S DISEASE

Albin Quito, age 28, is a nurse manager in a large teaching hospital. Lately, he has noticed that he is more tired than usual, often wakes up at night covered with sweat, and just does not feel well. He attributed his symptoms to "a touch of the flu" and to his busy work schedule. Yesterday morning, he noticed a large swollen area on the right side of his neck. He made an appointment with his primary health provider. At that appointment, a large cervical lymph node was found, and blood was drawn. A biopsy of the node and a computed tomography (CT) scan of the chest were scheduled.

Assessment David Herzog, the clinic nurse, obtains a nursing assessment on Mr. Quito. His physical exam is normal, with the exception of the enlarged node, which is not painful to touch. When Mr. Quito is weighed, he says that he has lost 7 lbs. (3.2 kg) in the past 2 months. Test results include mild anemia and an increased neutrophil count. Reed–Sternberg cells are found in the lymph node biopsy. The physician makes the diagnosis of Hodgkin's disease and tells Mr. Quito that his prognosis is very good. After learning about treatment options, Mr. Quito decides to undergo radiation therapy.

Diagnosis Mr. Herzog identifies the following nursing diagnoses:

- Anxiety related to malignancy and uncertainty about ability to continue working in his present position
- Risk for Infection related to impaired immunologic function
- Fatigue related to the effects of the cancer and planned treatment

Expected Outcomes The expected outcomes in the plan of care specify that Mr. Quito will:

- Verbalize a decrease in anxiety.
- Remain free of infection.
- Use methods to preserve energy.

Planning and Implementation The following nursing interventions are planned and implemented:

- Encourage to discuss treatment schedule with supervisor to plan release time.
- Encourage to join a support group for people with cancer.
- Provide information about illness and radiation therapy.
- Discuss ways to decrease the risk of infection.
- Discuss energy management strategies such as:
  - Take a short nap once or twice a day to provide total body rest.
  - Do not overexert during weekends.
  - Maintain a well-balanced diet.

Evaluation When Mr. Quito returns to begin radiation, he brings his friend Nancy. He asks Mr. Herzog to discuss his treatment with her. Mr. Quito says, "I am still really scared, but being able to talk about this with Nancy will help a lot." Mr. Quito has made arrangements for a leave of absence from work, with the understanding that his job will be held for him. He states that he will have some money problems but is working them out. He also says he feels that taking a nap is silly but he'll try it. They have found a cancer support group and plan to attend the next meeting.

 Critical Thinking in the Nursing Process

1. Review radiation and chemotherapy in Chapter 8. How do each of these treatments work to kill malignant cells?
2. What information will you give Mr. Quito about preventing infection while he is at home?
3. How might the psychological and socioeconomic effect of the diagnosis of cancer differ in a young adult versus an older adult?

Nursing Interventions Classification

The following Nursing Interventions (McCloskey & Bulechek, 2000) may be considered when planning care for clients with hematologic disorders:

- Bleeding Precautions
- Blood Products Administration
- Emotional Support
- Energy Management
- Environmental Management: Safety
- Infection Protection
- Nutrition Management
- Oral Health Restoration
- Teaching: Disease Process

(*Note:* The bibliography listings for this and all chapters have been compiled at the back of the book.)

Chapter Review

key terms by topic

Use the CD-ROM disk enclosed with your textbook to hear the pronunciation of the key terms in the chapter.

Hematologic disorders
erythrocytes, leukocytes, platelets

Red blood cell disorders
hemoglobin, hemolysis, anemia, poly-cythemia

Platelet and coagulation disorders
thrombocytopenia, hemostasis, petechiae, hemophilia

White blood cell disorders
agranulocytosis, leukemia, multiple myeloma

Lymphatic system disorders
lymphatic system, lymphadenopathy, malignant lymphomas

key points

■ Because blood is the transport medium for oxygen, nutrients, and other substances, disorders that affect the blood often have widespread effects on other organs and systems.

■ The primary function of RBCs is oxygen transport to the cells. Anemia, lack of RBCs and hemoglobin, is a common disorder. It has a variety of causes, including nutritional deficiencies, genetic disorders, inadequate RBC production, and loss of RBCs through bleeding or abnormal destruction. Too few RBCs or inadequate hemoglobin can lead to cellular hypoxia, causing weakness and fatigue.

■ Polycythemia (too many RBCs) usually develops secondarily to chronic hypoxia, for example, in clients with chronic lung disease. Too many RBCs increase the viscosity or "stickiness" of the blood.

■ Platelets are vital to the process of blood clotting (coagulation) and control of bleeding. Clients with thrombocytopenia (low platelet count) are at significant risk for bleeding.

■ Hemophilia is a clotting disorder that is genetically transmitted on the X chromosome from mother to sons. In hemophilia, lack of a specific clotting factor interrupts the clotting cascade. Again, this leads to a significant risk for bleeding with minor injuries.

■ The primary function of WBCs is to fight off infection, destroy foreign matter, and eliminate damaged or abnormal cells in the body. Too few WBCs affects immune function.

■ Leukemia is a malignancy in which abnormal WBCs multiply, gradually replacing normal bone marrow and impairing the ability to form normal blood cells and fight off infection. The risk factors, treatment, and prognosis for different types of leukemia vary.

■ Multiple myeloma also is a WBC malignancy. It, however, affects B lymphocytes called plasma cells. These cells proliferate and invade bone marrow, lymph nodes, and other tissues. Clients with multiple myeloma have bone pain and a high risk for pathologic fractures.

■ The lymphatic system also is involved in the immune response. Lymph nodes often swell during infections. Painless swelling of a lymph node, however, may indicate a malignancy such as Hodgkin's disease, non-Hodgkin's lymphoma, or others.

Medialink

Additional interactive resources for this chapter can be found on the Companion Website at www.prenhall.com/burke. Click on Chapter 24 and "Begin" to select the activities for this chapter.

For NCLEX review questions and an audio glossary, access the accompanying CD-ROM in this book.

for further study

For more information about blood transfusions, see Chapter 10.

For more information about corticosteroids, see Chapter 13.

For more information about radiation therapy, see Chapter 8.

For more about loss and grieving, see Chapter 9.

For more information about immunity, see Chapter 13.

For more information about kidney damage and renal failure, see Chapter 21.

For more information about potassium, see Chapter 5.

Critical Thinking Care Map

Caring for a Client with Acute Myelocytic Leukemia
NCLEX-PN Focus Area: Safe, Effective Care Environment

Case Study: Catherine Cole is a 37-year-old secretary. About 2 months ago, she began to tire easily and experience night sweats and an intermittent fever. She also noticed that her skin was pale, she bruised easily, and she was having heavier menstrual periods. After seeing her primary care physician, Mrs. Cole is admitted to the hospital for a bone marrow biopsy.

Nursing Diagnosis: Ineffective Protection

COLLECT DATA

Subjective

_____
_____
_____
_____
_____
_____

Objective

_____
_____
_____
_____
_____
_____

Would you report this data? Yes/No

If yes, to: _____

Nursing Care

_____
_____
_____
_____
_____
_____
_____
_____

How would you document this? _____
_____
_____

Data Collected
(use those that apply)

- States "I'm so tired, and I have these bruises all over me. I'm so afraid of the results of the bone marrow test. I don't know what we will do if I have cancer."
- 5'4" inches (156 cm) tall, weighs 106 lb (48.1 kg)
- Vital signs T 100° F; P 102; R 22; BP 130/82
- Night sweats and intermittent fever for past 2 months
- Numerous petechiae scattered over trunk and arms
- Ecchymoses lower right arm and right calf
- Relates menstrual periods heavier than normal
- Oral mucosa red, with several small ulcerations in buccal areas
- Low RBC count; low hemoglobin and hematocrit; low platelets; high WBC count; myeloblasts present

Nursing Interventions
(use those that apply)

- Place in a private room.
- Limit visitors to husband and daughter.
- Verbally and in writing remind staff, family, and client to practice good hand washing. Post a sign in the room as a reminder, and discuss the importance of hand washing with Mrs. Cole and her family.
- Take and record vital signs every 4 hours.
- Frequently assess for and report signs of bleeding such as increased bruising, joint pain, occult blood in body fluids, and menstrual pad count.
- Assist with oral hygiene every 2 to 4 hours, using a soft-bristle toothbrush or a sponge. Offer warm saline or dilute hydrogen peroxide mouth rinses.
- Encourage to alternate activity with rest.
- Teach about the bone marrow biopsy. Allow time for questions.
- Refer to oncology nurse specialist.

NCLEX-PN Exam Preparation

1. A 19 year old client is admitted in sickle cell crisis. The FIRST nursing action would be to:
   a. administer pain medications
   b. obtain blood samples for analysis
   c. administer antibiotics
   d. insert Foley catheter

2. A client is admitted with a diagnosis of pernicious anemia. Priority nursing care would include:
   a. prevention of infection
   b. increasing iron intake
   c. providing rest periods
   d. increasing fluid intake

3. An LPN is assigned to a client with thrombocytopenia. A priority goal of nursing care is:
   a. prevention of infection
   b. prevention of injury
   c. prevention of dehydration
   d. prevention of nutritional deficit

4. A 19 year old client with hemophilia A wants to join an athletic team in college. Which of the following would be most appropriate?
   a. hockey
   b. golf
   c. basketball
   d. baseball

5. The nurse establishes a nursing diagnosis of Impaired Oral Mucous Membrane for a client with leukemia who is experiencing stomatitis. Client teaching would include avoiding:
   a. warm saline as a mouth rinse
   b. application of petroleum jelly to the lips
   c. citrus fruit juice
   d. cool liquids for hydration

6. A client developed disseminated intravascular coagulation (DIC) following injuries sustained in an automobile collision. Which of the following, if observed, requires intervention by the nurse?
   a. The knee gatch on the bed is elevated.
   b. The client is resting on her right side.
   c. The client has oxygen per nasal cannula at 5 L/min.
   d. The client has cool compresses to her knees.

7. The priority nursing care focus for a client diagnosed with multiple myeloma is:
   a. prevention of injury and pain control
   b. balanced nutrition and prevention of injury
   c. safety and preservation of mental status
   d. control bleeding and preserve energy

8. A client develops lymphedema of her left arm following a left radical mastectomy. Discharge teaching would include:
   a. removing antiembolic stockings or pressure devices daily
   b. elevating extremity when seated or in bed
   c. inspecting skin every other day
   d. adding low potassium foods to diet

9. A client is evaluated for possible Hodgkin's disease. Which of the following assessment findings would be expected?
   a. enlarged cervical lymph node
   b. absent Reed–Sternberg cells
   c. negative Epstein–Barr virus
   d. immovable, painful inguinal lymph nodes

10. The nurse develops a nursing diagnosis of Risk for Infection for a client with leukemia. The BEST action by the nurse would be to:
    a. require visitors with colds or flu to wear masks
    b. wash hands when leaving the room
    c. document signs of infection in the medical record
    d. maintain prescribed protective isolation protocols at all times

chapter

25

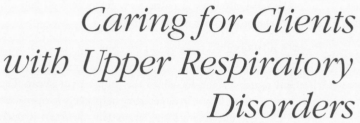

Caring for Clients with Upper Respiratory Disorders

CARING tip

❝There are many professions within the nursing arena, so look for ways to challenge yourself throughout your career.❞

Rosemary Brown, BSN, RN-C • Nursing Instructor • Idaho State University • Pocatello, Idaho

LEARNING outcomes

After completing this chapter, you will be able to:

- Describe the structure and functions of the upper respiratory tract.
- Describe assessment and data collection for upper respiratory function.
- Describe common disorders affecting the upper respiratory tract and their manifestations.
- Discuss the nursing implications for diagnostic tests, medications, and treatments ordered for clients with upper respiratory disorders.
- Provide care for clients having surgery involving the upper respiratory system.
- Identify nursing care needs for the client with a tracheostomy.

MediaLink

 www.prenhall.com/burke

Use the above address to access the free, interactive Companion Website created for this textbook. Get hints, instant feedback, and textbook references to chapter-related multiple choice questions. Link to other interesting sites.

The primary function of the respiratory system is to provide the cells of the body with oxygen and to eliminate carbon dioxide (a waste product of cellular metabolism). Air moves into the lungs and carbon dioxide moves out of the body through the upper respiratory tract.

The upper airway cleans, humidifies, and warms air. An open upper airway is needed for effective breathing. Upper respiratory disorders may affect the nose, sinuses, pharynx, tonsils, and larynx. They range from minor colds to life-threatening conditions like laryngeal obstruction. When swelling, bleeding, or secretions affect breathing, the client may become frightened and anxious. Nursing care focuses on managing the airway and symptoms, communicating effectively, and providing psychological support for the client and family.

Structure and Function of the Upper Respiratory System

THE NOSE AND SINUSES

The respiratory system begins at the *nose* (Figure 25-1A ◆). Cartilage and the facial bones give the nose structure. The nostrils *(nares)* are two cavities in the nose, separated by the *nasal septum.* They open into the nasal portion of the pharynx. Nasal hairs just inside the nares filter air as it enters the nose. The air is warmed by mucous membranes lining the nares. Mucous membranes contain scent receptors and cells that secrete thick mucus. The mucus traps dust and bacteria and contains an enzyme that destroys bacteria. The mucus and trapped debris are moved to the pharynx and then swallowed. Ridges within each nasal cavity (called *turbinates*) help trap heavier particles of debris.

The *sinuses* are openings in the facial bones (Figure 25-1B). Sinuses lighten the skull, assist in speech, and produce mucus that drains into the nasal cavities and helps trap debris.

THE PHARYNX

The *pharynx* (throat) is a passageway for both air and food. It is divided into three regions: the nasopharynx, oropharynx, and laryngopharynx.

The *nasopharynx* starts at the nose. Air, mucus, and trapped debris move through the nasopharynx, where the *tonsils* and *adenoids* (masses of lymphoid tissue in the back wall of the nasopharynx) trap and destroy infectious agents. The *eustachian* tubes also open into the nasopharynx, connecting it with the middle ear.

The *oropharynx* lies behind the oral cavity. It carries both air and food. During swallowing, the soft palate (see Figure 25-1A) rises to prevent food from entering the nasopharynx. The lining of the oropharynx protects it from damage by friction and from chemicals in food and fluids.

The *laryngopharynx,* a passageway for both food and air, connects the oropharynx to the larynx.

THE LARYNX

The *larynx* (voicebox) connects the laryngopharynx with the trachea and routes air and food into the proper passageway. The larynx is protected by cartilages that help keep it open (see Figure 25-1A). The inlet to the larynx (the *epiglottis*) is open when air is moving through it; during swallowing, the epiglottis tips down to cover the opening of the larynx. The larynx also contains the vocal cords, which help produce speech. If anything other than air enters the larynx, a cough reflex is initiated to expel the foreign substance before it can reach the lungs.

CLINICAL alert

The cough reflex does not work if the person is unconscious.

Upper Respiratory Infections and Inflammations

The upper respiratory tract is constantly exposed to infectious and inflammatory agents in the environment. Most upper respiratory infections (URIs) and inflammations are minor illnesses. However, complications may result. In the frail older adult, the risk of serious problems following a URI can be significant.

Figure 25-1. ◆   (A) The upper respiratory system. (B) The sinuses.

PATHOPHYSIOLOGY

Most upper respiratory infections are caused by easily spread viruses. When the virus or an allergen enters the airway, it may cause acute inflammation of the upper airway, including the sinuses, pharynx, or larynx. The airway mucosa swells and secretes clear, yellow, or greenish exudate. A bacterial infection may develop following the viral infection. URIs occur more frequently during the fall and winter.

Rhinitis

Rhinitis, inflammation of the nasal cavities, is the most common upper respiratory disorder.

Acute viral rhinitis (the common cold) is highly contagious. Most adults experience two to four colds each year. More than 200 strains of virus can cause the common cold, including rhinovirus, respiratory syncytial virus, and adenovirus. These viruses are spread by hand-to-hand contact and by inhaling the virus. The virus can be spread to others for a few days *before* and *after* symptoms appear (Table 25-1 ◆).

Allergic rhinitis (hay fever) results from an allergic response to substances such as plant pollens, mold, or animal dander. Allergic rhinitis tends to occur seasonally. Histamine and other immune mediators are released in response to contact with the allergen. This causes vasodilation and increased leakiness of capillaries in the mucosa (see Table 25-1). The sinuses may become congested, causing a headache. Chronic allergies may lead to postnasal drip and snoring.

Influenza

Influenza (flu) is a highly contagious viral respiratory disease. It often occurs in epidemics. Yearly outbreaks of influenza affect about 48 million Americans each winter. Influenza and

BOX 25-1

population FOCUS

Risk of Influenza in Older Adults

Older adults who get influenza have a high risk of developing pneumonia. Respiratory function changes with aging: The cough is less effective and residual lung volume increases. These changes increase the risk for pneumonia. Pneumonia is a serious complication of influenza that may be fatal. (See Chapter 26 for more information about pneumonia.)

Reye's syndrome is a rare but potentially fatal complication of influenza. It is more likely to affect children but also has been identified in older adults. It usually develops within 2 to 3 weeks after the influenza. Clients with Reye's syndrome often develop liver failure and brain dysfunction.

its complications (primarily bacterial pneumonia) cause about 20,000 deaths yearly. Older adults with influenza have an increased risk of complications (Box 25-1).

Influenza viruses are transmitted by airborne droplet and direct contact. The incubation period is short, and the manifestations develop rapidly (see Table 25-1). Fever and acute manifestations last up to a week; cough and fatigue may persist for several weeks.

Sinusitis

Sinusitis is an inflammation of the mucous membranes of the sinuses (see Figure 25-1B). Sinusitis is usually caused by a bacterial infection, and often follows a URI.

When drainage from the sinuses is obstructed, mucus secretions caught in the sinus cavity become a bacterial

TABLE 25-1 RHINITIS VERSUS INFLUENZA

	ACUTE VIRAL RHINITIS	ALLERGIC RHINITIS	INFLUENZA
LOCAL MANIFESTATIONS	Nasal mucosa red, swollen, and congested Clear, watery secretions with **coryza** (runny nose) Sneezing and coughing	Nasal mucosa pale, swollen, and congested Thin, watery nasal discharge Itchy, watery eyes Sneezing	Coryza Sore throat Dry, nonproductive cough; may become productive Substernal burning
SYSTEMIC MANIFESTATIONS	Low-grade fever Headache Malaise Muscle ache	Headache	Chills and fever Headache Malaise Muscle ache Fatigue and weakness
COURSE AND POSSIBLE COMPLICATIONS	Lasts few days to 2 weeks Mild and self-limited Secondary infections (e.g., sinusitis, otitis media) may follow	Occurs with exposure to allergens (pollen, mold, animal dander) Chronic congestion may cause snoring, postnasal drip	Abrupt onset 1- to 2-week duration Cough and fatigue may last several weeks Secondary infections (sinusitis, otitis media, pneumonia, bronchitis) may follow

growth medium. This infection causes an inflammatory and immune response, leading to more swelling and pressure. Sinusitis may become chronic if the infection is not adequately treated. Clients who smoke, have allergies, or habitually use nasal sprays also may develop chronic sinusitis.

Sinusitis causes pain and tenderness across the infected sinuses, headache, fever, and malaise. The pain usually increases with leaning forward. Pain also may be referred to the upper teeth. The nasal mucous membrane is red and swollen in clients with sinusitis. The client may complain of nasal congestion, purulent nasal discharge, bad breath, fever, malaise, and fatigue. Symptoms often worsen after awakening and then become less severe in the afternoon and evening as secretions drain.

Sinus infection may spread to surrounding structures, causing complications such as abscess or cellulitis, meningitis, sepsis, or hearing loss.

Pharyngitis and Tonsillitis

Pharyngitis (acute inflammation of the throat) is common. It is usually viral but may also be bacterial. *Group A beta-hemolytic Streptococcus* (strep throat) is the most common bacterial cause. Streptococcal infection also may cause **tonsillitis** (acute inflammation of the tonsils). Streptococcal infections usually occur between late fall and spring, especially in cold climates. Pharyngitis and tonsillitis are contagious and are spread by droplet nuclei. Incubation varies from a few hours to several days.

Pharyngitis causes pain and fever. Throat discomfort may vary from scratchiness to pain and **dysphagia** (difficulty swallowing). The manifestations of acute viral and bacterial pharyngitis are listed in Box 25-2.

In tonsillitis, the tonsils are bright red and swollen with white exudate. The uvula may also be red and swollen. Cervical lymph nodes are usually tender and enlarged. The client with tonsillitis complains of a sore throat, difficulty swallowing, general malaise, fever, and *otalgia* (pain in the ear). The infection may extend to the ear through the eustachian tubes, causing acute otitis media. (See Chapter 31 for more information about otitis media and other disorders of the ear.)

Peritonsillar abscess (*quinsy*) is a potential complication of tonsillitis. In a peritonsillar abscess, pus forms behind the tonsil, causing marked swelling and deviation of the uvula toward one side. The client may be unable to swallow anything but liquids. Drooling and contraction of the muscles used in chewing may also occur.

Rare but serious complications of streptococcal pharyngitis and tonsillitis include acute glomerulonephritis and rheumatic fever. These potential complications are caused by an abnormal immune response to the bacteria. They can develop 1 to 5 weeks after the acute infection. (See Chapter 21 for more information about acute glomerulonephritis, and Chapter 22 for more information about rheumatic fever.)

BOX 25-2
MANIFESTATIONS OF ACUTE PHARYNGITIS

VIRAL PHARYNGITIS
- Gradual onset
- Low-grade fever
- Sore throat
- Mild hoarseness
- Headache
- Throat bright pink to red

STREPTOCOCCAL PHARYNGITIS
- Abrupt onset
- Fever of 101° F (38.3° C) or higher
- Severe sore throat
- Dysphagia
- Malaise, muscle aches
- Tender, enlarged cervical lymph nodes
- Throat bright red
- Patches of creamy exudate may be seen on oropharynx and tonsils

Epiglottitis

Acute epiglottitis (inflammation of the epiglottis) is uncommon. It is, however, a medical emergency. Clients with epiglottitis have difficulty swallowing food (*odynophagia*) and have manifestations of pharyngitis. The epiglottis appears red, swollen, and edematous.

CLINICAL alert

Constantly monitor clients with epiglottitis for signs of respiratory distress: nasal flaring, restlessness, **stridor** (a high-pitched, harsh sound heard during inspiration), use of accessory muscles, and decreased oxygen saturation measurements. Do not insert a naso- or oropharyngeal airway as this can cause spasm and total airway obstruction. Nasotracheal intubation may be necessary to maintain the airway. Be prepared for emergency intubation of the client at any time.

Epiglottitis is frightening for both the client and the nurse. Maintain a calm, reassuring manner to help relieve anxiety.

Laryngitis

Laryngitis (inflammation of the larynx) is common. Laryngitis may occur alone or with other disorders of the upper respiratory tract. It is commonly associated with viral URI and may also occur in clients with bronchitis, pneumonia, or other respiratory infections. Excessive use of the voice, sudden changes in temperature, or exposure to dust or pollutants can also cause laryngitis. It is more common in the winter and in colder climates.

In laryngitis, the mucous membrane lining the larynx becomes inflamed and the vocal cords may be swollen. The primary manifestation of laryngitis is a change in the voice. Hoarseness or *aphonia* (complete loss of the voice) may occur. Clients complain of a sore, scratchy throat and may have a dry, harsh cough.

COLLABORATIVE CARE

Most acute URIs are self-limiting, and clients are encouraged to provide self-care. Medical management focuses on establishing an accurate diagnosis, providing symptomatic relief, and preventing complications. Bacterial URIs such as sinusitus and streptococcal pharyngitis are treated to speed recovery and reduce the risk of complications.

Laboratory and Diagnostic Tests

A *throat swab* is obtained when streptococcal pharyngitis is suspected. Nurses are often responsible for obtaining the culture (Procedure 25-1). Tests such as the LA antigen and ELISA allow rapid identification of the bacteria (as little as 10 minutes) but are not highly sensitive. If the test is positive, treatment for strep throat is started. If the test is negative, the swab is cultured to determine if streptococcus is present.

A *complete blood count (CBC)* may be done. The white blood cell (WBC) count is usually normal or low in viral infections and elevated in bacterial infections. A *chest x-ray* may be done to rule out complications such as pneumonia.

Nasal swabs or *radiologic studies* (x-ray or computed tomography [CT] scan) may be ordered if sinusitis is suspected. CT scans are more sensitive in detecting the inflammatory changes of sinusitis.

Pharmacology

INFLUENZA. Yearly immunization with influenza vaccine is the most important measure to reduce the risk of influenza.

Polyvalent influenza virus vaccine (containing antigens of several viral strains) is about 85% effective in preventing influenza infection for up to a year. Although the vaccine is readily available and inexpensive, only about a third of people at risk get the vaccine each year. The vaccine should be given annually to:

- People over the age of 50
- Residents of nursing homes
- Pregnant women
- Adults and children with chronic heart or lung disorders or chronic metabolic diseases (e.g., diabetes)
- Health care workers
- Family members of at-risk clients

Because the vaccine is produced in eggs, it should not be given to people with an allergy to eggs. About 5% of those vaccinated may develop low-grade fever, malaise, or muscle aches after vaccination. Serious adverse reactions include anaphylaxis (an acute allergic response) and Guillain–Barré syndrome, an acute neurologic disorder that can cause temporary paralysis. An intranasal vaccine will soon be available.

Several drugs are available to prevent or shorten the duration of influenza in unvaccinated people who are exposed to the virus. Zanamivir (Relenza) and GS4104 reduce the severity and duration of influenza. These drugs attack the virus itself, reducing its spread in the body. Amantadine (Symmetrel) and rimantadine (Flumadine) also may be used to prevent or decrease symptoms.

BACTERIAL INFECTIONS. Bacterial infections such as sinusitis, strep pharyngitis, and tonsillitis are treated with antibiotics. Treatment is continued for at least 10 days. The client is no longer contagious after 24 hours of antibiotic therapy.

PROCEDURE 25-1   Obtaining a Throat Swab

- Obtain a sterile cotton swab or throat swab kit.
- Identify the client, explain the procedure, and provide for privacy.
- Place the client in a sitting position if possible.
- Use standard precautions.
- Ask the client to open the mouth, extend the tongue, and say "ah."
- Quickly swab the tonsils, reddened areas of the oropharynx, and any exudate.
- Insert the swab into the specimen container. Avoid contaminating the outside of the container or the swab.
- Label the container.
- Send the specimen and requisition to the laboratory.

■ SAMPLE DOCUMENTATION

10/27/02	Oropharynx red, patches of white exudate noted on tonsils and oropharynx. Throat swab (oropharynx, tonsils, and exudate) obtained and sent to lab for culture.
	_____ S. Doene, LPN.

Antibiotics also are used to treat sinusitis. Antibiotic therapy is continued for a full 2 weeks; a longer course may be prescribed to prevent relapse. If the client's sinusitis does not improve, hospitalization and intravenous antibiotic therapy may be required.

RHINITIS. A number of drugs, many available without prescription, provide symptomatic relief of viral URIs. Mild decongestants may help relieve the manifestations of coryza and nasal congestion. Oral or topical (nasal spray) decongestants are also prescribed for clients with sinusitis to reduce mucosal edema and promote sinus drainage. See Box 25-3 for how to administer nose drops. Topical nasal steroids may be used after antibiotic therapy has been initiated, in the later stages of treating subacute or chronic sinusitis, and for prophylaxis of recurrent problems.

CLINICAL alert

Decongestant nasal sprays should be used for no more than 3 to 5 days. When used for a longer time, they can cause *rebound congestion,* which causes the client to use the spray more frequently and in larger doses.

Decongestants and antihistamines help relieve the manifestations of allergic rhinitis. Many decongestants and antihistamines are available without a prescription, including long-acting nonsedating antihistamines. Inhaled steroids or cromolyn, a mast cell stabilizer, may be prescribed if nonprescription drugs are ineffective. (See Table 25-2 ◆.)

Warm salt-water gargles, throat lozenges, or mild analgesics may be used for sore throat. Over-the-counter analgesics such as aspirin, acetaminophen, or NSAIDs help relieve fever and muscle ache. Antitussives may decrease cough and promote rest. Systemic mucolytic agents such as guaifenesin help liquefy secretions and promote sinus drainage.

Complementary Therapies

Complementary therapies and practices are appropriate for treating many URIs. Herbal remedies such as echinacea and garlic have antiviral and antibiotic effects. Taken at the first sign of infection, echinacea may reduce the duration and symptoms of a common cold or influenza. The recommended dose of echinacea varies, depending on the part of the plant

BOX 25-3
NURSING CARE CHECKLIST

ADMINISTERING NOSE DROPS

To administer nose drops:
☑ Tilt the client's head backward and to the side on which the drops are to be instilled.
☑ Have the client remain in position for 5 minutes to allow the drops to reach the posterior nares.

used in the preparation. It should not be used for longer than 2 weeks. Echinacea is contraindicated for women who are pregnant or lactating. It should not be used by people who have an autoimmune disease such as multiple sclerosis or rheumatoid arthritis.

Aromatherapy with essential oils such as basil, cedarwood, eucalyptus, frankincense, lavender, marjoram, peppermint, or rosemary can reduce congestion, enhance comfort, and promote recovery from a URI. Caution clients that these essential oils should be used only for inhalation and must not be taken internally.

Surgery

Clients with sinusitis, tonsillitis, or peritonsillar abscess may require surgery. *Irrigation* of an infected sinus (*antral lavage*) can be performed in the physician's office under local anesthesia. The sinus is irrigated with saline solution to wash out purulent exudate and promote drainage. *Endoscopic sinus surgery* may be performed to relieve obstruction of the opening to the sinus and restore ventilation and drainage of the sinus. Nasal packing is left in place for 24 to 48 hours following surgery. On discharge, the client is instructed to:

- Use a humidifier or normal saline spray.
- Avoid blowing the nose, straining, lifting, and stenuous exercise for a week.
- Sneeze with the mouth open.
- Avoid smoking, air pollutants, and nasal trauma.
- Notify the physician for a temperature greater than 101° F, severe pain, or excessive bleeding.

Tonsillectomy (surgical removal of the tonsils) is done to treat recurrent or chronic infections, enlarged tonsils that may obstruct the airway, peritonsillar abscess, or malignancy. The most significant postoperative complication of tonsillectomy is hemorrhage. If hemorrhage develops, the client returns to surgery, where the bleeding vessel is *ligated* (tied off). A peritonsillar abscess may be drained by *needle aspiration* or by *incision and drainage (I&D)* under local anesthesia. Tonsillectomy follows the I&D, either immediately or 6 weeks later.

NURSING CARE

Education is the primary nursing role in caring for most clients with acute or chronic URIs. Self-care is appropriate for most clients with viral infections. Unless the problem is recurrent or a complication occurs, medical treatment is rarely required. Clients need to be able to recognize the difference between acute, self-limiting disorders and those that require medical treatment.

ASSESSING

Assessment data collected by the nurse helps determine the effects of an upper respiratory problem on the client's life, can

TABLE 25-2 NURSING IMPLICATIONS FOR PHARMACOLOGY: CLIENTS WITH UPPER RESPIRATORY INFECTIONS			
CLASS/DRUGS	**PURPOSE**	**NURSING RESPONSIBILITIES**	**CLIENT TEACHING**
Decongestants ■ Phenylephrine (Neo-Synephrine, others) ■ Phenylpropanolamine (Comtrex, Ornade, Triaminic, others) ■ Pseudoephedrine (Sudafed, Actifed, others)	Decongestants constrict blood vessels, reducing inflammation and edema of nasal mucosa and relieving nasal congestion. Very effective when applied topically (by nasal spray) due to rapid onset of action. Duration of effect is short, followed by vasodilation and rebound congestion. May be habit forming.	Assess for contraindications such as high blood pressure or chronic heart disease. These drugs constrict blood vessels, increasing the blood pressure and heart rate. Do not give the drug if the client is taking antihypertensive medications or a monoamine oxidase (MAO) inhibitor.	Do not use more than the recommended dose. Check with your doctor before taking these drugs if you are taking any prescription medications or are being treated for high blood pressure or heart disease. Do not use nasal sprays for more than 3–5 days. Increase fluid intake to relieve mouth dryness. These drugs may cause nervousness, shakiness, or difficulty sleeping. Stop the drug if these effects occur.
Antihistamines ■ Brompheniramine (Dimetane, others) ■ Chlorpheniramine (Chlor-Trimeton, others) ■ Clesmastine (Tavist) ■ Dexchlorpheniramine (Dexchlor, others) ■ Triprolidine (Actidil, Myidil) Nonsedating ■ Cetirizine (Zyrtec) ■ Fexofenadine (Allegra) ■ Loratadine (Claritin)	Antihistamines are widely available without prescription. They are frequently combined with decongestants in over-the-counter cold and allergy preparations. Other than the nonsedating forms, most antihistamines cause some drowsiness.	Before giving or recommending these drugs, ask about possible contra-indications, such as: a. Acute asthma or chronic respiratory disease b. Glaucoma (increased intraocular pressure) c. Impaired gastrointestinal function or obstruction d. An enlarged prostate gland or other urinary tract obstruction e. Heart disease	Do not drive or operate machinery while taking antihistamines that are known to be sedating. Stop the drug and notify your doctor immediately if you become confused or very drowsy or sleepy, or you experience chest tightness, wheezing, bleeding, or easy bruising. Do not use alcohol or other CNS depressants while taking antihistamines. Hard candy, gum, ice chips, and liquids help relieve mouth dryness caused by antihistamines.

identify risk factors for complications, and can suggest whether the problem is appropriate for self-care or for medical treatment. Box 25-4 lists subjective and objective data to collect.

DIAGNOSING, PLANNING, AND IMPLEMENTING

Nursing care for clients with significant manifestations or complications of URI focuses on maintaining airway clearance, breathing patterns, and adequate rest.

INEFFECTIVE BREATHING PATTERN

■ Monitor respiratory rate and pattern for changes from base-line. *Tachypnea or rapid, shallow respirations may result from*

fever and muscle ache. Shallow respirations may lead to decreased ventilation of alveoli or to atelectasis (lack of ventilation of an area of lung).

■ Pace activities to allow rest periods. *Tachypnea increases the work of breathing and is fatiguing.*

■ Elevate the head of the bed. *The upright position reduces the work of breathing and improves lung expansion.*

INEFFECTIVE AIRWAY CLEARANCE

■ Monitor the effectiveness of cough and ability to remove airway secretions. *Fatigue and general malaise may decrease the ability to cough effectively and move secretions. Changes in the respiratory system associated with aging also affect the older adult's ability to maintain a clear airway effectively.*

BOX 25-4
ASSESSING CLIENTS WITH UPPER RESPIRATORY INFECTIONS

SUBJECTIVE DATA

- Pain: Location (nose, face, throat, or chest); character, timing, aggravating factors, and relief measures
- Cough: Type (dry or productive), timing
- Sputum and/or nasal drainage: Amount, color, odor
- Shortness of breath or *dyspnea* (difficult or labored breathing)
- Difficulty swallowing or smelling, or altered taste
- Past medical history: Known allergies, chronic respiratory problems; surgery or trauma of the upper respiratory tract; chronic diseases, such as diabetes or heart disease; smoking history and/or exposure to environmental pollutants or allergens

OBJECTIVE DATA

- Observe for difficulty breathing, pausing while talking, hoarseness, and cough; respiratory rate, note depth and symmetry of chest movement
- Inspect nares: Color, moisture of mucosa; presence of swelling; presence, color, and amount of drainage
- Inspect oropharynx: Color, moisture; presence of swelling, exudate, or post-nasal drainage
- Percuss (lightly tap) over frontal and maxillary sinuses for tenderness
- Auscultate lung sounds and note any *adventitious* (abnormal) sounds (see Chapter 4 for more details about assessing clients).

- Following tonsillectomy, position with head to the side for drainage of secretions from the mouth and pharynx. Leave the nasopharyngeal airway in place until the client can swallow and the gag reflex returns. *This prevents aspiration and maintains the airway.*
- Apply an ice collar as ordered. *The ice collar reduces swelling and provides a mild analgesic effect.*
- Immediately report excessive bleeding (large amounts of bright red drainage, choking on drainage, or vomiting of bright red blood) to the charge nurse and physician. *The client may need to return to surgery to stop the hemorrhage.*
- Maintain adequate hydration. Assess mucous membrane moisture and skin turgor. *Fever, rapid respiratory rate, and decreased fluid intake may lead to dehydration and thick, sticky secretions that are more difficult to expectorate.*
- Increase the humidity of inspired air with a bedside humidifier. *Increasing the water content of inhaled air helps loosen secretions and soothe mucous membranes.*
- Teach the client how to cough effectively. Administer analgesic medications as ordered. *The huff technique of coughing increases the cough's effectiveness and spares energy (See Chapter 26 for client teaching of this technique.) Relieving muscle ache increases the ability to cough effectively.*

DISTURBED SLEEP PATTERN

- Assess sleep using subjective and objective information. *Decreased ability to rest increases fatigue and prolongs recovery time.*
- Place in a semi-Fowler's or Fowler's position for sleep. *Elevating the head of the bed decreases the work of breathing and may allow better rest.*
- Provide antipyretic and analgesic medications at bedtime or shortly before. *These medications promote comfort by reducing fever and relieving muscle aches.*
- If necessary, request a cough suppressant medication for nighttime use. *Cough suppressants are not recommended during the day because coughing promotes airway clearance, but at night they may allow the client to rest.*

IMPAIRED VERBAL COMMUNICATION

- Encourage the client with laryngitis to rest the voice and to use alternate methods of communicating such as writing. *Resting the voice speeds recovery and decreases throat discomfort.*
- Instruct to use throat lozenges or sprays, or to gargle with a warm antiseptic solution. *These measures soothe the throat.*
- If the client smokes, encourage quitting. *Cigarette smoke is an irritant that increases the risk for laryngitis and delays healing.*

EVALUATING

To evaluate the effectiveness of care for a client with URI, collect data such as the following:

- Rate and depth of respirations
- Ability to effectively manage secretions
- Knowledge/understanding of effective medication use
- Duration of manifestations
- Absence of complications

Discharge Considerations

Because many URIs are appropriately treated at home, planning and teaching for home care is vital. Box 25-5 lists assessment data to collect when planning for discharge.

Encourage rest during the acute phase of the illness. Stress the importance of staying well hydrated. Teach clients to use disposable tissues to cover the mouth and nose while coughing or sneezing to prevent airborne spread of URI. Instruct the client to blow the nose with both nostrils open to prevent infected matter from being forced into the eustachian tubes. Remind clients to wash hands frequently, especially after coughing or sneezing, to help prevent spreading the disease to others. Clients can limit their incidence of URIs by avoiding exposure to crowds. Teach the client that although becoming chilled or going out in the rain does not cause colds and influenza, physical or psychological stress does make the

BOX 25-5
ASSESSING FOR DISCHARGE

UPPER RESPIRATORY INFECTIONS

Client

- Self-care: Ability to independently manage activities of daily living (ADLs), self-administer prescribed or recommended medications
- Knowledge: Recommended activity level; prescription and over-the-counter medications and their appropriate use; indications for seeking medical care
- Home environment: Appropriate heating and cooling; access to clean water for drinking and handwashing; indoor pollutants such as cigarette smoke, dust, and allergens such as pets

Family

- Members of household: Small children; individuals at high risk for complications of URI
- Caregivers: Availability and willingness to provide care as needed, assist with shopping, transportation, and caring for dependents
- Financial resources: Income; availability of sick leave; resources for drugs and medical care required

Community

- Immunization clinics or low-cost immunization options
- Access to health care resources

---

body more susceptible to URIs. Maintaining good general health and stress-reduction activities supports the immune system and helps prevent acute URIs.

Teaching about influenza focuses on prevention. Stress the importance of yearly influenza vaccination for clients in high-risk groups and their families. Teach clients how the disease is spread, including how to reduce risk by avoiding crowds and people who are ill.

Discuss appropriate use of over-the-counter medications for relief of manifestations (see Table 25-2). Teach clients to limit their use of nasal decongestants to every 4 hours for only a few days at a time. Suggest that clients avoid using aspirin or acetaminophen unless needed to relieve muscle aches and promote rest, because these medications may actually prolong acute viral URIs. Encourage warm saline gargles or throat lozenges for symptomatic relief of sore throat.

Help the client with allergic rhinitis identify possible allergens and strategies to avoid contacting them. Discuss the possible benefits of skin testing to identify allergens and, if necessary, immunotherapy to reduce the allergic response.

Stress the importance of completing the entire course of prescribed antibiotics for bacterial infections. Discuss the pre-

scribed antibiotic and help develop a schedule that helps the client remember to take all doses. If the course of therapy will be prolonged, discuss measures to prevent superinfections such as vaginitis or oral thrush. Unless contraindicated, suggest that the client eat 8 ounces daily of yogurt containing live bacterial cultures while on antibiotics.

Teach about possible complications of influenza and other URIs and their manifestations. Emphasize that complications should be reported promptly to the physician.

Nursing Process Case Study
■ CLIENT WITH UPPER RESPIRATORY INFECTION

Monica Wunderman is a 27-year-old woman who was recently treated for tonsillitis caused by group A *Streptococcus*. She presents to the emergency department (ED) 10 days later appearing acutely ill. She states that her throat is so sore that she has difficulty swallowing even liquids. Barbara Ironhorse, the ED nurse, completes an assessment of Ms. Wunderman.

Assessment T 102° F (38.8° C). On inspection of her mouth, an acutely swollen and reddened area of the soft palate is noted. Yellow exudate is present. CBC reveals an elevated WBC of 16,000 per mm^3. A diagnosis of peritonsillar abscess is made. Needle aspiration of the abscess is performed.

Diagnosis The following nursing diagnoses are identified for Ms. Wunderman:

- Pain related to swelling
- Risk for Ineffective Airway Clearance related to pain and swelling
- Deficient Fluid Volume related to fever and difficulty in swallowing fluids

Expected Outcomes The expected outcomes for the plan of care are that Ms. Wunderman will:

- Experience minimal or no pain.
- Maintain a patent airway as demonstrated by normal respiratory rate and rhythm.
- Maintain optimal fluid intake as evidenced by ability to consume fluids and semiliquid foods, appearance of moist mucous membranes, normal skin turgor, and a decrease in temperature.

Planning and Implementation Ms. Ironhorse implements the following interventions to prepare Ms. Wunderman for home care:

- Advise to drink ice-cold fluids, as they may be easier to swallow and may provide a local analgesic effect. Instruct to avoid citrus juices, hot or spicy foods, and rough-textured foods for 1 week.
- Teach pain-relief measures such as applying an ice collar as desired and gargling with warm saline solution every 1 to 2 hours for the first 24 to 48 hours after aspiration of the abscess.
- Instruct to take all medications as prescribed.

Evaluation When Ms. Ironhorse contacts Ms. Wunderman by telephone 2 days after her visit to the emergency room, she reports complete relief of symptoms. She is afebrile, takes fluids without difficulty, and has had no problems with her breathing. She has not experienced any pain.

 Critical Thinking in the Nursing Process

1. Describe common manifestations of upper respiratory infections and measures to promote comfort.

2. Describe common pharmacologic interventions for these clients.

3. While Ms. Wunderman developed a complication that required medical intervention, many clients present in the emergency department or urgency care clinics with uncomplicated URI. What can nurses do to reduce this unnecessary use of emergency departments and urgency care clinics?

Upper Respiratory Trauma or Obstruction

Epistaxis

The nose has a rich blood supply. **Epistaxis,** or nosebleed, may begin in many ways: trauma (picking the nose or getting hit), drying of nasal mucous membranes, local or systemic infection, substance abuse (e.g., cocaine), arteriosclerosis, and hypertension. Nosebleed may result from bleeding disorders, severe liver disease, or treatment with an anticoagulant or antiplatelet medication. In adults, men have more nosebleeds than women.

PATHOPHYSIOLOGY

Ninety percent of all nosebleeds arise from a rich vascular area in the anterior nasal septum. These vessels are the most susceptible because of their location. Posterior nosebleed may also be caused by trauma, but more often occurs secondary to systemic disorders like hypertension or diabetes. Posterior epistaxis tends to be more severe and occurs more frequently in the older adult.

COLLABORATIVE CARE

The goal of treatment for epistaxis is to identify and control the source of bleeding. Anterior bleeding can usually be managed by simple first-aid measures, such as pressure (pinching the nose toward the septum) for 5 to 10 minutes and applying ice packs to the nose and forehead to cause vasoconstriction. The sitting position decreases blood flow to the head and reduces venous pressure. Having the client lean forward reduces drainage of blood into the nasopharynx and lessens the chance the client will swallow it. The client should spit out the blood. This allows a better estimate of the amount of bleeding and prevents nausea and vomiting resulting from swallowed blood. If applying pressure does not control the bleeding, pharmacologic interventions, nasal packing, or surgery may be necessary.

Pharmacology and Nasal Packing

Topical vasoconstrictors such as cocaine (0.5%), phenylephrine (Neo-Synephrine) (1:1000), or adrenaline (1:1000) may be applied by nasal spray or on a cotton swab held against the bleeding site. The bleeding vessel may be cauterized using a chemical such as silver nitrate or Gelfoam.

One-inch gauze impregnated with antibiotic ointment or a Foley catheter with the balloon inflated may be used as nasal packing. The packing is placed directly against the bleeding site (anterior or posterior) (Figure 25-2 ◆).

Surgery

Surgical cautery procedures may be used to seal bleeding vessels. The resulting scab must be left undisturbed until the mucosa has healed, or further bleeding may occur. Some

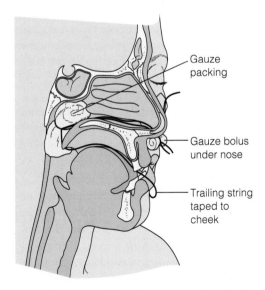

Figure 25-2. ◆ Posterior nasal packing. Ties exiting through the nose and mouth are used to stabilize the packing in position and remove it when it is no longer needed.

clients with posterior bleeding require surgery to tie off the bleeding artery. Nasal packing is inserted and left in place for at least 24 hours, during which time the client is monitored for bleeding.

NURSING CARE

Nosebleeds can be frightening, particularly when they occur spontaneously, without preceding trauma. Support, reassurance, and education are important roles for nurses caring for clients with epistaxis.

ASSESSING

In clients with epistaxis, data collection occurs while measures to stop the bleeding are implemented. Subjective data includes information about when the nosebleed started, how long it has continued, and measures that have been taken to stop the bleeding. The client's medical history, including chronic diseases and current medications, may provide clues. Objective data to obtain include the client's vital signs and the extent of bleeding. Inspect the oropharynx using penlight and tongue depressor for further evidence of bleeding.

DIAGNOSING, PLANNING, AND IMPLEMENTING

ANXIETY

- Maintain an attitude of calm encouragement. *This reassures the client that the nosebleed is not life threatening. If epistaxis has occurred spontaneously, the client may fear that it indicates a major health problem.*
- Have the client pinch the nares together at the bridge of the nose. *Ninety percent of nosebleeds originate in the front of the nose where direct pressure usually stops the bleeding. Having the client put pressure on the nose provides focus and helps restore a sense of control. This reduces anxiety.*
- Encourage to breathe slowly and deeply through the mouth. *Controlled mouth breathing maintains lung ventilation and reduces anxiety.*
- Assess the client with nasal packing frequently for adequate oxygenation (e.g., mental status, oxygen saturation measurements). Maintain supplemental oxygen as ordered. *Cerebral hypoxia produces a sense of apprehension and fear.*

RISK FOR ASPIRATION

The highly anxious client who has blood draining into the nasopharynx is at risk for aspirating blood into the trachea. The client with nasal packing is unable to breathe through the nose, increasing the risk of aspirating food or fluids when eating.

- Position upright with the head forward. Provide a basin for the client to expectorate blood. *This reduces the risk of aspiration and nausea from swallowed blood.*

- Apply ice or a cold compress to the nose. *Cold constricts blood vessels and reduces bleeding.*
- Place the client with nasal packing with the head elevated and on one side when asleep. *This position reduces the risk of aspiration of oral secretions.*

EVALUATING

In order to evaluate care for the client with epistaxis, check for additional bleeding (be sure to check the oropharynx for blood running down the throat). Evaluate the client's understanding of instructions, including when to return for removal of nasal packing and measures to prevent future nosebleeds.

Discharge Considerations

Following an episode of epistaxis, teaching focuses on measures to prevent further nosebleeds. Advise the client to avoid strenuous exercise for several days or weeks, depending on the severity of the nosebleed and its treatment. Instruct clients not to blow the nose or do things like heavy lifting or bending that could increase pressure and dislodge the crust. Caution to sneeze with the mouth open to avoid increasing pressure in nasal vessels.

Suggest lubricating nasal mucosa with petroleum jelly, a water-soluble lubricant, or bacitracin ointment to reduce the risk of spontaneous bleeding in clients with anterior nose bleeds. Recommend using a humidifier or vaporizer to minimize dryness of the mucous membranes. Instruct clients not to blow the nose forcefully or pick the nose. Encourage the client who has experienced spontaneous epistaxis to seek medical evaluation for possible underlying problems like hypertension or bleeding disorder.

Nasal Trauma or Deviated Septum

The nose is the most commonly broken bone of the face. A *nasal fracture* (broken nose) usually results from a sports injury or from trauma related to violence or motor vehicle wrecks.

PATHOPHYSIOLOGY

One or both sides of the nose may be broken. A fracture that involves only one side of the nose rarely causes displacement or deformity. It is usually not serious, although swelling can obstruct the airway. Bilateral fractures are more common. Complex fractures may involve other nasal structures and frontal bones of the face as well as soft tissue. The manifestations of bilateral nasal fracture are listed in Box 25-6.

Hematoma, infection or abscess, perforation or deviation of the septum, and leakage of cerebrospinal fluid (CSF) may complicate nasal fractures. The client with a nasal fracture may also have fractures of other facial bones, particularly when facial trauma is severe.

BOX 25-6
MANIFESTATIONS OF NASAL FRACTURE

- Epistaxis
- Deformity (flattening, depression, S or C shape) or displacement to one side
- *Crepitus* (a grating sound or sensation)
- Soft-tissue trauma (periorbital edema, bruising, black eye)
- Instability of nasal bridge

COLLABORATIVE CARE

The major goals of treatment for nasal fractures are to maintain a patent airway and prevent deformity. X-rays of the head and face are done to identify the fracture and to assess for other facial fractures. The nasal cavity is examined to rule out septal hematoma. If a CSF leak is suspected, additional diagnostic tests such as a CT scan may be performed.

Simple reduction of a nasal fracture may be done in the emergency room using local anesthesia. An external splint may then be applied for 7 to 10 days to maintain proper alignment until healing takes place. Ice may be gently applied to the face and nose to control edema and bleeding. Nasal packing may be used to control epistaxis.

Complex nasal fractures, fractures that do not heal properly, or a persistent CSF leak may require surgical repair of the fracture or realignment of the nasal bones. The most common procedure used is rhinoplasty with concurrent septoplasty.

Rhinoplasty (surgical reconstruction of the nose) is done to relieve airway obstruction and repair visible deformity of the nose following fracture. Using an intranasal incision, the framework of the nose is reshaped. Prosthetic implants may assist in reshaping the nose. Rhinoplasty is usually an outpatient procedure. Following surgery, nasal packing is left in place for up to 72 hours to minimize bleeding and provide tissue support. A plastic splint molded to the shape of the nose is removed in 3 to 5 days. The splint protects the reshaped nose and helps to control swelling. Most swelling and bruising subside within 10 to 14 days; normal sensation may take several months to return.

NURSING CARE

Nursing care for clients with nasal fracture focuses on airway management; controlling pain, bleeding, and swelling; and providing necessary teaching.

ASSESSING

Ask the client with a suspected nasal fracture how and when the injury occurred. Carefully observe respiratory status and call for help immediately if the airway is compromised. Inquire about pain, bleeding, and difficulty breathing. Inspect the nose and face for apparent deformity, swelling, and *ecchymosis* (bruising). Gently palpate the nose for *crepitus* (a grating sound or sensation).

DIAGNOSING, PLANNING, AND IMPLEMENTING

INEFFECTIVE AIRWAY CLEARANCE

- Monitor for signs of respiratory distress such as tachypnea, dyspnea, shortness of breath, tachycardia, and use of accessory muscles. Monitor oxygen saturation levels. *Swelling and deformity may obstruct the airway. If the fracture is malpositioned during healing, resulting deformity can also impair nasal airway clearance. Abnormal signs and declining oxygen saturation levels may indicate airway obstruction.*
- Have suction equipment available. *Suctioning of the oropharynx may be necessary to remove blood and secretions and maintain a clear airway. Avoid suctioning the nasopharynx; this could cause additional tissue trauma.*
- Monitor cough effectiveness and ability to manage airway secretions. *Pain, edema, and nasal bleeding may affect the client's ability to cough effectively.*
- Maintain adequate hydration. *Decreased fluid intake or active bleeding may cause dehydration and increase the viscosity of secretions, making them harder to spit out.*

RISK FOR INFECTION

- Assess for evidence of a CSF leak (clear fluid leaking from the ear or nose). If noted, test drainage for glucose. CSF will test positive for glucose on a dextrostrip. Report to the charge nurse or physician. *A CSF leak indicates a higher risk for ascending infection and meningitis.*
- Avoid suctioning if possible. *Suction catheters could cause additional trauma and introduce microorganisms.*
- Monitor vital signs every 4 hours. *A rise in temperature may indicate infection.*
- Administer antibiotics as ordered. *Antibiotics are often prescribed to prevent infection because nasal mucosa are populated with many bacteria.*

EVALUATING

Evaluate the effectiveness of nursing care by collecting data related to patency of the airway, comfort, and absence of infection. As the fracture heals, evaluate the position of the nasal septum and appearance of the nose.

 Discharge Considerations

When a nasal fracture is suspected, the client should seek medical evaluation and treatment as soon as possible.

Encourage the client to elevate the head of the bed with blocks and apply ice or cold packs to the nose for 20 minutes four times a day to reduce swelling. Inform the client that while swelling will subside within days, bruising may persist for several weeks. Reassure that the final cosmetic outcome following a nasal fracture cannot be determined until swelling has subsided.

Instruct the client who has a CSF leak to rest in bed with the head elevated or in a recliner chair. Fluids may be restricted; with the client, explore ways to distribute allowed fluids throughout the day. Instruct to avoid straining, blowing the nose, sneezing, or vigorous coughing. Discuss manifestations of infection, including stiff neck, headache, and fever. Instruct the client to contact the physician immediately if these manifestations occur.

Laryngeal Obstruction or Trauma

Laryngeal obstruction is a life-threatening emergency. The larynx is the narrowest part of the upper airway. It can be partially or fully obstructed by aspirated food or foreign objects. **Laryngospasm** (spasm of the muscles of the larynx) or laryngeal edema due to inflammation, injury, or anaphylaxis also can obstruct the larynx. The most common cause of obstruction in adults is ingested meat that lodges in the airway (the "café coronary"). Risk factors for food aspiration include ingesting large boluses of food and not chewing them enough, consuming excess alcohol, and wearing dentures. Laryngospasm may be caused by repeated or traumatic attempts at intubation, chemical irritation, or hypocalcemia. An acute type I hypersensitivity response may cause anaphylaxis and severe laryngeal edema.

The manifestations of laryngeal obstruction include coughing, choking, gagging, obvious difficulty breathing with use of accessory muscles, and inspiratory stridor. As the airway is obstructed, signs of asphyxia are seen. Respirations are labored and noisy with wheezing and stridor. The client may become *cyanotic* (blue). Respiratory arrest and death may result without prompt intervention.

Trauma to the larynx can occur in motor vehicle wrecks or assaults (e.g., blows to the neck or attempted strangulation). Trauma may cause cartilage fractures and loss of airway patency. Soft-tissue injuries can cause swelling that impairs the airway further. The client with laryngeal trauma may have *subcutaneous emphysema* (air under the skin), a change in the voice, dysphagia, inspiratory stridor, *hemoptysis* (bloody sputum), and a cough.

The goal of treatment is to maintain an open airway. If airway obstruction is partial and the client is able to cough and breathe, diagnostic tests may be done to locate the foreign body. An endotracheal tube may be inserted to maintain the airway that is in spasm or for laryngeal edema. For the client in anaphylaxis, epinephrine is given to reduce laryngeal edema and relieve obstruction.

CLINICAL alert

When airway obstruction is complete, the Heimlich maneuver must be performed immediately to clear the obstruction. Perform the maneuver by administering forceful thrusts to the upper abdomen or lower chest, continuing until the obstruction is relieved or more definitive care can be given (Figure 25-3 ◆).

Closely monitor clients at risk for laryngeal obstruction (e.g., newly extubated clients and clients receiving medications that may cause anaphylaxis, such as intravenous antibi-

Figure 25-3. ◆ (A) The Heimlich maneuver performed on a conscious victim who is sitting or standing. (B) The Heimlich maneuver performed on an unconscious victim.

otics or radiologic dyes) for manifestations of obstruction, including dyspnea, nasal flaring, tachypnea, anxiety, wheezing, and stridor. Laryngeal obstruction is a medical emergency requiring immediate intervention to open the airway and prevent brain damage or death. Suction the airway as needed; small aspirated foreign bodies may be removed by suctioning. Be prepared to assist with emergency intubation or tracheotomy as needed. If obstruction is complete, initiate a cardiopulmonary arrest procedure (code).

Client and family teaching focuses on preventing aspiration and teaching techniques to relieve obstruction. Clients who wear dentures should be cautioned to take small bites, chewing carefully before swallowing. Discuss the relationship between excess alcohol intake and food aspiration. Promote training of the general public in cardiopulmonary resuscitation (CPR) and the Heimlich maneuver. The more people who are adequately trained in emergency procedures, the more likely it is that emergency procedures will be initiated in a timely manner. Advise clients with a known risk for anaphylaxis (such as people with a previous anaphylactic response and those allergic to bee venom) to wear a Medic-Alert tag and carry a bee-sting kit to prevent severe laryngeal edema.

Figure 25-4. ◆ In obstructive sleep apnea, the pharynx is obstructed by the soft palate and tongue.

Sleep Apnea

Sleep apnea, the temporary absence of breathing during sleep, is common. Sleep apnea affects men more than women, and is more common in older adults. Obesity, enlarged tonsils, and using alcohol or sedatives before sleep contribute to sleep apnea.

Obstructive sleep apnea is the most common form. The upper airway is obstructed as muscles of the pharynx relax and the tongue falls back (Figure 25-4 ◆). In *central* sleep apnea, no effort to breathe is seen; the respiratory muscles remain relaxed.

Common manifestations of sleep apnea include loud snoring, frequent nighttime waking, daytime sleepiness, headache, and irritability. Other problems may follow, such as hypertension, morning headache, irritability, and impotence.

Clients may show personality changes, impaired memory, and inability to concentrate.

Sleep apnea is diagnosed in a sleep laboratory. The treatment plan includes measures to reduce airway obstruction, prevent apneic episodes, and provide psychological support. Weight loss often is the first intervention prescribed. Strict avoidance of alcohol and hypnotic medications also is vital.

Continuous positive airway pressure (CPAP) therapy is often prescribed for sleep apnea. The client wears a tightly fitting nasal mask. An air compressor blows air into the back of the throat, preventing the airway from collapsing.

Nursing care for clients with sleep apnea focuses on teaching the client and family how to use respiratory equipment and other management measures. Discuss the relationship of obesity, alcohol, and sedatives to the syndrome and provide instruction and referral to programs such as Weight Watchers and Alcoholics Anonymous.

Upper Respiratory Tumors

Tumors of the upper respiratory tract are relatively uncommon. They can, however, obstruct the airway and interfere with breathing. The larynx is the upper airway structure most often affected by tumors.

Benign Laryngeal Tumors

Benign tumors may develop on the vocal cords of the larynx, particularly in clients who chronically shout, project, or vocal-ize in a very high or low tone. Vocal cord nodules are often called "singer's nodules"; cheerleaders and public speakers may also develop them. Cigarette smoking and chronic irritation from pollution contribute to their development. Hoarseness and a breathy voice are manifestations of vocal cord nodules.

Correcting the underlying problem (e.g., voice training or quitting smoking) may correct benign tumors. If necessary, the tumors may be surgically removed.

If surgery is performed, observe closely for signs of airway obstruction, such as labored breathing or inspiratory stridor. Apply cold packs to the neck area to reduce the risk of swelling. To prevent aspiration, do not give food or fluids until the cough and gag reflexes have returned.

When teaching the client and family, stress the importance of voice rest. Refer clients, particularly singers, to a speech therapist for voice training. Emphasize the need to keep the voice within its normal range to reduce vocal cord stress. Talk to the client about quitting smoking, particularly if the client is also a singer.

Laryngeal Cancer

Cancer of the larynx is uncommon, but can be devastating. If found early, it can be cured, especially when it is limited to the vocal cords. The disease usually affects older adults; men are affected more often than women. Laryngeal cancer is more common in African Americans than in whites (Box 25-7). The two major modifiable risk factors for laryngeal cancer are prolonged use of tobacco and alcohol. Other modifiable risk factors include poor nutrition and occupational exposure to wood dust, paint fumes, chemicals, and asbestos.

PATHOPHYSIOLOGY

Changes in laryngeal mucosa occur when it is continually subjected to noxious irritants such as cigarette smoke. White, patchy precancerous lesions known as *leukoplakia* develop first, followed by the appearance of red, velvety patches called *erythroplakia,* a later stage of tumor development. Laryngeal cancer spreads both by direct invasion of surrounding tissues and by metastasis.

Laryngeal cancer may occur in any of the three areas of the larynx: the glottis, the supraglottis, and the subglottis. Lesions of the true vocal cords or *glottis* are more common than cancers of other areas of the larynx (Figure 25-5 ◆). Fortunately, these cancers tend to be slow growing.

The primary manifestation of *glottic* cancer is a change in the voice; the tumor prevents complete closure of the vocal cords during speech. The *supraglottic* (above the glottis) area includes the epiglottis and false vocal cords. A tumor may be large before manifestations such as painful swallowing, a sore

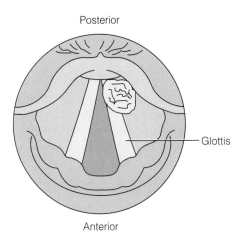

Posterior

Anterior

Glottis

Figure 25-5. ◆ Cancer of the larynx. Most lesions form along the edges of the glottis.

throat, or a feeling of a lump in the throat develop. As the tumor grows, difficulty breathing, foul breath, a palpable lump in the neck, and pain that radiates to the ear may occur. *Subglottic* tumors (below the vocal cords) are the least common laryngeal cancers and often have no early symptoms. As the tumor enlarges, manifestations of airway obstruction develop. Common manifestations of laryngeal cancer are summarized in Box 25-8.

COLLABORATIVE CARE

Most small cord lesions can be cured with early diagnosis and treatment. Left untreated, however, 90% of clients die within 3 years. Treatment (surgical removal, radiation, chemotherapy) is determined by the stage of the cancer. (See Chapter 8 for discussion of cancer staging.)

Laboratory and Diagnostic Tests

Direct or indirect *laryngoscopy* is performed when the client has manifestations of laryngeal cancer. Suspicious lesions are biopsied. Other diagnostic tests may include x-rays of the head, neck, and chest, as well as CT or magnetic resonance imaging (MRI) scan. A needle biopsy of enlarged lymph nodes helps

BOX 25-7

population
FOCUS

Laryngeal Cancer

Laryngeal cancer is about 50% more common in African Americans than it is in whites. Teach African American clients how to reduce their risk for laryngeal cancer by stopping smoking, abstaining from alcohol or drinking only moderately, and managing other risk factors (exposure to fumes, etc.). Discuss the early manifestations of laryngeal cancer, and stress the importance of seeking treatment promptly.

**BOX 25-8
MANIFESTATIONS
OF LARYNGEAL CANCER**

- Hoarseness or voice change that lasts more than 2 weeks
- Persistent cough
- Persistent sore throat
- Difficult or painful swallowing
- Dyspnea
- Foul breath
- Palpable lump in neck
- Persistent earache
- Unintended weight loss

confirm the diagnosis. A barium swallow may be done to evaluate swallowing and tumor extension into the esophagus.

Chemotherapy

Chemotherapy is not the treatment of choice, although it may be used to treat tumors that have metastasized beyond the head and neck or for tumors that are too large to be surgically removed. A multiple-drug treatment regimen often is used to maximize effectiveness. (See Chapter 8 for more information about chemotherapy.)

Radiation

Radiation therapy is often the treatment of choice for early laryngeal cancer. Radiation disrupts the DNA of the cell, causing it to die. External beam radiation is most often used. Radiation therapy is often combined with surgery, but it may be used alone in the early stages of laryngeal cancer or when the client refuses (or is not a candidate for) surgery. In advanced cancer, it may be used following laryngectomy to treat cervical lymph nodes.

Surgery

Surgery may be performed to remove the tumor and maintain an open airway. Carcinoma in situ and vocal cord polyps may be treated on an outpatient basis, using a laser to vaporize the tumor. Early cancers may be treated with *cordotomy* (removal of the tumor from the vocal cord) or *cordectomy* (removal of the affected vocal cord). These surgeries may be performed by laser. The voice is preserved after these procedures, although total voice rest is prescribed, with only whispering allowed for at least a week following surgery.

Laryngectomy, removal of the larynx, may be necessary for some clients. With a partial laryngectomy (removal of one half or more of the larynx), the client is able to resume normal speaking, breathing, and swallowing. In total laryngectomy, the entire larynx is removed, along with the surrounding tissues; normal speech is lost, and a permanent **tracheostomy** (a surgical opening into the trachea) is created. The tracheostomy tube inserted during surgery may be left in place for several weeks and then removed, leaving a natural stoma, or it may be left in place permanently. Because the trachea and the esophagus are permanently separated by this surgery (Figure 25-6 ◆), there is no risk of aspiration during swallowing.

If cervical lymph nodes contain cancer cells, a *radical neck dissection* may be done along with total laryngectomy. In a radical neck dissection, cervical lymph nodes, the sternocleidomastoid muscle, internal jugular vein, cranial nerve XI (spinal accessory), and submaxillary salivary gland are removed on the tumor side of the neck. After surgery, the client may have difficulty lifting and turning the head because of muscle loss. The shoulder on the affected side drops. Postoperative neck exercises can help reduce shoulder drop and increase range of motion on the affected side.

Speech Rehabilitation

Various techniques may be used to restore speech after a total laryngectomy. *Esophageal speech* uses swallowed air and con-

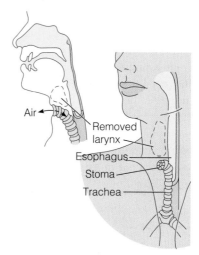

Figure 25-6. ◆ Following a total laryngectomy, the client has a permanent tracheostomy. No connection between the trachea and esophagus remains.

trolled belching to create sound and form words. The client uses muscles of the mouth and tongue normally involved in speech. This form of speech takes practice, and many clients are unable to resume speaking fluently.

A surgical procedure, the *tracheoesophageal puncture (TEP),* creates a small *fistula* (passage) between the posterior tracheal wall and the anterior esophagus (Figure 25-7 ◆). A small, one-way valve in the fistula allows the client to force air from the lungs into the mouth by covering the tracheostomy stoma with a finger. The air creates vibration and sound, and the client uses the tongue, lips, teeth, and palate to articulate the words. The one-way valve prevents food from entering the trachea.

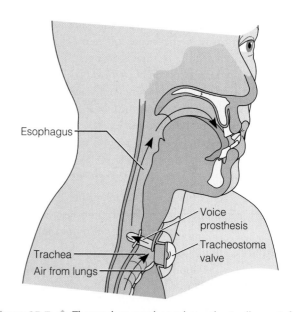

Figure 25-7. ◆ The tracheoesophageal prosthesis allows air from the trachea to be diverted through the prosthesis into the esophagus and oropharynx, producing speech when the tracheostomy stoma is occluded. A one-way valve prevents food from entering the trachea.

Figure 25-8. ◆ (A) The client holds the vibrating tip of the speech generator against the throat, using the mouth to form words. (B) A plastic tube on the handpiece of the speech aid device produces an audible tone. The client holds the tube against the roof of the mouth when forming words.

Several *speech generators* are available for the laryngectomy client. One type is held against the neck; it transmits vibrations to the neck and into the mouth. Muscles of the mouth and tongue form vibrations into words. (Figure 25-8A ◆) Another device delivers a tone into the mouth through a plastic tube (Figure 25-8B). The lips, tongue, and mouth muscles then form the sound into words.

NURSING CARE

ASSESSING

Nurses can help to identify clients at risk for or with early manifestations of laryngeal cancer. Because manifestations of the disease often do not occur until the cancer is advanced, obtaining good subjective data from the client is vital. Box 25-9 lists assessment data to collect.

DIAGNOSING, PLANNING, AND IMPLEMENTING

The client with laryngeal cancer has multiple nursing care needs. The risk for impaired verbal communication exists, whether or not a total laryngectomy is planned. Clients may experience dysphagia that interferes with swallowing and nutrition before treatment. Radiation, chemotherapy, or surgery also may interfere with nutrition. The diagnosis of cancer is frightening for most clients, no matter what the potential for cure is with treatment. Problems related to communication, nutrition, and anticipatory grieving are

included in this section. Nursing care specific to the client undergoing a laryngectomy is included in Box 25-10. Nursing care of the client with a tracheostomy is reviewed in Procedure 25-2.

BOX 25-9
ASSESSING CLIENTS WITH LARYNGEAL CANCER

SUBJECTIVE DATA

- Recent and/or persistent voice changes (hoarseness, breathiness); difficulty or pain with swallowing, persistent sore throat, cough, or ear pain; difficulty breathing; sensation of a lump in the throat
- Recent unintended or unexplained weight loss
- Smoking history: Packs smoked per day; number of years smoked. Alcohol consumption: Amount per day or week; number of years of alcohol use
- Chronic diseases; occupation

OBJECTIVE DATA

- General appearance: Apparent health, skin color
- Difficulty breathing or swallowing, hoarseness, changes in voice quality, and cough
- Inspect: Neck for asymmetry or masses; mouth and oropharynx for white or red patches
- Palpate: Lips, cheeks, and tongue for masses; neck for symmetry, masses, lymph node enlargement, and tenderness

> ## BOX 25-10
> ## NURSING CARE CHECKLIST
>
> ### TOTAL LARYNGECTOMY
>
> #### Before Surgery
>
> ☑ Provide routine preoperative care and teaching (see Chapter 7).
> ☑ Assess anxiety level and provide psychological support.
> ☑ Discuss postoperative communication stategies. Emphasize that total laryngectomy results in a loss of speech and that the client will breathe through a permanent stoma in the neck.
>
> #### After Surgery
>
> ☑ Provide routine postoperative care (see Chapter 7).
> ☑ Monitor respiratory status at least every 1 to 2 hours, including airway patency; respiratory rate, depth, and pattern; and lung sounds.
> ☑ Monitor oxygen saturation levels. Report levels of less than 95% (or established parameters) to the charge nurse or physician.
> ☑ Place the call light within easy reach at all times; answer the call light promptly.
> ☑ Encourage family members to stay with the client whenever possible.
> ☑ Encourage deep breathing and coughing.
> ☑ Elevate the head of the bed.
> ☑ Maintain humidification of inspired gases.
> ☑ Maintain fluid intake (initially intravenously, then orally).
> ☑ Perform tracheal suctioning using sterile technique as needed.
> ☑ Provide tracheostomy care as needed (see Procedure 25-2).
> ☑ Teach to support the head when moving in bed.
> ☑ Assist out of bed and with ambulation as soon as allowed after surgery.
> ☑ Teach to protect the stoma from particulate matter in the air with a gauze square or other stoma protector.
> ☑ Maintain intravenous fluids and/or enteral feedings until able to take adequate amounts of food and fluids orally.
> ☑ Prior to initiating feeding, assist to begin performing mouth rinses.
> ☑ When able to resume oral intake, begin with soft foods, not liquids.
> ☑ Reassure the client that choking is not possible, because there is no connection between the esophagus and trachea.
> ☑ Provide for privacy during initial attempts at eating.
> ☑ Encourage the client and family members to express their fears and anxieties.

IMPAIRED VERBAL COMMUNICATION

Removing the larynx results in voice loss. Before surgery, discuss alternate methods of communication, both short and long term, with the client and family members. Ultimately, the choice is the client's; some may choose to forgo laryngectomy to avoid voice loss when the chance for long-term success and cancer cure is minimal.

■ Before surgery, assess for additional obstacles to communication. *Hearing loss, illiteracy, previous stroke, or weakness may affect the ability to use alternate communication strategies.*
■ Provide alternate ways to communicate (pencil and paper, magic slate, an alphabet board) and encourage practice. *Having the client choose what to practice helps lessen anxiety and increases the sense of control.*
■ Encourage the client to consult a speech therapist before surgery if possible. *The client may be a candidate for esophageal speech, TEP, or a speech generator.*
■ Assess frequently. Place the call bell at hand when leaving. *The presence and availability of a caring nurse decrease anxiety and promote communication.*

IMBALANCED NUTRITION: LESS THAN BODY REQUIREMENTS

Large tumors may affect the ability to eat. The client with cancer often requires additional calories because of the effects of the disease. After surgery, enteral or parenteral feedings often are ordered until the client is able to eat. After a total laryngectomy, the client initially loses the senses of taste and smell. The client may partially recover the sense of taste but may complain that eating no longer holds pleasure.

■ Assess nutritional status using height and weight charts, reported weight loss, and body mass indicators such as skin folds. *A complete assessment aids in planning to meet current and anticipated calorie needs.*
■ Evaluate current diet, preferred foods, and understanding of nutrition. *Providing a diet that takes the client's preferences into account will encourage adequate intake.*
■ Monitor intake and output and food consumption. *Monitoring food and fluid intake is necessary to determine if the client is consuming adequate calories and fluids for healing.*
■ Weigh daily. *The daily weight provides a measure of both nutritional status and fluid balance.*
■ Contact the dietitian for further evaluation, planning, and education. *A professional can identify nutritional needs and help plan a diet to meet them.*
■ Encourage experimentation with foods of different textures and temperatures. *Cold foods or foods with a soft texture are easier to swallow.*
■ Encourage frequent, small meals rather than three large meals per day. *The client who has difficulty swallowing is likely to consume more food this way.*

PROCEDURE 25-2 Tracheostomy Care Checklist

- Gather all supplies
- Provide for privacy. Explain the procedure and provide for communication (e.g., eye blinking or raising a finger to indicate distress).
- Place in semi-Fowler's or Fowler's position.
- Use standard precautions and sterile technique as indicated.
- Assess lung sounds; suction as needed using sterile technique.
- Wearing clean gloves, remove the tracheostomy dressing.
- Wearing sterile gloves, use sterile applicators or gauze 4 × 4s moistened with normal saline to clean the incision.
- If the tracheostomy tube has an inner cannula that can be removed for cleaning, remove the tube and soak it in sterile saline.
- Cleanse the tracheostomy tube flange (collar) in the same manner as the incision.
- Clean the inner cannula using a small brush or cotton-tipped applicators. Rinse thoroughly in normal saline and tap it gently to remove excess liquid.

- Suction the outer cannula using sterile technique.
- Replace the inner cannula into the tracheostomy tube.
- Replace the dressing. Do not cut the dressing or use a cotton-filled dressing because fibers may be aspirated into the respiratory tract.
- Apply clean tracheostomy ties.
- Once the clean ties are secured, remove the old ties.
- Assess breathing and tolerance of the procedure.
- Dispose of supplies and used solutions. Wash hands.

■ SAMPLE DOCUMENTATION

0830	Trach care provided. Suctioned for moderate amount of thin, yellow sputum. Lung sounds clear after suctioning. Incision clean, no evidence of inflammation. Healing well. Tolerated procedure well.
	S. Doene, LPN.

- Recommend liquid supplements such as Ensure as needed to increase calorie intake. Provide information about where to obtain supplements. *Liquid dietary supplements provide balanced nutrition and added calories. They are available in major supermarkets.*
- Provide mouth care prior to meals and supplemental feedings. For the client with stomatitis or esophagitis related to radiation or chemotherapy, provide a topical anesthetic such as viscous lidocaine before eating. *Bad breath or a foul taste in the mouth suppresses appetite. Inflamed mucosa may make eating uncomfortable. A topical anesthetic can relieve discomfort and promote food intake* (see Stomatitis, Chapter 18).
- Provide an antiemetic 30 minutes before eating if nausea is a problem. *An antiemetic can relieve nausea and make eating possible.*

ANTICIPATORY GRIEVING

The client with laryngeal cancer faces the diagnosis of cancer, the prospect of mutilating surgery, and loss of both a body part and an important function, speech. Loss of speech affects social interactions, one's career, and the ability to get help when necessary. A radical neck dissection changes the appearance and function of the neck, altering body image and self-concept.

- Provide opportunities for the client and family members to express feelings of grief, anger, or fear about the diagnosis of cancer, the impending surgery, and the anticipated loss of speech. *The client needs the opportunity (and permission) to grieve anticipated losses in order to move toward coping and acceptance of the loss.*
- Be calm and supportive. Provide privacy and emotional support for client and family to work through the grieving process. *It is important for the client and family to know that their feelings of loss are real and accepted by caregivers.*
- Help the client and family discuss the potential impact of the loss on family structure and function. *Discussion helps family members to understand and support one another.*
- Refer the client and family for counseling as appropriate. *Counseling may be necessary to prevent a sense of defeat and hopelessness.*
- Help the client and family identify additional resources for coping, such as strategies they have used in the past to deal with crises. *This identifies strengths they can use to deal with the present situation.*

EVALUATING

Collect the following data to evaluate the effectiveness of nursing interventions for the client with laryngeal cancer:

- Airway remains patent; experiences no difficulty breathing
- Communicates care needs effectively
- Anxiety remains within a manageable level
- Maintains weight
- Demonstrates willingness to participate in speech therapy

Discharge Considerations

In the community, teach about the risk factors and early warning signs of laryngeal cancer, so it can be recognized and treated early. After diagnosis of laryngeal cancer, provide information and clarify treatment options, discussing the risks and benefits of each. Stress the importance of early intervention to reduce the risk of local spread and metastasis. If a total laryngectomy is the treatment of choice, discuss options for communication after surgery. Present the options realistically. Clients may have difficulty manipulating the tracheoesophageal puncture device for speech; only about 30% of clients master esophageal speech.

Teach the client undergoing radiation therapy about the treatments, care of the skin and secretions during therapy, and expected side effects. (See Chapter 8 for further discussion about managing the effects of radiation therapy.)

Assess the client's and family's resources and ability to provide home care following surgery (Box 25-11).

Teach the client and family members how to care for the tracheostomy and provide the opportunity for redemonstration of care. The client uses clean technique rather than sterile technique in providing stoma care. Once the stoma is fully healed, the tracheostomy tube may no longer be needed. Teach the following:

- Use a humidifier or vaporizer in the home to add humidity to inspired air.
- Increase fluid intake to maintain mucosal moisture and loosen secretions
- Shield the stoma with a stoma guard (such as a gauze square) to prevent particles from entering the lower respiratory tract.
- Promptly remove secretions from skin surrounding the stoma to prevent irritation and skin breakdown.
- Protect the stoma with a cupped hand or washcloth while showering or bathing; don't submerge the neck or head.
- Do not participate in water sports. All other activities are allowed, but lifting may be more difficult because of the inability to hold the breath (the Valsalva maneuver).

Encourage the client to work with a physical therapist to regain function and mobility of the neck and shoulder if a radical neck dissection has been done.

BOX 25-11
ASSESSING FOR DISCHARGE

LARYNGEAL CANCER
Client

- Self-care: Ability to perform ADLs independently, care for tracheostomy, manipulate TEP device or electronic speech device
- Knowledge: Treatment plan; dealing with adverse effects of radiation or chemotherapy; preventing respiratory infections; using communication techniques; maintaining nutritional status; indications for seeking medical intervention
- Motivation: Smoking cessation, abstinence from alcohol consumption
- Home environment: Access to clean water for handwashing and tracheostomy care; indoor pollutants such as cigarette smoke, dust, and allergens such as pets

Family

- Caregivers: Availability and willingness to provide care as needed; assist with shopping, transportation, and caring for dependents; willingness to avoid smoking inside the home
- Financial resources: Income; availability of sick leave; impact of diagnosis and treatment options on career and income; resources for drugs, medical supplies, and medical care required

Community

- Access: Health care resources and supplies; transportation; support groups and services such as laryngectomy groups, hospice services
- Air quality: Presence of industrial or agricultural polutants such as smoke, smog, or dust

Both the client and family need emotional and motivational support through this trying time. Provide referral to local support groups such as a laryngectomy club or lost cord club. Encourage the client to discontinue the use of cigarettes and alcohol. Discuss ways to achieve good nutrition. If the client and family are having difficulty adjusting to the diagnosis of cancer and the effects of treatment, provide referral to counseling. (See the Critical Thinking Care Map at the end of this chapter.)

Nursing Interventions Classification

The following nursing interventions (McCloskey & Bulechek, 2000) may be useful for clients with upper respiratory disorders:

- Airway Management
- Fever Treatment
- Immunization/Vaccination Administration
- Airway Suctioning
- Caregiver Support

- Communication Enhancement: Speech Deficit
- Incision Site Care
- Nutrition Management

(*Note:* The bibliography listings for this and all chapters have been compiled at the back of the book.)

Chapter Review

key terms by topic

Use the CD-ROM disk enclosed with your textbook to hear the pronunciation of the key terms in the chapter.

URI and inflammations
rhinitis, influenza, sinusitis, coryza, pharyngitis, tonsillitis, dysphagia, stridor, laryngitis, tonsillectomy

Trauma or obstruction
epistaxis, rhinoplasty, laryngospasm, sleep apnea

Tumors
laryngectomy, tracheostomy

key points

- A patent airway and unobstructed airflow is vital to sustain life and function. While upper airway disorders often are minor, many potentially can affect airway patency and become life threatening.
- Most upper respiratory infections are relatively minor and appropriate for self-care.
- While many decongestants and antihistamines are available without a prescription, these drugs are not appropriate for all people. They may cause drowsiness, increased blood pressure, or problems for people who have glaucoma, intestinal problems, or urinary retention.
- Bacterial complications such as pneumonia, sinusitis, and peritonsilar abscess may follow viral URI. These complications do require medical treatment, often antibiotic therapy.
- Acute epiglottitis and laryngeal spasm, edema, or obstruction are medical emergencies that require immediate treatment to maintain an open airway and sustain life.
- Most nosebleeds occur in the anterior portion of the nose and can be controlled by putting pressure and ice on the nose. Older adults are at risk for posterior nosebleeds. Posterior nosebleeds are more difficult to control and often require medical treatment.
- The primary risk factors for laryngeal cancer are smoking and excess alcohol use. Discuss these lifestyle factors with all clients, especially those who have other risk factors for laryngeal cancer.
- Persistent hoarseness or voice change is a common manifestation of laryngeal cancer. Prompt clients to seek medical assessment if this occurs. Stress that with early intervention, laryngeal cancer is curable and the ability to speak is preserved.

Medialink

Additional interactive resources for this chapter can be found on the Companion Website at www.prenhall.com/burke. Click on Chapter 25 and "Begin" to select the activities for this chapter.

For NCLEX review questions and an audio glossary, access the accompanying CD-ROM in this book.

for further study

For more information on care and teaching of the surgical client, see Chapter 7.

For more information on cancer staging, chemotherapy, and radiation therapy, see Chapter 8.

For further study about acute glomerulonephritis, see Chapter 21.

For discussion of rheumatic fever, see Chapter 22.

For more about pneumonia and about the huff technique of coughing, see Chapter 26.

For more information about otitis media and other ear disorders, see Chapter 31.

Critical Thinking Care Map

Caring for a Client with Total Laryngectomy
NCLEX-PN Focus Area: Reduction of Risk Potential

Case Study: David Tom is a 61-year-old divorced man with two grown children. He has smoked two packs of cigarettes daily since high school. He drinks three or four cocktails every evening. Mr. Tom was recently diagnosed with laryngeal cancer after he sought care for a sore throat and hoarseness that persisted for a few months. He has been admitted to the surgical care unit from the intensive care unit (ICU) 2 days post total laryngectomy.

Nursing Diagnosis: Risk for Ineffective Airway Clearance

COLLECT DATA

Subjective

_____
_____
_____
_____
_____
_____

Objective

_____
_____
_____
_____
_____
_____

Would you report this data? Yes/No

If yes, to: _____

Nursing Care

_____
_____
_____
_____
_____
_____
_____
_____

How would you document this? _____
_____
_____

**Data Collected
(use those that apply)**

- PB 146/84; P 92 and regular; R 18; T 100° F (37.7° C) per rectum
- Tracheostomy tube present
- O_2 per tracheostomy collar
- Oxygen saturation 94%
- Rates pain in neck and right shoulder at 6 on a scale of 1 to 10
- Continuous tube feeding per nasogastric tube
- Two Hemovac wound drains in the right neck draining 15 and 35 mL serosanguinous fluid
- Complains that head "feels heavy"
- Ambulatory within the room without assistance
- Using Magic Slate to communicate

**Nursing Interventions
(use those that apply)**

- Assess respiratory rate, lung sounds, and cough effectiveness every 2 hours.
- Monitor quantity, color, and odor of secretions.
- Encourage to deep breathe and cough hourly.
- Assess pain at least every 2 to 3 hours and administer analgesics as ordered.
- Up at bedside and ambulating at least four times per day.
- Provide written information as requested.
- Monitor intake, output, and daily weight.
- Arrange for a dietary consultation to determine calorie needs.

NCLEX-PN Exam Preparation

TEST-TAKING TIP

The NCLEX-PN is a timed test. Pace yourself. Be aware of your remaining time. Use all of the time allotted, if needed. You will have 5 hours to complete the test.

1. After teaching a client about the antihistamine Chlor-Trimeton, which statement indicates that further instruction is necessary?
   a. "I'm not going to drive today. My sister will pick me up."
   b. "I will stop at the grocery store for a bag of hard peppermint candy."
   c. "I'm going to a wine-tasting party tonight."
   d. "I'll call my doctor if I have trouble breathing."

2. In order to most effectively anticipate the needs of a client who has undergone a tonsillectomy, the nurse would plan to:
   a. apply a warm compress to the neck
   b. place the patient in a supine position
   c. remove the nasopharyngeal airway immediately
   d. place a humidifier by the bedside

3. Which of these laboratory tests is the most definitive diagnostic test for streptococcal pharyngitis?
   a. CBC
   b. nasal swabs
   c. ELISA test
   d. throat culture

4. A resident of a nursing home will be receiving the influenza injection. Which information would be the most important for the care of this client?
   a. allergy history
   b. name of insurance company
   c. medical history
   d. respiratory status

5. The nurse understands that the most important intervention for the client with a noncomplicated upper respiratory viral infection is:
   a. obtaining throat cultures
   b. teaching self-care
   c. monitoring vital signs
   d. antibiotic medication teaching

6. In teaching a client about laryngitis, it is important to focus on:
   a. resting the voice
   b. effective coughing techniques
   c. increased fluids
   d. use of a cough suppressant at bedtime

7. A client presents to the emergency department with severe bleeding from the anterior nasal septum. The nurse's first response should be to:
   a. apply ice packs to the nose
   b. give the client an emesis basin to spit out the blood
   c. pinch the nose toward the septum
   d. ask what precipitated the incident

8. Which of these statements, if made by a client diagnosed with sleep apnea, would indicate an understanding of this condition?
   a. "I'm going to sleep on my back for the next 2 weeks."
   b. "I would like to see the dietitian about my weight."
   c. "Please ask the doctor to order a sleeping pill for me."
   d. "I won't snore so loud if I drink a glass of wine before bedtime."

9. A client at a blood pressure clinic tells the nurse that his voice has been hoarse for "about a month now." He denies sore throat or difficulty swallowing. The appropriate response by the nurse is:
   a. "Since you don't also have a sore throat, it really isn't anything to worry about."
   b. "Persistent hoarseness is a sign of voice strain. You should rest your voice for a couple weeks and see if it improves."
   c. "Try using warm salt-water gargles three to four times a day. This sounds like persistent laryngitis."
   d. "Persistent hoarseness can be an early sign of laryngeal cancer. Please tell your doctor about this."

10. A client who has had a total laryngectomy and permanent tracheostomy is afraid to eat for fear of choking. The nurse's response is based on the knowledge that:
    a. choking is a significant risk following total laryngectomy
    b. choking can be prevented by closing the tracheostomy stoma with a finger while swallowing
    c. the trachea and esophagus are not separate, so choking is not a risk
    d. oral intake should begin with water only until the client learns to swallow without choking

Answers for Review Questions, as well as discussion of Case Study Critical Thinking questions, appear in Appendix V.

Caring for Clients with Lower Respiratory Disorders

chapter **26**

LEARNING outcomes

After completing this chapter, you will be able to:
- Identify the structures and function of the lower respiratory system.
- Explain the mechanics of respiration.
- Describe the pathophysiology and manifestations of common lower respiratory system disorders.
- Discuss nursing implications for medications and treatments used for lower respiratory system disorders.
- Provide appropriate care for a client having thoracic surgery.
- Use the nursing process to assess, plan, and implement individualized care for clients with lower respiratory system disorders.
- Reinforce teaching and learning for clients with lower respiratory system disorders and their families.

Disorders of the lower respiratory system are common, affecting people in the community, acute care, and long-term care facilities. Lower respiratory system disorders have both local and systemic effects. Local effects include cough, excess mucus production, **dyspnea** (difficulty breathing), **hemoptysis** (bloody sputum), and chest pain. Systemic effects may include fever, anorexia and malaise, **cyanosis** (a bluish-gray skin color), edema, clubbing of fingers and toes, and other manifestations of impaired gas exchange.

Structure and Function of the Lower Respiratory System

The lower respiratory system includes the lungs and the bronchi. Its function is to provide oxygen to the cells of the body and to eliminate carbon dioxide, a waste product of metabolism. This process, called **respiration,** includes:

- *Ventilation* (breathing): Air moves into and out of the lungs.
- *External respiration:* Oxygen and carbon dioxide are exchanged between the alveoli and the blood.
- *Gas transport:* Blood transports oxygen and carbon dioxide to and from the lungs and the cells of the body.
- *Internal respiration:* Oxygen and carbon dioxide are exchanged between the blood and the cells.

THE LUNGS

The lungs fill both sides of the chest, separated by the mediastinum. The heart, great blood vessels, bronchi, trachea, and esophagus sit in the *mediastinum* (Figure 26-1 ◆). The *apex* of each lung is just below the clavicle, and the *base* of each lung rests on the diaphragm. The lungs are soft and spongy, composed of elastic connective tissue.

The right lung has three lobes; the left is smaller, with only two lobes. Each lobe is further divided into segments.

BRONCHI AND ALVEOLI

The trachea divides into *right* and *left mainstem bronchi.* The mainstem bronchi enter the lungs at the *hilus.* The bronchi branch into smaller bronchi, then into smaller and smaller *bronchioles,* ending in the tiny *alveoli* (Figure 26-2 ◆). During inspiration, air moves through these passageways to the alveoli, where gas exchange occurs.

There are millions of alveoli in each lung, providing a huge area for gas exchange. Alveoli have extremely thin walls, made of a single layer of cells over a very thin connective tissue membrane. The outer surface of the alveolus is covered with pulmonary capillaries. Oxygen and carbon dioxide easily diffuse across the walls of the alveoli and capillaries. The alveoli contain cells that secrete *surfactant,* a detergent-like substance that helps keep them open.

PULMONARY CIRCULATION

The pulmonary circulation includes the pulmonary arteries, which deliver oxygen-poor blood to the lungs, and the pulmonary veins, which return oxygenated blood to the heart. In the lungs, the vessels branch into a pulmonary capillary network that surround the alveoli. Vessels enter and exit the lungs at the hilus.

THE PLEURA

The *pleura* is a double-layered membrane that covers the lungs (see Figure 26-1). The *parietal pleura* lines the chest wall and mediastinum. The *visceral pleura* covers the outer lung surfaces. The layers of the pleura hold the lungs out to the chest wall, sliding against one another during breathing. The potential space between the layers of the pleura contains a small amount of serous fluid to lubricate and reduce friction during breathing. There is a slight negative pressure in the pleural space.

RIB CAGE AND INTERCOSTAL MUSCLES

The lungs are protected by the rib cage and the intercostal muscles. There are 12 pairs of ribs. The spaces between the ribs (the *intercostal spaces*) are named for the rib immediately above (e.g., the space between the third and fourth ribs is the third intercostal space). The *intercostal muscles* between the ribs, along with the diaphragm, are *inspiratory muscles.*

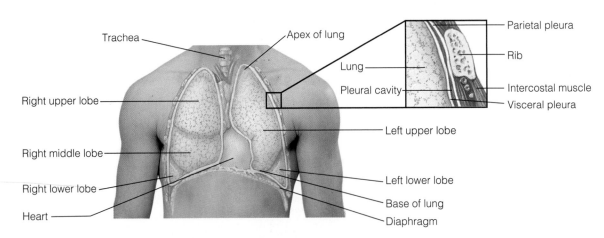

Figure 26-1. ◆ **The lower respiratory system, showing the lungs and layers of visceral and parietal pleura.**

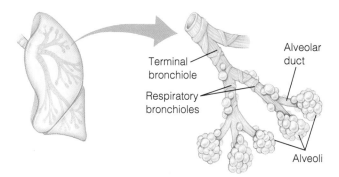

Figure 26-2. ◆ The functional tissue of the lungs, including the respiratory bronchioles and alveoli.

MECHANICS OF RESPIRATION

Ventilation, air movement into and out of the lungs, has two phases: *inspiration,* as air flows into the lungs, and *expiration,* when gases flow out of the lungs. The two phases make up a breath, and normally occur 12 to 20 times per minute. Inspiration lasts about 1 to 1.5 seconds; expiration lasts about 2 to 3 seconds.

During inspiration, the diaphragm contracts and flattens out and the intercostal muscles contract to increase the size of the chest cavity (Figure 26-3A ◆). The lungs stretch and their volume increases. This reduces pressure within the lungs to slightly less than atmospheric pressure. Air rushes into the lungs as a result.

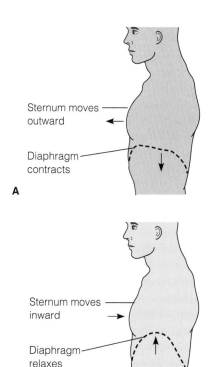

Sternum moves outward

Diaphragm contracts

A

Sternum moves inward

Diaphragm relaxes

B

Figure 26-3. ◆ (A) During inspiration, the diaphragm contracts and flattens, and the intercostal muscles contract, moving the chest wall up and outward. This increases the volume of the chest cavity. (B) During expiration, the muscles relax, the diaphragm rises, and the lungs recoil.

Expiration is primarily passive. The inspiratory muscles relax, the diaphragm rises, the ribs descend, and the lungs recoil (Figure 26-3B). Pressures in the chest cavity increase, compressing the alveoli. The pressure within the lungs is higher than atmospheric pressure, and gases flow out of the lungs.

FACTORS AFFECTING RESPIRATION

Breathing is controlled by respiratory centers in the brain and by chemoreceptors in the brain, aortic arch, and carotid arteries. These centers and receptors respond to changes in the amount of oxygen, carbon dioxide, and hydrogen ions in arterial blood. For example, increased carbon dioxide or a drop in pH stimulate the respiratory centers, and the respiratory rate increases.

Other factors affect ventilation and the work of breathing:

- *Airway resistance* is created by friction as gases move through the airways. Resistance is increased by airway constriction or edema, excess mucus, or by tumors that narrow the airways. As resistance increases, gas flow decreases.
- *Compliance* is the *distensibility* (stretchiness) of the lungs. It depends on both lung tissue and the rib cage.
- *Elasticity* is the tendency of lung tissue to return to its uninflated size and shape.

CLINICAL alert

A balloon is a good example of compliance and elasticity. When a balloon is brand new, it is very elastic and not very compliant—it takes a lot of work to begin inflating it (poor compliance). When the air is released, it returns to its previous shape (good elasticity). After it has been blown up a few times, it becomes increasingly compliant, and easier to inflate. However, it doesn't return to its original shape, because some of its elasticity has been lost.

- Alveoli contain a liquid film that creates *surface tension,* drawing the walls of the alveolus closer together. *Surfactant* reduces this surface tension, prevents the alveoli from collapsing between breaths, and reduces the work of breathing.

LUNG VOLUME AND CAPACITY

Lung volume and capacity are measured with *pulmonary function tests (PFTs).* Lung volume and capacity (Figure 26-4 ◆) are affected by sex, age, weight, and health status.

The *total lung capacity (TLC),* is the total volume of the lungs at their maximum inflation. It is calculated by adding the: (1) *tidal volume (VT),* the air (about 500 mL) exchanged during normal quiet breathing; (2) *inspiratory reserve volume (IRV),* the air (about 2,100 to 3,100 mL) that can be inhaled over and above a normal inspiration; (3) *expiratory reserve volume (ERV),* the air (about 1,200 mL) that can be forced out following a normal exhalation; and (4) *residual volume (RV),*

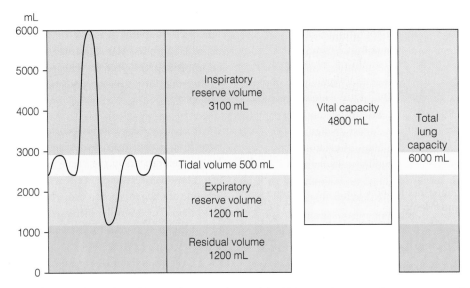

Figure 26-4. ◆ The relationship of lung volumes and capacities. Volumes shown are for an average adult male.

the air (about 1,200 mL) remaining in the lungs after maximal exhalation. The *vital capacity (VC)*, about 4,500 to 4,800 mL in healthy adults, is the sum of the VT, IRV, and ERV.

About 150 mL of air remains in the airways with each breath, never reaching the alveoli. This is called *anatomical dead space volume.*

Infectious and Inflammatory Disorders

The lower respiratory system is protected from infection by a number of defenses. If an organism makes it past the upper respiratory tract, it is usually trapped in mucus of the lower respiratory tract. *Cilia* (small hairs) that line the airways and the cough reflex then push it out. Organisms that make it past all these barriers usually are killed rapidly in the alveolus by the immune defenses of the body. When these defenses are impaired, the risk of infection increases. For example, chronic lung disease impairs the mucus and ciliary responses to invasion. Older adults have a higher risk of lower respiratory infections (Box 26-1). Even in healthy clients, pathogens can enter the lungs, causing an infectious or inflammatory response.

Acute Bronchitis

Bronchitis (inflammation of the bronchi) can be either acute or chronic. Acute bronchitis is relatively common among adults. Chronic bronchitis is a component of chronic obstructive pulmonary disease (COPD) and is discussed in that section of this chapter.

Acute bronchitis typically follows an upper respiratory infection. People with impaired defense mechanisms and smokers have a higher risk for bronchitis. Viruses, bacteria, and toxic gases or chemicals can cause bronchitis. The inflam-

matory response leads to vasodilation and edema of the bronchial linings. Mucus production increases, stimulating the cough reflex.

The cough is initially nonproductive, but later becomes productive. The cough often occurs in *paroxysms* (uncontrollable bursts), and may be aggravated by cold, dry, or dusty air.

BOX 26-1

population
FOCUS

Lower Respiratory Tract Infections in Older Adults

Changes associated with aging and disease affect respiratory function and airway clearance, increasing the risk of infections. The number of cilia decreases, and the cough weakens. Gag and cough reflexes diminish. Residual volume increases, and vital capacity decreases. The older adult is at risk for dehydration, leading to thick, sticky mucus that is difficult to expectorate. Immune function declines with aging. Limited mobility, a smoking history, surgery, multiple medications, malnutrition, and chronic diseases also may increase older adults' risk for respiratory infections.

Substernal chest pain is common. Other symptoms include fever and general malaise.

Acute bronchitis usually is diagnosed by the history and examination. A *chest x-ray* may be ordered to rule out pneumonia, because the manifestations can be similar. Treatment includes rest, increased fluid intake, and mild analgesics to relieve fever and malaise. An antibiotic such as erythromycin or penicillin may be prescribed. An expectorant cough medication is recommended for daytime, and a cough suppressant at night to facilitate rest.

Clients with acute bronchitis are rarely hospitalized, so nursing care focuses on teaching. Advise that bed rest is not often necessary. Activities of daily living (ADLs) can be maintained with adequate rest. Instruct to increase fluid intake. Discuss the use and effects of ordered drugs. Stress the importance of smoking cessation. Instruct to contact primary care provider if symptoms do not improve within a week or if they become worse.

Pneumonia

Pneumonia is inflammation of the respiratory bronchioles and alveoli. It is a leading cause of death in the United States, particularly among older adults and people with debilitating diseases. Pneumonia may be either infectious or noninfectious. Bacteria, viruses, fungi, protozoa, and other microbes can lead to infectious pneumonia. Noninfectious causes include aspiration of gastric contents and inhalation of toxic or irritating gases.

PATHOPHYSIOLOGY

The microbes causing infectious pneumonia usually enter the lungs when secretions from the oral and nasopharynx are aspirated. *Streptococcus pneumoniae* (pneumococcal pneumonia) is the most common pathogen; others include *Haemophilus influenzae,* some gram-negative bacteria, and the influenza virus.

Pneumonia is classified by its cause (acute bacterial or viral), or by its location (lobar or bronchial) (Table 26-1 ◆).

Acute Bacterial Pneumonia

When bacteria invade the lungs, an inflammatory response follows. Inflammation causes the alveoli to become edematous and fill with fluid. Blood cells and bacteria collect in the alveoli and respiratory bronchioles, leading to *consolidation* (solidification) of lung tissue. The lower lobes of the lungs are usually affected because of gravity. Consolidation of a large portion of an entire lung lobe is known as *lobar pneumonia. Bronchopneumonia* is patchy consolidation involving several lobules. Eventually, macrophages digest and remove the fluid, bacteria, and damaged cells from the infected lung.

The onset of bacterial pneumonia typically is acute, with shaking chills, fever, and cough productive of rust-colored or purulent sputum. Chest pain (aching or sharp and localized) is common. Diminished breath sounds and fine crackles are heard over the affected lung area. If the involved area is large, respiratory distress is evident. The older adult may have fewer respiratory symptoms, presenting with fever, tachypnea, and altered mental status.

TABLE 26-1	FEATURES OF INFECTIOUS PNEUMONIAS		
TYPE	**ONSET**	**RESPIRATORY MANIFESTATIONS**	**OTHER MANIFESTATIONS**
Pneumococcal or lobar pneumonia	Abrupt	Cough productive of purulent or rust-colored sputum Chest pain Decreased breath sounds and crackles over affected area Possible dyspnea and cyanosis	Chills and fever
Bronchopneumonia	Gradual	Cough, scattered crackles Minimal dyspnea and shortness of breath	Low-grade fever
Legionnaires' disease	Gradual	Dry cough Dyspnea	Chills and fever Malaise, headache Muscle and joint pain Confusion
Viral pneumonia	Sudden or gradual	Dry cough	Flulike symptoms
Atypical pneumonia	Gradual	Dry, hacking, nonproductive cough	Fever, headache Muscle and joint pain
Pneumocystis carinii pneumonia	Abrupt	Dry cough Tachypnea and shortness of breath Respiratory distress	Fever

The most common complication of pneumococcal pneumonia is *pleuritis* (pleurisy), painful inflammation of the adjacent pleura. Pneumonias can cause extensive lung damage, leading to necrosis, abscess, and *empyema* (a collection of pus in the pleural cavity).

Pneumocystis carinii Pneumonia

The majority of people with acquired immunodeficiency syndrome (AIDS) develop pneumonia caused by *Pneumocystis carinii,* a common parasite. Most people are immune to *P. carinii,* but it is an *opportunistic* organism that can cause an infection when the immune system is suppressed.

Infection with *P. carinii* causes affected alveoli to thicken, become edematous, and fill with foamy, protein-rich fluid. Gas exchange is severely impaired as the disease progresses. Respiratory distress can be significant. (See also Chapter 13.)

Aspiration Pneumonia

Aspiration of gastric contents into the lungs causes a chemical and bacterial pneumonia known as *aspiration pneumonia.* The risk for aspiration pneumonia is highest during emergency surgery and when cough and gag reflexes are depressed or swallowing is impaired. Older adults and clients receiving tube feedings are also at risk for aspiration pneumonia.

Vomiting may not be obvious; silent regurgitation of gastric contents may occur if the level of consciousness is reduced. The low pH of gastric juice causes severe inflammation in the lungs. Pulmonary edema and respiratory failure may result.

COLLABORATIVE CARE

With early diagnosis and treatment, most clients with pneumonia recover fully. However, pneumonia has a significant mortality, especially among the old and weak.

Diagnostic Tests

- *Sputum Gram stain* and *culture and sensitivity* are done to identify the organism and appropriate antibiotic therapy. It is important to obtain sputum for culture from the lower respiratory tract, not the mouth and nasal passages (Procedure 26-1).
- *Complete blood count (CBC)* with *white blood cell (WBC) differential* shows an elevated WBC count with more immature WBCs in an acute bacterial pneumonia.
- *Arterial blood gases (ABGs)* may be done to evaluate gas exchange.
- *Pulse oximetry* is used to monitor arterial oxygen saturation. The SaO_2 is the percentage of arterial hemoglobin that is saturated or combined with oxygen; it normally is 95% or

---

PROCEDURE 26-1   Obtaining a Sputum Specimen

■ BEFORE THE PROCEDURE

- Gather all supplies.
- If possible, obtain specimen before starting oxygen and/or antibiotic therapy.
- Unless otherwise specified, obtain specimen early morning, just after awakening.
- Increase fluid intake prior to obtaining specimen to help liquefy secretions.

■ PROCEDURE

- Use standard precautions.
- Provide for privacy.
- Provide mouth care to reduce contamination by oral flora.
- Instruct to cough deeply several times, expectorating mucus into container.
- To obtain specimen by suctioning:
  - Use aseptic technique.
  - Attach sterile mucus trap between suction catheter and tubing.
  - Perform tracheal suctioning.
  - Detach and close mucus trap. Clear suction catheter and tubing, and dispose of suction equipment appropriately.

- Close container securely using aseptic technique.
- Label container (name and other identifying data, time and date, and any special conditions).
- Enclose container in clean plastic bag, and send to laboratory.

■ AFTER THE PROCEDURE

Provide mouth care. Document the time and date the specimen was obtained, and note its color, consistency, and odor.

■ SAMPLE DOCUMENTATION

8/13/03	0630	Specimen of moderate amount thick green odorless sputum obtained by deep coughing. Sent for culture and sensitivity.
		_____ S. Hamilton, LVN

higher. An SaO$_2$ of less than 95% may indicate impaired gas exchange or ventilation.

■ *Chest x-ray* helps identify the extent and pattern of lung involvement. Fluid, consolidated lung tissue, and *atelectasis* (areas of alveolar collapse) can be identified.

■ *Fiberoptic bronchoscopy* may be done to obtain a sputum specimen or remove secretions from the bronchi (Figure 26-5 ◆). A bronchoscope is used to view tissues and collect specimens. Nursing care for the client undergoing a bronchoscopy is summarized in Box 26-2.

Immunization

Pneumococcal vaccine is recommended for people over age 65; those with chronic cardiac or respiratory conditions, diabetes mellitus, alcoholism, or other chronic diseases; and immuno-comprised people. Annual influenza vaccine is also recommended for vulnerable populations such as those listed above, health care workers, and residents of long-term care facilities.

Pharmacology

Medications used to treat pneumonia may include antibiotics to eradicate causative organisms and bronchodilators to reduce bronchospasm and improve ventilation. Bronchodilators and their nursing implications are discussed in more detail in the section of this chapter on asthma.

An agent to "break up" mucus or reduce its viscosity may be prescribed. Guaifenesin, a common ingredient in expectorant cough syrups, helps to liquefy mucus, making it easier to expectorate.

Oxygen Therapy

Oxygen may be ordered when pneumonia interferes with gas exchange. The *nasal cannula* delivers 24% to 45% oxygen

Figure 26-5. ◆ Fiberoptic bronchoscopy.

BOX 26-2
NURSING CARE CHECKLIST

BRONCHOSCOPY
Before the Procedure

☑ Provide routine preoperative care as outlined in Chapter 7.
☑ Reinforce teaching.
☑ Remove dentures and partial plates; provide mouth care just prior to the procedure.

After the Procedure

☑ Keep resuscitation and suction equipment at the bedside.
☑ Closely monitor vital signs and respiratory status.
☑ Maintain NPO status until cough and gag reflexes have returned.
☑ Provide emesis basin and tissues for expectorating sputum and saliva.
☑ Monitor color and character of respiratory secretions. Sputum may be blood-tinged for several hours; notify physician if sputum is grossly bloody.

Client and Family Teaching

☑ The procedure takes about 30 to 45 minutes, and may be done in the room, in a procedure room, or in surgery.
☑ You will have little pain or discomfort. You will receive an anesthetic. You will be able to breathe, but not talk.
☑ You may have a sore throat and hoarse voice after the procedure. Throat lozenges or warm saline gargles can help relieve sore throat.
☑ You may have a fever during the first 24 hours after the procedure.
☑ Report persistent cough, bloody or purulent sputum, wheezing, shortness of breath, difficulty breathing, or chest pain to your doctor.

(room air is 21% oxygen) with flow rates of 2 to 6 liters per minute (Figure 26-6 ◆). A *simple face mask* can deliver 40% to 60% oxygen. Up to 100% oxygen can be delivered by the *nonrebreather mask,* the highest concentration possible without mechanical ventilation. When the amount of oxygen delivered must be carefully regulated, a *Venturi mask* is used. The percentage of oxygen delivered by Venturi mask can be precisely regulated, from 24% to 50%. A severely hypoxic client may require intubation and mechanical ventilation. Endotracheal intubation and mechanical ventilation are discussed in the section on respiratory failure.

Other Therapies

Increasing fluid intake to 2,500 to 3,000 mL per day helps liquefy secretions, making them easier to cough up and expec-

A

B

C

Figure 26-6. ◆ (A) Nasal cannula. (B) Simple face mask. (C) Nonrebreather mask.

torate. If oral intake is inadequate, intravenous fluids and nutrition may be required.

When mucus secretions are thick and viscous or the cough is weak, percussion, vibration, and postural drainage may be ordered. *Percussion* is done by rhythmically striking or clapping the chest wall with cupped hands (Figure 26-7 ◆). Cupping traps air between the palm and the skin, causing vibrations that loosen respiratory secretions. The trapped air also provides a cushion, preventing injury. A mechanical percussion device also may be used. The breasts, sternum, spinal column, and kidney areas are avoided during percussion.

Vibration helps loosen and move secretions into larger airways. Vibrations are produced by tensing and vibrating the arm muscles while keeping firm pressure on the chest wall with the hands.

Percussion and vibration are performed along with postural drainage. *Postural drainage* uses gravity to help remove secretions from a particular lung segment. The client is positioned with the lung area to be drained above the trachea or mainstem bronchus. Drainage of all lung segments requires a variety of positions (Figure 26-8 ◆); however, few clients need all segments drained. Postural drainage should be done before meals to avoid nausea and vomiting.

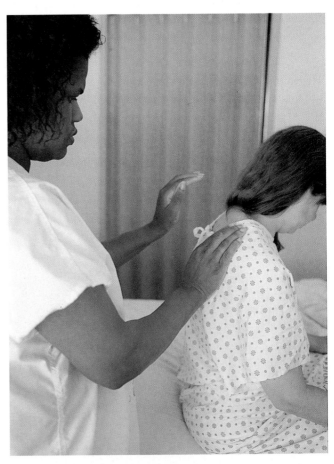

Figure 26-7. ◆ Percussing the upper posterior chest. Note the cupped position of the nurse's hands.

Figure 26-8. ◆ Positions for postural drainage.

![icon] # NURSING CARE

ASSESSING

Collecting assessment data is important not only to monitor the progress of clients with pneumonia, but also to identify possible manifestations of pneumonia in clients with other problems. Nurses often identify clients in the community, long-term care, and acute care settings who are at risk for pneumonia. Box 26-3 outlines assessment data related to pneumonia.

DIAGNOSING, PLANNING, AND IMPLEMENTING

INEFFECTIVE AIRWAY CLEARANCE

Airway inflammation, edema, and secretions interfere with air movement and airway clearance in clients with pneumonia.

- Assess respiratory status, including vital signs, breath sounds, and cough and sputum at least every 4 hours. *The client with acute pneumonia can quickly develop respiratory distress; frequent assessment allows early intervention.*
- Notify the physician if oxygen saturation falls below 92% or ordered level. *Airway obstruction can interfere with alveolar ventilation and gas exchange, leading to tissue hypoxia.*
- Place in Fowler's position. Encourage frequent position changes, sitting at the bedside, and ambulation as allowed. *These measures promote lung expansion and facilitate the movement of secretions.*
- Assist to cough, deep breathe, and use the incentive spirometer. *Coughing and deep breathing help clear airways.*
- Provide at least 2,500 to 3,000 mL of fluid per day. *A liberal fluid intake helps liquefy secretions, promoting their clearance.*
- Assist with pulmonary hygiene measures, such as postural drainage, percussion, and vibration. *These techniques help mobilize and clear secretions.*

BOX 26-3
ASSESSING CLIENTS WITH PNEUMONIA

SUBJECTIVE DATA

- Chest pain (location, character, timing, duration, aggravating or relieving factors); shortness of breath or difficulty breathing; cough (type, timing, productive or nonproductive); type and amount of sputum
- History of chronic diseases; allergies, asthma, or other respiratory conditions; heart failure; medications used
- Smoking history or exposure to environmental or occupational polutants; use of alcohol and/or other drugs such as heroin, cocaine, or marijuana

OBJECTIVE DATA

- Vital signs including temperature and apical pulse
- Skin color (lips, nail beds, nose, ears, and tongue)
- Level of consciousness and mental status
- Respiratory status, including respiratory rate and depth, dyspnea, cough; symmetry of chest movement; lung sounds including any adventitious sounds such as:
  - *Crackles:* Short, discrete, crackling, or bubbling sounds
  - *Wheezes:* Musical sounds caused by narrowed airways due to inflammation, constriction, or excessive mucus
  - *Friction rub:* A loud, dry, creaking sound caused by inflammation of the pleura

---

- Administer ordered medications, and monitor their effects. *If the ordered medications are ineffective or have adverse effects, a different drug may need to be prescribed.*
- Administer oxygen as ordered. *Oxygen promotes alveolar gas exchange.*

INEFFECTIVE BREATHING PATTERN

Chest pain can lead to rapid and shallow breathing that causes fatigue and does not fully ventilate all areas of the lungs.

- Place in an upright or semi-upright position. *This position promotes lung expansion and ventilation as well as comfort.*
- Provide for periods of rest. *Rest reduces fatigue and the work of breathing.*
- Assess and document chest pain. Provide analgesics as ordered. *Adequate pain relief allows better lung ventilation.*
- Reassure the client who is experiencing respiratory distress. *Hypoxia and respiratory distress cause anxiety. Anxiety increases the respiratory rate and fatigue, and decreases ventilation.*
- Teach use of slow abdominal breathing. *This promotes lung expansion.*
- Teach relaxation techniques, such as visualization and meditation. *These techniques help reduce anxiety and slow breathing.*

ACTIVITY INTOLERANCE

- Assess for any increase in pulse, respirations, dyspnea, diaphoresis, or cyanosis with activity. *These findings may indicate limited activity tolerance.*
- Assist with self-care activities as needed. *Assistance with ADLs reduces the client's energy demands.*
- Schedule activities, planning for rest periods. *Rest periods minimize fatigue and improve activity tolerance.*
- Provide assistive devices, such as an overhead trapeze. *Assistive devices help reduce the energy required to move and change positions.*
- Enlist support persons to help minimize stress and anxiety. *Stress and anxiety increase metabolic demands and can decrease activity tolerance.*
- Provide emotional support and reassurance that strength and activity level will return to normal when pneumonia has resolved. *The client may be concerned that fatigue will continue after the acute infection is resolved.*

EVALUATING

To evaluate the effectiveness of nursing care, reassess the client's respiratory status, ability to clear secretions, and ability to gradually increase activity levels.

Discharge Considerations

Teaching focuses on prevention of pneumonia as well as its treatment. Discuss the benefits of immunizations against influenza and pneumococcal pneumonia with clients in high-risk groups. Pneumococcus vaccine usually provides immunity to pneumococcal pneumonia. Annual influenza vaccine helps prevent pneumonia, because viral infection often precedes pneumonia.

Many clients with pneumonia are managed in the community, unless their respiratory status is significantly compromised. Stress the importance of taking ordered medications and completing the entire prescription. Provide information about side effects and their management. Teach to identify adverse effects that should be reported to the primary care provider.

Instruct to limit activities and increase rest to conserve energy. Encourage to maintain fluid intake to keep mucus thin for easier expectoration. Explain that small, frequent meals reduce the energy demand for eating and may be better tolerated. Recommend that the client and household members avoid smoking to prevent further irritation of the lungs. Complementary therapies (Box 26-4) may be used to relieve chest congestion and promote comfort.

Tell the client and family to report increasing shortness of breath, difficulty breathing, temperature, fatigue, headache, sleepiness, or confusion to the physician as these may indicate worsening condition. Stress the importance of keeping all follow-up appointments to ensure cure of the disease.

COMPLEMENTARY THERAPIES

BOX 26-4

Pneumonia and Bronchitis

The aromas of cedarwood and frankincense or inhaling the steam of water containing eucalyptus or sage may help relieve chest congestion. Massaging the chest with lavender also may help. Licorice root can be used to relieve congestion and as a cough suppressant. Licorice interacts with some drugs used to treat high blood pressure and heart disease and should be used with caution. Its use is contraindicated during pregnancy. Tea tree oil (applied topically or a few drops on a handkerchief) has anti-infective properties and may be used together with conventional treatment of pneumonia.

Pleural effusion

Figure 26-9. ◆ Thoracentesis. A needle is inserted between the ribs into the pleural space to withdraw excess pleural fluid.

Pleuritis

Pleuritis (pleurisy) is inflammation of the pleura that covers the lung surface and lines the inner chest wall. Pleuritis usually results from another process, such as a viral infection, pneumonia, or rib injury.

The onset of pleuritis is often abrupt, with characteristic *pleuritic* pain. Pleuritic pain is sharp or stabbing and usually very localized. Deep breathing, coughing, and movement aggravate the pain. Breathing is rapid and shallow, and breath sounds are diminished. A *pleural friction rub* or harsh, grating sound, may be heard over the affected area.

Treatment of pleuritis includes analgesics and nonsteroidal anti-inflammatory drugs (NSAIDs) to relieve the pain. Codeine may be ordered to relieve pain and suppress the cough.

Nursing care focuses on promoting comfort. Positioning and splinting the chest while coughing can be helpful. Wrapping the chest with 6-inch-wide elastic bandages may help relieve pain; care must be taken, however, to ensure that the lungs are still fully ventilated.

Advise that pleuritis usually lasts only a short time and resolves spontaneously. Instruct to report symptoms such as increased fever, productive cough, difficulty breathing, or shortness of breath to the physician. Discuss appropriate use of and precautions when taking NSAIDs and recommended analgesics.

Pleural Effusion

Pleural effusion is a collection of excess fluid in the pleural space. Pleural effusions result from respiratory disorders (e.g., pneumonia, lung cancer, or trauma) or from systemic diseases such as heart failure or kidney disease.

A large pleural effusion presses on lung tissue, causing dyspnea and shortness of breath. Breath sounds are diminished or absent, and the affected area may sound dull when percussed. Chest wall movement may be limited.

When pleural effusion interferes with breathing, a *thoracentesis* may be done to remove the fluid. A large needle is inserted into the pleural space to remove the excess fluid (Figure 26-9 ◆). Thoracentesis may be done at the bedside. Local anesthesia is used. The procedure requires less than 30 minutes to complete. Nursing care for the client undergoing a thoracentesis is outlined in Box 26-5.

Nursing care focuses on supporting respiratory function and assisting with procedures such as thoracentesis. With a large pleural effusion, Impaired Gas Exchange and Activity Intolerance are high-priority nursing problems. Following thoracentesis, it is important to monitor for complications such as pneumothorax.

Teaching focuses on symptoms of recurrent effusion or complications after thoracentesis that should be reported to the physician. Instruct to report increasing dyspnea or shortness of breath, cough, hemoptysis, or pleuritic pain.

Lung Abscess and Empyema

Lung abscess and empyema are potential complications of pneumonia and other respiratory infections. A *lung abscess* is local lung destruction or necrosis and pus formation. Aspiration pneumonia is the most common cause of lung abscess. *Empyema* is pus in the pleural cavity. Bacterial pneumonia, rupture of a lung abscess, and infection due to chest trauma are the major causes of empyema.

Manifestations of these disorders typically develop about 2 weeks after the initiating event (aspiration, pneumonia, etc.). Signs of an acute infection with chills and fever, pleuritic chest pain, malaise, and anorexia develop. The cough may be productive of foul-smelling, purulent, and even blood-streaked sputum. Breath sounds are diminished, and crackles may be heard in the region of the abscess. Rupture and drainage of an abscess into a bronchus is a frightening complication.

BOX 26-5
NURSING CARE CHECKLIST

THORACENTESIS

Before the Procedure

- ☑ Verify a signed consent for this procedure.
- ☑ Reinforce teaching.
- ☑ Administer cough suppressant if ordered.
- ☑ Bring supplies to the client's room: Thoracentesis tray, sterile gloves, local anesthetic, antiseptic solution, dressing, and an extra overbed table or mayo stand.
- ☑ Position client sitting on side of bed, leaning forward with arms and head supported on an anchored overbed table.
- ☑ Advise that pressure may be felt when the needle is inserted, but no pain should be experienced.

During the Procedure

- ☑ Support and assist client to remain still and in position during the procedure.
- ☑ Provide psychological support as needed.
- ☑ Monitor respirations, pulse, and color, informing the physician of any changes.

After the Procedure

- ☑ Apply dressing to puncture site.
- ☑ Position client on unaffected side for 1 hour.
- ☑ Label any specimens (name, date, source, and diagnosis); send to laboratory for analysis.
- ☑ Record vital signs, breath sounds, and cough and assess for bleeding or crepitus at puncture site every 15 minutes × 4, every 30 minutes × 2, then every 2 to 4 hours or as indicated.
- ☑ Obtain chest x-ray.
- ☑ Allow resumption of normal activies after 1 hour if no complications develop.

Intravenous antibiotic therapy is ordered. Postural drainage may be done to relieve obstruction and promote drainage. In some cases, bronchoscopy is used to drain an abscess. A chest tube may be used to drain an empyema. See the section on pneumothorax for further discussion of chest tubes.

Most clients recover fully with appropriate treatment. Nursing care needs relate primarily to maintaining a patent airway and adequate gas exchange. When teaching, emphasize the importance of completing the prescribed antibiotic therapy. Antibiotic therapy may be continued for up to one month or more. Stress the need to contact the physician if symptoms do not improve or if they become worse: infection from lung abscess can spread to lung and pleural tissue, and also via the blood, causing systemic sepsis.

Tuberculosis

Tuberculosis (TB) is a chronic, recurrent infectious disease that usually affects the lungs. Tuberculosis also can involve other organs. This disease, caused by *Mycobacterium tuberculosis,* is an important health problem worldwide. It is common in developing countries of Asia, Africa, the Middle East, and Latin America.

In the United States, TB usually affects immigrants, people with HIV, and disadvantaged populations, such as the homeless. People with altered immune function, including older adults, are at particular risk for tuberculosis. Some strains of tuberculosis have become resistant to the drugs used to treat the disease.

PATHOPHYSIOLOGY

M. tuberculosis is a slow-growing, slender, rod-shaped, acid-fast organism. It has a waxy outer capsule that increases its resistance to destruction. It is transmitted by *droplet nuclei,* airborne droplets produced when an infected person coughs, sneezes, speaks, or sings. Infection develops when a susceptible host breathes in droplet nuclei and the contaminated particle evades the normal defenses of the upper respiratory tract to reach the alveoli. A small, poorly ventilated or crowded environment and prolonged exposure increase the risk of infection. The risk also is increased by impaired immune function.

Pulmonary Tuberculosis

Droplet nuclei containing the bacillus implant in an alveolus or respiratory bronchiole, usually in an upper lobe. An immune response brings WBCs to the site. These cells phagocytize and isolate the bacteria but cannot destroy them. A sealed-off colony of bacilli, called a *tubercle,* is formed.

Usually, scar tissue forms around the tubercle, and the bacilli remain isolated. These lesions can be seen on x-ray. If the immune system is impaired, primary tuberculosis can progress, destroying lung tissue. A previously healed lesion may be reactivated. This is known as *reactivation tuberculosis.* It occurs when the immune system is suppressed by age (Box 26-6), disease, or immunosuppressive drugs. About 5% of infected people develop active primary disease; another 5% develop reactivation tuberculosis at a later time (Figure 26-10 ◆).

Manifestations of tuberculosis develop gradually. They include fatigue, weight loss, anorexia, low-grade afternoon fever, and night sweats. The cough is dry initially and later

population
FOCUS

**BOX
26-6**

Tuberculosis in Older Adults

Up to 30% of newly diagnosed tuberculosis affects people over age 65. Most cases are due to reactivation of dormant bacteria as cell-mediated immunity declines with aging. Living in long-term care facilities also increases the risk for tuberculosis.

Presenting symptoms of tuberculosis in an older adult may be vague, such as coughing, weight loss, anorexia, or periodic fevers. Yearly tuberculin skin testing with purified protein derivative (PPD) is recommended for long-term care residents.

Interior of alveolus

Pulmonary capillary

Alveolar walls

Ingested tubercle bacillus

Alveolar macrophage

Bronchiole

Interior of alveolus

Tubercle bacilli that reach the alveoli of the lung are ingested by macrophages but often survive.

Early tubercle

Tubercle bacilli multiplying in macrophages attract additional macrophages into the area, forming an early tubercle.

Tubercle bacilli

Caseous center

Lymphocyte

After a few weeks, many of the macrophages die, releasing tubercle bacilli into the center of the tubercle, which is surrounded by a mass of macrophages and lymphocytes. The disease may become dormant after this stage.

Outer layer of mature tubercle

Tuberculous cavity

Tubercle bacilli

In a mature tubercle, a firm outer layer surrounds the mass of macrophages and lymphocytes.

Rupture of bronchiole wall

With reactivation, the bacilli multiply within the tubercle until it ruptures, allowing bacilli to spill into a bronchiole and disseminate throughout the respiratory system and to other organs.

Figure 26-10. ◆ The pathogenesis of tuberculosis.

becomes productive of purulent or blood-tinged sputum. It is often at this stage that the client seeks medical attention.

Extrapulmonary Tuberculosis

Colonies of *M. tuberculosis* can develop in other organs. These distant sites may be active or dormant. The kidney and genitourinary tract are common sites for extrapulmonary tuberculosis. The large, weight-bearing joints, such as the hips and knees, are most often affected by *tuberculous arthritis*. *Miliary tuberculosis* occurs when the bacilli spread throughout the body. *Tuberculosis meningitis* results when tuberculosis spreads to the subarachnoid space.

COLLABORATIVE CARE

Collaborative care for tuberculosis focuses on: (1) early detection; (2) effective treatment; and (3) preventing its spread to others.

Clients with active tuberculosis rarely need hospitalization. With appropriate treatment, they become noninfective to others fairly rapidly. When a client with tuberculosis is hospitalized, respiratory isolation is maintained to reduce the risk of infecting other clients and health care workers.

Tuberculosis is a potential threat to public health. As such, it must be reported to local and state public health departments. The client's contacts are then identified and examined. People who share living or work environments should receive testing and prophylactic treatment.

Screening Methods

The *tuberculin test* is used to screen for tuberculosis. People exposed to TB develop an immune response to the bacillus within 3 to 10 weeks after infection. Injection of a small amount of purified protein derivative (PPD) of tuberculin activates this response, causing local inflammation. The Mantoux test is commonly used to screen for TB; 0.1 mL of PPD is injected intradermally into the dorsal aspect of the forearm (Figure 26-11 ◆). The test is read within 48 to 72 hours, and recorded as the diameter of induration (raised area) in millimeters. The area of induration is used to determine infection (Table 26-2 ◆). A positive response indicates that the client has developed an immune response to the bacillus; it does *not* mean that the client has active TB or is currently infectious.

Diagnostic Tests

■ A series of three consecutive early morning sputum specimens are sent for *acid-fast bacilli smear* and *culture* (see Procedure 26-1). The acid-fast smear is a rapid test for the tubercle bacillus. Use personal protective devices when obtaining sputum specimens that may carry TB. Collect the specimens in a room equipped with air flow control devices, ultraviolet (UV) light, or a combination of these. If air flow or UV protection is not available, wear a special mask that can filter the droplet nuclei.

■ *Chest x-ray* is used to diagnose and evaluate TB.

■ *Fiberoptic bronchoscopy* and bronchial washing may be used to obtain culture specimens if necessary. Review Box 26-2 for

Figure 26-11. ◆ (A) Intradermal injection of PPD. (B) A local inflammatory response to PPD. (C) Measuring induration produced by the inflammatory response.

	TABLE 26-2 INTERPRETING TUBERCULIN TEST RESULTS	
AREA OF INDURATION	**SIGNIFICANCE**
< 5 mm	Negative response
5–9 mm	Positive for people who: ■ Are in close contact with someone who has active TB ■ Have an abnormal chest x-ray ■ Have HIV infection
10–15 mm	Positive for people with other risk factors: ■ Born in a high-incidence country ■ Low socioeconomic status ■ Injection drug use ■ Resident in a long-term care facility
> 15 mm	Positive for all people

nursing care of the client undergoing fiberoptic bronchoscopy.

Pharmacology

Antituberculosis drugs are used to prevent and treat tuberculosis. Clients with a recent skin test conversion from negative to positive are started on prophylactic treatment, especially when other risk factors are present. Daily isoniazid (INH) for 6 to 12 months is commonly used to prevent active TB.

The tuberculosis bacillus readily becomes drug-resistant when only one anti-infective agent is used. Active disease is always treated with at least two antibacterial medications. Because the organism is protected by the tubercule, 6 or more months of treatment is required to eliminate it. Three antitubercular drugs may be used for the first 2 months of treatment. All three drugs are given daily by mouth. For the remainder of the treatment period, the drugs may be given twice weekly. (See Table 26-3 ◆.)

Antitubercular medications have many undesired effects. Most are toxic to the liver. Warn clients to avoid alcohol and other liver toxins (such as acetaminophen) while taking these drugs. Report manifestations of adverse effects to the physician.

TABLE 26-3

NURSING IMPLICATIONS FOR PHARMACOLOGY: CLIENTS RECEIVING ANTITUBERCULOSIS DRUGS

DRUG	ACTION	NURSING RESPONSIBILITIES	CLIENT AND FAMILY TEACHING
Isoniazid (INH, Laniazid, Nydrazid)	Isoniazid is used alone to prevent tuberculosis, and in combination with rifampin, ethambutol, or both to treat active disease.	Give 1 hour before or 2 hours after eating if tolerated; may be given with meals to reduce GI effects. Report adverse effects: a. Numbness and tingling of the extremities b. Abnormal liver function studies or jaundice c. Rash, drug fever, anemia, or abnormal bleeding Monitor responses to other medications, as INH may interfere with their metabolism, causing toxicity.	Take as ordered for the entire course of treatment. Take on an empty stomach; take with meals if nausea and vomiting occur. Call your doctor if you develop anorexia and jaundice (yellowing of skin and eyes). Take pyridoxine as ordered to prevent neurologic effects. Avoid alcohol and other liver toxins while taking INH. Call your doctor if you develop a rash, fever, bruising, bleeding gums, or fatigue. Use birth control while taking INH; this drug may harm the fetus.
Rifampin (RMP, Rifadin, Rimactane)	Rifampin is commonly used in combination with INH and other antitubercular drugs. It is relatively low in toxicity. Rifampin increases the rate of metabolism of many drugs, decreasing their effectiveness.	Give on an empty stomach. Report abnormal CBC, liver function studies, and renal function studies to the physician. Monitor the effectiveness of drugs administered concurrently.	Rifampin causes sweat, urine, saliva, and tears to turn red-orange. This is not harmful, but may permanently stain soft contact lenses. Do not take aspirin with rifampin. Report fever, flulike symptoms, fatigue, sore throat, or unusual bleeding to your doctor. If you use oral contraceptives, use supplemental birth control while taking this drug.

(continues)

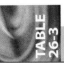

	NURSING IMPLICATIONS FOR PHARMACOLOGY: CLIENTS RECEIVING ANTITUBERCULOSIS DRUGS (CONTINUED)		
DRUG	**ACTION**	**NURSING RESPONSIBILITIES**	**CLIENT AND FAMILY TEACHING**
Pyrazinamide (PZA, Tebrazid)	Pyrazinamide often is given during the first 2 months of treatment. It is toxic to the liver. It also increases serum uric acid levels, but rarely causes gout.	Give with meals to reduce GI side effects. Report changes in liver function studies and serum uric acid levels to the physician.	Call your doctor if you develop anorexia, nausea, vomiting, jaundice, or a painful, red, hot, swollen joint. Avoid using alcohol or other liver toxins while taking this drug.
Ethambutol (EMB, Myambutol)	Ethambutol reduces bacterial resistance to other drugs. It is reversibly toxic to the optic nerve. Signs include decreased visual and color acuity. This drug may be safe for use in pregnancy.	Schedule eye exams as recommended during treatment. Give with meals to reduce GI effects. Report changes in liver and renal function tests and neurologic status to the physician.	Monitor vision daily by reading newspapers and looking at the same blue object. Notify your doctor if changes in vision or color perception occur.
Streptomycin (SM)	Streptomycin is a highly effective antibiotic. Resistance may develop if it is used alone. It must be given parenterally because it is not absorbed in the GI tract. It also has toxic effects on the kidneys and ears.	Inject deep IM into a large muscle mass, rotating sites. Report significant changes in urine output, weight, and renal function studies to the physician. Maintain fluid intake of 2,000–3,000 mL/day. Assess hearing and balance often. Schedule audiometric testing as indicated.	Drink at least 2½ –3 quarts of fluid daily. Weigh yourself on the same scale at least twice a week; report significant weight gain to your doctor. Call your doctor if your hearing declines, or you develop dizziness or ringing or buzzing sensations in the ear.

Compliance with the prescribed regimen may be a problem. Medications often are given under direct supervision, with a public health nurse watching the client take and swallow the drug.

NURSING CARE

Tuberculosis presents a greater threat to public health than it does to the individual. When the treatment regimen is followed, more than 90% of clients become noninfective within 3 months. Relapse is uncommon; the main cause of treatment failure is noncompliance.

RISK FOR INFECTION

■ Place in a private room with ventilation that prevents air in the room from circulating into the hallway or other rooms (a negative flow room). *A negative flow room with frequent fresh-air exchanges reduces droplet nuclei in the room and prevents their spread to other areas.*

■ Use standard precautions and TB isolation as recommended by the Centers for Disease Control and Prevention (CDC). Wear a mask and gown when caring for clients who do not cover mouth when coughing. *These measures are important to prevent the spread of TB to others.*

■ Use personal protective devices during care (HEPA-filtered respirator) to protect against occupational exposure to TB. *Surgical masks do not filter droplet nuclei; protective devices capable of filtering bacteria and particles smaller than 1 micron are necessary.*

■ Discuss the importance of respiratory isolation during initial treatment. Instruct to avoid crowds and close physical contact, and to maintain ventilation in living facilities during the first 3 weeks of treatment. *These measures help protect others when sputum is still likely to contain bacilli.*

■ Place a mask on the client when transporting within the facility for diagnostic or treatment procedures. *Covering the mouth during transport reduces air contamination and the risk to visitors and personnel.*

- Communicate the diagnosis to all personnel in contact with the client. *This allows personnel to take appropriate precautions.*
- Assist visitors to mask prior to entering the room. *Providing appropriate masks or respirators reduces the risk of infection.*
- Teach to cough and expectorate into tissues, then personally dispose of tissues in a closed bag. *This reduces potential contact with the bacilli by others.*
- Teach to collect sputum specimens, stepping outside to do so if necessary. *This reduces the risk of exposure to health care personnel, allows rapid dilution of droplet nuclei produced, and exposes them to UV light (which kills the bacteria).*

DEFICIENT KNOWLEDGE

- Assess knowledge, learning ability and interest, developmental level, and obstacles to learning. *Assessment allows teaching tailored to the client's needs and abilities.*
- Include significant others in teaching. *This allows clarification and reinforcement of teaching and learning.*
- Use teaching strategies and learning aids such as written and visual materials appropriate for age, level of education, and intellect. *Teaching tailored to the client is more effective and results in better learning.*
- Teach about TB and its treatment, including:
  - Nature of tuberculosis
  - Purpose of treatment and ordered follow-up
  - Preventing TB spread to others
  - Importance of maintaining good general health by eating a well-balanced, nutritious diet, balancing rest and exercise, and avoiding exposure to infection
  - Names, doses, purposes, and side effects of prescribed drugs
  - Importance of avoiding alcohol and other liver toxins while taking antituberculosis drugs
  - Fluid intake needs of 2½ to 3 quarts of fluid per day
  - Symptoms to report to the physician: chest pain, hemoptysis, or difficulty breathing; manifestations of drug toxicity (see Table 26-3)

  This information is necessary for the client to effectively manage TB and its treatment.
- Document teaching and learning. Reinforce as needed. *Several teaching–learning sessions may be needed due to the amount and complexity of information.*

INEFFECTIVE THERAPEUTIC REGIMEN MANAGEMENT

- Assess self-care abilities and support systems. *Assessment helps predict the ability to follow the ordered regimen.*

- Help identify barriers or obstacles to managing the ordered treatment. *Identifying potential barriers allows planning for solutions.*
- Assist to develop a plan for managing treatment. *A plan increases the sense of control and ownership and considers personal, cultural, and lifestyle factors.*
- Provide clear, written instructions at the client's level of literacy, knowledge, and understanding. *Written directions provide support and reinforcement.*
- Refer to smoking cessation programs, alcohol treatment and Alcoholics Anonymous, drug treatment and Narcotics Anonymous, and other support groups as appropriate. *Counseling, support groups, and other community resources provide additional assistance and support in managing TB and its treatment.*
- For homeless clients, arrange shelter placement or other housing and ongoing follow-up by easily accessed health care providers. *Active intervention for necessary services helps ensure compliance with treatment.*
- Refer to public health department for management and follow-up as indicated. *Public health follow-up often is required to prevent the spread of TB to other people.*

EVALUATING

To evaluate the effectiveness of nursing care for a client with TB, collect data related to the client's knowledge and understanding of TB and its treatment, ability and willingness to follow instructions for preventing the spread of TB to others, and compliance with the ordered treatment.

 # Discharge Considerations

Tuberculosis is a public health problem that requires a focus on the community as well as on the individual. Teach community members and people with TB how to reduce its spread:

- Cover the mouth when coughing or sneezing
- Use disposable tissues to contain respiratory secretions

Because the client with TB may be infective long before the disease is diagnosed, teach these measures to all people. Encourage people at high risk for TB to have regular screening. Discuss prophylactic treatment for people in close contact with a client who has active TB.

Explain the effect, dose, and timing for all medications. Emphasize the importance of long-term therapy to cure TB. Discuss precautions and possible side effects of the drugs that should be reported to the health care provider:

- Isoniazid (INH) may cause numbness, tingling, or burning in the extremities. Pyridoxine (vitamin B_6) often is ordered to prevent this effect.
- Avoid alcohol while taking INH or rifampin as these drugs may affect the liver. Report nausea, anorexia, jaundice, a

change in urine or stool color, or pain in the upper right quadrant.
- Rifampin may change the color of saliva, tears, and urine.
- Streptomycin can affect hearing and balance; promptly report any changes.
- Ethambutol may affect vision and color perception. Use

caution when driving or walking in unfamiliar areas. Promptly report any vision changes.

Refer to community services and agencies as appropriate. See the Critical Thinking Care Map at the end of this chapter for an opportunity to use the nursing process to plan care for a client with tuberculosis.

Obstructive Airway Disorders

Many diseases affect the airways and air flow. Air flow decreases when: (1) secretions obstruct the airway; (2) airway walls are edematous or swollen; (3) smooth muscle of the airways constricts, reducing their size; (4) the lungs lose elasticity, making exhalation more difficult; and (5) supportive tissue is lost, allowing airways to collapse.

Decreased air flow increases the work of breathing and causes air trapping in the lungs. Inhaled air mixes with trapped air, and less oxygen is available for gas exchange in the alveoli.

Asthma

Asthma is a chronic inflammatory airways disorder characterized by recurrent episodes of wheezing, breathlessness, chest tightness, and coughing. Although it is more common in children than adults, about 5% of adults have asthma. It is becoming more common and is causing an increasing number of deaths.

PATHOPHYSIOLOGY
A variety of factors can trigger an acute inflammatory response in asthma. Inflammation causes airway constriction, secretion of excess mucus, and edema of airway mucosa. The airways narrow, airflow is reduced, and the work of breathing increases. The sequence of events is outlined in Figure 26-12 ◆.

Either *external* or *internal* stimuli can trigger an asthma attack. Childhood asthma is often triggered by allergens, such as pollen, animal dander, or household dust. Pollutants such as tobacco smoke can provoke asthma. Respiratory infection is a common internal stimulus for an asthma attack. Exercise-induced asthma is also an internal stimulus; exercise in cold, dry air increases the risk in clients with this type of asthma. Emotional stress can trigger an asthma attack. Drugs such as aspirin and other NSAIDs, sulfites (used as preservatives in wine, beer, fresh fruits, and salad), and beta blockers can prompt an attack in some clients. The frequency and severity of attacks vary. Some clients have infrequent, mild attacks, while others have nearly continuous symptoms.

An attack of asthma is characterized by chest tightness, difficulty breathing, wheezing, and cough. Associated symptoms include tachypnea, tachycardia, anxiety, and apprehension.

Status asthmaticus is severe, prolonged asthma that does not respond to routine treatment. Without aggressive treatment, status asthmaticus can lead to respiratory failure. The client may require intubation and mechanical ventilation.

COLLABORATIVE CARE
Asthma is diagnosed by the client's history and manifestations. Diagnostic tests are used to identify possible triggers and to evaluate respiratory function during and between acute attacks. *Pulse oximetry* and *arterial blood gases* evaluate oxygenation during an acute attack. *Peak expiratory flow rate* assesses airflow restriction and the effectiveness of treatment. *Skin testing* may be done to identify specific allergens that may trigger asthma attacks.

Treatment focuses on controlling symptoms and preventing acute attacks. When an acute episode occurs, therapy focuses on restoring airflow and alveolar ventilation.

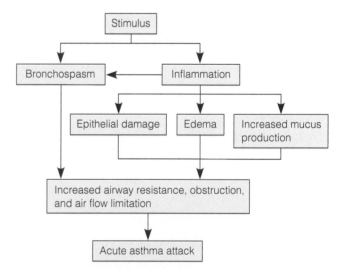

Figure 26-12. ◆ The sequence of an acute episode of asthma.

Preventive Measures

Asthma attacks often can be prevented by avoiding allergens and other triggers. Modifying the home environment (e.g., controlling dust, removing carpets, covering mattresses and pillows to reduce dust mites, and installing air filtering systems) may help. Pets may need to be removed from the household. Eliminating tobacco smoke in the house is also important. For exercise-induced asthma, wearing a mask that retains humidity and warm air when exercising in cold weather may prevent an attack. Early treatment of respiratory infections is vital.

Pharmacology

Drugs are used to prevent and control asthma symptoms, reduce the frequency and severity of attacks, and reverse airway obstruction. Drugs used for long-term control are taken daily. These include anti-inflammatory agents, long-acting bronchodilators, and leukotriene modifiers. Quick-relief medications used to relieve bronchoconstriction and airflow obstruction include rapid-acting bronchodilators, anticholinergic drugs, and systemic corticosteroids (Table 26-4 ◆).

NURSING CARE

ASSESSING

Good nursing assessment is vital to determine the effects of an acute asthma attack, initiate early interventions when needed, and evaluate the effectiveness of treatment. Box 26-7 summarizes assessment data to collect from clients with asthma.

DIAGNOSING, PLANNING, AND IMPLEMENTING

This section focuses on the priority nursing care needs for a client experiencing an acute attack of asthma.

TABLE 26-4   NURSING IMPLICATIONS FOR PHARMACOLOGY: CLIENTS RECEIVING ASTHMA DRUGS

DRUG	ACTION	NURSING RESPONSIBILITIES	CLIENT AND FAMILY TEACHING
Beta-Adrenergic Agonists ▪ Epinephrine ▪ Isoproterenol (Isuprel) ▪ Metaproterenol (Alupent, Metaprel) ▪ Terbutaline (Brethine) ▪ Isoetharine (Bronkosol) ▪ Albuterol (Proventil) ▪ Bitolterol (Tornalate) ▪ Pirbuterol (Maxair) ▪ Salmeterol (Serevent)	These drugs stimulate sympathetic nervous system (SNS) receptors in the lungs, causing bronchodilation. Given orally, parenterally, or by metered-dose inhalers (MDIs), they are used to prevent and treat acute attacks. Their side effects include nervousness, irritability, tachycardia, and dysrhythmias, particularly when given parenterally or by mouth.	Use with caution in clients with hypertension, cardiovascular disease, hyperthyroidism, or diabetes. When given by MDI, wait 1–2 minutes between puffs to allow airways to dilate, permitting the second dose to reach distal airways. Chart response. Desired effect is reduced dyspnea and wheezing; anxiety, irritability, insomnia, and tremor are common side effects.	Use your inhaler or nebulizer as instructed. If you are taking this drug with another medication by inhalation, use this drug first to open airways. Rinse your mouth after using inhalers to reduce systemic effects. Keep a log of your use; if drug becomes less effective, or you need it more often, contact your doctor. Report irregular pulse and other side effects to your doctor.
Anticholinergics ▪ Atropine ▪ Ipratropium bromide (Atrovent)	Anticholinergics dilate the bronchi. Atropine is used infrequently because it tends to dry secretions and has other side effects. Ipratropium bromide is available as an inhaler and has fewer side effects than atropine.	Assess for possible contraindications to the drug, including glaucoma, an enlarged prostate, or urinary retention. Provide ice chips, fluids, or hard candy to relieve dry mouth.	Take no more than the ordered number of doses per day. If the drug becomes less effective over time, notify your doctor. A dosage adjustment may be needed.

(continues)

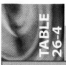

| | **NURSING IMPLICATIONS FOR PHARMACOLOGY: CLIENTS RECEIVING ASTHMA DRUGS (CONTINUED)** | | |

DRUG	ACTION	NURSING RESPONSIBILITIES	CLIENT AND FAMILY TEACHING
Corticosteroids ▪ Beclomethasone dipropionate (Vanceril, Beclovent) ▪ Triamcinalone acetonide (Azmacort) ▪ Flunisolide (AeroBid) ▪ Dexamethasone sodium phosphate (Decadron Phosphate Respihaler)	These are potent anti-inflammatory drugs used to prevent and treat acute episodes. They reduce the frequency and severity of attacks and allow lower doses of other drugs. Giving these drugs by inhalation reduces systemic side effects.	Give inhaler doses after bronchodilators to improve transit of the drug to distal airways. Report common side effects: Sore throat, hoarseness, and oropharyngeal *Candida albicans* infection.	Rinse your mouth after taking the drug; use good oral hygiene to reduce the risk of fungal infections. Do not use these drugs to treat an acute attack. The desired effect may not be noticed for several weeks. Call your doctor if you gain weight, retain fluid, or have muscle weakness, mood changes, or an appearance change.
Mast Cell Stabilizers ▪ Cromolyn sodium (Intal, Nasalcrom) ▪ Nedocromil (Tilade)	These drugs reduce inflammatory airway responses and prevent airway constriction in response to cold air. They have a wide margin of safety.	Report potential adverse effects of wheezing and bronchoconstriction.	Use these drugs only to prevent asthma attacks; do not use to treat an acute attack. Several weeks may be required before a beneficial effect is noted.
Leukotriene Modifiers ▪ Zafirlukast (Accolate) ▪ Zileuton (Zyflo)	Leukotriene modifiers interfere with airway inflammation, improving airflow and decreasing asthma symptoms. They are used to prevent asthma attacks; they are not used to treat an acute attack.	Give at least 1 hour before or 2 hours after meals. These drugs affect warfarin metabolism. Monitor for bleeding. Monitor liver enzymes, as these drugs may be toxic to the liver.	Take as ordered on an empty stomach. Call your doctor if you notice a change in color of stools or urine, or if jaundice develops.

INEFFECTIVE AIRWAY CLEARANCE

▪ Frequently assess respiratory status (see Box 26-7). Notify the charge nurse or physician of significant changes. *Respiratory status can change rapidly during an acute asthma attack.*

CLINICAL alert

Slow, shallow respirations; faint breath sounds; decreased wheezing; and an ineffective cough may indicate exhaustion and possible respiratory failure. Immediate intervention is vital.

▪ Assess skin color and temperature and level of consciousness (LOC) every 1 to 2 hours or as indicated. *Cyanosis; cool,* *clammy skin; and changes in LOC (such as agitation, lethargy, or confusion) indicate worsening hypoxia.*

▪ Report abnormal or significant changes in oxygen saturation levels and ABG results. *Oxygen saturation and ABG values indicate gas exchange and the effectiveness of treatment.*

▪ Place in Fowler's, high Fowler's, or orthopnic (with head and arms supported on the overbed table) position. *These positions reduce the work of breathing and increase lung expansion.*

▪ Administer oxygen as ordered. If a mask is used, monitor for feelings of claustrophobia or suffocation. *Supplemental oxygen reduces hypoxemia. Although the mask is very effective for delivering oxygen, it may increase anxiety.*

▪ Administer nebulizer treatments and provide humidification as ordered. *Bronchodilators and other drugs are given by nebulizer; humidity helps loosen secretions.*

ASTHMA

Subjective Data

- Complaints of shortness of breath, difficulty breathing, fatigue, apprehension
- History of asthma, allergies; known exposure to a trigger
- Current medications, effectiveness, when last used

Objective Data

- Respiratory status, including peak expiratory flow rate, oxygen saturation, ability to converse without pausing for breath; dyspnea; nasal flaring, chest expansion, use of accessory muscles, presence of retractions; lung sounds throughout chest, adventitious sounds; presence and effectiveness of cough, sputum production
- Vital signs, skin color
- Level of consciousness and mental status
- State of anxiety, apprehension

- Assist with chest physiotherapy, including percussion and postural drainage. *Percussion and postural drainage facilitate airway clearance.*
- Increase fluid intake. *Increasing fluids helps thin secretions.*
- Monitor effects of prescribed medications. *Medications used to improve airway status and facilitate breathing also may have significant adverse effects.*

FATIGUE

- Assist with ADLs as needed. *This allows energy conservation.*
- Provide rest periods between activities and treatments. *Rest helps prevent fatigue and reduce oxygen demands.*
- Assist with breathing and relaxation techniques to control breathing pattern. *Pursed-lip breathing helps keep airways open, abdominal breathing improves lung expansion. Relaxation techniques reduce anxiety and help slow the respiratory rate.*

ANXIETY

An acute asthma attack causes significant anxiety with a fear of suffocation. Hypoxia contributes to the sense of anxiety.

- Help identify coping skills that have been successful in the past. *Coping skills can help the client regain control.*
- Provide physical and emotional support. Remain present during periods of acute anxiety. Schedule time with the client every 1 to 2 hours, and reassure about a prompt response to the call light. *The severely anxious client may fear that he or she will die if someone is not on hand. Reassurance of readily available assistance and the presence of the nurse reduces anxiety.*

- Listen actively to concerns; do not deny or negate the fear of dying or of being unable to breathe. *Active listening promotes trust and helps the client express concerns.*
- Provide clear, concise directions and explanations. Avoid presenting too much information. *Anxiety interferes with learning. Explanations may need to be repeated frequently.*
- Reduce excessive stimuli, and maintain a calm demeanor. *This promotes rest.*
- Allow supportive family members to remain with the client. *Significant others provide additional support and can help reduce anxiety.*
- Assist with relaxation techniques such as guided imagery, muscle relaxation, and meditation. *These techniques help reduce anxiety and restore a sense of control.*

INEFFECTIVE THERAPEUTIC REGIMEN MANAGEMENT

- Assess understanding of asthma and prescribed treatment. Reinforce teaching as indicated. *Assessment helps identify misperceptions about asthma and its management that may contribute to acute attacks.*
- Discuss the effect of asthma and its management on lifestyle. *Discussion can help identify conflicts between lifestyle and the treatment regimen.*
- Help identify factors that contributed to the acute attack. *Awareness of contributing factors helps identify ways to prevent future attacks.*
- Assist to identify ways to integrate daily treatment into lifestyle. *Asthma management can impact significant others as well as the client, for example, eliminating smoking and pets in the household, removing carpets, and measures to reduce dust mites.*
- Provide verbal and written instructions. *Written instructions reinforce learning and allow future reference.*
- Refer to counseling, support groups, or self-help organizations. *Services such as these can help with required lifestyle changes and the demands of treatment.*

EVALUATING

To evaluate the effectiveness of nursing care, collect data related to:

- Respiratory status and breathing pattern
- Fatigue and activity tolerance
- Anxiety level
- Knowledge and understanding of measures to prevent future asthma attacks

Discharge Considerations

Teach about prescribed drugs. Provide information verbally and in writing, including:

- The drug name, its frequency, dose, and how to use it

■ The desired effect and purpose of the drug

■ Potential adverse effects and their management, including those that should be reported to the physician

■ Potential interactions with other medications (including over-the-counter medications) or with foods

■ What to do if the medication becomes less effective or is needed with increasing frequency over time

See Box 26-8 for teaching related to using a metered dose inhaler (MDI).

If specific triggers for asthma attacks have been identified, help identify ways to avoid these triggers. Because exercise, particularly in cold weather, often triggers an attack,

BOX 26-8
TEACHING FOR DISCHARGE

USING A METERED-DOSE INHALER

• Firmly insert the metered-dose inhaler (MDI) canister into holder.
• Shake vigorously for 3 to 5 seconds.
• Exhale slowly and completely.
• Close lips around mouthpiece or hold mouthpiece directly in front of mouth.
• Press and hold canister down once while inhaling deeply and slowly for 3 to 5 seconds (see figure).

• Hold breath for 10 seconds. Release pressure on container and remove from mouth, then exhale.
• Wait 20 to 30 seconds (or as directed) before repeating for a second puff.
• Rinse mouth after using inhaler.
• Rinse mouthpiece at least once a day.

HOME CARE RESOURCES FOR CLIENTS WITH ASTHMA
BOX 26-9

American Lung Association
1740 Broadway
New York, NY 10019
800-LUNG-USA (800-586-4872)
www.lungusa.org

Asthma and Allergy Foundation of America
1125 15th Street, NW, Suite 502
Washington, DC 20005
800-7-ASTHMA (800-727-8462)

Asthma Information Center
www.mdnet.de/asthma/

National Asthma Education and Prevention Program
National Heart, Lung, and Blood Institute Information Center
P.O. Box 30105
Bethesda, MD 20824-0105
301-251-1222

instruct to warm up slowly before exercise and wear a mask to retain air warmth and humidity while exercising. If necessary, help identify alternate indoor exercises. Discuss measures to prevent respiratory infections and support immune function, including adequate rest, good nutrition, and stress management. Recommend yearly influenza vaccine and immunization against pneumococcal pneumonia. Help identify stress management techniques to incorporate into lifestyle. Refer to a local or regional agency for further teaching and support as needed. See Box 26-9 for home care resources.

Chronic Obstructive Pulmonary Disease

Chronic obstructive pulmonary disease (COPD) is characterized by chronic and progressive obstruction of air flow in the lungs. It usually affects middle and older adults. Smoking is the most common cause of COPD. Other risk factors are secondhand smoke exposure, air pollution, occupational pollutants, and family history of COPD.

PATHOPHYSIOLOGY

In COPD, the airways are narrowed and gradually obstructed by inflammation, excess mucus production, and loss of elastic tissue and alveoli. Two different processes, chronic bronchitis and emphysema, cause these airway and lung tissue changes (Figure 26-13 ◆). Alveolar ventilation is impaired, as is gas exchange between the alveoli and the blood.

By the time COPD is diagnosed, the client may have had a productive cough, dyspnea, and exercise intolerance for as

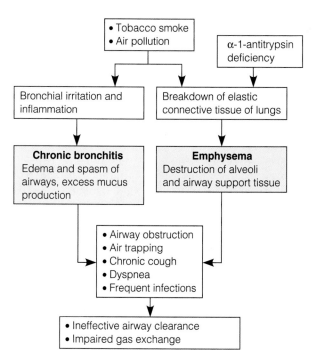

Figure 26-13. ◆ The process of COPD.

Figure 26-14. ◆ Typical appearance of a client with emphysema.

long as 10 years. The cough usually occurs in the mornings ("smoker's cough"). Dyspnea becomes worse as the disease progresses. Periodic episodes of increased sputum and difficulty breathing are common, often caused by respiratory infection.

Chronic Bronchitis

Chronic bronchitis is a chronic inflammatory airway disorder that causes excessive secretion of thick, tenacious mucus and a productive cough lasting 3 or more months. Narrowed airways and excess secretions obstruct air flow. The primary cause of chronic bronchitis is cigarette smoke.

Emphysema

Emphysema is destruction of alveolar walls leading to large, abnormal air spaces in the lungs. As in chronic bronchitis, cigarette smoking is its major cause. Deficiency of alpha-1-antitrypsin, an enzyme that normally prevents lung tissue destruction, also causes emphysema.

When alveolar walls are destroyed, air spaces enlarge and the surface area for gas exchange decreases. Think about an apple and an equal size bunch of grapes: the skin (surface area) of the apple is much smaller than the combined surface area of all the grapes in the cluster.

The alveoli become less elastic and airways tend to collapse during exhalation. This causes air trapping in the lungs. Over time, the anterior–posterior chest diameter increases, and the client develops a *barrel chest* (Figure 26-14 ◆). The manifestations of chronic bronchitis and emphysema are summarized in Table 26-5 ◆.

COLLABORATIVE CARE

Avoiding—never starting or stopping—smoking is the only way to prevent COPD and to slow its progression. Early in the disease, airway obstruction can be reversed and disability minimized. Treatment focuses on reducing symptoms and maintaining optimal function.

Diagnostic Tests

The following tests are used to help diagnose COPD, assess the client's status, and monitor the effectiveness of treatment.

■ *Pulmonary function testing* is used to evaluate lung ventilation and function. See the earlier section of this chapter on lung

TABLE 26-5   MANIFESTATIONS OF CHRONIC BRONCHITIS AND EMPHYSEMA

	CHRONIC BRONCHITIS	EMPHYSEMA
Onset	After age 35; recurrent respiratory infections	After age 50; progressive shortness of breath
Cough	Persistent, productive of copious, thick sputum	Absent or mild, nonproductive
Appearance	Often obese Edema and cyanosis Distended neck veins	Thin and *cachectic* (malnourished) Barrel chest Use of accessory muscles of respiration
Chest auscultation	Wheezing and rhonchi	Distant or diminished breath sounds

volumes and capacities. Instruct to avoid tobacco products, bronchodilators, or eating a heavy meal prior to testing.

- *Serum alpha-1-antitrypsin* levels may be drawn to screen for a deficiency of this enzyme.
- *ABGs* are drawn to evaluate the effect of COPD on gas exchange. During an acute episode, a low PO_2 (hypoxemia), high PCO_2 (hypercapnia), and low pH (respiratory acidosis) may be seen.

CLINICAL alert

Clients with COPD may have chronic hypercapnia. This reduces the effect of PCO_2 and pH on the respiratory drive; instead, breathing is driven by a drop in arterial oxygen levels. These clients may develop sleep apnea and respiratory arrest when given oxygen, because their drive to breathe is suppressed.

- *Pulse oximetry* is used to measure oxygen saturation *(O_2 sats)* of the blood. These levels may be used to continuously assess the need for supplemental oxygen.
- Other diagnostic tests may include *ventilation/perfusion scanning,* to evaluate the match between ventilation and perfusion of lung tissue; a *chest x-ray,* or a *computed tomography (CT) scan* of the chest.

Pharmacology

Medications are used to help manage COPD symptoms and slow progression of the disease.

Immunization against pneumococcal pneumonia and yearly influenza vaccine are recommended. A broad-spectrum antibiotic is ordered if infection is suspected. A bronchodilator such as ipratropium (Atrovent) or theophylline may be ordered. Theophylline also improves cardiac and respiratory muscle function. Review the nursing implications for bronchodilators as outlined in Table 26-3. Corticosteroids may be given to reduce inflammation and edema of the airways. Cough suppressants and sedatives are avoided. Alpha-1-antitrypsin may be given when this enzyme is deficient.

Oxygen Therapy

Clients with COPD may need home oxygen therapy. Oxygen may be used intermittently, at night, or continuously. Home oxygen is available as liquid oxygen, compressed gas cylinders, or oxygen concentrators. During an acute episode, oxygen and ventilatory assistance using a continuous positive airway pressure (CPAP) mask or mechanical ventilation may be required. CPAP is discussed in Chapter 25; mechanical ventilation is discussed later in this chapter. Careful observation is vital when oxygen is given without ventilatory support, as the drive to breathe may be inhibited, leading to respiratory arrest.

Other Therapies

Smoking cessation is vital. Nicotine chewing gum or patches may be prescribed, and referral made to a clinic, group, or counselor. Clients are advised to avoid other airway irritants and allergens. When air pollution is significant, the client may need to remain indoors. Air filtering systems or air conditioning may be useful.

Increased fluid intake, effective cough, percussion, and postural drainage help clear secretions. A liberal fluid intake keeps secretions thin. Forceful coughing is often less effective than leaning forward and repeatedly "huffing," with relaxed breathing between huffs. Percussion and postural drainage help clear secretions when they are thick or tenacious. Breathing exercises slow the respiratory rate and reduce fatigue. *Pursed-lip breathing* helps slow respirations and keep airways open during exhalation by keeping positive pressure in the airways. *Abdominal breathing* helps reduce the work of accessory muscles of respiration. (See Box 26-11.)

A lung transplant or lung reduction surgery may be done in end-stage COPD. Lung reduction surgery reduces the volume of the lung, reshapes it, and improves elastic recoil. It improves pulmonary function and exercise tolerance, and reduces dyspnea. (See Box 26-13 for nursing care of the client with lung surgery.)

NURSING CARE

ASSESSING

Clients with COPD need careful and frequent assessment (Box 26-10).

BOX 26-10
ASSESSING CLIENTS WITH COPD

SUBJECTIVE DATA
- Complaints of shortness of breath, difficulty breathing; onset and duration; fatigue; cough, amount and character of sputum
- Recent respiratory infection
- Smoking history; history of chronic lung disease, asthma, pneumonia, allergies
- Current medications, effectiveness, when last used; home oxygen

OBJECTIVE DATA
- Respiratory status, including peak expiratory flow rate, oxygen saturation; dyspnea, chest expansion, nasal flaring, use of accessory muscles; cough, sputum produced; lung sounds throughout chest, adventitious sounds such as wheezes, fine or course crackles
- Vital signs including apical pulse and capillary refill; neck vein distention
- Skin color; clubbing of nails
- Level of consciousness and mental status
- Level of anxiety, apprehension
- Height and weight; general nutritional status

DIAGNOSING, PLANNING, AND IMPLEMENTING

Because of the obstructive nature of COPD, airway clearance is a high-priority nursing problem. This chronic disease affects all areas of life as it progresses, making psychosocial issues a concern in planning nursing care.

INEFFECTIVE AIRWAY CLEARANCE

- Frequently assess respiratory status (see Box 26-10), skin color, and mental status. Report changes such as diminished breath sounds, ineffective cough, increasing cyanosis, or altered mental status to the charge nurse or physician. *Changes may indicate a decline in the client's condition.*
- Report oxygen saturations of less than 95% (or identified parameters). *Decreasing oxygen saturation levels may indicate airway obstruction and impaired alveolar ventilation.*
- Encourage fluid intake of at least 2,000 to 2,500 mL per day unless contraindicated. *Adequate fluid intake helps keep secretions thin.*
- Place in Fowler's, high Fowler's, or orthopnic position. Encourage activity to tolerance. *An upright position improves lung ventilation. Activity helps mobilize secretions and prevent them from pooling.*
- Assist to cough at least every 2 hours while awake. *Coughing helps mobilize secretions and maintain open airways.*
- Provide tissues and a paper bag to dispose of sputum. *This infection control measure reduces the spread of respiratory organisms to others.*
- Assist with percussion and postural drainage as needed. *Percussion helps loosen secretions in airways; postural drainage facilitates movement of these secretions out of the respiratory tract.*
- Provide rest periods between treatments and procedures. *Rest conserves energy and reduces fatigue.*
- Give expectorant and bronchodilator medications as ordered. *Using expectorants and bronchodilators before coughing, percussion, and postural drainage improves airway clearance.*
- Provide humidified oxygen as ordered. *Oxygen helps maintain blood and tissue oxygenation. Humidification decreases the drying effects of oxygen on respiratory tissues.*
- Prepare for transfer to intensive care if condition is deteriorating. *Respiratory failure is a possible complication of COPD that requires aggressive intervention to preserve life.*

IMBALANCED NUTRITION: LESS THAN BODY REQUIREMENTS

- Obtain diet history, weight and height, and skinfold measurements. *This data is used to evaluate nutritional status.*
- Observe and document food intake, including types and amounts consumed. *This provides information about possible need for supplements.*
- Monitor serum albumin and electrolyte levels. *These values provide information about nutritional status.*
- Consult with a dietitian to plan meals and supplements. *High-protein, high-calorie foods help maintain nutrition and reduce fatigue.*
- Provide frequent, small feedings with between-meal supplements. *Frequent, small meals help maintain intake and reduce fatigue associated with eating.*
- Assist to choose preferred foods from menu; encourage family members to bring food from home if allowed. *Providing food preferences encourages eating.*
- Keep snacks at bedside. *Snacks provide additional caloric intake.*
- Provide mouth care before meals. *This improves appetite.*

INEFFECTIVE COPING

- Assess interactions and the effect of the illness on the family. *Assessment helps identify effective and disruptive behaviors.*
- Help identify strengths for coping with the situation. *Identifying strengths helps the client and family regain a sense of control.*
- Encourage expression of feelings. Avoid judging the feelings as "good" or "bad," "right" or "wrong." *Active listening without judging promotes trust.*
- Help identify behaviors and attitudes that may hinder effective treatment, such as continuing to smoke in the house when the client is present. *Family members may be unaware of the effect of their behavior on the client's ability to change habits and cope with a disabling disease.*
- Encourage participation in care. *This helps develop skills for use at home.*
- Refer to available support groups, pulmonary rehabilitation programs, and community agencies or services such as home health, homemaker services, or Meals-on-Wheels as appropriate. *Support groups, community services, and structured rehabilitation programs provide additional support and enhance coping abilities.*

DECISIONAL CONFLICT: SMOKING

- Encourage to express feelings; acknowledge concerns, values, and beliefs. *This demonstrates acceptance of the client's right to make the decision. The nurse needs to avoid imposing personal values and beliefs about smoking on the client.*
- Help plan a course of action for quitting smoking. *When the client develops the plan, he or she has more ownership and interest in making it work.*
- Demonstrate respect for decisions and the right to choose. *Respect supports self-esteem and ability to cope.*
- Refer to a counselor or other professional as needed. *Counselors or other people trained to assist with smoking cessation can help with the decision and plan.*

EVALUATING

To evaluate the effectiveness of nursing care, collect assessment data related to airway clearance and respiratory status, nutritional status and diet intake, demonstrated coping behaviors by the client and family, and a commitment to smoking cessation.

Discharge Considerations

Teach the client with COPD effective coughing and breathing techniques (Box 26-11), how to prevent exacerbations, and management of the treatment regimen.

Advise client to maintain a fluid intake of at least 2 to 2½ quarts of fluid daily. Instruct to avoid respiratory irritants such as cigarette smoke (primary and secondary), other smoke sources, dust, aerosol sprays, air pollution, and very cold dry air. Teach to avoid large crowds and people with known infections to prevent infection. Instruct to obtain yearly influenza immunization. Discuss the exercise program, and encourage a balance of rest and activity as tolerated. Aerobic physical exercise (e.g., walking for 20 minutes at least three times weekly) improves exercise tolerance. Activities that strengthen the muscles used for breathing and ADLs, such as swimming and golf, also are helpful. Stress the importance of maintaining food intake, eating small frequent meals and using nutritional supplements as needed. If a salt-restricted diet is ordered, teach about foods to avoid and suggest seasonings to improve taste without salt.

Instruct to promptly report early signs of infection or exacerbation of the disease to the physician: fever, increased sputum, purulent (green or yellow) sputum, upper respiratory infection, increased shortness of breath or difficulty breathing, decreased activity tolerance or appetite, increased need for oxygen.

Reinforce teaching about prescribed medications, including purpose, use, and expected effects. Instruct to avoid over-the-counter medications unless approved by the physician. Teach about other treatment measures, such as home oxygen, percussion, postural drainage, and nebulizer treatments. If special equipment is required, be sure to discuss its use, cleaning, and maintenance.

Finally, advise clients with COPD to wear an identification band and carry a list of their medications at all times.

Nursing Process Case Study
■ CLIENT WITH COPD

Anna "Happy" Mercurio is an 83-year-old widow who lives with her two grown sons. Over the past 15 years, she has become more short of breath and has developed a chronic cough. Ten years ago, emphysema was diagnosed. She is in the hospital with possible pneumonia and an acute exacerbation of COPD.

Assessment Mrs. Mercurio denies smoking but says that her husband and two sons have been smokers "for practically their whole lives." She reports that she now must rest after just a few minutes of activity. Her cough is productive of moderate to large amounts of sputum, particularly in the mornings. Her dyspnea and sputum became worse 2 days ago; this morning, she was unable to get dressed without resting.

Mrs. Mercurio's skin is very warm and dry, her color dusky. She pauses frequently while talking to catch her breath. Respiratory rate 36, fairly shallow. Frequent cough productive of large amounts of thick, tenacious green sputum. Vital signs: P 115, irregular; BP 186/60; T 102.4° F (39° C). Weight 96 lbs. (43.6 kg), height 5′3″ (160 cm). Appears barrel-chested with moderate kyphosis. Chest hyperresonant to percussion. Distant breath sounds with scattered wheezes and rhonchi throughout lung fields. Chest x-ray shows patchy infiltrates. Laboratory results include high RBC count, low serum albumin, and oxygen saturation of 83%.

Admitting orders include sputum for culture; intravenous penicillin G, 2 million units every 4 hours; ipratropium (Atrovent) inhaler, 2 puffs every 6 hours; beclomethasone (Vanceril) inhaler, 2 puffs every 6 hours; bed rest with bathroom privileges; oxygen per nasal cannula at 2 L continuously; regular diet.

Diagnosis The following nursing diagnoses are identified for Mrs. Mercurio:

■ Ineffective Airway Clearance related to pneumonia and COPD

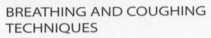

BOX 26-11
TEACHING FOR DISCHARGE

BREATHING AND COUGHING TECHNIQUES

Pursed-Lip Breathing
1. Inhale through nose with mouth closed.
2. Exhale slowly through pursed lips, as though whistling or blowing out a candle. Exhale twice as long as inhalation.

Diaphragmatic or Abdominal Breathing
1. Place one hand on abdomen, the other on the chest.
2. Inhale, concentrating on pushing abdominal hand outward while chest hand remains still.
3. Exhale slowly, while abdominal hand moves inward and chest hand remains still.

Controlled Cough Technique
1. After using bronchodilator, inhale deeply, and hold breath briefly.
2. Cough twice, first to loosen mucus, then to expel secretions.
3. Inhale by sniffing to prevent mucus from moving back into deep airways.
4. Rest.

Huff Cough Technique
1. Inhale deeply while leaning forward.
2. Exhale sharply with a "huff" sound. This helps keep airways open while mobilizing secretions.

- Impaired Gas Exchange related to lung disease
- Risk for Impaired Spontaneous Ventilation related to oxygen therapy and respiratory muscle fatigue
- Impaired Home Maintenance related to activity intolerance

Expected Outcomes   The expected outcomes specify that Mrs. Mercurio will:

- Expectorate secretions effectively.
- Return to her previous level of respiratory function.
- Maintain oxygen saturation greater than 92%.
- Maintain spontaneous respirations without excess fatigue.
- Express willingness to allow help with household tasks.

Planning and Implementation   The following interventions are planned and implemented:

- Assess respiratory status and level of consciousness every 1 to 2 hours until stable, then at least every 4 hours.
- Monitor O_2 saturation continuously.
- Increase fluid intake to at least 2,500 mL/day.
- Provide bedside humidifier.
- Keep head of bed elevated to at least 30 degrees.
- Provide mouth care after inhaler treatments.
- Provide uninterrupted rest periods after respiratory therapy and other procedures.
- Refer to home health for nursing follow-up.
- Refer to social services for assistance with home maintenance.

Evaluation   Mrs. Mercurio's condition gradually improves. At discharge, she is able to provide self-care with less fatigue and dyspnea. She is using oxygen only at night, admitting that it is just for security. Although scattered wheezes are present, her sputum is thinner, white, and easily expectorated. She will continue oral penicillin V for an additional 10 days at home. She will continue to use Atrovent and Vanceril inhalers at home. Mrs. Mercurio's sons have agreed to smoke only in the garage or outside. A home health nurse will visit three times weekly. A housekeeper will clean and do laundry weekly. Mrs. Mercurio is glad to go home and grateful for the help she will receive.

 Critical Thinking in the Nursing Process

1. Mrs. Mercurio had long-term exposure to secondhand smoke. How does secondhand smoke contribute to lung disease in adults and children?
2. The nursing care plan included the nursing diagnosis: Risk for Impaired Spontaneous Ventilation related to oxygen therapy and respiratory muscle fatigue. Review the respiratory drive and describe how chronic hypercapnia affects this process.

 Cystic Fibrosis

Cystic fibrosis (CF) is an inherited disorder of childhood that causes excess mucus secretion. Its most damaging effects are to the lungs. Today, many people with CF live into adulthood.

The genetic defect of CF causes excess mucus production in the lungs. Thick mucus plugs small airways and impairs normal airway clearing mechanisms. This leads to *atelectasis,* infection, *bronchiectasis,* and airway dilation. The lungs become scarred and stiff. Over time, COPD, *pulmonary hypertension* (increased pressures in the pulmonary vascular system), and right heart failure develop. The other primary features of CF are lack of pancreatic enzymes and impaired digestion, and increased sodium and chloride in sweat.

The signs and symptoms of CF include dyspnea, chest congestion, and a chronic cough productive of large amounts of thick, sticky sputum. A barrel chest and clubbing of the fingers and toes may be seen. Digestive problems cause abdominal pain and *steatorrhea* (bulky, foul-smelling stool).

Treatment goals for CF include preventing or treating respiratory complications and maintaining adequate nutrition.

A *pilocarpine iontophoresis sweat chloride test* is used to diagnose CF. Pilocarpine and a small electric current are used to increase sweating. The sweat is collected and analyzed.

Dornase alfa, an enzyme that helps liquify mucus in CF, is given to improve airway clearance. This drug is given by aerosol. Prophylactic antibiotics often are given to prevent recurrent respiratory infections.

Chest physiotherapy with percussion, vibration, postural drainage, and coughing is essential for airway clearance. Oxygen therapy may be necessary. A liberal fluid intake helps liquify mucus secretions. Lung transplantation currently is the only definitive treatment for CF. Single-lung, double-lung, and heart–lung transplants have been successful in CF clients.

Nursing care for the client with CF is similar to that for COPD. The genetic component of CF and the client's age are important considerations. Many adults with CF are just entering their productive years and face a shortened life span.

Reinforce teaching for respiratory care techniques, including percussion, postural drainage, and controlled cough techniques. Stress the importance of avoiding respiratory irritants, such as cigarette smoke and air pollution. Discuss prevention of respiratory infection by maintaining immunizations, good general health, and avoiding large crowds and infected people.

Discuss the genetic transmission of CF. Refer for genetic testing if desired. Help sort through the impact of CF on future pregnancies and generations. Remember that the risk of CF may present an ethical dilemma about future pregnancies for clients and their families. Provide support as needed.

 Atelectasis

Atelectasis is partial or total lung collapse and airlessness. It may be acute or chronic. The usual cause of atelectasis is obstruction of the airway to affected area of lung. It may affect a small segment of a lung or an entire lobe. Atelectasis also may result from compression of the lung (e.g., a tumor) or an inability to keep alveoli open. The manifestations of atelectasis include absent or diminished breath sounds over the affected area, tachycardia, tachypnea, and dyspnea.

Prevention is the primary treatment for atelectasis. Clients with risk factors such as COPD, smokers undergoing surgery, and prolonged bed rest, need vigorous chest physiotherapy to keep airways open. Frequent respiratory assessment is important for early detection and treatment. Position on the unaffected side, with the involved side up to promote drainage. Move frequently, and encourage coughing and deep breathing. Encourage oral fluids to help liquefy secretions.

Bronchiectasis

Bronchiectasis is permanent dilation and destruction of large airways. It is usually due to repeated respiratory infections. Inflammation and airway obstruction weaken and dilate bronchial walls, causing secretions to pool and further infection and inflammation.

Bronchiectasis causes a chronic cough productive of large amounts of sputum. Other manifestations include hemoptysis, recurrent pneumonia, wheezing and shortness of breath, malnutrition, right-sided heart failure, and cor pulmonale (see the section of this chapter on pulmonary vascular disorders).

Treatment is similar to that for COPD. Antibiotics are ordered at the first sign of infection and may be used prophylactically. Inhaled bronchodilators also may be ordered. Chest physiotherapy is a vital part of care. Percussion and postural drainage help mobilize secretions. Oxygen may be ordered. If lung destruction is local, the affected segment may be surgically removed.

Nursing care of the client with bronchiectasis is much the same as for COPD. Airway clearance is a primary problem, as is ineffective breathing pattern. Teaching is vital to help the client and family manage the disease and prevent progression.

Interstitial Lung Disorders

Many lung diseases damage the interstitial or connective tissue of the lung. Occupational lung diseases and sarcoidosis fall into this group of disorders. Toxic drugs and radiation also cause interstitial damage.

In these disorders (Table 26-6 ◆), inflammation damages the alveoli and interstitial tissue of the lung. Normal lung tissue is replaced by fibrotic (scar) tissue. As a result, the lungs become stiff and noncompliant (difficult to inflate).

The onset of interstitial lung disease may be acute or gradual. A dry cough and dyspnea on exertion are common symptoms of interstitial lung diseases. Respirations are often rapid and shallow. Fine inspiratory crackles at the lung bases may be heard. Clubbing of the fingers and toes may develop.

Occupational Lung Disease

Occupational lung diseases are directly related to inhaling noxious substances in the work environment. There are two major classifications:

1. *Pneumoconioses,* caused by inhaling *inorganic* dusts and particulates

TABLE 26-6	COMMON INTERSTITIAL LUNG DISORDERS AND THEIR CAUSES	
DISORDER	**CAUSE**	**HIGH-RISK POPULATION**
Pneumoconioses ◾ Silicosis ◾ Asbestosis ◾ Black lung disease	Inorganic dusts ◾ Silica ◾ Asbestos ◾ Coal	Hard rock miners, foundry workers, sandblasters, pottery makers, granite cutters People involved in mining, milling, manufacturing, and application of asbestos products Coal miners
Hypersensitivity pneumonitis	Organic dusts	People exposed to cotton dust, moldy sugar cane fiber; farmers; people who raise birds
Sarcoidosis	Unknown	Young adults; African Americans

2. *Hypersensitivity pneumonitis,* allergic responses to inhaled organic dusts

When a noxious substance is inhaled, the body's response depends on: the size of the particles; whether it is organic or inorganic; where it lands in the respiratory tract; and the individual. Normal lung defenses attempt to remove foreign matter, however these defenses may be impaired by smoking, alcohol, or allergic reactions.

Sarcoidosis

Sarcoidosis is a systemic disease of unknown cause. Lesions develop in the lungs, lymph nodes, liver, eyes, skin, and other organs. These lesions may heal or cause scarring. It can cause significant lung damage and eventual disability.

COLLABORATIVE CARE
Prevention is important for all occupational lung diseases. Containing dust and wearing personal protective devices that limit the amount of inhaled particles are essential for people who work in industries with known risks.

Diagnostic testing shows restricted ventilation, with reduced vital capacity and total lung capacity. Gas exchange is affected, leading to low oxygen saturation and hypoemia, especially with exercise. The chest x-ray shows interstitial lung damage. A bronchoscopy may be done to obtain tissue for biopsy. Specialized lung scans can show the extent of scarring.

Management of interstitial lung disease includes measures to identify and remove the cause, reduce inflammation, prevent progression, and support current lung function. Treatment is nonspecific. Anti-inflammatory drugs, such as corticosteroids, may reduce the inflammatory response and slow the progression of the disease. Generally, care is supportive, similar to that for clients with COPD.

NURSING CARE

Nursing care for clients with interstitial lung diseases is much the same at that for a client with COPD.

Activity intolerance is a common problem. The client's ability to perform ADLs may be significantly impaired. Nursing measures to reduce energy use and provide rest are essential. Caregiver role strain, either actual or potential, must be considered when the client with severe disability is being cared for at home.

Ineffective coping may also be a priority nursing diagnosis. Many occupational lung diseases develop after 20 to 30 years of exposure to the hazardous material. Clients who began working after high school may develop signs of disease in their 40s and face the possibility of changing occupations or becoming disabled. The resulting role strain affects all family members.

 ## Discharge Considerations

Teach clients at risk for occupational lung diseases how to reduce this risk. Nurses in industrial and public health settings should be alert to potential dangers. Teach workers about measures to reduce dust in their work area and the use of personal protective devices such as masks. Educate children of people with occupational lung disease about the risks associated with the occupation.

Teach how to avoid further lung damage, for example, avoid respiratory irritants such as cigarette smoke and heavy air pollution. Recommend influenza and pneumococcal pneumonia immunizations. Yearly tuberculin testing is recommended for clients with silicosis.

Teach pulmonary hygiene measures, such as maintaining fluid intake, coughing, and deep-breathing exercises. If oxygen therapy is ordered, teach about its use and care of the equipment. Always include teaching about the use and effects of any ordered medications.

If corticosteroid therapy is prescribed, stress the importance of taking the medication as prescribed and not stopping it abruptly. Include information about managing the side effects of corticosteroids by limiting sodium and increasing potassium in the diet, taking the medication with food or milk to minimize gastric irritation, and identifying early signs of infection. See Chapter 13 for more information about corticosteroid drugs.

 # Lung Cancer

Lung cancer is the leading cause of cancer deaths in the United States. It has a grim prognosis: Most people with lung cancer die within one year of the diagnosis.

Cigarette smoking is the most important cause of lung cancer. About 85% of lung cancer is related to smoking. The disease is 10 to 30 times more common in smokers than nonsmokers. The more the person smokes and the longer the person smokes, the greater the risk. Other risk factors for lung cancer are radiation exposure and inhaled irritants, asbestos in particular.

PATHOPHYSIOLOGY

Most primary lung tumors arise in the cells lining the airways. These tumors differ by cell type, incidence, presentation, and manner of spread (Table 26-7 ◆).

Lung cancer tends to be aggressive and locally invasive, and metastasize widely. Tumors begin as mucosal lesions that grow to obstruct the bronchi or invade adjacent tissue.

Tumors frequently spread via the lymph system to nodes and other organs. Lung cancer usually is well advanced when diagnosed, with tumor cells in lymph nodes and distant metastasis.

Initial symptoms often are blamed on smoking or chronic bronchitis. In addition to manifestations of the tumor and cancer (Box 26-12), lung cancers often produce hormone-like substances that cause indirect symptoms. These are known as *paraneoplastic syndromes* or manifestations.

Lung cancer metastasizes to the lymph nodes, brain, bones, liver, and other organs. Confusion, impaired balance, headache, and personality changes may be symptoms of brain

TABLE 26-7

LUNG CANCER CELL TYPES

	CELL TYPE	LOCATION AND MANIFESTATIONS	SPREAD
	Small-cell (oat cell) carcinoma	Central mass; may cause endocrine symptoms or thrombophlebitis	Distant metastasis common at diagnosis
	Adenocarcinoma	Peripheral mass; few symptoms	Early metastasis to CNS, bone
	Squamous cell carcinoma	Central mass; cough, dyspnea, atelectasis, wheezing	Spreads by local invasion
	Large-cell carcinoma	Large peripheral lesion; may cause gynecomastia or thrombophlebitis	Early metastasis

BOX 26-12 MANIFESTATIONS OF LUNG CANCER

LOCAL
- Cough, hemoptysis
- Wheezing and dyspnea
- Chest pain, hoarseness or dysphagia

GENERAL
- Anorexia, weight loss
- Fever

PARANEOPLASTIC
- Fluid and electrolyte imbalances
- Cushing's syndrome
- Peripheral neuropathy, muscle weakness
- Thrombophlebitis
- Anemia, disseminated intravascular coagulation (DIC)

metastasis. Tumor spread to the bone causes bone pain, pathologic fractures, and possible spinal cord compression. When the liver is affected, symptoms may include jaundice, anorexia, and upper right quadrant pain.

Superior vena cava syndrome, partial or complete obstruction of the superior vena cava, is a potential complication. Symptoms such as edema of the neck and face, headache, dizziness, vision changes, and syncope may develop abruptly or gradually. Veins of the upper chest and neck are dilated, and the skin is flushed or cyanotic. Laryngeal edema may cause dyspnea.

COLLABORATIVE CARE
Prevention of lung cancer should be a primary goal for all health care providers. Reducing tobacco use will have a greater impact on the death rate from lung cancer than treatment advances.

Diagnostic Tests
- *Chest x-ray* often shows the first evidence of lung cancer.
- Malignant cells may be identified by *sputum cytology.* This test requires a sputum sample on arising.
- A *CT scan* is used to evaluate tumor size and location.
- *Bronchoscopy* may be done to visualize the tumor and obtain a specimen for biopsy. A cable-activated instrument is used to obtain a biopsy specimen. (Review nursing care of the client undergoing a bronchoscopy in Box 26-2.)
- A *percutaneous needle biopsy* or aspiration of pleural fluid by *thoracentesis* may be done if the tumor is in the periphery of the lung.

Pharmacology
Combination chemotherapy is the primary treatment for some types of lung cancer. It is used as an adjunct to surgery or radiation for other types. It may lengthen survival when metastases are present. (See Chapter 8 for more information about chemotherapy.)

Other medications that may be ordered include bronchodilators to reduce airway obstruction and antibiotics to treat infection. Analgesics are ordered after surgery and for pain management in advanced cancers.

Surgery
Surgery is the only real chance for a cure in most lung cancers. At the time of diagnosis, however, most tumors are beyond the stage at which they can be completely removed. The goal of surgery is to remove all tumor cells, including involved lymph nodes.

The type of surgery depends on the location and size of the tumor, as well as the client's health status (Table 26-8 ◆). As much functional lung as possible is preserved. Nursing care of the client having lung surgery is outlined in Box 26-13.

Radiation Therapy
Radiation therapy is used alone or in combination with surgery or chemotherapy. Before surgery, it is used to shrink tumors. When surgery is not an option, radiation therapy may

TABLE 26-8   TYPES OF LUNG SURGERY

PROCEDURE	DESCRIPTION	USED FOR
Laser bronchoscopy	Bronchoscopy used to guide laser to resect tumor	Tumors localized in a main bronchus
Thoracotomy	Incision into the chest wall	Gain access to the lung for surgery
Wedge resection	Removal of a small section (wedge) of lung tissue	Small, peripheral lesions
Segmental resection	Removal of a single bronchovascular segment of a lobe	Localized peripheral lung tumors
Lobectomy	Removal of a single lung lobe	Tumors confined to a single lobe
Pneumonectomy	Removal of an entire lung	Tumors throughout a lung, in the main bronchus, or fixed to the hilum

BOX 26-13
NURSING CARE CHECKLIST

LUNG SURGERY
Before Surgery

☑ Provide routine preoperative care and teaching (see Chapter 7).

☑ Obtain baseline assessment data, particularly respiratory and cardiovascular status.

☑ Reinforce teaching, allowing time to practice breathing and coughing techniques.

☑ Establish a way to communicate if an endotracheal tube will be in place after surgery.

☑ Introduce to intensive care unit and policies if client will return there after surgery.

After Surgery

☑ Assess and provide routine postoperative care (Chapter 7).

☑ Frequently assess respiratory status (color, rate and depth, chest expansion, lung sounds, and oxygen saturation). Promptly report changes to the charge nurse or physician.

☑ Assist with coughing, postural drainage, and incentive spirometry. Suction as needed while intubated.

☑ Maintain chest tube drainage system. Initially measure output hourly, then every 2 to 4 or 8 hours as indicated. Notify physician if output exceeds 70 mL/hr and/or is bright red, warm, and free flowing.

☑ Assist to move in bed and ambulate as soon as possible.

be the treatment of choice. Complications such as superior vena cava syndrome may be treated with radiation. (Radiation therapy is discussed further in Chapter 8.)

Other Therapies

Pleural effusion is a frequent complication of lung cancer. As fluid collects, the lung cannot fully expand and ventilation is impaired. A *thoracentesis* may be done to remove the excess pleural fluid. (Review Box 26-5 for nursing care related to a thoracentesis.)

NURSING CARE

ASSESSING

Obtain complete respiratory assessment data. Include smoking history and the duration of current symptoms. Obtain data related to both respiratory and cardiovascular status, especially if surgery is anticipated.

Assess for concerns related to lung function, the cancer itself, and the planned treatment.

DIAGNOSING, PLANNING, AND IMPLEMENTING

INEFFECTIVE BREATHING PATTERN

■ Assess and document respiratory status at least every 4 hours; more frequently as indicated. *Early identification of altered respiratory function is important to maintain tissue oxygenation.*

■ Report abnormal oxygen saturation levels and blood gas results to the charge nurse or physician. *Changes in blood oxygen levels may indicate respiratory compromise.*

■ Elevate the head of the bed to 60 degrees. *Elevating the head of the bed promotes lung expansion.*

■ Assist to turn, cough, deep breathe, and use incentive spirometer. Help splint the chest with a pillow or blanket when coughing. *These measures promote airway clearance.*

■ Administer oxygen as ordered. *Supplemental oxygen improves alveolar oxygenation and gas exchange.*

■ Suction as needed. *Pharyngeal suctioning may be required when the client is unable to clear secretions by coughing.*

■ Assist with percussion and postural drainage as ordered. *Percussion and postural drainage help clear airways and maintain effective respirations.*

■ Provide reassurance and emotional support. *Relief of anxiety promotes a more effective breathing pattern.*

ACTIVITY INTOLERANCE

Loss of functional lung tissue due to the tumor or surgery affects the ability to maintain normal activities.

■ Document responses to activity, including pulse, respiratory rate, dyspnea, and fatigue. *Tachycardia, tachypnea, dyspnea, or fatigue with activities is a sign of activity intolerance.*

■ Plan rest periods interspersed with activities and procedures. *Rest periods reduce oxygen demands and fatigue.*

■ Assist to increase activities gradually. *Gradual increases in activity improves exercise tolerance.*

■ Teach energy conservation measures, such as sitting while showering and dressing and wearing slip-on shoes. *These measures reduce oxygen demand and promote independence.*

■ Keep frequently used objects within easy reach. *This helps conserve energy.*

■ Encourage to remain as active as possible. *Maintaining activity levels improves physical and emotional well-being.*

■ Allow family members to provide assistance as needed. *This helps the client conserve energy and allows the family to feel useful.*

PAIN

■ Assess and document pain. *Remember that pain is subjective; however, reluctance to cough or move may indicate unreported pain.*

■ Provide analgesics as needed to maintain comfort. *Adequate pain relief promotes postoperative recovery and coping. Good pain management is vital to improve recovery from surgery and to allow a peaceful death for the terminal cancer client.*

■ For cancer pain, maintain a continuous medication schedule using opiates, NSAIDs, and other drugs as ordered. *Addiction is not a concern for the terminal cancer client; adequate pain relief that does not allow "breakthrough" pain is vital.*

■ Use adjunctive pain relief measures, such as massage, positioning, distraction, and relaxation techniques. *These techniques promote relaxation and enhance pain relief.*

■ Encourage activities that distract from pain such as reading, television, and social interactions. *Distraction helps the client focus away from the pain.*

■ Allow significant others to remain with the client. *Physical presence provides emotional support.*

ANTICIPATORY GRIEVING

■ Spend time with the client and family. *Time is necessary to develop a trusting, therapeutic relationship.*

■ Answer questions honestly; do not deny the probable outcome of the disease. *Honesty reinforces reality and promotes a sense of control over decisions to be made.*

■ Encourage expression of feelings, fears, and concerns. *Open communication helps promote understanding and acceptance.*

■ Assist to understand the grieving process and to accept responses as normal. *Explanation enhances understanding of the grieving process and the ability to cope.*

■ Help identify strengths and effective coping measures. *Past successes in coping with crises can help with the present situation and develop a sense of control.*

■ Encourage use of other support systems, such as spiritual and social groups. Refer to support groups, social services, and hospice care as indicated. Provide American Cancer Society literature and information as appropriate. *These support systems can help the client and family cope with the diagnosis.*

■ Discuss advance directives (the living will and durable power of attorney for health care). *These documents give more control over treatment when the client is no longer able to express his or her own wishes.*

EVALUATING

Collect data related to the client's respiratory status, ability to complete ADLs and other activities, pain control, and acceptance of the probable outcome of the disease to evaluate the effectiveness of nursing care.

Discharge Considerations

Provide honest information about lung cancer, the expected outcome, and planned treatment. Do not promote false hope.

Stress the importance of stopping smoking, especially if surgery has been done. The client with lung cancer may have difficulty recognizing the need to stop smoking. Include information about the effects of nicotine and the tars in ciga-rette smoke on healing and already compromised lung tissue (Box 26-14).

Provide information about planned treatments, explaining expected effects and usual side effects of each. Help identify ways to cope with noxious effects. If surgery has been done, discuss activities and exercises to improve strength and regain function. Stress the need to continue coughing and deep-breathing exercises at home. Provide information about symptoms to report to the physician: fever, increasing dyspnea, cough, increased or purulent sputum, redness, pain, swelling, or incisional drainage.

Discuss medication use, including desired and adverse effects and interactions with other drugs or foods. Teach how to use analgesics and other pain relief measures.

BOX 26-14
TEACHING FOR DISCHARGE

CIGARETTE SMOKING

Tobacco was first used in religious ceremonies and to offer friendship. At one time, it was thought to help cure many common diseases. Tobacco is now known as the leading preventable cause of illness in the world.

Cigarette smoke contains about 4,000 chemicals, including nicotine. Nicotine is highly addictive, producing a feeling of well-being. Tar, the particulate matter in cigarette smoke, causes most of its ill effects in the lungs. Smoke paralyzes cilia, reducing clearance of tars from the bronchial tree.

To help the client quit smoking:

• Help identify barriers and obstacles to quitting.
• Teach about nicotine's addictive properties.
• Explain that withdrawal may cause anxiety, irritability, headache, and insomnia.
• Help develop a plan with a target date to quit and ways to deal with obstacles, withdrawal symptoms, and the temptation to resume smoking.
• Offer self-help material at an appropriate reading level.
• Refer to a counselor, physician, or smoking-cessation clinic.
• Reassure that relapse is common. Continue to provide support and encouragement, helping avoid further relapses.

In addition, help prevent children and teens from starting to smoke:

• Provide education programs to help them avoid smoking.
• Reduce minors' access to tobacco, especially cigarettes and chewing tobacco (often the first product used by teenage boys).

Provide information about hospice services, home health, cancer support groups, and American Cancer Society services.

Nursing Process Case Study
■ CLIENT WITH LUNG CANCER

After coughing up bloody sputum, James Mueller, 68 years old, sees his physician. A chest x-ray shows a mass in his right lung. He is admitted for diagnostic tests.

Assessment In the nursing history, Mr. Mueller describes himself as "pretty healthy," except for a smoker's cough. He has a 50 pack-year smoking history (a pack per day for 50 years, since age 18). He says he quit after a small heart attack 3 years ago but started again after 4 months. His cough has become productive and he admits he is more short of breath than usual with activity.

Vital signs are BP 162/86; P 78, regular; R 20; and T 98.4° F (36.9° C). Color good, skin warm and dry. Wheezes noted in right chest; good breath sounds throughout. A sputum specimen sent for cytology is positive for small-cell bronchogenic cancer. The CT scan shows a central mass with mediastinal and subclavicular lymph node involvement. A small mass is also seen on Mr. Mueller's lumbar spine. After talking with his physician and an oncologist, Mr. Mueller decides on a trial course of chemotherapy.

Diagnosis The following nursing diagnoses are identified for Mr. Mueller:

■ Ineffective Airway Clearance related to tumor
■ Risk for Imbalanced Nutrition: Less Than Body Requirements related to side effects of chemotherapy
■ Risk for Ineffective Coping related to lung cancer diagnosis
■ Deficient Knowledge about lung cancer and aids for smoking cessation

Expected Outcomes The expected outcomes specify that Mr. Mueller will:

■ Maintain a patent airway.
■ Maintain current weight.
■ Express feelings and concerns about the effect of cancer on the family.

■ Participate in care.
■ Contact appropriate support groups.
■ Verbalize an understanding of his disease, its treatment, and prognosis.
■ Develop a plan to stop smoking.

Planning and Implementation The following interventions are planned and implemented:

■ Teach measures to promote airway clearance.
■ Instruct to report: Increased dyspnea or hemoptysis, severe wheezing, chest pain.
■ Discuss nausea relief measures, including premedication with an antiemetic.
■ Teach about lung cancer and its effects.
■ Encourage a family conference with children and grandchildren.
■ Refer to local cancer support group.
■ Refer to home health for follow-up and teaching.
■ Help develop a plan to stop smoking.
■ Ask physician for a prescription for nicotine patches or gum.

Evaluation After 3 months of chemotherapy, Mr. Mueller's tumor has not regressed, and a liver scan shows further metastasis. He and his wife decide to stop treatment, a decision with which the children reluctantly agree. The Muellers are referred to hospice services. With their help, Mr. Mueller is able to remain at home. His pain is managed initially with oral MS Contin, and later with a morphine infusion. Mr. Mueller dies at home with his family at his side 9 months after his diagnosis of lung cancer.

Critical Thinking in the Nursing Process

1. Describe how chemotherapy drugs work against cancer cells, and discuss the reason for using a combination of drugs as opposed to single-drug treatment (see Chapter 8).
2. Develop a care plan to deal with the common side effects of chemotherapy.
3. How could the nurse help if a client decided to stop cancer treatment but the family disagreed with the decision?

Pulmonary Vascular Disorders

The cardiovascular and respiratory systems are closely linked. A good match of air flow and blood flow is essential to maintain gas exchange and oxygen delivery to all body tissues and organs. Disorders previously discussed in this chapter affect air flow; this section discusses disorders that affect blood flow to the lungs.

Pulmonary Embolism

A **pulmonary embolism** is blockage of a pulmonary artery that disrupts blood flow to the lung. *Thromboemboli*, or blood clots, are the most common pulmonary emboli. Tumors, bone marrow fat, amniotic fluid, and foreign matter also can become emboli. Because a large pulmonary embolism can be fatal, prevention is the best treatment.

PATHOPHYSIOLOGY

Most pulmonary emboli begin as clots in the deep veins of the legs or pelvis. The risk factors are those for deep vein thrombosis: impaired venous blood flow, blood vessel damage, and altered coagulation. Prolonged immobility is the primary risk factor; others are discussed in Chapter 23.

Deep vein thrombosis may not be suspected until pulmonary embolism occurs. When the clot breaks loose from the vein wall, it travels through vessels that become gradually larger until it reaches the right side of the heart and enters the pulmonary artery. The pulmonary arteries and arterioles become smaller and smaller, and the clot is trapped, obstructing blood flow. No blood flows through capillaries beyond the occlusion, so no gas exchange occurs in that portion of the lung. A large clot can obstruct blood flow to a major part of the lung, causing sudden death.

The symptoms of a pulmonary embolism depend on its size and location (Box 26-15). Small emboli may go unnoticed; larger emboli cause manifestations similar to a myocardial infarction (heart attack).

Fat emboli may occur after a long bone fracture (e.g., the femur) as bone marrow fat is released. Fat emboli cause a sudden onset of dyspnea, tachypnea, tachycardia, confusion, delirium, and decreased level of consciousness. *Petechiae* may be seen on the chest and arms.

COLLABORATIVE CARE

Preventive measures include elastic stockings (TED hose), pneumatic compression devices, and early ambulation to prevent venous stasis. Elevating the legs of immobilized clients and leg exercises also help prevent venous stasis and pulmonary emboli.

When a pulmonary embolism is suspected, a *lung scan* may be ordered. Albumin tagged with a radioisotope is injected intravenously. As the tagged albumin moves through pulmonary blood vessels, the lungs are scanned to show its distribution (Figure 26-15 ◆). *Pulmonary angiography* uses a radiocontrast dye to evaluate pulmonary circulation. This procedure has a higher risk than the lung scan.

Treatment of a pulmonary embolis is supportive. Oxygen is given, and analgesics may be ordered to relieve pain and anxiety. Pulmonary artery and wedge pressures are monitored with a balloon (Swan–Ganz) catheter (see Chapter 22). The client is monitored for dysrhythmias.

Pharmacology

A thrombolytic drug (e.g., streptokinase, urokinase, or t-PA) may be given to disintegrate a large pulmonary embolus and

> ### BOX 26-15
> ### MANIFESTATIONS OF PULMONARY EMBOLISM
>
> - Abrupt onset of dyspnea, chest pain
> - Anxiety, apprehension
> - Cough
> - Tachycardia, tachypnea
> - Diaphoresis
> - Cyanosis

restore pulmonary blood flow. The primary risk of thrombolytic therapy is bleeding, particularly intracranial bleeding. See Chapter 22 for more information about thrombolytic therapy and its nursing implications.

Anticoagulants are ordered to prevent further clotting and embolization. Low-dose heparin is given to prevent DVT. When pulmonary embolus has occurred, an intravenous heparin infusion is ordered. The activated partial thrombo-

A

B

Figure 26-15. ◆ (A) A normal lung scan showing perfusion of all areas of the lungs. (B) A lung scan showing impaired blood flow to the right lung due to pulmonary embolus.

Figure 26-16. ◆ Example of a vena caval filter to prevent emboli from reaching the lungs.

plastin time (APTT) or PTT is monitored, and the client is assessed for signs of abnormal bleeding. Heparin is continued until oral anticoagulant (warfarin) therapy is fully effective, 5 to 7 days after its initiation. Anticoagulants are continued for 2 to 3 months or longer. Bleeding is a risk for any client taking anticoagulants. (See Table 23-6 for nursing implications of anticoagulants.)

Surgery

An umbrella-like filter may be inserted into the inferior vena cava of clients who have recurrent pulmonary emboli. This device traps large emboli while allowing blood to flow through the vena cava (Figure 26-16 ◆).

NURSING CARE

When a pulmonary embolus occurs, the client has urgent nursing care needs and may be transferred to intensive care for close observation and monitoring.

RISK FOR INEFFECTIVE TISSUE PERFUSION: CARDIOPULMONARY

- Encourage early ambulation following surgery or illness.
- Apply elastic stockings or pneumatic compression devices as ordered.
- Assist with leg exercises.
- Discourage using pillows under the knees.
  These measures promote venous return from the legs, reducing venous stasis and the risk for DVT and pulmonary emboli.

IMPAIRED GAS EXCHANGE

- Frequently assess respiratory status, including rate, depth, effort, and lung sounds. *Maintaining optimal ventilation facilitates gas exchange in well-perfused areas of the lung.*
- Report changes in level of consciousness, mental status, and skin color to the charge nurse or physician. *A change in LOC or mental status and/or cyanosis may indicate hypoxemia.*
- Place in Fowler's or high-Fowler's position. *This position promotes lung expansion and ventilation.*

- Start oxygen by nasal cannula or mask as ordered. *Supplemental oxygen increases alveolar and arterial oxygenation.*
- Report low oxygen saturation levels and abnormal arterial blood gas results. *ABGs and pulse oximetry are used to assess gas exchange and the effect of interventions.*
- Maintain bed rest. *Bed rest reduces oxygen demands.*

DECREASED CARDIAC OUTPUT

A large pulmonary embolus can affect cardiac output and tissue perfusion.

- Assess vital signs every 15 to 30 minutes initially, then every 2 to 4 hours as indicated. *Frequent assessment is important during the early, unstable period following pulmonary embolus.*
- Record hourly urine output. *Decreased urine output may indicate impaired renal perfusion.*
- Assess skin color, temperature, and capillary refill. *These assessments are used to evaluate tissue perfusion.*
- Monitor cardiac rhythm. *Monitoring allows early detection and treatment of dysrhythmias.*
- Assess for and report neck vein distension and peripheral edema. *Right-sided heart failure may result from pulmonary embolism due to increased pulmonary pressures.*
- Maintain intravenous and arterial lines. *The client may be unstable and critically ill, requiring immediate interventions to maintain life.*
- Provide frequent skin care. *Impaired peripheral perfusion and tissue oxygenation increase the risk of skin breakdown.*
- Instruct to report chest pain or other symptoms. *Decreased cardiac output and an increased workload may cause angina.*

ANXIETY

- Reassure and provide emotional support. Accept fear of dying, and reassure that treatment usually restores respiratory function. *The fear of death is very real; reassurance helps relieve excess anxiety.*
- Remain with the client as much as possible. *This helps reduce anxiety.*
- Explain procedures and treatments, using short, simple sentences. *Simple explanations reduce fear of the unknown.*
- Reduce environmental stimuli, and use a calm, reassuring manner. *These measures help reduce anxiety in both the nurse and the client.*
- Allow family members to remain present as much as possible. *Calm, supportive family members provide further reassurance.*
- Administer morphine as ordered. *Morphine reduces both pain and anxiety.*

 Discharge Considerations

Teach clients to reduce the risk for DVT and pulmonary embolism:

- On automobile trips, stop every 1 to 2 hours for a brief stretch and walk to restore venous circulation.
- During long flights, get up every hour or so, and do leg exercises while seated.
- Do not cross legs.
- Exercise regularly (e.g., walking).
- Wear elastic hose when standing for prolonged periods. Avoid hose that bind around the knee or thigh.

Teach about prescribed anticoagulants, including symptoms of bleeding to report to the physician. Instruct to use a soft toothbrush and avoid taking aspirin (unless prescribed) and other over-the-counter drugs without the doctor's approval. Stress the importance of wearing an identification bracelet or tag to alert medical personnel about anticoagulant use.

Pulmonary Hypertension

Arterial pressure in the pulmonary system normally is low (25/8) compared with the systemic BP (120/80). **Pulmonary hypertension** is an abnormal elevation of the pulmonary arterial pressure. It can develop with no obvious cause, or may occur as a result of chronic lung disease or another problem. Long-standing pulmonary hypertension can lead to *cor pulmonale,* with right ventricular hypertrophy and failure. COPD is the usual cause of cor pulmonale.

Manifestations of pulmonary hypertension include increasing dyspnea, fatigue, angina, and syncope (fainting or light-headedness) with exertion. Clients with cor pulmonale have a chronic productive cough, progressive dyspnea, wheezing, and signs of right heart failure (peripheral edema and distended neck veins). The skin is warm, moist, and dusky red.

Supplemental oxygen and drugs such as calcium channel blockers may be ordered for pulmonary hypertension. Rapid-acting direct vasodilators such as inhaled nitric oxide may be ordered. Salt and water intake may be restricted. Bilateral lung or heart–lung transplant may be done for primary pulmonary hypertension.

Nursing care is supportive, focusing on the underlying lung disease. *Impaired gas exchange* is a significant problem, as are problems such as *activity intolerance, anxiety, fatigue,* and others. See nursing assessment and interventions for COPD and for heart failure.

Provide information about pulmonary hypertension and cor pulmonale as appropriate. Include the disease process, and manifestations to report to the physician, including change in activity tolerance, increased edema, and signs of respiratory infection or exacerbation. Discuss the importance of planned rest periods between activities and ways to conserve energy, such as using a shower chair. Stress the importance of not smoking due to its effects on the lungs and blood vessels. As always, teach about the purpose, use, and effects of medications.

Pneumothorax and Hemothorax

A closed chest cavity with negative pressure in the pleural space is necessary for breathing. Excess fluid, air, or blood in the pleural space interferes with lung expansion and breathing. Chest and lung injury can result from penetrating or blunt trauma or inhalation injury. Assessment of airway, breathing, and circulation (ABCs) is vital in these disorders.

Pneumothorax

Accumulation of air in the pleural space is called **pneumothorax.** Pneumothorax can occur without apparent cause, due to chronic lung disease, or as a result of trauma.

PATHOPHYSIOLOGY

When the pleura is breached, air enters the pleural space. Pressure in the pleural space is no longer negative, and the lung on the affected side collapses. A small portion of the lung or the entire lung may be affected, depending on the amount

and rate of air accumulation. Table 26-9 ◆ illustrates and summarizes the major types of pneumothorax.

When a bleb on the lung surface ruptures *(spontaneous pneumothorax),* air moves freely into and out of the pleural space. As a result, the pneumothorax often is small. A gunshot wound or stab wound to the chest causes a *traumatic open pneumothorax (sucking chest wound)* that allows air to move freely through the chest wall. In a *tension pneumothorax,* injury to the chest wall or lungs allows air into the pleural space but prevents it from escaping. Air accumulates rapidly, and the lung on the affected side collapses. The heart, great vessels, and trachea shift to the unaffected side of the chest, placing pressure on the opposite lung.

CLINICAL alert

Tension pneumothorax is a medical emergency requiring immediate intervention to maintain the airway, breathing, and circulation.

TABLE 26-9

TYPES OF PNEUMOTHORAX

	TYPE	PATHOPHYSIOLOGY	MANIFESTATIONS
Normal lung / Pleural space (A)	Spontaneous	Rupture of a bleb (blister) on lung surface allows air from lungs into pleural space. ▪ *Primary* occurs in previously healthy people, usually young men. Smoking a risk factor. ▪ *Secondary* affects people with COPD and other chronic lung diseases.	Abrupt onset Pleuritic chest pain Shortness of breath Tachypnea, tachycardia Unequal chest movement Decreased breath sounds on affected side Hyperresonant percussion tone
Puncture wound through chest wall (B)	Traumatic	Result of chest trauma. ▪ *Open* due to penetrating trauma that allows air from outside to enter pleural space. ▪ *Closed* occurs when torn visceral pleura allows air from lung to enter pleural space; rib fracture a common cause. ▪ *Iatrogenic* due to laceration of visceral pleura during a procedure such as central line insertion.	Pain Dyspnea Tachypnea, tachycardia Decreased chest movement Absent breath sounds Air movement through an open wound
Mediastinal shift to unaffected side / Wound in chest wall allows air to enter pleural space but not to escape (C)	Tension	Air enters pleural space through chest wall or from lungs but is unable to escape. Air accumulates rapidly causing collapse of lung on affected side. Heart, great vessels, trachea, and esophagus shift toward unaffected side.	Hypotension, shock Severe dyspnea Tachypnea, tachycardia Decreased chest wall movement Absent breath sounds Trachea deviates toward unaffected side

COLLABORATIVE CARE

Treatment of pneumothorax depends on its severity. Clients with a small simple pneumothorax may simply be monitored with x-rays. Air is gradually reabsorbed, and the lung reexpands. With a larger pneumothorax, the air is removed from the pleural space to allow the collapsed lung to reexpand. A

thoracentesis may be done, inserting a needle into the pleural space to withdraw the air. Review Box 26-5 for nursing care of a client having a thoracentesis. A catheter with a one-way valve may be inserted into the pleural space. The one-way valve allows air to leave the pleural space but prevents it from entering.

Figure 26-17.   ◆   A closed chest drainage system.

Chest Tubes

The usual treatment for pneumothorax is *chest tubes* connected to a closed-drainage system. The drainage system has a one-way valve or a "water seal" that prevents air from entering the chest cavity during inspiration and allows air to escape during expiration. Applying low suction to the system helps reestablish negative pressure, allowing the lung to reexpand.

Several closed-drainage systems are available. Some use water to prevent air from entering the pleural space and to regulate suction (Figure 26-17 ◆). Others are "dry" systems that include a mechanical one-way valve to prevent air entry and a suction regulator. Chest tube drainage collects in a graduated chamber that allows easy measurement. To ensure system function, it is important to prevent damage and maintain the integrity of all tubes and connections. Box 26-16 outlines nursing care for a client with chest tubes.

NURSING CARE

Restoring ventilation and gas exchange is the highest priority of care for the client with a pneumothorax.

ASSESSING

Collect assessment data from clients with risk factors for pneumothorax, such as chest or abdominal trauma (e.g., motor vehicle crash or fall from a height), COPD, or procedures such as central line insertion or thoracentesis. Assess clients with known pneumothorax for the effect of treatment measures.

Ask about chest pain or difficulty breathing. Inquire about previous history of pneumothorax or chronic lung disease. Obtain smoking history.

Assess respiratory status, including dyspnea, rate and depth of respirations, chest wall movement, and lung sounds. Note level of consciousness and skin color. Observe neck veins for distention and position of trachea.

BOX 26-16
NURSING CARE CHECKLIST

CHEST TUBES
Before the Procedure

☑ Verify a signed consent for the procedure.
☑ Reinforce teaching. Local anesthesia will be used; pressure may be felt during insertion. Breathing will improve when the chest tube is in place.
☑ Gather supplies as indicated: Thoracostomy tray, local anesthetic, sterile gloves, drainage system, sterile water to fill water seal and suction chambers.
☑ Position as ordered for the procedure.

During the Procedure

☑ Assist as needed. Provide physical and psychological support.
☑ Notify physician of changes in respiratory rate and effort, pulse, and color.

After the Procedure

☑ Document vital signs, breath sounds, oxygen saturation, color, and respiratory effort at least every 4 hours.
☑ Maintain closed system. Tape all connections; secure chest tube to chest wall.
☑ Keep collection device below chest level.
☑ Check tubes frequently for kinks or loops.
☑ If water seal system is used:
  ☑ Frequently check water seal chamber. The water level should fluctuate with respiratory effort; if it does not, the system may not be patent or intact. Periodic air bubbles in water seal chamber are normal and indicate that trapped air is being removed from the chest.
  ☑ Keep the device upright.
  ☑ Add water to the suction control chamber as needed.
☑ Measure drainage every 8 hours, marking level on drainage chamber. Do not empty chamber. Report drainage that is cloudy, in excess of 70 mL/hr, or red, warm, and free flowing.
☑ When chest tube is removed, immediately apply sterile occlusive dressing.

DIAGNOSING, PLANNING, AND IMPLEMENTING

IMPAIRED GAS EXCHANGE

When the lung collapses, gas exchange no longer occurs in the affected part of the lung.

- Document vital signs, oxygen saturation, and respiratory status at least every 4 hours. *Frequent assessment is necessary to monitor response to impaired lung function and treatment.*
- Place in Fowler's or high Fowler's position. *This position facilitates lung expansion.*
- Administer oxygen as ordered. *Supplemental oxygen improves blood oxygen levels.*
- Provide emotional support. *Dyspnea and hypoxemia are frightening and produce anxiety.*
- Assist with frequent position changes and ambulation. *Movement promotes lung ventilation.*
- Provide rest. *Rest conserves energy and reduces oxygen demands.*

RISK FOR INJURY

- Assess chest tube and drainage system at least every 2 hours. *The system must remain patent and intact to function effectively. Inadvertent removal of a chest tube or damage to the closed drainage system allow air and pathogens to enter the chest cavity.*
- Secure chest tubes to chest wall and prevent tension on the tubes during care and ambulation. *Chest tubes are minimally secured with a suture and can be dislodged during activity.*
- Secure drainage tubing to sheet or gown. *Looping the drainage tubing prevents direct pressure on the chest tube itself.*
- Prevent kinking or occlusion of chest or drainage tube during repositioning. *This maintains the patency of the tubing.*
- Teach to keep drainage system below chest when sitting or ambulating. Suction usually can be disconnected during ambulation. *Ambulation promotes lung ventilation and reexpansion. Keeping the system below chest promotes drainage.*
- Observe insertion site for redness, swelling, pain, or drainage. Report fever or signs of infection to the physician. *Disruption of skin integrity increases the risk for infection.*
- Immediately reconnect any disrupted connections. *A closed system is vital to prevent air from entering the pleural space.*

- If the tube is inadvertently removed, promptly seal the wound with a sterile occlusive dressing. If a sterile dressing is not available, use other occlusive material such as foil or plastic wrap. Tape dressing on three sides only. *An occlusive dressing taped on three sides allows air to escape through the wound but prevents air from entering the wound on inhalation.*

EVALUATING

Frequently assess respiratory status and oxygenation to evaluate the effectiveness of nursing care.

Discharge Considerations

Clients who have had a spontaneous pneumothorax have a 50% risk of recurrence. Stress the importance of quitting smoking to reduce the risk. Advise avoiding activities that can increase the risk, such as mountain climbing, flying in unpressurized aircraft, scuba diving, and possibly contact sports.

Instruct to gradually increase exercise and activity to previous levels. Stress the importance of follow-up care and monitoring. Advise to report the following to the physician: Upper respiratory infection; fever, cough, or difficulty breathing; sudden, sharp chest pain; or redness, pain, swelling, tenderness, or drainage from the chest tube puncture wound.

Hemothorax

Hemothorax, blood in the pleural space, usually results from chest trauma or surgery. When blood collects in the pleural space, pressure on the affected lung impairs ventilation and gas exchange.

Hemothorax causes symptoms similar to those of a pneumothorax. Lung sounds are decreased. A dull percussion tone is heard over the collection of blood, usually at the lung base. Chest x-ray is used to confirm the diagnosis of hemothorax.

Thoracentesis or chest tubes are used to remove blood from the pleural space. With significant hemorrhage (e.g., following trauma or surgery), the blood may be collected for reinfusion.

Nursing care focuses on maintaining respirations, gas exchange, and cardiac output. In a large, slow-developing hemothorax, respiratory status is the primary concern. Nursing diagnoses and interventions are similar to those for pneumothorax. When hemothorax develops rapidly and hemorrhage is significant, shock is a risk (see Chapter 10).

Chest and Lung Trauma

Rib Fracture

Simple rib fracture, usually of a single rib, is the most common chest wall injury. This usually is a minor injury. In older adults or people with chronic lung disease, however, it can lead to problems such as pneumonia, atelectasis, and respiratory failure. If the fracture is displaced, bone can tear the pleura and cause pneumothorax.

A rib fracture causes pain on inspiration and coughing. Bruising may be seen over the fracture site. Crepitus (a grating sensation) may be felt with breathing. Breath sounds are diminished, especially in the bases, because of splinting.

FLAIL CHEST

When two or more adjacent ribs are broken in several places, part of the chest wall becomes free-floating. This is a *flail chest*. The flail segment moves inward during inspiration and moves outward with expiration. This is called *paradoxic movement* (Figure 26-18 ◆). Flail chest affects lung expansion and increases the work of breathing. The lung under the flail segment often is damaged.

In addition to paradoxic chest movement, flail chest causes pain and dyspnea. Chest expansion is unequal, and crepitus is present. Breath sounds are diminished, and crackles may be heard.

Pulmonary Contusion

Pulmonary contusion, or lung tissue injury, frequently occurs with chest trauma. When the chest is rapidly compressed and then decompressed (e.g., being thrown against the steering wheel then back in a motor vehicle crash), alveoli and pulmonary vessels rupture, causing tissue hemorrhage and edema. After the initial injury, inflammation further impairs breathing and gas exchange.

Manifestations of pulmonary contusion include shortness of breath, restlessness, apprehension, and chest pain. Copious sputum, possibly blood-tinged, is present. Tachycardia, tachypnea, dyspnea, and cyanosis develop as well.

Smoke Inhalation

Smoke inhalation is the leading cause of death in burn injury. Smoke inhalation is common when a burn occurs in a closed space, and is suspected with burns on the face or upper torso or singed nasal hairs.

Smoke inhalation can lead to burns of airways, carbon monoxide or cyanide poisoning, and lung damage from noxious gases. Manifestations of smoke inhalation include dyspnea, wheezes or crackles, and possibly ashlike material in sputum. Carbon monoxide is a colorless, odorless gas that binds readily with hemoglobin, reducing its ability to carry oxygen to cells of the body. The manifestations of carbon monoxide poisoning are listed in Box 26-17. Survivors of severe carbon monoxide poisoning may have permanent neurologic damage. Cyanide inhalation can be fatal; other toxic chemicals can cause bronchospasm and edema of the airways and alveoli.

Near-Drowning

Aspiration and oxygen deprivation are the primary problems in near-drowning. Significant hypoxemia and loss of con-

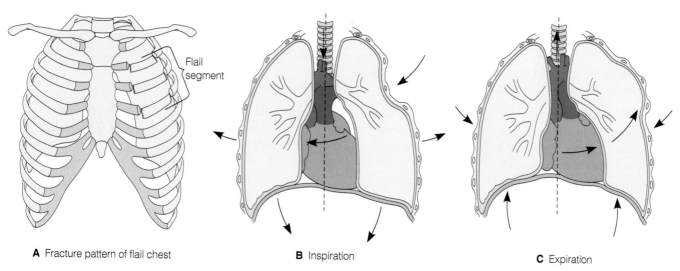

A Fracture pattern of flail chest   **B** Inspiration   **C** Expiration

Figure 26-18. ◆ Flail chest with paradoxic chest movement.

BOX 26-17
MANIFESTATIONS OF CARBON MONOXIDE POISONING

LOW LEVELS
- Headache, dizziness
- Dyspnea
- Nausea
- "Cherry-red" skin and mucous membranes

HIGHER LEVELS
- Confusion, irritability, hallucinations
- Visual disturbance
- Hypotension
- Seizures, coma

sciousness can occur within 3 to 5 minutes of immersion; death can occur within 5 to 10 minutes. Immersion in very cold water may prolong survival.

The near-drowning victim who aspirates either fresh or salt water can develop pulmonary edema and respiratory failure. Fresh-water drowning also causes blood cell hemolysis and electrolyte imbalances. In near-drowning, inhaled microorganisms and debris can lead to pneumonia.

Manifestations of near-drowning include altered consciousness, restlessness, and apprehension. The client may be hypothermic and complain of headache or chest pain. Other signs include vomiting, cyanosis, apnea, tachypnea, and wheezing. Pink froth may be seen in the mouth and nose. Shock and cardiac arrest may occur.

COLLABORATIVE CARE

Diagnostic tests to determine injury and lung function include:

- *Serum electrolytes* and *ABGs* to evaluate fluid and electrolyte and acid–base balance and oxygenation.
- *Carboxyhemoglobin* if carbon monoxide poisoning is suspected.
- *Chest x-ray* to evaluate chest wall injury and lung damage.
- *Bronchoscopy* for suspected pulmonary contusion or smoke inhalation.

Simple rib fractures typically heal uneventfully. Analgesia is ordered to facilitate breathing, coughing, and movement. An intercostal nerve block may be done. Rib belts, binders, and taping ribs are *not* recommended, because they can interfere with ventilation. With a flail chest, however, taping may be done to stabilize the chest wall.

Initial treatment of inhalation injury is removing the victim from the fire or water and providing effective cardiopulmonary resuscitation (CPR). Immediate restoration of effective breathing and circulation is key to preserving life. Oxygen is given as soon as available.

CLINICAL alert

When the victim is hypothermic, resuscitation is continued until the body temperature is about 90° F (32° C). "He's not dead until he's warm and dead" is a basic rule in hypothermia.

All clients with inhalation injury need supplemental oxygen. Coughing and suctioning are important to remove secretions and debris. Percussion and postural drainage may be done.

Intubation and mechanical ventilation may be ordered for flail chest, pulmonary contusion, and inhalation injuries as these clients often are critically ill. Intubation and mechanical ventilation are discussed in the next section of this chapter.

NURSING CARE

IMPAIRED AIRWAY CLEARANCE

- Frequently assess respiratory status. Note the amount, color, and consistency of sputum. *The client often is unstable; frequent assessment is necessary to rapidly detect changes.*
- Elevate head of bed. *This promotes alveolar ventilation.*
- Instruct to cough, deep breathe, and change position every 1 to 2 hours. Encourage to use incentive spirometer. Assist with percussion and postural drainage as needed. *These measures help remove secretions and debris, and prevent atelectasis or pneumonia following chest trauma.*
- Teach to splint affected area with a blanket or pillow when coughing. *Splinting improves ventilation and reduces pain.*
- Suction as needed. *Suctioning may be required when cough is ineffective or when intubated.*
- Stabilize endotracheal tube with tape and ties. *Stabilizing the tube prevents its displacement into a mainstem bronchus, which could result in ventilation of only one lung.*
- Report decreased breath sounds, increased adventitious sounds, pink, frothy or purulent sputum; chills or fever; or changes in vital signs or mental status. *Changes in respiratory status, vital signs, or mental status may indicate a complication such as pulmonary edema or pneumonia.*

IMPAIRED GAS EXCHANGE

- Report changes in skin color, oxygen saturation, and arterial blood gases. *Alveolar damage and pulmonary edema can significantly impair gas exchange.*
- Assess for anxiety or apprehension, restlessness, confusion or lethargy, or complaints of headache. *These may indicate hypoxia or hypercapnia.*
- Monitor intake and output; weigh daily. Maintain ordered fluid restriction. *Fluid volume excess can increase pulmonary edema and further impair with gas exchange.*
- Maintain oxygen and mechanical ventilation as ordered. *Oxygen and/or mechanical ventilation improve gas exchange.*

- Administer sedation as needed. *Sedation may be required to maintain effective mechanical ventilation.*
- Provide frequent mouth care. *Oxygen dries mucous membranes. Mouth care promotes comfort and helps prevent damage.*
- Restrict activity and allow periods of uninterrupted rest. *These measures reduce oxygen consumption.*

PAIN

- Frequently assess pain, using a pain scale. *Pain interferes with lung expansion and coughing.*
- Provide analgesics as ordered or on a schedule. *Regular analgesia controls pain more effectively than PRN doses.*
- Assess for respiratory depression related to narcotic analgesia. *Although pain control is important to maintain ventilation, narcotics can depress the respiratory center.*

INEFFECTIVE TISSUE PERFUSION: CEREBRAL

Inhalation injury can affect cerebral perfusion and oxygenation. Increased intracranial pressure (ICP) may develop after near-drowning.

- Frequently monitor neurologic status. Report changes promptly. *Change in level of consciousness or behavior is the earliest sign of increased ICP.*
- Place in Fowler's position. Keep the head in a neutral position. *Elevating and keeping the head straight promotes blood and CSF circulation.*
- Maintain effective ventilation and oxygenation. *Hypercapnia and hypoxemia increase cerebral edema.*

Discharge Considerations

The most effective treatment for chest trauma and lung injury is prevention. Teach use of seat belts with shoulder restraints to help prevent lung and chest injuries in motor vehicle crashes.

A working smoke detector (with functioning batteries) could prevent most deaths from smoke inhalation. Instruct to regularly check smoke detectors and replace batteries yearly. Encourage families to develop a fire escape plan and to use fire drills to rehearse the plan. Smoldering cigarettes are a leading cause of house fires; help develop a plan to stop smoking. Teach to drop and roll should clothing catch fire. (Fire rises, increasing the risk of respiratory injury when standing.)

To prevent drowning, life preservers and flotation vests or jackets need to be worn, not stored in the boat hold. These devices are designed to keep the head above water. Encourage to always wear life vests when boating, water-skiing, or windsurfing. Wet suits help prevent hypothermia in very cold water. Advise never to swim alone, when fatigued, or immediately after a meal. Advise to cover or fence swimming pools, hot tubs, and ponds to prevent inadvertent entry and drowning. Just as alcohol and driving do not mix, neither do alcohol and boating or other water sports.

A population well trained in effective CPR provides the best second line of defense. Rapid restoration of breathing is essential to prevent brain damage. Encourage everyone to be trained and maintain current CPR certification. Work with communities to increase the number of trained individuals. Refer to local chapters of the American Red Cross or the American Heart Association for classes.

For a minor chest wall injury, discuss pain control and its importance in preventing complications. Teach to splint the rib cage during coughing. Stress the importance of coughing and deep breathing. Explain the reasons to avoid taping or wrapping the chest continuously. Describe complications to report to the physician: chills and fever, productive cough, purulent or bloody sputum, shortness of breath or difficulty breathing, and increasing chest pain. Emphasize the importance of avoiding respiratory irritants, such as cigarette smoke and pollutants.

A large pulmonary contusion can lead to long-term respiratory compromise. This can require changes in activities and possibly occupation.

Respiratory Failure

Many of the conditions discussed in this chapter can lead to **respiratory failure.** In respiratory failure, the lungs are unable to oxygenate blood and remove carbon dioxide to meet the body's needs, even at rest. COPD is the usual cause of respiratory failure. Other lung diseases, trauma, neuromuscular disorders, and heart disease can also lead to respiratory failure.

PATHOPHYSIOLOGY

Respiratory failure is not a disease; it results from severe respiratory dysfunction. Blood oxygen levels are very low; the P_{O_2} may be less than 50 to 60 mm Hg (hypoxemia). Carbon dioxide levels rise as the lungs are unable to eliminate it. Tissue hypoxia and high P_{CO_2} levels (hypercapnia) lead to acidosis. See Chapter 5 to review acid–base balance.

> ### BOX 26-18
> ### MANIFESTATIONS OF
> ### RESPIRATORY FAILURE
>
> #### DUE TO HYPOXEMIA
> - Dyspnea, tachypnea
> - Cyanosis
> - Restlessness, anxiety, confusion
> - Tachycardia, dysrhythmias
> - Hypertension
> - Metabolic acidosis
>
> #### DUE TO HYPERCAPNIA
> - Dyspnea, respiratory depression
> - Headache, drowsiness, coma
> - Tachycardia, hypertension
> - Heart failure
> - Respiratory acidosis

The manifestations of respiratory failure are caused by hypoxemia and hypercapnia (Box 26-18). Hypercapnia causes vasodilation and depresses the central nervous system. As carbon dioxide levels increase, the respiratory center may be depressed. When this occurs, the usual carbon dioxide stimulus to breathe is lost, and low blood oxygen levels provide the only stimulus to breathe. Providing oxygen without mechanical ventilation may remove any drive to breathe, with dire results.

The prognosis for acute respiratory failure depends on the underlying disease. Acute respiratory failure due to an uncomplicated drug overdose usually resolves quickly and completely. Respiratory failure due to chronic lung disease often has a prolonged course and less favorable outcome.

Acute Respiratory Distress Syndrome

Acute respiratory distress syndrome (ARDS) is a severe form of acute respiratory failure. It can follow direct or indirect lung injury. Smoke inhalation and near drowning are direct lung injuries that may lead to ARDS; shock and sepsis cause indirect lung damage and can precipitate ARDS.

A massive inflammatory response damages the lungs. This damage occurs rapidly, often within 24 hours of the initial insult. Damage to the alveolar–capillary membrane allows plasma and blood cells to leak into the interstitial space and alveoli. Alveolar surfactant is inactivated, and the cells that produce it are damaged. Alveoli collapse, the work of breathing increases, and gas exchange is impaired. Hypoxemia develops and the PCO_2 rises.

The manifestations of ARDS usually develop 24 to 48 hours after the initial insult. Dyspnea and tachypnea are initial symptoms. Breath sounds are initially clear. Increasing respiratory distress and *refractory hypoxemia* (low oxygen saturation and PO_2 levels that do not improve with supplemental oxygen) develop. As respiratory failure progresses, the client may become agitated and confused or lethargic.

The prognosis for ARDS varies. Many clients recover fully. However, sepsis and multiple organ dysfunction syndrome (MODS) may develop. When this occurs, the prognosis is poor.

COLLABORATIVE CARE

Treatment focuses on the underlying cause or disease process, as well as supporting ventilation and correcting hypoxemia and hypercapnia.

Diagnostic tests include *arterial blood gases (ABGs)*. The arterial PO_2 may be less than 50 to 60 mm Hg, and the PCO_2 often is high, usually more than 50 mm Hg. The pH is low, indicating acidosis. In ARDS, *chest x-ray* shows diffuse infiltrates and a "white out" pattern as lung tissue collapses and fibrosis develops.

Pharmacology

Bronchodilators may be given to reverse airway spasm and constriction. Infection is treated with antibiotics. Corticosteroids may be ordered to reduce airway edema and inflammation. Surfactant therapy may be ordered for clients with ARDS. Other drugs used to treat ARDS may include inhaled nitric oxide and drugs to block the inflammatory response.

Clients on mechanical ventilation often require sedation to reduce anxiety and analgesics to relieve pain. Benzodiazepines such as midazolam (Versed) provide sedation, and intravenous analgesics such as morphine relieve pain. These drugs also reduce the respiratory drive, facilitating mechanical ventilation. Occasionally, a neuromuscular blocking agent may be given to paralyze the respiratory muscles and allow the ventilator to control the client's respirations. These clients require intensive care management.

Oxygen Therapy

Oxygen therapy is vital to treat the hypoxemia of acute respiratory failure. Clients with chronic COPD may need only 1 to 3 liters by nasal cannula; higher flow rates often are necessary for other clients. High oxygen concentrations (40% to 60% or higher) are used only for short periods to avoid oxygen toxicity. Oxygen toxicity reduces lung compliance, increasing the work of breathing. A tight-fitting mask with continuous positive airway pressure (CPAP) may be used to improve alveolar ventilation and allow lower oxygen concentrations.

Airway Management

Clients who need mechanical ventilation are intubated with an endotracheal tube (ETT) extending from the mouth or nose into the trachea (Figure 26-19 ◆). Most ETTs have an air-filled or foam cuff just above the end of the tube that prevents air from escaping back into the upper airways during ventilation. A tracheostomy may be done if mechanical ventilation is needed for more than 3 or 4 weeks (see Table 26-10 ◆). Box 26-19 outlines nursing care for the client with an ETT.

Figure 26-19.   ◆   Nasal endotracheal intubation.

Endotracheal intubation increases the risk for infection as defenses of the upper airway are bypassed. ETTs pass through the larynx, so talking is not possible. Enteral or parenteral nutrition are required, because eating is not possible when an ETT is in place. A nasogastric feeding tube, gastrostomy, or jejunostomy may be used for enteral nutrition.

When the ETT is removed, the client is placed on humidified oxygen and closely observed for respiratory distress (nasal flaring, dyspnea, wheezing, anxiety, decreased oxygen saturation levels). Reintubation may be necessary. Sore throat and a hoarse voice are common following extubation. Oral intake is restarted slowly, with careful assessment of swallowing.

Mechanical Ventilation

Clients with respiratory failure may require mechanical ventilation. *Positive-pressure ventilators* are commonly used in acute respiratory failure (see Table 26-11 ◆). Positive pressure ventilation increases lung volume and reduces the work of breathing and oxygen demand.

TYPES, MODES, AND SETTINGS. Positive-pressure ventilators can be set for a number of different modes or patterns of ventilation (Table 26-12 ◆). In addition to the mode of operation,

BOX 26-19
NURSING CARE CHECKLIST

ENDOTRACHEAL TUBE (ETT)

☑ Frequently assess respiratory status. Report changes to charge nurse or physician.

☑ Monitor vital signs, skin color, LOC, and mental status at least every 4 hours.

☑ Secure ETT with tape and/or ties. Mark tube placement in relation to the mouth or nose. Notify charge nurse or physician if the tube becomes displaced.

☑ Provide oral and nasal care every 2 hours; assess oral and nasal mucosa for redness and irritation. Move oral ETT to opposite side of mouth every 8 hours.

☑ Using sterile technique, suction ETT as needed to remove secretions. Using clean technique, suction oropharynx as needed.

☑ Closely monitor ETT cuff pressure, maintaining recommended pressure.

☑ Provide humidified air or oxygen.

☑ Ensure that all ventilator alarms are in "on" position.

☑ Establish communication using hand signals, eye movement, a note pad, magic slate, or picture board.

four other settings are used when a volume-cycled ventilator is used:

- The rate or number of breaths per minute
- The tidal volume, or milliliters of air delivered with each breath
- Oxygen concentration of delivered air (FIO_2)
- Positive end-expiratory pressure (PEEP)

For most adults, the *rate* is initially set between 12 and 15 breaths per minute. It is adjusted based on the PCO_2. If the PCO_2 falls below 40 mm Hg, the client is being hyperventilated so the rate is reduced. An increased PCO_2, above 40 mm Hg, indicates hypoventilation; in this case, the rate is increased.

TABLE 26-10

ADVANTAGES AND DISADVANTAGES OF ENDOTRACHEAL AIRWAYS

AIRWAY	ADVANTAGES	DISADVANTAGES
Oroendotracheal	Rapidly inserted Larger endotracheal tube can be used	Uncomfortable Difficult to stabilize Can interfere with mouth care
Nasoendotracheal	Better tolerated Easier to stabilize	Smaller tube may be difficult to clear of secretions Risk of pressure necrosis of nares Risk of otitis media (can impair eustachian tube drainage)
Tracheostomy	More comfortable Easily stabilized Allows oral food intake	Requires surgical procedure

	TYPES OF MECHANICAL VENTILATORS	
TYPE	**FUNCTION**	**EXAMPLES**
Positive-pressure ventilators	Push air into the lungs	Bird
■ Pressure-cycled ventilators	Deliver air until a set airway pressure is reached	Bennett
		Bennett
■ Volume-cycled ventilators	Deliver air until a set volume has been reached	Ohio
		Bear

TABLE 26-11

The *tidal volume (VT)* setting controls the amount of air delivered with each breath. For adults, the tidal volume is set at 650 to 1,000 mL, depending on the client's size. Excess tidal volumes can cause lung trauma.

The oxygen percentage of delivered air can be adjusted. The FIO_2 is set at the lowest possible level to maintain the PO_2 and oxygen saturation at desired levels. For most clients, the goal is to maintain an oxygen saturation greater than 90%.

When oxygen concentrations of 50% or higher cannot maintain the PO_2 or oxygen saturation within the desired range, *PEEP* is added to improve oxygenation. PEEP prevents airway pressure from falling below a preset level, even at the end of expiration.

TABLE 26-12   MODES OF VENTILATOR OPERATION

MODE	DESCRIPTION
Control	Ventilator controls rate, volume or pressure, and flow rate of all breaths.
Assist-control	Client can trigger ventilator with inspiratory effort; breaths will be delivered at a preset rate if client fails to breathe.
Synchronized intermittent mandatory ventilation (SIMV)	Ventilator delivers a set number of mandatory breaths (synchronized with client's breathing) per minute; client can breathe on own between ventilator-assisted breaths.
Positive end-expiratory pressure (PEEP)	Used together with other ventilator modes; positive pressure is maintained in airways throughout respiratory cycle.
Pressure support ventilation (PSV)	Pressurized inspiratory flow supports inspiratory effort, reducing work of breathing.

COMPLICATIONS. Although endotracheal intubation and mechanical ventilation can be life-saving, they also carry a risk for injury.

The intubated client may develop pressure necrosis of the nose, lip, or trachea. Less saliva is produced, and mouth care can be difficult. If the tube is dislodged, ventilation of one or both lungs may be affected. Infection is a significant risk; sterile technique must be used when suctioning to avoid introducing bacteria into the respiratory tract. Condensed moisture in ventilator tubing is always drained toward the ventilator (away from the client), to further reduce the risk of infection. Secretions often become thick and tenacious, increasing the risk of atelectasis.

Mechanical ventilation can cause *barotrauma* (lung injury due to pressure). Pneumothorax and subcutaneous emphysema may result. Decreased cardiac output is a risk. GI bleeding is another potential complication. Many of these complications can be prevented by careful ventilator management and ETT care.

WEANING. *Weaning* is the process of removing the ventilator. Clients who have needed mechanical ventilation for a brief period may be taken off the ventilator and extubated rapidly. A more gradual weaning process is used if mechanical ventilation has been used for a longer time. The client is closely monitored during weaning. Vital signs, respiratory rate, dyspnea, oxygen saturation, and arterial blood gases are frequently assessed. If the oxygen saturation or PO_2 fall below specified limits, mechanical ventilation may be restarted.

Terminal weaning, gradual withdrawal of mechanical ventilation from a client who is not expected to survive, may be done for a terminal illness or irreversible condition. The client is moved to a quiet room or even home prior to removing the ventilator. Family members are encouraged to stay throughout the process. Ventilator support is gradually withdrawn, while analgesia and sedation are given to maintain comfort.

Other Therapies

A pulmonary artery catheter is inserted to monitor pressures and cardiac output. Fluid replacement is carefully monitored to avoid either hypovolemia or fluid overload. Enteral or parenteral feeding is provided to maintain nutritional status. The client with ARDS may be placed in prone position to improve oxygenation.

NURSING CARE

ASSESSING

Clients in respiratory failure often are critically ill. They need both intensive medical care and intensive nursing care. Frequent monitoring and assessment are vital. Obtain subjective data such as complaints of dyspnea and a history of COPD or acute pneumonia. Identify any recent episode of shock, sepsis, or other critical condition.

Carefully assess respiratory status, including rate, depth, ease of breathing (retractions, use of accessory muscles, nasal flaring). Auscultate breath sounds for depth, equality, and adventitious sounds. Assess mental status, including level of consciousness and level of anxiety. Obtain complete vital signs, including apical pulse and oxygen saturation. Document color of skin and mucous membranes, peripheral pulses, and capillary refill.

DIAGNOSING, PLANNING, AND IMPLEMENTING

IMPAIRED SPONTANEOUS VENTILATION

- Assess vital signs and respiratory status every 15 to 30 minutes. Report changes. *The client in respiratory failure is critically ill; frequent assessment is vital to detect changes and evaluate interventions. Respiratory failure increases the work of breathing and can lead to fatigue and inadequate ventilation. This may occur before mechanical ventilation is established or during the weaning process.*
- Promptly report changes in arterial blood gases and oxygen saturation. *These are important indicators of gas exchange and respiratory status.*
- Administer oxygen as ordered. Observe closely for respiratory depression. *Supplemental oxygen may suppress the respiratory drive.*
- Place in Fowler's position. *Fowler's position improves lung ventilation and decreases the work of breathing.*
- Promote rest. Assist with care, space procedures and activities, and allow uninterrupted rest periods. *Rest reduces oxygen and energy demands.*
- Unless intubated and mechanically ventilated, avoid sedatives and respiratory depressant drugs. *These medications can further depress the respiratory drive, worsening respiratory failure.*
- Prepare for endotracheal intubation and mechanical ventilation:
  - Obtain intubation tray with sterile endotracheal tubes and laryngoscope with a variety of adult blades.
  - Set up endotracheal suction and bring sterile catheter and glove kits and sterile normal saline to bedside.
  - Notify respiratory therapy department to set up ventilator.

- Request portable chest x-ray to verify tube placement when procedure completed.

The client with respiratory failure may require emergency intubation and mechanical ventilation to sustain respirations.

- Explain procedure, reassuring client that this is a temporary measure to reduce the work of breathing and allow rest. Instruct that endotracheal tubes interfere with talking, and establish a way to communicate. *Thorough explanations help relieve anxiety.*

INEFFECTIVE AIRWAY CLEARANCE

- Frequently assess respiratory status. *Increasing respiratory rate, crackles and rhonchi, frequent coughing or setting off ventilator alarms, and increasing restlessness or anxiety may indicate impaired airway clearance and a need for suctioning.*
- Suction as needed to maintain patent airway. Procedure 26-2 outlines the steps for endotracheal suctioning. *Suctioning removes secretions the client is unable to clear.*
- Obtain specimen for culture if sputum appears purulent or becomes odorous. *Sputum culture and sensitivity are done to identify pathogens and appropriate antibiotics to treat infection.*
- Perform percussion, vibration, and postural drainage as ordered. *These techniques help loosen secretions and move them into larger airways, where they can be cleared.*
- Firmly secure endotracheal or tracheostomy tube. Prevent tension on tube during turning, positioning, transferring, or getting out of bed. If necessary, loosely restrain hands. *These measures help prevent displacement or inadvertent removal of the endotracheal tube or tracheostomy.*
- Maintain fluid intake. Monitor intake and output. Weigh daily. *Adequate hydration helps liquefy secretions but preventing fluid overload is important for lung function.*

RISK FOR INJURY

The client in respiratory failure is at risk for injury due to altered level of consciousness, endotracheal intubation, and mechanical ventilation.

- Assess frequently, including a head-to-toe assessment. *Frequent assessment allows early identification of potential problems.*
- Maintain low pressure in the ETT cuff. *Low cuff pressures reduce the risk of damage to the trachea.*
- Do not bypass or turn off any ventilator alarms. *The intubated client cannot call out for help. The client who has received a neuromuscular blocker cannot breathe without ventilator support and cannot use the call bell.*
- Report changes such as increasing air leak around ETT cuff and decreased breath sounds or chest movement. *These may indicate tracheal necrosis, migration of the ETT into the right mainstem bronchus, pneumothorax, or atelectasis.*
- Turn and reposition frequently, stabilizing the ETT while moving. *Frequent position changes help prevent skin and tissue breakdown due to pressure.*
- Keep skin and linens clean, dry, and wrinkle-free. Protect bony prominences with padding. *Because the client may not*

PROCEDURE 26-2 Endotracheal Suctioning

- Use standard precautions.

■ BEFORE THE PROCEDURE

- Obtain all supplies.
- Identify client; provide for privacy.
- Explain procedure. Suctioning is not painful, but is uncomfortable. During suctioning, breathing will be difficult. This lasts only a brief time (up to 10 seconds). Suctioning causes coughing, helping to clear the lungs.
- Establish a way to communicate during suctioning (e.g., raising a finger if unable to tolerate suctioning).

■ PROCEDURE

1. Regulate suction to no more than 80 to 120 mm Hg of suction.
2. Open sterile saline, leaving cap loosely in place.
3. Put on personal protective wear.

■ WITH AN IN-LINE CATHETER

- Attach catheter to suction tubing.
- Adjust the oxygen (FIO_2) to 100%; allow three breaths.
- Manipulating catheter through plastic shield (to maintain sterility), insert the catheter with no suction until resistance is met; slowly withdraw catheter while applying suction.
- Apply suction for no more than 10 seconds (count seconds or watch clock—the time passes quickly), then allow rest for three to five breaths. Repeat as needed for a total of no more than three times.
- Disconnect suction tubing from catheter, clear tubing, and turn off suction.

■ WITH A SEPARATE CATHETER-AND-GLOVE KIT

- Open suction catheter/glove kit. Remove saline cup, and fill with sterile saline.

- Put on sterile gloves. Attach catheter to suction tubing, keeping dominant hand sterile; lubricate catheter with sterile saline.
- Use nondominant hand to adjust oxygen (FIO_2) to 100%; allow three breaths.
- Using nondominant hand, disconnect ventilator tubing from endotracheal tube.
- Holding suction catheter with dominant (sterile) hand and suction control valve with nondominant hand, insert catheter, with no suction, until resistance is met. Apply suction while slowly withdrawing catheter.
- Suction for no more than 10 seconds. Reconnect ventilator, and allow rest for three to five breaths; clear suction tubing with sterile saline.
- Repeat as needed for a total of three times.
- Reconnect ventilator.
- Clear suction tubing; turn off and disconnect catheter, discarding it with the gloves.
- Provide three additional breaths at 100% oxygen, then readjust to previous ordered level.

■ AFTER THE PROCEDURE

- Assess lung sounds and tolerance of the procedure.

■ SAMPLE DOCUMENTATION

6/15/04	2100	Suctioned via endotracheal tube for moderate amount of thick, greyish sputum. Tolerated procedure well. Good breath sounds noted in all lung fields; scattered coarse crackles cleared with suctioning.
		_____ S. Evans, LVN.

---

perceive pain and pressure or move voluntarily, good skin care is mandatory.

- Perform passive range-of-motion (ROM) exercises every 4 to 8 hours. *These exercises maintain joint flexibility and help prevent contractures associated with long-term immobility.*
- Keep side rails up and use soft restraints as needed. *These measures help prevent falling, inadvertent disconnection of the ventilator, or pulling out the ETT.*

- Administer H_2-blockers and antacids as ordered. *Stress gastritis and GI hemorrhage are common, preventable complications of mechanical ventilation.*

DECREASED CARDIAC OUTPUT

- Monitor vital signs every 1 to 2 hours. *Positive-pressure ventilation decreases cardiac output; applying PEEP further reduces cardiac output. This drop can increase tissue damage and cause dysrhythmias. Frequent assessment allows early detection of decreased cardiac output.*

- Measure urinary output hourly; report if less than 30 mL/hr. *A fall in urine output is an early sign of decreased cardiac output.*
- Assess level of consciousness every 2 to 4 hours. *A change in LOC may indicate cerebral hypoxia.*
- Report changes in hemodynamic pressures to the charge nurse or physician. *Changes in hemodynamic pressures may indicate a drop in cardiac output.*
- Weigh daily. *Daily weight is the best indicator of fluid status; decreased cardiac output may cause fluid retention.*
- Provide frequent skin care, keeping skin clean and dry and protecting pressure points. *Tissue hypoxia increases the risk of skin breakdown, infection, and sepsis.*
- Maintain intravenous fluids as ordered. *Intravenous fluids are given to maintain vascular volume and prevent dehydration.*

ANXIETY

- Stay with the client as much as possible. *The presence of a caregiver provides reassurance that help is readily available.*
- Explain all monitors, procedures, unusual sounds, and machinery. *Understanding the equipment and the meaning of beeps, buzzers, and alarms reduces anxiety.*
- Provide a simple means of communicating, such as a slate, picture board, or alphabet board. If a muscle-paralyzing drug has been given, use methods such as looking to the right for "yes" and left for "no." Reassure that the ability to speak will return once the ETT is removed. *The inability to speak and call out for help is frightening. Providing an alternate means of communication helps reduce anxiety.*
- Encourage family members to visit frequently and remain with the client if possible. Assist family to provide as much care as possible. *Family visits help reduce anxiety and feelings of abandonment. Allowing family members to participate in care helps reduce their anxiety as well as the client's.*
- Provide distraction with radio or television if allowed. *Distraction helps reduce the focus on machines and unusual sounds of monitors and alarms.*
- Reassure clients that intubation and mechanical ventilation are temporary measures and that they will be able to breathe independently again. *Clients may fear continued dependence on mechanical ventilation.*
- Provide sedation and antianxiety medications as needed, especially when a neuromuscular blocker has been used. *The client whose voluntary muscles have been paralyzed remains mentally alert.*

EVALUATING

To evaluate the effectiveness of nursing care for the client with respiratory failure, collect assessment data related to breathing, respiratory status, and cardiac output; freedom from injury, tissue damage, and complications of immobility; and level of anxiety.

 Discharge Considerations

Prior to discharge, discuss factors that precipitated respiratory failure and measures to prevent it in the future. Discuss the importance of avoiding respiratory irritants. Encourage to remain indoors with an air filter or air conditioning when pollution levels are high, obtain influenza and pneumonia immunizations, and avoid exposure to cigarette smoke. Teach effective coughing and measures such as percussion, vibration, and postural drainage.

For the client with ARDS, explain that ARDS did not result from their actions, but results from serious illness. Reassure that clients who survive the initial insult of ARDS generally recover without significant long-term adverse effects. Advise that recovery may be prolonged, however. Stress the importance of avoiding cigarette smoking.

Nursing Interventions Classification

The following Nursing Interventions (McCloskey & Bulechek, 2000) may apply to care for clients with lower respiratory disorders:

- Airway Management
- Airway Suctioning
- Anxiety Reduction
- Artifical Airway Management
- Chest Physiotherapy
- Cough Enhancement
- Infection Control
- Medication Administration: Inhalation
- Oxygen Therapy
- Respiratory Monitoring
- Smoking Cessation Assistance
- Tube Care: Chest
- Ventilation Assistance

(*Note:* The bibliography listings for this and all chapters have been compiled at the back of the book.)

Chapter Review

key terms by topic

Use the CD-ROM disk enclosed with your textbook to hear the pronunciation of the key terms in the chapter.

Structure and function
dyspnea, hemoptysis, cyanosis, respiration

Infectious and inflammatory disorders
bronchitis, pneumonia, atelectasis, pleural effusion

Obstructive airway disorders
asthma, chronic obstructive pulmonary disease (COPD), atelectasis

Pulmonary disorders
pulmonary embolism, pulmonary hypertension, pneumothorax, hemothorax, respiratory failure, acute respiratory distress syndrome

key points

- Effective lung ventilation and gas exchange can be affected by a number of disorders, including infectious diseases, airway restriction, structural changes of the lung tissue or chest wall, acute or chronic inflammatory disorders, and tumors.

- Pneumonia, although treatable, remains a leading cause of death, particularly in older adults. Pneumonia interferes with gas exchange in the alveoli. It may be caused by bacteria, viruses or other infectious organisms, or by aspiration of gastric contents.

- Tuberculosis (TB) is a chronic infectious disease that can remain asymptomatic and undetected for years. The tuberculin test is used as a screening tool for TB. A combination of antituberculosis drugs are given for 6 to 12 months to treat active TB. Controlling the spread of TB and promoting compliance with therapy are primary nursing responsibilities.

- Asthma is a chronic inflammatory airway disease that affects both children and adults. It often can be controlled with medications and by avoiding triggers for acute attacks. Acute asthma can cause severe airway restriction, interfering with ventilation of alveoli and gas exchange.

- Chronic obstructive pulmonary disease (COPD) is a progressive disorder that gradually obstructs airflow into and out of the lungs. Lung tissue is destroyed. Cigarette smoking is the primary risk factor for COPD. Nursing care focus is on maintaining optimal lung function.

- As with COPD, cigarette smoking is the primary risk factor for lung cancer. Lung cancer often is advanced by the time it is diagnosed, so its prognosis is poor. Surgery offers the best hope for cure.

- Prevention of venous stasis and deep vein thrombosis (DVT) is the best treatment for pulmonary embolism. Elastic hose, early ambulation, and leg exercises are nursing care measures to prevent DVT.

- An intact chest wall and pleural membrane are necessary to maintain effective lung ventilation. Pneumothorax (air in the pleural space) and hemothorax (blood in the pleural space) interfere with lung expansion and ventilation. Chest tubes are inserted to restore negative pressure in the pleural space.

- Shoulder strap seat belts, floatation vests, and working smoke detectors are vital preventive measures for chest and lung trauma.

- Respiratory failure is the inability of the lungs to exchange oxygen and carbon dioxide to meet the needs of the body. It is a critical condition. Clients often require intensive care management with endotracheal intubation and mechanical ventilation.

Medialink

Additional interactive resources for this chapter can be found on the Companion Website at www.prenhall.com/burke. Click on Chapter 26 and "Begin" to select the activities for this chapter.

For NCLEX review questions and an audio glossary, access the accompanying CD-ROM in this book.

for further study

For in-depth discussion of shock, see Chapter 10.

For more about nursing implications of corticosteroid drugs, and for more information about *Pneumocystis carinii* pneumonia, see Chapter 13.

For discussion of deep venous thrombosis and of methods of measuring arterial pressure, see Chapter 23.

For further study related to continuous positive airway pressure (CPAP), see Chapter 25.

Critical Thinking Care Map

Caring for a Client with Tuberculosis
NCLEX-PN Focus Area: Physiological Integrity, Reduction of Risk Potential

Case Study: Harry Facée, a 53-year-old man, arrives at a community clinic in a large metropolitan city. He complains of aching chest pain that has lasted for the past few days and says that now his sputum is bloody. He is afraid he might have lung cancer, so he feels he should see a doctor.

Nursing Diagnosis: Risk for Noncompliance

COLLECT DATA

Subjective _____

Objective _____

Would you report this data? Yes/No

If yes, to: _____

Nursing Care

_____

_____

_____

_____

_____

_____

_____

_____

How would you document this? _____

_____

_____

Data Collected
(use those that apply)

- Homeless for past 10 years; uses shelters only during very cold or wet weather
- Complains of chronic cough that now is productive of pink sputum
- Often wakes up drenched with sweat in the middle of the night
- Complains of increasing fatigue
- Vital signs: BP 152/86; P 92; R 20; and T 100.2° F (37.8° C)
- Clean; answers questions appropriately and intelligently
- Very thin, almost emaciated
- Sputum Gram stain positive for acid–fast bacillus

Nursing Interventions
(Use those that apply)

- Provide verbal and written information about tuberculosis.
- Teach about prescribed medications, possible adverse effects, and importance of completing the entire prescribed regimen.
- Emphasize importance of continued follow-up.
- Teach and demonstrate sputum and droplet control measures.
- Refer to local incentive shelter program for directly observed medical therapy and meals.

NCLEX-PN Exam Preparation

1. The nurse is reviewing the medical history of a client with chronic bronchitis. Based on her knowledge of this condition, the nurse would expect to find that the client:
   a. has worked in a cotton mill for 40 years
   b. smoked unfiltered cigarettes for 25 years
   c. received a pacemaker at the age of 55
   d. had a father who died of lung cancer

2. Your client had a tuberculin skin test with a positive result. The husband is concerned that he may also have TB. You explain that a positive skin test indicates that:
   a. an allergic reaction to the antigen has occurred
   b. the husband has been exposed and should also be tested
   c. tuberculosis is a bloodborne disease and the husband does not have to worry
   d. the husband definitely has contracted the disease and should begin medications

3. The nurse is caring for a client with acute asthma. When reporting to the next shift, it is most important for the nurse to describe:
   a. medication effectiveness
   b. intake and output results
   c. lung assessment findings
   d. level of consciousness

4. When teaching use of a metered dose inhaler (MDI), the nurse instructs her client to:
   a. take quick shallow breaths in rapid succession while holding the canister down
   b. use the inhaler containing the anti-inflammatory drug first, then the bronchodilator
   c. use the anti-inflammatory drug as needed to treat acute episodes of wheezing
   d. rinse the mouth after using the inhaler to reduce systemic absorption of the drug

5. Which of the following statements best represents a nurse's understanding of the relationship between COPD and supplemental oxygen?
   a. Because oxygen is flammable, the client should not smoke.
   b. Oxygen is used only at night for clients with COPD.
   c. The flow rate should be set at 8 L/min.
   d. The client needs to be closely monitored for signs of respiratory depression.

6. Which of these statements by the client would indicate that further instruction in preventing atelectasis is needed?
   a. "It is too painful to walk in the hallway today."
   b. "I need to drink extra water for lunch."
   c. "I don't need any pain medication right now."
   d. "I would like to have a laxative before I go to sleep."

7. When assisting with a thoracentesis, the nurse knows that the physician will insert the needle into the:
   a. thoracic cavity
   b. pleural space
   c. mediastinum
   d. visceral space

8. A client with a chest tube trips while ambulating, accidentally pulling his chest tube out of the chest. The first thing the nurse should do is:
   a. call the physician
   b. place an occlusive dressing over the wound
   c. reinsert the tube
   d. empty the collection device

9. The nurse evaluates her teaching as effective when a client with COPD:
   a. develops a realistic plan to stop smoking
   b. verbalizes the necessity of restricting her activity
   c. states that she will get a pneumococcal pneumonia immunization at age 65
   d. promises to smoke only outdoors and when she is symptom free

10. The nurse caring for a client with COPD recognizes which of the following as an early sign of possible respiratory failure?
    a. restlessness and tachypnea
    b. deep coma
    c. hypotension and tachycardia
    d. decreased urine output

chapter

27

Caring for Clients with Musculoskeletal Trauma

CARING tip

❝Accept that we are all flawed. Daily to weekly, look at yourself in one situation that went poorly. Ask yourself, 'How did I close off (or did I) in this situation?'❞

Carole J. Kendall, RN, BSN • Vocational Nurse Director • Copper Mountain College • Joshua Tree, California

LEARNING outcomes

After completing this chapter, you will be able to:

- Describe the structure and function of bones, joints, muscles, ligaments, and tendons.
- Discuss factors that lead to musculoskeletal trauma.
- Relate risks for and manifestations of musculoskeletal trauma.
- State how fractures are classified.
- Discuss collaborative interventions for clients who have experienced musculoskeletal trauma.
- Discuss common complications of fractures and nursing strategies to prevent them.
- Discuss psychological effects unique to amputation.
- Describe the difference between skin and skeletal traction.
- Provide individualized care for clients who have experienced musculoskeletal trauma.

MediaLink

www.prenhall.com/burke

Use the above address to access the free, interactive Companion Website created for this textbook. Get hints, instant feedback, and textbook references to chapter-related multiple choice questions. Link to other interesting sites.

Structure and Function of the Musculoskeletal System

The musculoskeletal system includes bones and joints of the skeleton, connective tissues such as tendons and ligaments, and the skeletal muscles. The musculoskeletal system allows us to remain upright and to move and protects our vital organs.

BONES

The human skeleton has 206 bones (Figure 27-1 ◆). Bones provide structure and support soft tissues. They protect vital organs from injury. Bones are classified by shape (Figure 27-2 ◆):

- *Long bones,* such as those in the arms and legs, have a shaft, called a *diaphysis,* and two broad ends, called *epiphyses.*
- *Short bones* include those of the wrist and ankle.
- *Flat bones,* including skull bones, the sternum, and ribs, are thin and flat; most are curved.
- *Irregular bones* vary in size and shape. They include the vertebrae, the scapulae, and the bones of the pelvis.

Bone cells include *osteoblasts* (cells that form bone), *osteocytes* (cells that maintain bone), and *osteoclasts* (cells that resorb bone). Bones also contain collagen (a type of connective tissue) and minerals (primarily calcium and phosphate). Bones are covered with *periosteum,* a double-layered connective tissue that contains blood vessels and nerves.

There are two types of bone: *Compact bone* is smooth and dense, whereas *spongy bone* contains spaces. Both types are found in almost all bones of the body. Compact bone forms the shaft of long bones and the outside layer in other types of bones. The spongy sections of bones contain bone marrow. *Red bone marrow,* found mostly in flat bones such as the sternum, ribs, and ileum, makes blood cells and hemoglobin. *Yellow bone marrow,* found in the shaft of long bones, primarily contains fat and connective tissue.

Bones that are being used and subjected to stress (such as weight-bearing activity) are constantly remodeled. In this process, bone is resorbed and new bone is deposited. Bone remodeling is regulated by hormones, the effects of gravity, and mechanical stress from the pull of muscles. Without activity and stress on the bones, more bone is resorbed and less new bone is formed.

JOINTS, LIGAMENTS, AND TENDONS

Joints, also called *articulations,* are where two or more bones meet. Joints hold the skeleton together while allowing the body to move. The three primary types of joints are:

1. *Synarthrosis*—immovable joints (e.g., such as skull sutures)
2. *Amphiarthrosis*—slightly movable joints (e.g., vertebral joints)
3. *Diarthrosis* or *synovial*—freely movable joints (e.g., shoulders, hips)

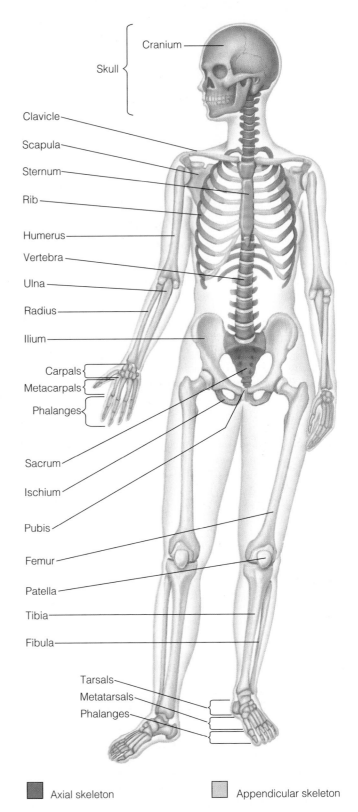

Axial skeleton   Appendicular skeleton

Figure 27-1. ◆ Bones of the human skeleton.

Synovial joints are found at all limb articulations. The surfaces of synovial joints are covered by cartilage, and the joint cavity is enclosed by a tough, fibrous capsule. This cavity is lined with synovial membrane and filled with synovial fluid. Synovial fluid lubricates the joint, facilitating smooth

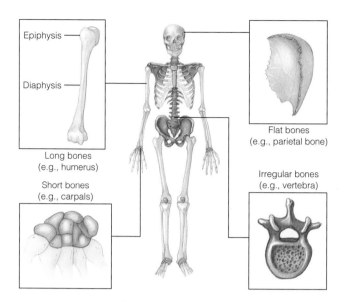

Figure 27-2. ◆ Classification of bones by shape.

Epiphysis

Diaphysis

Long bones
(e.g., humerus)

Short bones
(e.g., carpals)

Flat bones
(e.g., parietal bone)

Irregular bones
(e.g., vertebra)

TABLE 27-1 MOVEMENT OF SYNOVIAL JOINTS	
MOVEMENT	**DESCRIPTION**
Abduction	Move away from the midline of the body
Adduction	Move toward the midline of the body
Extension	Straighten limb at a joint
Flexion	Bend limb at a joint
Dorsiflexion	Bend ankle to bring top of foot toward shin
Plantar flexion	Straighten ankle to point toes down
Pronation	Turn forearm to place palm down
Supination	Turn forearm to place palm up
Eversion	Turn out
Inversion	Turn in
Circumduction	Move in a circle
Internal rotation	Move inward on a central axis
External rotation	Move outward on a central axis

movement of the articulating bones. Synovial joints allow many different kinds of movements (Table 27-1 ◆).

Ligaments are bands of connective tissue that connect bones to bones. Ligaments either limit or enhance movement, provide joint stability, and enhance joint strength. *Tendons* are fibrous connective tissue bands that connect muscles to bones and enable the bones to move when skeletal muscles contract. *Bursae* are small sacs of synovial fluid that cushion and protect bony areas that are at high risk for friction, such as the knee and the shoulder.

MUSCLES

There are three types of muscle tissue: skeletal muscle, smooth muscle, and cardiac muscle. *Skeletal muscle,* also known as *voluntary muscle,* allows voluntary movement. Both *smooth muscle* and *cardiac muscle* are involuntary; their movement is controlled by internal mechanisms. The muscles of the bladder wall, gastrointestinal system, and bronchi are smooth muscle. Cardiac muscle is in the heart.

Skeletal muscles are thick bundles of parallel fibers. Each muscle fiber is a bundle of smaller structures called *myofibrils.* Myofibrils are strands of smaller repeating units called *sarcomeres,* which allow the muscle to contract. Skeletal muscle contracts when motor neurons release acetylcholine, a neurotransmitter. This produces an action potential that causes muscle contraction. The more fibers that contract, the stronger the muscle contraction.

Nerve impulses maintain muscle tone. Lack of use causes muscle atrophy, whereas regular exercise increases the size and strength of muscles. Prolonged strenuous activity can cause a buildup of lactic acid and muscle fatigue.

Musculoskeletal Trauma

Musculoskeletal **trauma** occurs when tissues are subjected to more force than they are able to absorb. The severity of trauma depends on both the amount of force and the location of impact, because different parts of the body can withstand different amounts of force. For example, small bones in the hand cannot absorb as much energy as the femur. Many external sources can cause trauma, and the force can vary in severity. A step off the curb, a fall, being tackled in a football game, and a motor vehicle crash are a few examples.

Musculoskeletal trauma ranges from mild to severe, for example, soft tissue injury, fracture, or complete amputation. Musculoskeletal trauma often affects surrounding tissues. A bone fracture can affect the function of muscles, tendons, and ligaments that attach to it.

Nurses can play a major role in trauma prevention. Teach children and young adults the importance of using safety equipment—such as automobile seat belts, bicycle helmets, football pads, proper footwear, protective eyewear, and hard hats—to prevent or decrease the severity of injury from trauma. Older clients are at higher risk for musculoskeletal trauma due to falls. Assess the home for potential hazards such as poorly lighted stairs or no hand railings. Encourage removing throw rugs and clutter from travel areas. Discuss using bath mats and installing grab bars in bathrooms. Advise wearing shoes with good treads to decrease the risk of slipping.

Soft Tissue Trauma

Sprains, strains, and other soft tissue injuries are common injuries. The lower back and cervical spine are the most common sites for muscle strains. The ankle is the most commonly sprained joint, usually caused by inversion of the foot.

PATHOPHYSIOLOGY

A **contusion,** the simplest musculoskeletal injury, is bleeding into soft tissue resulting from blunt force. With significant bleeding, a **hematoma** forms. A contusion causes swelling and discoloration (a bruise), which initially appears purple or blue ("black-and-blue"). As blood cells break down and are reabsorbed, the mark becomes brown, then yellow, and finally disappears.

A **sprain** is a ligament injury. Sprains are caused by a twisting motion that overstretches or tears the ligament. Sprains are graded by the extent of damage:

- Grade I—overstretching with mild bleeding and inflammation
- Grade II—severe stretching and some tearing with inflammation and hematoma
- Grade III—complete tearing of the ligament
- Grade IV—the bony attachment of the ligament is broken away.

A **strain** is a microscopic tear in the muscle that causes bleeding into the tissues. A strain (or "pulled muscle") occurs when a muscle is forced to extend past its elasticity. Strains may be caused by inappropriate lifting or by a sudden acceleration–deceleration injury, like a motor vehicle crash. The characteristics of sprains and strains are compared in Box 27-1.

COLLABORATIVE CARE

Soft tissue trauma is treated with measures that decrease swelling, alleviate pain, and encourage rest. The client is instructed to avoid using the injured area. A splint may be applied. Ice is applied for the first 48 hours, after which heat can be applied. A compression dressing, such as an Ace bandage, may be applied. The injured extremity should be elevated to the level of the heart to increase venous return and decrease swelling. If the lower extremity is injured, crutches are provided. A knee injury also requires a knee immobilizer. If the upper extremity is injured, a sling is provided.

BOX 27-1
CHARACTERISTICS OF SPRAINS AND STRAINS

SPRAIN
- Ligament injury
- Joint instability
- Pain, swelling, discoloration
- Increased pain with joint use

STRAIN
- Muscle tear
- Swelling, local tenderness
- Sharp or dull pain
- Increased pain with muscle contraction

Nonsteroidal anti-inflammatory drugs (NSAIDs) and analgesics, including narcotics, may be ordered to manage pain and reduce the inflammatory response.

NURSING CARE

ASSESSING

To assess soft tissue injury, collect both subjective and objective data. Ask about the mechanism of injury and when it occurred. Ask about any protective devices that were being used at the time of injury (e.g., seat belt or airbag). Obtain specific information about pain, including location, character, intensity, and aggravating and relieving factors. Ask about the effect of the injury or pain on use of the extremity and ability to bear weight. Ask about movement and sensation distal to the injury, especially numbness, tingling, or inability to move. Also inquire about previous injuries and self-care measures that have been used for this injury (e.g., analgesics, ice or heat, wrapping, or rest).

Inspect the injured area for redness, swelling, or deformity. Assess active range of motion of affected joints.

CLINICAL alert

Do not attempt to move an injured joint beyond the point of comfort. If fracture is suspected, immobilize the joint and do not assess range of motion until the fracture has been ruled out. This is especially important when there is a risk of cervical spine fracture.

Palpate for swelling, warmth, tenderness, deformity, and crepitus (a grating sensation or sound). Check movement and sensation distal to the injury.

DIAGNOSING, PLANNING, AND IMPLEMENTING

PAIN

The pain of soft tissue injuries is caused by tissue damage and edema.

- Instruct to rest the injured extremity. *Rest allows the injured muscle or ligament to heal.*
- Apply ice to the injury. *Ice causes vasoconstriction and decreases swelling in the injured area. Ice may also numb the tender area.*
- Maintain compression dressing, such as an Ace bandage. *A compression dressing decreases swelling, edema, and pain.*
- Elevate the extremity 2 inches above the heart. *Elevating the extremity promotes venous return and decreases swelling.*
- Teach the acronym RICE to remember acute injury care: rest, ice, compression, elevation. *Acronyms help memory. Knowing the treatment plan decreases anxiety and pain.*
- If pain continues after several days, instruct to apply heat. *Heat increases blood flow and venous return, decreasing edema and pain.*
- Advise to take aspirin or NSAIDs on a regular basis (around the clock as recommended) with food. *When a blood level is maintained, these drugs reduce inflammation, relieving pain. Taking the drug with food reduces gastrointestinal upset.*
- Instruct to use analgesics (over-the-counter or prescribed) to maintain comfort, preventing pain from becoming severe. *Severe pain increases muscle tension and can make it more difficult to relieve pain with medications.*

IMPAIRED PHYSICAL MOBILITY

- Teach correct use of crutches, canes, or slings if prescribed. *Using correct technique increases the safety and effectiveness of these devices.*
- Remind to rest injured extremity. *Using the extremity can delay healing and increase the risk of further injury.*
- Encourage follow up with primary care provider. *Severe sprains may require further treatment such as a brace or surgical intervention.*

EVALUATING

To evaluate the effectiveness of nursing care, assess pain, safety when ambulating, and knowledge of home care.

 Discharge Considerations

Teach about ordered medications, splints, dressings, and assistive devices. Always observe use of assistive devices. If the device is inappropriate, the risk of falling can be increased. Older adults often have less muscle mass in the upper extremities; a walker may be safer than crutches. Specify when to schedule a follow-up appointment with the physician. Explain that activity limitations will be evaluated at the follow-up appointment. Reinforce the RICE acronym (rest, ice, compression, elevation). Emphasize the importance of rest to allow complete healing. Instruct to report any complications, such as numbness, coolness of the limb, or severe pain, to the physician immediately. Warn that severe swelling can lead to compartment syndrome, discussed in the next section of this chapter.

 Fractures

A **fracture** is a break in the continuity of a bone. Fractures vary in severity according to the location and the type of fracture.

PATHOPHYSIOLOGY

A fracture occurs when bone is subjected to more force than it can absorb. Fractures may result from a direct blow, a crushing force *(compression),* a sudden twisting motion *(torsion),* a severe muscle contraction, or disease that has weakened the bone *(pathologic fracture).*

Types of Fractures

Fractures are classified in a number of different ways (Table 27-2 ◆). A *closed* or *simple fracture* is the most common. *Open* or *compound fractures* disrupt the skin over the fracture, allowing bacteria to enter the wound. This increases the risk of complications. *Complete fractures* involve the entire width of the bone, whereas *incomplete fractures* do not. In a *stable (nondisplaced) fracture,* the pieces of bone remain in alignment. In an *unstable (displaced) fracture,* the bones move out of correct alignment.

The direction of the fracture line is also used to classify fractures. The fracture line may be *oblique,* at a 45-degree angle to the bone, *spiral,* or along the lengthwise plane of the bone *(greenstick fracture).*

Fracture Healing

Fracture healing is affected by age, physical condition, and the type of fracture. When a bone fractures, blood vessels tear and a *hematoma* forms between the fractured bone ends and around bone surfaces. Bone and tissue damage causes a local inflammatory response. Clotting factors within the hematoma form a fibrin meshwork. Within 48 hours, fibroblasts and new capillaries growing into the fracture form *granulation tissue* that gradually replaces the hematoma. Phagocytes remove cell debris. Bone-forming cells called *osteoblasts* migrate to the fracture site, where they build a web of collagen fibers from both sides of the fractured bone. Chondroblasts lay down patches of cartilage as a base for bone growth. This *fibrocartilaginous callus* connects bone fragments, splinting the fracture. Osteoblasts continue to form collagen fibers and bone matrix, which are gradually mineralized with calcium and mineral salts to form *bony callus.* Osteoblasts promote new bone formation. *Osteoclasts* migrate to the repair site to remove damaged and excess bone in the callus. This process usually continues for 2 to 3 months. In the final phase of healing, excess callus is removed and new bone is laid down along the fracture line. As

TABLE 27-2 TYPES OF FRACTURES	
FRACTURE TYPE	**DESCRIPTION**
Closed (simple)	Skin over fracture remains intact.
Open (compound)	Broken bone protrudes through skin.
Comminuted	Bone fragments into many pieces.
Compression	Bone is crushed.
Impacted	Broken ends of bone are forced together.
Depressed	Broken bone is pressed inward (e.g., the skull)
Spiral	Jagged break due to twisting force.
Greenstick	Incomplete break along the length of the bone.

the bone heals and again is subjected to the mechanical stress of everyday use, osteoblasts and osteoclasts remodel the repair site along the lines of force.

Healing time varies with the individual. An uncomplicated fracture of the arm or foot can heal in 6 to 8 weeks. A

> ### BOX 27-2
> ### MANIFESTATIONS OF FRACTURES
>
> - Deformity
> - Swelling, ecchymosis (bruising)
> - Pain
> - Tenderness, guarding
> - Numbness
> - Crepitus
> - Muscle spasms

fractured vertebra takes at least 12 weeks to heal. A fractured hip may require 12 to 16 weeks.

Common manifestations of fractures are listed in Box 27-2. Fractures are frequently accompanied by soft tissue injuries that involve muscles, arteries, veins, nerves, or skin. The extent of soft tissue injury depends on the amount of energy or force transmitted to the area.

While most fractures are uncomplicated, serious complications can develop. A fractured pelvis or femur may cause significant bleeding and hypovolemic shock. Up to 4½ liters of blood can be lost with a pelvic fracture, for example. Open fractures may be complicated by infection. Blood flow to a portion of fractured bone may be disrupted, causing necrosis. Blood vessel damage and immobility increase the risk for developing deep vein thrombosis (DVT) (see Chapter 23). Other serious complications such as compartment syndrome, fat embolism, and delayed union are discussed below.

COMPARTMENT SYNDROME. A *compartment* is a space enclosed by a fibrous membrane or fascia. Compartments within the limbs may enclose and support bones, nerves, and blood vessels. **Compartment syndrome** occurs when excess pressure restricts blood vessels and nerves within a compartment. It may be caused by bleeding or edema within the compartment, or by external compression of the limb by a too-tight cast. Nerve damage occurs within 30 minutes. Impaired tissue perfusion may lead to necrosis. Unless promptly relieved, compartment syndrome may result in loss of the limb and sepsis. Compartment syndrome usually develops within the first 48 hours of injury, when edema is at its peak. Manifestations of compartment syndrome are shown in Box 27-3. Use the "5 Ps" to help remember these manifestations.

CLINICAL alert

Closely monitor for manifestations of compartment syndrome with forearm and tibia fractures. Notify the physician promptly if symptoms develop. Immediate intervention is necessary to preserve limb function.

If compartment syndrome develops, pressure is relieved by removing the tightly fitting cast or performing a *fasciotomy,*

BOX 27-3
MANIFESTATIONS OF COMPARTMENT SYNDROME

- Pain unrelieved by narcotic analgesics
- Pallor and decreased capillary refill
- Paresthesias (numbness and tingling)
- Paresis (weakness) or paralysis
- Pulselessness (pulse may be normal early)

a surgical procedure to relieve pressure within the compartment.

FAT EMBOLISM. *Fat emboli* occur when fat globules lodge in a pulmonary vessel or the peripheral circulation. When a bone breaks, fat globules can leave the bone marrow and enter the bloodstream. In the bloodstream, fat globules combine with platelets and travel to the brain, lungs, kidneys, and other organs, blocking small vessels and causing tissue ischemia. Fracture of a long bone, the femur in particular, is the primary risk factor for fat emboli.

Manifestations of fat emboli usually develop within a few hours to a week after injury. The symptoms result from occluded blood flow to the tissues and from fatty acids in the circulation. Altered cerebral perfusion causes confusion and changes in level of consciousness. If pulmonary circulation is affected, chest pain and acute shortness of breath develop. Manifestations of pulmonary edema and acute respiratory distress syndrome (ARDS) may occur (see Chapter 26). Normal clotting is disrupted, and petechiae develop on the skin and mucous membranes.

DELAYED UNION. *Delayed union* is prolonged healing of bones beyond the usual time period. Bone healing may be impaired by factors such as delayed fracture reduction, inadequate immobilization, infection, and age. Delayed union may lead to *nonunion* with persistent pain and movement at the fracture site.

COLLABORATIVE CARE

A fracture requires prompt treatment. The fracture is *reduced* (the normal alignment of bone restored) and immobilized as soon as possible.

Emergency Care

When fracture is suspected, the extremity or affected body part is immobilized. The neck and back are immobilized using a rigid cervical collar and backboard if a vertebral fracture is suspected. The joint above and below a suspected extremity fracture are immobilized. Pulses, color, movement, and sensation of the extremity are checked both before and after splinting. Open wounds are covered with a sterile dressing.

On arrival in the health care setting, x-rays of the affected body part are usually obtained to confirm the diagnosis of a fracture.

Fracture Reduction

Before the fractured bone is stabilized for healing, **reduction** (restoration of normal alignment) must be done. In *closed reduction,* external manipulation is used to reposition the bone. The fracture is then immobilized with a splint, cast, or traction. An x-ray may be done to verify proper position, and neurologic and circulatory status are assessed distal to the fracture. An *open reduction* is done in surgery. The bone is exposed and realigned; nails or screws may be used to maintain its position.

Casts

A *cast* is a rigid device used to immobilize broken bones and promote healing. Casts may be made of plaster or fiberglass. The joints above and below the fracture are immobilized by the cast so the bone will not move during healing. The cast is applied over a thin cushion of padding and molded to the normal contour of the body. Until the cast is completely dry, care is taken to avoid placing pressure on it; simply palpating a wet cast with the fingertips can leave dents that may cause pressure sores. A plaster cast may need up to 48 hours to dry, whereas a fiberglass cast dries in less than 1 hour. The type of cast applied depends on the location of the fracture (Figure 27-3 ◆). Nursing care and teaching for clients with casts is outlined in Box 27-4.

Significant swelling under the cast can impair blood flow and damage nerves and tissues of the extremity. If this occurs, the cast may be *bivalved,* or split down both sides, to relieve the pressure (Figure 27-4 ◆). The two halves of the cast are then held in place with velcro straps to keep the fracture immobilized.

Traction

Muscle spasms can pull bones out of alignment after a fracture. **Traction** uses a straightening or pulling force to return or maintain the fractured bones in normal position. Various types of traction may be used:

1. *Manual traction* is applied by physically pulling on the extremity. Manual traction often is used to reduce a fracture or dislocation. Other types of traction use ropes, pulleys, and weights to maintain alignment of the bones.
2. *Skin traction* applies the pulling force through the client's skin. Skin traction is noninvasive and is relatively comfortable for the client.
3. In *skeletal traction,* the pulling force is applied directly through pins inserted into the bone. Skeletal traction allows use of more weight to maintain bone alignment. The risk of infection is greater, however, and it may cause more discomfort.
4. *Straight traction* applies a pulling force in a straight line to the injured body part. The body provides a counterweight or opposing force to the traction. The most common type

A Short arm cast

B Shoulder spica cast

C Long leg cast

D One-and-one half hip spica cast

Figure 27-3. ◆ **Common types of casts.**

of straight traction is *Buck's traction* (Figure 27-5A ◆), in which the pulling force is applied to the skin of the affected leg.

5. *Balanced suspension traction* uses more than one force of pull to raise and support the injured extremity off the bed and maintain its alignment (Figure 27-5B and C). Balanced

---

BOX 27-4
NURSING CARE CHECKLIST

CAST CARE

☑ Support drying cast on pillows; do not cover.
☑ Use the palms of the hands to handle a drying cast.
☑ Frequently assess pulses, color, movement, and sensation of the affected extremity.
☑ Promptly report increased or severe pain; changes in pulses, color, movement, or sensation distal to the cast; or a "hot spot" or drainage on the cast.
☑ Pad or tape rough cast edges to reduce skin irritation.
☑ Use plastic wrap as needed to keep the cast clean and dry.

Client and Family Teaching

☑ The cast dries from the inside out; do not use a blow dryer to speed drying; do not cover the cast while it is drying.
☑ A sensation of warmth during drying is normal.

☑ Keep the cast clean and dry.
☑ If a fiberglass cast gets wet, dry it with a blow dryer on cool setting.
☑ Notify your doctor immediately if you develop increased pain, coolness, color changes, increased swelling, or loss of sensation in the injured limb.
☑ Do not put anything into the cast.
☑ Use a blow dryer on cool setting to relieve itching by blowing cool air into the cast.
☑ A sling may help distribute the weight of the cast evenly around the neck; do not roll the sling as this may impair circulation.
☑ Use crutches as taught to prevent weight bearing on the affected leg.
☑ The cast will be removed with a cast saw. You will feel its vibration, but the saw will not cut the skin.

Figure 27-4. ◆ Bivalving a cast.

suspension traction increases mobility while maintaining bone position. It also makes it easier to change linen and perform back care. Box 27-5 outlines nursing care for clients in traction.

Surgery

Surgery may be required to align and stabilize a fractured bone. In the simplest form of surgery, an external fixator device is applied to immobilize the fracture. An *external fixator* uses a frame connected to pins inserted into the bone (Figure 27-6 ◆). The pins require care similar to that of skeletal traction pins. The client is monitored for infection, and frequent neurovascular assessment is performed.

Internal fixation is usually done in a surgical procedure called an *open reduction and internal fixation (ORIF).* In this procedure, the fracture is directly reduced, and a nail, screws, plates and screws, or pins are inserted to hold the bones in place (Figure 27-7 ◆). Open fractures and hip fractures are frequently repaired with ORIF. Nursing considerations for a client with ORIF are outlined in Box 27-6.

Line of pull

Footplate

A

Pearson attachment

B

C

Figure 27-5. ◆ Examples of traction. (A) Buck's traction, a straight, skin traction. (B) Balanced suspension traction for a femur fracture. (C) Skeletal traction to stabilize a fractured humerus.

BOX 27-5
NURSING CARE CHECKLIST

TRACTION

☑ Maintain the pulling force and direction:
  ☑ Center client on the bed; maintain body alignment with the direction of pull.
  ☑ Ensure that nothing is lying on or obstructing the ropes.
  ☑ Tape knots; do not allow knots to come in contact with the pulley.
  ☑ Ensure that weights hang freely and do not touch the floor.
☑ *For skin traction:*
  ☑ Frequently assess pulses, color, sensation, and movement distal to wrappings; notify physician or rewrap (if ordered) as necessary.
  ☑ Remove weights only if intermittent traction has been ordered and to rewrap bandages.
  ☑ Frequently assess skin, bony prominences, and pressure points for irritation or breakdown.
  ☑ Protect pressure sites with padding and protective dressings.
☑ *For skeletal traction:*
  ☑ Never remove weights.
  ☑ Frequently assess neurovascular status, skin, and pin insertion sites.
  ☑ Provide pin site care as ordered (or per protocol).
  ☑ Report signs of infection, such as redness, drainage, and increased tenderness.
  ☑ Report manifestations of complications of immobility, including pressure ulcers, deep vein thrombosis, atelectasis or pneumonia, paralytic ileus, and constipation.

Figure 27-6. ◆ An external fixator device used to stabilize a fractured tibia and fibula.

NURSING CARE

ASSESSING

Assess pain in the injured extremity using a standard pain scale. Assess the effectiveness of analgesia in relieving pain. Remember also that pain may be an early symptom of compartment syndrome. Assess distal pulses beginning with the unaffected extremity. Then compare the quality of pulses in the affected limb to those of the unaffected limb. Assess sensation proximal and distal to the fracture. Ask about changes in sensation (paresthesias). Check skin color and temperature in the extremity. Coolness may indicate arterial compromise, whereas warmth and a bluish tinge may indicate venous blood

Other Interventions

Analgesics and NSAIDs are ordered to relieve pain following a fracture. Parenteral analgesics or patient-controlled analgesia (PCA) may be used for the first 24 to 48 hours. (See discussion of PCA in Chapter 6.)

Stool softeners may be given and dietary fiber increased to decrease the risk of constipation secondary to narcotics and immobility. An antiulcer drug such as a histamine blocker or antacid may be ordered to prevent gastrointestinal bleeding. Antibiotics may be given, particularly with open or complex fractures.

Electrical bone stimulation may be used to treat fractures that are not healing appropriately. An electrical current is used to increase the migration of osteoblasts and osteoclasts to the fracture site. Mineral deposition increases, promoting bone healing.

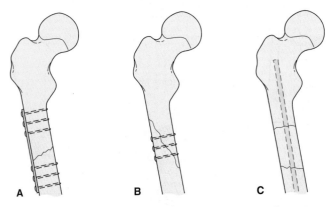

A   **B**   **C**

Figure 27-7. ◆ Internal fixation devices. (A) A plate and screws used to stabilize an oblique fracture. (B) Screws inserted through the fracture. (C) A medullary nail inserted into the bone to stabilize a segmental fracture.

BOX 27-6
NURSING CARE CHECKLIST

ORIF

Before Surgery

☑ Provide routine preoperative care as outlined in Chapter 7.
☑ Maintain skin traction as ordered.
☑ Reinforce teaching.

After Surgery

☑ Provide routine postoperative care (Chapter 7).
☑ Frequently assess neurovascular status; promptly report changes to charge nurse or physician.
☑ Assess wound drainage (on dressing and in surgical drain such as Hemovac).
☑ Maintain alignment of affected extremity as ordered.
☑ Encourage and assist with mobility as soon as allowed.

pooling. Assess motion distal to the fracture site. Limited range of motion (ROM) may indicate such problems as nerve damage and paralysis.

DIAGNOSING, PLANNING, AND IMPLEMENTING

The nursing diagnoses and interventions that follow may be used for any client with a fracture. The nursing implications of specific bone fractures are listed in Table 27-3 ◆.

PAIN

- Administer analgesics as ordered on a regular basis to prevent intense pain. *Pain is more effectively relieved if analgesics are given before pain becomes severe.*
- Splint and support the injured area. *Splinting helps relieve pain by immobilizing the fracture.*
- Elevate the injured extremity above the heart. *Pain is caused by the fracture itself as well as muscle spasms and swelling. Elevating the extremity promotes venous return and decreases edema, which decreases pain.*

TABLE 27-3

NURSING IMPLICATIONS OF SPECIFIC FRACTURES

FRACTURE	USUAL TREATMENT	NURSING IMPLICATIONS	CLIENT TEACHING
Clavicle	Figure-8 or clavicular strap (see Figure 27-8 ◆)	Frequently assess neurovascular status of injured arm.	Applying a figure-8 splint or strap; skin care Wrist and elbow ROM exercises
Humerus	Hanging arm cast, traction, or ORIF, depending on location and severity	Frequently assess neurovascular status of injured arm.	Cast care, sling application Finger and shoulder ROM exercises as indicated
Wrist and hand	Posterior plaster splint and sling; short arm cast; or finger splint	Frequently assess neurovascular status of injured hand. Compartment syndrome is a risk.	Manifestations of complications to report Elevate arm Finger exercises
Femur	Skeletal traction followed by external fixator, ORIF, or cast brace that allows limited weight bearing	Frequently assess vital signs and neurovascular status of affected leg. Bleeding may lead to shock. Assess respiratory status; fat embolism is a risk.	Analgesic use Reporting signs of complications ROM exercises of lower legs, feet, and toes Pin site or incision care
Tibia and fibula	Long leg cast for 3–4 weeks, followed by short leg cast. External fixation device or ORIF may be used.	Frequently assess neurovascular status; blood vessels or nerves may be damaged. Compartment syndrome is a risk. Assess knee; bleeding into joint may occur.	Weight bearing restrictions as ordered Pin or incision site care Crutch walking
Ankle and foot	Closed reduction and short leg cast	Assess neurovascular status of distal foot and toes.	Cast care, crutch walking

(continues)

TABLE 27-3   NURSING IMPLICATIONS OF SPECIFIC FRACTURES (CONTINUED)

FRACTURE	USUAL TREATMENT	NURSING IMPLICATIONS	CLIENT TEACHING
Skull	Observation for simple fracture; surgical elevation of depressed skull fracture	Frequently assess neurologic status: LOC; mental status; pupil response to light; extremity movement and strength; vital signs. Promptly report changes. See Chapter 29.	Observations for altered mental or neurologic status Prescribed activity restrictions Preventing future head injuries
Face	Monitoring; ORIF if severely displaced	Monitor airway and breathing. Monitor neurologic status as noted above. Promptly report changes.	Analgesic use Effect of swelling on appearance and expected changes Indications or options for plastic surgery
Spine	Immediate immobilization. For nondisplaced fractures, cervical collar, halo immobilizer, thoracic brace, or body cast. For displaced fractures, surgical stabilization and/or skeletal traction.	Frequently assess extremity movement and sensation. Promptly report changes to the physician. Maintain spinal immobilization and alignment. Provide good skin care. See Chapter 30.	Skin care under the brace Pin site care Length of immobilization Preventing complications of immobility See Chapter 30
Rib	Analgesia and respiratory care to prevent atelectasis or pneumonia. Fracture of two or more adjacent ribs in two or more places causes *flail* chest (see Chapter 26).	Frequently assess respiratory status (rate, depth and equality of chest movement, breath sounds). Provide adequate pain relief to encourage deep breathing. Encourage use of incentive spirometer.	Analgesic use Avoid rib belt or tape unless ordered by physician Splint chest with hand or pillow to cough and deep breathe Use of incentive spirometer Contact doctor if fever or shortness of breath develops
Pelvis	Bed rest on firm mattress. If unstable or displaced, pelvic sling followed by surgery.	Closely monitor for bleeding and shock. Monitor neurovascular status of lower extremities. Report hematuria, rectal bleeding, or blood in feces. Log-roll for comfort.	Analgesic use Activity restrictions Contact doctor for blood in urine or feces, difficulty voiding or defecating Report numbness, tingling, or weakness of lower extremities to doctor

- Apply ice. *Ice causes vasoconstriction, decreasing swelling. It may also numb the area.*
- Move gently and slowly. *Gentle movement reduces the risk of muscle spasms.*
- Encourage distraction and other adjunctive pain relief measures such as meditation and visualization. *These measures promote relaxation and reduce the intensity of pain.*

IMPAIRED PHYSICAL MOBILITY

- Assist with active ROM exercises of the unaffected limbs. *ROM helps prevent muscle atrophy and maintain strength and joint function.*

Figure 27-8. ◆ A clavicular strap to immobilize a fractured clavicle.

- Teach isometric exercises, and encourage them every 4 hours. *Isometric exercises help prevent muscle atrophy.*
- Encourage ambulation when able; provide assistance as needed. *Ambulation maintains and improves circulation and helps prevent muscle atrophy and bone loss.*
- Reinforce teaching and observe use of assistive devices (canes, crutches, walkers, slings, etc.). *Proper use of devices maintains safety and helps prevent falls and complications of immobility.*
- Encourage flexion and extension exercises of the lower extremities. *Flexion and extension exercises promote venous return, helping prevent deep vein thrombosis.*
- Turn the client on bed rest every 2 hours. If in traction, teach client to shift weight hourly. *Turning and weight shifts increase circulation and help prevent skin breakdown.*

RISK FOR INEFFECTIVE TISSUE PERFUSION

Tissue perfusion can be affected by bleeding, edema, compartment syndrome, and immobility.

- Assess the 5 Ps (pain, pallor, pulse, paresthesias, and paresis) every 1 to 2 hours. *Unrelenting pain, pallor, diminished distal pulses, paresthesias, and paresis are indicators of compartment syndrome. Notify the physician immediately. (Note that pulses may not change with compartment syndrome.)*
- Assess cast for tightness. *Edema can cause the cast to become too tight; a tightly fitting cast affects distal circulation.*
- If the cast is too tight, prepare to assist with bivalving (see Figure 27-4). *Bivalving (splitting the cast) relieves pressure caused by a too-tight cast.*
- Elevate the injured extremity above the heart. *Elevating the extremity increases venous return and decreases edema.*
- Administer anticoagulant as ordered. *Anticoagulants may be ordered to reduce the risk for deep vein thrombosis.*
- Apply antiembolism stockings or pneumatic compression boots. *These devices increase venous return, decrease blood pooling, and the risk of DVT.*

EVALUATING

To evaluate the effectiveness of nursing care, collect data related to pain and the effectiveness of analgesia, safety and mobility, and tissue perfusion.

Discharge Considerations

The needs for teaching and home care vary, depending on the type and severity of the fracture and its location. For example, a client with a simple fracture of the tibia may need only teaching about cast care and crutch walking. An older client who has surgery to repair a hip fracture has more teaching needs, including using an abduction pillow and restrictions on weight-bearing and hip flexion. Referrals to visiting nurses and community services are more likely in older clients. Teach measures to reduce the risk of falls and fractures (see Box 27-7).

Teach about ordered activity restrictions. If a cast has been applied, discuss cast care and dealing with irritants such as itching. Instruct about slings, crutches, or a walker as appropriate. Instruct to elevate the extremity to reduce swelling. Ice may be applied initially to reduce both pain and edema. Instruct to perform range-of-motion exercises of affected extremity as allowed. Teach the importance of eating well-balanced meals to promote healing. Stress the importance of follow-up care, and provide information about manifestations of complications to report to the physician.

Suggest resources for clients who need an extended period of immobilization or limited activities:

- Home care agencies for wound care and monitoring healing
- Physical therapy to evaluate home safety and suggest modifications as needed, and to teach crutch walking, limited weight bearing, transferring, and other activities
- Local medical suppliers for equipment and supplies such as slings or braces, crutches, walkers, wheelchairs, overhead trapeze units, shower chairs, elevated toilet seats, grab bars, and bedside commodes

BOX 27-7

population
FOCUS

Reducing Fractures in Older Adults

Falls are the most common cause of fractures in older adults. Hip fractures are the leading cause of hospitalization for injuries in older adults. The clavicles and wrists are also commonly fractured. Fractures in older adults can lead to loss of functional ability or death. Fall-related deaths are usually related to complications from prolonged immobility, not the act of falling.

A number of measures can reduce the risk of falling and fracture:

- Encourage children, adolescents, and younger adults to maintain an adequate calcium intake to prevent osteoporosis (see Chapter 28).
- Remove scatter rugs and obstacles in traffic areas of the home.
- Paint a contrast stripe on the edge of stairsteps.
- Provide night-lights and transition lighting between bedroom and bath.
- Install grab-bars in the bath and railings on stairs.
- Teach to turn using a series of small steps.
- Instruct to wear well-fitting shoes or hard-soled slippers when ambulating.
- Encourage regular aerobic and strength-training exercises.
- Review medication regimen with the physician.
- Teach safe use of assistive devices such as canes and walkers.

- Local pharmacies for dressing supplies
- Fitness equipment suppliers for rehabilitation needs such as hand or ankle weights for strengthening exercises

Hip Fracture

Hip fractures are a significant problem, especially in older adults. Hip fracture often leads to loss of independence and restricted activity, even after healing is complete.

PATHOPHYSIOLOGY

A hip fracture is a break of the femur at the head, neck, or trochanteric regions (Figure 27-9 ◆). Fractures of the head or neck of the femur are called *intracapsular fractures; extracapsular fractures* are fractures of the trochanteric region. Most hip fractures occur in the neck or trochanteric regions. When the head or neck of the femur is involved, impaired blood supply to the bone increases the risk of poor healing and *avascular necrosis.*

Manifestations of a hip fracture include pain, and shortening and external rotation of the affected lower extremity.

COLLABORATIVE CARE

A hip fracture usually is diagnosed by the history, physical examination, and an x-ray of the affected hip. Buck's traction may be applied to reduce muscle spasm until surgery can be done.

An open reduction and internal fixation (ORIF) is performed to promote mobility, decrease pain, and prevent complications. Fixation is accomplished by securing the femur with pins, screws, nails, or plates (Figure 27-10A ◆). ORIF works well for fractures in the trochanteric area. If the femoral head or neck is fractured, a prosthesis is inserted to replace the femoral head (Figure 27-10B). This procedure is called an *arthroplasty.* If both the femoral head and the hip socket (the acetabulum) must be replaced, a *total hip replacement* or *arthroplasty* is performed. (See Chapter 28 for more information about total joint replacement.)

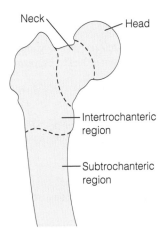

Figure 27-9. ◆ The *head* of the femur fits into the socket of the pelvis. The *neck* is the narrower area below the head. The *trochanteric* region is below the neck.

Figure 27-10. ◆ (A) A surgical nail or screw used to stabilize an intertrochanteric hip fracture. (B) A hip prosthesis used if the femoral head is damaged.

NURSING CARE

ASSESSING

Careful assessment is vital both before and after surgery. Monitor vital signs frequently, and report changes from baseline. Monitor temperature, reporting any elevation. Increased temperature may indicate wound infection, respiratory infection, or sepsis. Assess color, temperature, capillary refill, pulses, and movement and sensation of affected leg, comparing findings with unaffected leg. Report changes to the charge nurse or physician. If surgery has been performed, assess the wound for healing, drainage, and signs of infection or inflammation. Promptly report shortening and internal rotation of the affected leg, which could indicate dislocation of the affected hip.

DIAGNOSING, PLANNING, AND IMPLEMENTING

Nursing care of a client with a hip fracture is challenging. After age 50, the risk of hip fracture increases every year. Many clients with a hip fracture are older and have several underlying health problems. Nursing care focuses on relieving pain, maintaining circulation to the injured extremity, and increasing mobility.

PAIN

- Ask about location and nature of pain. *It is important to differentiate pain caused by the fracture or surgery from pain of other causes such as angina, a respiratory infection, or intestinal ileus.*
- Ask to rate pain using a standardized pain scale before and after any intervention. *The pain scale provides a means of evaluating the effectiveness of pain relief measures.*
- Apply Buck's traction as ordered. *Buck's traction immobilizes the fracture before surgery, reducing pain and additional trauma.*
- Administer analgesia as ordered. A PCA pump may be ordered. *Analgesics relieve pain and reduce muscle tension and*

spasm. PCA pumps allow more effective pain control with lower total doses of analgesia.

■ Move gently and slowly. *Gentle turning prevents severe muscle spasms.*

■ Encourage distraction, deep breathing, relaxation, and other adjunctive pain relief measures. *Adjunctive measures improve the effectiveness of analgesics.*

IMPAIRED PHYSICAL MOBILITY

Maintaining mobility is important to prevent complications of immobility (such as atelectasis, pressure sores, and deep vein thrombosis), especially in older adults.

■ Turn clients on bed rest at least every 2 hours. Encourage hourly weight shifts when in traction. *Turning and weight shifting increase circulation and help prevent skin breakdown.*

■ Place a pillow between the legs when in bed and during turning. *A pillow prevents adduction of the affected hip, which could lead to dislocation.*

■ Encourage isometric exercises and flexion and extension exercises of the feet, ankles, elbows, shoulders, and knees every 4 hours. *These exercises help maintain muscle tone and promote venous return from the extremities.*

■ Work with physical therapy to promote activities as allowed. *The physical therapist can help mobilize the client when weight bearing is limited, and can provide assistive devices and teaching about their appropriate use.*

■ Assist to a hip chair at the bedside. *A hip chair prevents excess hip flexion. Sitting at the bedside several times per day improves circulation and lung expansion.*

■ Assist and encourage ambulation per physician's orders. *Ambulation helps prevent muscle atrophy and other complications of immobility.*

■ Apply antiembolism (TED) hose or pneumatic compression devices (PCDs) as ordered. Remove hose or the PCD at least every 8 hours to inspect the skin. *TED hose and PCDs promote venous return from the lower extremities, reducing the risk of deep vein thrombosis.*

■ Administer anticoagulants as ordered and monitor for adverse effects (bleeding). *Anticoagulants may be ordered to reduce the risk of DVT. While the risk for bleeding is low, it is important to monitor for abnormal bleeding of the wound, gums, GI tract, or other sites.*

IMPAIRED SKIN INTEGRITY

■ Use sterile technique for dressing changes. *Sterile technique reduces contamination of the wound by infectious organisms.*

■ Assess wound color, healing, and the presence of any drainage. *Redness, swelling, and purulent drainage may indicate infection.*

■ Administer antibiotics as ordered. *Prophylactic antibiotics may be ordered to prevent wound infection.*

■ Promptly report any temperature elevation, tachycardia, or signs of wound infection to the physician. *Prompt identification and treatment of a wound infection promote healing and may prevent the development of osteomyelitis (see Chapter 28).*

Collect data regarding level of pain and pain relief, ability to resume physical mobility, wound healing, and skin integrity to evaluate the effectiveness of nursing care for the client with a fractured hip.

Discharge Considerations

Hip fracture in the older adult can lead to loss of independence and long-term disability. Box 27-7 outlines teaching to help prevent hip fractures. Helping the client regain independence in activities of daily living (ADLs) is a priority in planning for discharge. Box 27-8 outlines assessment data to help determine an older adult's ability to return to his or her previous living situation after a hip fracture.

Explain activity restrictions. Teach how to limit the amount of weight placed on the affected extremity. Discuss the importance of sitting in a high, firm chair to minimize hip flexion; a high toilet seat can be added to a regular toilet seat. Encourage equipping a shower with a rail to aid stability and prevent falls. If a walker is needed, teach how to use it. Explain that the walker should not be carried. Instruct client

---

BOX 27-8
ASSESSING FOR DISCHARGE

HIP FRACTURE
Client

● Self-care: Ability to independently perform ADLs, and to use assistive devices such as a walker, elevated toilet seat, grab-bars, shower seat

● Knowledge: Cognitive function; understanding of activity and weight bearing limitations; understanding of complications to report to physician

● Psychosocial: Acceptance of help from others

● Home environment: Adequate lighting, grab-bars in bathroom, level floors; barriers to independence (stairs, small bathrooms, or deep tubs for bathing)

Family and Caregivers

● Cognitive status of primary caregiver; ability and willingness to assist with ADLs and household chores; understanding of activity restrictions

● Resources for medications and treatments, in-home caregivers, or long-term care if necessary

Community

● Availability of home health services and long-term care facilities as needed; access to public transportation, medical services, pharmacies to lift it, advance it, and then take two steps. If a cane is needed, teach how to use it to reduce weight bearing on the affected side. Stress the importance of well-balanced meals, and explain all ordered medications.

The client who is cognitively impaired does not learn as effectively and is less able to independently perform ADLs following hip fracture. The stress of the injury and surgery also may worsen manifestations of dementia. Teaching needs to be very focused, presented in brief sessions, and repeatedly reinforced. Temporary or permanent placement in a long-term care facility may be necessary following a hip fracture. This also may be the case if the primary caregiver is cognitively impaired. Discharge planning needs to begin on admission to the hospital. Provide information and referrals for home care services or long-term care facilities as appropriate. Recommend facilities that provide physical therapy and structured activities to promote independence and recovery.

Nursing Process Case Study
■ CLIENT WITH HIP FRACTURE

Stella Carbolito, 74 years old, lives alone. She depends on a pension check and Social Security for her income. While walking to the market, Mrs. Carbolito falls and breaks her left hip. She is transported by ambulance to the nearest hospital.

Assessment On admission, Mrs. Carbolito's left leg appears shorter than her right, and it is externally rotated. Distal pulses are present and strong bilaterally; both legs are warm. Mrs. Carbolito complains of severe pain but denies any numbness or burning. She can wiggle the toes on her left leg and has full movement of her right leg. Her vital signs are: T 98.0° F (36.6° C); P 100; R 18; BP 120/58. X-ray shows a fracture of the left femoral neck. Mrs. Carbolito is admitted with an order for 10 lbs. of straight leg traction. An ORIF is planned for the following day.

Diagnosis Mrs. Carbolito's nurse, Maria Davis, identifies the following nursing diagnoses:

- Pain related to fracture and muscle spasms
- Impaired Physical Mobility related to bed rest and left hip fracture
- Risk for Ineffective Tissue Perfusion related to fracture and swelling

- Risk for Disturbed Sensory Perception related to risk of nerve impairment

Expected Outcomes The expected outcomes for Mrs. Carbolito's care specify that she will:

- Verbalize adequate pain control.
- Relate an understanding of the purpose of traction and surgery.
- Demonstrate exercises as taught.
- Report increased pain, numbness, tingling, or weakness to the nurse.

Planning and Implementation The following nursing interventions are planned and implemented:

- Assess pain using a standard scale before and after giving analgesics.
- Give analgesics on a regular basis as ordered to control pain.
- Document color, pulses, temperature, movement, and sensation in left leg every 2 to 4 hours.
- Apply straight leg (Buck's) traction as ordered.
- Teach deep breathing and relaxation techniques, as well as isometric and flexion/extension exercises.
- Discuss the purpose of traction and surgery to repair the hip fracture.

Evaluation Two days after surgery, Mrs. Carbolito is out of bed and in a hip chair. Her pain is effectively managed with the ordered analgesic and relaxation exercises. She does isometric and flexion/extension exercises when reminded. Plans are being made for Mrs. Carbolito's discharge to her daughter's home. A community nurse and physical therapist will visit, and the hospital social worker has ordered a trapeze for her bed, an elevated toilet seat and cushion for her chair, and a walker.

Critical Thinking in the Nursing Process

1. What preoperative teaching does Mrs. Carbolito need before the planned ORIF of her left hip?
2. Explain why Mrs. Carbolito was placed in traction when she was going to the operating room anyway.
3. List all the departments in the hospital that will be involved in Mrs. Carbolito's care. Describe their roles.

Joint Dislocation or Subluxation

Joint dislocations and subluxations usually result from trauma, although they also may occur spontaneously. A **dislocation** is separation of contact between two bones of a joint. Traumatic dislocations result from sudden force; joint disease can cause a spontaneous dislocation. A *subluxation* is partial separation of the bones of a joint. While any joint may be affected, shoulder and hip dislocations are the most common. Joint dislocations often are recurring injuries for clients actively participating in contact sports and other vigorous physical activities.

The manifestations of a dislocation include pain, change in shape of the joint, change in length of the extremity, immobility, and change in the axis of the bone.

Manual traction is used to reduce the dislocation (**reduction** restores the usual relationship of the bones). Narcotic analgesics, muscle relaxants, or conscious sedation may be given before the dislocation is reduced. (See Chapter 7 for more information about conscious sedation.)

When the shoulder is dislocated, it is placed back in the joint by manual traction and then is immobilized in a sling for 3 weeks. A rehabilitation program is then initiated.

A dislocated hip requires immediate reduction. If a displaced hip is not reduced within 6 hours of injury, necrosis of the femoral head may result. The dislocated hip also threatens the sciatic and femoral nerves. Movement, sensation, pallor, and pulses must be assessed frequently. After reduction, the hip is immobilized with bed rest and a cast or traction. Immobilization allows the tendons and ligaments to heal.

When joint dislocation or subluxation is suspected, carefully assess for manifestations of the disorder and possible complications such as neurovascular trauma. Assess pain, including location, severity, character, timing, and factors that aggravate or relieve it. Assess color, warmth, pulses and capillary refill, sensation and movement of the affected extremity. Compare the affected extremity with the corresponding unaffected extremity. Promptly report any changes or abnormal findings to the charge nurse or physician.

If traction is required, maintain the alignment of the affected extremity. Carefully assess for and implement nursing care to prevent complications of immobility (such as impaired skin integrity or atelectasis).

Stress the importance of following recommendations for immobilization. Discuss skin care and suggest ways to prevent skin-to-skin contact, particularly in the axillary area. Advise rehabilitation exercises to strengthen muscles and other supportive structures in the shoulder, decreasing the risk of future dislocations. Discuss activities that may precipitate recurrent dislocations and suggest alternatives.

When a hip dislocation has occurred, weight bearing may be limited for up to 6 months. Provide instructions or refer to physical therapy for teaching about crutch walking or using a walker. Discuss cast and skin care if a cast is applied after reduction (see the fracture section of this chapter). Suggest lining the edges of the cast in the groin area with plastic to avoid soiling. Teach the client in traction or a spica cast about possible complications of immobility, and measures to reduce their risk. Provide referrals to physical and occupational therapy and home health services as needed.

Repetitive Use Injuries

Repetitive use injuries can result from repeated twisting and turning of the wrist, pronating and supinating of the forearm, kneeling, or raising the arms over the head. Common repetitive use injuries include carpal tunnel syndrome, bursitis, and epicondylitis. These injuries can result in significant disability and lost work time.

PATHOPHYSIOLOGY
Carpal Tunnel Syndrome
The carpal tunnel is a canal through which tendons and the median nerve pass from the wrist to the hand. *Carpal tunnel syndrome* is one of the most common work-related injuries. It occurs more commonly in women. It develops when the tunnel narrows, compressing and irritating the median nerve. This usually results from inflammation and swelling of structures in the wrist joint. Numbness and tingling of the thumb, index finger, and middle finger of the affected hand develop. The affected hand is weak, and "falls asleep" at night, with pain that is relieved by shaking or massaging the hand and fingers. The client may have difficulty holding utensils or performing precise activities with the affected hand.

Bursitis
Bursitis is inflammation of a bursa. A *bursa* is a closed, fluid-filled sac found in areas where there is friction, for example, where a tendon passes over a bony prominence. Bursae in the shoulder, hip, leg, and elbow often become inflamed due to friction between the bursa and surrounding tissue. Manifestations of bursitis include local tenderness and pain with joint movement. The client guards the joint to decrease pain.

Epicondylitis
Epicondylitis is inflammation of a tendon where it inserts into the bone. Epicondylitis is also called *tennis elbow* or *golfer's elbow*. Repeated trauma that causes tears, bleeding, and

Figure 27-11. ◆ Phalen's test. The wrist is flexed 90 degrees with the fingers extended. Finger numbness during the test may indicate carpal tunnel syndrome.

inflammation of the tendon can lead to epicondylitis. Its manifestations include point tenderness, pain radiating down the forearm, and a history of repetitive use.

COLLABORATIVE CARE

Repetitive use injuries are diagnosed by history and physical examination. History may reveal an occupation that involves computer work, jackhammer operation, mechanical work, gymnastics, or percussive devices. Leisure activities or participating in sports such as tennis, golf, softball, or baseball also increase the risk for these disorders. Fractures of the arm or wrist, or diseases such as rheumatoid arthritis, increase the risk of carpal tunnel syndrome. When carpal tunnel syndrome is suspected, the *Phalen test* (see Figure 27-11 ◆) may be done to help make the diagnosis.

Initial treatment for repetitive use injuries is rest and immobilization of the involved joint. The joint may be splinted, and ice applied in the first 24 to 48 hours to decrease pain and inflammation. After this period, heat may be applied every 4 hours.

NSAIDs are usually given to reduce inflammation. In some cases, corticosteroids may be injected into the joint.

For carpal tunnel syndrome, surgery may be necessary. In carpal tunnel surgery, the carpal ligament is resected to enlarge the tunnel and relieve pressure on the nerve.

 NURSING CARE

Nursing care for repetitive use injuries usually occurs in a community-based care setting. Teaching is a primary focus of nursing care.

PAIN

- Encourage use of an appropriate splint or joint immobilizer. *Splinting maintains joint alignment and reduces pain and inflammation.*
- Teach safe application of ice or heat to the affected joint as indicated. *Ice causes vasoconstriction and numbs the tender area; heat decreases swelling by increasing venous return. Inappropriately applied, both ice and heat can damage tissues.*
- Instruct about using NSAIDs as ordered. *Taken on a regular basis (not as needed for pain), NSAIDs decrease swelling and inflammation, reducing pain.*
- Instruct not to discontinue treatment abruptly. *Stopping treatment abruptly may cause the injured joint to become reinflamed.*

IMPAIRED PHYSICAL MOBILITY

- Refer to physical therapy for appropriate exercises. *The physical therapist can teach exercises to maintain joint mobility.*
- Suggest occupational therapy. *Occupational therapy can help the client learn new ways to perform tasks to prevent recurring symptoms.*

EVALUATING

To evaluate the effectiveness of nursing care, assess the client's knowledge and understanding of the disorder and its treatment.

 Discharge Considerations

Teach about repetitive use injury and its causes and treatments. Rehabilitation may be necessary to restore independence. Help identify ways to avoid activities that increase risk of injury. Suggest that an environmental risk manager or ergonomic specialist evaluate the client's work station and recommend measures to reduce the risk of repetitive use injuries. Wrist supports or an ergonomic keyboard may be useful for the client who uses a computer extensively. Appropriate desk and chair height also are important in maintaining correct anatomical position while working. Provide information about sources for braces or other assistive devices.

Amputation

Amputation is partial or total removal of a body part. Amputation may be done to treat bone cancer, may be the result of a chronic condition (like peripheral vascular disease or diabetes), or it may occur due to trauma. Regardless of the cause, amputation is devastating to the client. The loss of a limb has significant physical and psychosocial effects on the client and family. Adapting to amputation may take a long time and significant effort.

Peripheral vascular disease (PVD) is the major cause of lower extremity amputation (see Chapter 23). Peripheral neuropathy in clients with diabetes also increases the risk for amputation.

Trauma is the major cause of upper extremity amputation. Most traumatic amputations result from motor vehicle crashes or accidents involving machinery at work.

PATHOPHYSIOLOGY

Impaired blood flow and untreated infection that causes **gangrene** (tissue death) can lead to amputation. In PVD, circulation to the extremities is impaired. This leads to edema and tissue damage. Healing also is impaired. Minor injuries and stasis ulcers can become infected as altered immune function allows bacteria to invade and proliferate. In peripheral neuropathy, loss of sensation frequently leads to unrecognized injury and infection. Untreated infection can lead to gangrene and amputation.

A limb may be partially or completely severed by acute trauma. In some cases the severed limb may be reattached. Extensive tissue damage, however, may make reattachment impossible.

Level of Amputation

The level of amputation is determined by the extent of tissue damage and remaining healthy tissue. When possible, joints are preserved for better function of the extremity. Figure 27-12 ◆ illustrates common sites of amputation.

Complications

Potential complications of amputation include infection, delayed healing, and contracture.

INFECTION.   As with all surgeries, infection is a risk following amputation. The client who is older, has diabetes, or has PVD is at a particularly high risk for infection. Local manifestations of infection include drainage, odor, redness, positive wound cultures, and increased discomfort at suture line. Systemic manifestations include chills and fever, tachycardia, and possibly a fall in blood pressure. If any of these manifestations develop, immediately notify the charge nurse or physician. Pneumonia may develop, with a productive cough, pain on deep inspiration, and malaise. Provide good skin care, maintain aseptic technique during dressing changes, and encourage coughing and deep breathing to prevent infection.

DELAYED HEALING.   Delayed healing is healing that occurs at a slower rate than expected. Infection or impaired circulation can lead to delayed healing. It is a particular risk in older clients who are more likely to have chronic diseases such as diabetes or PVD. Poor nutrition and smoking also are risk factors for delayed healing. Notify the physician if the wound is not healing appropriately or if the stump is cool to the touch.

CONTRACTURES.   A **contracture** is abnormal flexion and fixation of a joint caused by muscle atrophy and shortening. Contracture of the joint above the amputation is a common

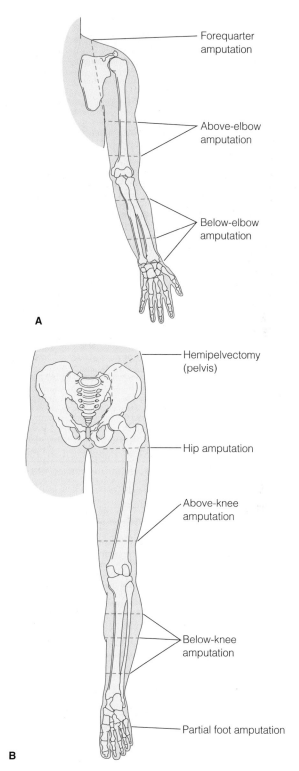

Figure 27-12. ◆ Common sites of amputation. (A) The upper extremities; (B) the lower extremities.

complication. Measures to prevent contractures are outlined in Box 27-9.

PHANTOM PAIN.   **Phantom pain** is felt along nerves of the body part that has been amputated. It is caused by trauma to the nerves serving the amputated part. The missing extremity feels numb, crushed, trapped, twisted, or burning.

BOX 27-9
NURSING CARE CHECKLIST

PREVENTING CONTRACTURES AFTER AMPUTATION

☑ Encourage joint extension.

☑ With above-knee amputation, place in prone position several times daily; do not elevate stump on pillows after the first 24 hours.

☑ For below-knee amputation, elevate foot of bed, keeping knee extended.

☑ Position upper extremities using the same principles.

☑ Provide active or passive ROM exercises every 2 to 4 hours for all joints.

☑ Use trapeze on bed frame to encourage frequent position changes.

☑ Teach importance of moving and ROM exercises.

☑ For a thigh or above-knee amputation, avoid sitting for prolonged periods.

☑ Teach postural exercises to compensate for loss of weight on affected side.

Figure 27-13. ◆ With an above-knee amputation, a figure-8 bandage is wrapped around the waist, then brought down over the stump and back up around the hips.

COLLABORATIVE CARE

Following amputation, the wound may be open (*guillotine*) or closed (*flap*). Open amputations are done when an infection is present. The end of the stump (remaining portion of the limb) is left open to drain. Continuous skin traction is applied to the limb. When the infection has cleared, the wound is closed.

In a closed amputation, a flap of skin is formed to cover the end of the wound. A rigid plaster shell or a soft compression dressing is applied to the stump after amputation to reduce edema, prevent infection, and promote healing. The rigid dressing helps mold the stump to fit a prosthesis. A soft compression dressing (gauze covered by an elastic wrap) is used when frequent wound checks are necessary. The elastic wrap helps prevent edema and form a conical shape to the stump. The bandage is applied from distal to proximal (Figure 27-13 ◆). After the wound is dressed, the client is encouraged to toughen the stump skin by pushing it into first soft and then harder surfaces.

The client with a closed amputation may return from surgery with a temporary prosthesis. Limited weight-bearing may be allowed within 24 to 48 hours after surgery. Once the stump is completely healed, a *prosthetist* (a professional who makes and fits artificial limbs) discusses available prosthetic options with the client. The prosthesis is custom made and fitted to the client. Some clients may have several prostheses made for different functions, depending on their age, occupation, and activity level. Options available for arm amputees include:

■ A shoulder harness with cables attached to a hook. The hook functions as a hand and fingers, activated by chest and shoulder muscle contraction.

■ A cosmetic hand, also activated by shoulder and chest muscle contractions.

■ A myoelectric arm operated by battery-powered motors. The motors are activated by electrodes, which transmit neuromuscular impulses.

Physical and occupational therapy are provided to help regain optimal function. The client with a leg amputation is taught how to use crutches or a walker for ambulation. The client with an arm amputation may need to relearn how to perform many ADLs such as bathing, dressing, and eating.

A member of the clergy, psychologist, or social worker may help the client cope with the loss of a limb and the grieving process.

NURSING CARE

ASSESSING

Initial assessment focuses on responses to surgery and identifying potential complications. Frequently assess vital signs and pain. Report significant changes in vital signs (such as a fall in blood pressure, tachycardia, or difficulty breathing) to the charge nurse or physician. Monitor temperature every four hours, reporting an elevation. Monitor urine output, reporting an output of less than 30 mL per hour.

Have client describe location and character of pain, and rate the pain using a pain scale. Report pain unrelieved by analgesics or that changes in location or character.

Assess wound and dressing, reporting excessive or bright red drainage that could indicate hemorrhage. Monitor wound healing, assessing for redness, swelling, purulent drainage, or evidence of a hematoma.

Observe the client's responses to the wound and amputated limb. The client may initially refuse to look at the affected limb, but should gradually begin taking interest in the limb and wound care.

DIAGNOSING, PLANNING, AND IMPLEMENTING

Nursing care goals are to relieve pain, promote healing, prevent complications such as infection, promote mobility, and support the client and family as they grieve and adapt to the loss of a limb. Box 27-10 describes special considerations for the older adult with an amputation.

PAIN

- Administer analgesics as ordered. A PCA pump may be used initially. *Postoperative pain can be compounded by muscle spasms, swelling, and phantom pain. PCA pumps increase client control over and allow early relief of pain before it intensifies.*
- Splint and support injured area. *Splinting reduces muscle spasm and decreases edema, relieving pressure and pain.*
- Unless contraindicated, elevate the stump for 24 hours. *Elevating the stump promotes venous return and decreases edema, which will decrease pain.*
- Frequently reposition, turning slowly and gently. *Repositioning relieves pressure on tissues. Slow, gentle turning helps prevent severe muscle spasms.*
- Encourage distraction, meditation, deep breathing, and relaxation exercises. *These adjunctive measures help client refocus, reducing the intensity of pain, including phantom pain.*

RISK FOR INFECTION

- Change wound dressing as ordered, using aseptic technique. *Aseptic technique prevents contamination of the wound with bacteria.*

BOX 27-10

population
FOCUS

The Older Adult with an Amputation

Holistic nursing care is especially important for the older client with an amputation.

- Renal and liver function decline with aging, increasing the risk of adverse and toxic drug effects. Closely monitor response to medications.
- Altered circulation prolongs wound healing, and immune function often declines with aging, increasing the risk for infection. Monitor for local and systemic signs of infection.
- Slowed reflexes and gait alterations may disrupt balance. Introduce assistive devices in stages.
- A walker may be more appropriate than crutches, because older clients have less upper body strength. Address safety issues, such as the risk for falling.
- Assess the need for in-home assistance and make appropriate referrals to visiting nurses and home health aides.

- Protect wound and dressing from contamination by urine or feces. *A high above-knee (AK) or hip amputation wound can be contaminated during toileting, increasing the risk for infection.*
- Administer antibiotics as ordered. *Antibiotics inhibit bacterial growth and help prevent or eliminate infection.*
- Teach stump-wrapping techniques. *Correctly wrapping the stump improves circulation, reducing the chance of infection.*
- Report elevated WBC count. *The WBC count rises as the body tries to rid itself of infection.*

RISK FOR DYSFUNCTIONAL GRIEVING

- Encourage verbalization of feelings, asking open-ended questions. *Open-ended questions allow discussion of feelings and communicate a willingness to listen.*
- Maintain eye contact and actively listen. *Eye contact and active listening communicate respect for the client and his or her feelings.*
- Reflect on the client's feelings. *Reflection statements, such as "You seem angry," allow the client to recognize feelings and validate their presence.*
- Allow unlimited visiting hours, if possible. *Unlimited visiting hours promote increased social supports.*

DISTURBED BODY IMAGE

- Encourage verbalization of feelings, and validate that feelings are real and appropriate. *This allows communication of fears and lets the client know the nurse is willing to listen.*
- Allow to wear clothing from home. *Familiar clothing provides emotional comfort and helps the client retain a sense of identity.*
- Encourage looking at the stump. *Looking at and touching the stump helps the client face fear of the unknown and move from denial to acceptance.*
- Encourage participation in stump care. *Active participation in care increases self-esteem and independence.*
- Offer visitation by another amputee. *A support person who has experienced the same change provides hope for regaining independence.*
- Encourage active participation in rehabilitation. *Active participation in rehabilitation increases independence and mobility.*

IMPAIRED PHYSICAL MOBILITY

- Perform ROM exercises on all joints. *ROM exercises help prevent contractures that limit mobility.*
- Maintain postoperative dressing (rigid or compression). *Postoperative dressings help mold the stump and promote healing.*
- Frequently turn and reposition. Place the client with a lower extremity amputation in prone position every 4 hours. *Repositioning increases blood flow to muscles. Prone position helps prevent hip contracture.*
- Teach crutch walking or the use of assistive devices. *These devices allow more rapid resumption of activity.*
- Encourage active participation in physical therapy. *Physical therapy may initially be fatiguing; continuing participation increases energy level and activity tolerance.*

EVALUATING

To evaluate the effectiveness of nursing care for the client with an amputation, assess pain and the effectiveness of relief measures. Note the presence or absence of wound infection or a complication such as pneumonia. Note the client's and family's response to the wound and the loss of a body part. Assess physical mobility and participation in physical therapy.

Discharge Considerations

Assess knowledge of care needs, activity restrictions or special needs, and resources for home care. Discuss home management—who is responsible for household activities such as cleaning and cooking. Inquire about arrangements that have been made for home care activities and ADLs. Evaluate use of prescription and nonprescription medications, paying particular attention to interactions and drugs that may affect balance, mental alertness, or appetite. Ask about social habits, such as cigarette smoking, alcohol use, or other drug use, that may affect healing or the ability to provide self-care.

Assess the home environment for potential safety hazards and access to care needs, such as:

- Scatter rugs
- Stairs between living areas of the house
- Grab bars to facilitate toileting and bathing
- Clean water and other needs for wound care

Teach stump bandaging to prepare for fitting the prosthesis. Discuss positioning to prevent contractures. Teach stump exercises to maintain joint mobility and muscle tone of the affected limb. Encourage resumption of physical activities as soon as possible. Discuss household modifications to promote independence, such as grab bars in the bathroom, faucets with single-handle controls for water flow and temperature, and handheld shower heads and shower chairs for bathing. Encourage to contact local and national agencies and support groups such as:

American Amputee Foundation
P.O. Box 250218 Hillcrest Station
Little Rock, AR 72225
501-666-2523

National Rehabilitation Information Center
8455 Colesville Road, Suite 935
Silver Spring, MD 20919-3319
800-346-2742

Nursing Interventions Classification

The following nursing interventions from the Nursing Interventions Classification (NIC) (McCloskey & Bulechek, 2000) may be useful for clients with musculoskeletal trauma:

- Amputation Care
- Cast Care: Wet
- Cast Care: Maintenance
- Exercise Therapy: Joint Mobility
- Positioning
- Splinting
- Traction/Immobilization Care

(*Note:* The bibliography listings for this and all chapters have been compiled at the back of the book.)

Chapter Review

 key terms by topic

Use the CD-ROM disk enclosed with your textbook to hear the pronunciation of the key terms in the chapter.

Musculoskeletal trauma
contusion, hematoma, sprain, strain, fracture, compartment syndrome, reduction, traction

Joint dislocation or subluxation
dislocation, amputation, gangrene, contracture, phantom pain

key points

- Musculoskeletal injury, from minor strains to amputation, affects comfort and interferes with mobility and maintenance of ADLs. An extended period of recovery and rehabilitation may be required to recover previous function.

- Common complications of immobility, such as pneumonia and deep vein thrombosis, are a risk for clients with musculoskeletal injuries.

- With all musculoskeletal injuries, assessment of circulation, movement, and sensation distal to the injury is important both initially and as part of continuing care.

- Fractures may be stabilized for healing with a cast, surgical insertion of pins or plates, or using traction. Skin and wound care are important to prevent infection and complications of immobility.

- Compartment syndrome is a serious complication of fracture that requires immediate attention. Remember the 5 Ps: pain, pallor, paresthesias, paresis, and possible pulselessness. Do not assume, however, that compartment syndrome is not developing if the client has a strong pulse distal to the injury.

- Hip fractures are a significant risk in older adults, and can lead to loss of independence. Provide meticulous nursing care focusing on rehabilitation from the time of hospital admission to full recovery.

- Carpal tunnel syndrome is a common repetitive use injury that can impair fine motor function of the hands. Prevention is the best treatment.

- Amputation due to trauma or disease is traumatic both physically and psychologically. Loss of a body part causes grieving and disturbs body image. Many ADLs need to be relearned following amputation.

 Medialink

Additional interactive resources for this chapter can be found on the Companion Website at www.prenhall.com/burke. Click on Chapter 27 and "Begin" to select the activities for this chapter.

For NCLEX review questions and an audio glossary, access the accompanying CD-ROM in this book.

for further study

For more information on deep vein thrombosis, see Chapter 23.

For more about manifestations of pulmonary edema and acute respiratory distress syndrome, see Chapter 26.

For discussion of patient-controlled analgesia (PCA), see Chapter 6.

For information about about total joint replacement, see Chapter 28.

For further study about prevention of osteomyelitis, see Chapter 28.

For more information about conscious sedation, see Chapter 7.

For discussion of peripheral vascular disease (PVD), see Chapter 23.

Critical Thinking Care Map

Caring for a Client with Below-Knee Amputation
NCLEX-PN Test Focus Area: Psychosocial Integrity: Coping and Adaptation

Case Study: John Rocke is a 45-year-old divorced man with a history of poorly controlled diabetes mellitus. He lives alone in a second-floor apartment. Two days ago, Mr. Rocke underwent a left below-knee amputation as a result of gangrene of his left foot, a consequence of his diabetes.

Nursing Diagnosis: Ineffective Individual Coping

COLLECT DATA

Subjective	Objective
_____	_____
_____	_____
_____	_____
_____	_____
_____	_____
_____	_____

Would you report this data? Yes/No

If yes, to: _____

Nursing Care

_____
_____
_____
_____
_____
_____
_____

How would you document this? _____
_____
_____

Data Collected
(use those that apply)

- Vital signs stable
- Stump splinted; covered by soft dressing
- Wound healing without signs of infection
- Refuses ROM exercises and turning
- Complaining of severe pain
- Yells "Get out! I don't want anyone to see me like this" when anyone enters room
- Tolerating 1,800-cal American Diabetes Association (ADA) diet

Nursing Interventions
(use those that apply)

- Encourage verbalization of feelings.
- Contact the physician for a referral to a psychologist or social worker.
- Request a change from PRN analgesia to a PCA pump.
- Teach the importance of moving and ROM exercises to prevent contractures.
- Encourage turning and lying prone.

NCLEX-PN Exam Preparation

1. The nurse is caring for a client who has a new cast. How should the cast be handled while it is drying?
   a. only with the fingertips
   b. with the entire hand and finger
   c. not at all
   d. only with the palms of the hands

2. When caring for a client with an above-knee amputation (AKA), it is important for the nurse to encourage the client to spend time in:
   a. the prone position
   b. the supine position
   c. a flexed position
   d. a position of comfort

3. The nurse is caring for a client who has just had an ORIF of the right hip. It is important for the nurse to keep the hip in a position of:
   a. comfort
   b. adduction
   c. flexion
   d. abduction

4. The nurse is caring for a client who has just had surgery to repair a fracture of the tibia. The client's leg is in a cast and he is receiving PCA morphine for pain. He continues to complain of severe pain and paresthesia in his foot. The nurse should:
   a. elevate the leg above the heart.
   b. bivalve the cast.
   c. immediately notify the physician.
   d. request an increase in the dose of morphine.

5. When educating the client with a sprained ankle about home care, the nurse should teach the client the acronym:
   a. BRAT
   b. RICE
   c. RACE
   d. ROSE

6. The nurse is caring for a client who earlier in the day had surgery to repair a fractured femur. The client's temperature has been elevated since the previous shift. Current assessment findings include a temperature of 101.5° F, facial petechiae, and confusion. The nurse recognizes these as manifestations of:
   a. hemorrhage
   b. infection
   c. compartment syndrome
   d. fat embolism

7. The nurse is caring for a client who has recently had a below-knee amputation (BKA) of the left leg. The nurse knows that the most common cause for amputation of the lower extremities is:
   a. motor vehicle accidents
   b. accidents involving machinery at work
   c. bone cancer
   d. peripheral vascular disease (PVD)

8. When caring for a client in traction, the nurse should make sure the client is in:
   a. a position of comfort
   b. body alignment with the direction of pull
   c. semi-Fowler's position
   d. Fowler's position

9. When caring for a client who has a sprained ankle, the application of ice is used to:
   a. cause vasodilation
   b. promote venous return
   c. cause vasoconstriction
   d. allow the injured muscle to heal

10. Which of the following types of traction increases the client's mobility while maintaining appropriate bone position?
    a. balanced suspension
    b. straight traction
    c. skin traction
    d. skeletal traction

Cultural Care STRATEGIES

Considering Cultural Variations Related to Space

A 25-year-old male Cuban-American client says to the nurse, "Everybody in this culture is so cold. When I talk up to them they are always backing away. I think the nurses think I'm going to attack them sexually or something. They keep backing away from me. It's especially noticeable if I'm in line waiting for something. I may be standing close to the person in front of me, and they turn around and glare."

All verbal communication occurs in the context of space (Giger & Davidhizar, 1999). *Personal space* is the area needed by an individual to maintain intimacy and safety in relationships. Since health care providers frequently invade a person's space when providing direct care, understanding the cultural perceptions of space is important. For example, among Americans and most Europeans, personal space is highly valued, and an unannounced invasion will often result in the client's becoming suspicious and tense (Bechtel & Davidhizar, 1988).

Proximity to Others

Hall (1966) established three different dimensions of personal space: *intimate zone* (0–18 inches), *personal zone* (18 inches to 3 feet), and the *social zone* (3 to 6 feet). The intimate zone is used for close, personal encounters like comforting, counseling, and direct care activities. Invading this area without the client's acknowledgment may lead to suspicion and hostile feelings.

For most interactions not involving direct care or intimate conversation, the personal zone is considered most appropriate. In presenting client education and information, a distance of 18 inches to 3 feet is close enough for privacy yet far enough away to avoid intimate touch. Health care providers who have the respect of their clients and families are often able to interact well in this zone.

Individuals are frequently not conscious of their personal space requirements, although they react to invasion of their territory. The nurse should always be aware of clients' and families' body language during interactions. Signs that suggest the client's personal space is being invaded include stepping back, looking uncomfortable and tense, and not facing the nurse during communication.

Objects in the Environment

Objects in the environment can have great meaning for clients of different cultures, and the client may feel uncomfortable when the nurse discards or moves these objects.

Objects can also affect client care and teaching. For example, when the nurse sits behind a desk, a position of authority is assumed. This may be appropriate in some cases, but usually communication is improved by sitting across from or at a 90-degree angle to the client.

Removal of a client's personal items can create distrust. For example, it may be necessary to remove a wedding ring prior to treatment, but the client may feel this takes away a strong sense of support. Likewise, placing a Roman Catholic person's rosary on a table out of reach can cause anxiety.

Items that may seem worthless to the caregiver can be of great significance to the client. For example, some clients collect plastic medicine cups to symbolize the adversities overcome in the treatment plan. If the nurse discards the medicine cups, the client may lose track of how much success has taken place and may not be as motivated to comply with treatment.

Nursing Implications

1. **Provide information about the need to invade a client's space.** When it is necessary to invade a client's space the nurse should provide information about what will be done and how long it will take. This information will enhance compliance and increase the client's comfort.
2. **Assess the client for degree of comfort when invading personal space.** Personal space boundaries vary from individual to individual. While most individuals are comfortable in a conversational space of 3 to 6 feet, some individuals need more space. It is important to be alert for reactions of clients during close physical contact.
3. **Provide privacy for clients during close physical care.** Use of privacy curtains, keeping the client covered whenever possible, exposing only the necessary body part, and asking other persons to leave the room during close physical care can increase feelings of security.

Self-Reflection Questions

1. What space do you need to feel comfortable during interactions with strangers?
2. What space do you prefer when you are with friends?
3. What do you do when your personal space is invaded?
4. How can you assist clients to accept your care when you must invade their personal space?

Caring for Clients with Musculoskeletal Disorders

chapter **28**

CARING tip

❝ Remember that learning is a life-long task. Remember to teach your patients. ❞

Patricia Noonan, RN, BSN • Instructor • Shawsheen School of Practical Nursing • Billerica, Massachusetts

LEARNING outcomes

After completing this chapter, you will be able to:
- Relate the effects of common musculoskeletal disorders to the normal structure and function of the musculoskeletal system.
- Identify manifestations of impaired musculoskeletal function.
- Describe the pathophysiology of common musculoskeletal disorders.
- Discuss collaborative care measures to diagnose and manage musculoskeletal disorders.
- Provide individualized nursing care for clients with musculoskeletal disorders.
- Provide appropriate nursing care for clients undergoing musculoskeletal surgery.
- Provide teaching and home care for clients with musculoskeletal disorders.

MediaLink

www.prenhall.com/burke

Use the above address to access the free, interactive Companion Website created for this textbook. Get hints, instant feedback, and textbook references to chapter-related multiple choice questions. Link to other interesting sites.

The tissues and structures of the musculoskeletal system may be affected by a variety of disorders. When these problems occur, clients may experience impaired physical mobility, altered body image, discomfort or pain, and the inability to perform self-care. Many musculoskeletal conditions are chronic. Nursing care focuses not only on physical care needs, but also on teaching and providing psychosocial support for the client and family.

Structural and Bone Disorders

Scoliosis and Kyphosis

Scoliosis and kyphosis are the two most common deformities of the spinal column. **Scoliosis** is a lateral curvature of the spine. **Kyphosis** is exaggeration of the normal posterior curve of the thoracic spine (Figure 28-1 ◆).

PATHOPHYSIOLOGY
Scoliosis

Scoliosis is usually diagnosed in adolescence. It affects girls much more often than boys. In most cases it is *idiopathic* (has no identified cause). The lateral curve of scoliosis is usually seen in the thoracic, lumbar, or thoracolumbar regions of the spine. As it develops, the muscles and ligaments shorten on the concave side of the curvature. In scoliosis, the shoulders and hips are not level, and the creases of the waist are asymmetric. A lateral curvature and rotation of the spine is seen on x-ray. Severe scoliosis causes back pain and possible dyspnea, anorexia, and nausea as internal organs are crowded.

Kyphosis

Kyphosis often is caused by structural changes in the spine from congenital disorders, Paget's disease, osteoporosis, or osteomalacia. The manifestations of kyphosis include moderate back pain and increased curvature of the thoracic spine as viewed from the side ("hunchback"). Impaired mobility and respiratory problems may occur in cases of severe curvature.

COLLABORATIVE CARE

Diagnosis of scoliosis and kyphosis is made by inspection and x-rays of the spine. The client stands with the arms relaxed and hanging freely at the sides while the examiner evaluates the client from both the back and the front for symmetry of the shoulders, scapulae, waist creases, and the length of the arms. The client then bends forward, and the examiner

| A | Normal spine | Scoliosis | B | Normal spine | Kyphosis |

Figure 28-1. ◆ (A) Scoliosis, a lateral curvature of the spine. (B) Kyphosis, exaggerated posterior curvature of the thoracic spine.

observes for prominence of the scapula or hip. The client is then viewed from the side while the screener looks for increased thoracic rounding or lumbar swayback.

Conservative treatment of scoliosis and kyphosis may include weight loss, active and passive exercises, and braces for support. Clients with severe scoliosis or kyphosis may require surgery.

NURSING CARE

RISK FOR INJURY

- Assess the environment for safety hazards. *Some braces may not allow bending or twisting of the spine.*
- Advise to use the handrail on stairways and take precautions when walking on slippery surfaces, throw rugs, and so on. *A brace may increase the risk of falling and impair the ability to prevent falls.*
- Instruct to wear a smooth cotton T-shirt or cotton tube under the brace, change undergarments at least daily, and wash them with a mild soap. Avoid lotion and body powders. *The brace can irritate the skin and increase the risk of skin breakdown.*
- Advise to loosen brace during meals and for the first 30 minutes after each meal. *Loosening the brace promotes food intake and comfort while eating.*
- Teach how to apply the brace, and explain any activity restrictions. *Prolonged sitting may be restricted. The brace is worn when ambulating.*

Discharge Considerations

Reassure clients with scoliosis or kyphosis that the condition was not caused by poor posture. If a brace is ordered, provide verbal and written instructions for wearing the brace, such as the number of hours per day it is to be worn and activity restrictions to follow when wearing or not wearing the brace. Teach how to protect and care for skin under the brace.

If scoliosis or kyphosis restricts respiratory excursion, discuss the importance of not smoking and of avoiding respiratory infections. Encourage these clients to obtain pneumococcal and influenza immunizations.

Osteoporosis

Osteoporosis, literally defined as "porous bones," is a bone disorder in which bone mass is lost. Bones become more fragile, increasing the risk of fractures. Osteoporosis usually is associated with aging. Eighty percent of those affected are women, and most are over the age of 60.

Although the cause of osteoporosis remains unclear, several risk factors have been identified. Some risk factors cannot

be changed; others can be changed. Box 28-1 lists the risk factors for osteoporosis.

PATHOPHYSIOLOGY

The reduced bone mass of osteoporosis is caused by an imbalance of the processes that influence bone growth and maintenance. Peak bone mass is achieved at about age 35. After that time, bone formation does not keep pace with resorption, and bone mass is lost.

Two types of osteoporosis have been identified. *Type I osteoporosis* occurs in postmenopausal women between ages 51 and 75 and is caused by estrogen deficiency. *Type II osteoporosis,* or *senile osteoporosis,* affects both men and women over age 70. It develops more slowly and is associated with calcium deficiency.

The usual manifestations of osteoporosis are loss of height, progressive curvature of the spine, low back pain, and fractures.

Height is lost as vertebral bodies collapse. Characteristic dorsal kyphosis and cervical lordosis develop, causing the "dowager's hump" often associated with aging. The abdomen tends to protrude and knees and hips flex as the body attempts to maintain its center of gravity (Figure 28-2 ◆).

A fracture may be the first obvious sign of osteoporosis. Some fractures are spontaneous. Others may result from everyday activities (twisting, bending, lifting, rising from bed). These are known as **pathologic fractures,** fractures that occur with minimal or no trauma. Wrist and vertebral fractures are common. Hip fractures associated with osteoporosis often interfere with the ability to maintain normal activity and live independently.

COLLABORATIVE CARE

The care of the client with osteoporosis focuses on stopping or slowing the process, relieving the symptoms, and preventing complications. Proper nutrition and exercise are important components of treatment.

BOX 28-1
RISK FACTORS FOR OSTEOPOROSIS

RISK FACTORS THAT CANNOT BE CHANGED
- Age, female gender
- Race (Caucasian or Asian)
- Family history
- Endocrine disorders

RISK FACTORS THAT CAN BE CHANGED
- Calcium deficiency
- Estrogen deficiency
- Smoking, excess alcohol intake
- Sedentary lifestyle
- Medications

Height

5'6"

5'3"

5'

4'9"

4'6"

4'3"

Age 40 60 70

Figure 28-2. ◆ Changes in height, posture, and spinal curves caused by osteoporosis.

Bone density measurements can help predict the risk for fracture; x-rays may not show osteoporotic changes until more than 30% of the bone mass has been lost. A baseline bone density exam is now recommended for premenopausal women in their 40s.

Calcium

Calcium is vital to preventing osteoporosis. Adequate calcium intake in the older adult may slow bone loss. Adequate calcium intake before age 30 to 35 increases peak bone mass and reduces the risk of osteoporosis later in life. Calcium needs change over the lifetime (see Table 28-1 ◆ for National Institutes of Health calcium intake recommendations). Box 28-2 lists foods high in calcium.

Calcium supplements are available in many forms. A combination of calcium with vitamin D is recommended, particularly for older adults who may have limited sun exposure.

Pharmacology

Estrogen or hormone replacement therapy (HRT) or selective estrogen receptor modulators (SERMs) may be ordered to prevent or treat bone loss in postmenopausal women. These drugs are discussed in Chapter 33. Other drugs that may be used to prevent or treat osteoporosis include:

■ Alendronate (Fosamax) and risedronate (Actonel) to inhibit bone resorption.

■ Calcitonin, a hormone.
■ Sodium fluoride, a mineral.

Table 28-2 ◆ outlines the nursing implications of these drugs.

TABLE 28-1	NIH RECOMMENDED DAILY CALCIUM INTAKE	
AGES	**MILLIGRAMS OF CALCIUM**
0–6 months	400
6 months–1 year	600
1–5 years	800
6–10 years	800–1,200
11–24 years	1,200–1,500
25–50 years	1,000
Pregnant or lactating	1,200–1,500
51–64 years: Women on HRT and men	1,000
51+ years: Women not on HRT	1,500
65 and older	1,500

BOX 28-2

FOODS HIGH IN CALCIUM

- Dairy products (best source):
  - Milk, yogurt
  - Cheese
- Tofu
- Sardines, with bones
- Clams, oysters
- Canned salmon
- Spinach, greens
- Broccoli, cauliflower, bok choy
- Green beans
- Dark molasses

NURSING CARE

Nursing care focuses on preventing osteoporosis itself, and preventing injuries in clients who have osteoporosis.

RISK FOR INJURY

- Keep bed in low position. Use side rails if indicated to prevent client from getting up alone. Provide nighttime lighting to toilet facilities. *Most falls are preventable, particularly in hospitals and long-term care facilities.*
- Avoid using restraints if at all possible. *Restraints may increase the risk of falling and the risk of injury due to a fall. Clients also may fracture osteoporotic bones when pulling against restraints.*
- Encourage weight-bearing exercises for 30 to 40 minutes at least three times a week. *Weight-bearing exercises such as walking or low-impact aerobics promote bone growth. Swimming (including walking on the bottom of the pool) is not a weight-bearing activity.*
- Encourage older adults to use assistive devices as needed to remain active and independent. *Walking sticks, canes, and other tools help the client engage in activities that promote bone growth.*
- Teach older clients about safety and fall precautions. *Helping identify and correct safety hazards in the home can reduce the risk of falls, fractures, and potential disability.*
- Evaluate medication regimen for drugs that may increase the risk of falling (some antihypertensives, anti-anxiety agents, antihistamines, or sedatives). *Many drugs may cause orthostatic hypotension or sedation, increasing the risk for falling.*

IMBALANCED NUTRITION: LESS THAN BODY REQUIREMENTS

- Teach all clients recommended calcium intake for their age (see Table 28-1). *An adequate calcium intake is vital to prevent and treat osteoporosis.*

- Provide a list of foods high in calcium (see Box 28-2), and help identify ways to include these foods in the diet. *Calcium obtained through the diet is an effective way to maintain adequate calcium levels in the body.*
- Teach clients using calcium supplements to take calcium carbonate supplement (e.g., Tums) 30 to 60 minutes before meals. Calcium citrate supplements should be taken with meals to prevent gastrointestinal (GI) distress. All supplements should be taken in divided doses (two to three times daily). *Taking calcium supplements at the appropriate time and in divided doses increases their absorption and effectiveness.*

PAIN

- Assess acute or new complaints of pain. *Acute pain usually results from a fracture, such as compression fracture of the vertebrae.*
- Give acetaminophen or anti-inflammatory drugs as indicated for pain. *Acetaminophen often is well-tolerated by older adults. Regular doses of nonsteroidal anti-inflammatory drugs (NSAIDs) can help manage chronic pain.*
- Apply heat to the painful area, being careful to avoid burning the client. *A controlled heating pad (e.g., Aqua-K) may offer temporary pain relief. To avoid the "rebound effect," remove the heat pad every 20 to 30 minutes.*
- Assist physical therapy to plan an exercise regime. *Exercise is vital to maintain bone mass, but modifications may be necessary to promote comfort.*

Discharge Considerations

Teaching about osteoporosis is important to prevent the disease and its consequences. Stress the importance of maintaining the recommended daily calcium intake. This is particularly important for adolescent girls and young adult women, who may avoid eating many high-calcium foods such as dairy products because of concerns about weight. Emphasize that low-fat (or nonfat) dairy products also contain calcium. For clients who avoid dairy products because of lactose intolerance or a vegetarian diet, suggest alternate sources such as sardines, salmon, broccoli, and dark green leafy vegetables. Refer to a dietitian for further teaching and diet planning.

Teach the importance of physical activity and weight-bearing exercise to prevent bone loss. Suggest regular exercise such as walking for at least 20 minutes four or more times a week. Inform that swimming and pool aerobic exercises are not as helpful to maintain bone density because of the lack of weight bearing.

Teach postmenopausal women about hormone replacement therapy (HRT) to prevent bone loss. Refer to primary care provider for more information about the risks and benefits of HRT.

Stress the importance of not smoking. Provide information about smoking cessation programs and support groups.

	TABLE 28-2	NURSING IMPLICATIONS FOR PHARMACOLOGY: CLIENTS WITH OSTEOPOROSIS

DRUG/CLASSIFICATION	DESCRIPTION	NURSING RESPONSIBILITIES	CLIENT TEACHING
Bisphosphonates ■ Alendronate (Fosamax) ■ Risedronate (Actonel)	The bisphosphonates inhibit bone resorption, increasing the bone density and reducing the risk of fractures. They are used to prevent and treat osteoporosis.	Give with water on arising, 30 minutes before food or other medications. Hold calcium supplements and foods high in calcium for 2 hours after giving the drug. Instruct to avoid lying down for 30 minutes after taking the drug. Report changes in renal function studies (BUN and creatinine) and serum electrolytes to physician.	Take with clear water only; avoid eating or drinking for 30 minutes. Do not lie down until after you have eaten breakfast. Report heartburn or difficult or painful swallowing to your PCP. Report tingling around the mouth or numbness and tingling of fingers or toes. Take calcium and vitamin D supplements as instructed.
Calcitonin ■ Calcitonin-salmon injection, synthetic ■ Calcimar ■ Miacalin (injection or nasal spray)	Calcitonin prevents further bone loss and increases bone mass in osteoporosis if adequate calcium and vitamin D are consumed. Calcitonin may be used by postmenopausal women who cannot or will not take estrogen.	Observe for possible anaphylactic reaction for 20 minutes after giving; have resuscitation equipment available. Alternate nostrils daily when giving by nasal spray. Report nausea and vomiting, anorexia, mild flushing of the hands or feet, and urinary frequency. Teach how to handle and inject the drug at home.	Take in the evening to reduce side effects. Warm nasal spray to room temperature before using. Rhinitis (runny nose) is common with calcitonin nasal spray. Nasal sores or itching may occur. Report nosebleed to your primary care provider. Nausea and vomiting will improve as treatment continues. Be sure to consume adequate calcium and vitamin D.
Fluoride ■ Slow-release sodium fluoride (Slow Fluoride)	Fluoride stimulates bone growth by stimulating the proliferation of osteoblasts.	Give with crackers or bread to reduce nausea. Monitor serum fluoride levels and report levels outside the normal range (95–185 ng/mL) to the primary care provider.	Take with crackers or bread to minimize nausea. Maintain adequate calcium intake. Keep follow-up appointments as directed.

Discuss the effect of heavy alcohol use on bone mass, and suggest it be used moderately, if at all.

Discuss safety and fall prevention with the client who has osteoporosis. Advise to remove scatter rugs and clutter from walkways in the house. Instruct to use a night light or graduated lighting from the bedroom to the bathroom to reduce the risk of nighttime falls. Discuss placing grab bars in strategic locations such as the shower and next to the toilet to reduce the risk of falling.

Provide a list of local and national resources, such as medical equipment supply retailers and osteoporosis support groups and foundations. The National Osteoporosis Foundation and the Osteoporosis and Related Bone Diseases National

Resource Center have many client information pamphlets and resources. Refer to a health care provider, social services, or occupational therapy as indicated for bone density testing, home care services, or rehabilitation.

Nursing Process Case Study
■ CLIENT WITH OSTEOPOROSIS

Nancy Bauer is a 53-year-old school teacher. She has smoked a pack of cigarettes a day for 30 years and drinks one to two glasses of wine with dinner each evening. She does not routinely exercise. Mrs. Bauer has had symptoms of menopause for 8 years, but she has never been on estrogen therapy. Both Mrs. Bauer's mother and her 60-year-old sister have osteoporosis.

Mrs. Bauer is having continuous low back pain unrelieved by mild analgesics. She frequently wakes up during the night because of the pain.

Assessment Mrs. Bauer's vital signs are all within normal limits. She has full range of motion of all extremities. She reports discomfort when bending over and returning to an upright position. She has a noticeable "hump" on her upper back and is 1 inch shorter than her stated height.

Diagnosis The nursing diagnoses for Mrs. Bauer include the following:

- Pain of the lower spine
- Imbalanced Nutrition: Less Than Body Requirements related to inadequate intake of calcium
- Risk for Injury related to effects of osteoporosis

Expected Outcomes The expected outcomes specify that Mrs. Bauer will:

- Relate a decrease in back pain.
- Be able to describe ways to treat her osteoporosis.
- Verbalize the benefits of stopping smoking to prevent further bone loss.
- Make an appointment with her women's health care provider to discuss hormone replacement therapy.
- Engage in regular physical activity.

Planning and Implementation The following interventions are planned and implemented for Mrs. Bauer:

- Teach back-strengthening exercises.
- Assess current knowledge base, and teach prevention and treatment of osteoporosis.
- Provide verbal and written information about dietary sources and calcium supplements.
- Assist in planning a program of physical exercise.

Evaluation On her return visit 6 months later, Mrs. Bauer reports that she feels much better. She is on hormone replacement therapy. She is eating more calcium-rich foods and taking a daily supplement of calcium with vitamin D. Mrs. Bauer has reduced her wine intake to one glass in the evening. She also states that since she stopped smoking, she has been walking 30 to 45 minutes every day.

Critical Thinking in the Nursing Process

1. Why is Mrs. Bauer shorter than she was as a young adult?
2. What foods would you encourage for clients at high risk for osteoporosis who also are at high risk for cardiovascular disease?
3. What physical activities could you plan to help prevent osteoporosis in a client who is wheelchair-bound or has limited mobility?

Osteomalacia and Paget's Disease

Osteomalacia and Paget's disease also affect the structure and integrity of bone.

Osteomalacia, also known as *adult rickets,* results from inadequate mineralization of bone. When insufficient amounts of calcium or phosphate are available, the bone matrix is not mineralized and the bone is unable to bear weight. This causes deformities of weight bearing bone and pathologic fractures. Osteomalacia is commonly caused by a lack of vitamin D. Vitamin D, obtained from certain foods and ultraviolet (UV) radiation from the sun, is necessary to maintain calcium and phosphate levels in the body. Osteomalacia can be corrected with treatment. For more information about the relationship of vitamin D, calcium, and phosphorus in the body, see Chapter 5.

In Paget's disease of the bone, the activity of *osteoclasts* (which break down and resorb bone) increases. This stimulates activity in *osteoblasts* (cells that form new bone) to replace lost bone. However, the new bone formed is soft and poorly mineralized, so it is prone to fractures. The cause of this disease is unknown. The manifestations of osteomalacia and Paget's disease are listed in Box 28-3.

Clients with osteomalacia often are placed on vitamin D supplements. Calcium and phosphate supplements also may be ordered. Drugs such as the biphosphonates and calcitonin are used along with calcium supplements for clients with Paget's disease. Review Table 28-2 for the nursing implications of these drugs.

BOX 28-3
MANIFESTATIONS OF OSTEOMALACIA AND PAGET'S DISEASE

OSTEOMALACIA

- Bone pain
- Difficulty changing positions (lying to sitting; sitting to standing)
- Muscle weakness
- Waddling gait
- Dorsal kyphosis
- Pathologic fractures

PAGET'S DISEASE

- Bone pain
- Deformity
- Pathologic fractures
- Chalk-stick fractures of lower extremities
- Compression fractures
- Kyphosis, loss of height
- Muscle weakness

Nursing care for clients with osteomalacia or Paget's disease is similar to that provided for clients with osteoporosis.

Osteomyelitis

Osteomyelitis is an infection of the bone. It is usually caused by *Staphylococcus aureus* bacteria, although other pathogens also can infect the bone. Osteomyelitis can occur at any age, but usually affects children under age 12 and adults over age 50. Box 28-4 lists risk factors for osteomyelitis. The older adult is at risk for several reasons: reduced immune function, chronic diseases, impaired circulation, and a higher risk of pressure ulcers.

PATHOPHYSIOLOGY

Pathogens usually enter the bone through an open wound, such as an open fracture or a gunshot or puncture wound. Bacteria also may spread to the bone from a local tissue infection. After entry, bacteria lodge and multiply in the bone, causing an inflammatory and immune system response. Phagocytes attempt to contain the infection. In the process, they release enzymes that destroy bone tissue. Pus forms, followed by edema and vascular congestion. Canals in the marrow cavity of the bone allow the infection to spread to other parts of the bone. If the infection reaches the outer margin of the bone (Figure 28-3 ◆), it raises the periosteum of the bone and spreads along the surface. Blood supply to the bone is disrupted, leading to ischemia and, eventually, necrosis of the bone. Blood and antibiotics cannot reach the bone tissue, making it difficult to treat the infection.

The diagnosis of osteomyelitis often is not made until the infection has become chronic. A surgical wound or fracture that does not heal may be the initial sign of infection. Box 28-5 lists the manifestations of osteomyelitis.

COLLABORATIVE CARE

Early diagnosis and treatment of osteomyelitis with antibiotic therapy is important to prevent bone necrosis.

Diagnostic Tests

Blood work shows an *elevated white blood count (WBC)* and *erythrocyte sedimentation rate (ESR)*, both nonspecific signs of

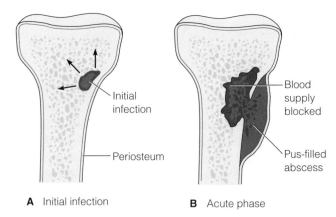

Figure 28-3. ◆ Osteomyelitis. (A) Bacteria enter and multiply in the bone. (B) The infection spreads to other parts of the bone. If the infection reaches the outer part of the bone, the periosteum separates from the surface of the bone.

infection. *Blood* and *tissue cultures* are obtained to identify the infecting organism. An *x-ray* of the affected bone may not detect the infection; *magnetic resonance imaging (MRI), computed tomography (CT) scan,* or *ultrasound* is more accurate for diagnosing osteomyelitis. A *bone scan* may be ordered to help identify active infection. Box 28-6 describes nursing care of a client having a bone scan.

Pharmacology

Antibiotics initially are given intravenously. This may be continued after discharge from the hospital, or an oral antibiotic may be used. Treatment is continued for 4 to 6 weeks.

Surgery

Surgery may be done to obtain a specimen for culture. It may also be done to **debride** the area (remove foreign material and dead or damaged tissue). In surgical debridement, the periosteum is excised and the *cortex* (outer portion of the bone) is drilled to release the pressure from accumulated pus. Following irrigation, drainage tubes connected to an irrigation system may be inserted to keep the cavity clean. After surgery, the nurse is responsible for instilling and removing dilute antibiotic solutions through the drainage tubes.

CLINICAL alert

Use strict sterile technique when caring for a wound irrigation to prevent additional contamination of the infected bone.

NURSING CARE

ASSESSING

The nurse can be instrumental in identifying early manifestations of osteomyelitis. Frequently and carefully assess at-risk

---

BOX 28-4
RISK FACTORS FOR OSTEOMYELITIS

- Open fracture
- Gunshot or deep puncture wound
- Orthopedic surgery
- Soft tissue infection
- Pressure ulcers
- Impaired immune function
- Venous stasis or arterial ulcers of the legs
- Diabetes mellitus

> ## BOX 28-5
> ## MANIFESTATIONS OF OSTEOMYELITIS
>
> - Chills and fever
> - General malaise, fatigue
> - Pain in the affected limb
> - Limited weight bearing in extremity
> - Redness, swelling, heat, tenderness over site
> - Purulent wound drainage, slowed healing

clients for manifestations (see Box 28-5). The older adult may have less specific symptoms, presenting instead with confusion and vague complaints.

DIAGNOSING, PLANNING, AND IMPLEMENTING

Priority nursing diagnoses for the client with osteomyelitis focus on comfort and limited mobility. Because osteomyelitis can be difficult to treat, it also is important to address emotional responses to the disease.

PAIN

■ Provide analgesics on a scheduled basis over 24 hours rather than as needed. *Scheduled analgesic doses allow maintenance of constant blood levels.*

> ## BOX 28-6
> ## NURSING CARE CHECKLIST
>
> ### BONE SCAN
> #### Before the Procedure
> ☑ Verify the presence of a signed consent for the procedure.
> ☑ Assess knowledge and reinforce teaching.
> ☑ Client may eat, drink, and ambulate.
> ☑ Remove all clothing and jewelry.
> ☑ Empty bladder.
>
> #### During the Procedure
> ☑ Radioactive material is injected intravenously.
> ☑ Instruct to drink four to six glasses of water after the injection and before scanning.
> ☑ Scanning takes 30 to 60 minutes to complete.
>
> #### After the Procedure
> ☑ Apply warm compresses to injection site if red or swollen.
> ☑ Increase fluid intake and activity to promote excretion of the radioactive material.
> ☑ No radioactive substance precautions are necessary.

■ Offer analgesic 20 to 30 minutes prior to tests, procedures, or exercises. *Premedicating allows time for the medication to take effect prior to a procedure.*

■ Splint or immobilize the affected extremity. *Splinting or immobilizing the involved extremity provides support and reduces pain caused by movement.*

■ Use adjunctive strategies (e.g., distraction, relaxation) for pain management. *Muscle or joint pain may be relieved with measures that promote relaxation and vasodilation, such as warm, moist packs; warm baths; or heating pads to the involved extremity.*

■ Provide assistive devices (such as a splint, walker or crutches) for ambulation. *Assistive devices help support the involved extremity and reduce weight bearing when ambulating.*

■ Handle the affected area gently. *Gentle handling and minimal manipulation help reduce pain.*

HYPERTHERMIA

■ Monitor temperature every 4 hours and during periods of chilling. Report fever to the charge nurse or physician. *A sudden rise in temperature or continued elevation may indicate a lack of response to treatment. Blood cultures may be ordered when an acute temperature elevation occurs.*

■ Keep environment cool and provide light clothing and bedding during fever. *A cool environment and light clothing promote comfort when the temperature is elevated.*

■ Promote fluid intake of 2,000 to 3,000 mL/day. *The client with an elevated temperature needs additional fluid to replace losses through perspiration.*

IMPAIRED PHYSICAL MOBILITY

■ Keep the affected limb in functional position when immobilized. *Keeping the affected extremity in functional position reduces the risk of contractures.*

■ Maintain rest. Avoid weight bearing on the affected extremity. *Stress on the weakened bone can lead to pathologic fractures.*

■ Assist with active or passive range-of-motion (ROM) exercises every 4 hours. *ROM exercises help maintain normal joint mobility.*

EVALUATING

Collect assessment data related to pain, fever, and fluid balance (urine output, skin turgor, and temperature) to evaluate the effectiveness of nursing care. Also assess physical mobility, strength, and skin condition when evaluating nursing care.

Discharge Considerations

Reinforce teaching about medications and wound management at home. Emphasize the importance of taking all antibiotics as prescribed. Instruct to use pain medications as needed to prevent pain from becoming severe. Discuss possible drug side effects, and provide information about managing these effects. For example, increase fluid and fiber intake to prevent constipation caused by many analgesics, and consume 8 ounces of live-culture yogurt to help prevent diarrhea and yeast infections (mouth or vagina) often associated with prolonged antibiotic therapy.

Teach wound care as needed. Refer for home health services as appropriate. Provide a list of resources for wound care supplies such as local medical suppliers. Teach general principles of infection control, including the importance of good handwashing, especially after toileting or contact with wound drainage.

Rest or limited weight bearing generally is ordered for the affected limb. Bed rest is recommended for vertebral osteomyelitis until back pain has eased enough to allow ambulation. Teach how to avoid complications of immobility. Suggest frequent position changes, keeping skin and linens clean and dry, and active ROM exercises for unaffected joints.

Emphasize the importance of good nutrition. An adequate supply of calories, protein, and other nutrients are necessary for immune function and healing. Suggest frequent small meals and using supplements such as Ensure.

Stress the need to keep all follow-up appointments to ensure complete eradication of the infection.

Bone Tumors

Bone tumors (or *neoplasms*) may be either benign or malignant, primary or secondary. Benign tumors are more common than malignant. *Primary* bone tumors are rare in adults, occurring more frequently in adolescents. *Metastatic* bone tumors (that is, seeded from a tumor elsewhere in the body) are more com-

---

> ### BOX 28-7
> ### MANIFESTATIONS OF BONE TUMORS
>
> - Deep bone pain; worse at night and at rest
> - Redness, warmth, swelling over the affected bone
> - Enlarging mass over affected bone
> - Muscle weakness or atrophy
> - Fever

mon in adults, often originating from tumors of the prostate, breast, kidney, thyroid, and lung.

PATHOPHYSIOLOGY

Primary bone tumors are classified by the tissue from which they arise: bone *(osteogenic)*, cartilage *(chondrogenic)*, collagen *(collagenic)*, and bone marrow *(myelogenic)* (Table 28-3 ◆).

Primary tumors cause bone breakdown *(osteolysis)*, which weakens the bone, resulting in fractures. Malignant bone tumors invade and destroy adjacent bone tissue by producing substances that promote bone resorption or by interfering with a bone's blood supply. Benign bone tumors, unlike malignant ones, have a symmetric, controlled growth pattern. As they grow, they push against neighboring bone tissue. This weakens the bone's structure until it is unable to withstand the stress of ordinary use and frequently causes pathologic fracture.

Bone tumors are usually identified when an injury brings the mass to the client's attention. Box 28-7 lists the common manifestations of bone tumors.

COLLABORATIVE CARE

Because symptoms are usually vague, tumor diagnosis may be delayed.

TABLE 28-3   COMMON PRIMARY BONE TUMORS

TUMOR ORIGIN	BENIGN TUMORS	MALIGNANT TUMORS	SITE
Bone (Osteogenic)	Osteoma	Osteosarcoma—most common malignant tumor of bone tissue	Long bones (femur, tibia), knee
Cartilage (Chondrogenic)	Osteochondroma—most common benign tumor		Pelvis, scapula, ribs
		Chondrosarcoma	Femur, pelvis, ribs, head of long bones
Collagen (Collagenic)		Fibrosarcoma	Femur, tibia
Bone marrow (Myelogenic)		Multiple myeloma—most common primary malignancy of the bone	Vertebrae, ribs, skull, pelvis
Unknown		Ewing's sarcoma—usually occurs in adolescence	Long bones; pelvis, ribs, scapula, sternum

Diagnostic Tests

Conventional *x-rays* show the location of the tumor and the extent of bone involvement. *CT scan* and *MRI* are used to identify the extent of tumor invasion into surrounding tissue. A *biopsy* is done to identify the type of tumor. In addition to the above diagnostic tests, the client with a malignant bone tumor will have elevated *serum alkaline phosphatase, red blood cell (RBC) count,* and *serum calcium* levels.

Chemotherapy

Chemotherapeutic drugs are given to shrink the tumor before surgery, to prevent recurrence after surgery, or to treat tumor metastasis. See Chapter 8 for further discussion of chemotherapy and its nursing implications.

Radiation Therapy

Radiation therapy may be used in combination with chemotherapy. Radiation therapy is frequently applied to metastatic bone lesions to control pain. It is also used to eliminate bony tumors or to eliminate any remaining tumor after surgery. Radiation therapy is discussed in Chapter 8.

Surgery

Surgery is performed to remove the tumor. The tumor itself may be excised, or the affected limb amputated. To avoid amputation, a bone graft from a cadaver or metal prostheses often are used to replace missing bone. Care of the client undergoing amputation is presented in Chapter 27.

NURSING CARE

Nursing care needs for the client with a bone tumor focus on both the physical aspects of care as well as the psychosocial effects of the diagnosis and its treatment.

PAIN

- Assess pain, including location, intensity (ask the client to rate the pain on a standard pain scale), quality or type, aggravating and relieving factors, and duration. *An accurate assessment of pain is necessary to help determine its cause and to evaluate the effectiveness of interventions.*
- Develop strategies for controlling both acute pain (from surgery, fracture, or inflammation) and chronic pain (from tumor growth and spread). *Effective pain management is based on the acuity and intensity of the pain. See Chapter 6 for more information about pain management.*
- Encourage use of both pharmacologic and nonpharmacologic methods to prevent pain from becoming intense. *Pain relief measures are more effective when used to control pain before it becomes intense.*
- Provide assistive devices (e.g., canes, walkers, crutches) when ambulating. *Assistive devices reduce pain by supporting weight bearing during ambulation.*
- Provide regular rest periods between scheduled treatments. *Rest reduces muscle tension and pain.*

IMPAIRED PHYSICAL MOBILITY

- Teach correct use of trapeze. *Using the trapeze helps strengthen the biceps of the arm and allows clients to reposition themselves, get out of bed, and perform other activities.*
- Begin muscle-strengthening and active and passive ROM exercises immediately after surgery. A continuous passive motion (CPM) machine may be used after surgery on an extremity. *Muscle strengthening and ROM exercises maintain joint function and prevent muscle wasting.*
- Assist the client who has leg surgery or amputation with exercises to strengthen the triceps muscles of the arms and with quadriceps and gluteal setting exercises and leg raises. *Muscle-strengthening exercises prepare the client for using assistive devices (e.g., crutches) for ambulation and other activities until a prosthesis is fitted.*
- Refer to physical or occupational therapy for fitting of and teaching about assistive devices such as a cane, crutches, or a walker. *Assistive devices promote mobility and reduce the risk of falling.*

DISTURBED BODY IMAGE

- Listen to and support the client who is grieving loss of a limb or other changes such as hair loss associated with treatment. *The client who has lost a body part or experienced a change in body image will go through a grieving process.*
- Allow time for open discussions of feelings about changes in body image and potential changes in social and personal life. *Open and accepting discussion helps the client work through grieving and begin coping with the changes.*

ANTICIPATORY GRIEVING

- Listen actively and encourage verbalization of feelings and concerns about the diagnosis and treatment. *Active listening promotes trust and provides an opportunity for the client and family to work through accepting the diagnosis.*
- Present information in a matter-of-fact manner, taking time to listen to and address concerns. Discuss expected effects and potential side effects of surgery, chemotherapy, and radiation therapy. *Accurate and appropriate information empowers the client and family to make decisions about treatment.*
- Refer to a counselor, the clergy, or, as appropriate, hospice services. *The client with a malignant bone tumor faces the very real possibility of dying as a result of the disease, particularly when the tumor is metastatic from another site. Trained professionals can help the client and family identify and express their feelings, and work through the grieving process.*

Discharge Considerations

Teach about the disease, its potential consequences, and treatment options. Provide information about how to minimize side effects. Depending on the location of the tumor and planned treatment, modifications of the home environment may be necessary. Discuss potential barriers to mobility, such as stairs or lack of access to transportation. Help identify a network of support people who can assist with coping, care, and treatment as needed. If surgery has been performed, teach wound care, demonstrating dressing changes and stump care (if amputation has occurred). Provide a list of local resources for obtaining supplies. Discuss activity and weight-bearing restrictions. Refer to physical therapy for teaching about ambulation and appropriate muscle-group strengthening exercises. Ensure that the client who has experienced an amputation is working with or has a referral to a prosthetic specialist. For the client with metastatic disease, discuss hospice services and support groups for clients with cancer.

 ## Common Foot Disorders

Hallux valgus and hammertoe are common foot disorders that cause pain or difficulty in walking. Wearing poorly fitting or confining shoes may contribute to these disorders.

HALLUX VALGUS

Hallux valgus, or *bunion,* is enlargement and lateral displacement of the great toe (Figure 28-4A ◆). They develop due to chronic pressure against the great toe. Heredity and joint disorders contribute, as does wearing pointed, narrow-toed shoes or high heels. The toe bends away from the midline of the body, and the metatarsophalangeal (MTP) joint becomes enlarged. Calluses develop over the joint. Hallux valgus is obvious on physical examination of the foot. The client may complain of pain and difficulty fitting into shoes.

HAMMERTOE

Hammertoe (claw toe) is a deformity of the toe characterized by flexion of the proximal interphalangeal (PIP) joint with hyperextension of the MTP and distal interphalangeal (DIP) joints. It may affect any toe, but the second toe is usually affected. The flexed PIP joint rubs against the shoe, causing painful corns to develop (Figure 28-4B).

COLLABORATIVE CARE

Corrective shoes often are ordered for clients with foot disorders. Orthotic devices that cushion and stretch the affected joints may be placed within shoes or between the toes. Analgesics may be ordered, or corticosteroid drugs injected into the affected joints to relieve acute inflammation. A bunionectomy may be done to treat hallux valgus. Surgery also may be done to correct hammertoe.

 # NURSING CARE

PAIN

- Instruct to wear appropriate or corrective footwear. *Shoes that fit well and provide enough foot space laterally and dorsally, such as running shoes, are recommended. In some cases, the client may need special shoes or orthotics.*
- Provide information about resources for obtaining a proper shoe fit. *Shoe stores and repair shops often can stretch a shoe at the pressure area. Fabric shoes are more comfortable for people with bunions because fabric stretches more readily than leather or synthetic materials.*
- Suggest protective pads to wear over bunions, calluses/corns, and the ball of the foot. *Protective pads help reduce pain and irritation when shoes are worn.*
- Instruct to remove pads and inspect skin every other day. Clients who have difficulty reaching or observing the foot should ask another person to do the inspection for them. *Skin inspection is particularly important if sensation has been lost in the feet due to diabetes or chronic peripheral vascular disease.*

RISK FOR INFECTION

Risk for infection following foot surgery may be increased because of impaired peripheral circulation and exposure of the feet to the environment.

- Teach proper care and cleaning of incision and exposed pins implanted during surgery. *Pins may be inserted to maintain the position of the bones and joints.*
- Instruct to wear a plastic bag over the cast or pins when bathing or walking in rain or snow. *When casts or pins are exposed in water, infection may result.*

Figure 28-4. ◆ (A) Hallux valgus (bunion). (B) Hammertoe.

 ## Discharge Considerations

Teach clients in all age groups the importance of well-fitting footwear. Discuss with women in particular the long-term effects of wearing high-heeled shoes with constricting toes.

Suggest alternatives for stylish footwear, and encourage clients to wear supportive and nonrestrictive footwear at all times. Discuss the possible effects of bunions on balance, and talk about safety measures to prevent falls and injury. Teach techniques to relieve pressure on affected joints as discussed in the nursing care section.

Joint and Connective Tissue Disorders

The term **arthritis,** which literally means inflammation of a joint, is often used for any disorder that causes pain and stiffness of the musculoskeletal system. *Rheumatism* is another term used to describe pain in the joints and related tissues. Some arthritic disorders are limited to the joint and surrounding tissues; others are more widespread systemic diseases. Several, such as rheumatoid arthritis and systemic lupus erythematosus, are *connective tissue disorders.*

Connective tissue is the most abundant and widely distributed body tissue. It connects body parts; provides support; forms bones, cartilage, and the walls of blood vessels; and attaches muscles to bones. Connective tissue diseases have diverse manifestations. Arthritic disorders, regardless of their cause, can create problems of mobility, deformity, and disability.

Osteoarthritis

Osteoarthritis (OA) is a degenerative joint disease characterized by progressive loss of joint cartilage in synovial joints. Osteoarthritis is the most common type of arthritis and is a leading cause of disability in older adults. It affects men and women equally. Risk factors for OA include age, repetitive joint use or trauma, heredity, obesity, and congenital or acquired defects.

PATHOPHYSIOLOGY

Osteoarthritis affects the entire joint: the cartilage, bone, synovial membrane, and the ligaments, muscles, and tendons that surround the joint. The joint cartilage loses its strength and elasticity and is gradually destroyed. As the cartilage erodes and ulcerates, the underlying bone is exposed. The bone thickens in exposed areas, and cysts develop. Cartilage-coated *osteophytes* (bony outgrowths) change the anatomy of the joint. As these spurs or projections enlarge, small pieces may break off, leading to mild inflammation of the joint.

The hips, knees, lumbar and cervical vertebrae, proximal and distal interphalangeal (PIP and DIP) joints of the fingers, wrist, and big toe joint of the foot are affected most frequently by osteoarthritis.

The onset of OA is usually gradual and insidious, and the course slowly progressive. Localized joint pain (**arthralgia**) is the most common symptom of OA. Following periods of immobility (e.g., on awakening in the morning or after an automobile ride), involved joints may stiffen. Range of motion of the joint decreases as the disease progresses, and grating or crepitus may be noted during movement. Bony overgrowth may cause joint enlargement. Enlarged joints are characteristically bony-hard and cool on palpation. The manifestations of OA are listed in Box 28-8.

Osteoarthritis of the spine may cause degeneration of disks between the vertebrae and narrowing of the joint spaces. Degenerative disk disease may be complicated by *herniated disk,* the protrusion of the nucleus pulposus of the disk. Herniation can compress nerve roots, causing severe pain and muscle weakness. See Chapter 30 for further discussion of disk disorders. Loss of cartilage between the processes of the vertebrae causes localized pain, stiffness, muscle spasm, and limited range of motion. Osteophytes may form on these processes, increasing pain and muscle spasm.

COLLABORATIVE CARE

The diagnosis of OA is based on the history and on physical and x-ray examination of affected joints. Initially, the joint space narrows. As the disease progresses, bone density increases, osteophytes are seen at the joint periphery, and bone cysts may be noted.

Clients with OA are encouraged to lose weight if obese and to remain physically active. Exercise helps maintain muscle tone and joint support, and promotes weight loss. Exercise in water (non–weight bearing) may help clients with OA of the knees or hips. Heat applied locally to affected joints can relieve discomfort. Box 28-9 provides selected complementary therapies that may be beneficial for clients with OA.

BOX 28-8
MANIFESTATIONS OF OSTEOARTHRITIS

- Deep, aching pain in affected joints
- Pain aggravated by use, relieved by rest
- Stiffness following immobility
- Limited ROM
- Crepitus with movement
- *Heberden's nodes* on distal interphalangeal (DIP) joints
- *Bouchard's nodes* on proximal interphalangeal (PIP) joints

BOX 28-9 COMPLEMENTARY THERAPIES

Osteoarthritis

Many complementary therapies may help relieve the discomfort of osteoarthritis and maintain mobility. Refer the client to a trained practitioner or naturopathic physician. Selected complementary therapies for OA include:

- Aromatherapy: Massage or compress of cypress or rosemary to affected joints
- Herbs: Glucosamine and chondroitin; natural anti-inflammatories such as willowbark
- Magnets over affected joints
- Reflexology
- Therapeutic touch
- Yoga

Pharmacology

The pain of OA often can be managed with mild analgesics such as aspirin or acetaminophen. Acetaminophen is preferred for use in older clients because it has fewer toxic side effects. Nonsteroidal anti-inflammatory drugs (NSAIDs) may also be ordered. These medications are discussed in more detail in the section of this chapter on rheumatoid arthritis. Capsaicin cream can reduce joint pain and tenderness when applied topically to affected joints such as the knees or hands. In some cases, a long-acting corticosteroid mixed with a local anesthetic may be injected directly into the affected joint. Although this procedure relieves pain, it can increase cartilage breakdown if done frequently.

Surgery

Surgery may be done when pain and limited joint motion interfere with ADLs. *Arthroscopy* may be done for osteoarthritis of the knee. Using an arthroscope, the joint is inspected, and damaged cartilage and osteophytes can be removed.

    Arthroplasty, reconstruction or replacement of a joint, is often done when the client has severely restricted mobility and pain at rest. In most cases, both surfaces of the affected joint are replaced with prosthetic parts in a procedure known as a *total joint replacement.* Joints that may be replaced include the hip, knee, shoulder, elbow, ankle, wrist, and joints of the fingers and toes.

    In a *total hip replacement,* the joint surfaces of the acetabulum and femoral head are replaced (Figure 28-5A ◆). The entire head of the femur and part of the femoral neck are removed and replaced with a prosthesis. In a *total knee replacement* (Figure 28-5B), the femoral side of the joint is replaced with a metallic surface, and the tibial side with polyethylene.

    Infection is the major complication of total joint replacement surgery. Infection impairs healing and can lead to failure and removal of the prosthesis. Box 28-10 outlines nursing care for the client undergoing total joint replacement. See Chapter

Figure 28-5. ◆ (A) Total hip replacement. (B) Total knee replacement.

7 for more information about caring for the client undergoing surgery.

NURSING CARE

OA frequently complicates pain management and interferes with mobility in both home and institutional settings. It rarely is the primary nursing care problem unless the client is having joint surgery for the effects of OA.

ASSESSING

Nursing assessment of the client with OA focuses on the effects of the disease on ADLs (functional assessment). Assessment data to collect for a client with OA are outlined in Box 28-11.

DIAGNOSING, PLANNING, AND IMPLEMENTING

CHRONIC PAIN

- Administer analgesic or anti-inflammatory medication as needed. *Analgesics reduce the perception of pain; anti-*

BOX 28-10
NURSING CARE CHECKLIST

TOTAL JOINT REPLACEMENT

Before Surgery

☑ Provide routine preoperative care and teaching. See Chapter 7.

☑ Reinforce teaching as indicated.

☑ Teach use of overhead trapeze for changing positions.

☑ Teach or provide ordered skin preparation such as shower, shampoo, and skin scrub with antibacterial solution.

☑ Administer intravenous antibiotic as ordered.

After Surgery

☑ Provide routine postoperative care (see Chapter 7).

☑ Assess neurovascular status (color, temperature, pulses and capillary refill, movement, and sensation) of the affected limb hourly for the first 12 to 24 hours, then every 2 to 4 hours. Report abnormal findings immediately.

☑ Empty and record wound suction drainage every 4 hours.

☑ Frequently assess for bleeding. Reinforce the dressing as needed. Report significant bleeding to the charge nurse or physician.

☑ Maintain extremity position using sling, abduction splint, brace, immobilizer, or other ordered device.

☑ Help shift position at least every 2 hours while on bed rest.

☑ Assist out of bed as soon as allowed (usually 24 to 48 hours postoperatively). Reinforce teaching about avoiding weight bearing on affected extremity; use overhead trapeze, pivot turning, and toe-touch.

☑ Initiate physical therapy and exercises as prescribed.

☑ Use sequential compression devices or antiembolism stockings as ordered.

☑ For total hip replacement, prevent hip flexion greater than 90 degrees and adduction of the affected leg. Provide a seat riser for toilet or commode.

☑ Report signs of hip prosthesis dislocation, including pain or shortening and internal rotation of the affected leg.

☑ For total knee replacement, use a continuous passive range-of-motion (CPM) device or range-of-motion exercises as prescribed.

☑ Reinforce teaching about postdischarge exercises and activity restrictions. Emphasize the importance of scheduled follow-up physician visits.

☑ Make referrals as needed to home health agencies and physical therapy.

BOX 28-11
ASSESSING CLIENTS WITH OSTEOARTHRITIS

SUBJECTIVE DATA

• Pain: Location and characteristics; effect on ADLs (occupation, household tasks, activities, self-care, sleep/rest); relief measures used (analgesics, heat or cold, splinting or wrapping, rest)

• Changes in mobility; usual activities and any limitations

• Patterns of sleep/rest

• Coping with effects of joint pain, stiffness, and limited mobility

OBJECTIVE DATA

• Mobility: Gait, ability to sit and rise from sitting, ability to step into and out of tub or shower, negotiate stairs

• Ability to perform ADLs: Manipulate clothing for toileting, perform hygiene and grooming activities, feed self

• Joint swelling, redness, tenderness, warmth; range of motion

• Effect on function; observe ability to:
  • Comb hair, pick up and hold a utensil with each hand, write
  • With each leg, run heel of one foot down shin of opposite leg; stand from sitting position and walk
  • In sitting position, bend down to tie shoes

■ Apply heat to painful joints using the shower, a tub or sitz bath, warm packs, hot wax dips, heated gloves, or *diathermy,* which uses high-frequency electrical currents to generate heat. *Heat reduces muscle spasm, relieving pain. Moist heat penetrates deeper than dry heat; diathermy delivers heat to deeper body tissues.*

■ Emphasize the importance of proper posture and good body mechanics for walking, sitting, lifting, and moving. *Good body mechanics and posture reduce stress on affected joints.*

■ Encourage the overweight client to reduce. *Excess weight places abnormal stress on joints, particularly the knees.*

■ Encourage use of nonpharmacologic measures such as progressive relaxation, meditation, visualization, and distraction. *These adjunctive pain-relief measures can reduce muscle tension and spasm, promoting comfort.*

IMPAIRED PHYSICAL MOBILITY

■ Teach active and passive ROM exercises as well as isometric, progressive resistance exercises. *These exercises help maintain muscle tone and strength and mobility of affected joints and prevent contractures.*

inflammatory drugs reduce local inflammation, swelling, and pain in affected joints.

■ Teach use of splints or other devices on affected joints as needed. *The pain of OA is often relieved by joint rest.*

- Encourage participation in low-impact aerobic exercises such as water aerobics. *Aerobic exercise improves endurance and cardiovascular fitness.*
- Provide analgesics or other pain-relief measures prior to exercise or ambulation. *With decreased pain, exercise tolerance improves.*
- Teach good body mechanics and encourage to avoid heavy lifting. *Good body mechanics reduce the stress on joints.*
- Encourage planned rest periods during the day. *Rest reduces fatigue, pain, and joint stress.*
- Teach use of ambulatory aids such as a cane or walker as ordered. *These devices help relieve some weight bearing and stress on affected joints.*

SELF-CARE DEFICIT

- Assist with ADLs as needed. *OA can significantly interfere with ADLs such as cooking, brushing hair, bathing, and toileting. Minimal assistance can promote self-esteem and as much independence as possible.*
- Refer to an occupational therapist for exercises and assistive devices. *The occupational therapist can identify measures that will help the client remain independent.*
- Help obtain assistive devices such as long-handled shoehorns, zipper grabbers, long-handled tongs or grippers for retrieving items from the floor, jar openers, and special eating utensils. *These devices can promote independence in performing ADLs.*

EVALUATING

In order to evaluate the effectiveness of nursing care, collect data regarding ability to manage pain, maintain mobility, and perform ADLs.

Discharge Considerations

With environmental modifications and assistive devices, the client with OA often can remain home and independent. Assess the home for hazards to mobility, such as scatter rugs. Identify the need for assistive devices such as handrails, grab bars, walk-in shower stall, or shower chair and handheld shower head. Help obtain and install assistive devices as indicated.

Teach ways to help maintain joint function and mobility:

- Exercise helps maintain joint mobility, and develops supportive muscles and tendons. Walking is an effective low-impact, aerobic exercise.
- Do not overuse or stress affected joints.
- Balance exercise with rest of affected joints.
- If obese, lose weight to decrease stress on weight-bearing joints.
- Sit in a straight chair without slumping; avoid soft chairs or recliners.
- Sleep on a firm mattress or use a bed board.

Teach about prescribed or over-the-counter medications for OA. Discuss their use, side effects, and any particular precautions specific to the medication. Discuss nonpharmacologic pain-relief measures such as heat, rest, massage, relaxation, and meditation.

If arthroplasty has been done, reinforce teaching about activity and weight-bearing. Teach use of splints, braces, slings, or other devices to maintain the desired limb position during healing. Discuss assistive devices such as overhead trapeze for getting out of bed, elevated toilet seats, and chairs to use and avoid when sitting. Encourage practice of prescribed exercises. Observe and reinforce teaching as needed for using crutches or a walker.

Discuss possible complications, including signs of infection or dislocation, and instruct to notify the physician promptly if these occur. Refer for home care, physical or occupational therapy, or other community resources as indicated. See the Critical Thinking Care Map at the end of this chapter for an opportunity to use the nursing process to plan care for a client with osteoarthritis and total hip replacement.

Rheumatoid Arthritis

Rheumatoid arthritis (RA) is a chronic, systemic inflammatory disorder that primarily affects the joints. It is a connective tissue disorder that affects more women than men, and usually develops between the ages of 30 and 50 years. Usually, multiple joints are affected. The disease has periods of remission and exacerbation. RA is an autoimmune disorder of unknown cause. See Chapter 13 for more information about autoimmune disorders.

PATHOPHYSIOLOGY

In rheumatoid arthritis, T lymphocytes (T cells) migrate to the joint and infiltrate the synovial membrane. An immune response is initiated, and IgG, an immunoglobulin, is produced. The body sees this as a foreign substance, and produces autoantibodies to the IgG. These autoantibodies, known as *rheumatoid factors,* bind with the IgG to form immune complexes. Complement is activated, and a variety of white blood cells are attracted to the area. These cells phagocytize immune complexes. In the process, they release enzymes that destroy joint tissue.

The resulting inflammation affects the joint and surrounding tissues. Affected joints are swollen, red, and painful. Joint tissue is destroyed by an extensive network of new blood vessels (vascular granulation tissue known as *pannus*) in the synovial membrane. Pannus erodes the cartilage and bone of affected joints and invades surrounding tissues, including ligaments and tendons (Figure 28-6 ◆).

Rheumatoid arthritis is a systemic disease. Symptoms such as fatigue, anorexia, weight loss, and nonspecific aching and stiffness often occur before typical joint changes are evident. Joint manifestations of rheumatoid arthritis often develop slowly and insidiously. Joint swelling with stiffness, warmth, tenderness, and pain are typical. The pattern of joint

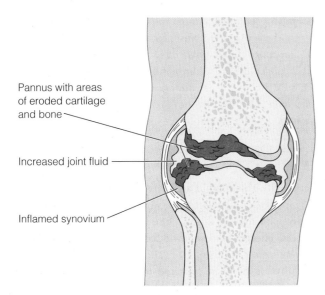

Figure 28-6. ◆ Joint inflammation and destruction in rheumatoid arthritis.

Pannus with areas of eroded cartilage and bone

Increased joint fluid

Inflamed synovium

involvement is usually *polyarticular* (involving multiple joints) and *symmetric*. The joint and systemic manifestations of RA are listed in Box 28-12. Clinical features of RA and OA are compared in Table 28-4 ◆.

The course of rheumatoid arthritis is variable and fluctuating. Early disease progression is more rapid than later in the disease. Destruction of affected joints and problems of immobility are the primary complications of RA (Figure 28-7 ◆).

COLLABORATIVE CARE

The diagnosis of rheumatoid arthritis is based on the history, physical exam, and diagnostic tests. There currently is no cure for RA. Treatment goals are to relieve symptoms, stop or reduce joint destruction, and maintain function. A multidisciplinary approach is used, with a balance of rest, exercise, physical therapy, and treatments to modify the disease process. For the older adult, less emphasis may be placed on

---

BOX 28-12
MANIFESTATIONS OF RHEUMATOID ARTHRITIS

JOINT

- Swelling, warmth, tenderness, and pain:
  - Usually affects proximal interphalangeal (PIP) and metacarpophalangeal (MCP) joints of fingers, wrists, knees, ankles, and toes
- Limited range of motion
- Morning stiffness lasting more than 1 hour
- Joint destruction and deformity (see Figure 28-7):
  - *Swan-neck deformity:* Flexion of DIP joint with hyperextension of PIP joint
  - *Boutonnière deformity:* Hyperextension of DIP joint with flexion of PIP joint
  - *Ulnar deviation* and *subluxation* of MCP joints
  - Carpal tunnel syndrome
  - Hallux valgus and hammertoe deformities of the foot

SYSTEMIC

- Fatigue, weakness
- Anorexia, weight loss
- Low-grade fever
- Anemia
- *Rheumatoid nodules:* Firm subcutaneous tissue nodules over elbow, MCP joints, toes

---

preventing joint deformity and more emphasis on maintaining function.

Diagnostic Tests

- *Rheumatoid factors (RF)* are present in most people with RA.
- *Erythrocyte sedimentation rate (ESR)* is typically elevated, often markedly. The ESR is an indicator of inflammatory activity.

TABLE 28-4

CHARACTERISTICS OF RHEUMATOID ARTHRITIS AND OSTEOARTHRITIS

FEATURE	RHEUMATOID ARTHRITIS	OSTEOARTHRITIS
Onset	Usually insidious, may be abrupt	Insidious
Course	Often progressive, with remissions and exacerbations	Slowly progressive
Pain and stiffness	On arising, lasting > 1 hour; following prolonged immobility	Following activity or periods of immobility; short duration
Affected joints	Red, hot, swollen; tender to palpation; decreased ROM Multiple joints affected	May be swollen; cool and bony hard to palpation; decreased ROM One or several joints affected
Systemic manifestations	Fatigue, weakness, anorexia, weight loss, fever, anemia	Fatigue

Figure 28-7. ◆ Typical hand deformities associated with rheumatoid arthritis.

■ *Synovial fluid* aspirated from inflamed joints is analyzed.
■ *X-ray* of affected joints shows characteristic joint changes as the disease progresses.

Rest and Exercise

During an acute disease flare, both joint and total body rest are ordered. Regular rest periods during the day are recommended. Inflamed joints may be splinted to provide local joint rest. Rest is balanced with physical therapy and exercise to maintain muscle strength and joint mobility. Range-of-motion exercises are ordered to maintain joint function and prevent contractures. Isometric, isotonic, and low-impact aerobic exercises such as swimming and walking also may be ordered.

Pharmacology

A variety of drugs and drug groups are used to manage RA. Aspirin and other NSAIDs and mild analgesics are used to reduce inflammation and manage the signs and symptoms of the disease (see Table 28-5 ◆). Corticosteroids may also be used to reduce acute pain and inflammation. A diverse group of drugs called disease-modifying or slow-acting antirheumatic drugs appear to alter the disease course and reduce joint destruction. These drugs include gold compounds, penicillamine, antimalarial agents, sulfasalazine, and immunosuppressive and cytotoxic drugs.

Surgery

Surgery may be done to relieve pain and repair or replace joints damaged by RA. *Arthrodesis* (joint fusion) may be used to stabilize joints such as cervical vertebrae, wrists, and ankles. Arthroplasty, or total joint replacement, may be necessary in cases of gross deformity and joint destruction. Total joint replacement and nursing care needs of clients undergoing this surgery are discussed in the previous section on osteoarthritis.

Other Therapies

Several newer treatments may be used to treat progressive RA. *Plasmapheresis* may be used to remove circulating antibodies,

moderating the autoimmune response. *Total lymphoid irradiation,* another option, decreases total lymphocyte levels.

For most clients with rheumatoid arthritis, an ordinary, well-balanced diet is recommended. Some clients may benefit from substituting usual dietary fat with omega-3 fatty acids found in certain fish oils.

NURSING CARE

Clients with rheumatoid arthritis have multiple nursing care needs involving all functional health patterns. In addition to its physicial manifestations, the disease also has many psychosocial effects. It is an incurable chronic disease that may lead to severe crippling. Pain and fatigue can interfere with the ability to perform expected roles, such as home maintenance or job responsibilities. Other people may not understand the systemic nature of the RA or realize the difference between rheumatoid arthritis and osteoarthritis.

ASSESSING

Assessment of the client with RA focuses on the progress of the disease and on its effect on functional abilities (see Box 28-13). To assess the status of the disease, collect data such as the following:

■ Pain level; number of affected joints
■ Duration of morning stiffness
■ Redness, heat, and swelling of affected joints
■ Other symptoms such as fatigue, weakness, anorexia, fever

DIAGNOSING, PLANNING, AND IMPLEMENTING

PAIN

The pain of active RA is constant. It affects self-care, ADLs, and contributes to fatigue.

■ Encourage to adjust activities according to pain level. *Pain is an indicator of stress on inflamed joints. Increasing pain indicates a need to decrease activity.*
■ Teach use of heat or cold for pain relief. A warm shower, tub bath, warm compresses or paraffin dips can be used to apply heat. If heat increases pain and swelling during periods of acute inflammation, cold packs may be more effective. *Both heat and cold have analgesic effects and can help relieve associated muscle spasms.*
■ Discuss the importance of taking anti-inflammatory medications as ordered, and the relationship between inflammation and pain. *Anti-inflammatory agents reduce chemical mediators of inflammation and swelling, relieving pain.*
■ Encourage use of other nonpharmacologic pain-relief measures such as visualization, distraction, meditation, and progressive relaxation techniques. *These techniques can reduce muscle tension and help the client focus away from the pain,*

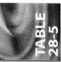

TABLE 28-5   NURSING IMPLICATIONS FOR PHARMACOLOGY: CLIENTS WITH RHEUMATOID ARTHRITIS

DRUG/CLASSIFICATION	DESCRIPTION	NURSING RESPONSIBILITIES	CLIENT TEACHING
Aspirin ▪ Acetylsalic acid, aspirin, Ecotrin, Empirin, others	Aspirin inhibits prostaglandin synthesis and activity, reducing inflammation. It also has an analgesic and antipyretic effect. It inhibits platelet aggregation and normal blood clotting. Doses of up to 3.6 to 4.8 g/day are required for the best anti-inflammatory effect.	Assess for contraindications such as allergy or bleeding disorders. Give crushed or whole with food or milk to prevent gastric irritation. Do not crush enteric-coated or sustained-release forms. Stop the drug and notify the doctor if rash, hives, or signs of gastrointestinal bleeding develop.	Always take with food or milk. If gastric upset or nausea develop, try enteric-coated aspirin. Do not substitute acetaminophen for aspirin as it does not have anti-inflammatory effects. Report dark stools, vomiting blood, abnormal bleeding, blurred vision, ringing in the ears, rashes, or difficulty breathing to your doctor. Check labels of other over-the-counter drugs carefully; many contain aspirin. Do not use alcohol while taking aspirin; it greatly increases the risk of gastrointestinal bleeding.
Other Nonsteroidal Anti-inflammatory Drugs (NSAIDs) ▪ Ibuprofen (Motrin, others) ▪ Indomethacin (Indocin) ▪ Ketoprofen (Orudis) ▪ Naproxen (Anaprox, Naprosyn) ▪ Piroxicam (Feldene) ▪ Sulindac (Clinoril) ▪ Tolmetin (Tolectin) ▪ Others	NSAIDs are used to manage arthritis and other causes of inflammation. Although each is different, all inhibit prostaglandin synthesis, reducing inflammation. All are more costly than aspirin. They may allow fewer daily doses to achieve their effect. For most, adverse effects are similar to aspirin.	Obtain baseline weight and vital signs. Carefully monitor clients who are elderly or have reduced kidney function for toxicity. Give with food or milk to minimize gastric effects. Report possible adverse effects such as GI bleeding; impaired renal function; and CNS effects.	Take as ordered to maintain a constant blood level for the best effect. It may take several weeks for the full effect to occur. Take with food or milk. Weigh weekly; report sudden weight gain of more than 3 to 5 pounds to your doctor. Report changes in vision, hearing, mood, urination; or bloody urine, bloody vomit; or blood in stool to your doctor. Avoid alcohol and aspirin while taking NSAIDs. Use acetaminophen as needed for pain relief.
Second-Generation NSAIDs: COX-2 Inhibitors ▪ Celecoxib (Celebrex) ▪ Rofecoxib (Vioxx)	COX-2 inhibitors are a new type of NSAID that suppress inflammation and pain with a lower risk of serious side effects such as gastrointestinal ulcers, bleeding, and kidney problems.	Assess for contraindications such as allergy to aspirin or other NSAIDs or advanced kidney disease Administer by mouth without regard to meals.	Take with a full glass of water; stay upright for 15–30 minutes after taking. Promptly notify your doctor if you develop abdominal pain, tarry stools, rash, edema, or unexplained weight gain. Notify your doctor if you are or plan to become pregnant.

decreasing the intensity of the pain experience. See Chapter 6 for further discussion of adjunctive pain-relief measures.

FATIGUE

- Encourage a balance of activity with periods of rest. Stress the importance of planned rest periods during the day. *Both joint and whole-body rest are important to reduce the inflammatory response.*
- Assist to prioritize activities, scheduling the most important ones early in the day. *Prioritizing allows the client to maintain activities that are meaningful and important.*
- Encourage to engage in regular physical activity in addition to ordered ROM exercises. *Aerobic exercise promotes a sense of well-being and restful sleep.*
- Help identify tasks that can be delegated to others. *Enlisting the help of family and friends can help the client maintain those activities that are important.*

INEFFECTIVE ROLE PERFORMANCE

- Discuss effects of the disease on career and other life roles. *Discussion helps the client accept changes and begin to identify strategies for coping with them.*
- Encourage discussion of feelings about the disease and its effect on client and family roles. *Open discussion helps family members identify and accept feelings about losses and changes.*
- Listen actively to concerns, acknowledging their validity. *Demonstrating acceptance of these feelings and concerns promotes trust.*
- Help identify strengths to use in coping with role changes. *Past coping strategies and family strengths can be used to deal with necessary role changes.*
- Encourage client to make decisions and assume personal responsibility for disease management. *Clients who assume an active role in managing their disease maintain a greater sense of self-control and self-esteem.*
- Encourage to maintain life roles to the extent possible. *Maintaining roles helps the client cope with this chronic and potentially crippling disease.*
- Refer to counseling or support groups. *Counseling and support groups can help the client and family develop effective coping strategies.*

DISTURBED BODY IMAGE

- Demonstrate a caring, accepting attitude. *This helps the client accept physical changes caused by RA and avoid feelings of hopelessness or powerlessness.*
- Encourage discussion about the effects of RA, both physical and psychosocial. *Verbalization helps the client identify feelings and provides an opportunity to validate these feelings.*
- Involve client in decision making and provide choices whenever possible. *Autonomy enhances the sense of control.*
- Discuss clothing and adaptive devices that promote independence. *Independence enhances self-esteem.*

- Provide positive feedback for self-care activities and adaptive strategies. *Positive reinforcement encourages the client to continue adaptive measures and maintain independence.*
- Refer to self-help groups, support groups, the Arthritis Foundation, and other agencies for assistive devices and literature. *These groups can help the client develop strategies to cope with the effects of RA, enhancing self-concept, body image, and independence.*

EVALUATING

To evaluate the effectiveness of nursing care for a client with RA, collect data such as: quality and quantity of rest; effective use of NSAIDs and analgesics; ability to maintain ADLs and usual roles; statements about body image and coping with disease effects.

Discharge Considerations

The client has the primary responsibility for managing rheumatoid arthritis. Assessment and teaching are vital to prepare for this responsibility. Box 28-13 outlines assessment data to collect related to home care.

BOX 28-13
ASSESSING FOR DISCHARGE

RHEUMATOID ARTHRITIS
Client

- Ability to perform ADLs; need for help or assistive devices; ability to cope with activity limitations and economic effects; acceptance of assistance from others
- Understanding of rheumatoid arthritis and its effects; prescribed medications; activity and rest recommendations; long-term prognosis
- Home environment: Stairs, environmental barriers that limit independence (e.g., small bathrooms, deep tubs for bathing); energy-saving features (such as easily loaded clothes washer and dryer, easy to clean floors)

Family and Caregivers

- Ability and willingness to assist with ADLs and household tasks; acceptance of rest needs and altered roles and relationships
- Financial resources for prescribed drugs and treatments

Community

- Availability of home health services; access to public transportation, medical services, pharmacies
- Support groups and other resources

Teach about the disease and its systemic effects. Stress the importance of following all aspects of the treatment plan. Encourage active involvement in planning care.

Help identify strategies to balance rest and exercise. Instruct to reduce exercise and increase rest if pain and stiffness increase. Teach to use heat and cold to promote comfort and activity.

Teach about prescribed medications. Emphasize the need to take NSAIDs as ordered, not on an as-needed basis for pain. Review Table 28-5 for additional client and family teaching about NSAIDs. Emphasize the importance of keeping regular follow-up appointments to monitor the disease and treatment.

Suggest assistive devices to maintain independence. Include ambulatory aids, such as canes and walkers, and self-care aids, such as hand-held showers, long-handled brushes and shoe horns, and eating utensils with over-sized or special handles. Discuss clothing options to help maintain independence, such as elastic waist pants without zippers, Velcro closures, zippers with large pull tabs, and slip-on shoes. Refer to local and community agencies as indicated.

CLINICAL alert

Remember that the client with rheumatoid arthritis is vulnerable to quackery and unproven alternative treatment strategies. Maintain open lines of communication to encourage discussion of these options and possible experimental therapies with the treatment team.

Nursing Process Case Study
■ CLIENT WITH RHEUMATOID ARTHRITIS

Janice James, 42 years old, first noticed vague joint pain, fatigue, poor appetite, and general malaise about 6 weeks ago. Her symptoms have continued, and she reports feeling very stiff in the mornings, often lasting until 10:00 or 11:00 A.M. She sees her nurse practitioner (NP) when she notices that her knuckles and finger joints are not just achy but also swollen and hot. The NP tentatively diagnoses rheumatoid arthritis and refers Mrs. James to a rheumatology clinic.

Assessment Mrs. James's past medical history reveals only the usual childhood diseases and three uncomplicated pregnancies and deliveries. Mrs. James states that she is allergic to penicillin.

Objective assessment data reveals swelling of PIP and MCP joints of both hands. The second and third PIP and second MCP joints on the right hand appear red and shiny, and are hot, spongy, and tender to palpation. Mrs. James can extend her fingers to 180 degrees but cannot make a complete fist with either hand. Her grip strength is weak bilaterally. Wrist ROM is limited in all directions. Mrs. James's knees also appear swollen, and flexion is slightly limited.

Blood work shows ESR 52 mm/hr and hematocrit 30%. She has a positive rheumatoid factor.

Diagnosis The following nursing diagnoses are identified for Mrs. James:

■ Pain related to joint inflammation
■ Impaired Home Maintenance related to fatigue
■ Activity Intolerance related to the effects of inflammation
■ Risk for Noncompliance with therapeutic regimen related to lack of information and understanding

Expected Outcomes The expected outcomes are that Mrs. James will:

■ Verbalize effective pain-management strategies.
■ Verbalize a plan to reduce her responsibilities for home maintenance.
■ Express a willingness to plan rest breaks during the day.
■ Demonstrate understanding of the prescribed treatment and the importance of compliance for both short- and long-term benefit.

Planning and Implementation The following nursing interventions are implemented over the first 6 weeks of Mrs. James's care at the rheumatology clinic:

■ Teach ways to relieve pain and morning stiffness, including:
   a. Take NSAIDs at equal intervals throughout the day.
   b. Take morning NSAID dose with milk and crackers about 30 minutes before arising.
   c. Perform ROM exercises in shower or bathtub.
■ Teach ways to minimize joint stress while performing ADLs.
■ Discuss delegation of household tasks to other family members.
■ Explore ways to incorporate 30-minute rest breaks into work schedule.
■ Reinforce teaching about disease process, prescribed drugs and their effects, and the importance of balanced rest and exercise.

Evaluation After 6 months, Mrs. James's "morning sickness" now lasts about 45 minutes, and her hand and wrist ROM have improved. She has had difficulty scheduling rest periods at work and has had to struggle to delegate household tasks. "I don't look sick to the kids, and they seem to think housecleaning is a terrible imposition on their time. It's often easier to just do it myself than to fight about it. Besides, that way it gets done right." Mrs. James has faithfully followed her treatment plan, keeping her scheduled appointments and maintaining contact with the treatment team.

Critical Thinking in the Nursing Process

1. Explain the normal inflammatory process and relate this to the inflammatory joint changes Mrs. James experienced. Discuss the systemic effects of inflammation on Mrs. James as well.
2. When Mrs. James experiences an acute exacerbation of her disease one year later, the rheumatologist orders prednisone, 40 mg daily. The effect is dramatic in relieving

Mrs. James's pain and stiffness. She asks why the physician did not prescribe this drug in the first place. How will you respond?

Systemic Lupus Erythematosus

Systemic lupus erythematosus (SLE) is a chronic inflammatory connective tissue disease. SLE affects multiple body systems. It can range in severity from mild and episodic to a rapidly fatal disease.

SLE is much more common in women than in men and in Asians and Hispanics. It is more common and severe in people of African ancestry. Its cause is unknown, but genetic, environmental, and hormonal factors play a role in its development.

PATHOPHYSIOLOGY

In SLE, autoantibodies are produced that target normal body cells and cell components such as DNA, blood cells, and proteins involved in normal coagulation. These autoantibodies react with their corresponding antigen to form immune complexes, which are then deposited in the connective tissue of blood vessels, lymphatic vessels, and other tissues. This causes an inflammatory response that damages the tissues. Immune complexes frequently are deposited in and damage the kidneys. Other affected tissues include the musculoskeletal system, brain, heart, spleen, lung, GI tract, skin, and peritoneum.

Early in the disease, the manifestations of SLE mimic those of rheumatoid arthritis, including fever, anorexia, malaise, weight loss, and joint pain, inflammation, and stiffness. Skin manifestations are common. SLE was named for its characteristic red *butterfly rash* across the cheeks and bridge of the nose (Figure 28-8 ◆). This rash was thought to resemble the bite of a wolf, hence *lupus* (wolf) *erythematosus* (red). Many

Figure 28-8. ◆ The butterfly rash of systemic lupus erythematosus.

clients with SLE are photosensitive. A diffuse rash on skin exposed to the sun is common. Because SLE affects many body systems, its manifestations can be diverse (Figure 28-9 ◆).

The course of SLE is mild and chronic in most clients, with periods of remission and exacerbation. The number and severity of exacerbations tend to decrease with time.

Clients with SLE often have difficulty carrying a pregnancy to term. They also have an increased risk for infections, which may be severe. Infections such as pneumonia and septicemia are the leading cause of death in clients with SLE, followed by the effects of kidney or central nervous system involvement.

COLLABORATIVE CARE

The diagnosis of SLE is based on the history and physical exam, along with diagnostic tests. As with RA, effective management requires teamwork, with active participation by the client and the health care team.

Diagnostic Tests
- *Antinuclear antibodies (ANA)* are identified. While virtually all clients with SLE have positive ANA tests, so do many clients who do not have SLE.
- *Anti-DNA antibody testing* is a more specific indicator of SLE.
- The *erythrocyte sedimentation rate (ESR or sed rate)* often is elevated, and the CBC shows anemia and low RBC, WBC, and platelet counts.
- *Urinalysis* and renal function studies such as the *serum creatinine* and *blood urea nitrogen (BUN)* may be ordered to assess for kidney damage.

Pharmacology
Aspirin and NSAIDs often are used to manage joint pain and inflammation, fever, and fatigue. Table 28-5 outlined nursing responsibilities for aspirin and NSAIDs. Antimalarial drugs such as hydroxychloroquine (Plaquenil) may be ordered. Hydroxychloroquine can damage the retina of the eye; for this reason, an ophthalmologic exam is done every 6 months during treatment.

Corticosteroid drugs are used to treat severe and life-threatening manifestations of SLE. Some clients require long-term corticosteroid therapy to manage symptoms and prevent major organ damage. These clients have a high risk for corticosteroid side effects, such as cushingoid effects, weight gain, hypertension, infection, accelerated osteoporosis, and hypokalemia. See Chapter 13 for more information about corticosteroid therapy and its nursing implications. Immunosuppressive agents may be used alone or in combination with corticosteroids. These drugs increase the risk for infection and malignancy, and have other toxic effects.

Other Therapies
Because of the photosensitivity associated with SLE, sun exposure should be avoided. Sunscreens with a sun protection factor (SPF) rating of 15 or higher are recommended when out of

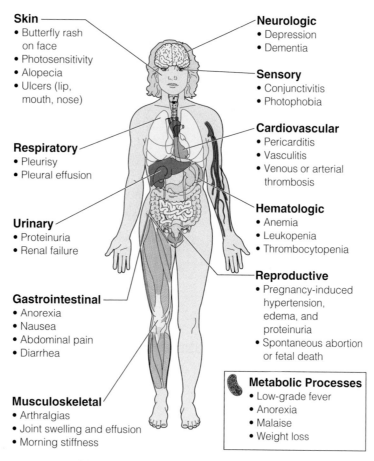

Skin
- Butterfly rash on face
- Photosensitivity
- Alopecia
- Ulcers (lip, mouth, nose)

Respiratory
- Pleurisy
- Pleural effusion

Urinary
- Proteinuria
- Renal failure

Gastrointestinal
- Anorexia
- Nausea
- Abdominal pain
- Diarrhea

Musculoskeletal
- Arthralgias
- Joint swelling and effusion
- Morning stiffness

Neurologic
- Depression
- Dementia

Sensory
- Conjunctivitis
- Photophobia

Cardiovascular
- Pericarditis
- Vasculitis
- Venous or arterial thrombosis

Hematologic
- Anemia
- Leukopenia
- Thrombocytopenia

Reproductive
- Pregnancy-induced hypertension, edema, and proteinuria
- Spontaneous abortion or fetal death

Metabolic Processes
- Low-grade fever
- Anorexia
- Malaise
- Weight loss

Figure 28-9. ◆ The multisystem effects of systemic lupus erythematosus.

doors. Some physicians recommend avoiding oral contraceptives, because estrogen can trigger an acute episode of SLE.

Clients with lupus nephritis who develop end-stage renal disease are treated with dialysis (hemodialysis or peritoneal dialysis) and kidney transplantation. These treatment strategies are discussed in Chapter 21.

NURSING CARE

Many of the nursing care needs for the client with SLE are similar to those for clients with rheumatoid arthritis. This section focuses on the needs related to dermatologic symptoms of lupus, the increased risk for infection, and health maintenance problems.

IMPAIRED SKIN INTEGRITY

Skin lesions are a common manifestation of SLE. They disrupt skin integrity and can be disfiguring.

- Discuss the relationship between sun exposure and disease activity, both dermatologic and systemic. *It is important for the client to understand that sun exposure can worsen both skin and systemic manifestations of SLE.*
- Help identify strategies to limit sun exposure:

a. Avoid being outside when sun is most intense (10:00 A.M. to 3:00 P.M.).
b. Use sunscreen with an SPF of 15 or higher.
c. Reapply sunscreen after swimming, exercising, or bathing.
d. Wear loose clothing with long sleeves and wide-brimmed hats when outside.
These strategies can help the client maintain a normal lifestyle while helping to prevent acute episodes.

- Keep skin clean and dry; apply therapeutic creams or ointments to lesions as ordered. *These measures promote healing and reduce the risk of infection.*

INEFFECTIVE PROTECTION

- Wash hands on entering room and before providing direct care. *Handwashing is the best defense against transmitting infection.*
- Use strict sterile technique in caring for intravenous lines and indwelling urinary catheters or performing any wound care. *Aseptic technique reduces the risk of contamination by microorganisms.*
- Monitor temperature and vital signs every 4 hours. Report signs of infection, including tenderness, redness, swelling, and warmth. *Prompt identification of an infection allows early initiation of appropriate treatment.*

■ Report abnormal laboratory values. *Increased WBCs may indicate infection; changes in liver or renal function studies, myocardial enzymes, or other laboratory values may indicate organ system involvement.*

■ If necessary, use protective isolation. *Treatment with corticosteroids or immunosuppressive agents impairs the ability to fight infection. Protective isolation may be necessary to prevent infection.*

■ Instruct family members and visitors to avoid direct contact with the client when they are ill. *A "minor" upper respiratory infection can be a significant illness for the client with SLE.*

■ Help ensure adequate food intake, offering supplementary feedings as indicated or maintaining parenteral nutrition if necessary. *Adequate nutrition is important for healing and immune system function.*

■ Teach the importance of good hand washing after using the bathroom and before eating. *Handwashing reduces the risk of infection with endogenous organisms.*

■ Provide good mouth care. *Good oral hygiene reduces the risk of infection from oral bacteria.*

Discharge Considerations

Teach about SLE and its potential effects. Both physical manifestations of SLE and psychosocial issues can affect the ability to effectively manage the disease. Encourage discussion about the impact of the disease. Refer the client and family to counseling as needed. Provide information about community and social service agencies, and local support groups.

Discuss the importance of skin care. Instruct to avoid irritating soaps, shampoos, or chemicals (e.g., hair dyes and permanent wave solution) to prevent excessive drying of the skin. Encourage use of hypoallergenic products. Stress the importance of limiting sun exposure, particularly between 10:00 A.M. and 3:00 P.M. Encourage use of appropriate sunscreen and to wear long sleeves and wide-brimmed hats. For clients with hair loss, discuss using wigs, turbans, or other head coverings. Remind that the hair will regrow during remission.

Stress the importance of avoiding exposure to infection. Encourage to avoid crowds and infectious people. Teach the importance of adequate rest and nutrition and avoiding stress to increase resistance to infection.

Teach about treatment plan, including rest and exercise, medications, and follow-up appointments. Stress the importance of contacting the physician promptly if symptoms of an exacerbation develop. Encourage to wear a medical alert bracelet or tag with their condition and therapy such as corticosteroids or immunosuppressives.

Discuss family planning. Oral contraceptives may be contraindicated; provide information about alternative means of birth control. Pregnancy is not contraindicated; however, the client should tell her women's health care practitioner of her SLE and notify her primary care physician of her pregnancy.

Gout

Gout is a metabolic disorder that leads to accumulation of urate crystals in joints and surrounding tissues. It affects more men than women, and its incidence increases with age.

Gout may be primary or secondary. *Primary gout* is a genetic disorder characterized by elevated serum uric acid levels. It is the most common form of gout. In *secondary gout,* uric acid levels increase due to another disorder or treatment with certain drugs. Disorders such as leukemia, chronic renal disease, and diabetic ketoacidosis can raise uric acid levels, as can drugs such as some diuretics and antituberculosis drugs. Alcohol ingestion also increases serum uric acid levels.

PATHOPHYSIOLOGY

Uric acid is the breakdown product of purine metabolism. Normally, a balance exists between the production and excretion of uric acid, with most of what is produced each day excreted via the kidneys and the rest in the feces. The serum uric acid level is normally between 3.4 and 7.0 mg/dL in men and 2.4 and 6.0 mg/dL in women. At levels greater than 7.0 mg/dL, urate crystals may form. Crystals tend to form in peripheral tissues of the body, where lower temperatures reduce the solubility of the uric acid.

Unless treated, gout may progress from *asymptomatic hyperuricemia,* with high serum uric acid levels but no symptoms, to *acute gouty arthritis.* The acute attack, usually affecting a single joint, occurs unexpectedly, often beginning at night. About half of initial attacks are in the joint of the great toe. The affected joint becomes red, hot, swollen, and exquisitely painful and tender. The client also may have fever, chills, and general malaise.

Acute attacks last from days up to several weeks and typically subside spontaneously. The interval between acute attacks is called the *intercritical period.* It may last years, although most people have another acute attack within 1 year. In *chronic tophaceous gout,* deposits of urate crystals known as tophi develop in cartilage, synovial membranes, tendons, and soft tissues. Tophi may be seen in the helix of the ear and on the extremities. The skin over tophi may ulcerate. Tophi can also develop in the tissues of the heart and spinal epidura. In some cases, uric acid stones may form in the kidney.

COLLABORATIVE CARE

The classic presentation of acute gout is so distinctive that the diagnosis often is based on the history and physical exam. *Serum uric acid* is nearly always elevated, usually above 7.5 mg/dL. Fluid aspirated from the inflamed joint shows typical needle-shaped urate crystals.

Treatment focuses on relieving an acute attack and preventing recurrent attacks.

Pharmacology

Nonsteroidal anti-inflammatory drugs (NSAIDs) are used to treat an acute attack of gout. Indomethacin (Indocin) is the most frequently used NSAID for gout. Aspirin is avoided because it may interfere with uric acid excretion. Review Table 28-5 for nursing implications for NSAIDs.

Colchicine, a drug that inhibits the deposition of urate crystals in tissues, also may be ordered to stop an acute attack. The use of colchicine, however, is limited by side effects such as abdominal cramping, diarrhea, nausea, or vomiting. Colchicine may be used in smaller doses (with fewer side effects) to prevent attacks of gout.

Drugs to promote uric acid excretion or block its production may be ordered to prevent attacks. *Uricosuric* drugs block reabsorption of uric acid in the kidney tubules, promoting its

excretion and reducing serum levels. Allopurinol affects purine metabolism, decreasing the production of uric acid (see Table 28-6 ◆).

Other Therapies

During an acute attack of gout, bed rest is ordered. It is continued for about 24 hours after the attack has subsided. The affected joint may be elevated, and hot or cold compresses may be applied for comfort.

A liberal fluid intake (3 or more liters per day) is ordered. Sodium bicarbonate or potassium citrate may be ordered to minimize the risk of uric acid renal stones.

TABLE 28-6

NURSING IMPLICATIONS FOR PHARMACOLOGY: CLIENTS WITH GOUT

DRUG/CLASSIFICATION	DESCRIPTION	NURSING RESPONSIBILITIES	CLIENT TEACHING
Colchicine	Colchicine prevents urate crystals from being deposited in tissues. It does not lower serum uric acid levels. It is available in combination with a uricosuric agent, probenecid. Plain colchicine is used to treat an acute attack of gout; combination therapy is used to prevent further attacks.	Assess for contraindications, such as serious GI, kidney, liver, or heart disease. Administer by mouth on an empty stomach. Report nausea, vomiting, or diarrhea to the physician; these side effects may require stopping the drug.	Drink 3–4 quarts of liquid per day. Report reactions such as GI distress, fatigue, bleeding, easy bruising, or recurrent infections to your doctor. Avoid using alcohol while you are taking this drug.
Uricosuric Drugs ▪ Probenecid (Benemid)	Probenecid inhibits the tubular reabsorption of urate, increasing the excretion of uric acid and decreasing serum uric acid levels.	Give after meals or with milk. Monitor intake and output. Increase fluid intake to at least 3 liters per day. Report adverse effects such as headache, dizziness, nausea and vomiting, flank pain, fever, hives, pruritus, and abnormal lab values.	Do not take aspirin or products containing aspirin while taking probenecid. Use acetaminophen for relief of mild pain. Drink at least 3 quarts of fluids per day.
▪ Sulfinpyrazone (Anturane)	Sulfinpyrazone improves uric acid excretion, reducing serum uric acid levels. It is used to prevent recurrent attacks of acute gout and treat chronic gout.	Give with meals or antacid. Monitor diabetic clients for hypoglycemia. Monitor for bleeding in clients receiving warfarin. Encourage fluid intake of at least 3 liters per day. Do not give concurrently with aspirin. Report signs of peptic ulcer disease to the physician promptly.	Drink at least 3 quarts of fluid per day. Take with meals to minimize gastric distress. Do not take aspirin; use acetaminophen for relief of mild pain. Report epigastric pain, nausea, or black stools to the physician promptly. Discontinue the drug immediately.

(continues)

	NURSING IMPLICATIONS FOR PHARMACOLOGY: CLIENTS WITH GOUT (CONTINUED)		
DRUG/CLASSIFICATION	**DESCRIPTION**	**NURSING RESPONSIBILITIES**	**CLIENT TEACHING**
Allopurinol (Zyloprim)	Allopurinol reduces uric acid production, lowering serum uric acid levels. It is used for clients with manifestations of primary or secondary gout.	Monitor intake and output. Increase fluids to 3 liters per day. Report adverse effects such as nausea, diarrhea, and rash. Give with meals. Report abnormal kidney and liver function tests, CBC, and prothrombin time or INR to the physician. Discontinue drug and notify the physician immediately if a rash develops.	Stop the drug and report skin rash, painful urination, bloody urine, eye irritation, or swelling of lips or mouth to your doctor. Take after meals. Drink 3–4 liters of fluid daily. Report abnormal bleeding, bruising, fatigue, pallor, sore throat, or frequent infections to your doctor. Acute gout may occur when you start this drug; continue drug as ordered. Do not take a double dose if you miss a dose. Use caution when driving, operating machinery, or performing other activities that require alertness; may cause drowsiness.

TABLE 28-6

CLINICAL alert

Carefully monitor clients receiving sodium bicarbonate or potassium citrate for fluid and electrolyte or acid–base imbalances (see Chapter 5).

Often, no specific diet is recommended. The obese client is advised to lose weight, but fasting is contraindicated. Alcohol intake and specific foods that tend to precipitate attacks are avoided.

NURSING CARE

ACUTE PAIN

Pain is a primary focus for nursing assessment and interventions during an acute attack of gout.

- Ask client to rate pain using a standard pain scale. Note the location and quality of the pain. *Acute gout causes exquisite tenderness of the affected joint. Accurate assessment of pain facilitates evaluation of treatment measures.*
- Position for comfort. Elevate the joint or extremity (usually the great toe) on a pillow, maintaining alignment. *Elevating the joint improves blood return, relieving some of the edema.*
- Protect the affected joint from pressure, using a foot cradle to keep covers off the foot. *Affected joints are so tender that even the weight of a sheet can be unbearable.*

- Administer prescribed anti-inflammatory and antigout medications as ordered. In the initial period, colchicine may be given hourly. *These medications reduce the acute inflammatory response, gradually relieving discomfort.*
- Administer analgesics as prescribed. *Analgesics often are ordered until the acute inflammation is relieved.*
- Monitor for desired and adverse effects of medications. Report adverse effects to the physician. *Anti-inflammatory and antigout medications can have significant side effects that may require a change of therapy.*
- Maintain bed rest. *Rest and immobilizing the affected joint help reduce joint inflammation.*

Discharge Considerations

Without appropriate treatment between episodes of acute gout, recurrences are likely. Teaching is a vital nursing responsibility for the client with gout.

Teach about the disease and its manifestations. Advise that initial attacks cause no permanent damage but recurrent attacks can lead to permanent damage and joint destruction. Discuss other potential effects of continued hyperuricemia, including tophaceous deposits in subcutaneous and other connective tissues. Discuss the risk for kidney damage and stones.

Teach about prescribed medications. Stress the need to continue medications until discontinued by the physician, even if there are no symptoms. Discuss potential side effects of the drugs, and their management. Instruct to drink about 3 quarts of fluid per day and to avoid using alcohol. Instruct to avoid over-the-counter medications without talking to the physician. Encourage to keep scheduled follow-up appointments.

Lyme Disease

Lyme disease is an inflammatory disorder caused by a spirochete, *Borrelia burgdorferi,* which is usually spread by ticks. It is the most commonly reported tick-borne illness in the United States. Although Lyme disease is usually seen in children, adults also can be affected. Geographically, Lyme disease is more common in the Northeast, Upper Midwest, and along the Pacific Coast. Ticks that act as vectors for Lyme disease are usually carried by mice or deer. The usual time of onset is the summer months.

Borrelia burgdorferi enters the skin at the site of the tick bite. After an incubation period of up to 30 days, it migrates outward in the skin, forming a characteristic lesion called *erythema migrans.* It may spread via lymph or blood to other skin sites, nodes, or organs.

Erythema migrans is the initial manifestation of Lyme disease. This flat or slightly raised red lesion at the site of the tick bite expands over several days (up to a diameter of 50 cm), with the central area clearing as it expands. Systemic symptoms such as fatigue, malaise, fever, chills, and muscle pain often accompany the initial lesion. As the disease spreads, secondary skin lesions develop, as do migratory musculoskeletal symptoms, including muscle and joint pain, and tendonitis. Headache and stiff neck are common. If untreated, the client may develop chronic arthritis, myocarditis, meningitis, encephalitis, and other neurologic manifestations.

A number of antibiotics may be used to treat Lyme disease. Treatment may be continued for up to 1 month to ensure that the organism has been eradicated. Aspirin or another NSAID may be prescribed to relieve arthritic symptoms. The affected joint may be splinted to rest the joint. When the knee is involved, weight bearing may be restricted and the client instructed to use crutches.

The nursing role in treating Lyme disease is primarily educational. Teach about the disease and its transmission. Emphasize the importance of completing the full course of antibiotic therapy. Discuss possible adverse effects of treatment and their appropriate management. Teach the client with arthritic manifestations about using NSAIDs, including the importance of maintaining a consistent schedule of doses rather than taking the medication only as needed for pain.

Nurses can take a major role in educating the public about Lyme disease and its prevention. Box 28-14 provides important information about preventing Lyme disease.

Ankylosing Spondylitis

Ankylosing spondylitis is a chronic inflammatory arthritis that primarily affects the spine, causing pain and progressive stiffening. The cause of ankylosing spondylitis is unknown. Heredity plays a role in its development. It affects men more often than women.

BOX 28-14
TEACHING FOR DISCHARGE

PREVENTING LYME DISEASE

- Avoid tick-infested areas, particularly tall grasses and dense brush.
- When walking or working in potentially infested areas, wear clothing that completely covers the extremities (e.g., long pants tucked into boot tops or long socks, and long-sleeved shirts tucked into pants).
- Use an insect repellent such as diethyltoluamide (DEET) or permethrin on skin and clothing.
- Inspect skin and clothing for ticks after you have been outside.
- Protect pets with tick collars and inspect them frequently for ticks.
- Remove any ticks found on the body or pets immediately. Grasp the mouth portion of the tick with fine tweezers where it enters the skin, and pull steadily and firmly until the tick releases. Do not twist or jerk.
- Put the tick in alcohol and save it for future examination in case you develop symptoms. Do not crush the tick.
- Wash the affected area thoroughly with soap and water; apply an antiseptic.
- If you develop flulike symptoms or a "bull's-eye" rash around the tick bite, notify a physician immediately.

The onset of ankylosing spondylitis is usually insidious. Clients may complain of persistent or intermittent bouts of low back pain. The pain is worse at night, followed by morning stiffness that is relieved by activity. Pain may radiate to the buttocks, hips, or down the legs. As the disease progresses, back motion is limited, the lumbar curve is lost, and the thoracic curvature is accentuated. In severe cases, the entire spine is fused, preventing any motion. Clients with ankylosing spondylitis may also develop arthritis in other joints, primarily the hip, shoulders, and knees. Systemic manifestations include anorexia, weight loss, fever, and fatigue. Many clients develop uveitis, inflammation of the iris and the middle, vascular layer of the eye.

Physical therapy and daily exercises are important to maintain posture and joint range of motion. NSAIDs relieve pain and stiffness and allow the client to perform necessary exercises.

As with other chronic arthritic disorders, the primary nursing role in ankylosing spondylitis is providing supportive care and education. Encourage to maintain a fluid intake of 2,500 mL or more per day. Suggest performing exercises in the shower because warm, moist heat prompts mobility.

Uveitis may cause photophobia and blurred vision in the affected eye. Provide indirect lighting and a darkened room for photophobia. If vision is significantly impaired, use appropriate measures such as:

■ Orient to surroundings; do not move furniture or place objects in usual pathways.

■ Introduce yourself verbally when entering the room. Tell client what you are doing during procedures.

■ Assist during ambulation by allowing client to hold your elbow.

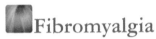

Fibromyalgia

Fibromyalgia, also known as *fibrositis,* is a common rheumatic syndrome of musculoskeletal pain, stiffness, and tenderness. Fibromyalgia usually affects women over the age of 50. It may be precipitated or aggravated by stress, sleep disorders, trauma, or depression.

The cause of fibromyalgia is unknown, and its pathophysiology is unclear. A gradual onset of chronic, achy muscle pain is typical. The pain may be localized or involve the entire body. The neck, shoulders, lower back, and hips are often affected. Tenderness is present, usually in small, localized trigger points. Local tightness or muscle spasm may also occur. Systemic manifestations of fibromyalgia include fatigue, sleep disruptions, headaches, and an irritable bowel. Pain and fatigue are aggravated by exertion.

This disorder may resolve spontaneously or become chronic and recurrent. The client with fibromyalgia needs reassurance of the benign nature of the disorder along with validation of its reality. Other therapeutic measures include local heat, massage, stretching and low-impact aerobic exercises, and sleep improvement. Amitriptyline, a tricyclic antidepressant, has been found to promote better sleep and relieve symptoms of fibromyalgia.

Nursing care for clients with fibromyalgia is supportive and educational, provided in community settings such as clinics and other primary care settings. It is important to validate concerns and reassure clients that their symptoms are not "all in the head." This syndrome is recognizable and manageable; its course is not progressive. Teach about the disorder. Provide verbal and written instructions about management strategies. Instruct to take prescribed medications at bedtime, because they may cause drowsiness. Caution about driving while taking the medication.

Low Back Pain

Acute or chronic low back pain usually is due to strains in the muscles and tendons of the back caused by abnormal stress or overuse. It involves the lumbar, lumbosacral, or sacroiliac areas of the back. Low back pain caused by degenerative disk disease and herniated vertebral disks is covered in Chapter 30.

PATHOPHYSIOLOGY

In general, there are five types of back pain:

■ *Local pain,* often caused by fractures, strains, or sprains. Tumors also may press on pain-sensitive structures, causing local pain.

■ *Referred pain* is caused by disorders of organs in the abdomen or pelvis, such as gastrointestinal or genitourinary disorders or an abdominal aortic aneurysm.

■ *Pain of spinal origin* is associated with pathology of the spine such as disk disease or arthritis.

■ *Radicular back pain* radiates from the back to the leg along a nerve root. It is sharp pain that may be aggravated by movement, such as coughing, sneezing, or sitting.

■ *Muscle spasm pain* is associated with many spine disorders. This type of back pain is dull and may be accompanied by abnormal posture and taut spinal muscles.

Low back pain may range from mild discomfort lasting a few hours to chronic, debilitating pain. Acute pain is usually caused by an activity such as lifting and bending or twisting.

COLLABORATIVE CARE

Low back pain usually is diagnosed by the history and physical exam. X-rays, CT scan, and MRI are ordered only when a potentially serious underlying condition is suspected.

Most clients with acute low back pain need only short-term treatment. Ice packs or ice massage can be applied or rubbed over the painful area for 15 minutes every hour or more. Moist, warm towels or a heating pad can be used as an alternative to ice therapy.

Prolonged rest is not recommended. In fact, increased activity helps to restore function and may increase endorphin levels. Exercise is initiated and increased gradually. Physical therapy frequently is used in combination with exercise. Diathermy (deep heat therapy), ultrasonography, hydrotherapy, and transcutaneous electrical nerve stimulation (TENS) units may be used to reduce the muscle spasms and relieve pain.

Other treatments include chiropractic manipulation of the spine to reduce spasms and pain. *Back school* is a rehabilitation program that teaches about the anatomy of the spine and ways to decrease the risk of recurring back injury.

Low back pain often can be managed with NSAIDs and analgesics. Muscle relaxants also may be ordered. For intense, intractable pain, a steroid solution may be injected into the epidural space. This helps decrease the swelling and inflammation of the spinal nerves.

NURSING CARE

INEFFECTIVE HEALTH MAINTENANCE

■ Teach appropriate body mechanics in lifting and reaching. Instruct to plan the lift, keep the object being lifted close to the body, and avoid twisting when lifting. Encourage to obtain help when lifting. *Using good body mechanics can prevent many back injuries.*

■ Encourage to avoid prolonged standing or sitting, lying prone, and wearing high heels. *These activities exacerbate back pain.*

■ Encourage an exercise program to strengthen abdominal and back muscles. Teach or refer for teaching about exercises such as partial sit-ups with the knees bent and knee–chest exercises to stretch hamstrings and spinal muscles. Instruct to do each exercise five times, gradually increasing to ten repetitions. Advise to stop any exercise that increases pain, and seek professional advice before continuing. *Prescribed back exercises, such as the pelvic tilt, partial sit-ups, and back rolls, strengthen back and abdominal muscles, reducing the risk of back injury and pain.*

■ Suggest workplace or environmental modifications to minimize stress on the lower back. *Lumbar supports in chairs, adjustment of chair or table height, and rubber floor mats help prevent back strain or injury.*

■ Encourage obese clients to lose weight. *Obesity changes the center of gravity, and increases the risk of injury when lifting.*

■ Encourage to stop smoking. *Smoking contributes to disk degeneration and the risk of injury.*

PAIN

■ Assess the quality, severity, and location of pain, as well as factors that tend to aggravate or relieve it. *Accurate assessment data can help identify the cause and type of pain.*

■ Instruct to take NSAIDs or analgesics on a routine schedule rather than as needed. *Maintaining a constant blood level of NSAIDs or analgesics reduces inflammation and improves pain relief.*

■ Instruct the client on bed rest to assume a side-lying position with the hips and knees flexed. Keep a pillow under or between the knees. Instruct to use a footstool when seated to support the weight of the feet. *These measures decrease pressure on intervertebral disks and spinal nerves.*

■ Teach about the "rebound phenomenon" of prolonged heat or ice therapy. *Ice remaining on the skin longer than 15 minutes or heat longer than 30 minutes causes a reverse effect known as the rebound phenomenon, and can increase inflammation and pain.*

Discharge Considerations

Back pain is a common problem. Nurses can make an impact on this significant problem by teaching health practices to prevent back pain. Teach safe lifing, bending, and turning during physical activity. Stress the importance of using large muscle groups of the legs to lift rather than bending and lifting with the smaller muscles of the back. Teach other aspects of good body mechanics, including posture, sleeping on a firm mattress, and sitting in chairs that provide good support. Discuss the positive effect of maintaining optimal body weight and good physical fitness.

In industrial and work settings, nurses should be alert for situations that increase the risk of back pain and injury. Office workers should have chairs with appropriate seat height and length and back support. Modifications of work space or machinery may be necessary for industrial workers to avoid excess stresses on back muscles. Finally, it is important to remember that back pain is a leading cause of lost work time for nurses themselves. Remind co-workers to use good body mechanics and to seek help when lifting or moving clients.

Muscular Dystrophy

Muscular dystrophy (MD) is a group of inherited muscular diseases that cause progressive muscle degeneration and wasting. The most common form of MD, *Duchenne's muscular dystrophy,* is inherited as a sex-linked recessive disorder, and is therefore transmitted from the mother to male children. This disorder affects males exclusively and occurs in 1 out of 3,500 live male births.

Muscle fiber atrophy, necrosis, regeneration, and fibrosis lead to progressive weakness of voluntary muscles in MD. The pattern of muscle weakness and the rate at which it progresses vary, depending on the type of MD. As the disease progresses, the person develops difficulty ambulating and eventually becomes wheelchair-bound and finally bed-bound.

There is no cure or specific treatment for MD. Care focuses on preserving and promoting mobility. A multidisciplinary approach, involving many members of the health care team, is necessary to meet the physical and psychological needs of these clients and their families.

Nursing care focuses on promoting independence and mobility and providing psychologic support. Teach about prescribed exercises such as stretching and counterposturing exercises. Discuss skin care and ways to prevent irritation under braces. Because the muscles of respiration may be affected, discuss ways to prevent respiratory infections, such as avoiding crowds during flu season and being immunized against pneumococcal pneumonia and influenza. Provide information about support services and organizations such as the Muscular Dystrophy Association.

Nursing Interventions Classification

The following Nursing Interventions (McCloskey & Bulechek, 2000) also may be helpful when caring for clients with musculoskeletal disorders:

■ Energy Management
■ Environmental Management: Safety
■ Exercise Promotion
■ Exercise Therapy: Joint Mobility
■ Fall Prevention
■ Pain Management
■ Positioning
■ Splinting
■ Teaching: Prescribed Medications

(*Note:* The bibliography listings for this and all chapters have been compiled at the back of the book.)

Chapter Review

key terms by topic

Use the CD-ROM disk enclosed with your textbook to hear the pronunciation of the key terms in the chapter.

Structural and bone disorders
scoliosis, kyphosis, osteoporosis, pathologic fracture, osteomyelitis, debride

Joint and connective tissue disorders
arthritis, osteoarthritis (OA), arthralgia, arthroplasty, rheumatoid arthritis (RA), systemic lupus erythematosus, gout, muscular dystrophy (MD)

key points

- Musculoskeletal system disorders affect comfort, mobility, ADLs, and safety. Education is a primary nursing role in all these disorders.

- Prevention is a key strategy for osteoporosis. Stress the importance of adequate calcium intake throughout the lifespan, and encourage menopausal clients to discuss preventive measures with their health care provider.

- Osteomyelitis, infection of the bone, is difficult to treat; prevention and early identification are vital. Promptly report general signs of infection, as well as redness, heat, wound drainage, continued pain , and refusal to use or bear weight on an extremity.

- Benign bone tumors and metastasis of tumors from other locations are more common than primary malignancy of the bone.

- Most people develop osteoarthritis as they age. The pain and joint effects of osteoarthritis are localized and are managed symptomatically with balanced rest and activity.

- Rheumatoid arthritis, on the other hand, is a systemic inflammatory disease. Its management is directed toward reducing inflammation and preventing joint destruction. Rheumatoid arthritis can have crippling effects. Stress the importance of a multidisciplinary treatment regimen to maintain function and mobility.

- Systemic lupus erythematosus also is a systemic connective tissue disease with symptoms similar to RA. It is less likely to cause joint crippling, but has more widespread effects than RA in many people. Reducing inflammation is a priority in both disorders.

- The arthritis of gout is caused by a disorder of purine metabolism and excess uric acid build-up in the body. It is not caused by eating too much rich food.

 ## Medialink

Additional interactive resources for this chapter can be found on the Companion Website at www.prenhall.com/burke. Click on Chapter 28 and "Begin" to select the activities for this chapter.

For NCLEX review questions and an audio glossary, access the accompanying CD-ROM in this book.

for further study

For more information about the relationship of vitamin D, calcium, and phosphorus in the body, see Chapter 5.

For in-depth discussion of care of the surgical client, see Chapter 7.

For radiation therapy related to bone cancer, see Chapter 8.

For more about care of the client undergoing amputation, see Chapter 27.

For further study about selective estrogen receptor modulators (SERMs), see Chapter 33.

Critical Thinking Care Map

Caring for a Client with Osteoarthritis and Total Hip Replacement

NCLEX-PN Focus Area: Physiological Integrity: Physiological Adaptation

Case Study: Robert Cerulli is a 72-year-old retired commercial fisherman who has significant degenerative changes in both hip joints. He is admitted for a right total hip replacement; a left total hip replacement is planned to follow in 6 to 12 months.

Nursing Diagnosis: Impaired Physical Mobility

COLLECT DATA

Subjective	Objective
_____	_____
_____	_____
_____	_____
_____	_____
_____	_____
_____	_____

Would you report this data? Yes/No

If yes, to: _____

Nursing Care

_____
_____
_____
_____
_____
_____
_____
_____
_____
_____
_____
_____
_____

How would you document this? _____
_____

Data Collected
(use those that apply)

- Takes carbidopa/levodopa (Sinemet 25-100) 4 times a day for Parkinson's disease
- No other chronic medical conditions
- No known medication allergies
- Does not smoke; consumes only small amounts of alcohol
- Alert and oriented
- Speech is soft but clear
- Vital signs: BP 116/64; P 68 regular; R 18; T 97.4° F (36.3° C) PO
- Color good, skin warm and moist
- Peripheral pulses strong and equal in upper extremities; slightly weaker but equal in lower extremities
- Feet cool to touch, good capillary refil
- Walks with a limp, favoring right hip; shuffling gait noted

Nursing Interventions
(use those that apply)

- Assess pain at least hourly during first 24 to 48 hours postoperatively, and as needed thereafter.
- Teach to use patient-controlled analgesia (PCA) and monitor effectiveness.
- Help change position at least every 2 hours; encourage use of overhead trapeze to shift positions frequently.
- Maintain sequential compression device and antiembolic stocking as ordered; remove for 1 hour daily.
- Remind to use incentive spirometer hourly for first 24 hours, then at least every 2 hours while awake.
- Assist out of bed three times a day after the first 24 hours.
- Maintain right hip abduction with abduction pillow.
- Perform passive ROM exercises of unaffected extremities every shift.
- Encourage frequent quadriceps-setting exercises and plantar and dorsiflexion of feet.
- Assess the surgical site frequently; report signs of excess bleeding or inflammation.
- Monitor temperature every 4 hours.
- Assess pulses, color, movement, and sensation of right foot hourly for the first 24 hours, then every 2 hours for 24 hours, then every 4 hours.

NCLEX-PN Exam Preparation

1. When caring for a client who sustained a gunshot wound to the femur 4 days ago, which of these assessments requires immediate nursing intervention?
   a. soiled dressing
   b. tenderness, swelling, redness over incision site
   c. increased capillary refill
   d. pain scale of 6

2. A client diagnosed with osteoporosis and a right hip replacement is preparing for discharge. Which of the following is the most important item on the discharge instruction sheet?
   a. use of walker and elevated toilet
   b. pain medication
   c. list of calcium enriched foods
   d. enrollment in a smoking cessation program

3. A nurse teaches the mother of a 4-year-old child how to prevent Lyme disease. Which of these statements indicates that further teaching is necessary?
   a. "We are going camping, but I'll make sure she stays out of the brush."
   b. "Even though it's warm, I'll make her wear long pants."
   c. "If a tick gets on my child, I'll pull it off immediately and squash it."
   d. "I'll buy some insect repellant before we leave on our vacation."

4. When assessing a client who has osteoarthritis, the nurse should expect to observe which of these findings?
   a. Superficial, sharp pain
   b. Stiffness following joint use
   c. Full ROM
   d. Crepitus with movement

5. Which of the following is an appropriate goal for teaching of a client with SLE?
   a. Will experience no joint pain or inflammation
   b. Will state rationale for maintaining vegetarian diet
   c. Will use SPF 15 or higher sunscreen when unable to avoid sun exposure
   d. Will relate necessity of splints to prevent joint damage

6. The nurse is teaching a client who is recovering from an acute gout attack about his prescription for sulfinpyrazone (Anturane). Which statement by the client would indicate an understanding of the instructions?
   a. "I'm going to drink less water so I won't swell up."
   b. "I'll take the Colchicine every day."
   c. "I'll let my doctor know if my stomach begins to hurt."
   d. "I will take my medicine on an empty stomach."

7. A client is diagnosed with chronic low back pain. The physician has asked the nurse to provide information related to this condition. Which of the following nursing diagnoses would the nurse be expected to address?
   a. Disturbed Body Image
   b. Ineffective Health Maintenance
   c. Hopelessness
   d. Acute Pain

8. Which of these nursing activities is the most important when caring for a client with muscular dystrophy?
   a. Neuromuscular/skin assessment
   b. Administering pain medications
   c. Respiratory assessment
   d. Cast care

9. The nurse admitted a client in the emergency department who sustained an injury to the right tibia while playing soccer. The physician becomes alarmed after the x-ray shows a mass in the tibia. A full body bone scan is ordered. While preparing the client for the procedure, the nurse would be accurate in stating:
   a. "Please try to hold your urine until after the procedure."
   b. "You will have to drink several ounces of a contrast medium."
   c. "I will ask the doctor to talk to you before you sign the consent form."
   d. "The procedure will only take a few minutes."

10. The student nurse is assisting with basic assessments at a local middle school. A young girl is noted to have a lateral curvature of the spine and asymmetry of the shoulders. The nurse recognizes this as a possible manifestation of:
    a. scoliosis
    b. kyphosis
    c. paget's disease
    d. osteomalacia

Answers for Review Questions, as well as discussion of Case Study Critical Thinking questions, appear in Appendix V.

chapter

29

Caring for Clients with Intracranial Disorders

CARING tip

❝Learning is a never-ending process. READ, READ, READ! Review the literature. Never be afraid to ask questions. Learn the standards of care and practice them. It could save your patient's life.❞

Peggy Bohannon, RN, MS • Director, Vocational Nursing Program • Lee College • Baytown, Texas

LEARNING outcomes

After completing this chapter, you will be able to:

- Describe the structure and functions of the central and peripheral nervous systems.
- Describe assessment and data collection techniques for neurologic function.
- Identify common manifestations of head injuries, increased intracranial pressure, tumors, cerebrovascular accident, seizures, and brain infections.
- Identify laboratory and diagnostic tests used to diagnose intracranial disorders.
- Describe the nursing care of clients with increased intracranial pressure.
- Discuss the nursing implications for medications ordered for clients with intracranial disorders.
- Identify the preoperative and postoperative care for clients undergoing a craniotomy.
- Use the nursing process to collect data, establish outcomes, provide individualized care, and evaluate nursing responses for the client with an intracranial disorder.

MediaLink

 www.prenhall.com/burke

Use the above address to access the free, interactive Companion Website created for this textbook. Get hints, instant feedback, and textbook references to chapter-related multiple choice questions. Link to other interesting sites.

The nervous system consists of the brain, spinal cord, and peripheral nerves. It is a very complex system that controls all motor, sensory, and autonomic activities of the body. It responds to changes within the body and to environmental stimuli. When the nervous system malfunctions, the person may experience acute or chronic disorders.

Structure and Function of the Nervous System

The nervous system is divided into the central nervous system (CNS) and the peripheral nervous system (PNS). The brain and spinal cord make up the CNS. The PNS consists of the cranial nerves, the spinal nerves, and the autonomic nervous system.

The **neuron** (basic cell of the nervous system) is made up of a dendrite, a cell body, and an axon (Figure 29-1 ◆). Dendrites are short, branch-like extensions on the cell body. They carry impulses to the cell body from other cells. The cell body controls the function of the neuron. At the other end of the neuron is a single, long projection known as the axon. It carries impulses away from the cell body. Many axons are protected and insulated by a white fatty substance called **myelin sheath.** Nerves covered with a myelin sheath are known as *myelinated* or white nerve fibers. Axons without myelin are unmyelinated or gray nerve fibers.

Neurons are responsible for neurotransmission. Nerve impulses move from one neuron to another neuron across a synapse (see Figure 29-1). A chemical **neurotransmitter** such as acetylcholine either helps the impulse cross the synapse or stops it. *Sensory* (or afferent) neurons carry impulses from the skin and muscles to the CNS. *Motor* (or efferent) neurons carry impulses from the CNS to the muscles for contraction and to glands in order to release secretions.

CENTRAL NERVOUS SYSTEM
The Brain
The brain is the control center of the nervous system. A rigid, bony skull protects the brain from external injury. Beneath the skull are three protective membranes or **meninges:** (1) dura mater, the outer layer; (2) arachnoid, the middle layer; and (3) pia mater, the inner layer directly attached to the brain (Figure 29-2 ◆ *inset*). Arterial blood vessels are located in the epidural space between the skull and dura mater. Cerebrospinal fluid (CSF) is found in the subarachnoid space between the arachnoid and the pia mater.

There are four major regions of the brain: cerebrum, diencephalon, brain stem, and cerebellum (see Figure 29-2).

CEREBRUM. The cerebrum is the largest area of the brain and is divided into a right and left hemisphere. Deep grooves called **fissures** separate the hemispheres and separate the cerebrum from the cerebellum. Nerve fibers in the corpus callosum connect the two hemispheres and allow them to communicate with each other. The right hemisphere controls the left side of the body while the left hemisphere controls the right side of the body. In every individual one hemisphere is more dominant than the other. The left hemisphere is responsible for speech, problem solving, reasoning, and calculations. The right hemisphere controls visual–spatial information such as art, music, and the surrounding physical environment.

The cerebrum consists of gray matter and white matter. The outer layer or cerebral cortex contains the gray matter, which is made up of neurons. The rest of the cerebrum is made up of myelinated nerve fibers called white matter. Each cerebral hemisphere is divided into four lobes: frontal, parietal, temporal, and occipital (Figure 29-3 ◆). They are separated by fissures.

DIENCEPHALON. The diencephalon contains the thalamus and hypothalamus. The thalamus relays all sensory information into the cortex. The hypothalamus regulates temperature, fluid balance, thirst, appetite, emotions, and the sleep–wake cycle.

BRAIN STEM. The brain stem consists of the midbrain, pons, and medulla oblongata. The midbrain is the center for auditory and visual reflexes. It serves as a nerve pathway between the cerebral hemispheres and lower brain. The pons controls respiration. The medulla oblongata is located at the base of the brain stem. It controls heart rate, blood pressure, respirations, coughing, swallowing, and vomiting.

CEREBELLUM. The cerebellum is connected to the midbrain, pons, and medulla. Like the cerebrum, it has two hemispheres.

A neuron

Figure 29-1. ◆ A neuron

Figure 29-2. ◆ The four major regions of the brain with an illustration of the meninges.

It coordinates involuntary muscle activity and fine motor movements as well as balance and posture.

CEREBROSPINAL FLUID. Four ventricles within the brain make and circulate CSF in the subarachnoid space of the brain and spinal cord. CSF is a clear, colorless liquid that protects the brain and spinal cord from trauma. It also provides a place for nutrient exchange and waste removal. The daily amount of

CSF is about 125 mL to 150 mL. CSF has a high glucose content with very few white blood cells and no red blood cells.

BLOOD SUPPLY TO THE BRAIN. The brain receives about 750 mL of blood each minute and uses approximately 20% of the body's cardiac output. This large oxygen demand is necessary for glucose metabolism, which is the brain's only source of energy. The brain cannot store oxygen or glucose so it needs a constant supply of both.

Two arterial systems supply blood to the brain: (1) internal carotid arteries and (2) vertebral arteries. Most of the cerebrum is supplied blood by the internal carotid arteries. The brain stem and cerebellum receive their blood supply from the vertebral arteries. These major arteries are connected by smaller arteries forming a ring called the *circle of Willis.* This circle protects the brain by providing alternative blood flow routes when an artery is blocked. Cerebral veins drain venous blood into the jugular veins.

BLOOD–BRAIN BARRIER. The blood–brain barrier protects the brain from harmful substances in the blood. It allows only the passage of glucose, some amino acids, respiratory gases, and water. Substances such as urea, some toxins, and most antibiotics cannot pass this barrier. However, brain injury may cause a local breakdown of the barrier.

The Spinal Cord

The spinal cord exits the skull through the foramen magnum and extends to the first or second lumbar vertebra, where it ends in the cauda equina. It is about 17 inches long and ¾ inch thick. The spinal cord is surrounded and protected by vertebral column. The column consists of 7 cervical, 12 thoracic, 5 lumbar, 5 sacral, and 4 fused vertebrae, which form the coccyx.

The inside of the spinal cord is H-shaped and consists of gray matter surrounded by white matter. The gray matter contains three specialized areas called horns: (1) the ventral horn

Figure 29-3. ◆ Cerebral lobes with their functions. **Frontal** controls voluntary motor control on the opposite side of the body and determines emotions, motivation, complex thinking, judgment, and personality. Broca's area promotes speaking ability. **Parietal** interprets sensations and determines right from left and where the body is in relation to the environment. **Temporal** processes taste, smell, and hearing stimuli; also important in long-term memory. Wernicke's area promotes understanding of spoken and written word. **Occipital** processes visual stimuli.

(motor neurons), (2) dorsal horn (sensory neurons), and (3) lateral horn (sympathetic neurons). The white matter forms ascending and descending pathways known as spinal tracts. These tracts carry messages to and from the brain: ascending sensory pathways and descending motor pathways.

THE PERIPHERAL NERVOUS SYSTEM

The peripheral nervous system links the CNS with the rest of the body. It receives and conducts information from the external environment. Spinal nerves, cranial nerves, and ganglia make up the PNS. The PNS is divided into the somatic and autonomic nervous systems. The somatic system connects the skin and muscles to the CNS. The autonomic nervous system controls visceral organs and some glands.

Spinal Nerves

There are 31 pairs of spinal nerves (Figure 29-4 ◆). These nerves are named by their location:

- Cervical: 8 pairs (C1 to C8)
- Thoracic: 12 pairs (T1 to T12)
- Lumbar: 5 pairs (L1 to L5)
- Sacral: 5 pairs (S1 to S5)

Each spinal nerve contains sensory and motor fibers. Sensory fibers are in the dorsal root with motor fibers in the ventral root. The dorsal and ventral root of each spinal nerve attach it to the spinal cord. Damage to the dorsal root causes loss of sensation while damage to the ventral root results in flaccid paralysis.

An area of skin supplied by a single spinal nerve is called a **dermatome.** The dorsal roots of the spinal nerves carry sensations from specific dermatomes. Dermatomes are useful for locating pain sites and neurologic lesions.

Spinal nerves are also involved in reflexes. A **reflex** is an involuntary motor response to a stimulus. Reflexes follow a pathway known as a **reflex arc.** The reflex arc consists of a receptor, an afferent sensory neuron, the response center in the spinal cord or brain, an efferent motor neuron, and an effector muscle or gland (Figure 29-5 ◆).

Common reflexes include stretch, deep-tendon, withdrawal, and superficial. *Stretch reflexes* control muscle tone and help maintain posture. *Deep-tendon reflexes (DTRs)* are assessed at the wrists, elbows, knees, and Achilles tendon with a reflex hammer. Abnormal DTRs mean additional medical evaluation. *Withdrawal reflexes* occur when a person expects pain and automatically withdraws the threatened body part. *Superficial reflexes* result from gently stimulating the skin. For example, the plantar reflex is elicited by stroking the sole of the foot. The normal response is to curl the toes downward.

Cranial Nerves

Twelve pairs of cranial nerves begin in the brain or brain stem (Table 29-1 ◆). They have sensory or motor functions or both. The vagus nerve extends into the thoracic and abdominal areas. The other cranial nerves control function in the head and neck areas.

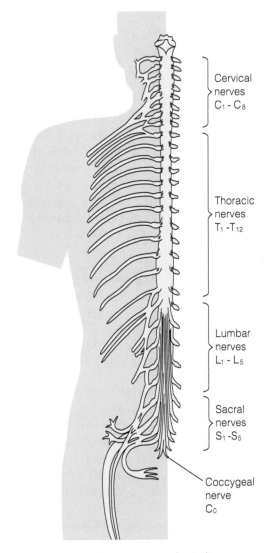

Figure 29-4. ◆ Distribution of spinal nerves.

Cervical nerves C₁ - C₈

Thoracic nerves T₁ -T₁₂

Lumbar nerves L₁ - L₅

Sacral nerves S₁ -S₅

Coccygeal nerve C₀

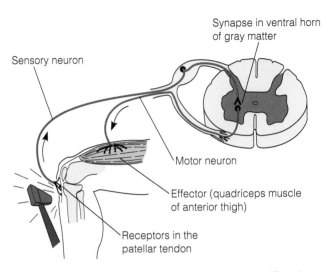

Figure 29-5. ◆ A typical reflex arc of the spinal nerve. The stimulus is transferred from the sensory neuron directly to the motor neuron at the point of synapse in the spinal cord.

Synapse in ventral horn of gray matter

Sensory neuron

Motor neuron

Effector (quadriceps muscle of anterior thigh)

Receptors in the patellar tendon

TABLE 29-1   THE CRANIAL NERVES

CRANIAL NERVE	FUNCTION
I Olfactory	Smell
II Optic	Vision
III Oculomotor	Pupil constriction Eyeball movement Raising of upper eyelid
IV Trochlear	Eyeball movement
V Trigeminal	Sensation of the scalp, nose, mouth, and cornea Chewing
VI Abducens	Lateral movement of the eyeball
VII Facial	Movement of facial muscles Secretions from lacrimal and salivary glands Taste in anterior two thirds of tongue
VIII Vestibulocochlear	Sense of hearing and equilibrium
IX Glossopharyngeal	Taste in posterior one third of tongue Sensation of pharynx and tongue Gag reflex Swallowing Secretions of parotid gland
X Vagus	Swallowing Controls parasympathetic nervous system activities (e.g., heart and respiratory rates, digestion) Sensation in pharynx and larynx
XI Accessory	Neck and shoulder movement
XII Hypoglossal	Tongue movement

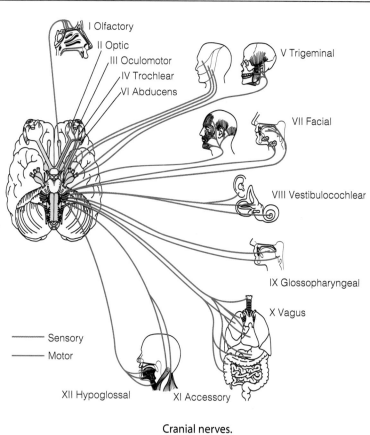

Cranial nerves.

THE AUTONOMIC NERVOUS SYSTEM

The autonomic nervous system (ANS) is part of the peripheral nervous system. It is responsible for maintaining the body's internal homeostasis. The ANS regulates respiration, heart rate, digestion, urinary excretion, body temperature, and sexual function.

There are two divisions: (1) the sympathetic nervous system (SNS) and (2) the parasympathetic nervous system (PNS). Fibers from both systems can affect the same structures. Generally when one system increases an action, the other system decreases the action. This process keeps the body in balance so that one action does not dominate.

The SNS prepares the body to handle stress. It plays a key role in the body's "fight-or-flight" response. The parasympathetic nervous system operates during nonstressful situations. It conserves the body's energy by regulating digestion, elimination, and other activities. (The actions of the SNS and PNS are shown in Figure 29-6 ◆.)

◆ Altered Intracranial Function

Intracranial disorders can be acute and life threatening or occur over a long period of time. These disorders often result in long-term problems that affect the client's and family's quality of life.

This chapter presents common head injuries followed by a discussion on increased intracranial pressure and altered level of consciousness. Additional topics include brain tumors, cerebrovascular accidents, seizures, brain infections, and headaches. Basic nursing care for the client having neurosurgery is described.

HEAD INJURIES

Head injuries are a leading cause of death and disability in the United States. Persons at an increased risk for head injuries are between the ages of 1 and 35 and the elderly. Traumatic brain injury affects more males than females. Motor vehicle accidents (MVAs) are a major cause of head injuries, followed by falls, sport injuries, and violent assaults. Elevated blood alcohol levels often increase the risk of an MVA.

Head injuries include scalp lacerations, skull fractures, concussion, contusion, and hematomas. Scalp lacerations often look worse than they are because they bleed profusely. A *skull fracture* is a break in the skull. It is usually caused by extreme force and can possibly result in brain damage. Skull fractures are either open from a tear in the dura or closed. There are four types of skull fractures:

1. *Linear*—a simple, clean break in the skull.
2. *Comminuted*—the skull is crushed into small, fragmented pieces.
3. *Depressed*—bone fragments may be pushed into the brain; usually caused by a powerful blow to the skull.
4. *Basilar*—occurs at the base of the skull. It involves the frontal or temporal lobe sinuses causing a CSF leak from the nose (**rhinorrhea**) or the ears (**otorrhea**). Other man-

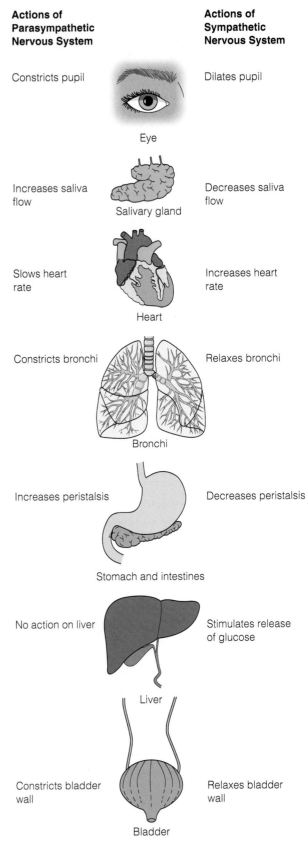

Actions of Parasympathetic Nervous System		Actions of Sympathetic Nervous System
Constricts pupil	Eye	Dilates pupil
Increases saliva flow	Salivary gland	Decreases saliva flow
Slows heart rate	Heart	Increases heart rate
Constricts bronchi	Bronchi	Relaxes bronchi
Increases peristalsis	Stomach and intestines	Decreases peristalsis
No action on liver	Liver	Stimulates release of glucose
Constricts bladder wall	Bladder	Relaxes bladder wall

Figure 29-6. ◆ Autonomic nervous system and the organs it affects. The right side shows the actions of the sympathetic nervous system. The left side shows the actions of the parasympathetic nervous system.

ifestations are *Battle's sign* (bruising over the mastoid process) and *periorbital ecchymosis,* sometimes called "raccoon eyes." If CSF leakage is present, the risk of infection is high.

Head injuries are classified as open or closed. *Open head injuries* involve an opening between the outside environment and the brain. Clients with this type of injury have a higher risk for meningitis. A *closed head injury* usually results from an acceleration–deceleration injury, also called the coup–contrecoup phenomenon (Figure 29-7 ◆). This causes bruising of the brain at two points resulting in extensive brain damage. Other closed head injuries are caused by a **concussion** or **contusion**. The amount of damage from a head injury relates to how the injury occurred, the type of injury, and its location. Brain damage develops from either direct trauma to the tissue or increased **intracranial pressure** and cerebral edema.

Intracranial hemorrhage is defined as bleeding within the skull. It is the most common serious complication of a head injury. Intracranial hemorrhage may result from the tearing of cerebral arteries or veins, or direct trauma. This bleeding leads to formation of a **hematoma** (an accumulation of blood). Blood accumulates in the epidural, subdural, or subarachnoid spaces, or within the cerebral lobes. Pressure on surrounding tissues leads to increased intracranial pressure. If the pressure is unrelieved, neurologic changes occur. Hematomas are classified by their location: epidural, subdural, or intracerebral (Figure 29-8 ◆). (Table 29-2 ◆ shows common brain injuries.)

INCREASED INTRACRANIAL PRESSURE

The cranium has three compartments: (1) the brain (80%), (2) blood (10%), and (3) cerebrospinal fluid (10%). Intracranial pressure (ICP) is the pressure exerted within the cranium by these contents. This pressure is measured by the CSF and ranges from 5 to 15 mm Hg. If the volume of one component increases, the volume of the other components must decrease to keep the pressure within its normal range. When this does not occur, increased intracranial pressure (IICP) develops. Normal activities such as coughing, sneezing,

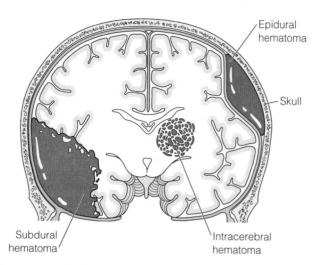

Figure 29-8. ◆ Three types of hematomas: epidural hematoma, subdural hematoma, and intracerebral hematoma.

straining, or bending forward can briefly increase ICP. Brief pressure increases are not harmful; however, prolonged increases can damage delicate brain tissue. IICP can develop with a head injury, brain surgery, or meningitis.

Cerebral blood flow is vital to deliver the required oxygen and glucose. For the brain to function properly, an adequate blood supply must travel to the brain. When ICP increases, cerebral blood flow decreases, causing ischemia. If ischemia lasts longer than 5 minutes, the result is irreversible brain damage. Cerebral blood flow is also affected by the amount of carbon dioxide and oxygen in the blood. Increased carbon dioxide levels ($PaCO_2$) and/or decreased oxygen levels (PaO_2) cause vasodilation of the cerebral arteries. Either one of these conditions will increase intracranial pressure.

Any increase in ICP causes neurologic changes in the client's level of consciousness (LOC), pupil response, speech, motor function, and vital signs. The changes become more dramatic as ICP increases. Manifestations may be labeled as early or late (Box 29-1). They develop slowly or rapidly. Not all manifestations occur in all clients. The location and cause of IICP will determine the symptoms. Often, the symptoms are subtle. The nurse must closely observe the client for any changes. Cushing's triad occurs late in the development of IICP. This is an ominous sign of impending death.

CLINICAL alert

The earliest sign of increasing ICP is a change in the level of consciousness.

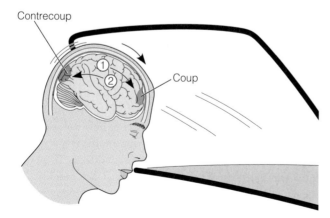

Figure 29-7. ◆ Coup–contrecoup head injury. Following the initial injury (coup), the brain rebounds within the skull and sustains additional injury (contrecoup) in the opposite part of the brain.

Cerebral Edema

Cerebral edema is an abnormal accumulation of fluid in the brain resulting in brain swelling. It may also be caused by vasodilation of the cerebral arteries. Cerebral edema often accompanies IICP. Brain injury, intracranial surgery, tumors, hemorrhage, and infections can cause cerebral edema. Edema

TABLE 29-2   COMMON BRAIN INJURIES WITH PATHOPHYSIOLOGY AND MANIFESTATIONS

BRAIN INJURY	PATHOPHYSIOLOGY	MANIFESTATIONS
Concussion	Brain injury is caused by violent shaking of the brain.	Immediate loss of consciousness for < 5 minutes. Drowsiness, confusion, dizziness. Headache, blurred or double vision.
Contusion	Bruising of the brain tissue caused by blunt trauma. More severe than a concussion because brain swelling occurs.	Vary with the size and location of the injury. Initial loss of consciousness; if LOC remains altered, the client may become combative. During unconsciousness, lies motionless; has pale, clammy skin; faint pulse; hypotension; shallow respirations; and altered motor responses.
Epidural hematoma	Severe blow to brain causes arterial bleeding that collects between the skull and dura mater. May be caused by skull fractures or contusion.	Brief loss of consciousness followed by a short period of alertness. Then the client rapidly progresses into a coma with decorticate or decerebrate posturing, *ipsilateral* (same-side) pupil dilation, and seizures.
Subdural hematoma	Major closed head injury causes venous blood to collect between dura mater and the subarachnoid layer.	Three types of subdural hematomas. *Acute:* Rapid deterioration from drowsiness and confusion to coma. Signs of compression are ipsilateral pupil dilation and contralateral hemiparesis.
	Subacute occurs from less severe head injury.	*Subacute:* Manifestations appear 48 hours to 2 weeks later; alert period followed by slow progression to coma.
	Chronic occurs most often in elderly, alcoholics, and those on long-term anticoagulant therapy.	*Chronic:* Manifestations develop weeks to months after initial injury. Slowed thinking, confusion, drowsiness; may progress to pupil changes and motor deficits.
Intracerebral hematoma	Bleeding into the brain tissue; may be caused by gunshot wound or a depressed skull fracture.	Decreasing level of consciousness; pupil changes, and motor deficits.

rises to its highest level within 48 to 72 hours, then gradually subsides. Without early recognition and treatment, the client's condition can deteriorate rapidly.

Frequently seen complications of IICP include an altered LOC, brain herniation, and brain death. The following information shows how these complications affect the client.

Altered Level of Consciousness

Consciousness means that the client is oriented to time, place, and person, and responds appropriately to external stimuli. To maintain normal consciousness, the brain must receive its constant supply of oxygen and glucose. It also requires an intact reticular activating system (RAS), located in the brain stem. The RAS keeps a person alert and responsive to the environment.

Many neurologic conditions alter the client's level of consciousness. Usually LOC is altered by IICP and cerebral edema. The following disorders will likely increase ICP and affect the person's ability to remain alert and oriented:

- Head injury
- Hematoma
- Cerebrovascular accident (CVA) or stroke
- Tumors
- Infections

Any condition that reduces oxygen and glucose levels in the brain may decrease LOC. Clients at an increased risk include those with poorly controlled diabetes and those with long-term cardiac or respiratory disease. Drugs such as alcohol, narcotics, sedatives, and anesthetics depress the CNS, which in turn alters consciousness. Seizures and toxins produced by liver or kidney failure may also alter LOC.

The client's altered LOC may be described using the terms in Box 29-2. However, it is best for the nurse to describe the client's actual behavior and response to stimuli instead of relying on a specific term. Altered LOC and behavior are early changes associated with IICP (see Box 29-1). As brain function deteriorates, more stimuli are needed to elicit a response from the client. Eventually, no response is obtained.

The Glasgow Coma Scale (Table 29-3 ◆) provides a quick guide for assessing LOC. It measures how well the client responds to eye opening and verbal and motor response. The lower the score, the worse the client's condition. To prevent permanent brain damage, the nurse must act quickly. The physician must be notified and measures started to lower IICP.

Brain Herniation

Brain herniation occurs late in the course of IICP. In an attempt to save brain tissue, the brain shifts from an area of

BOX 29-1
MANIFESTATIONS OF INCREASED INTRACRANIAL PRESSURE

	Early	Late
Level of consciousness	Irritability; personality changes; restlessness; short-term memory changes; disorientation to time, then to place and person; confusion	Decreasing LOC that progresses to coma No response to painful stimuli
Pupils	Pupils equal, round, and reactive to light	Pupils sluggish response to light then to fixed pupils. First, pupils may be dilated on one side (ipsilateral), then progress to bilateral dilation.
Vision	Decreased visual acuity, blurred vision, diplopia	Cannot assess due to decreasing LOC or coma
Motor function	Weakness in one extremity or side; hemiplegia on the opposite side	Decorticate or decerebrate positioning
Speech	Difficulty speaking	Cannot assess due to decreasing LOC or coma
Blood pressure	Elevated blood pressure	*Cushing's triad:* Increased systolic blood pressure, widening pulse pressure, bradycardia
Pulse	Slightly elevated pulse	
Respiration	Rate may increase	Decreased respiratory rate with altered respiratory patterns (e.g., Cheyne–Stokes)
Temperature	May be increased or decreased	Significantly elevated
Other symptoms	Headache worse on rising in the morning and with position changes	Continual headache Projectile vomiting Loss of pupil, corneal, gag, and swallowing reflexes

BOX 29-2
ALTERED LEVELS OF CONSCIOUSNESS

Full consciousness: Alert; oriented to time, place, and person; fully understands written and spoken words

Confusion: Disoriented to time, place, and person; unable to think clearly; short attention span; poor memory

Delirium: Motor restlessness; agitated and irritable; may have hallucinations; may be combative

Obtundation: Appears drowsy and lethargic; responds to verbal and tactile stimuli but quickly drifts back to sleep

Stupor: Generally unresponsive; may withdraw purposefully with vigorous or painful stimuli

Coma: Does not respond to stimuli

high pressure to low pressure. One common site is the foramen magnum (the hole at the base of the brain where the spinal cord exits). As pressure rises, the brain is pushed through the foramen magnum. This compresses the brain stem so that vital functions such as respiration cease. Without prompt recognition, the client eventually dies.

Brain Death
Brain death occurs when cerebral blood flow stops, resulting in irreversible loss of brain function. (The criteria for determining brain death can be found in Chapter 10, Box 10-14.) If organ donation is planned, the appropriate agencies are contacted.

COLLABORATIVE CARE
It is most important to identify and prevent IICP in any client with a neurologic problem. Medications are given immediately to lower ICP. Clients with severe head injuries need their ICP monitored. Uncontrolled intracranial bleeding requires immediate surgery.

TABLE 29-3 GLASGOW COMA SCALE

BEHAVIOR	RESPONSE	SCORE
Eye opening response	Spontaneously	4
	To speech	3
	To pain	2
	No response	1
Best verbal response	Oriented to time, place, and person	5
	Confused	4
	Inappropriate words	3
	Incomprehensible sounds	2
	No response	1
Best motor response	Obeys commands	6
	Moves to localized pain	5
	Flexion withdrawal from pain	4
	Abnormal flexion (decorticate)	3
	Abnormal extension (decerebrate)	2
	No response	1
Total score:		———
	Best response	15
	Comatose client	8 or less
	Totally unresponsive	3

Laboratory and Diagnostic Tests

The type and extent of neurologic deficits are often discovered during the history and physical examination. The following laboratory tests are ordered to determine the cause for the client's altered LOC:

■ *Blood glucose* is measured when hypoglycemia is suspected.
■ *Arterial blood gases* monitor pH and levels of oxygen and carbon dioxide. They can identify hypoxia and increased carbon dioxide levels.
■ *Toxicology screening* of blood and urine is done to identify alcohol or drug toxicity.
■ *Serum creatinine and BUN* are measured when renal failure is suspected.
■ *Liver function tests* (alanine transaminase [ALT], aspartate transaminase [AST]) can evaluate liver function.
■ *Complete blood count with differential* is used to assess for anemia or infectious disease.

The following diagnostic tests are ordered to determine the cause of IICP:

■ *Computed tomography (CT) scan* or *magnetic resonance imaging (MRI)* detects hemorrhage, edema, hematoma, or tumor.
■ *Cerebral angiography* provides x-ray views of cerebral blood flow and is used when a stroke is suspected.

■ *Lumbar puncture* provides a sample of CSF to analyze for possible meningitis.

Pharmacology

Medications play an important role in managing clients with IICP. The most frequently ordered drugs include: (a) osmotic diuretics, (b) loop diuretics, (c) corticosteroids, (d) anticonvulsants, (e) antipyretics, and (f) histamine antagonists.

Intravenous *fluids* are used to maintain the client's fluid and electrolyte balance and to prevent hypotension. Only 0.9% normal saline and lactated Ringer's solution are given because they can reduce cerebral edema while any other IV solution will increase it. They are infused at low rates such as 50 to 75 mL/hr. All IV solutions should be given using an intravenous pump to prevent volume overload.

Osmotic diuretics (e.g., Mannitol [Osmitrol]) draw water out of the edematous brain tissue to be excreted by the kidneys. Large or frequent doses of Mannitol cause dehydration and electrolyte losses. Loop diuretics decrease cerebral edema but cause less fluid and electrolyte losses.

Dexamethazone (Decadron), a *corticosteroid,* reduces cerebral edema but causes GI irritation and possibly gastric ulcers. Histamine H_2 antagonists like ranitidine (Zantac) or sucralfate (Carafate) or antacids are given to prevent gastric irritation. Antiemetics are used to prevent vomiting and the risk for aspiration.

Anticonvulsants may treat or prevent seizure activity associated with a head injury. Three anticonvulsants are ordered: (1) phenytoin (Dilantin), (2) diazepam (Valium), and (3) phenobarbital. Acetaminophen, an antipyretic, is used alone or in combination with a hypothermia blanket to treat hyperthermia. Hyperthermia raises cerebral metabolism and increases ICP.

Clients with severe head injuries and continually elevated ICP may be given *barbiturates.* Barbiturate therapy places the client in a coma, reducing metabolism of the injured brain. Lowering metabolism allows the brain time to heal without permanent damage. During this therapy, the client is closely monitored in the critical care unit.

ICP Monitoring

An ICP monitoring device is inserted into the skull to assess for IICP. This device is used only for clients in the critical care unit. Intracranial pressures are constantly monitored so that immediate treatment can be started before brain damage occurs. Because bacteria could enter the brain, the client is assessed for symptoms of meningitis.

Surgery

Cranial surgery is performed to reduce the client's ICP. In clients with head injuries, a bone flap is removed from the skull to allow room for the brain to expand. Emergency surgery is done to remove a blood clot or evacuate a hematoma. Surgery can also relieve the pressure of a brain tumor. Care of the client following a craniotomy is presented under the section on brain tumor.

NURSING CARE

ASSESSING

Clients with IICP need frequent nursing assessments. The nurse observes and reports immediately to the physician any sudden change in neurologic function. Subjective and objective findings help to identify the type of medical treatment the client will need (Box 29-3).

DIAGNOSING, PLANNING, AND IMPLEMENTING

The client with a head injury has multiple nursing needs. Besides preventing IICP, it is important to avoid its potential complications. If the client is unconscious, care is directed at maintaining the airway, nutrition, and skin integrity, as well as preventing problems from immobility and the risk of infection. Unconscious clients are usually cared for in the critical care unit. Persons with mild neurologic deficits are treated in the emergency department, then monitored at home.

INEFFECTIVE TISSUE PERFUSION: CEREBRAL

- Elevate the head of the bed 30 degrees and keep the head in a midline position. *These measures promote venous drainage from the head so that pressure does not build up.*
- Give oxygen as ordered. Use pulse oximetry to measure oxygen levels. Keep PaO_2 levels above 94% and $PaCO_2$ levels between 35 to 45. *The brain needs a constant supply of oxygen to prevent brain damage. Increased carbon dioxide levels can cause cerebral vasodilation, leading to cerebral edema.*
- Avoid Valsalva maneuver (e.g., coughing, straining during bowel movements); avoid hip flexion and abdominal distention. Give stool softeners as ordered. Monitor patency of nasogastric tube. *The Valsalva maneuver, hip flexion, gastric distention, and constipation can increase ICP. Stool softeners and a nasogastric tube may prevent IICP.*
- Monitor temperature every 2 hours for hyperthermia. Avoid rectal temperatures. *Temperature is monitored to prevent brain damage from an increased metabolic rate. Rectal temperatures can increase ICP.*
- Keep the client quiet; reduce noise and lights in the room; and space nursing activities over the shift. Speak softly and

BOX 29-3
ASSESSING CLIENTS WITH INCREASED INTRACRANIAL PRESSURE

SUBJECTIVE DATA

- Present health status:
  - When did change in LOC or memory occur first; onset slow or rapid?
  - Presence of headache, nausea, or vomiting
  - Visual changes such as double vision or blurring
  - Ringing in the ears; dizziness or feeling faint
  - Any numbness or tingling in extremities
- Past medical history:
  - History of trauma, infection, cranial surgery, seizures, or loss of consciousness
  - Medication and alcohol use

OBJECTIVE DATA

- Blood pressure, pulse, respirations, temperature
- Observe for memory lapses or altered thought processes.
- Assess orientation to time, place, and person and LOC. If client is unconscious, use the Glasgow Coma Scale (Table 29-3).
- Check pupil response to light by using a penlight. Normal response should be PERRLA: Pupils equal, round, reactive to light, and accommodation.
- Assess strength of hand grip and movement of extremities. Ask client to:
  - Squeeze your hands.
  - Push his or her feet against the resistance of your hands.
  - Raise both legs off the bed.
- Note nausea or vomiting.

- Note color and amount of drainage from ears and nose (halo sign); presence of racoon eyes or Battle's sign.

ADDITIONAL DATA FOR UNCONSCIOUS CLIENTS

- Note any change in breathing pattern.
- Assess for the Babinski reflex by stroking the bottom of the foot. An abnormal response in adults is when the big toe flexes upward and the other toes fan out.
- Assess corneal reflex by touching the corneal surface with a wisp of cotton. Normally, the client blinks.
- Assess the gag reflex by touching the back of the client's throat gently with a tongue blade. Normally, the client will show a gag reflex.
- Assess for abnormal posturing.

A

Decorticate Posturing

B

Decerebrate Posturing

calmly. *Loud noises and bright lights plus constant nursing care activities can increase ICP.*

- Turn client slowly and gently with a turn sheet. *Sudden movement can increase ICP.*

- Limit fluid over a 24-hour period. Monitor urine output every 1 to 2 hours. *Fluid restrictions may prevent and decrease cerebral edema. Urine output is monitored for signs of diabetes insipidus or syndrome of inappropriate antidiuretic hormone (SIADH).*

- If client is combative, avoid using restraints. Have nursing staff or family sit quietly with the client. *Restraining the client increases ICP. Family may provide a soothing atmosphere.*

- Monitor for seizure activity and maintain seizure precautions:
  - Keep oral airway and suction equipment at bedside.
  - Pad side rails with blankets.
  - Keep bed in low position with side rails up.
    Clients with neurologic injuries are prone to developing seizures and are at risk for injury.

INEFFECTIVE BREATHING PATTERN

- Monitor respiratory rate, depth, and rhythm for changes. *As ICP increases, the risk of respiratory distress rises. IICP is known to cause respiratory arrest. Unconscious clients may lose their cough reflex. Head injuries will decrease respiratory function.*

- Assess the client's ability to clear secretions. If unconscious or the client has a poor cough, suction the airway for less than 10 seconds. *Suctioning longer reduces oxygen levels and increases carbon dioxide levels, which can increase ICP.*

- Insert an oral airway as needed. *This prevents the tongue from obstructing the airway.*

- Turn the client from side to side every two hours; keep in a side-lying position with head of bed elevated. *Turning prevents pooling of secretions in one area of the lungs. Side positioning prevents the tongue from obstructing the airway.*

- If client is unconscious, keep NPO and provide oral hygiene. *Fluids are not given to the unconscious client to prevent aspiration. Oral hygiene removes secretions that could dry and be aspirated.*

RISK FOR IMBALANCED NUTRITION: LESS THAN BODY REQUIREMENTS

- Give tube feeding through a nasogastric or gastrostomy tube or total parenteral nutrition (TPN) as ordered. *Head injuries increase the client's metabolic rate and risk for malnutrition. Tube feedings or TPN are ordered to prevent malnutrition.*

- Before each tube feeding, check gastric residual. *Excess gastric residual means that the tube feeding is not being absorbed. This places the client at risk for malnutrition.*

- Monitor daily weights. *Daily weights help determine the client's nutritional status.*

RISK FOR IMPAIRED SKIN INTEGRITY

- Turn the client every two hours. Use a special mattress or bed as available. Lift rather than drag the client across the sheet. *Turning relieves pressure over bony prominences. Special mattresses (e.g., egg-crate cushion or beds) distribute the clients' weight more evenly. Dragging can cause skin tears.*

- Prevent skin breakdown by:
  - Keeping bed linens clean, dry, and wrinkle free
  - Bathing the client daily with mild soap
  - Cleansing the skin following urine and fecal soiling with a mild cleansing agent
  - Providing adequate hydration
    Keeping linens clean, dry, and wrinkle free decreases the risk of skin injuries. Daily hygiene keeps the skin soft and supple. Adequate hydration prevents the skin from drying out and cracking.

- Provide oral care and lubricate the lips every 2 to 4 hours. *This removes dried crusts and prevents drying and cracking of oral mucous membranes.*

- Keep the cornea moist by instilling methyl cellulose solution (0.5% to 1%). Apply protective eye shields if the corneal reflex is absent. *Proper eye care prevents corneal abrasion and irritation.*

IMPAIRED PHYSICAL MOBILITY

- Maintain extremities in position of function with support devices. Remove support devices every 4 hours for skin care. Place a pillow in the axilla area; use hand splints; use foam boots or high-top tennis shoes on the feet. *Pillows in the axilla area prevent abduction of the shoulder. Hand splints may prevent flexion contractures of the hands. Foam boots or high-top tennis shoes are used to prevent footdrop.*

- Perform passive range-of-motion (ROM) exercises at least four times per day. Do not perform on the client with IICP. *Unconscious clients are at a high risk for developing contracture. Passive ROM exercises done routinely maintain muscle tone and function, prevent additional disability, and restore impaired motor function.*

RISK FOR INFECTION

- Assess for a CSF leak and monitor for signs of infection. *Open head wounds such as a depressed skull fracture increase the risk for infection. They can be contaminated with dirt, hair, or other debris.*

- Test clear drainage from ear and nose for glucose by using a glucose reagent strip. *Clear drainage that tests positive for glucose indicates the presence of CSF.*

- Keep the nasopharynx and external ear clean. Place a sterile piece of cotton in the ear and loosely tape a 4″ × 4″ gauze under the nose to collect any drainage. Change the dressings when they become wet. *Bacteria can enter through these openings when wet dressings are present.*

- Remind client not to blow the nose, cough, or stop a sneeze. *Blowing the nose or coughing increases ICP. Stopping a sneeze can force bacteria up into the brain.*

- Use strict aseptic technique when changing head dressings or handling the ICP monitoring device. *Aseptic technique decreases the risk of introducing bacteria.*

EVALUATING

To evaluate the effectiveness of nursing care for a client with IICP, collect data such as the following:

- Alert and oriented to time, place, and person
- Absence of diplopia, tinnitus, dizziness, nausea, vomiting, or abnormal pupil response
- Strong hand grip, extremity movement, and steady gait

Discharge Considerations

The nurse assesses clients to determine whether they can manage their care at home or if they need to be transferred to a long-term care facility (Box 29-4). Clients with a mild head injury should be observed for at least 24 hours. If they are not hospitalized, they must be closely monitored at home. For example, with a linear skull fracture, family is taught to wake and observe the client every 2 hours during the first 8 hours after the accident. The client and family should return to the emergency department if the client develops any of the following manifestations:

- Increasing drowsiness, confusion, or slurred speech
- Difficulty waking the client
- Vomiting
- Blurred vision; one or both pupils dilated
- Prolonged headache
- Blood or clear fluid leaking from the nose or ears
- Weakness in arm or leg
- Seizures

　　Clients with a concussion may develop postconcussion syndrome. They may experience headache, poor concentration, dizziness, personality changes, and fatigue for weeks to months. Family support is important during this phase of recovery.

　　Clients with severe head injuries usually require extensive rehabilitation either as inpatient or outpatient. Rehabilitation may include physical, speech, and occupational therapy. Unconscious clients need placement in a nursing home. A social services department can help the family find a suitable facility and also assist with financial concerns. Because the prognosis of the client is uncertain, the family may need support services from counselors and the clergy.

Nursing Process Case Study
■ CLIENT WITH INCREASED INTRACRANIAL PRESSURE AND ALTERED LEVEL OF CONSCIOUSNESS

Martin Straton, 52 years old, fell during his daily run in the park. He hit his head on the right side and was knocked

BOX 29-4
ASSESSING FOR DISCHARGE

INTRACRANIAL DISORDERS
Client

- **Self-care:** Ability to perform ADLs as possible, perform appropriate physical exercises, use assistive devices as needed, plan rest periods; to self-administer medications; to prevent falls or other injuries; to follow discharge instructions
- **Knowledge:** Disease process; prescription and over-the-counter medications; indications for seeking medical care
- **Home environment:** Appropriate heating and cooling; access to clean water for drinking and handwashing; safe environment to minimize risk of injury; access for using assistive devices

Family

- **Members of household:** Ability to maintain a quiet, supportive environment
- **Caregivers:** Availability, willingness, and ability to provide short-term and long-term care, emotional stability, ROM exercises and positioning, skin care; to assist client with using assistive devices; to administer medications; to identify and manage potential complications (e.g., seizures); to transport to health care resources (e.g., physician, laboratory)
- **Financial resources:** Income, resources for medications, medical care, long-term care facility, and/or rehabilitation services as needed

Community

- Access to health care resources and rehabilitation services (e.g., physical, occupational, and speech therapies)
- Access to community support groups such as Meals-on-Wheels, Eldercare, and specialized support groups (e.g., stroke club)
- Access to respite care

unconscious. A bystander called an ambulance, which arrived in 10 minutes to transport him to the local hospital.

Assessment BP 150/90, P 60, R 14. He responds to verbal and tactile stimuli but quickly falls back asleep. His right pupil is dilated and does not react to light. He is unable to move his extremities on the left side. Oxygen is given by a face mask. CT scan shows an epidural hematoma on the right side with edema. The neurologist discusses the need for immediate surgery with Mr. Straton's wife. He was taken to surgery in the evening for burr holes to evacuate the hematoma. His surgery is successful, and he is transferred to the critical care unit.

Diagnosis   After surgery, the following diagnoses are made for Mr. Straton:

- Risk for Ineffective Tissue Perfusion: Cerebral related to increased intracranial pressure and edema
- Risk for Aspiration related to altered level of consciousness
- Risk for Impaired Skin Integrity related to immobility
- Risk for Imbalanced Nutrition: Less Than Body Requirements related to inability to eat

Expected Outcomes   The expected outcomes for the plan of care are that Mr. Straton will:

- Maintain adequate cerebral tissue perfusion.
- Demonstrate clear lung sounds.
- Maintain skin integrity.
- Maintain adequate nutritional status.

Planning and Implementation   The following interventions are planned and implemented for Mr. Straton:

- Perform neurologic and respiratory assessment with vital signs every two hours or as needed. Monitor pulse oximetry.
- Use measures to reduce cerebral edema such as:
  - Elevate head of bed 30 degrees; keep head in neutral alignment; avoid flexion of head and hips.
  - Provide calm environment and allow for rest periods.
- Assess ability to clear secretions; check gag reflex every shift; and suction posterior pharynx as needed.
- Turn side to side every 2 hours, and maintain side-lying position. Turn slowly with a turn sheet.
- Maintain NPO status and provide frequent oral hygiene.
- Assess skin over bony prominences every shift.
- Assess fluid status and document intake and output.

Evaluation   Twenty-four hours after surgery, Mr. Straton slowly starts to regain consciousness. His right pupil slowly reacts to light, and he moves his left extremities slightly. Mr. Straton continues to improve and is discharged to his home a week later.

 Critical Thinking in the Nursing Process

1. Mr. Straton was found unconscious. What assessments would you make and how could you maintain an open airway at the scene?
2. During the immediate postoperative period Mr. Straton becomes confused and tries to pull out his ICP monitoring device. You know you cannot restrain him. What other nursing interventions could you do?
3. Describe oral hygiene measures for clients who are unconscious.

Brain Tumor

Brain tumors are abnormal growths within the cranium. Their cause is unknown, but prolonged exposure to certain chemicals and radiation increases the incidence. Brain tumors occur at any age. The incidence is highest among young children and adults between the ages of 50 to 70.

Intracranial tumors are classified as either benign or malignant, based on tissue type and cell characteristics. The term *benign* can be misleading, because the tumor may be inaccessible by surgery, and as it grows, it presses on vital centers. If the compression increases, it leads to disability and death. Malignant tumors invade other areas of the brain and eventually cause death.

Brain tumors are also categorized as primary or secondary. Primary tumors develop from cells and structures within the brain. Secondary brain tumors develop in areas outside of the brain and metastasize to the brain. (The most common brain tumors are listed in Table 29-4 ◆.)

PATHOPHYSIOLOGY

Brain tumors invade, displace, and destroy brain tissue. As the tumor grows, it compresses tissue and nerves, eventually causing cerebral edema. When the brain fails to compensate for the increase in volume, the result is increased intracranial pressure. This will lead to the typical manifestations of IICP discussed earlier in the chapter. If untreated, the final result is brain herniation and death.

Manifestations are either local or generalized. Local manifestations relate to the location and function of that specific site (e.g., frontal lobe or temporal lobe) (Box 29-5). Knowing the tumor site helps the nurse plan the client's care. Tumors can press on cerebral blood vessels, decreasing their blood supply. This leads to complaints of dizziness. Generalized manifestations include headache that is usually worse in the morning, nausea, vomiting, changes in mental functioning, and seizures.

COLLABORATIVE CARE

A brain tumor is treated with chemotherapy, radiation therapy, surgery, or any combination of these. The choice of treat-

TABLE 29-4	CLASSIFICATION OF BRAIN TUMORS	
TUMOR	**CHARACTERISTICS**	
Glioma		
▪ Astrocytoma	Most common glioma	
	Graded I to IV according to degree of cell differentiation	
▪ Glioblastoma multiforme	Highly malignant	
	Fast-growing and highly invasive of other tissues	
Meningioma	Slow-growing tumor developing in the meninges	
Acoustic neuroma	Benign, slow-growing tumor of the acoustic nerve	
Metastatic brain tumors	Slow growing and malignant	
	Develop from primary sites in the lung and breast	

BOX 29-5
MANIFESTATIONS OF BRAIN TUMORS

FRONTAL LOBE TUMORS

- Personality changes, inappropriate behavior, impaired judgment, inability to concentrate
- Recent memory loss
- Motor deficits
- Expressive aphasia
- Seizures

PARIETAL LOBE TUMORS

- Sensory–perceptual deficits
- Seizures

TEMPORAL LOBE TUMORS

- Psychomotor seizures
- Receptive aphasia

OCCIPITAL LOBE TUMORS

- Visual deficits
- Headache

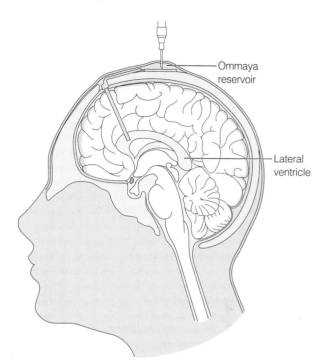

Figure 29-9. ◆ Ommaya reservoir for medication administration.

ment is based on the size and location of the tumor, the type of tumor, and the client's physical condition. The following tests aid in diagnosing a brain tumor:

- A *CT scan* or *MRI* is ordered to locate and define the size of the tumor.
- An *electroencephalogram (EEG)* is ordered if seizures are present.
- A *cerebral angiogram* is used to measure blood flow through the cerebral blood vessels.
- A *stereotactic needle biopsy* may be performed for some tumors.

Pharmacology

Chemotherapy may be used to treat a brain tumor. One way to administer the chemotherapy is by an Ommaya reservoir. This device is surgically implanted into the lateral ventricle of the brain (Figure 29-9 ◆). It allows the chemotherapy to be absorbed along with CSF. New timed-release chemotherapy wafers can be placed directly into the tumor cavity after the tumor is removed by surgery.

Radiation Therapy

Radiation therapy may be given to slow tumor growth or following surgery. The purpose is to destroy abnormal tumor cells that are more sensitive to radiation. Conventional external radiation may given daily, five times per week for 6 weeks. In special cancer treatment centers, a newer procedure called stereotaxic radiation or "gamma knife" is used for deep tumors. A stereotaxic frame is attached to the client's head. This allows a large, single dose of radiation to be directed at a small specific site so that normal cells are not harmed.

Intracranial Surgery

Surgery can remove a tumor, reduce its size (also known as **debulking**), or relieve symptoms. Some of the common intracranial surgeries are:

- *Burr hole:* A hole is drilled into the skull to remove a clot or to relieve pressure.
- *Craniotomy:* A surgical opening is made into the cranial cavity (Figure 29-10 ◆). A craniotomy is done by making a

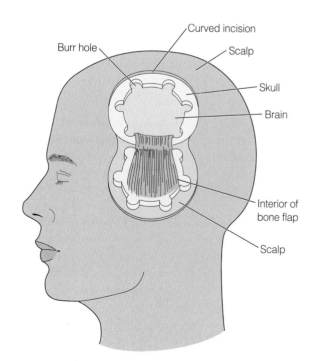

Figure 29-10. ◆ In a craniotomy, a portion of the skull and overlying scalp is removed to allow access to the brain.

series of burr holes. The bone between the holes (bone flap) is cut with a saw and then turned down. After the tumor is removed, the bone flap is sutured in place. A craniotomy is also used to repair defects following a head injury.

- *Supratentorial craniotomy* (above the tentorium) allows access to the frontal, temporal, occipital, and parietal lobes.
- *Infratentorial craniotomy* (below the tentorium) provides access to the cerebellum and brain stem.
- *Craniectomy:* Complete removal of a bone flap decreases cerebral edema.
- *Cranioplasty:* Synthetic material, a metal plate, or wire mesh is inserted where the skull was removed.

NURSING CARE

ASSESSING

Before delivering care, the nurse gathers information about the client's history and performs a basic neurologic examination. If the client is confused or has difficulty answering questions, the family should be included in the interview. Assessment data can identify how the brain tumor is interfering with the client's life (Box 29-6).

DIAGNOSING, PLANNING, AND IMPLEMENTING

The client with a brain tumor may have many nursing care needs. The diagnosis of a brain tumor is frightening. Clients and their families may face an uncertain future. In addition, the client may experience side effects from chemotherapy, radiation, or surgery. Following surgery, the client may develop an altered LOC, IICP, and seizures. The client will require intensive care in the immediate postoperative period. Nursing care following a craniotomy is found in Box 29-7. The client may also experience anxiety and an altered body image.

ANXIETY

- Explain diagnostic procedures and treatment methods to the client and family. Repeat information as needed. *The client and family need time to adjust to the diagnosis and its implications. If urgent treatment is necessary, they will not have time to adjust. Explaining the procedures and treatments may decrease anxiety.*
- Encourage client and family to express their feelings. *Talking about their feelings and fears can reduce anxiety.*
- Provide emotional support by listening and staying with the client. If the client prefers, arrange for a member of the clergy to visit. *Provide a calm environment. Listening and the nurse's physical presence may make the client feel calmer.*

DISTURBED BODY IMAGE

- Assess for signs and symptoms of a negative body image (e.g., refusal to look in the mirror, denial, and withdrawal

---

BOX 29-6
ASSESSING CLIENTS WITH BRAIN TUMORS

SUBJECTIVE DATA
- Present health status:
  - Change in memory, ability to concentrate, personality, or behavior
  - Describe frequency and location of headache
  - Difficulty speaking; double or blurred vision; ringing in the ears
  - Dizziness or changes in coordination or balance
  - Any numbness, tingling, or weakness in extremities
- Past medical history:
  - History of seizures or brain tumors

OBJECTIVE DATA
- Blood pressure, pulse, respirations, temperature
- Observe for orientation to time, place, and person, and memory lapses.
- Assess strength of hand grip and movement of extremities.
- Assess gait by asking the client to walk normally, then in a heel-to-toe fashion.
- Assess coordination.

---

from family and friends). *Physical changes; dependence on others for basic needs; and long-term speech, vision, and motor deficits can cause low self-esteem.*
- Provide or arrange for a client to have surgical cap, scarf, or turban. Assist the client to obtain a wig or hairpiece. Reinforce the fact that the hair will grow back. *These interventions can decrease the client's embarrassment about hair loss.*

EVALUATING

Collect the following data to evaluate the effectiveness of nursing interventions for the client following a craniotomy:

- Absence of neurologic deficits and signs of infection
- Anxiety remains at manageable level
- Knowledge of follow-up care

Discharge Considerations

Clients diagnosed with a brain tumor have short- and long-term needs. They may require chemotherapy or radiation treatments. If surgery is planned, the client and family need to discuss their fears about the potential side effects. Assess the client's and family's capabilities and resources to provide care after discharge. (See Box 29-4 for general discharge guidelines.)

BOX 29-7
NURSING CARE CHECKLIST

CLIENTS HAVING A CRANIOTOMY

Preoperative Care

See Chapter 7 for routine preoperative care.

☑ Assess understanding and level of anxiety of the planned surgery.

☑ Prepare the family for how the client will appear after surgery: A large dressing covering the head; possible swollen, bruised eyelids; and an endotracheal tube.

Postoperative Care

Refer to Chapter 7 for routine postoperative care.

☑ Review Nursing Care intervention for IICP.

☑ Monitor respiratory status every 1 to 2 hours and assess airway patency.

☑ Monitor oxygen saturation levels as needed.

☑ Position on the nonoperative side if a bone flap or large mass was removed, to decrease venous collection and pressure on the surgical incision.

☑ Apply cool cloth over client's eyes. Reduce noise and bright lights in the room.

☑ For pain, use non-narcotic analgesics or codeine.

☑ Assess and report CSF leak from ears, nose, or wound; a leak might indicate an opening in the dura that could allow bacteria into the brain.

☑ Provide interventions to prevent infection:
  ☑ Use strict aseptic technique when changing dressings and caring for wound drains and ICP monitor lines. Monitor for any purulent drainage.
  ☑ Administer prescribed antibiotics.
  ☑ Assess for manifestations of meningitis.
  ☑ After the head dressing is removed (usually 3 days post surgery), clean the incision with half-strength hydrogen peroxide to remove dried blood.

☑ If CSF leak is present, place a sterile dressing over the drainage area and change when damp.
  ☑ If CSF leaks from the nose, elevate head of bed 20 degrees unless contraindicated. Do not suction nasally; do not clean the nose; tell client not to put fingers in the nose.
  ☑ If CSF leaks from the ear, position client on side of leakage unless contraindicated. Do not clean the ear; tell client not to put fingers in the ear.

☑ Monitor for seizures and maintain seizure precautions.

If chemotherapy or radiation therapy is ordered, the following information should be given to the client and family:

- Importance of keeping appointments for chemotherapy or radiation therapy
- Adverse effects of chemotherapy or radiation
- Skin care with radiation therapy
- How to manage nausea or vomiting; nutritional support

Following a craniotomy, the client and family requires emotional support. The recovery process is lengthy. It involves adapting to body image changes and managing motor and sensory deficits. Encourage the family to be involved in the client's care. For example, they can assist the client with personal hygiene and meals. As clients are able, they should be encouraged to take an active role in their own care.

The client and family may need information about support groups and community resources. Clients with neurologic deficits are referred for physical, occupational, and speech therapy. Before the client is discharged home, the nurse should provide verbal and written information on the following topics:

- The use and side effects of anticonvulsant and anti-inflammatory medications
- Wound care:
  - Do not shampoo hair until the incision is healed, then pat the incision dry after shampooing. Avoid a curling iron or hair dryer on hot setting until hair has grown back.
  - When outside, wear a hat to prevent sunburn.
  - Protect the head until the wound is healed.
- Signs and symptoms to report:
  - Swelling at incision site; bloody, yellow, or clear drainage from ears, nose, or incision
  - Increased drowsiness
  - Changes in behavior
  - Stiff neck, severe headache, and elevated temperature
  - New sensory or motor deficits, vision changes, or seizures
- Safety precautions for motor deficits, sensory deficits, lack of coordination, seizures, and cognitive deficits
- Importance of follow-up appointments

Cerebrovascular Accident

A **cerebrovascular accident (CVA)** is also called a brain attack or stroke. It leads to neurologic deficits from decreased blood supply to a local area of the brain. CVAs are the third leading cause of death in the United States. They can occur at any age but occur most often in the elderly. There is a higher incidence in people with a family history of CVA. Other risk factors are listed in Box 29-8. Approximately 750,000 people suffer a CVA each year in the United States. CVAs can be fatal and frequently leave clients with some type of physical disability.

PATHOPHYSIOLOGY

A **transient ischemic attack (TIA)** (brief episode of reversible neurologic deficits) only last for several minutes, and usually last less than 24 hours. It is often a warning signal of a future CVA. The client may experience several TIAs before a CVA. The time between the TIA and a CVA ranges from hours to months. Manifestations include dizziness, visual

BOX 29-8
RISK FACTORS FOR CVA

- Hypertension
- Atherosclerosis
- Cardiac disease (coronary artery disease, congestive heart failure, rhythm problems [atrial fibrillation], rheumatic heart disease)
- High cholesterol
- Obesity
- Diabetes mellitus
- Smoking
- Excessive use of alcohol
- Drug use (cocaine)
- Oral contraceptives
- Persons over 65 years of age
- African Americans (twice the risk of Caucasians)
- Male gender (slightly higher risk)

loss in one eye, one-sided numbness or weakness of the fingers, arms or legs, or aphasia.

A CVA is the sudden loss of neurologic function. The three most common causes are: (1) thrombus, (2) embolus, and (3) hemorrhage (Table 29-5 ◆). Any one of these causes can partially or completely reduce blood flow to cerebral tissues. This decreases oxygen to the area of the brain supplied by the involved blood vessels. Initially, the brain cells are ischemic but quickly die resulting in a cerebral infarction. If the brain experiences **anoxia** (lack of oxygen to the brain) for more than 10 minutes, irreversible brain damage occurs. Adequate collateral blood supply can decrease the amount of damage. Large areas of infarction usually result in severe disability or death.

When cerebral blood supply is altered, there is temporary or permanent loss of neurologic function. The signs and symptoms of a CVA vary, depending on the area of the brain involved, the size of the area, and collateral blood flow. Typical manifestations alter movement, sensation, thought, memory, behavior, or speech (Table 29-6 ◆). However, the affects of a CVA are not limited to the nervous system. Complications of a CVA affect respiration, elimination, and muscle function.

Motor Deficits

A common manifestation following a CVA is motor deficits. Depending on the area of the brain involved, CVAs may cause weakness, paralysis, or spasticity. Because the sensory and motor nerves cross at the neck, sensory and motor deficits develop on the opposite side of the damage. For example, a CVA in the right hemisphere causes deficits in the left side of the body and vice versa. This is known as **contralateral** (opposite side) deficit. The deficits include:

- *Hemiparesis:* Weakness of the left or right half of the body.
- **Hemiplegia:** Paralysis of the left or right half of the body (Figure 29-11 ◆). Initially, the affected arm and leg are flaccid; they become spastic within 6 to 8 weeks. Spasticity can lead to adduction of the shoulder; flexion of the fingers, wrist, elbow, and knee; and external rotation of the hip. All of these problems limit the client's mobility and increase risk for complications of immobility (thrombophlebitis, orthostatic hypotension, aspiration and pneumonia, contractures, and decubitus ulcers).

Speech Deficits

Speech deficits usually result from a CVA affecting the dominant hemisphere. The left hemisphere is dominant in all right-handed people and most left-handed people. Strokes

TABLE 29-5   COMPARISON OF THE TYPES OF CVA (STROKE)

TYPE	CAUSE	ONSET	PATHOPHYSIOLOGY
Thrombotic CVA	Atherosclerosis of large cerebral arteries	During or after sleep	Atherosclerosis causes plaque to build up in cerebral arteries. If plaque is not removed or treated, a thrombus or clot develops. This leads to ischemia in the brain tissue supplied by the vessel.
Embolic CVA	Atrial fibrillation, congestive heart failure (CHF), rheumatic heart disease, Mitral valve disease Endocarditis	Sudden onset with immediate deficits	Embolus travels to a cerebral artery from a distant site, especially the heart. It usually lodges in a narrow portion of a cerebral artery causing necrosis.
Hemorrhagic CVA	Hypertension	Occurs suddenly, often during some activity	Hypertension weakens a cerebral blood vessel causing it to rupture. This leads to bleeding into the brain tissue or subarachnoid space.

	TABLE 29-6 MANIFESTATIONS AND COMPLICATIONS OF CEREBROVASCULAR ACCIDENT	

MANIFESTATIONS	POTENTIAL COMPLICATIONS
Motor Deficits	*Respiratory Problems*
▪ Hemiparesis	▪ Airway obstruction
▪ Hemiplegia	▪ Decreased ability to
▪ Facial droop	cough
	▪ Pneumonia
Speech Deficits	
▪ Expressive aphasia	*Gastrointestinal*
▪ Receptive aphasia	*Problems*
▪ Global aphasia	▪ Dysphagia
▪ Dysarthria	▪ Constipation
Visual Deficits	*Genitourinary Problems*
▪ Diplopia	▪ Incontinence
▪ Homonymous hemianopia	▪ Frequency
	▪ Urinary retention
Sensory–Perceptual Deficits	
▪ Agnosia	*Musculoskeletal*
▪ Apraxia	*Problems*
▪ Neglect syndrome	▪ Contractures
	▪ Muscle atrophy
Cognitive and Behavior	▪ Foot drop
Changes	▪ Shoulder adduction
▪ Memory loss	
▪ Short attention span	*Integumentary*
▪ Poor judgment	*Problems*
▪ Poor problem-solving ability	▪ Decubitus ulcers
▪ Emotional lability	
▪ Depression	

cause many speech and language problems. Among these problems are:

▪ *Expressive aphasia:* An inability to speak or write due to damage of Broca's area; the client usually can understand what is being said.

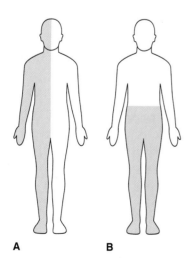

Figure 29-11. ◆ Types of paralysis. (A) Hemiplegia is paralysis of one half of the body. (B) Paraplegia is paralysis of the lower part of the body.

▪ *Receptive aphasia:* An inability to understand the spoken word due to damage of Wernicke's area. The client can speak but the words do not make sense.
▪ *Global aphasia:* A combination of expressive and receptive aphasia.
▪ *Dysarthria:* Difficulty in speech caused by paralysis of the muscles that control speech.

Visual Deficits

When a CVA damages the parietal and temporal lobes, vision is impaired. The client may experience diplopia or **homonymous hemianopia** (the loss of vision in half of the eye). The visual loss is opposite to the side affected by the stroke. The client sees only one half of the normal vision and must turn the head to see the environment (Figure 29-12 ◆).

Sensory–Perceptual Deficits

A CVA may alter sensation and perception. Manifestations can be as mild as numbness and tingling in the unaffected extremity or can be more involved. For instance, some clients do not recognize part of their body or know if an arm or leg is up or down. This increases the client's potential for injury. Common sensory–perceptual deficits include:

▪ *Agnosia:* The inability to recognize a familiar object such as a toothbrush
▪ *Apraxia:* The inability to carry out a familiar routine (e.g., brushing teeth or combing hair) even when paralysis is not present
▪ *Neglect syndrome* (or unilateral neglect): Client ignores the affected side of the body; tends to bump into walls, walk to one side, or fail to dress the affected side

Cognitive and Behavioral Changes

Clients who have had a CVA may have cognition changes. For example, they may experience a memory loss, decreased attention span, poor judgment, and an inability to solve problems. Behavioral changes include **emotional lability** (the client may laugh or cry inappropriately) or loss of self-control such as swearing or refusing to wear clothes. Depression is common, especially when there are functional and speech losses. Stress is poorly tolerated and is seen as uncontrolled anger.

Urinary and Gastrointestinal Problems

When the stroke damages only one hemisphere, bladder and bowel problems are usually short term. Initially, the client

Figure 29-12. ◆ Homonymous hemianopia. Loss of vision in the nasal field of the right eye and temporal field of the left eye.

may experience urinary frequency, urgency, or incontinence. These problems last longer when there are cognitive deficits. Constipation is not from the stroke but rather is a complication of immobility. Impaired swallowing or **dysphagia** (difficult swallowing) can interfere with the client's nutritional needs.

Right and Left Hemisphere Problems

Strokes usually occur in one hemisphere. Recent studies have shown that people who are left hemisphere dominant (right-handed) show certain symptoms. A comparison of right and left hemisphere strokes is given in Box 29-9.

COLLABORATIVE CARE

The client with a TIA receives medications or has surgery to prevent a stroke. Once a CVA has occurred, immediate medical attention is needed. At first, the medical team concentrates on diagnosing the type of CVA and preserving life. Drugs are ordered to reduce IICP and prevent neurologic deficits. Following the acute phase, care focuses on the client's rehabilitation.

Laboratory and Diagnostic Tests

The following diagnostic tests are used to detect the potential for a stroke or to identify physiologic changes once the CVA has occurred:

- CT scan identifies the size and location of the CVA. It is useful to differentiate between an infarction and hemorrhage. Nursing interventions for the client having a CT scan of the head are described in Box 29-10.
- MRI detects areas of infarction earlier than a CT scan.
- *Cerebral arteriography* identifies vessel abnormalities such as an aneurysm.

BOX 29-10
NURSING CARE CHECKLIST

CLIENTS HAVING CT SCAN OF THE HEAD
Preparation of Client

☑ Obtain a signed consent form.
☑ Check facility policy on withholding food and fluids. For A.M. test: NPO 8 hours before test. For P.M. test: May have a liquid breakfast.
☑ Give medications up to 2 hours before test.
☑ Identify for allergy to iodine dye (by asking about allergy to seafood).
☑ Remove hairpins, clips, and earrings.

Client and Family Teaching

☑ Follow the guidelines for not drinking or eating before the test.
☑ If contrast dye is injected, a warm sensation may be felt in the face or body.
☑ The exam lasts from 30 to 90 minutes.
☑ The CT scanner is a narrow circular enclosure with a round opening. You are strapped to a special table while the scanner revolves around your head. This test is painless, but the scanner makes a loud clicking noise.
☑ Someone is always immediately available during the test.

- *Doppler ultrasound* studies evaluate the flow of blood through the carotid arteries and identify if a vessel is partially or completely occluded.
- *Positron emission tomography (PET)* identifies the amount of tissue damage following a CVA.
- *Lumbar puncture* is used to obtain cerebrospinal fluid for examination (Box 29-11). It is performed only when there is no danger of IICP. (Removal of CSF during IICP greatly increases the risk of brain herniation.) Blood in the CSF indicates a hemorrhagic CVA. Nursing interventions for the client having a lumbar puncture are described in Box 29-11.

Pharmacology

Medications are given to prevent a CVA in clients with TIAs or a previous CVA. Antiplatelet medications are most frequently ordered. Platelets can collect in the cerebral arteries and potentially block a vessel. Daily use of low-dose "baby" aspirin effectively reduces clot formation. Other antiplatelet medications include dipyridamole (Persantine), ticlopidine (Ticlid), and clopidrogel (Plavix).

CVAs are now referred to as "brain attack" so that everyone realizes the urgency of seeking immediate medical help. If a thrombotic or embolic stroke is suspected, the client is given thrombolytic drugs such as alteplase (Activase r-tpa) or streptokinase (Streptase). These drugs dissolve blood clots, increase

---

BOX 29-9
RIGHT-HEMISPHERE VERSUS LEFT-HEMISPHERE CVA

Right-Hemisphere CVA	Left-Hemisphere CVA
Left hemiplegia	Right hemiplegia
Left visual field deficits	Right visual field deficits
Spatial–perceptual deficits	Aphasia
Denies or unaware of deficits	Aware of deficits
Easily distracted	Impaired intellectual ability
Poor judgment	Slow, cautious behavior
Impulsive	High level of frustration over losses

BOX 29-11
NURSING CARE CHECKLIST

CLIENTS HAVING LUMBAR PUNCTURE

Preparation of the Client

☑ Obtain a signed consent form.

☑ Obtain lumbar puncture tray and additional equipment requested by the physician.

☑ Have client empty the bowel and bladder before the procedure begins.

☑ Position the client in a lateral recumbent position on the side of the bed with the back toward the physician (see figure).

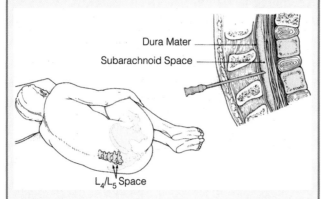

Dura Mater

Subarachnoid Space

L_4/L_5 Space

☑ Assist client to take slow, deep breaths and maintain position during the procedure.

Client and Family Teaching

☑ Reinforce and clarify information about the procedure.

☑ Explain the importance of not moving during the procedure.

☑ A Band-Aid will cover the place where the needle was inserted.

☑ After the procedure, remain flat in bed for 4 to 24 hours as ordered by the physician.

☑ If you have a headache or backache, ask for medications for pain.

After the Procedure

☑ Monitor vital signs and neurologic signs following facility policy.

☑ Monitor the puncture site for leakage of cerebrospinal fluid or hematoma formation.

☑ Encourage fluid intake to replace fluids lost (up to 3,000 mL in 24 hours).

☑ Give analgesics as prescribed for pain.

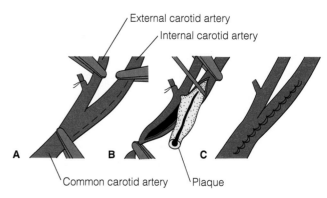

External carotid artery

Internal carotid artery

A   B   C

Common carotid artery   Plaque

Figure 29-13. ◆ Carotid endarterectomy. (A) The occluded area is clamped off and an incision is made in the artery. (B) Plaque is removed from the inner layer of the artery. (C) To restore blood flow through the artery, the artery is sutured or a graft is inserted.

Thrombotic strokes are treated with anticoagulant therapy. They do not dissolve an existing clot but prevent new clots from forming. Anticoagulants are never given to a client who is bleeding within the brain. The most common anticoagulants are heparin and warfarin (Coumadin). Newer low-molecular-weight heparin such as Lovenox may be ordered. Antiplatelet medications are started 24 hours after thrombolytic therapy.

During the acute phase, the client may receive antihypertensive drugs to control blood pressure. Hypertension can increase the area of infarction. If the client has IICP, mannitol or furosemide is used to decrease cerebral edema. An anticonvulsant such as phenytoin is given to prevent or control seizures.

Surgery

Surgery is performed to prevent a stroke. Persons with a history of TIAs or in danger of having another CVA may undergo a **carotid endarterectomy**. Surgery removes atherosclerotic plaque or a thrombus (Figure 29-13 ◆). Nursing care for the client following a carotid endarterectomy is described in Box 29-12. For the first 24 hours after surgery, the client is cared for in the critical care unit. Balloon angioplasty, a nonsurgical procedure, compresses plaque against the arterial wall. This increases blood flow to the cerebrum in hopes of preventing a CVA.

NURSING CARE

Clients with a CVA may fully recover or have numerous disabilities. Usually, the client has some residual effects from the stroke. It is common to find problems with mobility, speech, and swallowing and an inability to perform ADLs. As clients progress from the acute to the recovery phase, they are cared for in a long-term care facility, rehabilitation center, and the home.

ASSESSING

Subjective and objective information is obtained from the client with a suspected TIA or CVA. On admission to the hos-

blood flow, and prevent damage to the brain cells. To be effective, thrombolytics must be started within the first 3 hours after symptoms appear. They are not given when there is intracerebral bleeding.

BOX 29-12
NURSING CARE CHECKLIST

POST CAROTID ENDARTERECTOMY

☑ Place in a supine position with head and neck in mid-line alignment. Elevate the head of the bed 30 degrees unless contraindicated.

☑ Teach client to support the head with the hands when changing position.

☑ Maintain patency of wound drains.

☑ Monitor for *hemorrhage:* Assess for hematoma or bleeding at incision site. Assess neck size and check for drainage under the client's neck and shoulders.

☑ Monitor for *respiratory distress:* Assess respiratory rate, rhythm, depth, and effort. Assess for difficulty swallowing, tracheal deviation from the midline, and restlessness. Keep a tracheostomy set at the bedside.

☑ Monitor for *cranial nerve impairment:* Assess for facial drooping, hoarseness, dysphagia, tongue deviation, speech difficulty, or shoulder sag on one side.

☑ Monitor for *carotid artery occlusion* or *CVA:* Assess for confusion, dizziness, slurred speech, or hemiparesis.

☑ Monitor for *hypertension* or *hypotension:* Monitor blood pressure at least hourly. Report hypertension immediately because of the risk of CVA, artery rupture, or hypotension that could lead to myocardial ischemia.

BOX 29-13
ASSESSING CLIENTS WITH CVA

SUBJECTIVE DATA

- Present health status:
  - Change in memory or confusion
  - Any sudden severe headache
  - Difficulty speaking or understanding speech
  - Any visual changes such as double vision or blurring
  - Any dizziness, loss of coordination or balance
  - Any numbness, tingling, or weakness of the face, arm, or leg
- Past medical history:
  - History of hypertension, previous TIA or CVA, diabetes, arrhythmias, or cardiac disease
  - History of alcohol abuse, smoking
  - Use of antihypertensive, anticoagulant, or oral contraceptive medication

OBJECTIVE DATA

- Blood pressure, pulse, respirations, temperature
- Monitor for manifestations of IICP (see Box 29-1).
- Assess orientation and observe for memory lapses, flat affect.
- Assess for slurred speech, expressive or receptive aphasia.
- Test facial sensation by stroking face with cotton ball.
- Assess strength of hand grip, movement of extremities, and gait.
- Assess ability to swallow. If alert and oriented, ask client to swallow a small sip of water.
- Note presence of bowel and/or bladder incontinence. Palpate bladder for distention.

pital, the client is assessed for any neurologic deficits. If the client's condition is unstable, the respiratory and cardiac status are closely monitored. Box 29-13 suggests additional data to collect.

DIAGNOSING, PLANNING, AND IMPLEMENTING

Many nursing diagnoses are appropriate for the client with a CVA. Each person is affected differently, depending on the amount of brain damage and the area involved. The following problems are discussed: physical mobility, communication, sensory–perceptual deficits, bowel and urine elimination, and swallowing.

INEFFECTIVE TISSUE PERFUSION: CEREBRAL

The acute phase of a CVA is 24 to 72 hours after admission. If the CVA is extensive, the client is cared for in the critical care unit. ICP is monitored closely. See the section on IICP earlier in this chapter.

RISK FOR INEFFECTIVE AIRWAY CLEARANCE

■ Monitor respiratory status and airway patency. Suction the airway as necessary. Place the client in a side-lying position to prevent aspiration. Monitor respiratory status and give oxygen as ordered. *Breathing may be affected by the CVA. If*

the client is unconscious, suctioning is important to prevent airway obstruction. The client is at risk for developing atelectasis and pneumonia.

IMPAIRED PHYSICAL MOBILITY

■ Turn the client from side to side every 2 hours around the clock. Keep the body aligned and place extremities in proper position with pillows (Figure 29-14 ◆). *Mobility can be impaired by weak extremities, muscle wasting, or hemiplegia. Proper positioning and turning maintains joint function, decreases skin breakdown and dependent edema in the hands and feet. It also reduces the risk of other complications resulting from immobility.*

■ Monitor calves each shift for symptoms of thrombophlebitis: redness, warmth, and tenderness. *Clients on bed rest can develop thrombophlebitis.*

■ Do not use a footboard. Use hand splints as directed by the physical therapist. *Footboards are no longer recommended. Hand splints may prevent contractures of the fingers and wrist.*

A

B

C

Figure 29-14. ◆ Positioning the client with hemiplegia is important to prevent deformity of the affected extremities. (A) With the client in a supine position, place a pillow in the axilla (to prevent adduction) and under the hand and arm, with the hand higher than the elbow (to prevent flexion and edema). (B) When the client is lying supine, use a pillow from the iliac crest to the middle of the thigh to prevent external rotation of the hip. (C) When the client is in the prone position, place a pillow under the pelvis to promote hip hyperextension.

- Perform active ROM exercises on unaffected extremities and passive ROM exercises on affected exercises every 4 hours. *Active ROM exercises can improve muscle strength. Passive ROM exercises improve joint mobility.*
- Collaborate with the physical therapist to teach the client transfer and ambulation. *The physical therapist knows the correct transfer and ambulation techniques for the CVA client.*

IMPAIRED VERBAL COMMUNICATION

- Use the following guidelines when communicating with the client:
  - Speak to the client as an adult. Do not raise your voice when speaking to the client.
  - Allow adequate time for the client to answer.
  - Face the client and speak slowly.
  - When you do not understand the client's speech, be honest and say so.

  - Use short, simple statements and "yes" and "no" questions.
  - If clients cannot speak, ask them to nod the head or blink their eyes.
    Communication may be altered by expressive or receptive aphasia. All of these techniques can decrease the client's frustration and may motivate the client to communicate.
- Provide pad and pencil, magic slate, flash cards, computerized talking board, and/or picture board. *Other techniques may help the client communicate.*

DISTURBED SENSORY PERCEPTION

- Keep the environment free of clutter and well lit. Keep the bed in the low position with side rails elevated. *Clients with a CVA are at risk for injury.*
- Place items on the unaffected side. *Clients with a visual field deficit may ignore items on the affected side of the body.*
- Teach the client to turn the head and move the eyes toward the affected side of the body. *Clients with homonymous hemianopia cannot see half of their environment; turning the head and moving the eyes in one direction increases mobility and decreases the risk of injury.*
- Approach the client from the unaffected side and speak before touching. *These actions prevent startling the client.*
- If unilateral neglect is present, encourage client to handle affected extremities. *This increases the client's awareness of the affected side.*

IMPAIRED URINARY ELIMINATION AND CONSTIPATION

- Offer the bedpan or urinal, or assist client to bedside commode every 2 to 4 hours. *This reduces the risk of urinary incontinence and helps establish a regular voiding pattern.*
- Promote daily intake of 2,000 mL, but limit oral intake at night. *Adequate fluid intake may prevent urinary tract infection (UTI). Limiting intake may prevent incontinence at night.*
- Keep the skin dry and monitor for signs of redness. *Clients who are incontinent are at risk for skin breakdown.*
- Reinforce the client's pre-CVA bowel habits:
  - Drink 2,000 mL/day and eat a high-fiber diet.
  - Increase physical activity as tolerated.
  - Offer the bedpan or bedside commode at the same time each day; ensure privacy; and have the client sit in an upright position.
  - Give stool softeners as ordered.
    Increased fluids, fiber, and activity stimulates bowel activity. A regular daily time for bowel movements in the upright position and privacy promotes normal bowel elimination. Stool softeners help prevent hard stool that is more difficult to expel.

IMPAIRED SWALLOWING

- Place the client in an upright position for meals and 30 minutes afterward. Tilt the head slightly forward. *The client's swallowing reflex or ability to concentrate may be affected by a CVA. Upright position and tilting head forward prevent aspiration.*

- Provide oral care before meals. *Oral care stimulates saliva and eases swallowing.*
- Serve thickened liquids, pureed or soft food such as custard, canned fruits, and vegetables. *Thickened liquids and pureed and soft foods are easier to swallow and may prevent aspiration.*
- Encourage client to eat small bites of food and place food on the unaffected side of the mouth. *Small bites and using the unaffected side prevents food from collecting in the mouth and makes swallowing safer.*
- After eating, check the client's mouth for "pocketing" of food, especially on the affected side. *Accumulated food causes odor and tooth or gum disease.*
- Limit distractions during mealtime. *Distractions increase the risk of aspiration.*
- Have suction equipment available during mealtime. *Suction will be needed if the client starts to choke or aspirate.*

SELF-CARE DEFICIT

- Encourage the client to use the unaffected arm to bathe, brush teeth, comb hair, dress, and eat. *Self-care to the extent the client is able reduces their frustration, increases independence, and improves self-esteem. Using the unaffected arm will promote the client's feeling of independence.*
- Teach the client and family to put clothing on the affected extremity first and then dress the unaffected extremities. *This technique increases awareness of the affected extremity and promotes independence.*
- Consult with an occupational therapist to teach the client how to use assistive devices for eating, hygiene, and dressing. *An occupational therapist's role is to teach clients how to use their upper extremities and appropriate assistive devices.*

EVALUATING

Evaluate the effectiveness of nursing care of the client with a CVA by collecting data on the following:

- Airway remains patent
- Provides self-care or with assistance
- Communicates care needs effectively
- Copes with illness
- Demonstrates willingness to participate in rehabilitation
- Knowledge of medications

Discharge Considerations

After a CVA, the client and family face many changes. The middle-aged adult family member may become the caretaker for an older parent. An older adult may be unable to care for a spouse who has had a stroke. They may have to accept placement of the spouse in a long-term care facility.

Discharge planning includes assessing the client's and family's ability to care for the client (see Box 29-4). The client and family need teaching before the client can be sent home. The following topics should be included:

- Prevention of CVA; symptoms of TIA and CVA
- When to seek medical care (provide physician's name and emergency numbers)
- Complications such as aspiration, pneumonia, UTI, blood clots, and skin breakdown
- Medications: Use, dose, and side effects
- Equipment modifications in the home: For example, a raised toilet seat, grab bars in the bathroom, a bath chair, a vise-type jar lid opener, a long-handled shoehorn
- Safety measures to prevent falls
- Demonstration of feeding techniques and use of assistive devices
- Demonstration of ROM exercises and the use of any splints
- Physical care (ADLs, transfer techniques, skin care)
- Psychological support for client and family; respite care for the caregiver
- Community resources such as home health agency, Meals-on-Wheels, elder care (day care for adults); sources for special equipment (e.g., walker); support groups and stroke clubs

Rehabilitation is a lengthy process. The family will need to be patient as the client relearns ADLs. Emphasize that physical function may continue to improve for up to 3 months, and speech may continue to improve even longer.

Aneurysm

A cerebral **aneurysm** is an abnormal outpouching or dilation of a cerebral artery. It occurs at the point where the arterial wall is the weakest. The weakness is related to atherosclerosis, hypertension, or a congenital defect. Cerebral aneurysms usually develop in the Circle of Willis. There are several types of aneurysms: (a) berry, (b) saccular, (c) fusiform, and (d) dissecting (Figure 29-15 ◆). A ruptured cerebral aneurysm is the most common cause of a hemorrhagic CVA.

At first, the weakened portion of the artery enlarges and presses on nearby cranial nerves. Unless it affects cranial nerve function, the person is asymptomatic. As the aneurysm enlarges, it may periodically leak blood into the brain. The person complains of headache, nausea, vomiting, and pain in the neck and back. If the leak can spontaneously seal itself with a clot, the client again becomes asymptomatic. If the aneurysm keeps expanding, it is likely to rupture, forcing blood into the subarachnoid space at the base of the brain. This is known as a **subarachnoid hemorrhage.** Bleeding into the subarachnoid space causes meningeal irritation.

Manifestations of a subarachnoid hemorrhage include: (a) sudden, explosive headache; (b) stiff neck (*nuchal rigidity*); (c) change in consciousness; (d) photophobia; (e) nausea and vomiting; and (f) cranial nerve deficits. The major complications are rebleeding and vasospasm. Rebleeding can occur

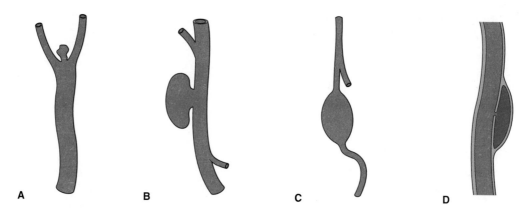

Figure 29-15. ◆ Types of aneurysms. (A) A berry aneurysm is a small sac on a stem or stalk. (B) A saccular aneurysm is formed from a distended small portion of the vessel wall. (C) A fusiform aneurysm is an enlarged area of the entire blood vessel. (D) A dissecting aneurysm is formed when blood fills the area between the tunica media and the tunica intima.

within the first 48 hours and later in 7 to 10 days. The later rebleeding occurs when the initial clot breaks down as part of the body's normal process. A *cerebral vasospasm* occurs when one or more cerebral arteries narrow, leading to ischemia and infarction. Both complications have a high mortality rate.

Diagnosis is made by a CT scan, angiography, and lumbar puncture. A *CT scan* of the brain shows the location and size of the aneurysm. *Cerebral angiography* is done to view the cerebral arteries, locate the aneurysm, and identify a vasospasm. The presence of blood in the cerebrospinal fluid during a *lumbar puncture* confirms a subarachnoid hemorrhage.

Several medications are given to avoid rebleeding and vasospasm until surgery is possible. Aminocaproic acid (Amicar) prevents the clot from being destroyed. A calcium channel blocker, such as nimodipine (Nimotop), decreases vasospasm. The client is given anticonvulsants to prevent seizures. Stool softeners prevent unnecessary straining that can increase intracranial pressure. Acetaminophen or codeine are used for pain control.

Surgery is the treatment of choice to prevent additional bleeding. It is preferred as soon as the client's condition is stable. The skull is opened and either a metal clip is placed at the neck of the aneurysm or the aneurysm is wrapped with synthetic material.

If the size or location of the aneurysm prohibits surgery, the client is managed conservatively. The nurse monitors the client for any signs of deterioration. Neurologic checks, blood pressure, pulse, and respirations are monitored hourly (more frequently if the client's condition worsens). The following aneurysm precautions are instituted to prevent an increase in ICP and the risk of rebleeding:

■ Place the client in a private, quiet, darkened room.
■ Limit visitors to two family members at any one time.
■ Elevate the head of the bed 15 to 30 degrees.
■ Keep on complete bed rest. Feeding and bathing may be allowed.
■ Avoid activities that increase ICP such as coughing, sneezing, straining, blowing the nose, moving self up in bed, or smoking.

Discharge teaching following a subarachnoid hemorrhage is similar to that for a CVA discussed earlier in this chapter. Clients with significant neurologic deficits are referred for rehabilitation services. The client and family need to follow postop craniotomy guidelines (see Box 29-7).

Seizure Disorder

The terms *seizure, convulsion,* and *epilepsy* are often used interchangeably. However, their meanings are very different. A **seizure** is a brief episode of abnormal electrical activity in the nerve cells of the brain. This electrical activity may involve all or part of the brain. A **convulsion** is involuntary muscle contraction and relaxation.

Seizures can occur as an isolated event. For example, it is not uncommon for a client to have a few seizures following a severe head injury. When seizures occur in a chronic pattern, the disorder is called **epilepsy** or *seizure disorder.* The cause of most seizure disorders is unknown. However, seizures beginning in adulthood usually result from other conditions such as a brain infection, CVA, or brain tumor.

PATHOPHYSIOLOGY

Neurons carry messages from the body by electrical impulses to the cerebral cortex. If a few unstable neurons continue sending electrical impulses, a seizure occurs. A group of abnormally firing neurons that start a seizure is called an **epileptogenic focus.** The part of the body controlled by these neurons performs abnormally. Certain conditions such as hypoglycemia, high fever, and hypoxia can trigger seizure activity. Seizures are classified as partial or generalized.

Partial Seizures

Partial (or focal) seizures start in one area of the cerebral cortex. There are two types of partial seizures:

1. *Simple partial seizures* cause uncontrolled jerking movements of a finger, hand, foot, leg, or the face. This motor activity may spread to other body areas and is known as the **jacksonian march.** Sometimes simple partial seizures

involve the sensory part of the brain. Symptoms include flashing lights, tingling sensations, or hallucinations. The seizure activity usually lasts 20 to 30 seconds, and the client does not lose consciousness.

2. *Complex partial seizures* are also known as psychomotor seizures. Manifestations include repetitive, nonpurposeful actions: lip smacking, aimless walking, or picking at clothing. These behaviors are called **automatisms** and last less than 1 minute. During the seizure, the person has an altered level of consciousness. Afterward, the client may be confused or not remember the seizure. The seizure can be preceded by an **aura** (a warning sign that something is going to happen). The aura may be an unusual smell, a sense of deja vu, or a sudden intense emotion.

Generalized Seizures

Generalized seizures involve both hemispheres of the brain and result in loss of consciousness. There are two common forms of generalized seizures:

1. *Absence seizures* are sometimes called *petit mal seizures* and occur more frequently in children. They are characterized by a brief change in consciousness such as a blank stare, blinking of the eyes, eyelid fluttering, and lip smacking. All motor activity is stopped during the seizure. Because the seizure lasts only 5 to 10 seconds, the client may unaware of it. Some clients can experience many seizures per day.

2. *Tonic–clonic seizures,* or *grand mal seizures,* are the most common seizure disorder in adults and children. Because these seizures can develop suddenly, the client risks potential injury such as head trauma, fractures, burns, or motor vehicle accidents. Tonic–clonic seizures follow a typical pattern: (a) aura, (b) epileptic cry, (c) tonic phase, (d) clonic phase, and (e) postictal phase.

The client experiences an aura such as a bright light, an odd taste in the mouth, or an unusual sound. He or she gives an epileptic cry, a loud cry caused by air being forced out of the lungs. At this time the client falls to the ground, loses consciousness, and has tonic contractions followed by clonic contractions (Figure 29-16 ◆). In **tonic contractions,** the body becomes rigid, with the arms and legs extended. The jaw is clenched and the eyes roll back. Breathing stops briefly, and the client develops cyanosis. During **clonic contractions,** movements are jerky as the muscles alternately contract and relax. In addition, tongue and cheek biting, as well as frothing from the mouth, may occur. Urinary and bowel incontinence are common. The entire seizure generally lasts about 1 to 2 minutes.

In the postictal phase, the client is unconscious for up to 30 minutes. The client regains consciousness slowly and may be confused and disoriented on waking. Individuals often experience headache, muscle aches, and fatigue following the seizure. Many people sleep for several hours afterwards. Amnesia of the events prior to the seizure is normal.

Figure 29-16. ◆ Tonic–clonic contractions in grand mal seizures. (A) Tonic phase. (B) Clonic phase.

Status Epilepticus

Status epilepticus is a continuous period of tonic–clonic seizures in which the client does not regain consciousness. Constant seizure activity can harm the brain's nerve cells and lead to permanent brain damage. It also causes physical exhaustion and respiratory distress. It is considered a life-threatening medical emergency. Status epilepticus can be triggered by abrupt discontinuation of anticonvulsant medication, by acute head injury, or by hypoxia.

COLLABORATIVE CARE

Initial treatment focuses on controlling the seizure. Long-term management involves identifying the cause and preventing future seizures. Collaborative care includes diagnostic testing, medications, and, in some cases, surgery.

Laboratory and Diagnostic Tests

A complete neurologic exam is done to identify the site of the seizures. The following diagnostic tests may be ordered:

■ *EEG* can determine the type of seizure and locate the seizure focus. See Box 29-14 for nursing implications with an EEG.

■ *Skull x-rays* may identify possible skull fractures.

■ *CT scan* or *MRI* may detect a tumor, CVA, or hemorrhage.

■ *Blood studies* are done to assess blood count, electrolytes, blood urea nitrogen (BUN), blood glucose, and to test for syphilis.

Pharmacology

Most seizure activity can be decreased or controlled with anticonvulsant medication. The goal is to use the lowest possible dose of medication with the fewest side effects. It takes several weeks to adjust the dose. Routine serum drug levels are drawn to determine effective doses and the potential for toxicity, as well as to identify clients who are not taking their medications. Each medication has a therapeutic and toxic level. Consult a drug handbook for the appropriate levels. If the client's seizures are not well controlled, a second medication is

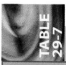

BOX 29-14
NURSING CARE CHECKLIST

CLIENTS HAVING AN ELECTROENCEPHALOGRAM (EEG)

Preparation of the Client

- ☑ Explain the procedure to the client.
- ☑ Withhold tranquilizer and depressant medications 24 to 48 hours before and caffeine-containing foods (e.g., coffee, tea, cola, and chocolate).
- ☑ Shampoo hair the night before.

Client and Family Teaching

- ☑ The test lasts from 1 to 2 hours.
- ☑ The test is painless. It is done while you lie on a stretcher or sit in a reclining chair.
- ☑ Electrodes are applied to the scalp with a thick paste.
- ☑ After the test, the nurse will help you remove the paste from your hair.

added. Many clients often need these drugs their entire life. Anticonvulsant drugs may interact adversely with other drugs. (Nursing implications are discussed in Table 29-7 ◆.)

Status epilepticus must be treated immediately. First, an airway is established. This is followed by intravenous administration of one or more anticonvulsant drugs. Diazepam (Valium) and lorazepam (Ativan) are the drugs of choice to stop seizure activity. Because these drugs are short acting, the dose may need to be repeated. For long-term control, phenytoin and phenobarbital are given.

Surgery

When medications do not control a client's seizures, surgery may be an option. New techniques allow the client to be awake during the surgery. While the client is awake, the surgeon can map the area of abnormal electrical discharges and remove it. It is important to identify the abnormal area of epileptogenic tissue clearly, so that normal brain tissue is not removed.

NURSING CARE

Nursing assessments and interventions focus on care during and immediately after a seizure. Once the client's condition is stable, client and family teaching are emphasized for discharge.

ASSESSING

The nurse collects subjective assessment data to determine the extent to which the seizure activity is interfering with the client's life and the type of medical intervention needed. Objective observations are made before, during, and after a seizure (Box 29-15).

DIAGNOSING, PLANNING, AND IMPLEMENTING

RISK FOR INEFFECTIVE AIRWAY CLEARANCE

- Loosen clothing around the neck. *Loosening clothing can maintain a patent airway.*
- Turn the client on the side. *During a seizure, the tongue may fall back and obstruct the airway. Secretions may pool at the back*

TABLE 29-7   NURSING IMPLICATIONS FOR PHARMACOLOGY: CLIENTS RECEIVING ANTICONVULSANT DRUGS

DRUGS	ACTIONS	NURSING IMPLICATIONS	CLIENT TEACHING
Clonazepam (Klonopin) Carbamazepine (Tegretol) Ethosuximide (Zarontin) Gabapentin (Neurotin) Lamotrigine (Lamictal) Phenobarbital Phenytoin (Dilantin) Fosphenytoin (Cerebryx) Primidone (Mysoline) Valproic acid (Depakene)	Anticonvulsant agents act in the motor cortex of the brain to prevent abnormal electrical discharges from the epileptic foci in this area. They control chronic seizures but do not cure seizure disorders. Also, they raise the seizure threshold so that a seizure cannot begin.	Give at the same time each day with meals to prevent gastric upset. Monitor for side effects (e.g., drowsiness, sedation, ataxia, diplopia, rash, or nystagmus). Check clients taking phenytoin for gingival hyperplasia. Monitor CBC, platelet count, and liver tests for adverse reactions. Monitor serum drug levels for therapeutic range.	Take at the same time each day with meals to prevent gastric upset. If omit a dose, call MD immediately. Do not drive a car or operate machinery when drowsy. If taking Dilantin, brush and floss daily. Report rash, bleeding, unsteady gait, or yellow eyes. Keep follow-up appointments with physician and lab for drug levels. Carry ID card identifying the type of seizures and the medications you are taking.

BOX 29-15
ASSESSING CLIENTS WITH SEIZURE DISORDERS

SUBJECTIVE DATA

- Present health status:
  - Describe where seizures begin in your body. What are you told happens during a seizure? How do you feel after the seizure? Do you have a warning sign (aura)?
- Past medical history:
  - History of birth or head injuries, brain tumor or infections, CVA, liver or renal disease, alcohol or drug addiction
  - Anticonvulsant medications

OBJECTIVE DATA

- Observe before, during, and after a seizure:
  - Precipitating factors; sudden onset or warning aura; length of seizure; presence of epileptic cry; urine or bowel incontinence; clenched teeth; foaming or bleeding from the mouth.
  - Where did the seizure begin; did it involve both sides? Were there tonic to clonic movements?
  - Loss of consciousness during and after seizure. How long?
  - Presence of automatisms (e.g., lip smacking, eyelid fluttering)
  - Rate, quality, or absence of respirations; presence of cyanosis
  - Amnesia about the seizure and events before it

of the mouth. Turning the client on the side allows secretions to drain from the mouth.

- Do not force anything into the client's mouth. *It is not recommended to place anything in the client's mouth during a seizure.*
- Give oxygen by mask as needed. *Seizures can cause hypoxia, so the client may need supplemental oxygen.*
- Provide suction at the bedside. *Suction is used to prevent aspiration.*

RISK FOR INJURY

- Maintain the bed in low position and keep side rails up. *A low bed position helps the client avoid falls and injuries. Side rails prevent the client from falling out of bed during a seizure.*
- Place blankets or protective pads over the side rails. *Padding decreases the risk of injury.*
- If the client is sitting or standing when the seizure begins, gently lower the client to the floor. *Loss of consciousness during a seizure would cause the client to fall.*
- If on the floor, place a folded towel or pillow under the client's head. *The head is protected to prevent injury.*
- Never restrain the client during a seizure. *Physically restraining the client could cause fractures of the arms or legs.*

- Clear the area of objects that could cause harm. *This provides an environment free of potential harm.*

ANXIETY

- Clients with a seizure disorder worry about having a seizure in public and fear rejection by others. Encourage the client to identify potential concerns and misconceptions. *The client needs time to accept the diagnosis and its effect on family, work, and future lifestyle. Misconceptions cause unnecessary worry and anxiety.*
- Provide information about community support groups. *Sharing information with other people with similar health problems may decrease the client's anxiety.*
- Refer the client to any local and state agencies for information about driving or operating dangerous machinery. *Accurate information decreases anxiety. The client needs to know there are legal limitations on driving until a person is proven free of seizures. A driver's license may be reinstated after a seizure-free period and a letter from a physician.*

EVALUATING

Collect the following data to evaluate the effectiveness of nursing care for the client with a seizure disorder:

- Seizures are controlled
- Free from injury
- Knowledge of medications

Discharge Considerations

Seizure disorders require lifelong management. Teach the client and family to understand the disorder, medications, and injury prevention. Refer to Box 29-4 for information to gather while planning the client's discharge.

Teach the care and observations necessary before, during, and after a seizure. Stress the importance of safety and keeping the airway patent. Teach the client and family ways to prevent injury at home by: (a) not smoking in bed or alone, (b) installing grab bars in the shower and tub area, (c) taking a shower rather than a tub bath to prevent drowning, and (d) keeping the bedroom and bathroom doors unlocked in case of an emergency.

The following points should be emphasized:

- Medication use, side effects, and the need to take at prescribed intervals.
- Record any seizure activity and medications taken daily.
- Avoid activities that require alertness and coordination until medication levels are stable.
- Importance of follow-up care and keeping appointments with physician and laboratory.
- Wear ID bracelet identifying seizure condition and medications.

- Limit intake of coffee; avoid alcohol.
- Avoid factors that may trigger a seizure: fatigue, fasting, excessive stress, flashing or blinking lights.
- Information on the Epilepsy Foundation of America.

Intracranial Infections

The most common inflammatory conditions of the brain are meningitis, encephalitis, and brain abscesses. They are caused by bacteria and viruses (Table 29-8 ◆). If untreated, these conditions may lead to long-term neurologic deficits or death.

MENINGITIS

Meningitis is an inflammation of the meninges of the brain and spinal cord. Bacterial meningitis may result from *Neisseria meningitidis* (meningococcal meningitis), *Streptococcus pneumoniae,* or *Haemophilus influenzae.* Organisms enter the brain by way of (a) the bloodstream, (b) the respiratory tract, or (c) penetrating wounds of the skull or cranial surgery. Most often, meningitis is secondary to another infection such as otitis media, an upper respiratory infection, or pneumonia. Viral meningitis, also called aseptic meningitis, is a less severe disease than bacterial meningitis. It is caused by several common viruses (see Table 29-8).

Once the bacteria or virus enters the central nervous system, it begins an inflammatory response in the meninges, CSF, and ventricles. The inflammatory process increases production of CSF. This can lead to cerebral edema and increase ICP. Although viral infection also triggers the inflammatory response, the course of the disease is shorter. Recovery is usually uneventful.

Manifestations show an irritation of the meninges, as outlined in Box 29-16. Two positive signs of meningeal irritation are Brudzinski's sign and Kernig's sign. In Brudzinski's sign, when the client's neck is flexed, the knees and hips flex. Kernig's sign is an inability to extend the leg when the hip is flexed at a 90-degree angle. The client may also show signs of IICP, including decreased LOC, seizures, and changes in vital signs and respiratory pattern.

Complications of meningitis may include seizures, sepsis, cranial nerve dysfunction, cerebral infarction, coma, and death. Meningitis may leave residual effects such as visual impairment, deafness, cranial nerve palsies, or paralysis.

Meningococcal meningitis can progress to the devastating complication of meningococcemia. This form of meningitis is spread by airborne droplets and is highly contagious. It can cause death within 10 to 12 hours after the client develops a high fever and petechial rash. Death results from an overwhelming septicemia, vascular collapse, and adrenal hemorrhage.

ENCEPHALITIS

Encephalitis is an acute inflammation of the white and gray matter of the brain and spinal cord. It is almost always caused by a virus, but it may also be caused by bacteria or fungi (see Table 29-8). Many of the viruses are associated with certain seasons of the year or particular geographic regions. The virus may be transmitted by ticks or mosquitoes.

Encephalitis ranges from a mild infection to a serious disease that could be fatal. There is widespread inflammation. Nerve cells may be extensively damaged. Edema and areas of

TABLE 29-8	COMPARISON OF INTRACRANIAL INFECTIONS	
INFECTION	**CAUSATIVE ORGANISM**	**SUSCEPTIBLE CLIENTS**
Bacterial meningitis		
▪ Pneumococcal meningitis	*Streptococcus pneumoniae*	Young adults and those over 40
▪ *Haemophilus influenzae* meningitis	*Haemophilus influenzae*	Children 2 months to 7 years
▪ Meningococcal meningitis	*Neisseria meningitidis*	Children under 5, adolescents, college students living in dormitories; higher incidence in males
Viral (aseptic) meningitis	Herpes simplex and zoster; mumps, Epstein–Barr virus; cytomegalovirus (CMV)	All ages
Encephalitis	St. Louis encephalitis virus, Eastern and western equine virus transmitted by ticks and mosquitoes; herpes simplex; rabies; after vaccination with measles, mumps, or rubella	All ages
Brain abscess	Secondary infection from streptococci, staphylococci, pneumococci	30 to 40 years old; higher incidence in men

BOX 29-16
MANIFESTATIONS OF MENINGITIS

- Headache
- High fever
- Photophobia
- Nausea, vomiting
- Nuchal rigidity (stiff neck)
- Positive Brudzinski's sign
- Positive Kernig's sign
- Restlessness and irritability
- Confusion, altered LOC
- Signs of IICP (elevated blood pressure, bradycardia, change in respiratory pattern, decreased LOC)
- Seizures
- Petechial rash (in meningococcal meningitis)

A   Brudzinski's Sign

B   Kernig's Sign

BRAIN ABSCESS

A **brain abscess** is a collection of purulent material within the brain. Many brain abscesses occur from an infection in the middle ear or nasal sinuses. They may develop after a head injury or intracranial surgery. Other sources include bacterial endocarditis; osteomyelitis; and lung, pelvic, or skin infections. Streptococci, staphylococci, and pneumococci are often the underlying causes.

The microorganisms in the brain tissue cause local inflammation. As the white blood cells destroy the organisms, pus forms. The body tries to protect the rest of the brain by forming a capsule around the pus. Unless the abscess is treated, the capsule enlarges and compresses nerves and brain tissue. Chronic inflammation can lead to edema and IICP.

Initially, the client complains of a headache. General symptoms associated with an acute infectious process include fever, chills, and malaise. As the abscess expands, nausea, vomiting, drowsiness, confusion, weakness on one side, and seizures develop.

COLLABORATIVE CARE

Bacterial meningitis is a medical emergency that could be fatal within days. Treatment focuses on a rapid diagnosis and starting antibiotic therapy immediately. Depending on hospital policy, the client may be placed in airborne precautions isolation. Management of viral meningitis focuses on relieving client symptoms with antipyretics and analgesics. Antibiotic therapy and specific isolation precautions are not indicated for viral meningitis

The treatment for encephalitis is similar to that for meningitis, with the exception of drug therapy. Antiviral medications are used. Isolation is not necessary, because encephalitis is not transmitted from person to person.

Treatment of the client with a brain abscess focuses on beginning antibiotic therapy promptly. Other manifestations are treated symptomatically. An abscess may be surgically drained or, if encapsulated, removed by a craniotomy. The decision to perform surgery is based on the client's general condition, as well as the stage and site of the abscess.

Laboratory and Diagnostic Tests

The diagnosis of bacterial or viral meningitis or encephalitis is based on clinical manifestations. Diagnosis of a brain abscess is more difficult because there are unclear symptoms. The following diagnostic tests may be ordered:

- *Lumbar puncture* is done to collect samples of CSF. The following findings indicate a positive diagnosis of bacterial meningitis: (a) CSF appears cloudy, (b) an elevated protein level and white blood cell count, (c) a decreased glucose level, and (d) elevated CSF pressure.
- *Culture and sensitivity* and *Gram stain* of the CSF can identify the bacteria or virus causing meningitis or encephalitis.
- *Cultures from the blood, urine, throat, and nose* are performed to identify the bacterial source of infection.
- *CT scan, MRI,* or *skull x-rays* may identify the infection source causing a brain abscess.

necrosis may lead to localized hemorrhage. IICP develops, progressing to brain herniation. Certain viruses seem to affect certain areas of the brain. For example, herpes simplex virus involves the frontal and temporal lobes.

Manifestations are similar to those of meningitis. Common symptoms include high fever, headache, stiff neck, and seizures. The client may be confused and disoriented or agitated and restless. As the disease progresses, the LOC deteriorates, and the client becomes comatose. Other manifestations include facial weakness, aphasia, visual disturbances, and hemiparesis.

Pharmacology

In cases of bacterial meningitis, high doses of penicillin, ampicillin, and third-generation cephalosporins are started immediately. The specific antibiotic is chosen after the culture and sensitivity report identifies the causative organism. Antibiotic therapy is given intravenously and in high doses so that it will cross the blood–brain barrier and reach the CSF. Drug therapy is continued from 7 to 21 days. Antibiotic therapy is also used to treat brain abscesses.

Anyone exposed to meningococcal meningitis is started on prophylactic antibiotic therapy immediately. The drugs of choice are rifampin (Rifadin) and ciprofloxacin (Cipro). All cases of meningitis must be reported to the local public health department.

Treatment for encephalitis consists of antiviral drugs such as vidarabine (Vira-A) and acyclovir (Zoviran). If started early in the disease course, they may decrease mortality. They are most effective if used before the client becomes comatose.

The following medications are given to relieve symptoms and to prevent complications from any one of the intracranial infections. Anticonvulsant medications prevent or control seizures. Antipyretics are used to reduce fever. Analgesics such as acetaminophen are given to relieve headache and neck pain. Osmotic diuretics and corticosteroids may decrease cerebral edema. The client initially may require antiemetics to control nausea and vomiting. Intravenous fluids may be necessary to prevent dehydration until the client is able to take oral fluids.

NURSING CARE

Clients with an intracranial infection are acutely ill. Depending on the extent of their illness, they may be cared for in the critical care unit or on a medical unit. If neurologic deficits are present, long-term nursing may be needed. The combination of fever, dehydration, and cerebral edema predisposes the client to seizures.

ASSESSING

An important aspect of care is to obtain a careful history and identify subjective and objective data. Box 29-17 outlines data to collect on the client with an intracranial infection.

DIAGNOSING, PLANNING, AND IMPLEMENTING

RISK FOR INEFFECTIVE TISSUE PERFUSION: CEREBRAL

- Monitor for altered neurologic function. See interventions for IICP discussed earlier in this chapter. *Inflammation from intracranial infections increases the client's risk for developing altered levels of consciousness, seizures, increased IICP, and cranial nerve dysfunction.*

BOX 29-17
ASSESSING CLIENTS WITH INTRACRANIAL INFECTIONS

SUBJECTIVE DATA

- Present health status:
  - Presence of nausea, vomiting, photophobia, or stiff neck
  - Confusion or headache
- Past medical history:
  - Exposure to mosquitoes or ticks
  - History of head injury, brain surgery, otitis media, or bacterial endocarditis

OBJECTIVE DATA

- Blood pressure, pulse, and temperature
- Assess orientation, LOC, memory, and response to stimuli.
- Assess for dizziness, diplopia, drooping eyelids, pupil changes, and hearing difficulty due to cranial nerve damage.
- Assess for Brudzinski's or Kernig's signs (see Figure 29-16A and B).
- Observe for any seizure activity, restlessness, and/or agitation.
- Inspect skin for presence of petechial rash over the body.

HYPERTHERMIA

- Monitor body temperature at least every 4 hours. *Clients with intracranial infections can spike high fevers, which could lead to seizures.*
- To reduce fever, remove unnecessary clothing and bed linen. Give antipyretic medications and tepid sponge baths as ordered. Apply a cooling blanket beneath the client. *Antipyretic drugs, tepid sponge baths, and a cooling blanket are used to reduce a fever. Removing unnecessary clothing and bed linen promotes cooling. The temperature is decreased slowly to prevent shivering which can raise the temperature higher.*
- Monitor for signs and symptoms of dehydration noting skin turgor, mucous membranes, and daily body weight. Measure and compare intake and output every 2 to 4 hours. Note urine concentration. *Fluids are restricted in clients with intracranial disorders to prevent cerebral edema. When a high fever exists, fluids are quickly lost. Both factors increase the client's risk for dehydration.*

ACUTE PAIN

- Reduce environmental stimuli; keep room quiet, and dim bright lights. *Environmental stimuli can increase the client's headache. Low lighting may decrease hallucinations and photophobia.*
- Provide gentle ROM exercises. *ROM exercises reduce joint stiffness and promote circulation.*

- Place client in position of comfort. *Positioning may decrease the client's muscle and joint aches.*
- Place a cool cloth over the client's eyes. *This may decrease the client's headache and the discomfort of photophobia.*
- Give a mild analgesic such as acetaminophen or codeine. *Meperidine and morphine sulfate are avoided because they can alter the size and reaction of the client's pupils.*

EVALUATING

Evaluate the effectiveness of the nursing care for a client with an intracranial infection by collecting the following data:

- Temperature within normal range
- Absence of headache and neurologic irritation
- No signs of IICP
- Knowledge of anti-infective therapy

Discharge Considerations

Following the acute phase of an intracranial infection, the client requires several weeks of convalescence. The client and family need to understand home management. The nurse assesses the client's and family's abilities and resources to provide care after discharge. See earlier discussion of discharge considerations in Box 29-4.

Include the following topics in the teaching session:

- Medications: Use, dose, and side effects. Emphasize the importance of taking all antibiotic or antiviral medication until completely gone to prevent new organisms from growing.
- Emphasize the importance of reporting fever, headache, or neck stiffness in people who had close contact with the client with meningitis.
- Encourage adequate rest and sleep as well as a well-balanced diet.
- Advise to increase physical activity gradually.
- Stress the importance of reporting any signs or symptoms of ear infection, sore throat, or upper respiratory infection.

The client with permanent neurologic deficits resulting from encephalitis is usually discharged to a rehabilitation setting or a long-term care facility. For infections transmitted by mosquitoes, the client and family need to know how to destroy breeding sites of insect larvae. They are also taught to avoid mosquito and tick bites by wearing protective clothing and insect repellents.

Headaches

Headache or **cephalalgia** is one of the most common symptoms people experience at all ages. Headaches may be caused by underlying conditions such as brain tumors, meningitis, or head injuries. They can also result from stress or muscle ten-

sion. Most headaches are mild and are relieved by a mild analgesic. Other headaches are chronic, intense, and recurring. Clinical manifestations vary according to the cause and type of the headache.

The cranium has many pain-sensitive structures. These include the skin, muscles, and periosteum of the skull; the nasal cavities and sinuses; parts of the meninges; cerebral blood vessels; and cranial nerves with sensory function. Stretching, inflammation, pressure, and dilation of the pain-sensitive structures can produce a headache. The most common types of headaches are migraine, cluster, and tension headaches (Table 29-9 ◆).

MIGRAINE HEADACHE

Migraine headaches are the most common type of vascular headache. Their exact cause is unknown. It is believed that at first the cerebral blood vessels constrict and then dilate, releasing serotonin, which causes the headache. Migraines differ in intensity, duration, and frequency from client to client, and episodes may be different in the same person (see Table 29-9).

CLUSTER HEADACHE

The cluster headache is a form of vascular headache. It typically begins 2 to 3 hours after the person falls asleep. The attacks usually occur in clusters of 1 to 8 daily for weeks or a few months; then they disappear for an extended period. Usually, the same side of the head is involved in each cluster of attacks. Cluster headaches are triggered by alcohol consumption.

TENSION HEADACHE

Tension headaches often result from prolonged muscle contraction of the head and neck. They are poorly localized with a gradual onset. Occupations that require a prolonged period of abnormal posture such as bending over a desk often precipitate tension headache. Slouching while reading or watching television can lead to muscle contraction. Most headaches are tension headaches.

COLLABORATIVE CARE

The first priority of care is to identify the underlying cause of the headache. If the cause is treatable, the headache symptoms should decrease or disappear. Migraine headaches are managed by drug therapy, client teaching, and controlling triggers. Eliminating alcohol may reduce the incidence of cluster headaches. Biofeedback and meditation are used to decrease the client's stress and the possibility of tension headaches. Improving poor posture and initiating comfort measures such as gentle massage or heat may also help.

A thorough history and physical examination are part of the diagnosis and treatment. A brain scan, MRI, x-ray studies of the skull and cervical spine, EEG, and lumbar puncture for CSF are used to rule out other neurologic problems. Serum metabolic screens and hypersensitivity testing also may be performed if systemic problems are suspected.

TABLE 29-9 TYPES OF HEADACHES

TYPE	RISK FACTORS	DESCRIPTION	MANIFESTATIONS
Migraine	More common in women	May be triggered by stress or crisis; foods such as alcohol, chocolate, caffeine, or nuts. Often correlates with menstrual cycle. May last hours to days. *Common:* May be associated with hereditary factors.	*Classic:* Preceded by aura; weakness in extremities, tingling in face or hands. Pulsating or throbbing pain on one side of the head, then spreads to other side. *Common:* No aura; occurs on one or both sides; may also cause nausea, vomiting, and diarrhea.
Cluster	More common in men	Series of headaches over a 2- to 3-month period, usually in spring or fall; then disappear for a long period of time.	Unilateral pain located around or behind the eye that can wake the client; also nasal congestion, tearing, facial flushing.
Tension	More common in women	May be triggered by stress, eyestrain, or poor posture. These triggers can cause muscle contraction in neck, face, and scalp.	Bilateral pain, tightness, pressure, or viselike feeling; pain is most common on awakening.

Pharmacology

The choice of medications for managing headaches depends on the specific type of headache. The goals are to reduce the frequency and severity of headaches and to limit or stop a headache when it occurs.

To reduce the frequency and severity of migraines, several prophylactic medications are ordered. Methysergide maleate (Sansert) decreases serotonin action and causes vasoconstriction. Propranolol (Inderal) prevents dilation of cerebral blood vessels. Verapamil (Isoptin) controls cerebral vasospasms. Amitriptyline (Elavil) blocks the uptake of serotonin and catecholamines.

Before a migraine becomes severe, ergotamine (Ergostat), ergotamine with caffeine, or dihydroergotamine (Migranal) may be used. They cause vasoconstriction of the cerebral blood vessels. These preparations may be given by the oral, sublingual, subcutaneous, intramuscular, intravenous, rectal, or intranasal route. When given at the first sign of an attack, ergotamine is effective in controlling up to 70% of acute attacks. Ergotamine tartrate may be given in suppository form at bedtime to prevent cluster headaches.

Sumatriptan (Imitrex) is effective in treating migraine and cluster headaches. It is available for oral, subcutaneous autoinjection, or intranasal use. This medication binds with serotonin and acts rapidly to stop the headache.

Once a migraine attack is in progress, a narcotic analgesic such as codeine or meperidine (Demerol) may be needed. Antiemetics such as promethazine (Phenergan) or metoclopramide (Reglan) are given to control nausea and vomiting.

Nonnarcotic analgesics such as aspirin or acetaminophen may be effective in relieving tension headaches. Additionally, tranquilizers such as diazepam may be employed to reduce muscle tension.

NURSING CARE

Nursing care begins by obtaining a history and description of the headache. It is important to identify the effects of recurring headaches on the client's daily life. Box 29-18 lists assessment data to collect. Nursing interventions focus on controlling the pain and discomfort of the headache.

PAIN

- Ask the client to rate the pain on a scale of 0 to 10 (10 = the worst pain) or provide a visual analog of faces that show different levels of discomfort. *Rating scales provide objective data about the client's subjective pain or discomfort. They can also evaluate the effectiveness of pain relief measures.*
- Minimize light, noise, and activity. Provide rest in a quiet, nonstimulating environment when the headache is present. *Reducing environmental stimuli may decrease pain.*
- Encourage the client to use deep breathing or relaxation techniques. *These strategies reduce tension and may help the client gain a sense of control over the pain.*
- Apply cold or warm cloth to the head and neck as ordered. *Cold causes vasoconstriction, which may reduce pain in vascular headaches. Heat reduces muscle tension and improves circulation.*
- Offer a back massage. *Massage promotes muscle relaxation, which is especially useful for tension headaches.*

Collect the following information to evaluate the effectiveness of providing care to the client with headaches:

- Decreased or absence of pain
- Understands medications
- Modifies lifestyle to reduce headaches

BOX 29-18
ASSESSING CLIENTS WITH HEADACHES

SUBJECTIVE DATA

- Present health status:
  - Describe headaches: Type of pain, frequency, duration, location, precipitating factors, time of day it occurs, relieving factors
  - Any light flashes or bright spots before the headache begins?
  - Does nausea, vomiting, or numbness accompany headache?
  - Interference with daily activities or associated with stress
  - Exposure to toxic chemicals at work
- Past medical history:
  - Family history of migraines
  - Medication and alcohol use
  - Any allergies

OBJECTIVE DATA

- Observe for facial flushing and tearing. (Present with cluster headaches.)
- Observe for pallor, diaphoresis, and one-sided weakness. (Present with migraines.)
- Note presence of nausea, vomiting, or diarrhea.
- Palpate neck and shoulder muscles for tightness (Present with tension headaches).

- Medication use, dosage, and side effects
- Importance of reporting ergotamine side effects (e.g., numbness and tingling in fingers and toes, leg weakness, and aching muscles)
- Eliminating caffeine, cured meats, monosodium glutamate (MSG), and foods containing tyramine (chocolate, red wine, aged cheese); avoiding smoking
- Participating in regular moderate exercise.
- Avoid fasting, fatigue, and irregular sleep patterns.
- Importance of keeping a headache diary.
- Identifying comfort measures during a headache: darkened, quiet room and applying a cool cloth to the forehead.

Nursing Interventions Classification

In addition, the following interventions developed by McCloskey and Bulechek (2000) may be appropriate for the client with intracranial disorders:

- Bed Rest
- Seizure Precautions
- Self-care Assistance: Bathing/Hygiene
- Caregiver Support
- Communication Enhancement: Speech Deficit
- Fall Prevention

(*Note:* The bibliography listings for this and all chapters have been compiled at the back of the book.)

Discharge Considerations

Because headaches are managed at home, client education is the main focus. Teach the client how to limit attacks and to reduce the effects of headaches. Clients with long-term or migraine headaches may be referred for stress reduction or biofeedback classes. The teaching session should include the following points:

Chapter Review

key terms by topic

Use the CD-ROM disk enclosed with your textbook to hear the pronunciation of the key terms in the chapter.

Structure and function of the nervous system
neuron, myelin sheath, synapse, neurotransmitter, meninges, fissures, dermatome, reflex, reflex arc

Head injuries
rhinorrhea, otorrhea, concussion, contusion, intracranial pressure, hematoma

Brain tumor
debulking

Cerebrovascular accident
CVA, transient ischemic attack (TIA), anoxia, contralateral, hemiplegia, aphasias (expressive, receptive, or global), homonymous hemianopia, emotional lability, dysphagia, carotid endarterectomy

Aneurysm
subarachnoid hemorrhage

Seizure disorder
seizure, convulsion, epilepsy, epileptogenic focus, jacksonian march, automatisms, aura, tonic contractions, clonic contractions, status epilepticus

Intracranial infection
meningitis, encephalitis

Headaches
cephalalgia

key points

- The highest incidence for head injuries is for people between the ages of 1 and 35 and the older adult. In the elderly, falls are a frequent cause of brain trauma.

- Increasing ICP is a medical emergency and must be treated immediately to prevent permanent brain damage or death.

- Subtle changes such as restlessness and drowsiness indicate a change in neurologic function and must be reported promptly.

- Intracranial surgery increases the risk of meningitis. It is extremely important to use aseptic technique when changing any wound dressing.

- Older adults often ignore the symptoms of a TIA mistakenly thinking it is part of the normal aging process because the symptoms disappear after a short time.

- The primary risk factors for a stroke are hypertension, atherosclerosis, cardiac disease, smoking, and age. Discuss potential lifestyle changes with high-risk clients.

- Clients with seizure disorders must understand their anticonvulsant medications and the importance of not discontinuing them without medical supervision.

- Meningococcemia, a complication of meningococcal meningitis, can cause death in 10 to 12 hours. Any client with a high fever and petechial rash must be seen by a physician immediately.

Medialink

Additional interactive resources for this chapter can be found on the Companion Website at www.prenhall.com/burke. Click on Chapter 29 and "Begin" to select the activities for this chapter.

For NCLEX review questions and an audio glossary, access the accompanying CD-ROM in this book.

for further study

For more about the signs of impending death, see Chapter 9.
For brain death criteria, see Box 10-14 in Chapter 10.
For in-depth discussion of antibiotic therapy, see Chapter 12.
For further study about impaired mobility, see Chapter 27.

Critical Thinking Care Map

Caring for the Client with a Cerebrovascular Accident
NCLEX-PN Focus Area: Physiological Integrity; Reduction of Risk Potential

Case Study: Mr. Boren, a 68-year-old African American male, had a CVA this morning. He is drowsy but responds to verbal stimuli by nodding his head to indicate "yes" when asked questions. He has flaccid paralysis in his left arm and left leg (he is left-handed). He shows visual field deficits that indicate homonymous hemianopia. A CT scan confirms the diagnosis of a right-brain CVA due to a thrombus of the middle cerebral artery. Mr. Boren is started on a continuous IV heparin infusion.

Nursing Diagnosis: Impaired Verbal Communication

COLLECT DATA

Subjective	Objective

Would you report this data? Yes/No

If yes, to: _____

Nursing Care

_____

_____

_____

_____

_____

_____

_____

_____

How would you document this? _____

_____

_____

Data Collected
(use those that apply)

- Lack of eye contact
- Left arm and leg flaccid
- Nods off while people speak to him
- Nods head to answer questions
- Makes a clenched fist of right hand when trying to speak
- Eyes look pleading

Nursing Interventions
(use those that apply)

- Provide a large marker and tablet.
- Place objects, call bell, and tissues on Mr. Boren's unaffected side.
- Use short, simple sentences when talking to Mr. Boren.
- Provide adaptive devices (silverware with thick handles and nonslip plates) for Mr. Boren to use.
- Contact speech therapy for consultation.
- Encourage Mrs. Boren to visit at mealtimes.
- Explain all health care procedures.
- Maintain a calm, unhurried manner.

NCLEX-PN Exam Preparation

1. In a case in which a client was accidentally struck in the head by a baseball bat, which condition should the nurse anticipate as a serious complication?
   a. clear fluid draining from the ears
   b. large hematoma at the impact site
   c. headache
   d. complaints of dizziness

2. The nurse recognizes that which factor in the client's history is the most common etiological factor in developing a CVA?
   a. surgery to repair a torn Achilles' tendon 3 months ago
   b. use of oral contraceptives for the past 10 years
   c. history of coronary artery disease (CAD)
   d. consumption of four beers per day

3. A client is scheduled for a lumbar puncture. Which nursing action is the most important prior to the procedure?
   a. Explain the importance of not moving during the procedure.
   b. Have the patient empty his bladder.
   c. Obtain a lumbar puncture kit.
   d. Ensure that the signed consent form is on the chart.

4. In evaluating the effects of the anticonvulsant drug, Dilantin, the nurse should monitor which lab value?
   a. complete blood count (CBC)
   b. platelet count
   c. liver enzymes
   d. serum blood levels of the drug

5. A client was admitted to your unit after a motorcycle accident. There is a large laceration on the right temporal region of the head. If the nurse monitors all of the following, which would indicate an early change in the client's condition?
   a. increased heart rate
   b. sluggish response by pupils to light
   c. irritability
   d. projectile vomiting

6. When documenting in the chart on a client with head trauma, which nursing note would be the most appropriate?
   a. Client is unresponsive but withdraws to painful stimuli.
   b. Client is observed to be in a stupor.
   c. Client's family is at the bedside.
   d. Physician has diagnosed client with head trauma, secondary to MVA.

7. Which nursing diagnosis has the highest priority for a client with status epilepticus?
   a. Anxiety
   b. Risk for Injury
   c. Risk for Ineffective Airway Clearance
   d. Risk for Ineffective Tissue Perfusion: Cerebral

8. A client is being discharged from the emergency room with a diagnosis of migraine headaches. It is most important to include which of the following teaching points?
   a. Keep a headache diary.
   b. Identify comfort measures during a headache.
   c. Refer client to stress reduction classes.
   d. Teach client how to eliminate attacks.

9. A client has been assessed by the physician. His notes indicate the following findings: positive Brudzinski's and Kernig's signs, increased ICP, sputum cultures positive for *Streptococcus pneumoniae*. Based on this information, the nurse can anticipate that the physician will diagnose this client with:
   a. encephalitis
   b. brain abscess
   c. bacterial meningitis
   d. subdural hematoma

10. A client begins to seize during your assessment. Which of the following interventions should be initiated first?
    a. Restrain the client's arms and legs to prevent injury.
    b. Loosen clothing around the neck.
    c. Turn client on the side.
    d. Place protective pads over the side rails.

Answers for Review Questions, as well as discussion of Case Study Critical Thinking questions, appear in Appendix V.

Caring for Clients with Degenerative Neurologic and Spinal Cord Disorders

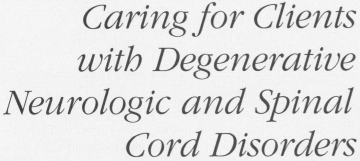

chapter 30

CARING tip

❝ On-the-job satisfaction comes from working with high standards and not changing them, even when others may pressure you to lower them. Don't be afraid to set your standards and not lower them. You will always go home feeling good about yourself. ❞

*Yazmin Mojica, RN, BSN, MA • Founder/President, National NCLEX®
Solutions • Educator/Consultant • Walnut, California*

LEARNING outcomes

After completing this chapter, you will be able to:

- Describe the pathophysiology of common degenerative neurologic disorders relating their manifestations to the disease process.
- Identify common manifestations of Alzheimer's disease, multiple sclerosis, Parkinson's disease, and myasthenia gravis.
- Identify laboratory and diagnostic tests used to diagnose degenerative neurologic disorders.
- Discuss the nursing implications for medications and treatments ordered for clients experiencing degenerative neurologic disorders.
- Describe the client's functional ability according to the level of damage to the spinal cord.
- Describe the nursing care needs of the client with quadriplegia.
- Provide nursing care for clients undergoing a laminectomy.
- Reinforce teaching to clients with a degenerative neurologic disorder.
- Use the nursing process to collect data, establish outcomes, provide individualized care, and evaluate responses for the client with degenerative neurologic and spinal cord disorders.

MediaLink

www.prenhall.com/burke

Use the above address to access the free, interactive Companion Website created for this textbook. Get hints, instant feedback, and textbook references to chapter-related multiple choice questions. Link to other interesting sites.

Degenerative neurologic disorders disrupt the central nervous system (CNS) and the peripheral nerves. They can cause devastating physical and emotional changes. The client and family will face lifestyle and role changes and may even experience financial difficulties. The exact cause of these disorders is uncertain. Some may have a genetic or autoimmune cause.

Spinal cord injuries and herniated disk problems are also discussed in this chapter. Permanent damage to the spinal cord can also present physical and psychological challenges to the client and caregiver.

Degenerative Neurologic Disorders

Common degenerative disorders of the CNS include Alzheimer's disease, multiple sclerosis, Parkinson's disease, myasthenia gravis, Huntington's disease, and amyotropic lateral sclerosis. Guillain–Barré syndrome is an example of a disorder affecting the peripheral nerves.

Cranial nerve disorders may be caused by trauma or inflammation. The pairs of cranial nerves are described in Chapter 29. The most common cranial nerve disorders affect the trigeminal (cranial nerve V) and the facial (cranial nerve VII) nerves.

A variety of nervous system disorders may have toxic or infectious causes. These disorders are rare but require significant nursing care when they occur. Rabies, tetanus, and Creutzfeldt–Jakob disease are presented in the last part of this section.

Alzheimer's Disease

Alzheimer's disease (AD) is a progressive, irreversible deterioration of the brain. It is characterized by a gradual loss of intellectual functioning. An estimated 4 million adults in the United States have Alzheimer's disease, the most common type of dementia. It affects adults in middle to late life. As one ages, the risk of developing AD increases. Genetic defects on chromosomes 1, 14, 19, and 21 are associated with Alzheimer's disease.

PATHOPHYSIOLOGY
Four pathologic changes are seen in the brains of AD clients: (1) loss of nerve cells, (2) reduced brain size, (3) presence of neurofibrillary tangles (Figure 30-1 ◆), and (4) neuritic plaques. A protein substance called amyloid causes the plaque formation. The neurofibrillary tangles and plaque lead to altered nerve impulse transmission. This results in loss of memory and cognition. There is also a decrease in acetylcholine, a neurotransmitter, that is essential for memory. AD affects the frontal lobe first and then involves the entire brain.

Alzheimer's disease is staged according to the client's symptoms and abilities (Box 30-1). It develops slowly over a long period of time, with the first sign being memory loss.

Memory deficits are subtle so that family and friends may not suspect a problem or deny that a problem exists. There is a progressive decline in cognition and judgment. The client exhibits **sundowning** (behavior characterized by increased agitation, disorientation to time, and wandering during afternoon and evening hours). In the last stage, the caregiver must meet the client's activities of daily living. Common complications include pneumonia, dehydration, malnutrition, and falls. Prognosis is poor, and death frequently occurs from pneumonia secondary to aspiration.

COLLABORATIVE CARE
Without the hope of a cure, the client and family face a long, devastating illness. They will need long-term follow-up and support.

Laboratory and Diagnostic Tests
Diagnosing AD begins by ruling out other causes for the client's symptoms such as depression. A complete blood count (CBC), thyroid studies, and electrolyte levels are used to exclude the following conditions: UTI or pneumonia, misuse of over-the-counter and prescription medications, hypothyroidism, and malnutrition and fluid or electrolyte imbalances. The following diagnostic tests are performed:

Figure 30-1. ◆ Neuron with neurofibrillary tangles seen in Alzheimer's disease.

BOX 30-1
MANIFESTATIONS OF ALZHEIMER'S DISEASE

STAGE 1 (EARLY)

- Short-term memory loss; forget location and names of objects
- Attempts to cover up memory loss
- Has difficulty learning new information or making decisions
- Decreased ability to concentrate
- Can be angry or depressed

STAGE 2 (MIDDLE)

- Unable to remember names of family members and gets lost in familiar locations
- Easily agitated and irritable
- Hides things due to paranoia
- Has difficulty using objects, reading, writing, and speaking
- Cannot follow a conversation
- Personal hygiene declines
- Unable to make decisions (e.g., choose clothing)
- Walks with unsteady gait, head down, shoulders bent, shuffles
- Paces aimlessly at night, manifested as "sundowning"; wandering behavior

STAGE 3 (LATE)

- Cannot recognize self or others
- Unable to communicate with words
- Has delusions and hallucinations
- Forgets to eat, bathe, swallow, walk, sit, and eventually becomes bedridden
- Bowel and bladder incontinence

- *Electroencephalogram (EEG)* may show a slowed brain wave pattern in the late stages.
- *Magnetic resonance imaging (MRI)* and *computed tomography (CT) scan* of the brain may show decreased brain size in the late stages.
- *Positron emission tomography (PET) scan* can show reduced glucose levels in the affected areas of the brain.
- *Mini-Mental Status Examination (MMSE)* shows the loss of memory and other cognitive skills over time.

Pharmacology

Anticholinesterase drugs, such as tacrine hydrochloride (Cognex), donepezil (Aricept), and rivastigmine (Exelon) block the breakdown of acetylcholine. They do not cure AD but seem to improve reasoning and memory in about 40% of the clients. Because they cause liver toxicity, liver function is monitored frequently. Antidepressants are given to treat depression. Antianxiety and tranquilizer medications are used to control behavioral symptoms.

NURSING CARE

ASSESSING

The nurse collects subjective and objective data to guide the type of care the client will need (Box 30-2).

DIAGNOSING, PLANNING, AND IMPLEMENTING

Nursing care focuses on assisting the client and caregiver to maintain the highest quality of life. Care can be as simple as altering the client's environment to full nursing assistance as the client declines.

DISTURBED THOUGHT PROCESSES

- Orient the client to person, place, and time frequently; place large, easy-to-read calendars and clocks within client's line of vision. *Orientation promotes reality and reduces confusion.*
- Keep the daily routine the same. Assign the same caregivers. *Daily routines and familiar staff decrease confusion and help the client cope.*
- Place client in a quiet environment with soft music. *A quiet environment is less distracting to a confused client and reduces agitation. Soft music may be soothing.*

BOX 30-2
ASSESSING CLIENTS WITH ALZHEIMER'S DISEASE

SUBJECTIVE DATA

- Present health status:
  - General health status
  - Change in memory
  - Difficulty concentrating
  - Difficulty making everyday decisions
  - Easily irritated or restless
  - Has difficulty using the correct word for an object
  - Frequency of nighttime wakening
  - Presence of incontinence
- Past medical history:
  - History of head trauma, CNS infection, or exposure to aluminum
  - Family history of Alzheimer's disease

OBJECTIVE DATA

- Observe client for lapses in memory or thought processes and ability to recognize family.
- Assess orientation to time, place, and person.
- Observe for unkept physical appearance in client's clothing and grooming.
- Note affect and ability to follow conversation.
- Note any deficits in speaking or reading.

- Schedule rest periods or quiet times throughout the day. *Fatigue contributes to confusion.*
- Keep familiar objects in the same place. *This will help them remember where objects are and decreases confusion.*

SELF-CARE DEFICITS

- Encourage the client to perform as much self-care as possible. *This promotes independence and activates the client's memory.*
- Demonstrate use of equipment (e.g., comb, toothbrush, eating utensils). *Visual cues help client remember prior tasks.*
- Perform daily bathing and hygiene measures as needed. *Clients in stages 2 and 3 often forget activities of daily living (ADLs) or fight bathing. Pressure ulcers may go unnoticed unless daily bathing is done.*
- Have family modify clothing with Velcro. Lay out daily clothing. *Velcro closures are easier for the client to use. Preselected clothing decreases frustration.*
- Encourage fluids during the day. *AD clients forget to drink fluids and may become dehydrated.*
- If hyperactive, provide a high-calorie diet. Encourage "finger foods" such as sandwiches and fruit. *Hyperactivity increases metabolism and the risk for malnutrition.*
- Limit the number of foods placed in front of the client at one time. Cut food into bite-size pieces. *Too many foods at one time can be confusing.*

CAREGIVER ROLE STRAIN

- Discuss the physical and emotional demands of caregiving with the caregiver and family. *Discussion allows the caregiver and family an opportunity to think about their future needs.*
- Teach the caregivers to take rest periods and avoid fatigue. *Caregivers feel overwhelmed by their responsibilities. They become physically and mentally exhausted and socially isolated.*
- Refer client and family to local AD support groups, national AD association, and home health. *Support groups and home health can assist in coping with the diagnosis.*
- Provide financial or social service referrals. *Referrals assist families in planning for long-term care.*

EVALUATING

Evaluate the effectiveness of nursing care by collecting data on the client's level of altered thought processes and self-care deficits. Also, evaluate the caregiver's physical and emotional endurance to care for the client.

Discharge Considerations

The nurse assesses the client's ability to stay in his or her home and the caregiver's ability to provide care (Box 30-3). Review the disease process and help identify potential support systems within the family and community. If the client will be cared for at home, address safety concerns (Box 30-4). Also, suggest the following strategies for helping the client:

BOX 30-3
ASSESSING FOR DISCHARGE

DEGENERATIVE NEUROLOGIC DISORDERS
Client

- Self-care: Ability to perform ADLs independently or with assistive devices; to plan physical activities, rest and sleep periods; to prevent potential injury; to self-administer prescribed medications as able
- Knowledge: Disease process; coping strategies, prescription medications; methods to limit fatigue; indications for seeking medical care
- Home environment: Appropriate heating and cooling; access to clean water for drinking and handwashing; adequate home lighting; presence of safety hazards such as throw rugs, and slick floors

Family

- Members of household: Ability to maintain a safe environment; avoid members with upper respiratory infections
- Caregivers: Availability and willingness to provide short-term and long-term care as needed; ability to provide emotional stability, to administer medications, to prepare meals; to provide ADLs, to identify potential home hazards, to prevent complications such as pneumonia, UTI, or skin breakdown
- Financial resources: Income; resources for adult day care, skilled nursing facility, rehabilitation center or services as needed; medications

Community

- Access to community resources such as Meals-on-Wheels, adult day care, specialized support groups
- Access to family and caregiver support groups
- Access to respite care

- Make a schedule of the client's daily activities.
- Label drawers containing client's clothes and label rooms.
- Use communication techniques to the client's level of ability.
- When the client is agitated, divert his or her attention by walking or rocking in a rocking chair.
- If the client wanders, have him or her wear a Medic-Alert bracelet or pendant.

Refer clients to social services for help with such legal matters as wills, advanced directives, and powers of attorney. Caregivers often feel alone as friends and family drift away. They become depressed and exhausted. When appropriate, recommend respite care. The need for a skilled nursing facility will cause the family many conflicting emotions. They need time to adjust to the idea but are often relieved to hand over the physical care to someone with more experience.

BOX 30-4
TEACHING FOR DISCHARGE

CLIENT WITH ALZHEIMER'S DISEASE

Safety Interventions

- Keep furniture in the same place and keep traffic areas free from clutter.
- Apply skidproof surface on stairs, install handrails, and mark stairs to show depth.
- Make sure that the client's shoes fit properly.
- Omit alcohol use, and limit medications that affect balance (e.g., antihypertensives).
- Use night-lights; provide ample lighting in hallways and on stairs.
- Lock cleaning solutions, pesticides, medications, and nonedible food in a cabinet.
- Protect the client from fire hazards; make matches, lighters, and cigarettes inaccessible. Modify the controls on the oven and stove.
- Install protective covers over electrical sockets, fans, and motors.
- Adjust the water heater to a safe temperature.
- Provide double lock systems to outside doors and fence the yard with a locked gate to prevent the client from wandering. Install alarms and bells on doors to sound when client attempts to exit.
- Have family or neighbor check on client at the same time every day.

Communication Techniques

- Face the client and talk directly to him or her; call the client by name.
- When first approaching the client, identify yourself.
- Use simple sentences and words with few syllables; repeat explanations as needed.
- Speak in a calm, low voice; have a relaxed approach.
- Ask one question at a time. Use questions that require only a yes or no response.
- Allow the client time to process what you are trying to say.

Nursing Process Case Study
■ CLIENT WITH ALZHEIMER'S DISEASE

Arthur and Ruth Joste have been married for 47 years; both are 73 years old. Their two children live in the same town. For the past 9 months, Arthur cannot remember friends' names and phone numbers. He miscalculates the checkbook balance and neglects his hygiene needs.

Assessment In the neurologist's office, Mr. Joste scores 20 out of a possible 30 points on the Mini-Mental Status Examination. His wife says that she covers up mistakes for her husband and that he wanders the house for several hours at night. After an evaluation, Mr. Joste is diagnosed with Alzheimer's disease. Both have feared this diagnosis and are overwhelmed.

Diagnosis Nursing diagnoses for Mr. Joste and his family include the following:

- Self-Care Deficit related to forgetfulness and declining physical abilities
- Risk for Injury related to decreased orientation
- Disturbed Sleep Pattern related to time disorientation and daytime sleeping

Expected Outcomes The Jostes are referred to Mr. Dixon Montane, a home health nurse. The expected outcomes of care specify that Mr. Joste will:

- Participate in grooming and hygiene activities as able.
- Remain free of injury.
- Obtain a minimum of 7 uninterrupted hours of sleep a night.

Planning and Implementation Mr. Montane makes a home visit to assess for potential hazards and to meet the Jostes' children. After touring the home, Mr. Montane recommends that Mrs. Joste remove throw rugs from hallways, and provide extra lighting in dark areas. He suggests that Mrs. Joste add a night-light in the bathroom and modify the doors with a safety lock system. He also suggests that Mr. Joste walk everyday and do simple chores, to decrease daylight sleep time and stimulate memory. He recommends labeling drawers with their contents. He reviews new communication techniques with the family.

A part-time homemaker will help Mrs. Joste with housekeeping chores. Mr. Montane also suggests hiring a home health aide to provide daily hygiene care. Mr. and Mrs. Joste will attend the weekly support group meetings for Alzheimer's disease for about 3 months.

Evaluation Six months later, Mr. Montane's follow-up visit finds that Mr. Joste has become increasingly confused. It seems unlikely that Mr. Joste will be able to remain at home and will need placement in a long-term care facility.

Critical Thinking in the Nursing Process

1. Identify several safety interventions to teach Mr. and Mrs. Joste.
2. List five interventions to decrease agitation in clients with AD.
3. A client with stage 2 Alzheimer's disease cannot focus on eating and is easily agitated. What strategies could you use to ensure that she eats enough to meet her needs?

Multiple Sclerosis

Multiple sclerosis (MS) is a chronic, degenerative disease that damages the myelin sheath surrounding the axons of the CNS. This disorder is marked by periods of exacerbation (symptoms appear) followed by periods of remission. In the end the person is chronically disabled and may become wheelchair bound.

MS affects Caucasian females more frequently between the ages of 20 and 40. A family history and living in the cold, damp, northern part of the United States increase the risk. The exact cause is unknown, but viral infections seem to trigger an autoimmune response. Emotional stress, fatigue, pregnancy, and acute respiratory infections tend to occur before the onset of MS.

PATHOPHYSIOLOGY

Myelin sheaths make up what is known as white matter in the CNS. Multiple sclerosis destroys the myelin sheath of the spinal cord, brain, and optic nerve and replaces it with *plaque.* The plaque can develop throughout the white matter of the CNS. This process is called **demyelination.** When the myelin is destroyed, nerve impulse conduction slows.

Manifestations vary according to the area of the nervous system affected (Figure 30-2 ◆). They may appear suddenly and last for days to months. As the disease progresses, exacerbations last longer and occur more often. When the nerve cells are finally destroyed, the manifestations become permanent. Fatigue is a common but often ignored symptom. Medical care is sought when the client develops diplopia, weakness, and tingling and numbness in the extremities. An unusual characteristic of MS is the worsening of motor symptoms after a hot shower or tub bath.

As the disease progresses, the client is prone to urinary tract infections, pressure ulcers, joint contractures, injuries from falls, pneumonia, and depression. Death often results from pneumonia and a debilitated condition.

COLLABORATIVE CARE

The treatment goal is to keep the client functioning for as long as possible. As the client becomes more disabled, speech, physical, and occupational therapists are consulted.

Laboratory and Diagnostic Tests

Manifestations are vague or mild, making an early diagnosis difficult. A positive diagnosis is based on the client's history, physical examination, and symptoms. Periodic diagnostic testing is done to follow the course of the disease. The following laboratory and diagnostic tests may be ordered:

■ *Cerebral spinal fluid (CSF) analysis* reveals an increased white blood cell (WBC) count. Elevated levels of

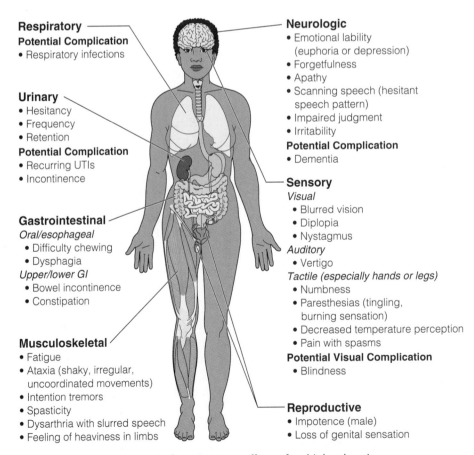

Respiratory
Potential Complication
• Respiratory infections

Urinary
• Hesitancy
• Frequency
• Retention
Potential Complication
• Recurring UTIs
• Incontinence

Gastrointestinal
Oral/esophageal
• Difficulty chewing
• Dysphagia
Upper/lower GI
• Bowel incontinence
• Constipation

Musculoskeletal
• Fatigue
• Ataxia (shaky, irregular,
  uncoordinated movements)
• Intention tremors
• Spasticity
• Dysarthria with slurred speech
• Feeling of heaviness in limbs

Neurologic
• Emotional lability
  (euphoria or depression)
• Forgetfulness
• Apathy
• Scanning speech (hesitant
  speech pattern)
• Impaired judgment
• Irritability
Potential Complication
• Dementia

Sensory
Visual
• Blurred vision
• Diplopia
• Nystagmus
Auditory
• Vertigo
Tactile (especially hands or legs)
• Numbness
• Paresthesias (tingling,
  burning sensation)
• Decreased temperature perception
• Pain with spasms
Potential Visual Complication
• Blindness

Reproductive
• Impotence (male)
• Loss of genital sensation

Figure 30-2. ◆ Multisystem effects of multiple sclerosis.

immunoglobulin G (IgG) in the CSF indicate increased immune system activity.

- *MRI* studies detect the plaque lesions in the white matter.
- *EEG* may show slowed brain activity during the acute stage of MS.

Pharmacology

The only drugs on the market to control MS are known as immune system regulators. They include *beta-interferon, glatiramer,* and *novantrone.* These medications do not cure MS but can decrease the number of exacerbations.

Steroids are given to decrease inflammation and increase periods of remission. Muscle spasms may be reduced with baclofen (Lioresal) and dantrolene (Dantrium). Fatigue is controlled with Amantidine (Symmetrel). Bethanecol (Urecholine) is used to control urinary retention and propantheline (Pro-Banthine) to control urinary frequency. Immunosuppressive agents are tried to decrease the immune system response.

Other Therapies

Physical therapists teach the client ways to maintain balance. For example, the client should stand with the feet slightly apart to give a wider base of support. The client with ataxia is taught to use a walker or cane. Spasticity is managed with stretching exercises, gait training, and the use of braces or splints. Severe spasticity and uncontrolled pain may be treated with surgical procedures like a neurectomy, rhizotomy, or cordotomy.

Plasmapheresis, or plasma exchange, is a procedure that removes plasma from whole blood. Its purpose is to remove T lymphocytes that cause inflammation. There has been some success with plasmapheresis causing a remission for clients with MS.

Nutrition

Diet therapy does not treat MS, but a well-balanced diet provides energy and strengthens the immune system. Reduced physical activity tends to cause weight gain and bone loss. Consult a dietitian about a diet low in calories but high in calcium and vitamin D. To prevent additional bone loss, encourage the client to perform weight-bearing activities (e.g., walking).

If the client has dysphagia, change the diet to make chewing and swallowing easier. For example, thickened drinks and small bites of food can prevent choking and fatigue. Avoid serving crackers, dry toast, or chips as they may cause choking.

 NURSING CARE

MS is a lifelong illness that the client and family can manage at home. When acute infections threaten the client's life, admission to a hospital may be necessary. As the disease advances, weakened muscle strength and spasticity increase the potential for complications from immobility. If the client becomes totally disabled and the family cannot provide care, a long-term care facility will be necessary.

Assessment data collected by the nurse can help identify the diagnosis, can determine the extent to which the disease is interfering with the client's life, and can indicate the type of treatment required at this stage of the disease (Box 30-5).

The client experiences fatigue, decreased mobility, urinary and bowel incontinence, and altered respiratory status. In addition, the client may be unable to perform ADLs. Coping with changes in lifestyle may cause depression.

FATIGUE

- Observe how fatigue affects the client's ability to perform ADLs. *Knowing how fatigue affects the client will assist in planning care.*
- Plan daily activities to include rest periods. *Rest is essential to decrease fatigue; rest periods can restore energy reserves.*
- Encourage the client to perform tasks in the morning hours. *Fatigue usually worsens in the afternoon.*

BOX 30-5
ASSESSING CLIENTS WITH MULTIPLE SCLEROSIS

SUBJECTIVE DATA

- Present health status:
  - Difficulty chewing or swallowing; weight loss
  - Mood swings: Depression to euphoria
  - Extreme fatigue
  - Diplopia or blurred vision
  - Muscle weakness or ataxia; numbness and tingling in extremities
  - Motor symptoms worsen after a hot shower or bath
  - Urinary frequency, retention, or incontinence; constipation
- Past medical history:
  - History of viral infections, living in northern United States, physical or emotional stress, or pregnancy
  - Use of steroid or immunosuppressant medications
  - Family history of multiple sclerosis

OBJECTIVE DATA

- Observe client for inattentiveness, difficulty finding the right word, poor coordination, muscle weakness, ataxia, and tremors.
- Note disheveled appearance or signs of incontinence.
- As the client speaks, listen for slurred speech or hesitating speech pattern.
- Auscultate for bowel tones; decreased bowel tones indicate slowed peristalsis.

SELF-CARE DEFICITS

- Encourage the client perform as much self-care as possible. *This promotes independence and decreases feelings of helplessness.*
- Allow adequate time to perform tasks. *Weak muscles and spasticity slow the client's ability to perform all tasks.*
- Provide adaptive devices such as arm or wrist braces, long-handled combs, or modified clothing. Provide shower chair or raised toilet seat. *Adaptive devices encourage the client to perform ADLs and may reduce fatigue.*

INEFFECTIVE COPING

- Encourage the client to state his or her feelings. Consult with a counselor or psychiatrist as needed. *Clients with MS feel helpless and isolated. They often believe they cannot effectively manage the symptoms of MS.*
- Refer to a support group and provide information about the National MS Society. *Support group and National MS Society can offer suggestions for coping with MS.*
- Refer to state vocational rehabilitation agency as needed. *Vocational rehabilitation agencies can assist the client with job retraining.*

EVALUATING

To evaluate the effectiveness of care for a client with MS, collect data on ability to perform ADLs; ability to cope with a chronic illness; and knowledge of medications, diet, and ways to prevent complications.

Discharge Considerations

Teaching topics are identified during the initial assessment (review Box 30-3). The newly diagnosed client is taught about the disease process, manifestations, prognosis, and treatment. The client and family should know how to prevent fatigue and exacerbations. The client should keep a diary about symptoms and activities in order to identify stressors. Discuss the following topics with the client and family:

- Avoiding stress, hot showers or baths, extremes of heat or cold, high humidity, physical overexertion, and infections
- Medications, side effects, and interactions with prescription or other drugs
- Adequate fluid intake, regular bowel and bladder elimination schedule, well-balanced meals, daily physical exercise, and weight control
- Ways to prevent complications: pressure ulcers, respiratory and urinary tract infections
- Ways to cope with pain, dysphagia, spasticity, and vision changes
- Importance of follow-up care with physician, nurses, and rehabilitation team

- Need for counseling if client is planning a future pregnancy

If the client is employed, discuss the availability of sick leave during periods of exacerbation. As the disease progresses, the client's home and lifestyle will require changes. The home health nurse can help evaluate the home. When the client becomes severely disabled, home assistance is recommended. Discuss support sources within their community.

Parkinson's Disease

Parkinson's disease (PD) is a chronic, progressive, degenerative neurologic disease that alters motor coordination. It is one of the most common neurologic disorders, affecting approximately 1 million people in the United States. Most people are diagnosed after the age of 50. It seems to affect Caucasian men more often than women.

The cause of Parkinson's disease is unknown. Parkinson-like symptoms called *parkinsonism* may develop in clients taking phenothiazines, haloperidol (Haldol), and methyldopa (Aldomet). The symptoms disappear when the drug is stopped. Parkinsonism is also caused by exposure to carbon monoxide or cyanide poisoning, repeated head trauma, or an illegal drug called MPTP (1-methyl-4-phenyl 6-tetrahydropyridine).

PATHOPHYSIOLOGY

Parkinson's disease results from a deficiency of **dopamine** (a neurotransmitter that inhibits voluntary motor function). An area of the basal ganglia, the substantia nigra, produces dopamine. Damage to this part of the brain causes an imbalance between dopamine and acetylcholine. When dopamine levels drop, acetylcholine is no longer inhibited. This means that acetylcholine causes constant excitement of the motor neurons. The client exhibits symptoms of impaired voluntary motor function.

Manifestations are subtle and may be mistaken as signs of normal aging (Figure 30-3 ◆). The onset is gradual and the disease progresses slowly. There are three cardinal signs: (1) tremor, (2) rigidity, and (3) **bradykinesia** (slowed voluntary movements and speech). The classic "pill-rolling" tremor occurs when the thumb and fingers move like they are rolling a pill. Tremors disappear during sleep and movement. Other manifestations are noted in Box 30-6.

COLLABORATIVE CARE

No specific laboratory or diagnostic tests exist for this disorder. Diagnosis is based on the client's history and the presence of two of the three cardinal symptoms.

Interventions vary with the extent of the client's manifestations and disability. The client may be treated with medication, surgery, and rehabilitation. The goal is to retain the highest level of function for as long as possible.

Pharmacology

Drug therapy does not cure Parkinson's disease. Its main purpose is to control symptoms. Drugs are chosen based on

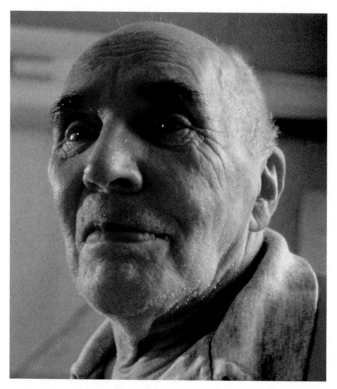

Figure 30-3. ◆ In Parkinson's disease, the client's face lacks expression.

the client's symptoms and individual response. Four different classes of drugs are used: *anticholinergics, monoamine oxidase inhibitors (MAOIs), dopaminergics,* and *dopamine agonists* (Table 30-1 ◆). The drugs prescribed depend on the client's symptoms and the length of effectiveness. For example, over time levodopa, a dopaminergic, loses its effectiveness, and side effects increase. Dopamine agonists are added to increase the effectiveness of levodopa. Eventually, drugs no longer control the symptoms, and the client's condition declines.

BOX 30-6
MANIFESTATIONS OF
PARKINSON'S DISEASE

- Tremor that moves from one arm to both arms and may involve lips, jaw, and head
- Rigidity of neck, shoulders, and trunk
- Bradykinesia:
  - Inability to initiate voluntary movements
  - Slurred speech, low amplitude
  - Decreased blinking
  - Masklike, expressionless face
- Drooling
- Excess sweating on face and neck
- Excessively oily skin
- Depression or memory loss

Surgery

Surgery is used to relieve symptoms. The two primary surgeries are a pallidotomy and stereotaxic thalamotomy. Both procedures are done under local anesthesia. In the *pallidotomy,* part of the globus pallidus is destroyed to control rigidity and tremors. *Stereotaxic thalamotomy* destroys part of the thalamus to reduce tremors; it is reserved for younger people with extreme unilateral tremor.

▐▐▐NURSING CARE

Clients with PD have complex needs. In the early stages, most clients remain at home with limited family assistance. As the client deteriorates and care increases, the family may want to consider placement in a long-term care facility. Throughout this illness, the client and family need continued support and counseling.

ASSESSING

Assessment should identify the client's symptoms and the extent to which the disease is affecting the client's daily life (Box 30-7). It is important to note the client's ability to function safely.

BOX 30-7
ASSESSING CLIENTS WITH
PARKINSON'S DISEASE

SUBJECTIVE DATA
- Present health status:
  - Difficulty making decisions
  - Mood swings; depression
  - Drooling or difficulty swallowing; weight loss
  - Arm or leg stiffness
  - Frequent falls
  - Loss of dexterity or ability to write
  - Insomnia
  - Urinary incontinence; constipation
- Past medical history:
  - History of head trauma, exposure to metals, carbon monoxide, or MPTP
  - Use of major tranquilizers

OBJECTIVE DATA
- Height and weight
- Observe client for infrequent blinking, expressionless face, slow slurred speech, stooped posture, shuffling gait, or depression.
- Assess for muscles that move in small jerky movements.
- Assess for tremors at rest that disappear with movement, or "pill rolling" tremor.
- Palpate skin for excessive sweating or oiliness; inspect for injury from falls.

TABLE 30-1 NURSING IMPLICATIONS FOR PHARMACOLOGY: CLIENTS WITH PARKINSON'S DISEASE

DRUG CLASS/DRUGS	ACTION	NURSING IMPLICATIONS	CLIENT TEACHING
Dopaminergics ■ Levodopa (Larodopa) ■ Carbidopa–Levodopa (Sinemet) ■ Amantadine (Symmetrel)	Levodopa is converted to dopamine in the brain and carbidopa prevents levodopa from being destroyed. Levodopa is the most effective drug for Parkinson's disease. Amantadine, an antiviral drug, raises dopamine levels.	Check for drug interactions before giving. Do not give to clients with angle-closure glaucoma. Monitor for nausea, hypotension, confusion, and dyskinesia. Assess for "on–off" effect—symptoms may appear or improve suddenly. Hold levodopa for 8 hours prior to giving Sinemet to avoid toxicity.	Take medication as directed. Do not alter dosages. Inform physician of other drugs you are taking. Change position slowly to avoid hypotension. Increase fluid intake and exercise regularly. Report the "on–off" effect, decreased motor movements, insomnia, and rapid heartbeat to your physician.
Dopamine Agonists ■ Bromocriptine (Parlodel) ■ Pergolide (Permax) ■ Pramipexole (Mirapex) ■ Ropinirole (Requip)	They are given to decrease tremor, rigidity, and bradykinesia.	Monitor for adverse reactions: nausea, orthostatic hypotension, and psychosis. See nursing implications under the dopaminergics.	Client teaching information is similar to that found under the dopaminergics.
Anticholinergics ■ Trihexyphenidyl (Artane) ■ Benztropine (Cogentin) ■ Biperiden (Akineton) ■ Procyclidine (Kemadrin)	They are given during the early stages of the disease or when the client can no longer take levodopa. These medications ease drooling, tremors, and rigidity.	Do not give to clients with glaucoma, cardiac dysfunction, and prostatic hypertrophy. Check for drug interactions. Monitor for side effects of dry mouth, blurred vision, constipation, urinary retention, and confusion. Taper off slowly to avoid parkinsonism.	Take the medication as prescribed. Check with physician before taking with other medications. Do not suddenly stop taking anticholinergics. Report blurred vision, constipation, difficulty urinating, rash, or increased temperature. Drink adequate amounts of fluid to prevent dehydration.
Monoamine Oxidase Inhibitor (MAOI) ■ Selegiline (Eldepryl)	It reduces tremor, rigidity, and bradykinesia.	Monitor for agitation, ataxia, insomnia, dizziness, or confusion.	Take the medication as directed. Report signs of insomnia, difficulty moving, or dizziness.

DIAGNOSING, PLANNING, AND IMPLEMENTING

Clients with PD develop problems similar to other degenerative neurologic disorders. Refer to previous nursing care sections in this chapter for discussions on fatigue, self-care deficits, and ineffective coping. This section focuses on mobility, communication, and nutrition. In later stages, the client may develop airway problems.

IMPAIRED PHYSICAL MOBILITY

■ Perform ROM exercises at least twice a day, emphasizing the trunk, neck, arms, hips, and legs. *ROM exercises promote joint function, strengthen muscles, and prevent contractures.*

■ Assist with ambulation at least four times a day. *Exercise fosters independence and self-esteem.*

- Use assistive devices such as canes, splints, or braces as needed. *Assistive devices improve balance and help the client maintain the correct position.*
- Consult with a physical therapist. *Physical therapy can help to improve coordination, balance, gait, and transfers. Exercise is also important in preventing contractures.*

IMPAIRED VERBAL COMMUNICATION

- Teach the client to face the listener and speak in short sentences. Allow extra time for self-expression. *These strategies reduce the client's frustration in communicating.*
- Provide a write-on, wipe-off slate; flash cards with common phrases; or pointing to objects. *Individualizing communication decreases anxiety and isolation.*
- Try to anticipate the client's needs. *This reduces the client's frustration.*

IMBALANCED NUTRITION: LESS THAN BODY REQUIREMENTS

- Place client in upright position for all meals and keep suction equipment at the bedside *to decrease the risk for aspiration.*
- Serve semi-solid or thickened liquid foods. Cut food into small pieces. *Food that is too liquid can be aspirated by the client. Smaller pieces are easier to swallow.*
- Massage the throat as the client swallows. *This helps the client to swallow.*
- Reduce distractions during mealtime. *This allows the client to focus on eating, chewing, and swallowing.*
- Obtain utensils that are easier for the client to grasp. *Modified utensils help the client eat and maintain a sense of self-esteem.*
- Increase daily fluid intake and fiber. *Fluids and fiber prevent constipation caused by several of the anti-Parkinson medications.*

EVALUATING

Evaluate the effectiveness of nursing care by collecting data related to ability to ambulate, chew, swallow, and communicate. In addition, evaluate for the absence of complications and knowledge of disease process and medications.

Discharge Considerations

Persons with PD face many complications. They may have skin breakdown from incontinence or immobility; they may fall; they may develop joint contractures. In addition, they may experience malnutrition, constipation, or infection. Assess and teach the client and caregiver ways to prevent these problems (review Box 30-3 for general guidelines).

Provide information about the disease, its management, and strategies for coping with tremors, dysphagia, and speech problems. Explain the purpose, side effects, and directions for taking each medication. Reinforce gait training, ROM exercises, and proper posture. Explain the importance of follow-up meetings with speech therapy, physical therapy, and occupational therapy. Refer the client to home health services so that the nurse can examine the home for risks of injury. The client may experience falls from poor vision, stooped posture, and confusion. Discuss safety measures. These include removing loose rugs and excess furniture, installing a raised toilet seat and handrails in the bathroom, and providing adequate lighting throughout the home and in outside areas. Refer to local support groups and the American Parkinson's Disease Association.

 # Myasthenia Gravis

Myasthenia gravis is a chronic, autoimmune disorder affecting women most often between the ages of 20 and 30. Clients experience periods of exacerbations and remissions. Stress, pregnancy, and secondary infections may trigger an acute onset.

For an unknown reason, the thymus gland produces antibodies that block or reduce the number acetylcholine receptors at each neuromuscular junction. Nerve impulses cannot be sent to the cranial nerves that control muscles of the face, lips, tongue, neck, and throat. This causes weakness of the facial, speech, and chewing muscles. Characteristic manifestations include eyelid ptosis, diplopia, slurred speech, nasal voice, difficulty chewing and swallowing, and fatigue. A smile appears as a snarl or grimace. There is progressive difficulty in performing fine motor tasks such as writing and progressive weakness of the respiratory muscles. The client faces the risk of aspiration and respiratory insufficiency. Onset is gradual, and manifestations may vary each day.

Two life-threatening emergencies are possible:

1. *Myasthenic crisis* is due to missed doses of medication or an infection. Clients suddenly develop increased muscle weakness, an inability to speak or swallow, and respiratory distress.
2. *Cholinergic crisis* is caused by overmedication with anticholinesterase (cholinergic) medications. The symptoms are similar to myasthenic crisis: severe muscle weakness plus nausea, vomiting, abdominal cramps, increased salivation, sweating, and bradycardia.

Either crisis requires immediate treatment and the possible need for mechanical ventilation.

A physical examination of the facial, oculomotor, laryngeal, and respiratory muscles is done. Diagnosis is confirmed by injecting edrophonium chloride (Tensilon), a short-acting anticholinesterase. Clients with myasthenia gravis show dramatic improvement in muscle strength, but the improvement lasts only about 5 minutes. *Electromyographic (EMG) studies* show increased muscle fatigue. *CT scan* of the chest may show a tumor of the thymus gland.

Pyridostigmine (Mestinon), an anticholinesterase medication, is the treatment of choice for myasthenia gravis.

Dosage is adjusted until the client's symptoms decrease. It is difficult to balance the correct dose without causing myasthenic or cholinergic crisis. The client is taught to record all signs and symptoms carefully so that medication doses can be adjusted (Table 30-2 ◆). Prednisone and cytotoxic agents, such as cyclosporine or azathioprine (Imuran), are added to block antibody production or decrease circulating antibodies.

CLINICAL alert

Administer anticholinesterase drugs on a strict time schedule. Clients with dysphagia may not be able to swallow the medication unless it is taken exactly on time. Doses taken too late may cause myasthenic crisis. Taking doses early may result in cholinergic crisis.

Along with drug therapy, a **thymectomy** (surgical removal of the thymus gland) may be performed to remove the source of the antibodies. A short-term treatment option involves plasmapheresis. This procedure removes the anti-acetylcholine receptor antibodies so that muscle weakness and fatigue decrease.

The nurse collects data about the client's muscle weakness; speech, chewing, or swallowing difficulties; and changes in vision. Nursing care focuses on decreasing or preventing respiratory and swallowing problems as well as reducing fatigue. The nursing diagnoses and interventions are similar to those presented earlier in caring for the client with MS or PD.

Once the client and family understand the disease and ways to cope with the physical and psychosocial problems, the client can be managed at home. Review home care assessment and strategies found under MS and PD. In addition, be sure the family knows cardiopulmonary resuscitation (CPR), and demonstrate how to insert an airway, suction, and use an Ambu bag.

Teaching should emphasize medication actions, side effects, scheduling, and symptoms of myasthenic and cholinergic crisis. Stress the importance of taking medications on an exact schedule. Advise the client to wear a Medic-Alert bracelet.

Refer the client and family to local support groups and provide information about the Myasthenia Gravis Foundation. Pregnancy should be discussed with the physician because it may cause manifestations to worsen. Also, medications such as neostigmine (Prostigmin) cross the placenta.

Huntington's Disease

Huntington's disease (HD) is a progressive, inherited neurologic disease. Men and women are affected equally between the ages of 35 and 45. It is transmitted as an autosomal-dominant genetic trait. Each child of a parent with HD has a 50% chance of inheriting the disease. There is no cure for this disease.

HD involves a lack of a neurotransmitter, gamma-aminobutyric acid (GABA). This causes acetylcholine levels to drop and dopamine levels to rise. Unlike PD in which a dopamine deficit slows movement, in HD the excess

TABLE 30-2   NURSING IMPLICATIONS FOR PHARMACOLOGY: CLIENTS WITH MYASTHENIA GRAVIS

DRUG GROUP/DRUGS	ACTION	NURSING IMPLICATIONS	CLIENT TEACHING
Anticholinesterase Drugs ■ Neostigmine (Prostigmin) ■ Ambenonium (Mytelase) ■ Pyridostigmine (Mestinon, Regonol) ■ For diagnosis: Edrophonium (Tensilon)	Anticholinesterase drugs prolong the action of acetylcholine to improve muscle contraction. Dose is adjusted to obtain maximum benefit with the fewest side effects. They are contraindicated in clients with urinary or GI tract obstruction, asthma, or hyperthyroidism.	Identify client's ability to swallow. Give the medication on a regular schedule at the exact time. Monitor for *myasthenic crisis:* Severe muscle weakness, difficulty breathing, swallowing, or speaking. Notify physician immediately. Monitor for *cholinergic crisis:* Excess salivation and sweating, bradycardia, nausea and vomiting.	Take drug as directed on a regular schedule at the exact time. Report symptoms of *myasthenic crisis* immediately: Severe muscle weakness, fast heartbeat, difficulty breathing, swallowing, or speaking. Report symptoms of *cholinergic crisis* immediately: Slow heartbeat, increased salivation or sweating, decreased blood pressure. Wear Medic-Alert ID. Be sure a family member is trained in CPR.

dopamine causes uncontrolled movement. Without GABA, there is premature death of basal ganglia and cerebral cortex cells. All of these changes develop slowly, affecting (a) personality, (b) intellectual function, and (c) movement. Emotional lability ranges from irritability and anger to depression. Delusions and hallucinations are not unusual. Memory and intellectual function decline to the point of dementia.

Chorea (constant, jerky, uncontrolled movements of the body) is a characteristic manifestation. The client exhibits mild fidgeting or writhing and twisting of the entire body. Motor symptoms are worse with emotional stress but decrease during sleep. Facial grimaces and tics affect speech, chewing, and swallowing, leading to choking and malnutrition. Bowel and bladder control is lost. As the chorea increases, the client is confined to bed. Prognosis is poor, with inevitable total dependence. Death is usually from aspiration pneumonia.

There is no specific test for this disease. Diagnosis is based on symptoms and family history. A PET shows changes in the brain. Offspring concerned about their chances of developing HD should have genetic testing.

Medications are given to control the symptoms of HD. The chorea movements may be modified by haloperidol (Haldol) or diazepam (Valium). Antidepressants and antipsychotics are prescribed in the early stage of the disease.

At first, the client and family can manage care at home. Refer them to local support groups or psychologist. The suicide rate is high when the client understands how drastically his or her life will change. As the client declines, care is similar to care for other deteriorating neurologic disorders. Eventually, skilled long-term care is needed.

Amyotrophic Lateral Sclerosis

Amyotrophic lateral sclerosis (ALS), named *Lou Gehrig's disease* after the famous baseball player who suffered from it, is a rapidly progressive, fatal neurologic disease. The exact cause is unknown. More men are affected between the ages of 40 and 70.

ALS involves loss of motor neurons in the spinal cord and brain stem. When electrical impulses cannot be sent from the brain to the voluntary muscles, they lose strength and atrophy. Although body function decreases, the person remains mentally alert.

This disorder is characterized by muscle weakness, **fasciculations** (involuntary contractions of the voluntary muscles, or twitching), and muscle wasting of the arms, legs, and trunk. Brain stem involvement causes speech and swallowing difficulties. Toward the end, clients develop breathing problems, and death is from aspiration pneumonia or respiratory failure. About 50% of clients die within 2 to 5 years of diagnosis.

Diagnosis is based on the client's symptoms. A series of different tests are done to rule out other conditions that mimic ALS. An EMG confirms muscle weakness. Muscle biopsies show loss of muscle fiber.

There is no cure for ALS. Only one medication, riluzole (Rilutek), seems to slow the destruction of motor neurons. Other medications include baclofen and diazepam to relieve muscle spasms. Psychological support is important for the client and family as the disease progresses.

For as long as possible, promote the client's independence in performing daily ADLs. The client and family should be referred to an ALS support group. Nursing care is similar to that for the client with MS, discussed earlier in this chapter. Before speech is lost, develop communication signals such as blinking for yes and no answers. When swallowing or breathing problems develop, anticipate enteral feedings and mechanical ventilation. In order to manage the client at home, the family is taught: (a) suctioning techniques and the Heimlich maneuver, (b) bowel and urinary catheter care, (c) enteral feedings, (d) skin care, and (e) turning and positioning the client.

Guillain–Barré Syndrome

Guillain–Barré syndrome (GBS), or *idiopathic polyneuritis,* is an acute, progressive inflammation of the peripheral nervous system (PNS). It is thought to be an autoimmune response that develops after a previous respiratory or gastrointestinal (GI) infection, or a recent vaccination. Most cases occur in people between the ages of 30 and 50.

Antibodies attack the myelin sheath covering the peripheral nerves. Without myelin, impulses are poorly conducted to the sensory and motor nerves. This causes rapid, muscle weakness, loss of reflexes, and paralysis.

Manifestations of GBS start in the lower extremities and move upward. The first symptoms are bilateral weakness and numbness and tingling in the legs. Within 24 to 72 hours, weakness extends to the arms and respiratory muscles and then progresses to paralysis. Cranial nerve involvement causes chewing, swallowing, and talking problems. If the autonomic nervous system is affected, blood pressure and pulse changes develop. Throughout this process, the person remains alert and oriented.

The most serious complication is respiratory failure. If this develops, a tracheostomy and mechanical ventilation are used for 2 to 3 weeks, but the time frame can vary. (See nursing care for the client with a tracheostomy in Procedure 25–2, and mechanical ventilation in Chapter 26.) Other complications, such as skin breakdown and deep vein thrombosis, relate to the length of time the client is paralyzed.

Most clients with GBS recover with few or no residual effects. Recovery time depends on how fast the myelin sheath can rebuild itself. Average rehabilitation is about 6 months but may take as long as 2 years. As the nerves recover, the client's symptoms improve in reverse order.

Diagnosis of GBS is based on clinical symptoms and a recent viral infection. A lumbar puncture shows elevated CSF protein levels. The results of EMG studies show a definite slowing of nerve conduction.

Medical management consists of plasmapheresis and intravenous immune globulin. Plasmapheresis removes the antibodies that caused GBS. It is beneficial when used within the first 2 weeks. Clients typically have five exchanges over 8 to 10 days. The action of intravenous immune globulin is unclear, but the effects are similar to plasmapheresis. Antibiotics are prescribed for urinary tract or respiratory infections. Anticoagulants are given to prevent deep vein thrombosis and pulmonary embolism.

Clients are acutely ill and are managed in a critical care unit. Nursing assessments are done every 1 to 2 hours. Nursing interventions focus on preventing immobility problems; promoting adequate hydration, nutrition, and respiratory function; and providing psychosocial support. It is important to anticipate the needs of the client and family. They are stunned by the rapid deterioration of function and fear permanent paralysis.

After the acute phase, the client is transferred to a skilled nursing facility or home. Those with extensive paralysis need inpatient or outpatient physical, occupational, and speech therapy. The caregiver may need help from a homemaker or home health aide. When recovery is long, the caregiver will need respite care.

Trigeminal Neuralgia

Trigeminal neuralgia *(tic douloureux)* involves two sensory branches of the trigeminal nerve: the maxillary and mandibular (Figure 30-4 ◆). Pain occurs along one or both of these branches. It affects women between the ages of 50 and 60. The cause may be injury from dental or surgical procedures, facial trauma, infection, or pressure on the nerve by a tumor.

Trigeminal neuralgia is characterized by severe, one-sided facial pain lasting a few seconds to a few minutes. The pain is described as stabbing or burning in the forehead, along the nose, lips, or cheek. Attacks occur for several weeks and then suddenly disappear. The client may remain pain free for days to years. With age, remissions become shorter.

Trigger zones on the face initiate an attack when they are stimulated. Simple actions like shaving, chewing, brushing the teeth, washing the face, change in temperature, or wind can set off an attack. An attack may cause wincing, grimacing, or tearing of the eye. To control pain, clients may refuse to wash, shave, eat, or talk.

Diagnosis is based on the characteristic location and type of pain. Anticonvulsants such as carbamazepine (Tegretol) and phenytoin (Dilantin) are given to control the attacks. Other drugs like baclofen (Lioresal) or clonazepam (Klonopin) may be added. If drug therapy fails, nerve blocks with local anesthetics are tried. Another option is a **rhizotomy** (the surgical severing of a nerve root to control pain). Only the sensory nerve root is destroyed. Motor function is preserved so that eating is unaffected. If the ophthalmic branch is damaged, the corneal reflex is lost.

Nursing care focuses on teaching self-care strategies including medications and potential side effects. Because this is a chronic condition, long-term use of narcotics is avoided. Discuss ways to avoid trigger points, such as using room-temperature water and soft cotton pads to wash the face. If the client refuses to eat during periods of pain attacks, encourage a soft high-protein and high-calorie diet.

After surgery, the client may lose sensation and corneal reflex on the involved side. Teach the client to chew on the unaffected side, to avoid hot foods or liquids, and to brush the teeth and check for food pockets between gums and cheek after every meal. Men should use an electric razor to shave. Clients should also protect the face from very cold or windy conditions, and, if necessary, wear a protective eye shield.

Bell's Palsy

Bell's palsy (facial paralysis) is associated with the herpes simplex virus. Inflammation causes edema and pressure on the facial nerve, resulting in necrosis. This leads to sudden weakness and paralysis on one side of the face. Paralysis distorts the affected side, causing ptosis of the eyelid, tearing, mouth drooping, drooling, an inability to smile, and difficulty chewing (Figure 30-5 ◆). There is also pain around or behind the ear. Most clients improve within a few weeks to months.

Diagnosis is based on the client's facial appearance. Treatment is a short-term course of steroids. Because it is linked to the herpes virus, clients are given antiviral drugs. Mild analgesics may reduce the facial pain. Nursing and home care is similar to that as the client with trigeminal neuralgia. (Review the strategies listed after surgery.) In addition, teach the client to apply warm, moist heat such as gel packs, which increases circulation and relieves pain. A facial sling may be applied during meals to prevent muscle stretching.

The loss of blinking increases the risk for corneal drying. Demonstrate how to instill artificial tears four times a day, and

Sensory distribution

Ophthalmic division

Maxillary division

Mandibular division

Motor distribution

Figure 30-4. ◆ Sensory and motor branches of the trigeminal nerve. There are three sensory branches: ophthalmic, maxillary, and mandibular.

Figure 30-5. ◆ The client with Bell's palsy shows the typical drooping of one side of the face.

to apply an eye patch at night. Be sure the client understands how to inspect the eye each day and to report eye pain, redness, swelling, or discharge. Recommend wearing dark glasses or goggles when outside or working in dusty conditions.

Rabies

Rabies is a viral infection of the CNS caused by an animal bite. The rabies virus is carried by wild and domestic animals, including bats, skunks, foxes, raccoons, cats, and dogs. The virus spreads from the wound to the peripheral nerves and eventually travels to the CNS. Incubation varies from 14 days to 3 months. Any animal that has bitten someone is observed for 1 to 2 weeks to detect rabies symptoms. Sick animals are euthanized and their brains examined for the rabies virus.

Clinical manifestations occur in three stages. In *stage 1,* the wound is painful, with a tingling sensation. The client experiences malaise, fever, headache, and sensitivity to light and loud noises. *Stage 2* develops within 24 to 72 hours. Any attempt at swallowing causes forceful spasms of the larynx. The person refuses to drink (*hydrophobia*). Swallowing problems lead to frothy drooling. Eventually, the sight or sound of water triggers the muscle spasms and excessive salivation. *Stage 3:* Without treatment, death occurs in about 7 days from cardiopulmonary arrest.

To prevent rabies, it is recommended that all household dogs and cats be immunized. Any animal bite and scratch is thoroughly cleaned with soap and water to remove the saliva and dilute the virus. The person is taken immediately to the emergency department to receive rabies immune globulin (RIg) as soon as possible after the bite. This is followed by five doses of inactivated human diploid cell rabies vaccine (HDCV) intramuscularly in the deltoid muscle on the day of exposure and on days 3, 7, 14, and 28 after exposure. Clients who show signs of rabies are cared for in the critical care unit with the room dark and quiet to decrease stimulation. Nursing care focuses on airway maintenance and seizure control. Standard precautions are essential, because the rabies virus is present in the saliva of the client. If an open wound of a health care provider is contaminated with infected saliva, the provider must receive postexposure immunizations.

Tetanus

Tetanus, or *lockjaw,* is a disorder of the nervous system caused by *Clostridium tetani.* This anaerobic bacillus produces spores that live in the soil and enter the body through open wounds contaminated with dirt, street dust, or feces. Most cases of tetanus occur in adults over 50 whose tetanus booster is older than 10 years. Incubation period averages 3 to 21 days but can be longer.

When the spores enter an open wound, two exotoxins are absorbed by the peripheral nerves and carried to the spinal cord. They interfere with the transmission of neuromuscular impulses leading to uncontrolled muscle spasms. Initially, the client exhibits pain at the wound site, stiffness of the jaw and neck, mild spasms, and difficulty swallowing. As it advances, the person has difficulty opening the jaw (**trismus**). Spasms of the facial muscles give the person a grinning expression. Painful seizures cause the back to arch. Despite these physical effects, the client remains alert and oriented. The mortality rate is high and usually due to asphyxia from spasms of the glottis and respiratory muscles.

There are no specific laboratory tests for tetanus. The diagnosis is based on the clinical manifestations. Active immunization can prevent tetanus. Children should receive tetanus toxoid as part of the diphtheria–tetanus–pertussis (DPT) immunization series. Adults should be given two doses of tetanus toxoid 4 to 6 weeks apart, with a third dose in 6 to 12 months. The Centers for Disease Control and Prevention (CDC) recommends a booster dose every 10 years.

If a wound is extensive or heavily contaminated or if the person's immunization status is unknown, give tetanus immune globulin (TIg) to destroy the tetanus toxins. This is followed by injections of tetanus toxoid according to the schedule mentioned before. All wounds, no matter how small, are thoroughly cleaned with soap and water. Foreign material is carefully flushed out or removed from a wound. Only hydrogen peroxide and iodine kill the tetanus organism.

Clients who develop tetanus are cared for in a critical care unit with minimal stimulation. They are given antibiotics to destroy the organism and anticonvulsants to stop any seizures. When muscle spasms and seizures are severe, paralytic agents are used. Airway obstruction is managed by mechanical ventilation. The recovery periods varies from 2 to 5 weeks.

Creutzfeldt–Jakob Disease

Creutzfeldt–Jakob disease (CJD) is a rare, progressive neurologic disease causing brain degeneration. The disease is transmissible and fatal within 6 to 12 months after diagnosis. It primarily affects adults over 60, with more cases in England, Chile, and Italy.

CJD destroys the brain's gray matter. On autopsy, the brain has numerous tiny holes resembling a sponge (called spongiform encephalopathy). The underlying cause seems to be an infective protein pathogen called a *prion*. It is resistant to normal chemical and physical sterilization methods. A few cases have been transmitted through corneal transplants and human growth hormone from cadavers.

Early manifestations include memory loss and personality and visual changes. Then the person rapidly develops dementia, muscle contractions, speech problems, and ataxia. Clients in the terminal stage are comatose until death.

Diagnosis is difficult because CJD mimics other degenerative neurologic diseases such as Alzheimer's disease. A thorough neurologic examination, EEG changes, and CT scan help confirm a diagnosis. However, the final diagnosis of CJD is made only by an autopsy.

No specific treatment exists for CJD. Medical and nursing care focus on providing support and comfort. Standard precautions are followed when handling all blood and body fluids. A 5% bleach solution seems to be most effective in disinfecting contaminated surfaces and equipment. It is not necessary to place the client in isolation.

Bovine spongiform encephalopathy (BSE), or "mad cow disease," is a form of spongiform encephalopathy that develops in animals. In the late 1990s, a CJD-like illness, known as *variant CJD*, appeared in younger clients. This seems to be linked to eating meat from animals infected with BSE. By late 2000, no cases of variant CJD have occurred in the United States.

Spinal Cord Disorders

The spinal cord, vertebrae, intervertebral disks, and spinal nerves are anatomically close to each other. For example, if the client suffers a thoracic vertebrae injury, pressure is applied to the spinal cord. Unless the pressure is relieved, the client could be paralyzed.

Spinal Cord Injury

A spinal cord injury (SCI) is usually due to trauma. Adolescent and young adult males experience most spinal cord injuries. Motor vehicle crashes cause most of the injuries, followed by violent acts, falls, and sports injuries.

The spinal cord provides a two-way path to conduct impulses between the brain and body. Nerves in the spinal cord connect to the body through nerve roots that exit the spinal column. These nerves provide motor and sensory information to the entire body below the head. Just like the spinal column, the spinal cord is divided into cervical, thoracic, and lumbar regions. The cervical region carries sensations from the head, neck, diaphragm, shoulders, and arms. The thoracic region supplies nerves to the chest that help in breathing and nerves of the sympathetic nervous system. The lumbar region supplies the legs, pelvis, and bowel and bladder.

PATHOPHYSIOLOGY

A number of factors cause spinal cord injuries. The neck can be forcibly bent forward or backward, compressing the vertebrae. Diving into shallow water also compresses the vertebrae and spinal cord (Figure 30-6 ◆). A bullet may penetrate the cord, or a fall may cause a fracture of the neck or back. Most injuries occur in the lumbar and cervical regions.

Spinal cord injuries (SCIs) are classified according to the level of injury and the amount of cord damage. An injury at the sixth cervical vertebra is called a C6 SCI. Cord damage is described as complete or incomplete. A complete SCI results in total loss of motor and sensory function below the level of injury. Incomplete injury causes varying degrees of function below the level of injury. The level of the injury determines whether the client develops paraplegia or tetraplegia (Figure 30-7 ◆). Damage at the thoracic level causes **paraplegia** (paralysis of the lower part of the body). High cervical injuries cause **tetraplegia**, formerly called quadriplegia. Tetraplegia is paralysis of the arms, trunk, legs, and pelvic organs.

As soon as bruising or compression occurs to the spinal cord, there is bleeding into the gray matter. At this point the damage may be reversible. However, the body's inflammatory response causes edema, hypoxia, and ischemia. This process actually expands the injury area and may cause more damage than the original injury. If the cord has not suffered irreversible damage, corticosteroids given within the first 4 to 6 hours after injury may stop the inflammation. Tissue repair occurs over a period of 3 to 4 weeks, but the spinal cord does not regenerate.

The client may have deficits in movement, sensation, and reflex activity. The level of the injury determines the client's deficits and potential for rehabilitation (Table 30-3 ◆). Complications occur either immediately after an injury or later on (Box 30-8). Clients with tetraplegia are prone to more complications than those with paraplegia.

SPINAL SHOCK

Spinal shock is a temporary loss of reflex activity below the level of spinal cord injury. It typically occurs 30 to 60 minutes after a complete SCI. There is loss of motor function, sensa-

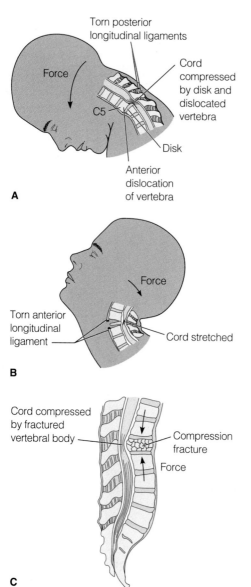

Figure 30-6. ◆ Spinal cord injury mechanisms. (A) Hyperflexion. (B) Hyperextension. (C) Cord compression.

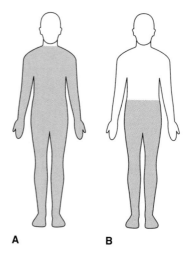

Figure 30-7. ◆ Types of paralysis. (A) Tetraplegia and (B) Paraplegia.

tion, spinal reflexes, and autonomic function. Other manifestations include (a) bradycardia, (b) hypotension, (c) loss of sweating and temperature control below the level of injury, (d) bowel and bladder dysfunction, (e) flaccid paralysis, and (f) **poikilothermia** (a condition found in spinal cord injury in which the client assumes the temperature of the environment). Spinal shock usually lasts from 1 to 6 weeks, and then reflex activity returns. Until it resolves, the client needs medical support, such as intravenous (IV) fluids.

Autonomic Dysreflexia

Autonomic dysreflexia is an exaggerated sympathetic response in clients with SCIs at or above the T6 level. Stimuli such as a full bladder or fecal impaction trigger a hypertensive crisis. The client develops severe hypertension (systolic up to 300 mm Hg); pounding headache; flushed, diaphoretic skin above the lesion and pale, cold, and dry skin below it; goose-

bumps; and anxiety. If untreated, autonomic dysreflexia can cause seizures, a cerebrovascular accident (CVA), or death.

This is a medical emergency. Elevate the head of the bed 45 degrees to lower the blood pressure. If this does not lower it, give antihypertensive medications as ordered. Monitor blood pressure every 2 to 3 minutes while at the same time assessing for the cause. If the client has a Foley catheter, check the tubing for kinks or irrigate the catheter to check for patency. When the client does not have a catheter, insert a straight catheter. If a fecal impaction is present, insert Nupercaine cream into the anus, wait 10 minutes, and manually remove the impaction.

COLLABORATIVE CARE

Care of the client with an SCI begins at the accident scene. All accident victims are treated as if they have an SCI. Moving a client at the scene can cause further damage to the spinal cord. If the client is moved incorrectly, pieces from a fractured vertebrae could penetrate the cord and cause permanent damage. Clients are not moved unless there is a life-threatening danger, such as being burned, crushed, or drowned.

Assess the client's airway, breathing, and circulation immediately. Next, assess the client for complaints of neck pain or changes in movement or sensation. Then immobilize the neck and place on a spinal backboard in a neutral position. When emergency personnel arrive, they apply a cervical collar.

In the emergency department, the client is assessed for other injuries, respiratory distress, and neurologic deficits. The neck and spine remain immobilized throughout assessment and diagnostic testing. Oxygen is given for clients with cervical or thoracic injuries. An intravenous line and fluids are started to prevent shock. Until the client's condition is stable, closely monitor for respiratory, cardiac, urinary, and GI complications. High-dose methylpredinisolone (Solu-Medrol), a corticosteroid, is started immediately to prevent spinal cord edema.

TABLE 30-3

FUNCTIONAL ABILITIES BY LEVEL OF SPINAL CORD INJURY

LEVEL	FUNCTION	ADL	ELIMINATION	MOBILITY
C1, C2, C3	No movement or sensation below the neck	D	D	Voice or sip-n-puff controlled electric WC
C4	Movement and sensation of head and neck; some partial function of the diaphragm	D	D	Chin-operated electric WC
C5	Controls head, neck, and shoulders; flexes elbows	WA	D	Electric WC
C6	Uses shoulder, extends wrist.	I or WA	WA	WC, self-transfer
C7–C8	Extends elbow, flexes wrist, some use of fingers	I	I	Manual WC
T1–T5	Has full hand and finger control, full use of thoracic muscles	I	I	Manual WC
T6–T10	Controls abdominal muscles, has good balance	I	I	Manual WC
T11–L5	Flexes and abducts the hips; flexes and extends the knees	I	I	Ambulates with leg braces, short braces, or canes
S1–S5	Full control of legs; progressive bowel, bladder, and sexual function	I	I	

D = Dependent, I = Independent, WA = With assistance, WC = Wheelchair

Laboratory and Diagnostic Tests

The following diagnostic studies are used to diagnose SCIs:

- *Cervical spine x-rays* show fracture or displacement of the vertebrae.
- *CT scan* or *MRI* shows damage to the vertebrae, spinal cord, and tissues around the cord.

Pharmacology

Corticosteroids are given for 1 to 2 weeks to decrease or control edema of the cord. Muscle spasms are treated with antispas-

---

BOX 30-8
COMPLICATIONS OF SPINAL CORD INJURY

- *Integument:* Decubitus (pressure) ulcers
- *Neurologic:* Pain, hypotonia, autonomic dysreflexia
- *Cardiovascular and peripheral vascular:* Spinal shock, orthostatic hypotension, bradycardia, deep vein thrombosis
- *Respiratory:* Limited chest expansion, pneumonia
- *Gastrointestinal:* Stress ulcers, paralytic ileus, stool impaction, stool incontinence
- *Genitourinary:* Urinary retention, urinary incontinence, neurogenic bladder, urinary tract infections, impotence, decreased vaginal lubrication
- *Musculoskeletal:* Joint contractures, muscle spasms, muscle atrophy, pathologic fractures, hypercalcemia

---

modics (Table 30-4 ◆). *Histamine H$_2$ antagonists* (e.g., ranitidine [Zantac]) are used to prevent stress-related gastric ulcers. Thrombophlebitis is prevented with *anticoagulants.* Stool softeners may be given as part of a bowel-training program.

Stabilization and Immobilization

Early management includes stabilizing and immobilizing the spinal cord. Thoracic and lumbar injuries are immobilized with braces or body casts. Cervical injuries are treated with cervical tongs or halo vest. Gardner–Wells tongs (Figure 30-8 ◆) are used for unstable cervical fractures. The tongs are inserted into the skull and attached to weights to keep the spine in correct alignment. The disadvantage is that the client must be monitored closely for displacement of the tongs. If traction is interrupted, the client faces additional spinal cord damage.

The halo vest (Figure 30-9 ◆) is used for stable cervical or thoracic fractures without cord damage. It allows greater mobility, self-care, and participation in a rehabilitation program. This device is secured through four pins inserted into the skull, two in the frontal bone and two in the occipital bone. The halo ring is then attached to a rigid plastic vest lined with sheepskin. Nursing care is described in Box 30-9.

Clients with cervical tongs and traction are placed on a kinetic bed, CircOlectric bed, or Stryker frame. These beds allow frequent turning to prevent immobility problems yet keep the spine aligned. Those with the halo vest can be placed in a regular bed.

TABLE 30-4	NURSING IMPLICATIONS FOR PHARMACOLOGY: CLIENTS RECEIVING ANTISPASMODICS IN SPINAL CORD INJURY		
DRUG GROUP/DRUGS	**ACTION**	**NURSING IMPLICATIONS**	**CLIENT TEACHING**
Baclofen (Lioresal) Diazepam (Valium) Dantrolene (Dantrium)	They are used to control muscle spasm and pain associated with acute or chronic musculoskeletal conditions. They are not always effective in controlling spasticity resulting from cerebral or spinal cord conditions.	Assess the client's spasticity and involuntary movements. Give with food to decrease gastrointestinal symptoms. Monitor for drowsiness and dizziness. Monitor for therapeutic effect.	Take with meals to decrease gastric irritation. These drugs may cause drowsiness or dizziness. If drowsy, avoid activities that require mental alertness or coordination. Check with physician before taking with other drugs. Do not stop the drug abruptly without discussing with your physician.

Surgery

Surgery is necessary when bone fragments or a hematoma compress the spine. It is also done to stabilize and support the spine. Different spinal surgeries may be performed such as a spinal fusion, decompression laminectomy, or insertion of metal rods. These surgeries are discussed later in the chapter.

NURSING CARE

Clients with an SCI need acute care in the hospital followed by rehabilitation. The care plan focuses on preventing complications of immobility, promoting self-care, and teaching the client and family.

ASSESSING

On arrival at the hospital the client is assessed from head to toe. Box 30-10 presents subjective and objective data to collect. During the acute phase, perform assessments at frequent intervals.

Figure 30-8. ◆ Cervical traction with Gardner–Wells tongs.

DIAGNOSING, PLANNING, AND IMPLEMENTING

Spinal cord injuries can affect all body systems. The nurse monitors for and plans interventions to prevent problems with breathing, physical immobility, bowel and bladder elimination, skin integrity, nutrition, and self-esteem.

INEFFECTIVE BREATHING PATTERN

- Monitor pulse oximetry levels. *It is important to measure oxygen levels in order to prevent respiratory problems.*
- Monitor for difficulty swallowing or coughing, respiratory stridor, and increased motor and sensory loss. *Injuries at C1 to C4 level alter respiratory function from paralysis of the respiratory, chest, and abdominal muscles. Edema of the cord can affect the client's ability to breathe spontaneously.*

Figure 30-9. ◆ Halo vest.

BOX 30-9
NURSING CARE CHECKLIST

CLIENTS IN HALO VESTS

☑ Inspect pins and traction bars for tightness; report loose pins to physician.

☑ Check for access to the front of the vest for emergency intervention.

☑ Never use the halo ring to lift or reposition the client.

☑ Assess the pin sites for redness, edema, and drainage.

☑ Clean pin sites daily.

☑ Inspect the skin under the vest for pressure areas.

☑ To provide skin care, loosen the sides of the vest. Wash and thoroughly dry the skin. Prevent the lining from becoming wet.

☑ Change the sheepskin lining when it is soiled or at least once each week.

☑ Turn the client every 2 hours.

☑ Provide mild analgesic for headache.

■ Turn, cough, and deep breathe at least every 2 hours. Suction PRN. *These measures decrease the risk for pneumonia and atelectasis.*

■ Increase fluids to 2,000 mL/day. *Increased fluids thin secretions, making them easier to expel and expectorate.*

IMPAIRED PHYSICAL MOBILITY

■ Perform passive ROM exercises to all extremities twice a day. *ROM exercises help prevent contractures and improve circulation.*

■ Use splints, trochanter rolls, and high-top tennis shoes *to prevent wrist drop, foot drop, and external rotation of the hips.*

■ Inspect skin daily for pressure ulcers. Use special bed if necessary. Turn client every 2 hours. *The lack of sensation along with immobility increases the risk for pressure ulcers.*

■ Provide diet high in protein, carbohydrate, and calories. *Stress from an SCI increases metabolism and the risk for malnutrition.*

■ Assess the lower extremities each shift for thrombophlebitis. Apply TED hose and remove for 30 to 60 minutes each shift. *Immobile clients are at risk for deep vein thrombosis (DVT). TED hose prevents blood from pooling in the lower extremities and reduces the risk for DVT.*

IMPAIRED URINARY ELIMINATION AND CONSTIPATION

■ During spinal shock, insert a Foley catheter or perform intermittent catheterization. After spinal shock, reinforce the bladder training program. A catheter prevents urinary retention and possible bladder rupture. *Clients have a high risk for urinary tract infection (UTI); the use of catheters is limited.*

■ Teach the client to use trigger voiding techniques such as stroking inner thigh, pulling the pubic hair, tapping on

BOX 30-10
ASSESSING CLIENTS WITH SPINAL CORD INJURY

SUBJECTIVE DATA

• Present health status:
  • General health status
  • Breathing difficulty
  • Loss of strength, movement, or sensation below level of injury
  • Numbness or tingling in extremities
  • Presence of fear, anger, or depression
• Past medical history:
  • History of traumatic injury: Car accident, sports injury

OBJECTIVE DATA

• Vital signs: Bradycardia and hypotension may indicate spinal shock.
• Monitor temperature. Clients with high cervical injuries may have poikilothermia.
• Assess respiratory rate, depth, and breath sounds; ability to cough; use of accessory muscles. Cervical injuries above C4 may cause respiratory distress or failure.
• Test motor strength: Ask the client to squeeze your hand, move legs, and wiggle the toes.
• Assess sensation: Ask the client to close his or her eyes; touch the body from the shoulder to the feet with a cotton ball. Note areas where the client cannot feel the touch.
• Palpate the bladder for fullness. Clients with cervical injuries cannot feel a full bladder.
• Auscultate bowel sounds. Decreased or absent bowel tones may indicate paralytic ileus.

the suprapubic area or abdomen. *These trigger voiding techniques cause reflex activity that may initiate voiding.*

■ Place the client on a bedside commode if possible. *Upright position facilitates complete bladder and bowel emptying.*

■ Monitor for cloudy, foul-smelling urine and increase fluid intake. *These clients have a high potential for UTI.*

■ Begin a bowel retraining program using stool softeners, rectal suppositories, and digital stimulation as needed. *These measures stimulate peristalsis and initiate bowel movements.*

SITUATIONAL LOW SELF-ESTEEM

■ Allow the client time to grieve or to express denial, depression, and anger over the changes in social, financial, and personal roles. *The client needs time to adjust to the lifestyle changes.*

■ Provide accurate information based on the physician's prognosis. *Accurate information helps the client understand his or her present and future needs.*

- Include family and significant others to treat the client as normally as possible. *These strategies can make the client feel worthy and of value.*
- Refer the client and family to support groups. *Support groups can help the client and family adjust to the changes.*

EVALUATING

To evaluate the effectiveness of care for a client with an SCI, collect data on bowel and bladder elimination, ability to manage ADLs, and absence of complications such as contractures, pressure ulcers, DVT, and infection.

 # Discharge Considerations

The nurse assesses the client's ability to live independently and, if necessary, the family's ability to provide care. In addition, it provides information about whether the client can live at home or will need care in a rehabilitation center (see Box 30-3).

The client's physical and emotional needs determine the type of rehabilitation program. Rehabilitation centers can offer specialized assistance but may not be near the client's home. These centers teach the client to function at the highest level possible.

Discharge responsibilities include teaching the client and family how to provide medications, ADLs, exercises, bowel and bladder programs such as urinary catheterization, and skin care. Discuss ways to prevent potential complications such as constipation, urinary retention, pressure ulcers, contractures, DVT, autonomic dysreflexia, and infections. Emphasize indications for notifying the physician. A physical therapist will demonstrate the use of any assistive devices such as wheelchair or crutches, and the need for position changes. Social services can arrange referral to a home health agency, transfer to a rehabilitation center, or a job retraining program. A home health nurse can evaluate for accessibility of the living area in the home.

Herniated Intervertebral Disk

A **herniated intervertebral disk,** also called *ruptured* or *slipped disk,* usually occurs in men between the ages of 30 and 50. Disk injury can develop from trauma, lifting incorrectly, sudden twisting of the spine, or degenerative changes due to arthritis. The majority of herniated disks occur in the lumbar (L4 or L5 to S1) or cervical regions. Herniated disks are a common cause of chronic back pain.

PATHOPHYSIOLOGY

The intervertebral disks are located between the vertebrae of the spinal column. They are made of an inner nucleus pulposus and an outer fibrous ring, the annulus fibrosus. The disks allow the spine to absorb compression by acting as shock

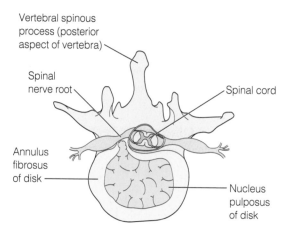

Figure 30-10. ◆ A herniated intervertebral disk. The herniated nucleus pulposus is applying pressure against the nerve root.

absorbers. A herniated intervertebral disk occurs when the nucleus pulposus protrudes through a weakened or torn annulus fibrosus (Figure 30-10 ◆). When the disk herniates or "slips," it compresses the nearby spinal nerve root and cause motor and sensory changes, pain, and altered reflexes (Box 30-11).

The herniation may be abrupt or gradual. Sudden straining of the back may cause immediate intense pain and muscle spasms. Gradual herniation resulting from degenerative changes and osteoarthritis has a slow onset of pain. The classic manifestation of a ruptured lumbar disk is recurrent low back pain. **Sciatica** describes pain that follows along the sciatic nerve. The pain ranges from mild to excruciating. It is increased by sitting, straining, coughing, sneezing, and walking. Sciatica is usually elicited when the client performs straight-leg raises.

BOX 30-11
MANIFESTATIONS OF HERNIATED INTERVERTEBRAL DISK

LUMBAR–SACRAL AREA (L4 TO L5 AND S1)
- Pain that radiates from hip down the leg, usually unilateral
- Muscle spasms
- Numbness and tingling of the leg and foot
- Decreased or absent knee and/or ankle reflexes

CERVICAL AREA (C5 TO C7)
- Neck stiffness
- Pain radiating from shoulder down arm to hand
- Numbness and tingling of neck, shoulder, arm, and possibly hand
- Decreased arm strength
- Decreased tricep reflex

COLLABORATIVE CARE

Medical care focuses on identifying the location of herniation and determining the type of treatment. Nursing care is directed toward preparing clients for diagnostic tests. The nurse also cares for the client following surgery and provides teaching for discharge.

Laboratory and Diagnostic Tests

A complete neurologic examination is part of diagnosing a herniated disk. Spinal *x-rays* can identify skeletal deformities and narrowing of the disk spaces. *CT scan* and *MRI* show the site of the herniation. *Myelography* is used both to rule out tumors and locate the herniation. Nursing implications for myelography are found in Box 30-12. *EMG* identifies specific spinal nerves that are affected by the pressure.

Pharmacology

Pain is managed with *nonsteroidal anti-inflammatory drugs (NSAIDs)* such as aspirin, ibuprofen (Motrin), and naproxen (Naprosyn). *Non-narcotic analgesics,* such as hydrocodone with acetaminophen (Vicodin) are given to control acute pain. Narcotics are avoided in clients with chronic pain as there is a risk of dependency. Muscle spasms are treated with *muscle relaxants. Transcutaneous electrical stimulation (TENS)* may relieve uncontrolled pain.

Medical Management

Besides medication, disk herniation is managed with bed rest for 1 to 2 days. This is followed by a physical therapy program. It may include proper body mechanics and positioning and exercises to strengthen the back. Clients should sleep on a firm mattress. Those with cervical injuries may need to wear a cervical collar or brace. Hot, moist compresses to the neck are useful to relieve muscle spasms. Most clients respond well to these conservative treatments.

Surgery

Surgery is necessary when conservative measures fail or there are serious neurologic deficits. The following surgical procedures may be used:

- *Diskectomy:* Removal of the herniated disk or disk fragments
- *Laminectomy:* Removal of the vertebral lamina to relieve pressure on the nerves. This is the most common surgical procedure. Nursing care is discussed in Box 30-13.

BOX 30-12
NURSING CARE CHECKLIST

CLIENTS UNDERGOING MYELOGRAPHY

☑ Check facility policy for client preparation.

Pretest Teaching

☑ Do not eat or drink for several hours before the test.
☑ You will be placed on a table that tilts so the dye can circulate in the spinal column.
☑ Dye is injected through a lumbar puncture. You may feel warmth or a burning sensation. Tell the physician if you feel pain.
☑ Stay in bed and follow the doctor's orders for position.
☑ Immediately report fever, stiff neck, or seizures.

Post-Test Nursing Care

☑ Monitor vital signs and assess neurologic status every 1 to 4 hours for 24 hours.
☑ Monitor lumbar puncture site for leakage of CSF or bleeding every 4 hours. Notify the physician of leakage or bleeding.
☑ Increase fluids to 2,400 to 3,000 mL in 24 hours. (This may reduce the headache.)
☑ Make sure that the client voids within 8 hours after the examination.
☑ Give analgesics and antiemetics as needed for pain, headache, or nausea.
☑ If water-soluble dye is used, elevate the client's head 45 degrees for 8 to 12 hours.

BOX 30-13
NURSING CARE CHECKLIST

CLIENTS HAVING A LAMINECTOMY
Before the Procedure

(See Chapter 7 for routine preoperative care.)
☑ Teach client logrolling technique.

After the Procedure

(See Chapter 7 for routine postoperative care.)
☑ After a cervical laminectomy:
  ☑ Place small pillow under the neck.
  ☑ Keep cervical collar in place.
☑ After a lumbar laminectomy:
  ☑ Keep the bed flat or elevate the head of the bed slightly.
  ☑ Place a small pillow under the head and a pillow under the knees.
☑ Logroll the client every 2 hours.
☑ Assess sensation and movement of arms and hands (cervical) and lower extremities and feet (lumbar). Report motor or sensory impairment immediately.
☑ Inspect dressing for drainage with halo sign; test for glucose.
☑ Palpate operative site for a hematoma. Maintain wound suction and patency of drains.
☑ For cervical laminectomy, assess for difficulty swallowing, hoarseness, increased swelling at neck, or labored breathing.

■ *Spinal fusion:* Insertion of bone graft (from iliac crest) between the vertebrae, which fuses the vertebra so they are more stable

■ *Chemonucleolysis:* Injection of the enzyme chymopapain into the nucleus pulposus to shrink or dissolve the protruding herniation

The surgical approach depends on the location and size of the ruptured disk. The posterior approach is used for lumbar surgery. An anterior or posterior approach is used for cervical disks.

After a successful surgery, the majority of clients are able to return to their jobs in about 6 weeks. They may experience a few small areas of permanent numbness in the involved leg.

NURSING CARE

Clients with a herniated disk experience pain and possibly reduced mobility. These problems can affect everyday life. Nursing care focuses on managing pain and preventing any further injury.

ASSESSING

The client is assessed for the degree to which a herniated intervertebral disk affects the client's daily life. Data can determine possible treatment options (Box 30-14).

DIAGNOSING, PLANNING, AND IMPLEMENTING

ACUTE PAIN

■ Maintain bed rest as prescribed. Teach to logroll when changing positions. *Restricting activity and proper positioning may prevent muscle spasms.*

■ Use a firm mattress or place a board under the mattress. *A firm bed supports the spinal column and muscles.*

■ Elevate the client's head and place a small pillow under the knees (for herniated lumbar disk) or under the neck (for herniated cervical disk). *Correct body positions can decrease intervertebral disk pressure.*

■ Give muscle relaxant and analgesic medications on a regular basis around the clock. *Giving the medications around the clock lessens periods of severe pain.*

■ Apply moist heat as ordered. *Moist heat increases blood flow and relaxes muscles.*

■ Do not refer to the client as an addict. *Clients with chronic pain develop a tolerance to pain medications and may require higher dosages.*

■ When chronic pain is unrelieved, refer to pain management clinic. *These clinics offer specialists in pain management techniques.*

BOX 30-14
ASSESSING CLIENTS WITH HERNIATED INTERVERTEBRAL DISK

SUBJECTIVE DATA
● Present health status:
  ● Pain radiating from hip to foot or neck to hand
  ● Muscle weakness or spasms
  ● Numbness and tingling of the leg, foot, or neck, shoulder, arm, or hand
  ● Neck stiffness
  ● Difficulty sleeping at night
● Past medical history:
  ● Falls, sudden straining of back, heavy lifting, or history of osteoarthritis
  ● History of myelogram

OBJECTIVE DATA
● Observe for abnormalities of the posture when standing.
● Assess ROM of affected extremity by asking client to perform straight-leg raises in the affected leg. Client feels pain when lifting the affected leg while dorsiflexing the foot. This indicates a lumbar injury.
● Assess level of muscle weakness in arm or leg.
● Assess location and type of pain, aggravating and relieving factors.
● Test patellar, Achilles, or tricep reflexes.
● Note changes in gait, for example, walking with a limp.

EVALUATING

To evaluate the effectiveness of nursing care for a client with a herniated disk, collect data related to absence of pain, muscle spasms, numbness, tingling, and neurological deficits.

Discharge Considerations

Preparing the client for care at home may involve teaching about pain control or follow-up after surgery. (Review Box 30-3 for guidelines.) Review medications and potential side effects. Teach the client and family about relaxation techniques. Listening to the client is important to determine the best methods for pain management. If needed, discuss referral to a pain management center with the physician.

The client is taught to maintain proper body positioning and body mechanics. The following are some of the guidelines to reinforce:

■ Sleep on a firm mattress or use a bedboard. Use a small pillow under the neck and sleep on the side with the knees flexed.

- Sit in straight-backed chairs.
- Avoid activities that flex the spine, such as bending or lifting, and do not twist the back.
- Follow the prescribed exercise program.
- Wear flat-heeled shoes that provide good support.
- Use proper body mechanics.

Following surgery, discuss incision site care and the symptoms of wound infection and healing. The client and family also need to understand the client's limitations. For example, driving is prohibited for the first 6 weeks. All activities that involve bending, twisting, and lifting are avoided. Clients should not lift more than 10 pounds. Review the use of a cervical collar, back brace, or corset. Reinforce indications for when to seek medical care.

Spinal Cord Tumor

Spinal cord tumors may be benign or malignant, primary or secondary. Primary tumors develop from a part of the cord. Secondary tumors start from lung, breast, or other cancer sites, then spread to the spinal cord. Spinal cord tumors are also classified as *intramedullary* (within the spinal cord) or *extramedullary* (outside the spinal cord). Most tumors occur in the thoracic and cervical areas.

Spinal cord tumors compress the cord, spinal nerve roots, and surrounding blood vessels. Manifestations relate to how fast or slow the tumor grows, the tumor site, and spinal nerve involvement. Slow-growing tumors allow the cord to adapt to the compression. Symptoms do not appear until the tumor is quite involved. Metastatic tumors usually grow quickly, causing symptoms to appear sooner.

Pain is often the first sign and is described as localized or radiating. Localized pain accompanies metastatic tumors involving the vertebrae. Radiating pain follows a path along the spinal nerve root. There is also motor and sensory deficits on one side of the body. Motor deficits include weakness and clumsiness; sensory deficits consist of numbness, tingling, and coldness in an extremity. Bladder involvement causes urinary frequency, urgency, and difficulty voiding.

The diagnosis of a spinal cord tumors begins with a history and neurologic exam. This is followed by a CT scan or MRI study to visualize the tumor. A lumbar puncture can identify the presence of tumor cells in the cerebrospinal fluid.

Spinal cord tumors are treated by surgical excision and radiation therapy. Surgery is most successful for extramedullary tumors. Intramedullay and metastatic tumors may be only partially removed due to their location or invasiveness of surrounding tissues. Surgery is followed with radiation therapy. Severe pain is managed by inserting an epidural catheter for continuous narcotic analgesic administration. Corticosteroids are given to control edema of the cord.

Assessments and nursing interventions are similar to those described for clients with an SCI or surgery for a herniated intervertebral disk. Care is different depending on whether the client has a benign or metastatic tumor. Discharge teaching includes how the family can provide physical care and manage pain (See Chapter 8 for cancer pain control methods.)

Nursing Interventions Classification

The following interventions by McCloskey and Bulechek (2000) may be appropriate for the client with degenerative neurologic and spinal cord disorders:

- Caregiver Support
- Respiratory Monitoring
- Urinary Incontinence Care
- Circulatory Care
- Family Support
- Sexual Counseling

(*Note:* The bibliography listings for this and all chapters have been compiled at the back of the book.)

Chapter Review

key terms by topic

Use the CD-ROM disk enclosed with your textbook to hear the pronunciation of the key terms in the chapter.

Degenerative neurologic disorders
Alzheimer's disease (AD), sundowning, multiple sclerosis (MS), demyelination, plasmapheresis, Parkinson's disease (PD),

dopamine, bradykinesia, myasthenia gravis, thymectomy, Huntington's disease (HD), chorea, amyotrophic lateral sclerosis (ALS), fasciculations, Guillain–Barré syndrome (GBS), trigeminal neuralgia, rhizotomy, Bell's palsy, rabies, tetanus, trismus, Creutzfeldt–Jakob disease (CJD)

Spinal cord disorders
paraplegia, tetraplegia, spinal shock, poikilothermia, autonomic dysreflexia, herniated intervetebral disk, sciatica, spinal cord tumor

key points

- Clients with advanced Alzheimer's disease must be monitored closely for disorientation and wandering to prevent injury.

- Multiple sclerosis is characterized by periods of exacerbation and remission with remissions occurring less often as the disease progresses.

- Early manifestations of Parkinson's disease are managed with the administration of levodopa medications.

- The client with myasthenia gravis and family are taught to identify the two life-threatening emergencies: myasthenic and cholinergic crisis.

- Clients with trigeminal neuralgia experience severe facial pain when their trigger zones are stimulated.

- Spinal cord injury at C4 or higher threatens the client's respiratory function. Report any symptoms of respiratory distress immediately to the physician.

- Clients with tetraplegia are at an increased risk for urinary tract infections and pneumonia. Any manifestation of these disorders should be treated immediately.

- Nursing care following a lumbar laminectomy focuses on logrolling the client every two hours until mobile. Immediately report any motor or sensory impairment.

Medialink

Additional interactive resources for this chapter can be found on the Companion Website at www.prenhall.com/burke. Click on Chapter 30 and "Begin" to select the activities for this chapter.

For NCLEX review questions and an audio glossary, access the accompanying CD-ROM in this book.

for further study

For the paired cranial nerves, see Chapter 29.

For care of a client with a tracheostomy, see Chapter 25.

For more information about mechanical ventilation, see Chapter 26.

For more about control of cancer pain, see Chapter 6.

Critical Thinking Care Map

Caring for the Client with Herniated Intervertebral Disk
NCLEX-PN Focus Area: Physiological Integrity

Case Study: A 50-year-old woman is thrown over the handlebars of her bicycle and sustains an intervertebral injury at C5 and C6. At the hospital a CT scan shows damaged ligaments and herniation of the C7 disk. She is sent home with a cervical collar to stabilize the area. Two weeks later she complains of insomnia, acute pain in her neck and shoulders, and numbness and tingling in her left hand. She is concerned about when she can return to work.

Nursing Diagnosis: Impaired Physical Mobility

COLLECT DATA

Subjective

_____

_____

_____

_____

_____

Objective

_____

_____

_____

_____

_____

Would you report this data? Yes/No

If yes, to: _____

Nursing Care

_____

_____

_____

_____

_____

_____

_____

_____

How would you document this? _____

_____

_____

Data Collected
(use those that apply)

• Insomnia
• Decreased ability to use left hand
• Pain in the neck and shoulders
• Concern about returning to work
• BP 110/78, P 68
• Complains of muscle weakness in left arm
• Unable to ride her bicycle at home
• Decreased reflexes in left arm

Nursing Interventions
(use those that apply)

• Consult with physical therapist for mobility plan.
• Increase fiber in the diet.
• Sleep on a firm mattress.
• Instruct her to keep the cervical collar on at all times.
• Give analgesics around the clock.
• Encourage six to eight glasses of water per day.
• Teach her to not lift objects or twist neck.

NCLEX-PN Exam Preparation

TEST-TAKING TIP

Be familiar with the relationship of functional abilities as they relate to specific levels of spinal cord injuries.

1. The nurse is caring for a client who has been hospitalized for evaluation of possible Alzheimer's disease. The client's symptoms include forgetfulness, difficulty making decisions, decreased ability to concentrate, and depression. The nurse knows that these are symptoms of:
   a. stage 1, early,
   b. stage 2, middle
   c. stage 3, late
   d. pre-Alzheimer's

2. The nurse is caring for a client with multiple sclerosis. Because urinary frequency is a manifestation of the disease, the nurse should expect which of the following medications to be prescribed?
   a. amantidine
   b. steroids
   c. dantrium
   d. pro-Banthine

3. When caring for the client with Parkinson's disease, it is important that the nurse:
   a. do everything for the client
   b. not assist the client
   c. not hurry the client
   d. encourage the client to do things quickly

4. The nurse is caring for a client who has sustained a spinal cord injury above the sixth thoracic vertebrae. Because the client is at risk for developing autonomic dysreflexia, the nurse should prevent the client from experiencing noxious stimuli such as:
   a. bladder distention
   b. a headache
   c. sneezing
   d. cold feet

5. If the client with a spinal cord injury above T6 does experience noxious stimuli, in addition to removing the noxious stimuli, the nurse should immediately place him in a:
   a. prone position
   b. supine position
   c. side-lying position
   d. semi-Fowler's position

6. In order to reduce the possibility of having the client experience autonomic dysreflexia, a nursing measure that can be implemented without a doctor's order includes:
   a. applying full-leg TED hose
   b. using pneumatic boots
   c. gradually lowering the lower extremities
   d. getting the client up quickly to ambulate

7. When caring for the client with a herniated lumbar disk, the nurse should:
   a. allow the client to remain in a comfortable position
   b. encourage the client to move as little as possible
   c. elevate the client's head and place a small pillow under the knees
   d. turn the client once a shift

8. The nurse is caring for a client with myasthenia gravis. When planning the client's care, the nurse knows that it is critical to:
   a. note any complaints by the client of changes in vision
   b. administer medications on a strict time schedule
   c. do the client's care quickly because they tire easily
   d. turn the client every 2 hours

9. When educating the client with trigeminal neuralgia who is taking Dilantin, it is important for the nurse to emphasize the need to:
   a. push fluids
   b. void frequently
   c. monitor caloric intake
   d. maintain good oral hygiene

10. The nurse is caring for a client who has just had a myelogram (water soluble dye was used). It is important for the nurse to encourage the client to:
    a. restrict fluids
    b. stay flat in bed for 8 to 12 hours
    c. drink plenty of fluids
    d. not eat for several hours

chapter

31

Caring for Clients with Eye and Ear Disorders

CARING tip

❝Work where there is a career ladder, so you have a motivator to achieve and set goals.❞

Rebecca Kelly, MSN, RN, CS • Coordinator, Practical Nursing • Greater Altoona Career and Technology Center • Altoona, Pennsylvania

LEARNING outcomes

After completing this chapter, you will be able to:

- Identify the major structures and functions of the eye and the ear.
- Describe changes in vision and hearing that occur with aging.
- Identify manifestations of eye and ear disorders.
- Describe the pathophysiology of common eye and ear disorders.
- Describe nursing implications for drugs prescribed for clients with eye and ear disorders.
- Provide safe nursing care for a client having eye or ear surgery.
- Use the nursing process to provide individualized care for clients with problems that affect vision or hearing.

MediaLink

 www.prenhall.com/burke

Use the above address to access the free, interactive Companion Website created for this textbook. Get hints, instant feedback, and textbook references to chapter-related multiple choice questions. Link to other interesting sites.

Vision and hearing are special senses that allow us to experience the world in which we live. The eyes allow us to see by providing a pathway for light, color and images to reach the brain. The ears allow us to hear by providing a pathway for sounds to reach the brain. The special senses warn us of danger and protect us from injury. In addition, specialized structures within the ear help maintain position sense and balance. Deficits in the special senses may limit self-care, mobility, independence, communication, and relationships with others.

Eye Structure, Function, and Disorders

The eyes are complex structures. The primary function of the eye is to convert patterns of light from the environment into a message that is transmitted via the optic nerve to the brain. The brain gives meaning to the message, allowing us to make sense of what we see.

The eye is protected and supported by the *accessory structures.* They include (Figure 31-1 ◆):

- The *eyelids* and *eyelashes,* which protect the eye, trap dirt and debris, regulate the amount of light entering the eye, and spread tears.
- The *conjunctiva,* a thin mucous membrane that covers the anterior surface of the eye and lines the inner surfaces of the eyelids.
- The *lacrimal apparatus,* which secretes and drains tears to cleanse and moisten the eye's surface. Tears are produced by the *lacrimal gland.* They contain an antibacterial enzyme that protects the eye from infections. Tears drain into the *lacrimal ducts* and from there into the nose.
- The *eye muscles* control eye movement and help maintain the shape of the eyeball.

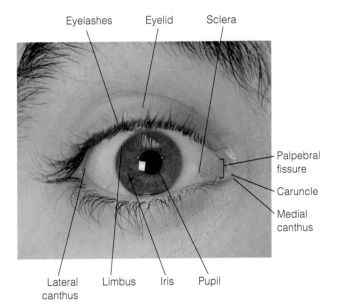

Eyelashes   Eyelid   Sclera

Palpebral fissure

Caruncle

Medial canthus

Lateral canthus   Limbus   Iris   Pupil

Figure 31-1. ◆ The external and accessory structures of the eye.

Each eye is a hollow sphere about 1 in. (2.5 cm) in diameter, surrounded and protected by bone and cushions of fat. The wall of the eyeball has three layers. The outermost layer consists of the white, fibrous *sclera,* and the transparent *cornea* (Figure 31-2 ◆). The sclera protects and gives shape to the eyeball. The border between the sclera and the cornea is called the *limbus* (see Figure 31-1). The cornea is a transparent window that allows light to enter the eye. It contains no blood vessels and is very sensitive to touch. When the cornea is touched, the eyelids blink (the *corneal reflex*) and tears are secreted.

The middle layer of the eyeball, the *uvea,* is very vascular. It includes the iris, the ciliary body, and the choroid. The *iris,* the colored part of the eye, regulates light entering the eye by controlling the size of the pupil. The *pupil* is the dark center of the eye through which light enters. The pupil constricts in bright light and dilates in dim light or darkness. The *ciliary body* encircles the lens. It controls the shape of the lens to focus light on the retina. The *lens* is a transparent structure behind the pupil that can change shape to focus light onto the retina. Like the cornea, the lens contains no blood vessels. The vascular *choroid* nourishes the other layers of the eyeball and absorbs light, preventing it from scattering within the eyeball.

The *retina* is the innermost lining of the eyeball. It contains millions of light receptors called rods and cones. *Rods* are very light sensitive and allow us to see in dim light. *Cones* allow us to see in color and provide a sharper image than rods. Most cones are located in the *macula,* the area where light passing through the pupil and lens focuses on the retina. The macula provides our central vision. In the center of the macula, the *fovea centralis* allows detailed color vision. The optic nerve enters the eye at the *optic disc.*

The hollow eyeball is divided into two interior cavities. The larger *posterior cavity* behind the lens contains the clear gelatinous *vitreous body.* The vitreous body shapes and supports the eye.

The *anterior cavity* is further divided into the *anterior chamber* (the space between the cornea and the iris) and the *posterior chamber* (the space between the iris and the lens). Aqueous humor, a clear fluid, circulates through the anterior cavity, nourishing the lens and cornea. Aqueous humor is constantly

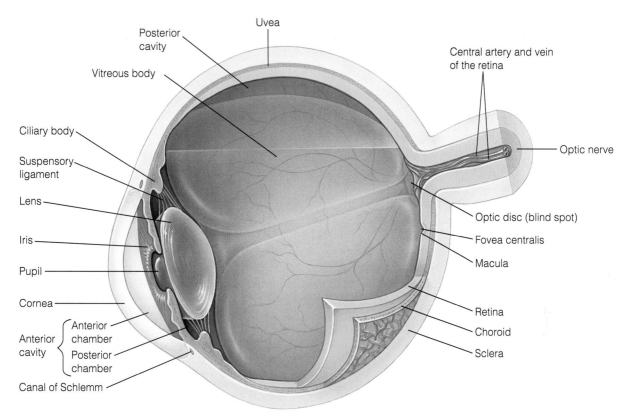

Figure 31-2. ◆ The internal structures of the eye.

formed and drained to maintain a relatively constant pressure within the eye. The drainage system for aqueous humor is the *canal of Schlemm,* a network of channels that circle the eye.

As light enters the eye, it is bent (or **refracted**), to focus on the retina. The cornea, aqueous humor, lens, and vitreous body bend light rays to focus the image. In order to change the point of focus from far to near, the lens changes shape, the pupil constricts, and the eyes converge. This is called *accommodation.*

The *optic nerves* are cranial nerves that meet at the *optic chiasma.* Here nerve fibers from the medial half of each retina cross to the opposite side to join nerve fibers from the lateral half of the other eye (Figure 31-3 ◆). The impulses generated in the retina travel to the *visual cortex* in the occipital lobe of the brain. The brain translates the impulses into the image we see, our *vision.*

The visual fields of each eye overlap considerably, and each eye sees a slightly different view. This allows *depth perception,* the ability to identify differences in distance between objects.

A number of changes in the eye and vision occur with aging. The lens becomes less elastic, affecting near vision. This is known as **presbyopia.** Clients with presbyopia may feel that their arms have become too short to read the newspaper comfortably.

Eyelid muscles may lose tone, causing the lower lid to turn out (*ectropion*) or the upper lid to droop (*ptosis,* Figure 31-4 ◆). The lid margin may turn inward (*entropion*), causing

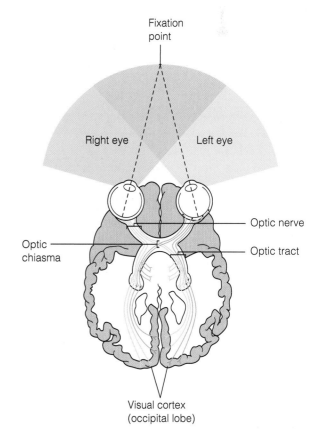

Figure 31-3. ◆ The visual fields of the eyes and the optic pathways.

Figure 31-4. ◆ Ptosis.

the lashes to irritate the eye. Tears are decreased, so the eyes may feel dry and scratchy. Other eye and vision changes commonly seen with aging are summarized in Table 31-1 ◆.

Infectious or Inflammatory Eye Disorders

The normally protective structures of the eye—the eyelids, eyelashes, and conjunctiva—may become inflamed or infected because they are constantly exposed to the environment.

DISORDERS AFFECTING THE EYELID

Blepharitis, inflammation of the eyelid, may be caused by an infection or by dermatitis. The eyelid is irritated and itchy. The eyelid margins are red, crusted, and scaly. A *hordeolum (sty)* is an infection of the sebaceous glands of the eyelid (Figure 31-5A ◆). A sty is red and painful. It may affect either

A

B

Figure 31-5. ◆ (A) Hordeolum (sty). (B) Chalazion.

the external or internal lid margin. *Chalazion* is a painless cyst or nodule of the eyelid (Figure 31-5B).

CONJUNCTIVITIS

Conjunctivitis (inflammation of the conjunctiva) is a common eye disease. It is usually caused by a bacterial or viral infection spread by direct contact (e.g., hands, tissues, towels). Acute conjunctivitis is usually mild, with redness, itching, tearing, and discharge of the eye (Figure 31-6 ◆).

Some infections, such as gonorrhea and trachoma, can damage the cornea, threatening vision. *Trachoma* is a major cause of blindness in parts of Africa, the Middle East, and Asia.

TABLE 31-1	AGE-RELATED CHANGES IN THE EYE AND VISION	

CHANGE	EFFECT ON VISION
Decreased corneal sensation and tear secretion	Increased risk of damage due to foreign body or trauma; increased risk of infection
Constriction of the pupil	Reduced light entering the eye; difficulty with night vision
Decreased elasticity and increased density of the lens	Difficulty focusing, especially for near vision Increased problems with glare Decreased color perception (especially blues, greens, and violet)
Loss of rods at periphery of retina	Decreased peripheral vision
Loss of fat and subcutaneous tissue around the eyes	Eyes appear sunken; decreased peripheral vision

Figure 31-6. ◆ An eye with acute conjunctivitis.

DISORDERS AFFECTING THE CORNEA

The clear cornea transmits and helps focus light and images onto the retina. It also protects the internal eye. The cornea has no blood supply. Scarring or ulceration of the cornea can lead to blindness.

Keratitis is inflammation of the cornea, usually caused by infection, lack of tears, or trauma. **Corneal ulcers** (Figure 31-7 ◆) may be caused by infection, trauma, or contact lens overuse. Herpes viruses such as herpes zoster (shingles) can cause corneal ulcers. Corneal ulcers may be superficial or deep. Scarring may occur, clouding the cornea. If the cornea is perforated, infection of the internal eye and vision loss may result.

Inflammation of the cornea causes discomfort, tearing, discharge, and **photophobia** (extreme sensitivity to light). *Blepharospasm* (spasm of the eyelid and inability to open the eye) may develop. Sudden, severe eye pain may indicate corneal perforation.

UVEITIS AND IRITIS

Uveitis is inflammation of the middle vascular layer of the eye. *Iritis* (inflammation of the iris only) is more common. The client complains of severe eye pain, photophobia, and blurred vision. The pupil is constricted, and the limbus (where the cornea meets the conjunctiva) is red.

COLLABORATIVE CARE

Prompt treatment of infectious or inflammatory eye disorders is important to preserve vision. Corneal ulcers are medical emergencies that must be referred to an ophthalmologist promptly for treatment.

Most of these disorders can be diagnosed by the history and examination of the eye. Usually, no diagnostic tests are required, although the following tests may be ordered:

■ *Fluorescein stain with slit lamp examination* will show corneal ulcers or abrasions, which appear green with staining.
■ *Conjunctival or ulcer scrapings* may be examined or cultured.

Pharmacology

Topical anti-infectives applied as eye drops or ointment often are ordered to treat eye infections. Antihistamines or corticosteroids may be prescribed when the eye is inflamed but no infection is present. Clients with uveitis may be given eyedrops to keep the pupil dilated and reduce discomfort.

Other Treatments

Eye irrigation may be ordered to remove purulent discharge associated with conjunctivitis. Local heat may be recommended for hordeolum or chalazion.

Corneal Transplant

When the cornea is scarred and opaque (see Figure 31-7), a corneal transplant can restore vision. Corneas may be taken from people who died as a result of acute trauma or a noninfectious illness. The client's scarred cornea is removed, and the graft is sutured in place. The sutures remain in place for up to a year. The eye is patched for 24 hours after surgery. The client must avoid activities that can increase intraocular pressure, such as straining to have a bowel movement, bending over, and lifting or pushing heavy objects. Eyedrops are ordered to reduce inflammation and prevent infection. Nursing care of the client undergoing eye surgery is discussed later in this chapter (see Box 31-2).

NURSING CARE

ASSESSING

Ask the client to describe the symptoms, their onset, and any relationship between the symptoms and an injury or exposure to an infection or allergen. Inquire about the effect on vision and any associated symptoms, such as chills or fever. Identify the date of the client's most recent eye examination. Ask about corrective lens use, including type of lenses. Obtain past medical history, especially any chronic diseases, previous eye problems, and current medication use.

Test vision (with client wearing corrective lenses if normally worn) using a Snellen chart (see Chapter 4, Figure 4-5) or Rosenbaum chart. The Rosenbaum chart (Figure 31-8 ◆) is held 12 to 14 inches from the eyes, with vision assessed in the same manner as with the Snellen chart. Inspect the eye, including the conjunctiva, lids, and surrounding tissues. Check pupil size and response to light and accommodation.

DIAGNOSING, PLANNING, AND IMPLEMENTING

The priority nursing diagnoses for clients with infectious and inflammatory eye disorders focus on the risk for impaired vision, pain, and risk for injury.

RISK FOR DISTURBED SENSORY PERCEPTION: VISUAL

■ Instruct to wash the hands thoroughly before inserting or removing contact lenses or instilling any eye medications. Teach to avoid touching or rubbing the eyes. *Handwashing*

Figure 31-7. ◆ Corneal ulcers.

Figure 31-8. ◆ Testing vision using a Rosenbaum eye chart.

is the single most important measure to prevent transmission of infection to the eye.

■ Emphasize the importance of proper contact lens care, including periodic lens removal and cleaning. *Improper cleaning and wearing contact lenses longer than recommended are major risk factors for infection and corneal damage.*

■ If the cornea perforates, place the client in the supine position, close the eye, and cover it with a dry, sterile dressing. Notify the physician immediately. *Corneal perforation can lead to loss of eye contents.*

PAIN

■ Administer analgesics routinely in the first 12 to 24 hours after corneal surgery. *The outer portion of the eye, the cornea in particular, is extremely sensitive. Giving analgesics on a schedule prevents pain from becoming severe.*

■ Patch both eyes if necessary. *Patching both eyes reduces eye movement and irritation of the affected eye.*

■ Teach the client to apply warm compresses for 15 minutes, three to four times a day. *Warm compresses reduce inflammation and promote comfort.*

■ Instruct to use dark sunglasses with ultraviolet (UV) protection when out of doors, even on cloudy days. *Bright light can cause eye pain in clients with an inflammation or infection.*

■ Advise to avoid excessive reading or other close tasks. *Eye rest also promotes comfort.*

RISK FOR INJURY

■ Discuss the effect of an eye patch on depth perception and peripheral vision. Teach the client to scan from side to side, and to be careful when judging distances or speed. *Patching one eye affects depth perception, increasing the risk for falling, traffic accidents, or other trauma.*

■ Instruct not to rub or scratch the eye. *Rubbing or scratching may spread infection or damage a corneal graft.*

■ Teach how to apply an eye shield at night. *An eye shield helps prevent inadvertent rubbing or trauma of the eye during sleep.*

■ Teach clients to use eye protection during activities that can damage the eye. *Trauma increases the risk of infection and scarring of the cornea.*

EVALUATING

Collect the following data to evaluate the effectiveness of nursing care:

■ Appearance of the eye
■ Vision (using a chart to measure visual acuity)
■ Demonstrates proper contact lens care
■ Demonstrates instillation of eye drops using appropriate technique

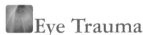

Discharge Considerations

Teach all clients about handwashing and proper eye care. Instruct clients to use a new, clean cotton-tipped swab or cotton ball for each eye when cleansing eyelids. Teach how to instill eye drops and ointments. If an eye patch is ordered, be sure the client or a family member knows how to apply it and where to obtain necessary supplies.

Teach contact lens users how to care for and clean the lenses. Stress the importance of periodically removing lenses, even extended-wear lenses. In general, lenses should be removed at night. Advise the client who has a corneal abrasion or keratitis to avoid wearing contact lenses until the cornea has healed completely.

Stress the importance of follow-up appointments after a corneal transplant. Reinforce teaching about how to prevent increased intraocular pressure (e.g., avoiding straining, vomiting, coughing, and lifting). Instruct the client and family to promptly report inflammation, graft cloudiness, or increased pain to the physician.

Eye Trauma

Any part of the eye, especially the exposed parts, can be affected by trauma. Foreign bodies, abrasions, and lacerations are the most common types of eye injury.

A *corneal abrasion* is a "scratch" of the cornea. Contact lenses, eyelashes, small foreign bodies, and fingernails often cause corneal abrasions. Corneal abrasions are extremely painful, causing photophobia and tearing. They usually heal rapidly without scarring.

Burns can affect the outer portion of the eye. Chemicals such as ammonia, oven and drain cleaners, and acids from car batteries commonly burn the eye. Thermal burns often occur in an explosion. UV light also can burn the eye (snowblindness or welder's-arc burn). A burn causes pain and affects vision. Eyelids are swollen and the conjunctiva is red and edematous; it may slough. The cornea often appears cloudy or hazy.

The eye may be *perforated* by metal flakes produced by high-speed drilling or grinding, glass shards, or weapons such as gunshots (including BBs), arrows, and knives. The layers of the eye can close after being penetrated by a small or sharp object. In these cases, the injury may not be apparent. Eye perforations cause pain, partial or complete loss of vision, and possibly bleeding or loss of eye contents.

Blunt eye trauma is often caused by sports injuries. The injury may be minor, such as lid *ecchymosis* (black eye) or *subconjunctival hemorrhage,* bleeding into the conjunctiva. These minor injuries typically do not need to be treated. *Hyphema,* bleeding into the anterior chamber of the eye, causes a reddish tint to the client's vision and visible blood in the anterior chamber. The eye orbit may be fractured by blunt trauma. The client experiences **diplopia** (double vision) and pain with eye movement. The eye appears sunken *(enophthalmos).*

COLLABORATIVE CARE

The extent of injury caused by trauma is determined by eye exam. Unless immediate treatment is required, as with a chemical burn, vision is evaluated with corrective lenses if normally worn. Eye movement is evaluated unless a penetrating object is present (Box 31-1). The lid and conjunctiva are inspected for foreign objects and lacerations. A topical anesthetic may be used to relieve eye pain and photophobia prior to inspection. *Fluorescein staining* can help identify the presence of foreign bodies and abrasions. *Ophthalmoscopic examination* is done to detect bleeding or trauma to the interior chamber.

BOX 31-1
ASSESSING CLIENTS:
THE CARDINAL FIELDS OF VISION

Eye movement is assessed using the *six cardinal fields of vision.* Ask the client to follow a pen or your finger while keeping the head still. Move the pen or your finger through the six fields one at a time, returning to the central starting point and pausing before proceeding to the next field (see figure). The eyes should move through each field without involuntary movements.

1 Penlight is to nurse's extreme left.   4 Penlight is to nurse's extreme right.

2 Penlight is left and up.   5 Penlight is right and up.

3 Penlight is left and down.   6 Penlight is right and down.

Six Cardinal Fields of Vision

Facial x-rays and computed tomography (CT) scans are used to identify orbital fractures or the presence of foreign bodies within the globe.

The eye is irrigated with sterile saline to remove small foreign bodies. Copious amounts of fluid are used to flush the eye when a chemical burn occurs. A special contact lens irrigating unit or a bottle of irrigant with intravenous tubing held to flush all eye surfaces may be used. During irrigation, fluid is directed from the inner canthus of the eye to the outer. The client's head is tipped slightly to the affected side to prevent contamination of the other eye. A sterile moistened cotton-tipped applicator or other instrument may be used to remove a foreign body. After the procedure, a topical antibiotic ointment is applied. An eye patch may be applied to keep the eye closed for approximately 24 hours.

Penetrating wounds usually require surgery. Narcotic analgesics, sedatives, and antiemetic drugs are given to relieve pain and anxiety and prevent vomiting (which increases intraocular pressure).

NURSING CARE

Nursing care for clients with eye trauma focuses on protecting the eye and preserving vision.

IMPAIRED TISSUE INTEGRITY: OCULAR

- Assess and record vision in each eye and both eyes, with and without corrective lenses. *The initial assessment provides a baseline and data about the effect of the injury on the client's vision.*
- Assess eye(s) and surrounding tissues for foreign bodies, burns, penetrating injury, or blunt trauma. *Eye trauma may be hidden by other injuries.*
- Immediately irrigate the eye if a chemical burn is suspected. *Irrigation to remove the chemical is of higher priority than assessment of the eye.*
- Remove loose foreign bodies using a moist, sterile, cotton-tipped applicator. *Prompt removal of foreign bodies may prevent corneal abrasion.*
- For a severe or penetrating injury, place the client on bed rest and stabilize the injured eye by applying an eye pad or gauze dressing loosely over both eyes. Stabilize any penetrating object if possible. *These measures reduce eye movement and can help preserve vision.*
- Following treatment, apply eye drops or ointment and an eye pad or shield as ordered. *An eye pad is often applied to the affected eye to reduce pain and photophobia and to promote healing.*

Discharge Considerations

Teaching people how to prevent eye injuries is an important nursing responsibility. Teach employees and people participating in high-risk sports and activities how and when to use eye protectors. Stress the importance of using seat belts and air bags to prevent eye injury in car crashes. Teach clients to immediately flush the eye with copious amounts of water if a chemical splash occurs. Loose, visible foreign bodies can be removed using a clean, moistened cotton-tipped swab. If an abrasion or penetrating or blunt injury is suspected, loosely cover the eye with sterile gauze and immediately seek medical attention. Instruct clients not to remove objects that penetrate the eye.

Following an injury, reinforce teaching about follow-up treatment. Discuss the ordered medications, including how to instill eyedrops and ointments. Stress the need to avoid rubbing or scratching the eye. Teach the client or family how to apply the eye pad or shield if ordered. If ordered, instruct the client to avoid activities that increase intraocular pressure, such as lifting, straining, or bending over to prevent further eye damage.

Refractive Errors

Changes in the shape of the cornea, lens, or the eyeball affect the focus of light on the retina. The result is blurred or indistinct vision. These *refractive errors* or defects are the most common cause of impaired vision. Common refractive errors include *myopia* (nearsightedness), *hyperopia* (farsightedness), and *astigmatism.* The causes and effects of these errors are summarized in Table 31-2 ◆.

Refractive errors often are detected through routine vision screening. The refractive error can usually be corrected with eyeglasses or contact lenses.

Several surgical procedures have been developed to correct refractive errors. *Radial keratotomy* uses a series of shallow

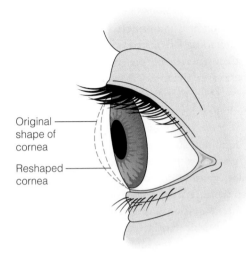

Original shape of cornea

Reshaped cornea

Figure 31-9. ◆ LASIK surgery corrects refractive error by flattening the cornea of the eye.

radial incisions in the cornea to flatten it. In a *photorefractive keratectomy (PRK),* a very thin layer of corneal tissue is shaved to reshape the cornea. *Laser in situ keratomileusis (LASIK)* is similar. A thin flap of the cornea is lifted, then the center of the cornea is shaved to flatten it (Figure 31-9 ◆). The flap is then replaced; it is held in place by the eye's natural stickiness. These surgeries require only minutes to complete and are done on an outpatient basis.

Nurses can help identify clients with refractive disorders and encourage them to seek treatment. Check the vision of clients who have difficulty reading printed material, identifying objects, or following visual directions using a standard eye chart. First test each eye, then test vision using both eyes (see

TABLE 31-2	COMMON REFRACTIVE ERRORS		
PROBLEM	**CAUSE**	**EFFECT**	**CORRECTION**
Myopia (nearsightedness)	Abnormally long eyeball	Light rays focus in front of the retina Distant objects are unclear Focus improves as object is closer to the eye	Concave corrective lenses Radial keratotomy Photoreceptive keratectomy (PRK) Laser in situ keratomileusis (LASIK)
Hyperopia (farsightedness)	Abnormally short eyeball	Light rays focus behind the retina Close objects are unclear Able to focus on distant objects through accommodation	Convex corrective lenses Laser thermakeratoplasty
Presbyopia	Impaired accommodation of the lens caused by aging		
Astigmatism	Irregularities in the curvature of the cornea and lens	Light rays are imperfectly focused on the retina	Requires correction only when refractive error affects vision

Chapter 4). Refer clients whose vision is poorer than 20/40 in either or both eyes to an optometrist or ophthalmologist for further evaluation. In addition to the obvious nursing diagnosis of Disturbed Sensory Perception, the following nursing diagnoses may be appropriate:

- Risk for Injury related to inability to clearly see traffic signs and directions
- Risk for Noncompliance related to financial or cosmetic concerns

Discuss the effect of eyeglasses on depth perception, and advise the client to be careful on stairs until he or she is used to the lenses. If contact lenses have been prescribed, teach and have the client demonstrate how to insert, remove, and care for them. Emphasize the importance of proper care to prevent eye infections or corneal abrasion. For clients who have had surgical correction of their vision, provide verbal and written instructions about postoperative care and follow-up. Teach the client and significant other how to instill prescribed eyedrops.

Cataracts

A **cataract** is clouding of the lens of the eye that impairs vision. Cataracts are common. Most people over age 65 have some cataract. The cataract affects vision in only a few of these people, however.

PATHOPHYSIOLOGY

Most cataracts are *senile cataracts,* caused by aging. As the lens ages, its cells become less clear. This usually first affects the edges of the lens, gradually spreading toward the center. Eventually, the entire lens may be clouded. When only a portion of the lens is affected, the cataract is called *immature.* A *mature cataract* involves the entire lens. Cataracts usually affect both eyes, but tend to develop at different rates. Risk factors for cataracts include exposure to sunlight (UV-B rays), cigarette smoking, heavy alcohol consumption, congenital conditions, eye trauma, diabetes mellitus, and drugs such as corticosteroids and chlorpromazine (Thorazine).

As a cataract matures, both near and distance vision are affected. Details become obscured. The clouded lens scatters light rays, causing problems with glare and difficulty adjusting between light and dark environments. With a mature cataract, the pupil appears cloudy gray or white rather than black.

COLLABORATIVE CARE

The diagnosis of a cataract is made based on the history and eye examination. As the cataract matures, the *red reflex* is lost. The location and extent of a cataract can be seen with ophthalmoscopic examination. No special diagnostic or laboratory procedures are required.

Cataracts are treated by surgical removal. This is an elective surgery, usually delayed until the cataract interferes with the client's activities of daily living and enjoyment of life.

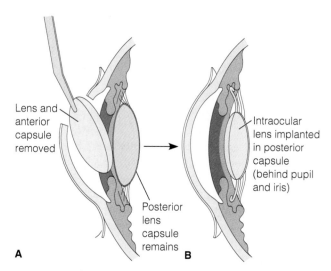

Figure 31-10. ◆ Cataract removal with intraocular lens implant. (A) The lens and anterior capsule are removed. (B) The intraocular lens is implanted within the posterior capsule behind the pupil.

Cataract surgery is usually done on an outpatient basis, using local anesthesia. The clouded lens is removed through a small incision in the cornea (Figure 31-10 ◆). An *intraocular lens* is implanted during the surgery to focus light and restore clear vision.

NURSING CARE

Nursing care for clients with cataracts focuses on teaching/learning needs in both the pre- and postoperative periods. Cataract surgery is usually done as an outpatient procedure, and the client is often discharged within 1 hour after surgery. Box 31-2 outlines nursing care of the client having eye surgery.

DEFICIENT KNOWLEDGE: CATARACTS

- Provide information about cataracts and their surgical removal. Explain that cataracts usually are removed only when they interfere with vision and activities of daily living (ADLs). *This helps the client decide about surgery.*
- Demonstrate a caring, understanding attitude toward concerns about vision. *Accepting the client's fears promotes trust and reduces anxiety.*

Discharge Considerations

Clients usually are discharged home within hours after cataract surgery. Provide verbal and written instructions about postoperative care and directions for follow-up appointments. Include a family member in the teaching. Teach the client and family how and when to instill the prescribed eyedrops. Instruct the client to avoid reading, lifting or strenuous activ-

BOX 31-2
NURSING CARE CHECKLIST

EYE SURGERY

Before Surgery

☑ Provide routine preoperative care as indicated (see Chapter 7).

☑ Assess understanding of the procedure. Clarify information as needed.

☑ Orient to the environment.

☑ Assess vision in the unaffected eye before surgery.

☑ Reinforce teaching about postoperative restrictions to prevent increased intraocular pressure: Avoid vomiting, straining at stool, coughing, sneezing, lifting more than 5 lbs., and bending over at the waist.

☑ Remove all eye makeup and contact lenses or glasses. Store them in a safe place.

☑ Administer preoperative medications and eyedrops or ointments as ordered.

After Surgery

☑ Assess and document vital signs, level of consciousness, comfort, and status of the eye dressing.

☑ Maintain the eye patch and shield as ordered.

☑ Place in semi-Fowler's or Fowler's position or as ordered.

☑ Approach client on unaffected side.

☑ Intervene as necessary to prevent vomiting, coughing, sneezing, or straining.

☑ Immediately report sudden, sharp eye pain to the physician.

☑ Place all personal articles and call bell within easy reach.

☑ Assist with ambulation when allowed.

☑ Administer eyedrops and other medications as ordered.

☑ Teach the client and family:

   a. How to instill eyedrops and about ordered medications

   b. How and when to apply eye patch and eye shield

   c. To avoid scratching, rubbing, touching, or squeezing the affected eye

   d. How to prevent constipation and straining, and about activity limitations

   e. Symptoms that should be reported to the physician, including eye pain or pressure, redness or cloudiness, drainage, decreased vision, floaters or flashes of light, or halos around bright objects

   f. To wear sunglasses with side shields when outdoors

   g. To make and keep recommended follow-up appointments

☑ Arrange or refer the client for assistance with other health care needs (such as insulin injections) as needed following discharge.

ity, to leave the eye dressing in place, and take prescribed medications during the initial 24-hour period. During the return visit, reinforce teaching about activity limitations to prevent increased intraocular pressure, protecting the operative eye, and symptoms of complications. Instruct to report eye pain, worsening of vision, headache, nausea, or itching and redness of the affected eye to the physician.

Glaucoma

Glaucoma is characterized by increased intraocular pressure and gradual loss of vision. It is a "silent" thief of vision: Peripheral vision is lost so slowly that it often is not noticed until late in the disease. This vision loss is permanent. Glaucoma is a leading cause of blindness worldwide.

PATHOPHYSIOLOGY

Aqueous humor fills the space between the lens and the cornea. It is produced by the ciliary body and flows through the pupil into the anterior chamber. From there, it drains through the trabecular mesh into the canal of Schlemm. The normal intraocular pressure of 12 to 20 mm Hg is maintained by a balance between aqueous humor production and drainage. When this balance is disrupted, intraocular pressure increases.

In *chronic simple glaucoma,* aqueous humor drainage through the trabecular meshwork is obstructed (Figure 31-11 ◆). The amount of fluid in the eye increases. As a result, intraocular pressure increases. The increased pressure damages retinal neurons and the optic nerve. Peripheral vision is gradually lost and the visual field narrows (Figure 31-12 ◆). Both eyes are usually affected. Untreated glaucoma eventually leads to blindness.

In *acute glaucoma,* the angle between the cornea and iris closes, completely blocking drainage of aqueous humor from the eye (see Figure 31-11B). Intraocular pressure rises abruptly, damaging the retina and the optic nerve. Box 31-3 lists the manifestations of chronic and acute glaucoma.

CLINICAL alert

Acute glaucoma is a medical emergency. Without prompt treatment, the affected eye will become blind. Immediately report manifestations of acute glaucoma to the charge nurse or physician.

Acute glaucoma usually affects one eye. Episodes often occur when the pupil dilates (in darkness or with emotional upset), closing the angle. Acute glaucoma can recur, therefore it is *vital* to avoid medications that can dilate the pupil.

COLLABORATIVE CARE

Although glaucoma cannot be cured, it can be controlled and vision preserved if it is diagnosed early. Routine eye examinations are recommended for early detection.

Diagnostic Tests

■ *Tonometry* is done to measure the intraocular pressure. Tonometry screening is recommended for all people over

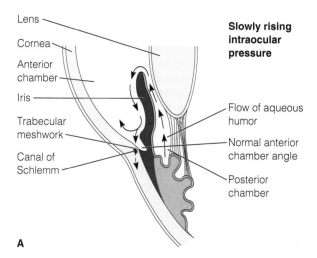

Slowly rising intraocular pressure

Lens

Cornea

Anterior chamber

Iris

Trabecular meshwork

Canal of Schlemm

Flow of aqueous humor

Normal anterior chamber angle

Posterior chamber

A

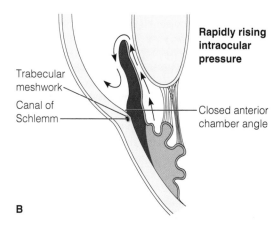

Rapidly rising intraocular pressure

Trabecular meshwork

Canal of Schlemm

Closed anterior chamber angle

B

Figure 31-11. ◆ Types of glaucoma. (A) Chronic simple glaucoma. Drainage of aqueous humor through the trabecular meshwork is impaired. (B) Acute glaucoma. The angle between the cornea and iris closes, completely blocking aqueous humor drainage.

the age of 60 (Box 31-4). The intraocular pressure is measured using a Schiøtz tonometer (Figure 31-13 ◆) or other tonometry instrument.

■ The angle of the anterior chamber of the eye is assessed with *gonioscopy.* The gonioscope measures the depth of the

Figure 31-12. ◆ Narrowing of the visual field with glaucoma. *(Courtesy National Eye Institute, National Institutes of Health.)*

BOX 31-3 MANIFESTATIONS OF GLAUCOMA

CHRONIC SIMPLE GLAUCOMA

• Painless
• Gradual loss of peripheral vision
• Difficulty adapting from light to dark
• Blurred vision
• Halos around lights
• Difficulty focusing on near objects

ACUTE GLAUCOMA

• Acute severe eye pain
• Blurred or cloudy vision
• Nausea and vomiting
• Halos around lights
• Affected eye red, cornea clouded
• Fixed (nonreactive) pupil

anterior chamber, and helps differentiate between chronic simple and acute glaucoma.

■ *Visual field testing* is used to identify loss of peripheral vision. The visual field is the entire area seen by the eye when focused on a central point.

Pharmacology

Drugs often are used to reduce intraocular pressure and preserve vision. They usually are administered as eyedrops. Several classes or groups of drugs are used, including drugs that affect pupil size or the production of aqueous humor. Table 31-3 ◆ outlines commonly used drugs and their nursing implications.

In acute glaucoma, diuretics may be given intravenously to lower intraocular pressure rapidly. Acetazolamide, a carbonic anhydrase inhibitor, and osmotic diuretics, such as mannitol, are used. Fast-acting miotic drops are also used to constrict the pupil and help open the angle.

Surgery

Surgery may be done to lower intraocular pressure in glaucoma. Laser surgery is used to open drainage into the canal of

population
FOCUS

BOX 31-4

Glaucoma

• Chronic simple glaucoma occurs more frequently and at an earlier age in African Americans. African Americans and people with a family history of glaucoma should be screened every 2 years over the age of 40.
• Acute glaucoma occurs more frequently in older adults and in people of Asian ancestry.

Figure 31-13. ◆ The Schiøtz tonometer for measuring intraocular pressure.

Schlemm by burning holes into the trabecular meshwork. A laser also may be used to destroy a portion of the ciliary body, reducing aqueous humor production. For acute glaucoma, the laser can be used to make a hole at the outside edge of the

iris. This allows aqueous humor to reach the canal of Schlemm.

NURSING CARE

ASSESSING

Nursing assessment related to glaucoma focuses on identifying clients at risk. Ask about vision, including recent changes, difficulty seeing at night, and halos around lights. Inquire about a family history of glaucoma or any previous episodes of acute glaucoma, and the date of the most recent eye examination.

Inspect the eye for possible redness or clouding of the cornea. Assess vision (with corrective lenses if worn) using a standard eye chart. Assess pupil response to light (see Chapter 4). Evaluate peripheral vision (Box 31-5).

DIAGNOSING, PLANNING, AND IMPLEMENTING

IMPAIRED HEALTH MAINTENANCE

The client with glaucoma may have other chronic conditions affecting the ability to manage the glaucoma. Reduced vision

---

TABLE 31-3

NURSING IMPLICATIONS FOR PHARMACOLOGY: CLIENTS WITH GLAUCOMA

DRUG/CLASS	DESCRIPTION	NURSING RESPONSIBILITIES	CLIENT AND FAMILY TEACHING

Miotic
■ Pilocarpine (Isopto Carpine, Ocusert-Pilo)
	Miotic drugs constrict the pupil and contract the ciliary muscle. This stretches and opens the trabecular meshwork, promoting aqueous humor drainage and reducing intraocular pressure. Pilocarpine is the most widely used of these drugs.	Report contraindications such as asthma, peptic ulcer disease, or urinary retention.
		After instilling drops, gently squeeze bridge of nose for 1–2 minutes to increase local effect and reduce systemic absorption.
		When using the Ocusert system:
		  a. Apply at bedtime.
		  b. Place Ocusert-Pilo in the conjunctival sac under the upper lid.
		  c. Report conjunctival irritation that does not clear within several days of use.
		  d. Remove and replace weekly.
		  e. Report side effects such as tearing, brow pain, and headache.
			To administer eyedrops:
			  a. Wash your hands.
			  b. Do not touch dropper.
			  c. Squeeze bridge of nose and keep eye closed for 1 minute after using drops.
			If using the Ocusert system, follow procedure at left.
			Avoid drugs such as over-the-counter cold and sleep medications.
			Vision may initially be blurred; this will clear.
			Night vision will be affected; use night lights in halls and baths, and avoid night driving.
			Report abdominal pain, wheezing, difficulty breathing, sweating, or flushing to your doctor.

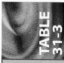

DRUG/CLASS	DESCRIPTION	NURSING RESPONSIBILITIES	CLIENT AND FAMILY TEACHING
Sympathomimetic ■ Epinephrine (Epitrate, Mytrate/Epifrin) ■ Dipivefrin (Propine) ■ Apraclonidine (Iopidine) ■ Brimonidine (Alphagan)	Sympathomimetic drugs reduce intraocular pressure by reducing aqueous humor production and increasing its absorption.	Monitor vital signs. Report adverse reactions such as acute glaucoma, hypertension, an irregular pulse, or chest pain. Report side effects such as anxiety, nervousness, and muscle tremors. Report itching, lid edema, and discharge from the eyes.	Report any change in vision or eye pain. Eye pain may indicate acute glaucoma; contact your doctor immediately. Avoid over-the-counter sinus and cold medications that may increase the risk of adverse effects of this drug.
Beta Blockers ■ Betaxolol (Betoptic) ■ Carteolol (Cartrol, Ocupress) ■ Levobunolol (Betagan) ■ Metipranolol (Opti-Pranolol) ■ Timolol (Timoptic)	Beta blockers are used to reduce intraocular pressure by reducing the production of aqueous humor in the ciliary body. Beta blockers do not affect vision like miotics and sympathomimetic drugs, and have a longer duration of action, allowing twice-a-day dosing.	Report contraindications such as asthma, chronic obstructive pulmonary disease (COPD), heart block, and heart failure. Hold pressure over bridge of nose after instilling drops to prevent systemic absorption. Report side effects such as bradycardia, hypotension, wheezing, and difficulty breathing.	Press on bridge of nose for 1 minute after instilling drops to keep the drug from entering your blood. Your vision may be blurred initially but will improve. Report worsening vision, difficulty breathing, reduced exercise tolerance, and sweating or flushing to your doctor.
Prostaglandin Analog ■ Latanoprost (Xalatan)	Latanoprost reduces intraocular pressure by improving the outflow of aqueous humor from the anterior chamber.	Administer once daily at bedtime. Report side effects such as burning, stinging, or redness of the eye.	Instill drops at bedtime, as your vision may be blurred after using the drops. The iris of your eye may darken while using this drug. This is not harmful. Report eye discomfort or redness to your doctor.
Carbonic Anhydrase Inhibitors ■ Acetazolamide (Diamox) ■ Dorzolamide (Trusopt)	Carbonic anhydrase inhibitors reduce aqueous humor production, lowering intraocular pressure. Intravenous acetazolamide is used to rapidly reduce intraocular pressure in acute glaucoma.	Topical ■ Squeeze the bridge of nose for 1–2 minutes after instilling the drug. ■ Report adverse or allergic effects, such as conjunctivitis or redness and itching of the lid. Systemic ■ Monitor fluid and electrolyte balance, daily weight, intake and output, and laboratory values. ■ Report laboratory value changes (electrolytes, renal and liver function tests) to the physician.	Topical ■ You may have eye stinging and a bitter taste in your mouth immediately after using the drops. ■ If your eye or lid become red, puffy, or itchy, stop using the drug and notify your physician. Systemic ■ Drink 2–3 quarts of fluid daily. ■ Change positions slowly because you may become dizzy on standing. ■ Notify your doctor of fever, sore throat, easy bleeding or bruising, numbness and tingling, tremors, flank pain, or a skin rash.

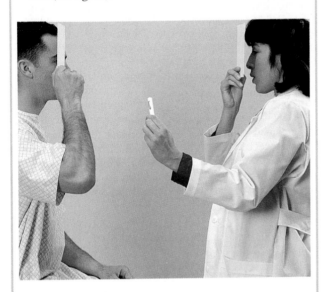

BOX 31-5
ASSESSING VISUAL FIELDS BY CONFRONTATION

- Face the client, seated about 2 feet apart.
- Instruct the client to cover the right eye and focus on your face.
- Cover your left eye, and focus on the client's face.
- Midway between the client and yourself, bring a light-colored object into the field of vision from the side (see figure).

- Ask the client to indicate when the object is seen.
- Check all visual fields of both eyes in this manner.

caused by the glaucoma can affect the ability to manage other conditions such as diabetes.

- Provide detailed verbal and written instructions about the ordered drugs. *Written instructions reinforce teaching and are a resource for the client.*
- Teach how to instill eyedrops, and have the client show you that he or she can do so. *Impaired vision, manual dexterity, or mobility may interfere with the ability to get drops into the eye. In some cases, a family member may need to do this for the client.*
- If taking other medications, ensure that the client can identify each and can take the appropriate dose if the drug is in injectable or liquid form. *Impaired vision and coexisting chronic diseases may make it difficult for the client to read medication labels, draw up or pour an accurate dose.*
- Emphasize the importance of keeping all follow-up appointments to monitor intraocular pressure and vision. *Inadequate treatment can allow vision loss to continue.*

RISK FOR INJURY

- Assess ability to provide self-care. Provide assistance as needed. *Clients may be reluctant to ask for help, believing that they should be able to perform these familiar tasks.*
- Provide a safe environment by removing furniture and other objects from traffic areas. Orient the client to the environment. Make frequently used items readily accessible. *These measures help ensure safety and promote independence.*
- Alert caregivers and housekeepers not to move items in the client's room. *Unexpected changes in the environment increase the risk for falls.*
- With the client's permission, raise the side rails on the bed. *The raised rails help remind the client to ask for help until the environment is familiar.*

ANXIETY

- Assess for evidence of anxiety. Repeated expressions of concern or denial that altered vision will affect the client's life are indicators of anxiety. *Identifying and acknowledging anxiety helps the client recognize and deal with it.*
- Discuss the effects of glaucoma and possible vision loss on lifestyle and roles. *This allows the client to express concerns and fears. It also provides an opportunity to suggest alternative activities and assistive devices.*

EVALUATING

Look at the following data to evaluate the effectiveness of nursing care for the client with glaucoma:

- Able to state the purpose, dose, time, and side effects of medications
- Can instill eyedrops as ordered
- Able to safely perform ADLs
- Relates the importance of follow-up care and can state the date of next vision exam

Discharge Considerations

Discuss the prescribed drugs, including the name, dose, timing, and possible adverse effects. Teach the client how to instill eyedrops. Stress the importance of continuing treatment and periodic eye examinations with intraocular pressure measurements.

Discuss the risks, warning signs, and management of future attacks with the client who has had an episode of acute glaucoma. If a permanent vision loss has resulted, discuss the effect of loss of vision on depth perception and safety.

If a significant amount of vision in both eyes has been lost, help identify changes in the home that can help the client remain safe and independent. Suggest removing scatter rugs and small items of furniture to allow the client to navigate safely in this already familiar environment. Refer to local and national resources that can help with assistive devices and modifications of the home.

Nursing Process Case Study
■ CLIENT WITH GLAUCOMA AND CATARACTS

Lila Rainey is an 80-year-old widow who lives alone in the family home. She has worn glasses for myopia since she was a young girl. Four years ago she was diagnosed with chronic simple glaucoma, for which she takes timolol maleate (Timoptic) 0.5%. Recently, she has had increasing difficulty reading and watching television. She no longer drives at night because the glare of oncoming headlights makes it very difficult for her to see. Mrs. Rainey is now being admitted to the day surgery unit for a cataract removal and intraocular lens implant in her right eye.

Assessment Mrs. Rainey is alert and oriented, though apprehensive about surgery. Vital signs are BP 134/72; P 86; R 18. Assessments of other body systems are essentially normal. Mrs. Rainey's pupils are round, equal, and react briskly to light and accommodation. Her conjunctivae are pink; sclera and corneas clear. The red reflex in the right eye is diminished. Her visual acuity is 20/150 OD (right eye) and 20/50 OS (left eye) with corrective lenses. Her intraocular pressures are 16 mm Hg OD and 12 mm Hg OS. The nurse reviews the operative procedure with Mrs. Rainey, answering her questions and telling her what to expect after surgery.

Diagnosis The following nursing diagnoses are identified for Mrs. Rainey:

■ Disturbed Sensory Perception: Visual related to myopia and lens extraction
■ Anxiety related to anticipated surgery
■ Deficient Knowledge related to a lack of information about postoperative care

Expected Outcomes The expected outcomes for the plan of care are that Mrs. Rainey will:

■ Regain sufficient vision to maintain ADLs, including reading and watching television for enjoyment.
■ Demonstrate a reduced level of anxiety.
■ Demonstrate eyedrop instillation postoperatively.
■ Verbalize postoperative care including signs of complications to be reported.

Planning and Implementation The following interventions are implemented for Mrs. Rainey:

■ Place call light and personal care items within easy reach.
■ Encourage expression of fears about surgery and its potential effect on vision.
■ Explain all procedures related to surgery and recovery.
■ Instruct her to avoid shutting eyelids tightly, sneezing, coughing, laughing, bending over, lifting, or straining to have a bowel movement.

■ Instruct to wear glasses during the day and an eye shield at night to prevent injury to the surgical site.
■ Explain and demonstrate the procedure for administering eyedrops.
■ Provide verbal and written instructions about postoperative care, including follow-up examinations, potential complications, and actions to take in response.

Evaluation Mrs. Rainey is discharged 3 hours after surgery. She is visibly relieved the following morning when the eye patch is removed and her vision is better than before surgery, even without her glasses. Mrs. Rainey instills her own eyedrops before discharge and relates an understanding of the postoperative care and safety precautions. Mrs. Rainey's daughter plans to visit her mother several times a week to help with household chores. Mrs. Rainey understands the chronic nature of her glaucoma and says that her vision is too important for her to neglect her timolol drops and routine eye exams.

 Critical Thinking in the Nursing Process

1. Mrs. Rainey was taught to hold pressure over the bridge of her nose for several minutes after instilling her timolol eye drops. Why?
2. Timolol drops are not appropriate for all clients. Which common chronic conditions would contraindicate the use of timolol drops and why?
3. What community resources would you suggest to Mrs. Rainey if she did not have a close family member to assist with housework?

Detached Retina

The retina contains neurons that allow us to see light and images. A *detached retina* is separation of the retina from the choroid, the vascular layer of the eye. Retinal detachments can occur spontaneously or result from trauma. The vitreous humor shrinks with aging, increasing the risk for detached retina.

PATHOPHYSIOLOGY

The retina can remain intact but separate from the choroid, or tear and fold back on itself (Figure 31-14 ◆). A break or tear in the retina allows fluid to seep between the retina and choroid, separating these layers. If the layers remain separated, the neurons of the retina become ischemic and die, causing permanent vision loss. For this reason, retinal detachment is a medical emergency that requires prompt treatment.

A detached retina is painless. The client may sense that a curtain or veil is being drawn across the vision. The affected area of vision relates to the area of detachment. Because light rays cross as they pass through the lens, a detachment in the upper part of the eye affects vision in the lower part of the visual field. Other common manifestations of a detached

Figure 31-14. ◆ Detached retina.

retina include floaters (irregular, dark lines or spots in vision) and flashes of light.

COLLABORATIVE CARE

A detached retina is diagnosed by the client's symptoms and examination of the eye. Until definitive treatment is available, the client's head is positioned so that the detached portion of the retina is lower than the rest of the eye.

Retinal detachment is often treated in an ophthalmologist's office. Several procedures may be used to reestablish contact between the retina and choroid. Air may be injected into the vitreous cavity, and the client positioned so that the air bubble pushes the detached portion of the retina against the choroid. Either laser therapy or cryotherapy, which uses a supercooled probe, may be used to initiate scarring that will "weld" the layers together. A surgical procedure, *scleral buckling,* creates an indentation or fold in the sclera, bringing the choroid into contact with the retina.

NURSING CARE

Early identification and treatment of a detached retina are vital to preserve sight. Carefully assess the client who complains of a sudden change in vision. Most eye disorders cause gradual loss of vision; those that cause a rapid loss are often medical emergencies. Promptly report rapid changes in vision to the charge nurse or physician. Remember that retinal detachment is painless; clients may seem to be more confused than concerned about what they are seeing. Review Box 31-2 for nursing care of the client undergoing eye surgery for a detached retina.

INEFFECTIVE TISSUE PERFUSION: RETINAL

■ Position client with area of detachment dependent. For instance, if vision is lost in the upper outer portion of the left eye, indicating an inferior medial retinal detachment of the left eye, place the client on the right side with the head

of the bed elevated. *Correct positioning allows the vitreous to press on the detached area, bringing the retina closer to blood vessels in the choroid and preserving retinal perfusion until treatment is available.*

ANXIETY

■ Maintain a calm, confident attitude while providing priority care. *Maintaining a calm but urgent manner helps reassure the client.*

■ Reassure the client a detached retina is treatable, usually on an outpatient basis. *Reassurance helps relieve the fear of permanent vision loss.*

■ Explain all procedures fully, including the reason for positioning. *Complete explanations help relieve anxiety and promote understanding.*

■ Allow supportive family members or friends to remain with the client as much as possible. *Additional support helps reduce anxiety.*

To evaluate the effectiveness of nursing care, collect the following data:

■ Did vision remain stable until treatment was provided?
■ Was vision fully or partially restored by treatment?
■ Did anxiety remain within acceptable limits?

Discharge Considerations

Following treatment for a detached retina, stress the importance of positioning as ordered. The client may be instructed to maintain a position with the affected area of the eye inferior to maintain contact between the retina and choroid.

The client who has had a spontaneous retinal detachment has an increased risk of future detachments. Discuss early symptoms, and emphasize the importance of seeking immediate treatment if they occur. Emphasize the need to maintain follow-up treatment with the ophthalmologist. If the retina remains detached, discuss safety measures to accommodate the loss of vision and changes in depth perception.

Macular Degeneration

Macular degeneration is a common cause of blindness in older adults. With aging, the neurons of the macula (the area of central vision) may atrophy or separate from the choroid.

When the macula is damaged, central vision becomes blurred and distorted, but peripheral vision remains intact. Distortion of vision in one eye is a common early symptom; straight lines appear wavy or distorted. Macular degeneration particularly affects activities that require close central vision, such as reading and sewing.

Laser treatment may slow macular degeneration, but often no effective treatment is available. Large-print books and magazines, the use of a magnifying glass, and high-intensity lighting can help the client to cope with reduced vision.

Promptly report new or rapid loss of central vision as early treatment may help preserve vision and slow the disease. Help clients with slowly progressive vision loss to adapt by recommending visual aids and other coping strategies.

Diabetic Retinopathy

Approximately 85% of diabetics develop *diabetic retinopathy,* a disorder affecting the capillaries of the retina. The capillaries are no longer able to transport blood and oxygen to the retina. Retinopathy affects clients with both Type 1 and Type 2 diabetes. Its extent seems to mostly relate to how long the client has had diabetes.

Initially, the venous capillaries dilate and develop microscopic aneurysms that may leak or rupture. These cause edema and small hemorrhages into the retina. As the disease progresses, large areas of the retina become ischemic, and new blood vessels form, spreading over the surface of the retina and into the vitreous body. These vessels are fine and fragile. They may leak or rupture, causing bleeding into the vitreous body. The vessels also increase the risk for a detached retina.

Yearly eye examination is recommended for all adults with diabetes. Laser treatment may be done to seal microaneurysms and destroy new, fragile blood vessels. Treatment slows the disease progress but does not cure it.

The nursing care focus for diabetic retinopathy is on education. Stress the importance of regular eye examinations for all clients with diabetes. Teach the client to report promptly any change in vision, including blurring; black spots (floaters), cobwebs, or flashing lights in the visual field; or a sudden loss of vision in one or both eyes. Emphasize that controlling blood glucose levels and maintaining blood pressure within normal limits will help limit diabetic retinopathy or slow its progress.

Enucleation

Occasionally, an eye must be removed. This procedure is known as *enucleation.* After the eye is removed, the conjunctiva and eye muscles are sutured to a round implant inserted into the orbit to maintain its shape. A permanent prosthesis is individually designed to closely resemble the client's other eye. The prosthesis can be fitted 1 to 2 months after surgery. Often, it is difficult to discern which eye is functional and which is the prosthesis.

CLINICAL alert

Don't make the mistake of charting, "Pupils equal, round, and react to light and accommodation (PERRLA)" on a client with an eye prosthesis!

Postoperative nursing care includes teaching, psychologic support, and observing for potential complications. The client may be instructed to apply warm compresses and instill antibiotic ointment or drops postoperatively.

Blindness

Blindness is defined as severely limited vision that cannot be corrected. Total blindness usually means the client cannot see light at all. In practical terms, a person who needs assistive devices or help from others for normal activities of daily living due to impaired vision is considered blind. Most blindness is preventable with early recognition and treatment of common eye disorders such as cataract and glaucoma.

Nurses can foster independence in the hospitalized client who is blind by doing the following:

- Orient to the environment verbally and physically. Describe the client's room using a central point such as the bed. Lead the client around the room, identifying chairs, sink, bathroom, and other landmarks. Be sure that objects such as chairs, personal items, and clothing are not moved within the room unless the client moves them. Leave doors either fully open or closed as the client wishes, but, to preserve safety, do not leave doors partially open. Keep the room and hallways free of clutter where the client will be ambulating.
- Use verbal communication freely. Describe activities going on around the client. Introduce yourself as you enter the room and let the client know when you are leaving.
- Provide other sensory stimuli such as radio and television as desired by the client.
- Orient to food trays, describing the position of food items on the plate and tray using the face of a clock as a reference (unless the client has always been blind and cannot visualize a clock face).
- When assisting with ambulation, allow the client to hold your arm as you walk slightly ahead. Do not hold the client's arm. Verbally describe the environment, such as "There will be two steps up 5 feet ahead."
- Do not be afraid to ask what assistance the client desires.
- For the client with a new loss of sight, refer for services as appropriate. Persons who are blind can receive mobility training, assistance with relearning self-care activities, education about communication tools, vocational and other forms of rehabilitation. State, local, and national agencies help coordinate services for the blind. Many assistive devices are available, including guide or pilot dogs, computer services, talking books and tape players, and low-vision aids.

Ear Structure, Function, and Disorders

The ear has two primary functions—hearing and maintaining balance. The ear is divided into three areas, the external ear, the middle ear, and the inner ear (Figure 31-15 ◆). All three areas are needed for hearing. The inner ear also helps maintain balance.

The *external ear* includes the auricle (or pinna), the auditory canal, and the tympanic membrane (eardrum). The *auricles* direct sound waves into the ear. The *auditory canal* is about 1 in. (2.5 cm) long. It focuses sound waves on the eardrum. Glands in the canal secrete *cerumen* (earwax), a yellow to brown waxy substance. Cerumen traps dirt and debris, protecting the tympanic membrane and middle ear from infection. The **tympanic membrane** (eardrum) separates the external ear and the middle ear.

The *middle ear* contains the auditory ossicles (bones): the malleus, the incus, and the stapes. These bones transmit vibrations from the tympanic membrane to the oval window of the inner ear. The middle ear is filled with air. It opens into the *eustachian* tube, which connects it with the nasopharynx. The eustachian tube helps equalize the pressure in the middle ear with atmospheric pressure.

The inner ear *(labyrinth)* is a maze of bony, fluid-filled chambers. The labyrinth has three regions: the vestibule, the semicircular canals, and the cochlea. The *vestibule* contains the oval window, and joins the cochlea and the semicircular canals. Receptors in the vestibule respond to changes in gravity and head position, helping maintain balance. The three *semicircular canals* also contain receptors that respond to head movements. The *cochlea* contains the *organ of Corti,* the receptor for hearing. The organ of Corti is sensory hair cells innervated by cranial nerve (CN) VIII (the vestibulocochlear nerve).

Hearing is the perception and interpretation of sound. Sound waves entering the external auditory canal cause the eardrum to vibrate. The ossicles transmit this vibration to the oval window, setting fluid within the vestibule into motion.

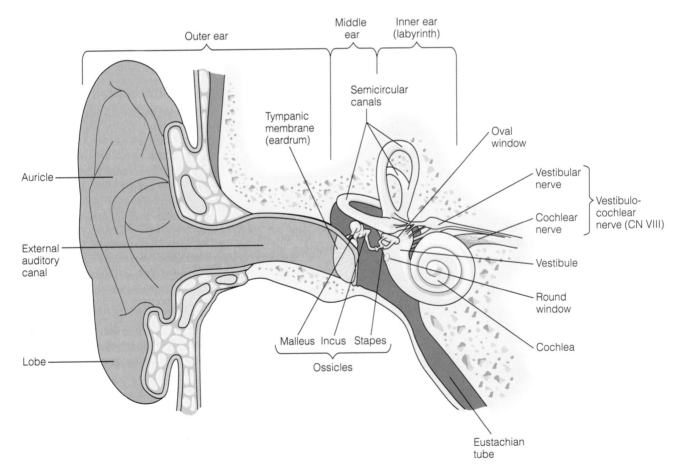

Figure 31-15. ◆ Structures of the external, middle, and inner ear.

The fluid movement stimulates receptors in the organ of Corti, which then send signals to the brain via CN VIII. Nerve fibers from each ear cross, so the auditory centers on each side of the brain receive impulses from both ears. The brain can receive and interpret a wide variety of sounds, as well as localize the source of the sound.

The inner ear also provides information to the brain about head position. This information is used to coordinate body movements so that *equilibrium* and *balance* are maintained. Changing head position sends different patterns of nerve impulses to the brain from the inner ear. The brain interprets these messages, stimulating motor centers to coordinate body movements.

External Otitis

Disorders of the external ear—like external otitis and impacted cerumen—can affect sound conduction and hearing. **External otitis,** or *swimmer's ear,* is inflammation of the ear canal. Swimmers, divers, and surfers are particularly prone to external otitis. Wearing a hearing aid or earplugs, which hold moisture in the ear canal, also is a risk factor.

PATHOPHYSIOLOGY

External otitis usually is caused by bacteria. **Cerumen** (earwax) is water repellent and has an antibacterial effect. Moisture, cleaning, or drying of the ear canal can remove earwax, increasing the risk of infection.

External otitis causes ear pain, which may be severe, and a feeling of fullness in the ear. Manipulating the outer ear increases the pain. Drainage may be present. The ear canal appears inflamed and swollen.

COLLABORATIVE CARE

Treatment of otitis externa usually includes:

- Thorough cleaning of the ear canal, particularly if drainage or debris is present
- Treating the infection with a topical antibiotic
- Topical corticosteroid drops (often combined with the antibiotic) to relieve the pain, itching, and swelling
- Teaching to prevent future episodes of swimmer's ear (see Box 31-6)

NURSING CARE

ASSESSING

When assessing a client with external otitis, ask about ear cleaning practices and participation in water sports or activities. Have the client describe ear pain, including its character, timing, aggravating factors (e.g., pulling or moving the auricle of the ear), and relieving factors. Assess hearing in both ears, using the whisper test (see Chapter 4) or an audiometer. Inspect the external ear for drainage, redness, or evidence of

---

> **BOX 31-6**
>
> **TIPS TO PREVENT EXTERNAL OTITIS**
>
> - Stay out of the water for 7 to 10 days or until completely healed.
> - When you resume water activities, use ear plugs, a tight-fitting swim cap, or wet suit hood to keep water out of the ears or protect the ear from cold water temperatures.
> - Use a hair dryer on the lowest setting to dry ear canals after swimming.
> - Do not insert cotton swabs or any other object into the ear canals.

trauma. Using an otoscope, insert the speculum just inside (no more than 1 cm) the canal to inspect for redness, swelling, drainage, or trauma.

DIAGNOSING, PLANNING, AND IMPLEMENTING

IMPAIRED TISSUE INTEGRITY

- Teach clients not to clean the ear canal with a toothpick, cotton-tipped applicator, or other tool. *This damages the skin and disrupts the protective cerumen, allowing infection to develop.*
- Teach how to instill prescribed ear drops (Box 31-7). *The medication is more effective when it is allowed to reach the inner portion of the ear canal.*
- Instruct to avoid getting water in the affected ear until it is fully healed. Cotton balls may be used while showering to prevent water from entering the ear canal. Instruct to avoid

> **BOX 31-7**
> **NURSING CARE CHECKLIST**
>
> **INSTILLING EAR DROPS**
> ☑ Wash hands.
> ☑ Warm the drops by holding the bottle or putting it in a pocket for about 5 minutes before instilling.
> ☑ Lie on the unaffected side or tilt the head toward the unaffected side.
> ☑ Partially fill the ear dropper with medication.
> ☑ Using the nondominant hand, straighten the ear canal by pulling the pinna of the ear up and back.
> ☑ Instill the prescribed number of drops into the ear canal.
> ☑ Remain on your side for about 5 minutes after putting in the drops.
> ☑ Loosely place a small piece of cotton in the opening to the ear canal for 15 to 20 minutes.

water sports and activities until allowed by the primary care provider. *Moisture in the ear canal can interfere with healing.*

EVALUATING

To evaluate the effectiveness of teaching related to external otitis, have the client demonstrate instilling ear drops. Review knowledge and willingness to avoid water sports until healing is complete. Ask to relate measures to prevent future episodes of external otitis.

Discharge Considerations

The client is ultimately responsible for following the prescribed treatment and preventing future episodes of external otitis. Provide verbal and written instructions for the prescribed medications. Teach the client how to prevent recurrent episodes. Inform all clients that ear canals rarely need cleaning beyond washing the external opening with soap and water. Teach clients of all ages not to clean ear canals with any implement.

Instruct the client to report any increase in pain, swelling, or redness around the ear, fever, malaise, or increased fatigue to the primary care provider.

Impacted Cerumen and Foreign Bodies

The ear canal is narrow and curved. It can become obstructed by earwax or foreign objects such as insects.

As earwax dries, it moves out of the ear canal. In some people, however, it accumulates. Older adults in particular are at risk for *impacted* (tightly wedged) cerumen. With aging, earwax becomes harder and drier. Attempting to remove earwax with cotton-tipped swabs often packs it more deeply into the ear canal.

Ear canal obstruction interferes with sound conduction and hearing. The client reports a sensation of fullness and **tinnitus** (ringing) in the ear. A foreign body or impacted cerumen can be seen using an otoscope.

Treatment focuses on clearing the canal. The canal may be irrigated to clear the obstruction. Impacted wax, objects, or insects may need to be removed using an ear curet, forceps, or other implement. Mineral oil or topical lidocaine drops are used to immobilize or kill insects before they are removed.

CLINICAL alert

If a foreign body such as a bean or an insect occludes the canal, do not irrigate with water. Water may cause the object to swell, making it more difficult to remove.

Teaching is important to prevent obstruction of the ear canal with earwax. Advise the client with impacted cerumen to use mineral oil or commercial products to soften wax and remove it by irrigating the canal with water. Stress the risk of impacting cerumen against the eardrum if cotton-tipped swabs are used to clean the ear canal. The swab also may break and lodge in the canal. If eardrops have been prescribed, teach the client and a family member how to instill them.

Otitis Media

Middle ear disorders can lead to permanent hearing loss without effective treatment.

Otitis media (inflammation or infection of the middle ear) is the most common middle ear disorder. It usually affects infants and young children but can occur in adults. While the eardrum protects the middle ear from the environment, the eustachian tube connects it with the nasopharynx. Organisms can enter the middle ear from the nose and throat through the eustachian tube.

PATHOPHYSIOLOGY

Upper respiratory infection (URI) and eustachian tube dysfunction are risk factors for otitis media. The tube is narrow and flat, normally opening only during yawning and swallowing. Allergies or URI can cause it to swell, impairing its function.

Serous otitis media occurs when the eustachian tube is obstructed. Air in the middle ear is gradually absorbed, causing negative pressure in the middle ear. The negative pressure draws serous fluid from the capillaries into the space.

Manifestations of serous otitis media include decreased hearing and a "snapping" or "popping" sensation in the affected ear. The eardrum moves less freely, and may appear retracted ("sucked in") or bulging. Fluid or air bubbles may be seen behind the drum. Changes in atmospheric pressure (e.g., flying or underwater diving) can cause acute pain, bleeding into the middle ear, or rupture of the eardrum.

Acute or *suppurative otitis media* usually follows URI. Drainage through the eustachian tube is impaired. Mucus and serous fluid collect in the middle ear. Bacteria enter from the nasopharynx, growing and multiplying in this fluid. The infection causes an immune response, and pus forms in the middle ear. The pus increases pressure in the middle ear and can rupture the eardrum.

Acute otitis media causes pain, often severe, in the affected ear. The client may have a fever, and complain of hearing loss, dizziness, **vertigo** (a sensation of whirling or rotation), and tinnitus. The eardrum is red and inflamed or dull and bulging (Figure 31-16 ◆). It does not move normally and may rupture, causing purulent drainage.

Complications

Acute mastoiditis may develop when acute otitis media is not effectively treated. Air cells in the mastoid process of the temporal bone (which is next to the middle ear) fill with pus.

Figure 31-16. ◆ A red, bulging tympanic membrane of otitis media.

Acute mastoiditis destroys these air cells. Manifestations of acute mastoiditis include recurrent earache and hearing loss on the affected side. The mastoid process (behind the ear) is tender and may be swollen, red, and inflamed. The client may complain of tinnitus, headache, and fever. Acute mastoiditis may lead to meningitis; an abscess also may develop.

Chronic otitis media is a permanent perforation of the eardrum. Middle ear infections are recurrent, and structures of the middle ear are destroyed. Severe conductive hearing loss may result.

COLLABORATIVE CARE

Otitis media is usually diagnosed by the client's history and the physical examination. A *pneumatic otoscope* is used to examine the eardrum. A puff of air is blown into the ear canal; this normally causes slight movement of the eardrum. In otitis media, the drum moves less freely. A diagnostic test called *impedance audiometry* may also be done to assess movement of the eardrum and middle ear structures.

Pharmacology

Decongestants are used to improve eustachian tube function and treat serous otitis media. (See Chapter 25 for more information about and the nursing implications of decongestants.) Acute otitis media is treated with antibiotics, often in combination with decongestants. Antibiotic treatment may be continued for 12 to 14 days. (See Chapter 12 for more information about antibiotic treatment.) Mild analgesics such as aspirin or acetaminophen are recommended to relieve pain and reduce fever.

Complementary Therapies

Complementary therapies may help promote comfort in the client with otitis media. A drop of lavender oil on cotton in the ear canal helps relieve discomfort. A warm cloth or a chamomile tea bag steeped in warm water can be used to apply heat to the side of the face or ear, reducing pain. A naturopathic practitioner may prescribe remedies such as pulsatilla, belladonna, or aconite.

Autoinflation

The client with eustachian tube dysfunction may learn to open the tube by performing the Valsalva maneuver, or by forcefully exhaling through the nose against closed nostrils.

Surgery

Surgery may be done to relieve pressure in the middle ear and prevent spontaneous eardrum rupture. In a *tympanocentesis,* a needle is inserted through the eardrum to draw fluid and pus out of the middle ear. *Myringotomy,* surgical drainage of the middle ear, may be done. *Ventilation (tympanostomy) tubes* may be inserted during myringotomy to allow ventilation and drainage of the middle ear during healing. The tube eventually comes out of the ear, and the eardrum heals. While the tube is in place, it is important to avoid getting any water in the ear canal. A *mastoidectomy,* removal of infected air cells, bone, and pus, may be done on a client with mastoiditis.

NURSING CARE

ASSESSING

Clients with otitis media are commonly seen and treated in community settings. Collect data about the onset and duration of symptoms, including pain, popping or snapping sensations in the ear, and any drainage from the ear. Ask about recent URI. Move the auricle of the ear, asking how movement affects the pain. The pain of otitis media usually does not change with manipulation of the external ear. Inspect the client's throat for redness, swelling, or drainage. Obtain the client's temperature. Assess hearing in both ears, using the whisper test or an audiometer. If trained, use an otoscope to inspect the ear canal and eardrum. Inspect and palpate the mastoid process for tenderness.

DIAGNOSING, PLANNING, AND IMPLEMENTING

Pain and the risk of damage to the middle ear are priority nursing care problems for the client with otitis media. Box 31-8 outlines nursing care of the client having ear surgery.

PAIN

- Advise using mild analgesics every 4 hours as needed to relieve pain and fever. *Nonprescription drugs help relieve pain and reduce fever.*
- Advise the client to apply heat to the affected side of the face and head unless contraindicated. *Heat dilates blood vessels, promoting fluid reabsorption and reducing swelling.*
- Instruct to promptly report abrupt pain relief to the physician. *Abrupt pain relief may mean the eardrum has ruptured, releasing pressure from the middle ear.*

BOX 31-8
NURSING CARE CHECKLIST

EAR SURGERY

Before Surgery

☑ Provide routine preoperative care as ordered (see Chapter 7).

☑ Assess hearing or verify that hearing has been assessed before surgery.

☑ Discuss postoperative communication strategies.

☑ Explain postoperative restrictions such as avoiding blowing the nose, coughing, and sneezing. Instruct to leave the mouth open if coughing or sneezing is necessary.

After Surgery

☑ Assess for bleeding or drainage from the affected ear. Note color, character, and amount of any drainage.

☑ Assess for nausea; administer antiemetics as ordered to prevent vomiting.

☑ Elevate the head of bed and position on the unaffected side.

☑ Assess for vertigo or dizziness, especially with movement. Avoid unnecessary movements such as turning. Ensure safety during ambulation.

☑ Assess hearing.

☑ Stand on the client's unaffected side to communicate. Use alternate strategies (such as writing) as needed.

☑ Remind to avoid coughing, sneezing, or blowing the nose.

☑ Provide instructions for home care.

   a. Avoid showers, shampooing, and immersing the head until approved by the physician.

   b. Keep the outer ear plug clean and dry, changing it as needed. Do not remove inner ear dressing until ordered by the physician.

   c. Avoid blowing the nose; if you need to cough or sneeze, keep mouth open.

   d. Do not swim, dive, or travel by air until allowed by the physician.

   e. You may need to take an antiemetic/antihistamine drug for up to 1 month after surgery.

   f. Notify the physician if you develop a fever, bleeding, increased drainage, increased dizziness, or decreased hearing.

DEFICIENT KNOWLEDGE: ANTIBIOTIC THERAPY

■ Stress the importance of completing the full course of antibiotic therapy. *Taking all of the ordered antibiotic is important to eliminate the infection and prevent antibiotic-resistant bacteria from developing.*

■ Discuss the desired and potential adverse effects of the prescribed antibiotic. Tell the client to report any adverse effects to the physician. *If the medication is ineffective or the client has an adverse reaction to it, a different antibiotic may be ordered.*

■ Inform the client that the antibiotic may cause diarrhea, vaginitis, or thrush. Unless contraindicated, instruct the client to eat 8 oz. of yogurt with live bacterial cultures daily during antibiotic therapy. *Antibiotics destroy normal body flora as well as infectious organisms. Live yogurt cultures help restore these beneficial microbes, preventing superinfection.*

■ Stress the importance of keeping follow-up appointments. *Follow-up is important to confirm cure of the infection and prevent complications.*

IMPAIRED TISSUE INTEGRITY

■ Instruct the client with ventilation tubes to avoid swimming, diving, or submerging the head while bathing. *Water can enter the middle ear through the ventilation tubes.*

■ Instruct the client to avoid air travel, rapid changes in elevation, or diving. *A rapid change in pressure can damage the inflamed middle ear.*

■ Encourage to rest, increase fluid intake, and eat a nutritious diet. *These general health measures improve immune function and promote healing.*

EVALUATING

Collect the following data to evaluate the effectiveness of care:

■ Knowledge of the treatment plan

■ Understanding of symptoms to report to the primary care provider

■ On follow-up visits, relief of symptoms, compliance with prescribed treatment, and hearing in both ears

Discharge Considerations

Teach about otitis media, its causes and prevention, and any specific treatment. Provide verbal and written instructions about the ordered antibiotic, its effects, recommended timing (with or without food, doses evenly spaced throughout the day), and possible side effects. Discuss the symptoms of allergic or adverse reactions that should be reported to the physician. Stress the importance of completing the full course of therapy.

If surgery has been performed, teach the client and family members about postoperative care. Discuss postoperative precautions, such as avoiding water in the ear canals and sudden changes in air pressure.

 Otosclerosis

Otosclerosis is a hereditary disorder that usually affects white females. Abnormal bone forms, immobilizing the stapes and causing a conductive hearing loss.

Hearing loss usually begins in adolescence or early adulthood. Both ears are affected. Air conduction of sound is lost. However, sound is conducted through bone. As a result, the client may be able to use a telephone but have difficulty conversing in person. The client also may experience tinnitus. Otosclerosis may be treated with surgical reconstruction of the middle ear.

Education and referral of the client to appropriate community agencies are important nursing care priorities for the client with otosclerosis. For the client who has surgery, nursing care is similar to that for other clients undergoing ear surgery (see Box 31-8).

Inner Ear Disorders

Inner ear disorders occur less frequently than other ear disorders. Labyrinthitis and Ménière's disease are the most common diseases of the inner ear.

PATHOPHYSIOLOGY

The inner ear (or labyrinth) contains the semicircular canals that help maintain balance, and the neural receptors for hearing. Inner ear disorders affect balance and may cause permanent hearing loss. **Vertigo,** a sensation of whirling or movement when there is none, is the key symptom of inner ear disorders.

CLINICAL alert

Vertigo is a disorder of equilibrium (balance). It can be disabling, causing falls, injury, and difficulty walking. Dizziness, on the other hand, is a feeling of unsteadiness, lack of balance, lightheadedness, or movement within the head. It is not as severe as vertigo.

Labyrinthitis

Labyrinthitis is inflammation of the inner ear. It may be caused by bacteria or viruses. Labrynthitis is uncommon. It causes severe vertigo, hearing loss, and nystagmus (rapid involuntary eye movements). Nausea and vomiting often accompany the vertigo. Falling is a significant risk if the client attempts to stand.

Ménière's Disease

Ménière's disease is a chronic inner ear disorder caused by excess fluid and pressure in the labyrinth of the inner ear. Its onset may be gradual or sudden. Clients with Ménière's disease have recurring attacks of vertigo with tinnitus and gradual hearing loss. The hearing loss usually affects one ear, although the other ear also may be affected. Attacks of severe vertigo occur abruptly and are unpredictable, lasting from minutes to hours.

COLLABORATIVE CARE

There is no cure for inner ear disorders. Treatment focuses on managing symptoms and preventing permanent hearing loss.

Several diagnostic tests may be done to identify inner ear disorders.

- Caloric testing is used to assess involuntary eye movements (nystagmus) in response to the stimuli of warm and cool water instilled into the ear canal.
- X-rays and CT scans of the inner ear structures may be done.
- A fast-acting diuretic may be given to decrease pressure in the inner ear. Hearing improves temporarily in clients with Ménière's disease.

Clients with labyrinthitis or an acute attack of Ménière's disease may need hospitalization to manage the vertigo and its effects. Drugs such a droperidol (Inapsine), meclizine (Antivert), prochlorperazine (Compazine), or hydroxyzine (Vistaril) are given to relieve vertigo and nausea. If nausea and vomiting are severe, intravenous fluids may be used to maintain fluid and electrolyte balance. Bed rest in a quiet, darkened room with minimal sensory stimuli and minimal movement provides the most comfort for the client.

The client with Ménière's disease may be placed on a low-salt diet and a diuretic to reduce the frequency of attacks. Tobacco, which can precipitate an attack, is avoided, along with alcohol and caffeine.

Surgery may be necessary to relieve excess pressure in the inner ear or to block transmission of stimuli related to balance and vertigo. There is a risk of hearing loss when surgery is required. Following surgery, the client is positioned to minimize ear pressure and vertigo. Movement is restricted, and the client is assisted during ambulation. Antiemetics and antivertigo drugs are used to manage the nausea and vertigo after surgery. Complications include infection and leakage of cerebral spinal fluid.

NURSING CARE

ASSESSING

Assess the effects of the disorder on balance and the ability to safely ambulate. Assess hearing, using the whisper test (see Chapter 4). Ask about tinnitus, including pitch, tone, quality, and duration. Refer for a complete hearing and ear examination if this has not been done. Assess for nystagmus (involuntary eye movement) by having the client follow an object through the six cardinal fields of vision (see Box 31-1). Nausea and vomiting may interfere with nutrition. Ask about usual food and fluid intake, and assess height and weight, skin color and condition, and for other signs of nutritional status. Discuss the effect of the disorder on the client's life. Unpredictable attacks of vertigo, tinnitus, and hearing loss can affect lifestyle, employment, sleep, rest, and ability to cope.

DIAGNOSING, PLANNING, AND IMPLEMENTING

RISK FOR TRAUMA

- Instruct to remain in bed during an acute attack of vertigo. Place the call light within easy reach. Ask the client not to get up without assistance. *Restricting movement during an acute attack reduces nausea, vomiting, and the risk of falling.*
- Teach the client to avoid sudden head movements or position changes. *Sudden movement may precipitate an attack of vertigo.*
- Administer drugs as ordered, including antiemetics, diuretics, and sedatives. *These medications may reduce the frequency, severity, and duration of attacks.*
- Teach the client who senses an oncoming attack to take the prescribed medication and lie down in a quiet, darkened room. *This decreases the risk of injury, and may reduce the duration and severity of the attack.*
- Instruct the client to pull to the side of the road and wait for the symptoms to subside if an attack occurs while driving. *This is vital to protect the safety of the client and others.*
- Discuss the importance of wearing a Medic-Alert bracelet or necklace. *A Medic-Alert bracelet or tag helps ensure appropriate treatment if the client is unable to answer questions or respond in an emergency.*
- Discuss the effect of one-sided hearing loss on the ability to identify sound direction. Encourage the client to use other senses as well (e.g., when crossing the street). *Sound perception and the ability to identify its direction change when hearing is lost in one ear.*

DISTURBED SLEEP PATTERN

Tinnitus can interfere with concentration, relaxation, and sleep.

- Discuss options for masking tinnitus:
   a. Ambient noise from a radio or sound system
   b. A masking device or white-noise machine
   c. A hearing aid that produces a tone to mask the tinnitus
   d. A hearing aid that amplifies ambient sound
   Masking the perception of tinnitus may allow the client to focus on something other than the sound.
- Suggest that the client discuss possible medications to treat tinnitus with the physician. *Drugs, including antidepressants such as nortriptyline (Aventyl, Pamelor), taken at bedtime may relieve tinnitus and promote rest.*

EVALUATING

To evaluate the effectiveness of nursing care, assess the safety measures. Discuss the client's and family's understanding of the disease and measures to reduce the frequency and severity of attacks. Discuss coping strategies the client will use to manage the effects of the disorder on his or her lifestyle.

Discharge Considerations

Safety is a primary focus of teaching for home care. Teach the client to change positions slowly, especially when ambulating. Turning the whole body rather than just the head helps to prevent vertigo. Because attacks can be unpredictable, the client should not ambulate alone unless in a safe environment. Instruct to sit down immediately when vertigo occurs and lie down if possible. Teach about prescribed medications, providing both verbal and written instructions about their use, desired effects, and possible adverse effects and precautions.

If the client has had surgery, provide information about postoperative care and follow-up. Teach techniques to minimize postoperative vertigo and associated nausea. Surgery may cause permanent hearing loss in the affected ear; discuss safety and communication strategies.

 Hearing Loss

Hearing loss impairs the ability to communicate in a world filled with sound and hearing individuals. Approximately 10 million adults in the United States are hearing impaired. Hearing loss is more common in older adults, affecting a quarter to a third of older adults. Up to 70% of long-term care residents have impaired hearing.

PATHOPHYSIOLOGY

Hearing loss is classified as conductive, sensorineural, or mixed, depending on what portion of the auditory system is affected. A hearing deficit can be partial or total, congenital or acquired. It may affect one or both ears. Some types of hearing loss affect the ability to hear specific frequencies of sound.

Conductive Hearing Loss

Anything that affects sound transmission from the external opening of the ear to the inner ear causes a *conductive hearing loss.* Obstruction of the ear canal (e.g., impacted cerumen) is the most common cause. Other causes of conductive loss include perforated eardrum, damage to the ossicles of the middle ear, fluid, scarring, or tumors of the middle ear. The client with a conductive hearing loss benefits from sound amplification by a hearing aid.

Sensorineural Hearing Loss

Disorders that affect the inner ear or the auditory pathways of the brain may cause a *sensorineural hearing loss.* Trauma, infection, diseases such as Ménière's disease, and ototoxic medications can lead to sensory hearing loss. In the United States, noise exposure is the major cause. Exposure to a high level of noise (e.g., standing close to the stage or speakers at a rock concert) damages the hair cells of the organ of Corti. Ototoxic drugs such as aspirin, furosemide (Lasix), and the aminoglycoside antibiotics also damage the hair cells. When ototoxic drugs are given together (e.g., when the client is getting both furosemide and gentamicin), the risk of sensory hearing loss increases.

Sensory hearing losses usually affect the ability to hear high-frequency sounds more than low-frequency sounds. This affects speech discrimination and communication, especially in a noisy environment. Hearing aids may not help.

Presbycusis

With aging, the hair cells of the cochlea degenerate, causing progressive hearing loss. Hearing begins to decline in early adulthood, progressing with time. **Presbycusis** is a type of sensorineural loss. Because hearing loss is gradual, the client and family may not realize the extent of the deficit. Hearing aids and other amplification devices are useful for most clients with presbycusis.

COLLABORATIVE CARE

Hearing evaluation includes gross tests of hearing (such as the whisper test), the Rinne and Weber tests, and audiometry.

- The *Rinne and Weber tests* (Box 31-9) compare sound conduction by air and through bone. Bone conduction of sound is better than air conduction with a conductive hear-

ing loss. With a sensory hearing loss, both air and bone sound conduction are affected.

- *Audiometry* is used to quantify hearing deficits. Specific sound frequencies are presented to each ear by either air or bone conduction to identify the type and pattern of hearing loss.

Amplification

A hearing aid or other amplification device can help many clients with hearing loss. These devices amplify sound, increasing the sound level so it can be heard by the client. This improves the perception and interpretation of the sound. Hearing aids must be individually prescribed by an audiologist. To be effective, proper design and fit as well as regular maintenance are necessary.

The least noticeable style of hearing aid fits entirely in the ear canal. It allows telephone use and can be worn during exercise. Because it is small, good manual dexterity is needed to insert it, clean it, and change the batteries. An in-ear hearing aid fits into the external ear (Figure 31-17A ◆). It is easier to handle and provides greater amplification than the in-canal style of hearing aid. With both the in-canal and in-ear style,

---

BOX 31-9
ASSESSING CLIENTS: THE RINNE AND WEBER TESTS

The Rinne and Weber tests are used to help determine if hearing loss is conductive or sensory.

- The Rinne test: Strike the tines of a tuning fork on the heal of your hand to start it vibrating (see figure A). Place the base of the tuning fork behind the ear, on the mastoid bone. Ask the client to tell you when the sound is no longer heard, then quickly move the tuning fork in

front of the ear canal. Ask if the client can hear the sound. If the client says yes, air conduction of sound is better than bone conduction, the normal finding.

- The Weber test: Place the base of a vibrating tuning fork on the middle of the top of the client's head (see figure B). Ask where the client best hears the sound. Sound is normally heard equally in both ears.

A   Rinne Test

B   Weber Test

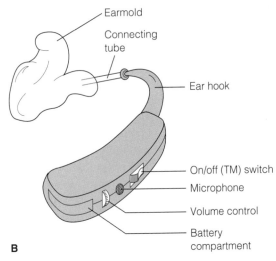

Figure 31-17. ◆ Types of hearing aids. (A) An in-ear hearing aid. (B) A behind-the-ear hearing aid.

cleaning is important. Small openings may become plugged with wax, interfering with sound transmission.

The behind-ear hearing aid is easier to manipulate (Figure 31-17B). For the client who wears glasses, it can be integrated into the earpiece of the eyeglasses.

Clients with profound hearing loss may require a body hearing aid. The microphone and amplifier of this aid are contained in a pocket-sized case that the client clips onto clothing, slips into a pocket, or carries in a harness. The receiver is attached by a cord to the case and clips onto the ear mold, which delivers the sound to the ear canal.

For the client who does not have a hearing aid, an assistive listening device, or "pocket talker," with a microphone and "Walkman"-type earpieces, is useful. Pocket talkers are available over the counter and are relatively inexpensive. The earpiece requires no special fitting, and the external microphone allows the client to focus on the desired sound rather than simply amplifying all sounds.

Surgery

Surgery may be done to correct damage to the middle ear. The client with a sensory hearing loss may require a cochlear implant to allow sound perception. Cochlear implants provide sound perception but do not restore normal hearing. The client can recognize warning sounds such as automobiles, sirens, telephones, and doors opening or closing. They also are

alerted to speech so they can focus on the person speaking. Many clients can learn to interpret the perceived sounds as words, especially with newer implant devices.

NURSING CARE

ASSESSING

Clients with a hearing loss often display signs that caregivers can recognize. Voice volume frequently increases, and the client positions the head with the better ear toward the speaker. Be alert for signs of impaired hearing such as cupping an ear, difficulty understanding verbal communication when the person cannot see the speaker's face, difficulty following conversation in a large group, and withdrawal from social activities. The client may appear unsociable or paranoid.

Inspect the external ear canal and eardrum, using an otoscope. Perform the whisper test and Rinne and Weber tests to evaluate hearing. Document findings, and recommend an audiologist for further evaluation if indicated.

DIAGNOSING, PLANNING, AND IMPLEMENTING

Priority nursing care problems for a client with a hearing loss include loss of a sensory function, impaired communication, and social isolation.

DISTURBED SENSORY PERCEPTION: AUDITORY

- Encourage the client to talk about the hearing loss and its effect on activities of daily living. *Listening to and providing support encourage the client to develop coping strategies.*
- Provide information about hearing loss and available services to the client and family. *Information about hearing aids, amplification devices, and other services helps the client plan ways to compensate for the loss.*
- Replace batteries in hearing aids on a regular and as-needed basis. *Hearing aid batteries last approximately 1 week.*
- If the hearing aid has a toggle switch for microphone/telephone, be sure it is in the appropriate position. Check hearing aids, cleaning out earwax as needed. *A hearing aid plugged with cerumen does not transmit sound well.*

IMPAIRED VERBAL COMMUNICATION

- Get the client's attention before beginning to speak. Use a wave of the hand or tap on the shoulder. *This allows the client to focus on the person speaking.*
- When speaking, face the client and keep the hands away from the face. Avoid making the client look into glare or standing so that your face is in shadow. Trim mustaches so the lips are visible. *People with a hearing loss often use lip-reading consciously or unconsciously to help understand spoken words.*

- When speaking, use a low voice pitch with normal loudness. The voice tends to become higher in pitch when loudness increases. *The ability to hear higher pitch tones often is lost; lowering the voice pitch allows the client to hear it more clearly.*
- Speak at a normal rate, and do not overarticulate. Use shorter sentences and pause at the end of each sentence. *Changing the pace of speech may make conversation more difficult to follow and to lip-read. Using short sentences and pausing gives the client time to interpret the message.*
- Reduce the noise in the environment before speaking with the client. *Excess noise interferes with the client's ability to focus on conversation.*
- Use nonverbal and written communication as needed. *Nonverbal cues and written messages may improve understanding.*
- Rephrase sentences as necessary. *Some words are more difficult to perceive than others; rephrasing often clarifies the message for the client.*
- Ask the client to repeat important information. *This helps ensure that the client understood the information.*
- Share information about the client's hearing loss and effective communication strategies with other staff. *Consistent use of effective communication strategies decreases the client's frustration.*

SOCIAL ISOLATION

- Help the client identify the extent and cause of social isolation. *Identifying the hearing deficit as a contributing factor to a sense of isolation may prompt the client to seek ways to improve hearing.*
- Encourage interaction with friends and family on a one-to-one basis in quiet settings. *Conversations in small groups and quiet settings are easier for the client to follow and participate in.*
- Treat the client with dignity. Remind friends and family that hearing loss does not mean loss of mental faculties. *Inappropriate responses to questions and comments can lead others to think of the client as "stupid" or demented.*
- Involve the client in activities that do not require acute hearing, such as checkers and chess. *Activities such as these allow social interactions without the stress of straining to hear.*
- Obtain a pocket talker or encourage the client and family to do so.
- Refer to an audiologist for evaluation and possible hearing-aid fitting.
- Refer to resources such as support groups and senior citizen centers. *These groups provide new social outlets.*

EVALUATING

Listen to the client's responses, and observe behavior, interactions with others, and signs of anxiety or stress to help determine the effectiveness of nursing interventions for the client with hearing loss.

Discharge Considerations

Teaching is vital to help prevent hearing loss. Teach all clients:

- How to safely clean ear canals
- The importance of preventing and treating ear infections
- To use ear plugs when swimming or diving
- To use ear protectors when operating loud equipment, shooting, or when exposed to constant high-pitched sound
- To avoid frequent exposure to loud noise such as extremely loud music

Help the client learn to manage and cope with hearing loss. Discuss evaluation by an audiologist to determine the usefulness of a hearing aid. Teach the client how to use, care for, and maintain a hearing aid. Encourage the client to acknowledge the deficit and ask people to speak clearly and repeat statements as needed. Voicing a preference for individual visits and small group interactions rather than large social functions can help the client to remain connected to friends and family.

Refer the client and family to national, state, and local agencies that provide education and assistance. Local and regional agencies are often listed in the telephone book. An audiology center may also have a list of local resources.

Nursing Interventions Classification

The following interventions (McCloskey & Bulechek, 2000) may also be useful for clients with eye or ear disorders:

- Ear Care
- Emotional Support
- Eye Care
- Fall Prevention
- Medication Administration: Topical
- Teaching: Disease Process
- Teaching: Prescribed Medication

(*Note:* The bibliography listings for this and all chapters have been compiled at the back of the book.)

Chapter Review

key terms by topic

Use the CD-ROM disk enclosed with your textbook to hear the pronunciation of the key terms in the chapter.

Eye function
refraction

Eye disorders
conjunctivitis, keratitis, corneal ulcer, photophobia, diplopia, cataract, glaucoma, presbyopia

Ear structure
cerumen, tympanic membrane

Ear disorders
external otitis (swimmer's ear), tinnitus, otitis media, vertigo, presbycusis

key points

- Glaucoma and cataracts, both very treatable conditions, are leading causes of blindness.

- Collect complete subjective and objective assessment data on clients who complain of changes in vision or a red, painful eye. While the cause may be minor and treatable, such as conjunctivitis, some conditions such as acute glaucoma may have similar symptoms and lead to permanent vision loss if not promptly treated.

- Teaching and maintaining client safety are primary nursing roles when caring for clients with eye or ear conditions.

- Most outer and middle ear conditions are minor and treatable, but can lead to conductive hearing loss if ignored.

- Vertigo, a sensation of movement, is a common manifestation of inner ear disorders. Clients with vertigo are at risk for falls, and often experience nausea and vomiting with the vertigo.

- Inspect the ear canal of clients who complain about recent hearing loss, especially if the client is older or wears a hearing aid or earplugs. Impacted cerumen can interfere with sound conduction and hearing.

Medialink

Additional interactive resources for this chapter can be found on the Companion Website at www.prenhall.com/burke. Click on Chapter 31 and "Begin" to select the activities for this chapter.

For NCLEX review questions and an audio glossary, access the accompanying CD-ROM in this book.

for further study

For assessment of pupil reflex and for more on hearing assessment, see Chapter 4.

For in-depth discussion of the client having surgery, see Chapter 7.

For nursing implications for antibiotics, see Chapter 12.

For more information about decongestants, see Chapter 25.

Critical Thinking Care Map

Caring for a Client with Age-Related Hearing Loss
NCLEX-PN Focus Area: Coping and Adaptation

Case Study: Carl Aaron is an 85-year-old retired logger who has been caring for his disabled wife in their home for the past 3 years. Mr. Aaron has osteoarthritis, which now makes it difficult for him to continue providing all the care his wife requires. They move into a care center where his wife can receive nursing care while he resides in the assisted living wing.

Nursing Diagnosis: Disturbed Sensory Perception: Auditory

COLLECT DATA

Subjective	Objective

Would you report this data? Yes/No

If yes, to:_____

Nursing Care

_____
_____
_____
_____
_____
_____
_____
_____

How would you document this? _____
_____
_____

Data Collected
(use those that apply)

- Proximal interphalangeal (PIP) and distal interphalangeal (DIP) joints swollen, cool and hard bilaterally
- Weber test, no lateralization
- Answers not always appropriate to the question
- Rinne test AC>BC
- Appears depressed
- Mental status exam is normal
- Frequently asks nurse to repeat questions
- Ear canals clean, no redness, small amount of dark earwax noted
- C/O hip pain when ambulating
- Audiometric testing reveals significant hearing loss consistent with presbycusis
- BP 144/86, P 78, R 18
- Expresses concerns about wife's care
- Ignores conversation at his table during meals about wife's care

Nursing Interventions
(use those that apply)

- Teach Mr. Aaron how to use and care for hearing aids.
- Provide a schedule of small group activities for Mr. Aaron.
- Supplement verbal with nonverbal communication strategies.
- Obtain a temperature-controlled heating pad to promote comfort.
- Use a pocket talker as needed until hearing aids are available.
- Ask Mr. Aaron's family to obtain headphones for radio and television use.
- Administer ordered nonsteroidal anti-inflammatory drug (NSAID) every 6 hours.
- Use effective communication techniques.
- Encourage Mr. Aaron to shower on arising to relieve morning stiffness.
- Face Mr. Aaron when speaking with him.
- Facilitate one-on-one interactions between Mr. Aaron and other residents.
- Speak distinctly in a low voice.

NCLEX-PN Exam Preparation

TEST-TAKING TIP

Do not read information into a test question. Choose the correct response based on the information presented and your nursing knowledge.

1. The nurse is working with a group of clients in a long-term care facility. All of the clients have moderate to severe hearing or visual impairment. When planning care for clients with sensory problems, the nurse should recognize that a priority is:
   a. establishing a support group for those with sensory deficits
   b. providing outside entertainment at least once a month
   c. encouraging their families to visit as often as possible
   d. maintaining a safe environment and preventing sensory deprivation

2. The nurse is caring for an elderly male client who wears eyeglasses to correct myopia. When planning the client's care, the nurse understands that the client's lenses are used to correct:
   a. nearsightedness
   b. farsightedness
   c. astigmatism
   d. nystagmus

3. A client with a middle ear infection is receiving instructions from the nurse about the correct method for administering eardrops. The nurse should instruct the client to:
   a. aim the eardrops directly at the eardrum
   b. pull the pinna (auricle) backward and downward
   c. pull the pinna (auricle) upward and backward
   d. saturate a cotton ball with the medication and place the cotton ball in the ear canal

4. The nurse is caring for a client who has a severe hearing impairment but is able to read lips well. An appropriate nursing goal would include:
   a. learning sight language as soon as possible
   b. increasing his physical activity by at least 25%
   c. investigating the purchase of a communication board
   d. participating in some type of social interaction at least once a week

5. A client calls the consulting nurse to report that she has accidentally splashed brake fluid in her eyes. The nurse advises the client to:
   a. call 911
   b. use nonprescription eyedrops and see a physician if she continues to have problems
   c. cover both eyes with warm compresses and rest for several hours
   d. immediately flush both eyes with large amounts of water and seek medical attention

6. The nurse is irrigating a client's eye with a sterile normal saline solution. The nurse should direct the flow of the solution from the:
   a. center of both eyes to the lower conjunctiva
   b. inner to the outer canthus
   c. lower to the upper conjunctiva
   d. outer to the inner canthus

7. The client states that because the pilocarpine drops prescribed for chronic simple glaucoma cause her eyes to burn and her vision to become blurry, so she has stopped using the medication. The nurse should tell the client:
   a. not to worry because most people who use the medication have the same complaint
   b. if she has discomfort, skip the medication a day before resuming the drops
   c. that although the drops may be uncomfortable, it is important to use them to retain her vision
   d. to lie down for at least 30 minutes after administering the drops

8. When educating the client about chronic simple glaucoma, the nurse describes the pathophysiologic process of the condition as:
   a. the vitreous humor cannot drain, thus causing pressure damage to the optic nerve
   b. the lens is damaged by excessive production of aqueous humor
   c. damage to the optic nerve
   d. the aqueous humor produced in the eye cannot adequately drain, thus causing pressure

9. During the nurse's initial assessment of an elderly woman with chronic simple glaucoma, what symptoms might the history reveal?
   a. light flashes in both eyes
   b. difficulty focusing and halos around lights
   c. watery drainage from both eyes
   d. sudden loss of vision in both eyes

10. When teaching the client about Ménière's disease, the nurse should instruct the client to avoid foods that are:
    a. low in sodium
    b. high in fat
    c. high in sodium
    d. high in potassium

Answers for Review Questions, as well as discussion of Case Study Critical Thinking questions, appear in Appendix V.

chapter

32

Caring for Male Clients with Reproductive System Disorders

LEARNING outcomes

After completing this chapter, you will be able to:

- Identify the major structures and functions of the male reproductive system.
- Describe the pathophysiology of common disorders of the male reproductive system.
- Identify diagnostic tests related to male reproductive function.
- List the manifestations of common disorders of the male reproductive system.
- Discuss nursing implications for medications used to treat disorders of the male reproductive system.
- Use the nursing process to provide care for clients with disorders of the male reproductive system.

MediaLink

www.prenhall.com/burke

Use the above address to access the free, interactive Companion Website created for this textbook. Get hints, instant feedback, and textbook references to chapter-related multiple choice questions. Link to other interesting sites.

The male reproductive system may be affected by structural and functional disorders, infectious and inflammatory disorders, and malignancies. Many of these disorders pose a risk to the client's fertility and sexuality, as well as urinary function.

Structure and Function of the Male Reproductive System

The reproductive organs function to provide sexual pleasure and produce children. Together with the endocrine system, the reproductive organs also produce hormones that direct development and sexual behavior. The reproductive organs also affect urinary function. The reproductive system in men includes the paired testes, the scrotum, ducts, glands, and penis (Figure 32-1 ◆).

TESTES AND SCROTUM

The *testes* produce sperm and testosterone. Sperm is produced in the *seminiferous tubules* of the testes. Leydig's cells produce testosterone.

The testes are suspended in the scrotum by the spermatic cord. The *scrotum* is a sac or pouch that regulates the temperature of the testes. The best temperature for producing sperm is about 2 to 3 degrees below body temperature. When the temperature is too low, the scrotum contracts to bring the testes up against the body. When the testes are too warm, the scrotum relaxes to allow the testes to lie further away from the body.

Spermatogenesis

Spermatogenesis is sperm production. This process begins with puberty and continues throughout a man's life, with several hundred million sperm produced daily. Spermatogenesis takes 64 to 72 days, and includes the following processes:

1. Sperm stem cells *(spermatogonia)* divide to produce daughter cells *(spermatocytes)* that have the same number of chromosomes (46) as the parent cell.
2. Spermatocytes further divide to produce *spermatids,* immature cells with half the number of chromosomes (23) as the spermatocyte.
3. Spermatids mature into sperm cells with a head and a tail. The head contains enzymes that allow the sperm to penetrate and fertilizate the ova. The tail allows the sperm to move. When the sperm and ova fuse, the resulting cell has the normal number of chromosomes (46).

Male Sex Hormones

The male sex hormones are called **androgens.** Most are produced in the testes, although a small amount is produced by the adrenal glands. *Testosterone,* the primary male sex hormone, is essential to develop and maintain sexual function. It also promotes metabolism, muscle and bone growth, and **libido** (sexual desire).

DUCTS AND SEMEN

Sperm mature and are stored in the *epididymis,* a long coiled tube that lies over the outer surface of each testis. When a man is sexually excited, the epididymis contracts to push the sperm through the *vas deferens* to mix with seminal fluid.

Seminal fluid is made of secretions from the seminal vesicles, the epididymis, the prostate gland, and Cowper's glands. Seminal fluid nourishes the sperm, provides bulk, and increases its alkalinity. (An alkaline pH is essential to mobilize the sperm and ensure fertilization of the ova.) Sperm mixed with this fluid is called *semen.* During **ejaculation** (expulsion of seminal fluid) semen enters the urethra for expulsion.

The total amount of ejaculate is about 2 to 4 mL. The sperm count of ejaculate in a healthy male is from 100 to 400 million.

PROSTATE GLAND

The *prostate gland* is about the size of a walnut. It encircles the urethra just below the urinary bladder (see Figure 32-1). Secretions of the prostate gland make up about one third of the volume of the semen. These secretions enter the urethra through several ducts during ejaculation.

PENIS

The penis is composed of a *shaft* and a tip called the *glans,* which is covered in the uncircumcised man by the *foreskin* (or *prepuce*). The shaft contains three columns of erectile tissue: The two lateral columns are called the *corpora cavernosa,* and the central mass is called the *corpus spongiosum.*

Erection occurs when a reflex triggers the parasympathetic nervous system to stimulate arteriolar vasodilation, filling erectile tissue with blood. The erection reflex may be initiated by touch, pressure, sights, sounds, smells, or thoughts of a sexual encounter. After ejaculation, the arterioles constrict, and the penis becomes flaccid.

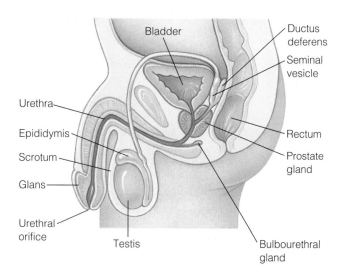

Figure 32-1. ◆ The male reproductive system.

Prostate Disorders

Benign Prostatic Hyperplasia

Enlargement of the prostate gland, **benign prostatic hyperplasia (BPH),** affects most men over the age of 50. The incidence of BPH increases with age: More than 90% of men over 70 years old have BPH. BPH tends to develop earlier in African Americans than in European Americans.

PATHOPHYSIOLOGY

Testosterone, the primary androgen, is converted to dihydrotestosterone (DHT) in the prostate gland. DHT stimulates growth of the prostate. Although testosterone levels decrease in aging, estrogen (produced in small amounts in men) levels increase. Estrogen appears to make the prostate more responsive to DHT, promoting its growth. Increases estrogen levels in relation to testosterone levels may contribute to BPH.

BPH develops in the central and transition zones of the prostate, next to the urethra. The expanding prostate compresses surrounding tissue, narrowing the urethra (Figure 32-2 ◆). Narrowing of the urethra causes the symptoms of BPH, summarized in Box 32-1. *Nocturia* (voiding more than once at night) is an early symptom.

If BPH is not treated, increased pressure in the bladder causes urine reflux into the ureters. This can eventually lead to *hydronephrosis,* which can affect kidney function (see Chapter 21). Fortunately, these complications are rare, because the symptoms associated with BPH force most men to seek help before they develop.

COLLABORATIVE CARE

Some men are diagnosed with BPH during a routine physical examination before symptoms develop. Others wait until the discomfort from dysuria, urgency, and urinary retention become almost unbearable before seeking care.

Diagnostic Tests

- A *digital rectal exam (DRE)* is done to assess the size and consistency of the prostate gland.
- A routine *urinalysis* is done; if the client has symptoms such as dysuria, a urine culture is also obtained.
- *Prostate-specific antigen (PSA)* levels are measured. PSA is produced by the prostate gland. Levels may be somewhat higher than normal (> 4 ng/mL) in BPH, but are significantly elevated with prostate cancer.
- *Uroflowmetry* measures the urine flow rate. If urine flow is severely obstructed, BPH is a probable diagnosis.

Pharmacology

Several drugs may be used to shrink the enlarged prostate and reduce the manifestations of BPH. Finasteride (Proscar) inhibits the conversion of testosterone to DHT in the prostate, causing the gland to shrink. It is most effective in men with significantly enlarged prostate glands. A small percentage of men taking this drug experience decreased libido.

Alpha-1 blockers such as terazosin (Hytrin), doxazosin (Cardura), and tamsulosin (Flomax) relax smooth muscle in the prostate, the urethra, and the bladder neck. Smooth muscle relaxation reduces urethral obstruction and improves urinary flow and symptoms of BPH.

Complementary Therapies

Saw palmetto is an herbal therapy that reduces the symptoms of BPH. Its effects are similar to those of finasteride, although its mechanism of action is unknown. It causes few side effects and is considered to be a safe herbal remedy.

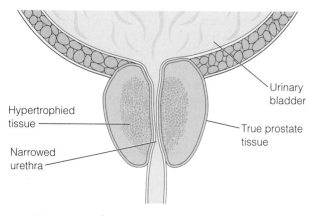

Figure 32-2. ◆ Benign prostatic hyperplasia (BPH).

> **BOX 32-1**
> **MANIFESTATIONS OF BENIGN PROSTATIC HYPERPLASIA**
>
> - Diminished force of urinary stream
> - Hesitancy in starting voiding
> - Dribbling after voiding
> - Sensation of incomplete emptying
> - Urinary retention
> - Frequency, urgency
> - Nocturia (early symptom)
> - Urge incontinence
> - Dysuria, hematuria

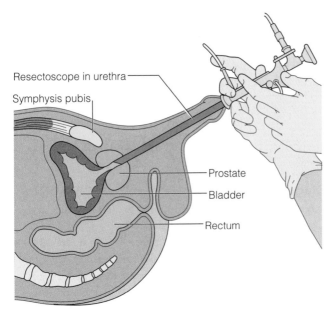

Resectoscope in urethra

Symphysis pubis

Prostate

Bladder

Rectum

Figure 32-3. ◆ Transurethral resection of the prostate (TURP). A resectoscope inserted through the urethra is used to remove excess prostate tissue.

Surgery

Clients with BPH may require surgery to relieve urinary obstruction. Only the portion of the prostate gland surrounding the urethra is removed in BPH. *Transurethral incision of the prostate* (TUIP) and *transurethral resection of the prostate* (TURP) are the most common procedures used. In the *TUIP* procedure, small incisions are made in the prostate and the bladder neck to widen the urethra. No tissue is removed, and this procedure can be done on an outpatient basis.

In a *TURP,* obstructing prostate tissue is removed using the wire loop of a *resectoscope* inserted through the urethra (Figure 32-3 ◆). Irrigating fluid carries resected tissue into the bladder to be flushed out on completion of the procedure. TURP is a relatively low-risk procedure with few complications. After surgery, *retrograde ejaculation* (discharge of seminal fluid into the bladder instead of through the urethra) is common. Fluid volume excess with hyponatremia, also known as *transurethral syndrome,* is a potential complication of TURP. Nursing care for the client having a TURP is outlined in Box 32-2.

Balloon urethroplasty or destroying excess prostate tissue with lasers or microwaves also may be used to treat BPH. These minimally invasive procedures can be done on an outpatient basis.

NURSING CARE

ASSESSING

Ask older men about difficulty voiding, including difficulty starting and stopping the flow of urine, the size of the urinary

---

BOX 32-2
NURSING CARE CHECKLIST

TRANSURETHRAL RESECTION OF THE PROSTATE (TURP)

Before Surgery

☑ Provide routine preoperative care and teaching (see Chapter 7).

☑ Inform client that he will return from surgery with a urinary catheter in place.

After Surgery

☑ Provide routine postoperative care (see Chapter 7).

☑ Assess and manage pain, which may include urethral discomfort, bladder spasms, and abdominal cramping due to gas.

☑ Use aseptic technique when managing urinary drainage and irrigation.

☑ Maintain accurate intake and output, including amounts of irrigating solution used. When allowed, encourage a liberal fluid intake.

☑ Frequently assess catheter patency; record color and character of urine.

☑ For the first 24 to 48 hours, monitor for hemorrhage (frankly bloody urine, large blood clots, decreased urinary output, increasing bladder spasms, decreased hemoglobin and hematocrit, tachycardia, and hypotension). Notify physician if manifestations occur.

☑ Explain that catheter may cause a sensation of needing to void. Instruct to avoid straining to void or when having a bowel movement.

☑ If a continuous bladder irrigation (CBI) is present, maintain irrigating fluid flow rate to keep the output light pink or colorless.

☑ Report changes in vital signs, mental status, and laboratory results.

☑ If CBI is not used, follow agency procedure and physician orders for irrigating the indwelling catheter (usually when the urine is frankly bloody or has numerous larger blood clots, or when bladder spasms increase).

☑ After catheter removal, assess amount, color, and consistency of voided urine. Explain that burning, dribbling, and small clots in the urine are common after catheter removal.

☑ Teach Kegel exercises (see Chapter 21) and to start and stop the urine stream several times during each voiding to reduce incontinence.

☑ Maintain antiembolic stockings and pneumatic compression devices as ordered. Assist with leg exercises and ambulation as ordered.

---

stream, and any symptoms such as burning, frequency, urgency, or nocturia. Monitor urine output, including amount (total and per voiding), color, clarity, and odor.

DIAGNOSING, PLANNING, AND IMPLEMENTING

INEFFECTIVE THERAPEUTIC REGIMEN MANAGEMENT

- Provide information about BPH and its treatment. Refer client to primary care provider or a urologist. *Most men are aware that BPH is very common, but are unsure of the function or exact location of the prostate gland. To make decisions, clients need to know about possible treatment options and their effects.*
- Advise to drink 2 to 3 liters of fluids daily, unless contraindicated by heart or kidney disease. *Fluids help prevent urinary tract infections and reduce dysuria.*
- Advise to restrict alcohol intake, especially late at night, to minimize problems with nocturia. *Nocturia can pose a safety risk for older men who may have age-related changes in vision, muscule strength, and coordination.*

EXCESS FLUID VOLUME

- Assess for manifestations of fluid volume excess and hyponatremia (see Chapter 5). *Transurethral syndrome, resulting from the large amounts of irrigating fluid used during and after surgery, can affect cardiovascular or pulmonary status, and lead to altered mental status.*
- Weigh daily. Monitor intake and output, including irrigating fluid used during and after surgery. Subtract the amount of irrigating solution used after surgery from the amount of output to determine the urine output. *Frequent assessments help identify fluid volume excess. Weight is an effective indicator of fluid volume status.*
- Restrict fluids and administer diuretics as ordered. *Fluid restriction conserves sodium, and diuretics decrease total fluid load.*

IMPAIRED URINARY ELIMINATION

- Change from leg drainage bag to a larger night drainage bag at bedtime. *A bag suspended from the bed frame at night permits gravity drainage of urine and prevents reflux of urine back into the bladder.*
- Avoid strapping the leg bag on too tightly. *Tight straps can decrease venous return and increase risk for thrombophlebitis and complications such as pulmonary emboli.*
- Place a soft cloth between the leg bag and thigh *to decrease friction and absorb dampness under the bag, reducing the risk of skin irritation.*
- Empty the leg bag every 3 to 4 hours *to prevent overfilling.*
- Promptly report any unexpected changes in urine color, consistency, or odor to the physician. Report continued hematuria, evidence of frank bleeding, or large blood clots, as well as a lack of or significant decrease in urine output. *These signs and symptoms may indicate a complication such as hemorrhage or infection.*

EVALUATING

Collect the following data to evaluate the effectiveness of nursing interventions for a client with BPH or who has had surgery to treat BPH:

- Urine output, including amount, color, clarity, and odor
- Ability to control urine flow without incontinence or dribbling
- Knowledge and understanding of treatment options
- Ability to manage home care, and understanding of when to contact the physician

 Discharge Considerations

Clients often are discharged within 2 days following a TURP. When TURP is done on an outpatient basis, the client may be discharged with an indwelling urinary catheter. Provide home care instructions as noted under Impaired Urinary Elimination above. Box 32-3 outlines discharge instructions after prostate surgery. Address concerns about sexuality following prostate surgery, providing referral to counseling or support services as indicated.

 Prostatitis

Prostatitis (inflammation of the prostate gland) is a relatively common problem in young and middle-aged men. While prostatitis may be caused by a bacterial infection, nonbacterial prostatitis is the most common type seen.

Acute bacterial prostatitis is often associated with lower urinary tract infections. The infecting organism is usually *Escherichia coli,* but other pathogens may also invade the prostate. Infected urine may reflux into the prostatic ducts, or perhaps organisms may ascend the urinary tract. There is evidence that contamination of the urinary *meatus* (opening of the urethra) during vaginal or anal sexual intercourse may play a role in ascending infections.

Nonbacterial prostatitis may be caused by organisms such as chlamydiae, mycoplasmas, and viruses, but its exact cause is unknown. Nonbacterial prostatitis may be a type of sexually transmitted disease or an autoimmune disorder. Manifestations of prostatitis are listed in Box 32-4.

It is often difficult to diagnose prostatitis. Urine and prostatic secretions are examined, and cultures are done to identify bacteria.

Bacterial prostatitis is treated with appropriate antibiotics. Extended antibiotic therapy may be necessary (up to 4 months) to eradicate the infection. Nonbacterial prostatitis is treated symptomatically. Nonsteroidal anti-inflammatory drugs (NSAIDs) are useful for pain, and anticholinergics may reduce voiding symptoms.

Instruct clients with prostatitis to increase fluid intake to about 3 liters daily and to void often. Advise them to maintain

BOX 32-3
TEACHING FOR DISCHARGE

PROSTATE SURGERY

Activity

Healing requires 4 to 8 weeks. Avoid strenuous activity and heavy lifting. Do not drive for 2 weeks. Take long walks, but take stairs slowly and carefully. Continue leg exercises (dorsiflexing the foot) to prevent blood clots in the legs. You can take showers, but avoid tub baths while the catheter is in place.

Bleeding

Bleeding may occur after a bowel movement, coughing, or increased exercise. If you notice blood in the urine, increase fluids and rest until urine is clear. If you have clots or are unable to urinate, call your doctor immediately. Avoid aspirin and nonsteroidal anti-inflammatory drugs (NSAIDs) for at least 2 weeks.

Bowel Movements

Keep bowel movements regular and soft to avoid pressure on the prostate area. Drink fruit juices and take stool softeners as ordered.

Diet

Resume your normal diet. Increase fluids to ten 8-ounce glasses daily. Avoid alcohol unless otherwise advised by your physician.

Sexual Intercourse

Do not have sex for 6 weeks after surgery to avoid bleeding. You may still have erections even with the catheter in place. When you resume sex, ejaculate may flow back into the bladder, so you express little or no semen.

Urination

After the catheter is removed, you may experience some burning, stinging, or leakage for several weeks, and you may pass small blood clots occasionally. These symptoms disappear as the area heals. Use pads to control leakage.

Work

If work is not strenuous, you may return in 4 weeks. Otherwise, wait 6 to 8 weeks.

Contact your doctor immediately if:

- You are unable to urinate.
- Bleeding is excessive or is not controlled by fluids and rest.
- You have chills and fever or severe abdominal pain.
- Your scrotum becomes swollen and tender.
- You have pain in one calf, chest pain, or difficulty breathing.

BOX 32-4
MANIFESTATIONS OF PROSTATITIS

- Pain, burning on urination
- Frequency, urgency
- Chills, fever
- Low back, perineal, or genital pain
- Pain following ejaculation
- Obstructed urine flow

regular bowel habits. These measures help decrease pain with voiding and defecation. Local heat, such as sitz baths, may help relieve pain and irritation. Stress the importance of finishing the course of antibiotic therapy to effectively treat the infection. In nonbacterial prostatitis, frequent ejaculation may help decrease congestion of the gland.

Frank discussion with the client is important. It may help to explain nonbacterial prostatitis as a chronic inflammatory disorder, similar to arthritis. Address misconceptions about the disease with the client and his partner. Sexual intercourse is actually helpful, and men cannot "infect" their partners.

Cancer of the Prostate

Cancer of the prostate is the most common type of cancer in North American men and the second leading cause of cancer death, following lung cancer. It is primarily a disease of older men, increasing in incidence with age and rarely occurring before age 40. In addition to age, race is a significant risk factor for prostate cancer (Box 32-5). Other risk factors include a family history of the disease. Occupational exposure to certain chemicals, a diet high in animal fat, and high serum testosterone levels also may contribute to the risk.

When diagnosed early, prostate cancer is curable. When the cancer is confined to the prostate at diagnosis, the 5-year survival rate is 100%. Prostate cancers may grow slowly or aggressively.

population
FOCUS

BOX 32-5

Prostate Cancer

At all ages, African American men have a higher incidence of prostate cancer than European American men. African Americans also are more likely to die of prostate cancer, with a mortality rate more than double that of other racial and ethnic groups. Increasing awareness of the risk for prostate cancer and screening procedures is particularly important in populations of African American men. To improve care and reduce the risk for advanced prostate cancer, recommend that all African American men have a yearly DRE and serum PSA from age 40 on.

PATHOPHYSIOLOGY

Prostate cancer is usually an *adenocarcinoma,* arising from glandular epithelial cells. It usually begins in the peripheral, posterior tissue of the gland. As the tumor grows larger, it may compress the urethra, obstructing urine flow. The tumor may spread locally to involve the seminal vesicles or bladder. It rarely invades the bowel.

Tumor metastasis is common. The pelvic lymph nodes are the most frequently involved. Distant metastasis usually affect bony tissue, especially the pelvic bones and spinal column. Prostate cancer may also spread to the liver and lungs.

In the early stages, prostate cancer usually causes no symptoms. As the tumor grows and spreads, manifestations of urinary obstruction, metastasis, and general symptoms of the disease develop, described in Box 32-6.

Compression fractures of the spine are common, potentially causing loss of mobility and bowel and bladder function. Tumors may eventually involve bone marrow, resulting in severe anemias and impaired immune function.

COLLABORATIVE CARE

Because prostate cancer is curable when diagnosed early, screening measures for early detection are vital to control the disease. The American Cancer Society recommends annual DRE and serum PSA check after age 50. Men at high risk, including African American males and men with a strong family history of prostate cancer, should receive annual screening exams including DRE and serum PSA beginning at age 40.

Many treatment options are available for prostate cancer. Watchful waiting may be the treatment of choice if the tumor is slow growing and the client is elderly.

BOX 32-6
MANIFESTATIONS OF PROSTATE CANCER

GENITOURINARY
- Dysuria, hesitancy, reduced urinary stream
- Frequency, nocturia, hematuria
- Erectile dysfunction
- Hard, enlarged prostate on DRE

MUSCULOSKELETAL
- Bone or joint pain
- Back pain

NEUROLOGIC
- Lower extremity weakness
- Bowel or bladder dysfunction

SYSTEMIC
- Weight loss
- Anemia, fatigue

Diagnostic Tests

- *DRE* is done as a screening measure and when an enlarged prostate is suspected. The posterior surface of the gland can be palpated using a gloved finger inserted into the rectum (see Figure 32-1).
- *Serum PSA levels* are measured. PSA levels increase significantly in prostate cancer.
- *Transrectal ultrasonography (TRUS)* is used to help differentiate prostate cancer from BPH. An ultrasonic probe is inserted into the rectum to examine the prostate gland. This test is not painful.
- A *tissue biopsy* is done to establish the diagnosis of prostate cancer. Tissue is obtained by either needle biopsy or transrectal ultrasound-guided biopsy. See Box 32-7 for nursing care of the client undergoing a transrectal ultrasound-guided biopsy.
- *Bone scan, magnetic resonance imaging (MRI),* or *computed tomography (CT)* scans may be performed to identify possible tumor metastasis.

Hormone Therapy

Hormone therapy is used to treat advanced prostate cancer. Hormone therapy can be accomplished by removing the testes (**orchiectomy**) or by using drugs. Drugs that block the effects

---

BOX 32-7
NURSING CARE CHECKLIST

TRANSRECTAL ULTRASOUND-GUIDED BIOPSY OF THE PROSTATE

Before the Procedure

☑ Reinforce teaching. The client will remain awake; a local anesthetic will be used. The client will have a feeling of rectal fullness, which may be very uncomfortable. A sharp pain (a "pinch") may be felt as the biopsy is obtained.

☑ Instruct to avoid aspirin products and nonsteroidal anti-inflammatory agents for a week before the biopsy.

☑ An enema is usually given prior to the examination.

☑ This procedure requires a signed consent.

After the Procedure

☑ Monitor vital signs and urine output for an hour following the procedure.

☑ Instruct to avoid strenuous activity for the rest of the day.

☑ Hematuria and some bloody streaks in the stool are expected for 24 to 48 hours after the procedure. Ejaculate also may contain blood for up to 2 weeks.

☑ Report unusual bleeding, such as blood clots in urine, bloody stools, or signs of infection, such as rectal pain, dysuria, and urgency.

of testosterone and other androgens inhibit tumor growth but do not cure prostate cancer. In advanced prostate cancer, hormone therapy may improve length and quality of life. The disadvantage of hormone therapy is side effects such as loss of libido, **erectile dysfunction (ED)** *(impotence),* hot flashes, and **gynecomastia** (breast enlargement). The client who has had an orchiectomy may have body image problems due to losing the testicles.

Radiation Therapy

Radiation therapy may be used to treat prostate cancer, avoiding many of the adverse effects of prostate surgery, such as impotence and urinary incontinence. Radiation may be delivered either by external beam or implants of radioactive seeds *(brachytherapy).* (See Chapter 8 for nursing care of the client receiving radiation therapy.)

Radiation therapy also may be used to reduce the size of bone metastasis, control pain, and restore function in clients with advanced prostate cancer.

Surgery

Prostatectomy, surgical removal of the prostate gland, may be done to treat prostate cancer. In a *simple prostatectomy,* only the prostate tissue is removed. A *radical prostatectomy* involves removal of the prostate, prostatic capsule, seminal vesicles, and a portion of the bladder neck. Prostatectomy may be done by several different approaches. Table 32-1 ◆ outlines different types of prostatectomy procedures with their specific nursing implications.

Most clients have problems with urinary incontinence and erectile dysfunction following radical prostatectomy. To prevent or treat urinary incontinence, an artificial urinary sphincter may be surgically implanted (Figure 32-4 ◆). The client with an artificial urinary sphincter must be able to manipulate the pump in the scrotum and to recognize when a problem with the appliance occurs.

Cryosurgery is a possible treatment option. Guided by ultrasound, a cryoprobe is inserted into the tumor. Prostate tissue is destroyed by intermittent freezing and thawing. This surgical treatment is associated with a risk of bladder outlet injury, urinary incontinence, impotence, and rectal damage.

NURSING CARE

ASSESSING

In most cases, nursing assessment of a client with prostate cancer is done on admission to a facility for radiation therapy or surgery. Refer to Chapter 8 for assessment data to collect prior to radiation therapy. For the client undergoing prostate surgery, see Chapter 7 for pre- and postoperative assessment data to collect. In addition, inquire about the client's understanding of his disease and the planned treatment.

DIAGNOSING, PLANNING, AND IMPLEMENTING

IMPAIRED URINARY ELIMINATION (RISK FOR INCONTINENCE)

- Assess the degree of incontinence and its impact on lifestyle. *Knowledge of the amount and type of incontinence and its effect on the client's life is used to plan appropriate nursing interventions.*
- Teach pelvic muscle exercises (Kegel exercises), and help plan a regular schedule to perform the exercises. *Pelvic muscle exercises can improve urine retention in the client with stress incontinence.*
- Refer to physical therapy or a continence specialist for additional measures. *Exercises, restricting some types of fluids, and other measures such as bladder training can often improve continence.*
- Teach methods to control dampness and odor.
  a. Advise maintaining a liberal fluid intake, only limiting fluids after dinner. *Restricting fluids does not prevent incontinence, although it may prevent nighttime episodes. Fluid restriction causes more concentrated urine, increasing odor problems.*
  b. Suggest using absorbent pads worn inside the underwear and changed as needed. *Most pads help control odor and dampness, increasing comfort.*
- Explore options such as an external collection device (external catheter or Texas catheter) for total incontinence. *This device, which collects urine as it leaves the urinary meatus, may improve self-esteem and allow resumption of social activities.*
- Encourage expression of feelings about the impact of incontinence on quality of life. *Listening to these concerns with sensitivity can help the client work through feelings and adapt to the inability to remain continent.*

SEXUAL DYSFUNCTION

- Encourage discussion of sexual function between the client, his partner, and his physician. *Most older men are active sexually and fully capable of sustaining an erection. Some men may refuse therapy because they fear the effect of treatment on sexuality. Open discussion of concerns assists with decision making about treatment options.*
- Discuss various treatment options and their effects on sexual function. *The incidence of erectile dysfunction varies with different therapies for prostate cancer.*
- Encourage the client to discuss concerns about sexuality with a counselor or therapist. *A therapist or counselor may be able to suggest alternative ways for expressing sexuality.*

PAIN

- Assess intensity, location, and quality of pain. *Because most clients with prostate cancer are over age 65, many have pain from other conditions such as osteoarthritis. Careful assessment helps identify its cause and direct treatment.*
- Teach pain-control methods, including pharmacologic and nonpharmacologic measures. (See Chapters 6 and 8 for

TABLE 32-1   APPROACHES TO PROSTATECTOMY

ILLUSTRATION	DESCRIPTION	NURSING IMPLICATIONS
Retropubic prostatectomy Symphysis pubis Prostate Bladder Rectum	The prostate gland is removed through an abdominal incision; the bladder is left intact.	Assess abdominal incision for urine drainage (none should be present) and signs of infection, such as redness, increased or purulent drainage, poor healing. Report to charge nurse or physician.
Suprapubic prostatectomy	The prostate gland is removed through an abdominal incision into the bladder.	Assess urine output from suprapubic and urethral catheters. Assess abdominal dressing for urine drainage; change saturated dressings frequently. Consult with a skin care specialist if necessary. Following urethral catheter removal, clamp suprapubic catheter as ordered and encourage voiding. Assess residual urine by unclamping the catheter and measuring urine output after voiding.
Perineal prostatectomy	The prostate gland is removed through a perineal incision between the scrotum and anus.	Assess perineal incision for drainage and evidence of infection. Avoid rectal temperatures or enemas. Use a T-binder or padded scrotal support to hold dressing in place. Following dressing removal, heat lamps or sitz baths may be used to promote comfort and healing. Teach perineal irrigation as ordered and after bowel movements.

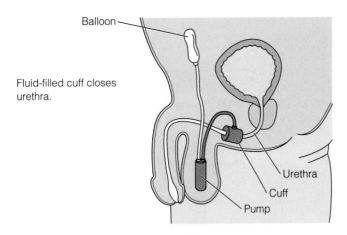

Balloon

Fluid-filled cuff closes
urethra.

Urethra

Cuff

Pump

To void, the pump is
squeezed, drawing fluid
from cuff to balloon. Urine
drains through open urethra.

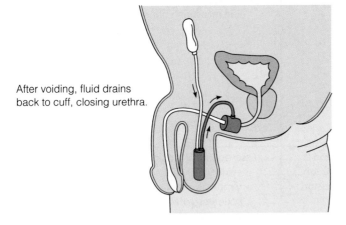

After voiding, fluid drains
back to cuff, closing urethra.

Figure 32-4. ◆ Operation of an artificial urinary sphincter.

more information about pain control in the client with cancer.) *Adequate pain management enhances quality of life and
allows the client to remain active.*

EVALUATING

To evaluate the effectiveness of nursing interventions for the
client with prostate cancer, collect data such as the following:

- Ability to control urination and remain continent
- If incontinent, ability to control odor and dampness; main-
  tain social activities
- Willingness to discuss sexuality and consider the effects of
  treatment on sexuality
- Pain level on a standard pain scale

See the Critical Thinking Care Map on caring for a client
with prostate cancer at the end of this chapter.

Discharge Considerations

Clients with prostate cancer face both the diagnosis of cancer
and a number of treatment options. The client and family
must deal with often conflicting advice from the urologist,
medical and radiation oncologists, friends, the media, and
advocate groups. Provide accurate information about available
treatments and their effects. Encourage discussion of concerns.
Provide information about prostate cancer support groups (if
available). Men struggling with treatment choices may learn
about the options from men who have experience.

Emphasize the importance of keeping appointments for
treatment and follow-up. Following treatment, yearly DRE
and PSA levels are done. Discuss early warning signs of metastasis to the spinal column, such as intermittent back pain that
is aggravated by activity. Other symptoms include leg weakness. Provide verbal and written instructions about prescribed
medications, including their purpose, dose, timing, and
expected and unintended effects.

If surgery has been done, provide postoperative instructions about catheter and dressing care, diet, activity resumption, and possible complications. Include family and significant others in teaching.

Provide information to all male clients about the importance of screening tests to detect prostate cancer early. The
American Cancer Society has free pamphlets about early detection of prostate cancer.

Disorders of the Testes and Scrotum

Structural and Inflammatory Disorders

CRYPTORCHIDISM

Cryptorchidism is failure of one or both testes to descend through the inguinal ring into the scrotum. In most cases, the testes descend without intervention in the first year of life. Cryptorchidism is primarily a childhood problem, although on rare occasions it is missed and discovered later in adolescent or adult life. When the problem continues into adolescence and adulthood, cryptorchidism increases the risk for testicular cancer and problems of fertility. Men who have a history of cryptochidism should be especially vigilant about testicular self-examination. Teach the client how to perform testicular self-examination (see Box 32-8 on page 897). Emphasize the importance of regular exams, and discuss findings that should be reported to the physician.

TESTICULAR TORSION

Testicular torsion, or twisting of the testes and spermatic cord, is a potential medical emergency. Boys and young men up to age 20 are at greatest risk for testicular torsion. Its cause is unclear, although elevated hormone levels and abnormal attachment of the testicles to the scrotum may contribute. Trauma to the scrotum may precipitate the condition in clients who are already predisposed.

Testicular torsion causes acute scrotal pain with a sudden onset. Nausea and vomiting frequently occur. The *cremasteric reflex* (retraction of the testicles when the skin on the inside of the thigh is stroked) may be depressed or absent.

Diagnostic studies such as testicular scanning may be used to evaluate blood flow to the testicle. Emergency surgery is done to relieve testicular and spermatic cord twisting and to fix the testicle within the scrotum. Impaired blood flow to the testicle can lead to testicular ischemia and necrosis. If the testicle is necrotic or severely damaged, it will be removed.

An episode of torsion is frightening for the adolescent male. He is usually very embarrassed by the problem and may imagine that early sexual activity or even fantasies that result in erections are responsible. Because adolescents are not likely to volunteer these concerns, the nurse should provide information to relieve some of these anxieties. Postoperative nursing care is similar to that for clients with scrotal surgeries, discussed below in the section on testicular cancer.

EPIDIDYMITIS

Epididymitis is inflammation of the epididymis. It is usually caused by an infection spread from the bladder, urethra, prostate gland, or seminal vesicles. In younger men, the cause is often a sexually transmitted organism such as *Chlamydia trachomatis* or *N. gonorrhoeae.* In older men, epididymitis usually is associated with a urinary tract infection or prostatitis. Early manifestations include pain and local swelling; the scrotum may swell to the extent that it interferes with walking. Fever and general malaise also may develop. Sterility is a potential complication of epididymitis. Antibiotics are prescribed to treat epididymitis. Nursing care focuses on relieving symptoms of the disorder. Ice packs may be applied to the scrotum to relieve pain. A scrotal support is usually applied. Discuss the possibility of infertility. The client may wish to seek evaluation for this problem at a later date.

ORCHITIS

Orchitis is inflammation of the testicle. It is commonly caused by an infection from other parts of the genitourinary tract. It also can occur as a complication of mumps; the mumps virus is excreted in the urine. Adult men with mumps are at highest risk for this complication. Trauma, including vasectomy and other scrotal surgeries, may cause inflammation of the testes. Manifestations of orchitis include severe testicular pain and swelling. Possible complications include hydrocele and abscess. These can lead to infertility or impotence. Bacterial orchitis is treated with antibiotics. Treatment for viral orchitis may be symptomatic. An abscess may require surgical drainage or orchiectomy. Nursing care is very similar to that of the client with epididymitis and other scrotal disorders.

Infertility

Infertility is the inability to conceive a child during a year or more of unprotected intercourse. *Sterility* is the absolute inability to conceive. When the sperm count drops below 20 million/mL, the client is likely to be infertile. Male infertility usually results from a testicular disorder, such as cryptorchism or orchitis. Less often, it may be caused by a systemic disease, hormonal disorder, or obstructed outflow of sperm from the testes. In many cases, no specific cause can be found for the infertility.

A sperm count is obtained to evaluate infertility in men. If an identifiable cause such as an endocrine disorder or varicocele (see next section) can be identified and treated, this may restore fertility. In many cases of male infertility, it is appropriate to counsel the client about options such as using a sperm donor or adopting a child.

Nursing care for the infertile male client focuses on providing information and psychologic support for the man and his partner.

Scrotal Masses and Trauma

Scrotal masses such as hydroceles, spermatoceles, and varicoceles (Figure 32-5 ◆) usually are benign and treatable.

SCROTAL MASSES

A *hydrocele* is a collection of fluid in the sac that encloses the testes. The cause is not always identifiable, but it may follow

Fluid-filled
mass in
scrotum

Hydrocele

Cystic
mass on
epididymis

Spermatocele

Dilation of
pampiniform
venous
complex

Varicocele

Figure 32-5. ◆ Common disorders of the scrotum

epididymitis, orchitis, injury, or a tumor. Scrotal enlargement may be the only manifestation of hydrocele, although it may cause pain or a tight sensation in the scrotum. Hydrocele is diagnosed by transillumination or ultrasound of the scrotum. Treatment is usually not necessary. If the hydrocele causes embarrassment or significant pain, a hydrocelectomy may be performed.

A *spermatocele* is a mobile, usually painless mass in the epididymis that contains dead sperm cells. The cause is thought to be leakage of sperm due to trauma or infection. Treatment is usually not necessary.

A *varicocele* is abnormal dilation of the spermatic veins above the testis. It is caused by incompetent or absent valves in the veins and almost always occurs on the left side. The dilated veins form a soft mass (often described as a "bag of worms") that can cause dull pain in the scrotum. This condition can decrease the sperm count and cause atrophy of the testicle, resulting in infertility. Varicoceles are usually treated, especially in younger clients.

SCROTAL TRAUMA

Scrotal trauma is usually minor, resulting in temporary hematomas caused by minor crushing or straddle-type injuries. More severe crush injuries can rupture the testicles. Occasionally, the client's clothing and scrotal skin can be trapped in moving machinery, resulting in avulsion injuries. Such an accident can tear the skin away from the penis and scrotum, sometimes releasing scrotal contents. Penetrating injuries of the scrotum due to knife or gunshot wounds also can occur. Treatment of scrotal trauma varies, depending on the extent of damage and the type of scrotal damage involved.

VASECTOMY-RELATED PROBLEMS

The most common surgery of the scrotum is **vasectomy**, a sterilization procedure in which a portion of the spermatic cord is removed. This surgery rarely causes long-term complications. However, some clients develop scar tissue that causes chronic pain. Other complications include chronic testicular pain and epididymal obstruction.

NURSING CARE

Obtain assessment data such as the following from clients who have a history of scrotal trauma, surgery, or who complain about scrotal swelling or pain:

- Ask about the onset, duration, and severity of symptoms.
- Inspect the scrotum for swelling, redness, and bruising or discoloration. Using a gloved hand, gently palpate each testis and epididymis for tenderness, warmth, or masses.

Teach the client with a scrotal disorder about the disorder and its treatment. If surgery is planned, discuss the client's fears about the surgery, pain management, and measures to reduce bleeding (see the section on testicular cancer that follows). Postoperatively, observe for swelling and discoloration of the scrotum. Report excessive swelling or discoloration to the physician, as this could indicate excessive bleeding. Discuss the possible effects of surgery on fertility, and actively listen to the client's concerns.

Testicular Cancer

Testicular cancer is the most common cancer in men between the ages of 15 and 35. Fortunately, it is one of the most treatable cancers, with a cure rate of greater than 90%.

Although its cause is unknown, risk factors for testicular cancer include the following:

- Age: Testicular cancer usually develops between ages 15 and 40, but may occur at any age.
- Cryptorchidism (undescended testicle)
- Family history
- Race and ethnicity: Men living in the United States, United Kingdom, and Scandinavia have a higher risk of developing testicular cancer than African and Asian men.

Unfortunately, most men who develop testicular cancer have no risk factors. Therefore, beginning at the age of 15, all men should perform monthly testicular self-examination (Box 32-8).

PATHOPHYSIOLOGY

Testicular cancer grows within the testicle, eventually replacing most of the normal tissue. Usually only one testicle is affected. Local spread is limited, but it often spreads rapidly through lymph and blood vessels to other organs. Spread by lymph vessels usually causes disease in retroperitoneal lymph nodes. Dissemination of the disease through the vascular system can lead to metastasis in the lungs, bone, or liver. The classic presenting symptom of testicular cancer is a painless hard nodule. Occasionally, the client may have a dull ache in the pelvis or scrotum. Acute pain related to the tumor is rare.

COLLABORATIVE CARE

Care focuses on diagnosing and eliminating the cancer and preventing or treating metastasis. Treatment depends on the stage of the cancer at diagnosis: Stage I is confined to the testicle; stage II includes regional lymph node involvement; in stage III, distant metastasis are present.

When testicular cancer is suspected, blood is drawn to identify tumor markers such as *alpha-fetoprotein (AFP), human chorionic gonadotropin (HCG), alkaline phosphatase,* and *lactic dehydrogenase (LDH).* Elevated levels indicate probable testicular cancer. These markers are also measured after surgery to help monitor the effectiveness of treatment.

An *ultrasound of the testicle* is performed to rule out other causes of the mass. *CT scans* are done to detect possible metastasis to the lungs or abdominal organs. Biopsy is often done at the time of surgery.

Pharmacology

Stage III testicular cancer is treated with a combination of surgery and chemotherapy. A combination of chemotherapy drugs is used. (See Chapter 8 for more information about chemotherapy for cancer and management of chemotherapy side effects.)

Surgery

Surgery to remove the affected testicle and spermatic cord (called a *radical orchiectomy*) is the primary treatment for early testicular cancer. This operation is performed through an incision in the inguinal area. Lymph nodes in the retroperitoneal area may also be removed, taking care to preserve the nerves necessary for ejaculation.

Radiation Therapy

Following surgery, radiation therapy is used to treat cancer in the retroperitoneal lymph nodes, the most frequent site of metastasis. The client may experience temporary diarrhea, nausea, or decreased bone marrow function. These problems are usually mild. (See Chapter 8 for more information about nursing care related to radiation therapy.)

NURSING CARE

ASSESSING

Nurses can be instrumental in identifying testicular cancer at an early, treatable stage. Ask men if they have noticed any

---

BOX 32-8
TESTICULAR SELF-EXAMINATION

- Examine your testicles during or just after a warm shower or bath. Soap on your hands and scrotum allows easy manipulation of tissue.
- Gently roll each testicle between your thumb and fingers. The testicles normally feel smooth, rounded, walnut-sized, and freely movable.

- If one testicle is significantly larger than the other, or if you feel any hard lumps, contact your health care provider immediately.
- Examine your testicles on the same day of each month (e.g., the first day of the month) to help you remember.

change in the size of their testicles. In some cases, the client's partner may notice a change in the size or feel of one testicle compared to the other. Palpate the scrotum and testicles, noting any difference in size or changes for the normal. Promptly report to the physician a testicle that is hard, irregular in shape, or is fixed (not movable within the scrotum).

DIAGNOSING, PLANNING, AND IMPLEMENTING

The client with an orchiectomy often is discharged on the day of surgery. Nursing care focuses on teaching and psychologic support.

DEFICIENT KNOWLEDGE

- Discuss using analgesics, ice bags, and a scrotal support to reduce postoperative pain. *Ice provides local analgesia and helps reduce scrotal swelling. A scrotal support is particularly helpful when the client ambulates. See Chapter 7 for routine pre- and postoperative care and teaching.*
- Instruct to contact the physician if complications develop: the incision gaps open, bleeding beyond slight oozing after 24 hours, or rapid scrotal swelling. *Because the client is usually discharged early, complications may not develop until after discharge.*

RISK FOR SEXUAL DYSFUNCTION

- Assess current sexual function. To do this, establish an atmosphere of openness and permission to discuss sexual concerns. *After the initial shock of the diagnosis, clients often have intense concerns about sexual and reproductive issues, which can be relieved only by information.*
- Help the client express his concerns about altered sexual function and appearance. *The ability to express sexuality and father children is a basic human need. The client may fear the loss of this ability, and will grieve its loss if treatment affects it.*
- Reinforce teaching about the expected effect of surgery on sexuality. Reassure that erectile and climactic function is rarely affected by testicular cancer and treatment. *If the treatment involves only an orchiectomy, there should be no lasting effects on sexual or reproductive function.*

- Discuss the option of preserving sperm in a bank prior to treatment. *This option may help relieve fears about the ability to father children in the future. Sperm banking must be done prior to treatment with surgery, chemotherapy, or radiation therapy.*

EVALUATING

To evaluate the effectiveness of nursing care for clients with testicular cancer, collect data such as the following:

- Ability to demonstrate and relate the importance of regular testicular self-examination
- Understanding of ways to reduce pain and swelling after surgery
- Knowledge of manifestations of complications and when to contact the physician
- Willingness to discuss or ask questions about effect of treatment on sexuality and reproduction

Discharge Considerations

Teach all young men how to perform testicular self-examination and stress the importance of establishing a routine. Shower cards that demonstrate testicular self-exam on one side and breast self-exam on the other are available through the American Cancer Society. These cards are a useful reminder.

Include families in teaching for the client with testicular cancer. If the client is sexually active, his partner needs information about the effects of treatment on sexuality and reproduction. If the client is a teenager, his parents often are involved in postoperative care. The client facing cancer needs the support of knowledgeable loved ones.

Teach postoperative care, including incision care, using ice and a scrotal support, and signs and symptoms of complications to report to the physician.

Discuss the need for continuing follow-up after treatment for testicular cancer. Surveillance includes periodic physical examinations, chest x-rays, tumor markers, and CT scans of retroperitoneal nodes for 5 to 10 years after orchiectomy.

Disorders of the Penis

Phimosis

Phimosis is constriction of the foreskin so that it cannot be pushed back over the glans penis. It may be congenital or may

follow infection or injury. Phimosis increases the risk of secondary infections, scarring, and perhaps cancer of the penis. Severe phimosis can interfere with urination. If the foreskin is forcibly retracted behind the glans, it may become trapped, impairing blood flow to the glans. Circumcision (removal of the foreskin) may be necessary to correct the condition. Teach clients and parents about the importance of hygiene measures to prevent infection and possible phimosis. Teach clients with phimosis to perform self-examination for cancer of the penis.

Priapism

Priapism is a sustained, painful erection that is not associated with sexual arousal. It is caused by impaired blood flow in the corpora cavernosa of the penis. Priapism may be idiopathic or be secondary to certain conditions or drugs (Box 32-9). The sustained erection of priapism often is painful and harder than normal. If the condition continues, there is a risk of tissue damage and impotence.

Initial treatment of priapism includes analgesia, sedation, and fluids. In clients with sickle cell disease, transfusion and oxygen are provided. Ice packs to the perineum may provide relief. If other measures are ineffective, surgery may be done to temporarily drain blood out of the penis.

Inspect the penis for degree of erection and color; palpate its firmness and degree of rigidity. Monitor urine output. Report oliguria or signs of acute urinary retention. Provide analgesics as ordered to manage pain. Address the client's anxiety about the condition, pain, treatment, and the threat to sexual function. Reassure the client that potency usually is maintained after surgical shunting. The client may be acutely embarrassed by the erection; address his concerns and reassure him that the erection is not within his control.

Cancer of the Penis

Cancer of the penis is rare in North America. Older men are most often affected. Its cause is uncertain. Phimosis, tightening of the foreskin that prevents retraction over the glans, is a significant risk factor. Penile cancer also is linked to viral infections, human papillomavirus (HPV) in particular. Other risk factors include exposure to ultraviolet (UV) light, unprotected sex with multiple partners, and cigarette smoking.

BOX 32-9
RISK FACTORS FOR PRIAPISM

ILLNESSES/CONDITIONS
- Sickle cell disease
- Leukemia
- Metastatic cancer
- Spinal cord trauma

DRUGS
- Papaverine
- Psychotropic drugs
- Alcohol
- Marijuana

PATHOPHYSIOLOGY

Squamous cell carcinoma accounts for 95% of all penile cancers. The tumor usually develops as a nodular or wartlike growth or a red velvety lesion on the glans or foreskin. The tumors tend to grow slowly. Penile cancer spreads to regional lymph nodes, and very late in the disease may spread to the bone, liver, or lungs. If the lesion is treated before nodes are involved, chances for a cure are good. Manifestations include a mass or persistent sore or ulcer at the distal end of the penis, involving the glans or foreskin. Most of these lesions are painless; however, they may ulcerate and bleed. Purulent, foul-smelling discharge may be noted under the foreskin.

COLLABORATIVE CARE

Cancer of the penis is diagnosed by biopsy of the lesion and any suspicious lymph nodes. Small, localized lesions may be treated with a topical chemotherapy drug, external-beam radiation, laser, or surgical excision. The penis may be partially or totally amputated if the cancer has spread into deeper structures. If a total *penectomy* is done, a perineal urethrostomy is created to preserve urinary continence. Clients with distant metastasis may be treated with chemotherapy.

NURSING CARE

When providing routine care, observe the penis for any visible lesions. If a lesion is noted, promptly report it to the physician. Following surgery, monitor the surgical site for healing and any signs of infection. Carefully monitor intake and output, and provide routine postoperative care. Inform the client that dribbling after voiding may occur for several weeks following surgery. Teach perineal care to reduce the risk of skin irritation and breakdown. Sitz baths may help relieve pain and promote healing. Carefully listen to concerns, being aware of the effect of a penectomy on body image, self-concept, and sexuality.

Discharge Considerations

To help prevent cancer of the penis, teach clients about the risks of unprotected sex, and encourage condom use. Inform clients about the possible link between UV rays and penile cancer, and encourage men to shield their genitals when sunbathing or using tanning salons. Discuss the importance of seeking prompt treatment for any lesion or abnormal drainage noted on the penis.

Erectile Dysfunction

Erectile dysfunction (ED) or **impotence** is the inability to attain and maintain an erection that allows satisfactory sexual intercourse. An estimated 10 to 15 million men in the United States have ED. Most are older than 65. This problem may involve total inability to achieve erection, an inconsistent ability to achieve erection, or the ability to sustain only brief erections.

There are many possible causes of ED, including many chronic diseases such as diabetes and atherosclerosis, and many drugs. In most men, the cause of ED is primarily physiologic. Psychological factors often contribute and are believed to cause 10% to 20% of cases of ED.

PATHOPHYSIOLOGY

A number physiologic mechanisms work together to cause an erection. For an erection to occur, the blood supply to the penis must be adequate, normal nervous system and hormonal actions are necessary, and appropriate psychological and social responses need to occur. Interruption of any of these factors and certain drugs can lead to impotence.

Atherosclerosis can interfere with the arterial blood supply to the penis. Surgeries such as radical prostatectomy or chronic diseases such as diabetes or multiple sclerosis can disrupt innervation. Decreased testosterone levels also can lead to erectile dysfunction. Many drugs, including antihypertensive medications, psychotropic drugs, hormones, and others, disrupt the normal mechanisms to achieve erection, leading to impotence.

COLLABORATIVE CARE

ED often can be effectively managed using drugs, mechanical devices, or surgery.

Diagnostic Tests

Diagnostic tests are done to help identify the cause of the problem.

■ *Blood tests* such as a chemistry profile and testosterone, prolactin, thyroxine, and PSA levels, are done to identify systemic disorders that may be causing the dysfunction.
■ *Nocturnal penile tumescence and rigidity (NPTR)* monitors erections that occur during rapid eye movement (REM)

sleep. This test may be done in a sleep laboratory or at home with a portable device.
■ *Cavernosometry* and *cavernosography* evaluate blood flow to and from the penis.

Pharmacology

Erectile dysfunction can be treated with drugs that work in a variety of ways. Sildenafil (Viagra) for ED was approved for use in 1998. Sildenafil does not directly cause an erection but enhances the natural response to sexual stimuli. At recommended doses, no effect occurs in the absence of sexual stimulation. Table 32-2 ◆ discusses nursing implications for this drug. Testosterone replacement also may be ordered for men with ED. Aldostadil (prostaglandin E_1) can be administered by inserting a semisolid pellet into the urethra or by direct injection into the penis. This drug stimulates an erection, but many men discontinue treatment because of the mode of delivery or dissatisfaction with lack of spontaneity. Transdermal nitroglycerin paste applied directly to the penis is another option to promote blood flow and erection.

Mechanical Devices

Men who cannot take sildenafil may use a *vacuum constriction device (VCD)* that draws blood into the penis with a vacuum, trapping it there with a constricting band at the base of the penis. This device, however, is cumbersome and may be an unacceptable option for many men.

Surgery

When ED does not respond to less invasive methods of treatment, a semirigid or inflatable prosthesis may be implanted (Figure 32-6 ◆). Clients are generally satisfied with the results of a penile implant. Partners are also more likely to report satisfaction, although the more firm erection can cause pain or prolong the duration of intercourse for an unacceptable period. Client and partner teaching is mandatory. Counseling

TABLE 32-2   NURSING IMPLICATIONS FOR PHARMACOLOGY: CLIENTS RECEIVING SILDENAFIL (VIAGRA)

DRUG/CLASS	ACTION	NURSING IMPLICATIONS	CLIENT AND FAMILY TEACHING
Sildenafil (Viagra)	Sildenafil is used to treat erectile dysfunction in men. Sildenafil works together with nitric oxide and an enzyme released during sexual stimulation to increase the firmness and duration of an erection. It may be taken once a day, about 1 hour before sexual activity.	Contraindicated for men taking any form of nitrate drug (including recreational nitrates); combination can cause significant hypotension. Relatively contraindicated for men who have cardiovascular disease. May cause priapism, especially in men with other risk factors. Approved only for use in men.	Take approximately 1 hour before sexual activity. Drug effect may diminish after 2 hours; do not take more than once a day. If you have high blood pressure or cardiovascular disease, check with your doctor before taking. Promptly report erection that lasts more than 4 hours, chest pain, or shortness of breath.

A Semirigid

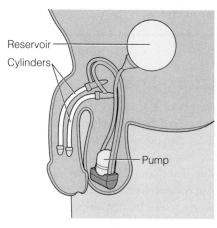

Reservoir
Cylinders

Pump

B Inflatable

Figure 32-6. ◆ Types of penile implants. (A) Semirigid rods implanted in the corpora cavernosa keep the penis in a constant state of semierection. (B) With an inflatable penile implant, the client compresses a pump in the scrotum to fill cylinders in the corpora cavernosa and achieve an erection. Pressing a release valve returns the fluid to a reservoir.

by a sex therapist may be needed to facilitate adaptation to the implant.

NURSING CARE

ASSESSING

Problems with erectile dysfunction often are revealed in the course of a health assessment interview. Ask about chronic diseases such as diabetes and thyroid conditions, hypertension and other cardiovascular disease, kidney failure, and neurologic conditions. Inquire about medications such as antihypertensive drugs (which often cause ED), antidepressants, tranquilizers, and sedatives. Explore psychosocial stressors that may contribute to ED. Discuss lifestyle and use of alcohol or street drugs. Finally, ask specific questions about sexual function, including a history of premature ejaculation, impotence, or other sexual problems.

DIAGNOSING, PLANNING, AND IMPLEMENTING

SEXUAL DYSFUNCTION

- Assess for risk factors such as a new medication or recent surgery. *Although most older men have at least one risk factor for ED, identifying specific risk factors can help focus treatment strategies.*
- Ask specific questions about sexual function and current sexual practices. *Men with ED and their partners often live in isolation with the problem for many years. The partner may be unaware of the problem or may believe the client has lost his attraction to the partner. The client may keep his problem secret because of an intense feeling of shame. Many clients greet the information about the high incidence of ED with a sense of relief that they are not alone.*
- Discuss previous methods of coping with ED. *Current coping strategies provide insight into the problem and help guide teaching.*
- Provide information about treatment options. *Information provides hope for successful resolution of the problem and helps the client and his partner identify acceptable treatment options.*
- Refer the client and his partner for counseling. *Although ED is primarily a physiologic problem, many clients benefit from counseling to address psychologic issues of ED.*

EVALUATING

To evaluate the effectiveness of nursing care for a client with erectile dysfunction, collect data such as the following:

- Willingness to discuss sexual function with a health care professional
- Willingness to share concerns with partner
- Knowledge of medical and surgical treatment options, their risks and benefits

Discharge Considerations

To reduce the risk of ED, advise clients to remain physically active, consume a low-fat diet, and avoid cigarette smoking and excess alcohol intake. Discuss the potential effects of high-risk medications on sexual function with clients during teaching. Provide information about various treatment options for ED, including their cost, intended benefit, and potential risks or drawbacks of each option. Stress the importance of contacting the primary care provider before taking any prescription or over-the-counter drug to treat ED. Encourage partners to be involved in the treatment plan.

Nursing Process Case Study
■ CLIENT WITH ERECTILE DYSFUNCTION

Donald Lawton, 68 years old, has been married for 40 years. At age 52, he was diagnosed with type 2 diabetes mellitus. He has had stable angina controlled with sublingual nitroglycerin for the past 5 years. Two years ago, he noticed that his erections were not as rigid as normal. Gradually, the problem has worsened until he can no longer attain an erection adequate for sexual intercourse. His libido remains unaffected. He relates shame and embarrassment, and is unable to discuss this problem with anyone, including his wife.

Assessment   Mr. Lawton talks to his doctor after his wife threatens to leave him, claiming neglect. He is referred to a urologist. Mr. Lawton says he values his relationship with his wife and that sexual intimacy has been important to them. He says their sexual activity has always been limited to foreplay and sexual intercourse, expressing mild distaste about other forms of sexual intimacy. He reports feeling as if he is no longer a man and that he is ashamed that he can no longer satisfy his wife. This has affected their entire relationship and communications.

Mr. Lawton's serum testosterone levels are normal. Nocturnal penile tumescence and rigidity monitoring in the sleep laboratory reveal an absence of erections during REM sleep. The urologist suggests a VCD and couples counseling.

Diagnosis   The following nursing diagnoses are identified for Mr. Lawton:

■ Sexual Dysfunction related to diabetes
■ Ineffective Sexuality Patterns related to lack of knowledge and poor communication patterns with wife
■ Disturbed Body Image related to change in erectile function

Expected Outcomes   The expected outcomes for the plan of care are that Mr. Lawton will:

■ Demonstrate the ability to discuss sexual concerns with his wife.
■ State acceptance of the change in his erectile function.
■ Demonstrate use of a VCD.

Planning and Implementation   The following interventions are planned and implemented for Mr. Lawton:

■ With permission, include his wife in discussions and teaching sessions.
■ Encourage couples counseling.
■ Listen to concerns about ED, and encourage communication.
■ Teach use of the VCD.

Evaluation   Mr. Lawton begins to discuss his sexual and relationship problems more freely. He and Mrs. Lawton begin to attend counseling. Mrs. Lawton states that she was afraid her husband no longer found her attractive and that he had found another woman. She greets the knowledge of the true nature of the problem with relief and concern. Privately, Mr. Lawton tells the nurse that he feels his marriage is improving and that even though "things" will never be the same, he is beginning

to look forward to some mutual exploration. Mr. Lawton masters the VCD with little difficulty, and 4 months later reports that he and his wife are "90% satisfied with the result."

 Critical Thinking in the Nursing Process

1. Mr. Lawton's ED was directly related to his diabetes. Describe the pathophysiology of diabetes-induced ED (see Chapter 17).
2. How does the nocturnal penile tumescence and rigidity test differentiate between physiologic and psychological causes of ED?
3. Discuss the importance of Mr. and Mrs. Lawton's lack of communication on the development of their sexual problems. Include possible reasons for their difficulty in discussing sexual concerns.

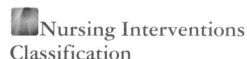Ejaculatory Dysfunction

There are many types of ejaculatory dysfunction. *Premature ejaculation* is often caused by psychological factors; diabetes also can cause premature ejaculation. *Delayed ejaculation* may be related to aging changes, such as decreased penile sensation or decreased libido. Ejaculation also can be affected by drugs to treat hypertension, depression, anxiety, and narcotic medications. *Retrograde ejaculation* (semen discharged into the bladder rather than through the urethra) is usually related to treatment of prostate disorders or testicular cancer.

Medical and nursing care for clients with ejaculatory problems focuses on assessing the problem and client teaching. Of these problems, premature ejaculation is most easily treated. Wearing a condom and techniques such as relaxation and guided imagery can delay sexual excitement and ejaculation. The client's partner can be taught how to avoid excessive stimulation until ejaculation. If the problem persists, referral to a specialist is appropriate.

Nursing Interventions Classification

The following selected nursing interventions may also be useful for male clients with reproductive problems (McCloskey & Bulechek, 2000):

■ Bladder Irrigation
■ Pelvic Floor Exercise
■ Teaching: Disease Process
■ Teaching: Procedure/Treatment
■ Tube Care: Urinary
■ Urinary Elimination Management

(*Note:* The bibliography listings for this and all chapters have been compiled at the back of the book.)

Chapter Review

key terms by topic

Use the CD-ROM disk enclosed with your textbook to hear the pronunciation of the key terms in the chapter.

Structure and function
androgens, libido, ejaculation

Prostate disorders
benign prostatic hyperplasia (BPH), orchiectomy, erectile dysfunction (ED), gynecomastia, prostatectomy

Disorders of testes and scrotum
infertility, vasectomy

Disorders of the penis
impotence

key points

- Prostate problems such as benign prostatic hyperplasia (BPH) and prostate cancer are the most common problems affecting the male reproductive system, especially in older adults.

- The manifestations of BPH and prostate cancer are similar: frequency, urgency, hesitency, a reduced urine stream, and nocturia. Physical examination and diagnostic testing are necessary to differentiate these disorders.

- In both BPH and prostate cancer, medications or "watchful waiting" may be appropriate treatment; surgery, however, is often the treatment of choice. Minimally invasive procedures such as balloon dilation, laser prostatectomy, or transurethral incision of the prostate (TUIP) may be used to treat BPH. Prostate cancer, on the other hand, is treated with a prostatectomy.

- Following a prostatectomy, the client is at risk for deep vein thrombophlebitis (DVT) and pulmonary embolism. Preventive measures such as leg exercises, elastic hose, pneumatic compression devices, and early ambulation are important to prevent these complications.

- Although testicular cancer is rare, its risk is highest in young men (15 to 35 years old). Teach all young men to perform testicular self-examination and stress the importance of doing it on a regular basis.

- Most clients with erectile dysfunction can be effectively treated with medication or an implanted prosthetic device.

Medialink

Additional interactive resources for this chapter can be found on the Companion Website at www.prenhall.com/burke. Click on Chapter 32 and "Begin" to select the activities for this chapter.

For NCLEX review questions and an audio glossary, access the accompanying CD-ROM in this book.

for further study

For more information about radiation therapy in the client with cancer, see Chapter 8.

For in-depth discussion of kidney function, see Chapter 21. For Kegel exercises, see Box 21-4.

Critical Thinking Care Map

Caring for a Client with Prostate Cancer
NCLEX-PN Focus Area: Safety and Infection Control

Case Study: William Turner is a 71-year-old African American man. He lives at home with his wife, who had a stroke two years ago. Mr. Turner has been in good health except for a "touch" of osteoarthritis in his hips and hands. He reports a gradual onset of urinary urgency over the past 2 years. During a routine physical examination, a hard nodule is palpated on his prostate gland, and his PSA level is found to be elevated. A radical retropubic prostatectomy is performed. He is discharged home several days later with an indwelling catheter in place. The home health nurse visits Mr. Turner 2 days after his discharge.

Nursing Diagnosis: Ineffective Health Maintenance

COLLECT DATA

Subjective	Objective
_____	_____
_____	_____
_____	_____
_____	_____
_____	_____
_____	_____

Would you report this data? Yes/No

If yes, to: _____

Nursing Care

_____
_____
_____
_____
_____
_____
_____
_____

How would you document this? _____
_____
_____

Data Collected
(use those that apply)

- History of osteoarthritis in hands and hips
- Home clean and neat
- Fully dressed, carrying large night urinary drainage bag
- Relates difficulty getting out of house to buy groceries due to embarrassment of being seen with drainage bag
- Reports inability to change from large drainage bag to leg bag due to arthritis
- VS within normal limits
- Pelvic incision healing well with no evidence of infection
- Lung sounds clear
- Urine pale yellow, not malodorous
- Uncertain about whether to continue pelvic muscle and dorsiflexion exercises at home
- Questions need for follow-up visits now that his cancer is cured

Nursing Interventions
(use those that apply)

- Discuss the possibility of stress incontinence after the catheter is removed.
- Reinforce the need for perineal muscle exercises while the catheter is still in place.
- Explore available support systems to identify people to assist with catheter care.
- Provide teaching for Mr. Turner and care assistants as appropriate.
- Discuss potential postoperative complications.
- Reinforce the importance of follow-up care to monitor the disease and healing.

NCLEX-PN Exam Preparation

TEST-TAKING TIP

When a question asks what you would do first, remember your priority-setting devices. Maslow's Hierarchy of Needs puts physiologic needs before psychological needs. Nursing process tells us to assess before we intervene. The ABCs guide us always to establish an airway first.

1. A common consequence following transurethral prostatectomy is:
   a. nocturia
   b. impotence
   c. decreased libido
   d. retrograde ejaculation

2. Following TURP surgery, bladder irrigation is done to:
   a. promote bladder tone
   b. clear blood clots and reduce spasms
   c. reduce the sensation to void
   d. prevent hyponatremia

3. A client is about to be discharged following TURP. What statement tells you he needs additional instruction?
   a. "It is okay to continue taking one regular daily aspirin for my heart."
   b. "It is all right to take showers even while the catheter is in place."
   c. "I should not have sex for 6 weeks."
   d. "I need to drink ten 8-ounce glasses of fluids a day."

4. Your client is 1 day postoperative from a TURP. Which complaint would you address first?
   a. pain
   b. leakage around the irrigation catheter
   c. blood clots in the fluid from the bladder irrigation
   d. pain in one calf and dyspnea

5. The client with nonbacterial prostatitis should be advised to:
   a. restrict fluids to avoid painful voiding
   b. have frequent sex
   c. wear a condom to avoid infecting their partner
   d. finish the antibiotic therapy

6. The most frequent cause of death in men in the United States is:
   a. lung cancer
   b. prostate cancer
   c. heart disease
   d. trauma

7. Removal of the testes (orchiectomy) may be used to treat:
   a. prostate cancer
   b. gynecomastia
   c. cryptorchidism
   d. penile cancer

8. Which of the following is an accurate statement regarding sildenafil (Viagra)?
   a. Sildenafil is helpful in patients who have cardiovascular disease.
   b. Sildenafil works better when combined with a nitrate drug.
   c. Sildenafil may cause priapism.
   d. Sildenafil is taken b.i.d. on an empty stomach.

9. Which of the following is a surgical emergency?
   a. phimosis
   b. cryptorchidism
   c. testicular torsion
   d. epididymitis

10. The classic presenting symptom of testicular cancer is:
    a. painful urination
    b. a painless hard nodule
    c. a tender, thickened area
    d. hematuria

Caring for Female Clients with Reproductive System Disorders

chapter **33**

LEARNING outcomes

After completing this chapter, you will be able to:

- Identify the major structures of the female reproductive system and discuss their functions.
- Identify and describe the functions of female sex hormones.
- Describe normal age-related changes in female reproductive system structure and function.
- Describe the pathophysiology of commonly occurring disorders of the breast and female reproductive system.
- Compare and contrast the manifestations of benign and malignant disorders of the breast and female reproductive system.
- Provide appropriate preoperative and postoperative nursing care for the client having gynecologic surgery.
- Use the nursing process when providing nursing care for female clients with disorders of the breast and reproductive system.

Disorders of the female reproductive system can occur at any point in a woman's adult life. They may affect her ability to bear children, her sexuality, and her sense of well-being as a woman. For many women, the ability to reproduce affects self-esteem, femininity, and general health. Women experiencing reproductive system problems may be asked to disclose personal, intimate information, which may be embarrassing and uncomfortable. Sensitivity on the part of the nurse is vital to establishing a caring, therapeutic relationship with the client.

Structure and Function of the Female Reproductive System

Although the reproductive organs in men and women are very different, they share common functions: providing sexual pleasure and producing children. The reproductive organs, in conjunction with the neuroendocrine system, also produce hormones that are important in biologic development and sexual behavior.

The female reproductive system includes the paired ovaries and fallopian tubes, uterus, vagina, the external genitalia, and the breasts. In women, the urethra and urinary meatus are separated from the reproductive organs; however, they are in such close proximity that a health problem with one often affects the other.

INTERNAL STRUCTURES

The internal organs of the female reproductive system include the ovaries, fallopian tubes, uterus, and vagina (Figure 33-1 ◆).

Ovaries and Ovulation

In adult women, the ovaries are flat, almond-shaped glands located below the ends of the fallopian tubes. The ovaries produce the female hormones estrogen and progesterone, and store immature ova called *oocytes*. A woman's total number of ova is present at birth.

The ovaries produce estrogens, progesterone, and androgens in a cyclic pattern. **Estrogens** are steroid hormones essential to the development and maintenance of secondary sex characteristics. Along with other hormones, estrogens also help prepare the female reproductive organs for growth of a fetus. Estrogens help maintain skin, bone, and blood vessel structure; affect serum cholesterol and high-density lipoprotein (HDL) levels; enhance blood clotting; and affect sodium and water balance. Estrogen secretion varies with the menstrual cycle (see below).

Progesterone primarily affects breast glandular tissue and the endometrium. During pregnancy, progesterone relaxes smooth muscle to decrease uterine contractions. It also increases body temperature. *Androgens* are responsible for normal hair growth patterns at puberty and also have metabolic effects.

The *ovarian cycle* has three phases lasting about 28 days. The *follicular phase* lasts from the 1st to the 10th day of the cycle. The *ovulatory phase* lasts from the 11th to the 14th day, ending with ovulation. The *luteal phase* lasts from the 14th to the 28th day (Figure 33-2 ◆).

Each ovary contains many small structures called *ovarian follicles*. Each follicle contains an immature ovum, called an oocyte. Each month, several follicles are mature, stimulated by *follicle-stimulating hormone (FSH)* and *luteinizing hormone (LH)*. The mature follicles (*graafian follicles*) produce estrogen, which stimulates development of endometrium. When the estrogen level is high enough to stimulate the anterior pituitary gland, a surge of LH is produced. LH stimulates development of the oocyte into a mature ovum and causes the ovarian follicle to rupture, releasing the ovum. This is the process of *ovulation*. The ruptured follicle then becomes a *corpus luteum*, which produces estrogen and progesterone to support the endometrium until conception occurs or the cycle begins again. If pregnancy does not occur, the corpus luteum degenerates, and its hormone production ceases. Falling progesterone and estrogen levels allow LH and FSH levels to increase, and a new cycle begins.

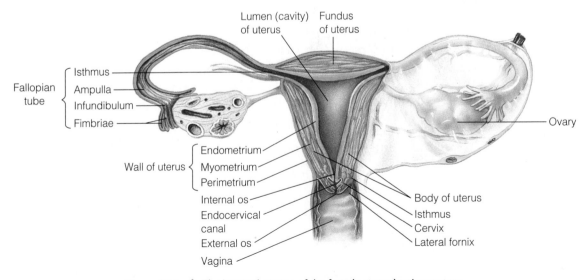

Figure 33-1. ◆ The internal organs of the female reproductive system.

A Ovarian cycle

B Uterine cycle

Figure 33-2. ◆ (A) Changes in ovarian follicles during the 28-day ovarian cycle. (B) Corresponding changes in the endometrium during the menstrual cycle.

Fallopian Tubes

The *fallopian tubes* (or uterine tubes) are thin tubes about 4 inches (10 cm) long and 1 cm in diameter. They are attached to the uterus on one end. The distal ends of the fallopian tubes are open, with projections called *fimbriae* that drape over the ovary. The fimbriae pick up the ovum after it is released from the ovary.

The fallopian tubes are made of smooth muscle and lined with cilia. Movement of the cilia and smooth muscle contractions move the ovum through the tubes toward the uterus. Fertilization of the ovum by sperm usually occurs in the outer portion of one of the fallopian tubes.

Uterus

The *uterus* is a thick-walled, pear-shaped muscular organ located between the bladder and rectum. Ligaments support it within the abdominal cavity. Its function is to receive the fertilized ovum and provide a site for growth and development of the fetus.

The uterine wall has three layers. The outer layer, the *perimetrium,* merges with the peritoneum. The middle layer, the *myometrium,* has muscle fibers that run in various directions, allowing expansion during pregnancy and contractions during the menses and childbirth. The *endometrium* lines the uterus. Its innermost layer is shed during menstruation.

The uterus is made up of three parts: the fundus, the body, and the cervix (see Figure 33-1). The cervix projects into the vagina. The uterine opening of the cervix is called the *internal os;* the vaginal opening is called the *external os.* The *endocervical canal* between the openings allows discharge of menstrual fluid and entrance of sperm. The cervix is a firm structure that softens in response to hormones during pregnancy.

The endometrium of the uterus responds to changes in estrogen and progesterone during the ovarian cycle to prepare for implantation of the fertilized embryo. The endometrium is receptive to embryo implantation for only about 7 days each month, during the time when the embryo would normally reach the uterus from the fallopian tube.

The menstrual cycle begins at the onset of menstruation (Figure 33-2B). During the *menstrual phase,* the inner endometrial layer detaches and is expelled as menstrual fluid. As the maturing follicle begins to produce estrogen, the *proliferative phase* begins. The inner endometrial layer is repaired and thickens, while spiral arteries proliferate and tubular glands form. Cervical mucus becomes thin, helping sperm move into the uterus. During the *secretory phase,* progesterone increases endometrial vascularity and prepares it to support the fertilized ovum. Cervical mucus thickens, blocking the internal os. If fertilization does not occur, hormone levels fall. Spasm of spiral arteries causes degeneration and sloughing of the inner endometrial layer, starting the process again.

Vagina

The vagina is a fibromuscular tube about 3 to 4 inches (8 to 10 cm) long located between the bladder and urethra and the rectum. The upper end contains the cervix in an area called the *fornix.* The mucous membrane walls of the vagina form folds, called *rugae.* Vaginal mucus is relatively acidic and bacteriostatic. Estrogen and normal vaginal flora help maintain its acid pH. The vagina is the birth canal, allows excretion of menstrual fluid, and is an organ of sexual response.

EXTERNAL GENITALIA

The external genitalia include the mons pubis, the labia, the clitoris, the vaginal and urethral openings, and glands (Figure 33-3 ◆).

The *mons pubis* is a pad of adipose tissue anterior to the symphysis pubis. After puberty, the mons is covered with hair.

The labia are divided into two structures. The *labia majora* are folds of skin and adipose tissue covered with hair

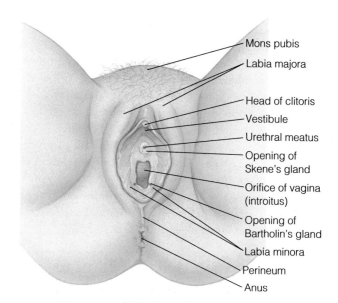

Figure 33-3. ◆ The female external genitalia.

that enclose the labia minora. The *labia minora* are hairless and contain some erectile tissue. The area between the labia is called the *vestibule.* It contains the openings of the vagina and urethra, as well as *Bartholin's glands.* These glands secrete lubricating fluid during sexual activities. *Skene's glands,* which open onto the vestibule on each side of the urethra, produce fluid to moisten the vestibule.

The *clitoris* is an erectile organ, analogous to the penis in the male. Like the penis, it is highly sensitive and distends during sexual arousal. The vaginal opening, called the *introitus,* is surrounded by a connective tissue membrane called the hymen, which determines the size and shape of the opening.

BREASTS

The *breasts* (or *mammary glands*) are supported by the pectoral muscles and are richly supplied with nerves, blood, and lymph (Figure 33-4 ◆). The areola, a pigmented area near the center of the breast, contains sebaceous glands and a nipple. The *nipple* usually protrudes and becomes erect in response to cold and stimulation. The primary purpose of the breasts is to supply nourishment for the infant.

The breasts are made of adipose, connective, and glandular tissue. Cooper's ligaments, which support the breast, extend from the outer breast tissue to the nipple, dividing the breast into 15 to 25 lobes. Each lobe contains *mammary glands* connected by ducts that open to the nipple.

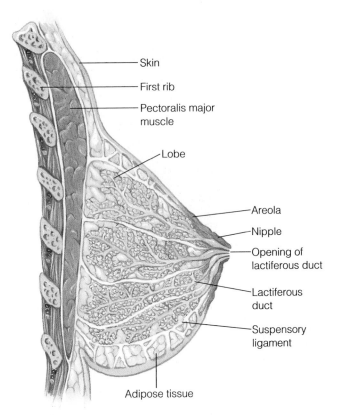

Figure 33-4. ◆ **Structure of the female breast.**

Breast Disorders

Breast disorders are common. Women are primarily affected, but men also can develop them. Breast tissue changes in response to hormones, nutrition, and physical and environmental factors. Most women notice increased tenderness and lumpiness prior to menses. More than half of all women who menstruate regularly find a lump in the breast; 80% of these lumps are not cancerous. When a woman discovers a breast lump, her first response is often fear: of breast cancer, of losing her breast, and perhaps of losing her life. Because American society views the breast as a significant part of feminine beauty, breast problems often threaten a woman's self-image.

Nurses play a critical role in teaching about normal breast tissue, common disorders, screening and risk factors for breast cancer, and breast self-examination.

Fibrocystic Breast Changes

Fibrocystic breast changes are noncancerous changes in breast tissue, causing swelling, pain, tenderness, and lumpiness. They

are thought to be caused by an excessive response to cyclic hormone changes. Fibrocystic changes are common in women 30 to 50 years old and rare in postmenopausal women.

PATHOPHYSIOLOGY

Fibrocystic changes are classified as nonproliferative or proliferative changes. *Nonproliferative* fibrocystic changes involve fibrosis of connective tissue, cyst formation, and inflammation (Figure 33-5 ◆). These changes do not increase the risk for breast cancer. *Proliferative* fibrocystic changes involve cell growth, with an increase in cell numbers, especially of epithelial gland cells. The risk for cancer is higher in clients with proliferative breast changes. Both forms of fibrocystic changes may be present.

Fibrocystic breast changes cause bilateral or unilateral breast pain or tenderness and a sense of fullness that increases just prior to menstruation. Lumps may be felt in the breasts, and discharge from the nipple may be noted. Multiple, mobile cysts can form, usually in both breasts. Fluid may be aspirated from these cysts.

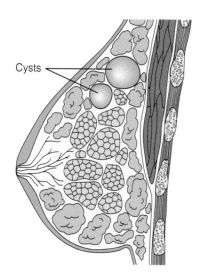

Figure 33-5. ◆ Fibrocystic breast changes.

COLLABORATIVE CARE

Diagnosis of fibrocystic breast changes is based on the history, physical exam, and mammography. A needle biopsy may be done to rule out malignancy.

Aspiration of a large cyst may relieve pain. A well-fitting supportive brassiere worn day and night helps relieve discomfort. Some women report that avoiding caffeine and chocolate relieves symptoms; both contain methylxanthines, believed to contribute to fibrocystic changes. Women who smoke report a reduction in breast lumps when they quit smoking. Mild analgesics and local heat or cold also are recommended. Vitamin E also may help relieve breast pain.

NURSING CARE

The nursing role for women with fibrocystic breast changes is primarily educational. Provide preoperative teaching and psychological support before breast biopsy. After the procedure, discuss home care and possible complications that should be reported to the physician. Reinforce teaching about measures to promote comfort. Suggest that although research has not confirmed the role of abstaining from caffeine or taking vitamin E to relieve discomfort, many women find these measures beneficial.

Mastitis

Mastitis is inflammation that causes tenderness, swelling, and redness of the breast. Mastitis usually affects lactating women, caused by organisms from the infant's nose and throat.

Mastitis is treated with antibiotics. Increasing fluid intake, wearing a supportive bra, and taking mild analgesics, such as aspirin or ibuprofen, help relieve symptoms. If lactating, the woman should continue to breast-feed from the unaffected breast and express milk from the affected breast.

Nursing care of the woman with mastitis includes teaching about the importance of handwashing, breast and nipple

care, and, in lactating women, regular, thorough emptying of the breasts to prevent engorgement.

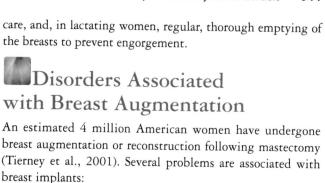

Disorders Associated with Breast Augmentation

An estimated 4 million American women have undergone breast augmentation or reconstruction following mastectomy (Tierney et al., 2001). Several problems are associated with breast implants:

- Scarring may occur around the implant, causing excessive firmness and distortion of the breast.
- The implant may rupture or bleed silicone gel through the capsule, causing local inflammation.
- While implants do not appear to increase the risk of breast cancer, they make early detection more difficult. Other disorders such as connective tissue disease and chronic fatigue syndrome have been linked with silicone breast implants, although a connection has not been proved. Most current implants are saline filled.

Nurses should reassure clients with implants that removing the implant is not recommended unless it has ruptured or the client has symptoms of an autoimmune disorder. Inform clients who have reconstructive breast surgery following mastectomy for cancer that local cancer recurrence usually is superficial and easily detected by palpation. Recurrent cancer is treated the same for clients with implants as for those without them.

Breast Cancer

Breast cancer is second only to lung cancer as a cause of cancer-related deaths among women. Breast cancer also strikes men, although rarely. While the incidence of breast cancer remains stable, mortality rates are decreasing (see Box 33-1).

Breast cancer is not one disease, but many, depending on the affected breast tissue, the effect of estrogen on the tumor, and the age of the person at onset. The two most significant risk factors for breast cancer are female gender and age over 50. Other risk factors for breast cancer are listed in Table 33-1 ◆.

TABLE 33-1	BREAST CANCER RISK FACTORS	
Gender	Female
Race	White
Age	Over 50
Family history	Breast cancer in mother or sister
Medical history	Cancer of other breast; endometrial cancer; proliferative fibrocystic breast changes
Menstrual history	Early menarche (before age 12); late menopause (after age 50)
Reproductive history	First birth after age 30; prolonged use of estrogen replacement therapy
Radiation exposure	Multiple chest x-rays or fluoroscopic exams, particularly before age 30
Lifestyle	More than two alcoholic drinks daily Obesity; smoking High economic status Breast trauma

PATHOPHYSIOLOGY

Breast cancer is unregulated growth of abnormal cells in breast tissue. It begins as a single transformed cell, which then multiplies. Breast cancer is hormone dependent: It does not develop in women without functioning ovaries who have never received estrogen replacement therapy. Most tumors occur in the ductal areas of the breast. Breast cancers are classified as noninvasive (in situ) or invasive. Invasiveness refers to penetration of the tumor into surrounding tissue. Two atypical types of breast cancer are inflammatory carcinoma and Paget's disease.

Noninvasive *(in Situ)* Carcinoma

In *noninvasive* breast cancer, malignant cells proliferate within the ducts or lobules of the breast without invading surrounding tissue. The nipple and the subareolar region are usually involved. Noninvasive cancers are typically diagnosed when the mass is seen on mammography rather than by a palpable breast mass or nipple discharge. Noninvasive cancers appear to increase the risk for invasive breast cancer.

Invasive Carcinoma

Most breast cancers are *invasive,* arising from the intermediate ducts of the breast. These tumors can be differentiated by cell type. However, the prognosis and treatment of the disease depend on the stage of the disease (see below), rather than on cell type. Invasive breast cancers spread to involve surrounding breast tissue, lymph, and blood vessels. The cancer can metastasize to distant sites through the bloodstream or lym-

phatic system. The common sites of metastasis of breast cancer are regional lymph nodes, bone, brain, lung, liver, and skin.

Inflammatory Carcinoma

Although rare, inflammatory breast cancer is the most malignant form of breast cancer. The client presents with a diffuse redness, warmth, and edema of the breast. A discrete mass may not be palpable. Metastases develop early and widely in clients with inflammatory carcinoma. The prognosis for this type of breast cancer is poor.

Paget's Disease

Paget's disease is a rare breast cancer that involves the nipple ducts. Initial symptoms are itching or burning of the nipple with superficial erosion, crusting, or ulceration.

Manifestations

Most breast tumors are discovered by the client as small, hard, and painless lumps or masses. The mass is usually found in the upper outer quadrant of the breast. Other symptoms are listed in Box 33-2. Skin changes such as dimpling, peau d'orange skin (Figure 33-6 ◆), and engorged vessels on the affected breast may occur.

Clients with bone metastasis may have pathologic fractures, chronic pain, and hypercalcemia. Clients with lung metastasis may have difficulty breathing, and brain metastasis can affect mental processes.

COLLABORATIVE CARE

Diagnosis of breast cancer begins with detection. The earlier breast cancer is detected, the more likely it is that treat-

Figure 33-6. ◆ Left, orange peel; right, peau d'orange skin.

ment will be effective in curing the disease or extending survival.

Breast Cancer Screening

Breast cancer screening includes breast self-exam, clinical examination, and mammography. These are usually used in combination.

Recommendations for breast cancer screening are:

- BSE monthly starting at age 20
- Clinical breast examination every 3 years from ages 20 through 39 and annually after age 40
- Baseline mammogram between age 40 and 49; annual mammogram after age 50

Figure 33-7. ◆ Teaching breast self-examination (BSE).

Step 1. Teach the client to observe her breasts in front of a mirror and in good lighting. Tell her to observe her breasts in four positions:

    With her arms relaxed and at her sides
    With her arms lifted over her head
    With her hands pressed against her hips
    With her hands pressed together at her waist, leaning forward

Instruct her to look at each breast individually, and then to compare them. She should observe for any visible abnormalities, such as lumps, dimpling, deviation, recent nipple retraction, irregular shape, edema, discharge, or asymmetry.

Step 2. Teach the client to palpate both breasts while standing or sitting, with one hand behind her head (Figure A). Tell her that many women palpate their breasts in the shower because water and soap make the skin slippery and easier to palpate. Show the woman how to use the pads of her fingers to palpate all areas of her breast, using the concentric circles technique (Figure B). Tell her to press the breast tissue gently against the chest wall, and to be sure to palpate the axillary tail.

A

Step 3. Instruct the client to palpate her breasts again while lying down, as described in Step 2. Suggest that she place a folded towel under the shoulder and back on the side to be palpated. The arm on the examining side should be over the head, with the hand under the head (Figure C).

B

Step 4. Teach the client to palpate the areola and nipples next. Show her how to compress the nipple to check for discharge (Figure D).

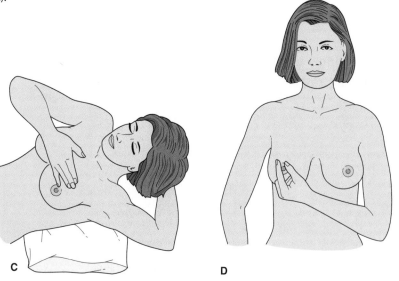

Step 5. Remind the client to use a calendar to keep a record of when she performs BSE. Teach her to perform BSE at the same time each month, usually 5 days after the onset of menses, when there is less hormonal influence on tissues.

C

D

BREAST SELF-EXAMINATION (BSE). BSE is an effective way of detecting breast cancer: Most breast cancers are found by the women themselves. All women should be taught to perform BSE monthly (Figure 33-7 ◆). Premenopausal women should perform BSE after their menstrual period, because hormonal changes increase breast tenderness and lumpiness prior to menses. Suggest that postmenopausal women perform BSE on the first day of each month.

CLINICAL BREAST EXAMINATION. In clinical breast examination, a trained health professional inspects and palpates the breasts and axillae, and checks for nipple discharge.

SCREENING MAMMOGRAPHY. Mammography is a low-dose x-ray of the breast used to detect breast lesions before they can be felt. Although mammography can detect breast tumors 2 years before they are palpable, most of these tumors have been present for 8 to 10 years. Mammography compresses breast tissue. It is uncomfortable to painful, depending on breast size and tenderness, and pain tolerance.

Box 33-3 discusses concerns about screening and treatment for older women.

Diagnostic Tests

■ *Diagnostic mammography* is done to visualize a palpable breast mass or identify a possible tumor in a client with other symptoms of breast cancer but no palpable mass.

■ *Ultrasonography* uses high-frequency sound waves to obtain a cross-sectional view of the breast. This technique can distinguish between solid and cystic masses.

■ *Computed tomography (CT) scans, magnetic resonance imaging (MRI),* and *positive emission tomography (PET) scans* may be done to locate and evaluate possible metastasis of breast cancer.

■ *Cytologic examination* of fluid from nipple discharge may reveal the presence of cancer cells.

■ *Tissue biopsy,* or examination of tissue from the lesion for cancer cells, is vital to diagnose breast cancer. Tissue for biopsy can be obtained in several ways:

a. Fine-needle aspiration biopsy uses a fine needle to remove fluid and cells from the breast lesion (Figure 33-8A ◆). Aspiration biopsy may be done using a stereotactic biopsy device; mammography and a computer are used to guide the needle.

b. Core-needle biopsy uses a large, hollow-core needle to remove one or more cores of tissue from the breast lesion.

c. Excisional biopsy is an open technique, in which the lesion is surgically removed and the tissue examined (Figure 33-8B).

Box 33-4 outlines nursing care for a client undergoing a breast biopsy.

■ In some centers, a *breast cancer risk profile* may be done to identify women who might benefit from aggressive therapy. This study subjects tumor cells to tests to determine their response to hormones, aggressiveness, and likelihood of recurring.

A Aspiration biopsy

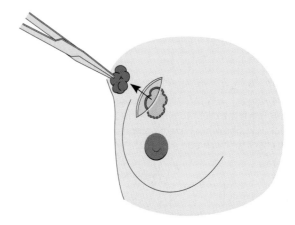

B Excisional biopsy

Figure 33-8. ◆ Types of breast biopsy. (A) In an aspiration biopsy, a needle is used to aspirate fluid or tissue from the breast. (B) In an excisional biopsy, the breast lesion is removed surgically, and its tissue is examined.

BOX 33-4
NURSING CARE CHECKLIST

BREAST BIOPSY

Before the Procedure

☑ Provide routine preoperative care as ordered (see Chapter 7).

☑ Provide psychological support.

Client and Family Teaching

☑ You will be notified of the results within a few days.

☑ Use a mild analgesic to relieve discomfort.

Fine-Needle Aspiration Biopsy

☑ Tissue and fluid are withdrawn from the lesion using a fine needle.

☑ This procedure takes only a few minutes and may be done in the physician's office.

Core-Needle Biopsy

☑ You will lie on a special table with your breast protruding through a hole.

☑ Local anesthesia will be used.

☑ Tissue from the lesion will be removed with a needle.

Excisional Biopsy

☑ The biopsy is done in ambulatory surgery with local anesthesia.

☑ The entire lesion and a small amount of surrounding tissue is removed.

☑ A nurse will explain what's happening, answer questions, and offer support during the biopsy.

☑ Tell the doctor if you have pain during the procedure.

☑ The incision is closed with sutures or tape and covered with a small dressing.

☑ Wear a well-fitting bra and apply ice packs to relieve discomfort and bruising after the procedure.

CLINICAL alert

Although tamoxifen reduces the risk for developing breast cancer, it increases the risk of endometrial cancer, deep vein thrombosis, and pulmonary embolism. Teach women taking tamoxifen the early warning signs of endometrial cancer. Stress the importance of yearly pelvic examinations. Emphasize the need to stop smoking.

When tamoxifen is ineffective or poorly tolerated, other hormone therapies may be used. In premenopausal women, the ovaries may be removed to reduce estrogen levels. Drugs such as diethylstilbestrol (DES), megestrol acetate (Megace), or aminoglutethimide (Cytadren) may be prescribed. However, these drugs have more side effects than tamoxifen.

Chemotherapy is commonly used to treat breast cancer when lymph nodes in the axilla are involved. It also is used to prolong life in late metastatic disease. (See Chapter 8 for more information about chemotherapy and its nursing implications.)

Radiation Therapy

Radiation therapy is typically used following breast cancer surgery to destroy any remaining cancer cells that could cause recurrence or metastasis. It is usually used in combination with lumpectomy for early-stage breast cancer. If a tumor is unusually large, radiation shrinks the tumor prior to surgery. Palliative radiation therapy is also used to treat chest wall recurrences and to help control pain and prevent fractures with bone metastases. Radiation is delivered by external beam or tissue implants.

Surgery

When breast cancer has not metastasized, the treatment of choice is surgery to remove the primary tumor combined with radiation therapy to reduce the risk of tumor recurrence or spread.

BREAST-CONSERVING SURGERY. Breast-conserving surgery involves removing the tumor and a disease-free margin surrounding the tumor (Figure 33-9A ◆). Lymph nodes under the arm (axillary nodes) are removed as well. Surgery is followed by whole breast radiation to destroy remaining cancer cells. This treatment is as effective as total mastectomy in treating breast cancer.

MASTECTOMY. Mastectomy (removal of the breast) is often done to treat breast cancer. *Radical mastectomy* is removal of the entire affected breast, underlying chest muscles, and lymph nodes under the arms. *Modified radical mastectomy* is the removal of the breast tissue and lymph nodes under the arm, leaving the chest wall muscles intact (Figure 33-9B). Box 33-5 outlines nursing care and teaching for the client undergoing a mastectomy.

Axillary node dissection usually accompanies breast cancer surgeries. This surgery can lead to long-term com-

Staging of Breast Cancer

Staging (classifying the tumor by size, lymph involvement, and metastasis) provides important information for deciding on treatment options. The choice of treatment also depends on age and the woman's preferences. Breast cancer tends to be more aggressive in premenopausal women (probably because of hormonal factors), requiring more aggressive treatment.

Pharmacology

Systemic therapy (tamoxifen, chemotherapy, or biologic therapy) is used to prevent breast cancer or to delay the recurrence of cancer in all client groups.

Tamoxifen (Nolvadex) interferes with estrogen activity. It is used to treat existing breast cancer and to reduce the risk for developing breast cancer in women who are at high risk. (See Table 33-2 ◆.)

TABLE 33-2 NURSING IMPLICATIONS FOR PHARMACOLOGY: CLIENTS RECEIVING TAMOXIFEN

DRUG CLASSIFICATION/ DRUGS	ACTION	NURSING IMPLICATIONS	CLIENT AND FAMILY TEACHING
Estrogen Blocker/Antineoplastic Agent ■ Tamoxifen (Nolvadex)	Tamoxifen inhibits tumor growth by blocking estrogen receptor sites of cancer cells. It is used to reduce the risk of breast cancer in high-risk women, prevent cancer recurrence after treatment, and as adjunctive therapy for advanced breast cancer. Tamoxifen increases the risk for endometrial cancer, deep vein thrombosis (DVT), and pulmonary embolism.	Assess for increased bone or tumor pain; provide analgesics as ordered. Monitor CBC, serum electrolytes, liver function tests, and thyroid hormone levels during treatment. Report abnormal results to the charge nurse or physician.	Use a diaphragm, condom, or other barrier contraception while taking this drug and for 1 month following. Weigh yourself weekly. Promptly report bone pain, weight gain, swelling, shortness of breath, nausea or vomiting, changes in mental status, headache, blurred vision, menstrual irregularities, or vaginal bleeding. This drug may cause hot flashes. Do not smoke while you are taking this drug.

plications, such as lymphedema, nerve damage, and adhesions. Exercises to promote optimal use of the affected arm are discussed in the discharge considerations section that follows.

BREAST RECONSTRUCTION SURGERY. Breast reconstruction is common following mastectomy. It may be done at the time of surgery or at a later date, depending on factors such as physical condition, need for additional therapy, and preference. An implant may be used under the muscle if sufficient tissue to cover the implant is available (Figure 33-10A ◆). Following radical surgery, muscle from the back or abdomen may be trans-

planted and used with or without an implant to reconstruct the breast (Figure 33-10B). A new nipple may be created by using tissue from the opposite nipple or other sites.

Metastatic Breast Cancer Treatment

If breast cancer has metastasized to other sites, the focus of treatment is *palliation* (symptom relief), extending life, and ensuring the comfort of the client. Therapies such as radiation therapy, hormone therapy, chemotherapy, or surgery may be used for palliative treatment, depending on the sites of metastases. Quality of life may take precedence over quantity of life.

A

B

Figure 33-9. ◆ Surgery for breast cancer. (A) In a lumpectomy, the tumor and a small margin of surrounding tissue are removed. (B) In a modified radical mastectomy, the entire breast and axillary lymph nodes are removed.

BOX 33-5
NURSING CARE CHECKLIST

MASTECTOMY

Before Surgery

☑ Provide routine preoperative care as outlined in Chapter 7.

☑ Reinforce teaching as needed.

☑ Allow access to support persons (significant others, religious or spiritual, or counselors).

☑ Offer emotional support.

After Surgery

☑ Provide routine postoperative care.

☑ Reinforce teaching about postoperative care and exercises (discharge may occur within hours or the day after surgery).

Client and Family Teaching

☑ Empty the drain and replace the dressing daily.

☑ Return for drain removal in 2 to 4 days or as ordered.

☑ Take the prescribed analgesic before pain becomes severe and before performing exercises.

☑ Report excessive bleeding to your doctor.

☑ Numbness and tingling in the axillary area are common.

☑ Begin arm and shoulder exercises to restore full mobility as recommended by your doctor.

☑ You may drive within 7 to 10 days and return to work within 4 to 6 weeks.

☑ Do not lift heavy objects with the arm on the operated side.

☑ Protect the affected arm from injury and infection: Wear rubber gloves when washing dishes, garden gloves when working outside; avoid having blood pressures taken or blood drawn on the operative side.

A Implant

B Latissimus dorsi myocutaneous flap

Figure 33-10. ◆ Breast reconstruction surgeries. (A) An implant is inserted under the pectoris muscle. (B) A latissimus dorsi flap is used to reconstruct the breast.

NURSING CARE

ASSESSING

Obtain subjective information from all women about their risk factors for breast cancer, such as a history of the disease in a close female relative (mother, grandmother, sibling), early menarche or late menopause, and childbearing. Ask about breast self-exam, including how they do it, how often, and their knowledge of abnormal findings and what to do if a lump is discovered. Ask about breast pain, nipple discharge, change in breast size, or a change in the appearance or skin of the breast.

With the client disrobed to the waist, inspect the breasts and nipples for size, symmetry, contour, skin color

and texture, venous patterns, and lesions. With the client supine and the arm behind the head, palpate each breast. Be sure to include the nipple and the axillary tail of breast tissue. Figure 33-7B shows one possible pattern for breast palpation. Note any palpable masses by location, size, shape, consistency, tenderness, mobility, and borders (sharp or poorly defined). Palpate each axilla for enlarged lymph nodes (Figure 33-11 ◆).

DIAGNOSING, PLANNING, AND IMPLEMENTING

DECISIONAL CONFLICT: TREATMENT OPTIONS

■ Discuss the disease process and treatment options. Provide an opportunity for questions. Answer as simply and directly as possible. Make eye contact with the client and

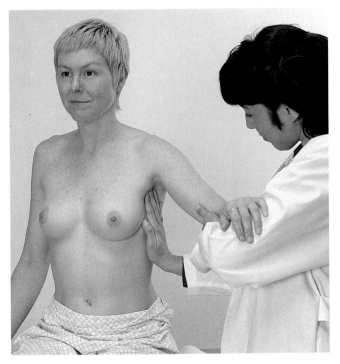

Figure 33-11. ◆ Palpating the axillary lymph nodes.

pay attention to body language. *Providing factual information and an opportunity to ask questions helps the client make an informed decision during a highly stressful time.*

■ Focus on immediate concerns, and provide up-to-date written material for review. *Stress and anxiety interfere with the ability to process information. Written materials can be reviewed later.*

■ Listen in a nonjudgmental manner during the decision-making process. *Nonjudgmental, empathic listening helps the client process information and make informed decisions.*

■ Provide opportunities to meet with other women who have had breast cancer surgery. *Breast cancer survivors often can answer questions the client is unable or unwilling to ask of care providers. They also can be a resource after surgery.*

ANTICIPATORY GRIEVING

■ Listen attentively to expressions of loss and observe for nonverbal cues (failure to make eye contact, crying, silence). *Breast surgery, even lumpectomy, alters the appearance of the breast. This loss is expressed through grief. Not all women grieve openly. Attending to nonverbal cues helps open discussion of feelings of loss and grieving.*

■ Spend time with the client. Do not rush interactions. *Taking time to be with the client communicates caring.*

■ Explain that periods of depression, anger, and denial after breast surgery are normal. *They are expected responses to loss and grieving.*

■ Enlist support from significant others to help the woman cope with her grief. *The client's family and friends can provide support during the grieving process.*

RISK FOR INFECTION

■ Assess dressings for bleeding, drainage, color, and odor every 4 hours for 24 hours. Circle any visible bleeding and drainage on the dressing as a baseline for subsequent assessment. *Excessive bleeding or drainage may indicate a postoperative complication that requires intervention.*

■ Observe incision and IV sites for pain, redness, swelling, and drainage. Assess the wound drainage system for patency; note the color and amount of drainage. *A local inflammatory response or wound drainage that is cloudy or malodorous may indicate an infection.*

■ Use aseptic technique when changing dressings, emptying wound drainage, and caring for intravenous tubing and sites. *Aseptic technique minimizes the risk of contamination with pathogens.*

■ Encourage a well-balanced diet. Refer to a dietitian as indicated. *Adequate nutrition promotes healing and immune function.*

■ Teach how to care for the incision and drainage system (cleansing, securing, and emptying). *The client is often discharged before the drainage system is removed, and needs teaching to provide self-care.*

■ Instruct to report fever, redness or hardness at the surgical site, or purulent drainage to the surgeon. *Early identification and treatment of infection can prevent more serious or long-term consequences.*

■ Instruct to avoid deodorants and talcum powder on the affected side until the incision is completely healed. *These substances may irritate the skin and impede healing.*

■ Discuss skin care during radiation therapy to reduce the risk of infection. *Radiation can cause dryness, itching, rash, or scaling of skin, increasing the risk of infection.*

RISK FOR INJURY

Removing axillary lymph nodes increases the risk for problems such as lymphedema and infection.

■ Use the nonsurgical side for blood pressures and blood samples. *Compression of the arm on the surgical side may cause lymphedema.*

■ Elevate the affected arm on a pillow. *Elevating the arm permits drainage, prevents swelling, and promotes circulation.*

■ Encourage range-of-motion (ROM) exercises of the affected arm. *Exercise helps develop new drainage channels.*

■ Teach protective measures: Avoid constricting sleeves, avoid lifting heavy objects, use a heavy oven mitt or potholder when cooking, and promptly apply antibiotic ointment to any cut or burn. Wear gloves when working in the yard or garden to prevent skin injury. *These measures help prevent infection and lymphedema.*

RISK FOR DISTURBED BODY IMAGE

■ Encourage verbalization of feelings. *Breast surgery can change body image. Talking about feelings of loss and change helps the client cope with the changes her body is experiencing due to surgery and treatment.*

- Explain that redness and swelling will fade with time. *Surgical changes may be compounded by side effects of chemotherapy or hormone therapy. Knowing that the scar will fade may help develop a more realistic view of the changes.*
- Include the partner (as desired) in discussions about physical changes caused by surgery and treatment. *The client may fear her partner's response to surgery. Open discussions facilitate adaptation of both partners to the changes.*
- Provide resources (pamphlets, books, referral to counselors or support groups) as appropriate. *Information and resources can assist with coping and adaptation to the changed body image.*
- Encourage the client to look at the incision when she feels ready. *Often, the reality is not as frightening as was imagined.*
- Reassure her that the decision about a prosthesis or reconstruction can be made at a later time. *Physical and emotional healing help the client make a better decision for long-term body image.*
- If the client is interested, provide written material about breast reconstruction and encourage meeting with a plastic surgeon and with women who have had reconstruction. *These steps allow the client to make a fully informed decision about available options.*

EVALUATING

To determine the effectiveness of nursing interventions, collect data such as the following:

- Makes an informed choice of treatment options based on extent of disease and personal preferences
- Expresses feelings of anger or sorrow related to potential consequences of breast cancer
- Looks at and touches incision; cares for incision and drainage system
- Remains free of infection or injury

Discharge Considerations

Limited postoperative exercises are started within 24 hours after surgery, beginning with ROM of the elbow, wrist, and hand. Encourage performance of activities of daily living (ADLs), such as eating, combing her hair, and washing her face. If wound drains are present, tell to avoid abducting the arm or raising the elbow above the shoulder height until drains are removed.

When wound healing is complete, abduction and external rotation of the upper arm may begin. Activities that require complete ROM include vacuuming and dusting. Forward and lateral elevation of the arms also increases function. Postmastectomy exercises such as wall climbing, overhead pulley, rope turning, and arm swings (Figure 33-12 ◆) should be discussed with the physical therapist.

Advise that adequate rest and emotional support are important to promote healing and recovery. Both radiation and chemotherapy can cause fatigue and other symptoms. Use measures (outlined in Chapter 8) to manage these symptoms.

Encourage participation in a breast cancer support group to share thoughts, feelings, experiences, and information about treatments, side effects, insurance problems, and other practical aspects of living with breast cancer. Discuss using online information services and bulletin boards for additional information and support.

Discuss manifestations of breast cancer recurrence, either as a second primary tumor or as metastasis from the original site. Advise to report signs and symptoms promptly (new breast lumps, a persistent cough or shortness of breath, jaundice or pain in the upper right quadrant of the abdomen, bone pain, or lumps around the collarbone or under the arm).

Advise a wholesome, balanced diet for healing and to deal with the effects of treatment, particularly chemotherapy. Maintaining body weight during chemotherapy can be difficult because of nausea and vomiting. Discuss potential solutions such as eating cold foods, which may be better tolerated than hot foods. Suggest complementary therapies such as guided imagery and meditation to help cope with adverse effects of treatment. Discuss the potential benefits of vitamin supplements (vitamins A, C, and E) to help promote healing and recovery.

Advise women who choose a prosthesis that a temporary lightweight prosthesis can be worn immediately after the drains and sutures have been removed. Because prostheses are expensive, advise not purchasing a permanent prosthesis until the wound has healed completely. Prostheses are available at medical suppliers and many larger department stores. Most private and government insurance policies pay for the first prosthesis.

Nursing Process Case Study
■ CLIENT WITH BREAST CANCER

Rachel Clemments is a 44-year-old divorced mother of two teenage girls. Because of a strong family history of breast cancer, she has been closely monitored (annual mammograms and clinical breast examination, monthly BSE) for the past 4 years. In spite of careful monitoring, however, 2 weeks ago she discovered a thickened area in her left breast. An incisional biopsy revealed invasive lobular carcinoma.

Assessment Ms. Clemments's history reveals that her mother, two aunts, and one sister had been diagnosed with breast cancer. Her mother and one of the aunts died before age 45. Physical assessment findings on admission include T 98.5° F (37.0° C); BP 110/62; P 65; R 14. Her weight is 120 lbs. (54 kg); she is 5′6″ (168 cm) tall.

Based on biopsy findings and her fear of future tumors, Ms. Clemments chooses to have a modified radical mastectomy and axillary node dissection. She is debating whether to have reconstructive breast surgery. Her oncologist has recom-

Figure 33-12. ◆ Postmastectomy exercises. (A) Wall climbing: Stand facing wall with toes 6 to 12 in. from wall. Bend elbows and place palms against wall at shoulder level. Gradually move both hands up the wall parallel to each other until incisional pulling or pain occurs. (Mark that spot on wall to measure progress.) Work hands down to shoulder level. Move closer to wall as height of reach improves. (B) Overhead pulley: Using operated arm, toss 6-foot rope over shower curtain rod (or over top of a door that has a nail in the top to hold the rope in place for the exercise). Grasp one end of rope in each hand. Slowly raise operated arm as far as comfortable by pulling down on the rope on opposite side. Keep raised arm close to your head. Reverse to raise unoperated arm by lowering the operated arm. Repeat. (C) Rope turning: Tie rope to door handle. Hold rope in hand of operated side. Back away from door until arm is extended away from body, parallel to floor. Swing rope in as wide a circle as possible. Increase size of circle as mobility returns. (D) Arm swings: Stand with feet 8 in. apart. Bend forward from waist, allowing arms to hang toward floor. Swing both arms up to sides to reach shoulder level. Swing back to center, then cross arms at center. Do not bend elbows. If possible, do this and other exercises in front of mirror to ensure even posture and correct motion.

mended a 6-month course of adjuvant chemotherapy, and she is concerned about side effects. One of her greatest concerns is how her illness will affect her ability to support and care for her daughters. She is afraid that treatment will limit her ability to keep her job and continue to meet her daughters' needs.

Since breast cancer seems part of the family legacy, she wonders, "When will it happen to my girls?"

Diagnosis The following nursing diagnoses are identified for Ms. Clements:

- Risk for Infection related to surgical incision
- Pain related to surgery
- Decisional Conflict about treatment related to concerns about risks and benefits
- Altered Family Processes related to effect of surgery and therapy on family roles and relationships
- Fear related to disease process/prognosis

Expected Outcomes The expected outcomes for the plan of care are that Ms. Clemments will:

- Remain free of infection.
- Relate adequate pain control during recovery.
- Evaluate the treatment options and decide on a course of action.
- Together with her daughters, acknowledge the need to change family roles and identify new coping patterns.
- Identify sources of fear and demonstrate behaviors that may reduce fears.

Planning and Implementation The following nursing interventions are planned and implemented for Ms. Clemments:

- Teach management of wound drain after discharge.
- Assess pain and provide analgesics as needed.
- Teach precautions and arm exercises for operated side.
- Suggest talking with a Reach to Recovery volunteer about concerns and feelings.
- Discuss chemotherapy management; refer to oncology nurse for further teaching.
- Provide educational resources about chemotherapy and breast reconstruction.
- Discuss using a temporary prosthesis until she decides about breast reconstruction surgery.

- Encourage discussion of reconstructive surgery with a plastic surgeon, emphasizing that it can be done at any time after mastectomy.
- Suggest attending breast cancer support group meetings for support and information.
- Refer to social services for consultation about family role changes.
- Encourage verbalization of fears about prognosis and future risks; refer for counseling as indicated.

Evaluation Ms. Clemments recovers from surgery without complications. She met with a Reach to Recovery volunteer, who provided a temporary prosthesis and booklets about postmastectomy exercises, chemotherapy, and breast reconstruction. The volunteer also referred her to a local breast cancer support group. Ms. Clemments has talked about her concerns related to breast reconstruction, as well as her fears about cancer recurrence and her daughters' risk for developing breast cancer in the future.

 Critical Thinking in the Nursing Process

1. What role could genetic counseling play in helping Ms. Clemments and her daughters better understand the daughters' risk of breast cancer?
2. Describe the types of breast cancer surgeries and their implications for nursing care.
3. What medications might help minimize the side effects of chemotherapy?

Disorders of Menstruation

Monthly menstruation often causes minor discomfort, such as breast tenderness, a feeling of heaviness and congestion in the pelvic area, cramping, and backache. Many women experience more serious effects, both physiologic and psychological. This section discusses premenstrual syndrome, dysmenorrhea, and abnormal uterine bleeding.

Premenstrual Syndrome

Premenstrual syndrome (PMS) is a symptom complex of irritability, depression, edema, and breast tenderness preceding menses. It may affect more than half of all women during their reproductive years. Risk factors for PMS include major life stressors, age greater than 30, and depression. The actual cause of PMS is unknown, but it is thought to involve imbalances of estrogen and progesterone.

PATHOPHYSIOLOGY

The pathophysiology of PMS is not clearly understood. Hormonal changes such as altered estrogen–progesterone ratios, increased prolactin levels and rising aldosterone levels during the luteal phase of the menstrual cycle (see Figure 33-2) are thought to contribute to the problem. Increased aldosterone levels cause salt and water retention and edema. Neurotransmitters such as monoamine oxidase and seratonin affect emotions and probably play a role in PMS.

Manifestations of PMS generally occur 7 to 10 days prior to the onset of the menstrual flow, and are relieved when the menstrual flow begins. The multisystem effects of PMS are shown in Figure 33-13 ◆. The manifestations of PMS and their intensity vary remarkably for each client.

COLLABORATIVE CARE

The goals of care for PMS are to relieve manifestations and help the client develop self-care strategies for episodes of PMS. The client is advised to keep a daily diary of symptoms for several months to evaluate their timing and severity.

Management focuses on diet, exercise, relaxation, and stress management. A diet high in complex carbohydrates with limited simple sugars and alcohol is recommended. Reduced salt intake helps to minimize fluid retention. Caffeine is restricted to reduce irritability. Increased intake of calcium, magnesium, and vitamin B_6 may be helpful. Exercise is beneficial, but adequate rest also is necessary. The client needs to balance periods of activity and rest. Techniques for

relaxation and stress management include deep abdominal breathing, meditation, muscle relaxation, and guided imagery.

If the manifestations of PMS are severe, drugs that affect hormone or neurotransmitter levels such as danazol (Danocrine), fluoxetine (Prozac), sertraline (Zoloft), or paroxetine (Paxil) may be prescribed.

Complementary therapies also may be used for PMS. These may include acupuncture, aromatherapy with various oils, herbs such as vitex or evening primrose oil, homeopathy, or reflexology.

NURSING CARE

Nursing care for the client with PMS focuses on teaching the client to manage manifestations of the disorder.

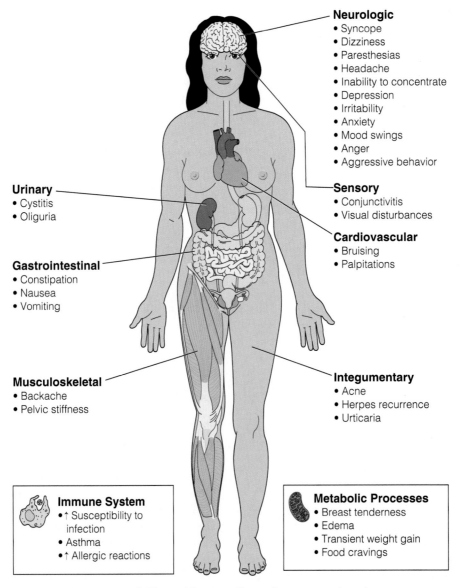

Figure 33-13. ◆ The multisystem effects of premenstrual syndrome.

EFFECTIVE THERAPEUTIC REGIMEN MANAGEMENT

- Encourage keeping a journal of menstrual cycle, physical symptoms, and mood changes. *Recognizing the signs and timing of PMS is the first step in developing ways to cope with the problem.*
- Review symptoms, relating them to diet, activity, and stress levels. *Identifying relationships helps develop strategies to reduce and manage the symptoms of PMS.*
- Explore self-care measures that have helped the client cope with mood alterations in the past. Encourage coping strategies such as relaxation techniques and exercise. *Using some drugs or alcohol to relieve PMS may actually make symptoms worse.*
- Review daily activities and suggest ways to balance rest periods and activity. *Rest decreases energy and oxygen consumption, increasing the amount available to muscles.*
- Explore ways to rearrange or reschedule activities during PMS symptoms. *Planning ahead provides more control and promotes effective coping.*
- Teach self-care measures to relieve pain: Heat application, relaxation techniques (such as breathing exercises, imagery techniques, or meditation), and exercise. *Heat relieves muscle spasms and dilates blood vessels, increasing blood supply to the pelvis and uterus. Relaxation and exercise promote release of naturally produced pain relievers (endorphins).*

Discharge Considerations

Teach the client that PMS is not a disease, but a response to hormone changes of the menstrual cycle. Understanding the condition allows the client to assume control, manage anxiety, and use appropriate strategies to reduce symptoms. Discuss dietary measures, relaxation techniques and exercise, stress reduction techniques, and support systems in teaching about PMS management.

Dysmenorrhea

Dysmenorrhea, pain associated with menstruation, is experienced by up to 75% of menstruating women. In *primary dysmenorrhea,* no disease process is identified. Prostaglandins stimulate muscles in the uterus to contract. These contractions can cause mild cramping to severe muscle spasms. As the muscles contract, blood flow to the uterus is restricted, causing ischemia and pain. Abdominal pain begins with the onset of menses and lasts 12 to 48 hours. Pain may radiate to the lower back and thighs. Other manifestations may include headache, nausea, vomiting, diarrhea, fatigue, or breast tenderness. Psychological factors, such as anxiety and tension, may contribute to dysmenorrhea. Childbirth tends to decrease the incidence and severity of symptoms.

Secondary dysmenorrhea is related to an underlying disorder that causes scarring or injury of reproductive organs.

Endometriosis, fibroid tumors, pelvic inflammatory disease, or ovarian cancer may cause painful menses. These conditions are discussed later in this chapter.

Care of the client with menstrual pain focuses on identifying its cause, and on managing pain. Drugs such as mild analgesics, prostaglandin inhibitors such as nonsteroidal anti-inflammatory drugs (NSAIDs), or oral contraceptives may be recommended to relieve pain. Nonpharmacologic measures include dietary changes, exercise, relaxation, and stress management. Dietary measures such as reducing intake of sodium, sugar, caffeine, and alcohol; decreasing fluid consumption; and increasing intake of protein, calcium, magnesium, and vitamin B_6 may be helpful. A balance of rest and exercise is important. Techniques for relaxation and stress management include deep abdominal breathing, meditation, muscle relaxation, and guided imagery. Use of a heating pad also helps reduce pain. As with PMS, complementary therapies such as aromatherapy, herbal preparations, reflexology, acupressure or massage may be helpful.

Nursing care focuses on helping the client develop effective coping strategies. Discuss using an NSAID such as ibuprofen on a regular basis during periods of menstrual pain. Teach nonpharmacologic pain relief measures, and encourage use of these as well for pain relief. Stress the benign nature of primary dysmenorrhea, being sure to validate the reality of the pain and discomfort. Discuss diet and exercise, as well as stress management techniques. Teach safe use of heat for pain relief. Provide information about engaging in sexual intercourse, explaining that orgasm may help relieve the client's symptoms.

Dysfunctional Uterine Bleeding

Dysfunctional uterine bleeding (DUB) is vaginal bleeding that is abnormal in amount, duration, or time of occurrence. Dysfunctional uterine bleeding is usually related to hormonal imbalances or pelvic tumors, either benign or malignant.

Amenorrhea is the absence of menstruation. It is usually caused by hormone imbalance. Because a certain percentage of body fat is required for menstruation to occur, anorexia nervosa or excessive athletic activity or training can also cause amenorrhea. Amenorrhea is a normal consequence of pregnancy, breast-feeding, and menopause, as well as removal of the uterus or ovaries.

Oligomenorrhea, scant menses, usually is related to hormonal imbalances. *Menorrhagia,* excessive or prolonged menstruation, may result from endocrine or reproductive system disorders. Clotting disorders and anticoagulant medications also can cause menorrhagia. Repetitive long or heavy cycles can lead to excessive blood loss, fatigue, anemia, hemorrhage, and sexual dysfunction.

Metrorrhagia, bleeding between menstrual periods, may be a sign of cervical or uterine cancer. For this reason, it is important to evaluate metrorrhagia promptly and thoroughly.

Mittleschmerz (midcycle spotting associated with ovulation) occurs in many women and is not considered metrorrhagia.

Postmenopausal bleeding may be caused by endometrial polyps, endometrial hyperplasia, or uterine cancer. The possibility of cancer makes early evaluation and treatment essential.

PATHOPHYSIOLOGY

Hormonal imbalance, especially progesterone deficiency with relative estrogen excess, causes endometrial tissue to proliferate. Unless this tissue is supported by adequate progesterone, sloughing occurs. Depending on ovarian function and the hormone imbalance, irregular, prolonged, or profuse vaginal bleeding may occur. *Anovulation,* absence of ovulation, is associated with both estrogen and progesterone deficiencies. Emotional upsets or stress also can cause hormonal imbalances and thus affect menstruation.

Pelvic tumors can also cause abnormal bleeding. They are discussed in later sections of this chapter.

COLLABORATIVE CARE

The care of the client with DUB focuses on identifying and treating the underlying disease. A careful history and physical examination are obtained. Abdominal and pelvic exams are done to rule out abdominal masses. The client may need to keep a menstrual history and basal body temperature chart for several months to relate ovulation to bleeding.

Diagnostic Tests

- *Complete blood count (CBC)* to evaluate the effects of DUB
- *Thyroid function tests* to rule out thyroid disorders such as hyper- or hypothyroidism as the cause of DUB
- *Serum estradiol (estrogen) and progesterone* levels to evaluate ovarian function
- *Serum hCG* and *LH* levels to evaluate pituitary function
- *Pap smear* to rule out cervical cancer
- *Pelvic ultrasound* to detect lesions such as fibroid or cancerous tumors. Box 33-6 describes nursing care for clients undergoing a pelvic ultrasound.
- *Laparoscopy* to visualize pelvic structures or hysteroscopy to detect abnormalities of the uterine cavity. Nursing care for the client undergoing a laparoscopy is outlined in Box 33-7.
- *Endometrial biopsy* may be done to examine endometrial tissues.

Pharmacology

For many clients, menstrual irregularities can be treated with hormones. Oral contraceptives or progesterone preparations may be ordered. Oral iron supplements may be prescribed to replace iron lost through menstrual bleeding.

Surgery

DUB is the leading cause of hysterectomy. However, the least invasive intervention that proves effective is preferred, beginning with a therapeutic dilation and curettage (D&C), then endometrial ablation, and, finally, hysterectomy.

> ### BOX 33-6
> ### NURSING CARE CHECKLIST
>
> #### PELVIC ULTRASOUND
> ☑ Force fluids and instruct not to void to ensure a full bladder.
> ☑ Explain procedure. Advise that transducer gel is cold but will be removed when the procedure is complete.
> ☑ For vaginal ultrasound, a transducer covered with a condom and coated with transducer gel is inserted into the vagina.
> ☑ Allow to empty bladder as soon as possible.

In a *therapeutic D&C,* the cervical canal is dilated and the uterine wall is scraped. D&C is used to diagnose and treat DUB and certain other disorders. It is contraindicated for any woman who has been taking anticoagulant drugs. Nursing care of the client undergoing D&C is outlined in Box 33-8.

Endometrial ablation permanently destroys the endometrial layer of the uterus by laser surgery or electrosurgical resection. It is done for women who do not respond to drug therapy or D&C. This procedure ends menstruation and reproduction.

In *uterine balloon heat therapy,* a specialized balloon is inserted through the cervix into the uterus, then inflated and heated. This outpatient procedure takes only 10 minutes and can be done using local anesthesia.

Hysterectomy, or removal of the uterus, may be done if other treatments are unsuccessful or malignancy is found, particularly if childbearing is no longer desired. In premenopausal women, the ovaries are usually left in place. In postmenopausal women, a total hysterectomy, or panhysterectomy, may be done, removing the uterus, fallopian tubes, and ovaries.

Hysterectomy may be done using an abdominal or a vaginal approach, or a vaginal approach with laparoscopic visualization of the pelvic cavity. Recovery is faster following vaginal or laparoscopic hysterectomy than with an abdominal hysterectomy. The abdominal approach, however, may be used when better access to and visualization of the pelvic cavity is needed. Nursing care of the client undergoing a hysterectomy is outlined in Box 33-9.

NURSING CARE

> ### ASSESSING

Nursing assessment focuses on subjective data related to the onset of symptoms, timing and amount of menstrual flow (in pads per day and duration of period), and associated symptoms such as pain or cramping, weakness, or excessive fatigue.

BOX 33-7
NURSING CARE CHECKLIST

LAPAROSCOPY
Before Surgery

☑ Instruct to douche with povidone–iodine (Betadine) solution and scrub around the umbilicus with pHisoHex or povidone–iodine the night before the procedure as ordered.

☑ Ask to empty bladder before procedure.

☑ Explain that shoulder pain or release of gas through the vagina may occur postoperatively. During the procedure, the abdomen is filled with carbon dioxide to facilitate visualization. The surgical table is tilted so the intestines fall away from pelvic organs (see figure). Some gas may remain in the abdomen after the procedure.

☑ Instruct to report excessive pain at once.

After Surgery

☑ Monitor vital signs. Report temperature greater than 101° F (38.3° C).

☑ Apply perineal pad. Instruct to change pad at least every 4 hours. Keep a pad count.

☑ Explain that hiccups may occur after surgery. If it becomes a problem, a drug may be ordered.

Laparoscope
CO_2 distends abdomen
Uterus
Light source
Ovary
Uterine tube

Laparoscopy. A flexible, lighted instrument (laparoscope) is inserted through a small incision to visualize the abominal and pelvic cavities.

DIAGNOSING, PLANNING, AND IMPLEMENTING

Dysfunctional uterine bleeding often causes anxiety, and may threaten self-image, sexuality, or reproductive potential.

INEFFECTIVE COPING

■ Discuss results of diagnostic tests and examinations with the client face-to-face. *This allows for open exchange of information.*

■ Provide information about causes, treatment, risks, long-term effects, and prognosis for DUB. *This allows the client to assume responsibility for her own health and become involved in her own treatment plan.*

■ Evaluate coping strategies and psychosocial support systems. Teach appropriate coping strategies if indicated. *The possibility of surgery or cancer may be a crisis for the client and her support system. Effective coping strategies help in dealing with this situational crisis.*

SEXUAL DYSFUNCTION

■ Discuss sexual intercourse during menstruation. Explain that orgasm may help relieve symptoms, but that it is nec-essary to use contraception to prevent pregnancy even during menstruation. *Orgasm frequently provides at least temporary relief of symptoms. Some women mistakenly believe that birth control measures are unnecessary during menstruation.*

■ Provide an opportunity to express concerns related to effect of DUB on lifestyle and sexual functioning. *Some women abstain from sexual activity due to symptoms of DUB. Encouraging verbalization of concerns can assist to develop strategies to minimize the impact of DUB on sexuality and lifestyle.*

■ Encourage frequent rest periods. *This conserves energy and may allow sexual function to resume.*

■ Provide information about alternative methods of sexual expression. *Methods of sexual expression other than vaginal intercourse may satisfy the needs of both partners.*

EVALUATING

Collect data related to the following to evaluate the effectiveness of nursing interventions:

■ Verbalizes ability to cope with symptoms and treatment of disorder.

BOX 33-8
NURSING CARE CHECKLIST

DILATION AND CURETTAGE (D&C)

Before Surgery

☑ If ordered, ask to come in the day before surgery for insertion of a laminaria tent to absorb cervical secretions and slowly dilate the cervix.

☑ Provide routine preoperative instructions (see Chapter 7).

After Surgery

☑ Monitor circulation and sensation in the legs; avoid placing a pillow under the knees.

☑ Instruct to use perineal pads and avoid tampons for 2 weeks.

☑ Explain that the the next menstrual period may be delayed.

☑ Instruct to avoid intercourse until after follow-up visit and cessation of vaginal discharge.

☑ Advise rest, avoiding heavy lifting for several days, and to report bright red or excessive bleeding (more than a normal menstrual period).

BOX 33-9
NURSING CARE CHECKLIST

HYSTERECTOMY

Before Surgery

☑ Assess understanding and reinforce teaching as needed. Provide emotional support.

☑ Instruct to cleanse abdominal and perineal areas as ordered.

☑ If ordered, administer a small cleansing enema and have client empty bladder.

☑ Provide routine preoperative care as ordered (Chapter 7).

After Surgery

☑ Provide routine postoperative care (see Chapter 7).

☑ Report excess bleeding, especially following a vaginal hysterectomy.

☑ Monitor for potential complications, such as infection, ileus, thrombophlebitis, and pulmonary embolus.

☑ Assess vaginal drainage; teach perineal care.

☑ Advise to restrict physical activity for 4 to 6 weeks, and avoid heavy lifting, stair climbing, douching, tampons, and sexual intercourse.

☑ Instruct to shower, avoiding tub baths, until bleeding has stopped.

☑ Instruct to report the following to the physician:
   a. Temperature greater than 100° F (37.7° C)
   b. Vaginal bleeding greater than a typical menstrual period or that is bright red
   c. Urinary incontinence, urgency, burning, or frequency
   d. Severe pain

☑ Encourage expression of feelings and concerns.

☑ If appropriate, provide information about hormone replacement therapy.

☑ Reinforce the importance of regular gynecologic examinations even after hysterectomy.

■ Discusses acceptable and satisfying sexual practices with partner.

Discharge Considerations

Provide support, reassurance, and information to help the client and her family understand her disorder and its treatment. Teach self-care measures to help minimize the effects of DUB on activities of daily living.

Discuss using ordered drugs, including oral contraceptives, iron supplements, or other agents, including dosage and side effects. Encourage to take iron supplement with orange juice to improve absorption, and avoid taking it with foods high in calcium (such as milk), which interfere with its absorption. Provide information about maintaining a balanced diet, increasing iron-rich foods, such as eggs, beans, liver, beef, and shrimp. Encourage a fluid intake of 2,000 to 3,000 mL a day.

Emphasize the need to report recurring episodes of DUB (particularly in postmenopausal women) to the health care provider immediately.

 Menopause

Menopause (or the *climacteric*) is the period during which menstruation permanently ceases. It marks the natural biologic end of reproduction. Perimenopause includes the 4 or 5 years surrounding menopause, during which estrogen production declines, and the menses permanently ceases due to loss of ovarian function. It extends for 1 year after the final menstrual period. At this point, a woman is said to be postmenopausal.

Menopause is a normal physiologic process. However, the hormonal changes that occur can lead to unpleasant side effects. These side effects may vary from simply annoying to disruptive and difficult.

In the United States, menopause occurs usually between ages 45 and 55. *Surgical menopause* occurs when the ovaries are removed in premenopausal women. Certain health risks increase after menopause, including heart disease, osteoporosis, and breast cancer.

PHYSIOLOGY

During menopause, the number of ovarian follicles declines significantly, and the follicles that remain are less sensitive to FSH and LH. (Review the ovarian cycle at the beginning of the chapter.) As follicles cease to develop, ovarian estrogen production ceases. The ovaries continue to produce androgens, and small amounts of a less active form of estrogen are produced by the adrenal glands. This remaining estrogen is insufficient to maintain the female secondary sexual characteristics. This causes a loss of breast tissue, body hair, and subcutaneous fat. The ovaries and uterus shrink in size. The skin becomes less elastic, and vaginal and perineal tissues atrophy. Vaginal lubrication decreases.

An imbalance between estrogen and FSH from the pituitary gland causes vasomotor instability. This instability can lead to night sweats and hot flashes, palpitations, and headaches. The woman may have an increased incidence of vaginitis, as well as **dyspareunia** (pain during sexual intercourse). Menstrual cycles become irregular and eventually stop. Other common manifestations of menopause include possible irritability, anxiety, insomnia, difficulty concentrating, and depression.

COLLABORATIVE CARE

Care related to menopause focuses on managing symptoms, teaching about menopause, and discussing postmenopausal health risks.

Pharmacology

Hormone replacement therapy (HRT) is often used to relieve unpleasant manifestations of menopause and reduce the risks associated with estrogen deficiency. HRT relieves hot flashes and night sweats. It also decreases vaginal dryness and perineal tissue atrophy, which can lead to painful intercourse and urinary incontinence. Long-term benefits of HRT include:

1. May reduce risk of coronary heart disease by up to 60%
2. Helps prevent bone loss, osteoporosis, and fractures
3. May help prevent or delay onset of Alzheimer's disease

HRT, however, is not without risk. Nausea, vomiting, weight gain, breast tenderness and engorgement, and vaginal bleeding are common side effects of HRT. Fluid retention may be a problem. Long-term estrogen replacement increases the risk of endometrial cancer and ovarian cancer. A combination of estrogen with progestin reduces the risk of these cancers, but may contribute to bloating and irritability. HRT may increase the risk of breast cancer. Clients on HRT also may develop gallbladder disease. Table 33-3 ◆ provides nursing implications and client teaching related to HRT.

Women for whom HRT is inappropriate or who choose not to use HRT may take drugs known as selective estrogen receptor modulators (SERMs), such as raloxifene (Evista), to prevent some of the long-term effects of menopause. SERMs act like estrogen in some tissues but not in others, and appear to reduce the risk of breast cancer and osteoporosis significantly in menopausal women. They do not prevent the manifestations of menopause.

Complementary Therapies

A number of complementary therapies may be used to help relieve the symptoms of menopause. These include aromatherapy with geranium, rose, or fennel; herbs such as black cohosh, vitex, ginseng, and dong quai; meditation; and supplements such as vitamins D and E and soy protein.

TABLE 33-3   NURSING IMPLICATIONS FOR PHARMACOLOGY: CLIENTS RECEIVING HORMONE REPLACEMENT THERAPY

DRUG CLASSIFICATION/ DRUGS	ACTION	NURSING IMPLICATIONS	CLIENT AND FAMILY TEACHING
■ Conjugated Estrogens/ Medroxyprogesterone Acetate (Prempro, Premphase) ■ Estradiol/norethindrone acetate (Combipatch)	These drugs replace lost estrogen to minimize the manifestations of menopause and potentially reduce the long-term risks of menopause. Progesterone is added to the estrogen to reduce the risk of endometrial cancer.	Notify physician of contraindications to HRT: Pregnancy, breast cancer, undiagnosed vaginal bleeding, thrombo-phlebitis, or history of stroke. Women currently using any form of HRT should complete current cycle before changing products.	This replaces hormones lost during menopause. Do not use if you think you may be pregnant. You may have spotting or irregular menstrual bleeding while on HRT. Have yearly Pap smear and mammogram. Talk to your doctor about continuing HRT every 6 months; visit annually. Promptly report unusual bleeding, abdominal pain, or other adverse effects to your doctor.

NURSING CARE

ASSESSING

Collect subjective assessment data such as date of the last menstrual period, timing and regularity of the menstrual cycle, and duration and amount of menstrual flow. Ask the client if there is any risk that she could be pregnant. Inquire about menopausal symptoms such as night sweats, hot flashes, vaginal irritation or discomfort with intercourse, and measures that she has taken to relieve symptoms.

DIAGNOSING, PLANNING, AND IMPLEMENTING

The nursing role during menopause focuses on education.

DEFICIENT KNOWLEDGE: MENOPAUSE

■ Discuss symptoms the client is experiencing, and suggest strategies for coping (see Discharge Considerations). *Appropriate information helps both understanding and decision making. Many effects of menopause can be managed with lifestyle and other nondrug strategies.*

■ Provide information about the benefits and risks of HRT. *Information helps the client decide whether HRT is right for her.*

■ Recommend a daily calcium intake of 1,500 mg for clients not on HRT and 1,000 mg for clients on HRT. *Adequate calcium is important to help reduce the risk of osteoporosis associated with menopause.*

■ Emphasize the importance of aerobic and weight-bearing exercise. *Exercise reduces the rate of bone loss, helps maintain optimal weight, and reduces cardiovascular risk.*

SEXUAL DYSFUNCTION

■ Encourage the woman to express feelings and concerns about the effects of menopause on her sex life. *The client may not be comfortable expressing her feelings until the nurse shows comfort with the topic and encourages her.*

■ Suggest spending more time in foreplay and using water-soluble gels (e.g., Replens) for vaginal lubrication. *These measures can prevent vaginal pain and irritation and improve the quality of the sexual experience for the client and her partner.*

RISK FOR SITUATIONAL LOW SELF-ESTEEM

■ Encourage expression of fears and concerns related to changes in interpersonal and family roles. *Some women associate aging with "uselessness" and unattractiveness.*

■ Encourage volunteer activities or employment for the woman who has extra time. *This promotes a sense of usefulness and contribution to society. Activities involving young people can help reduce anxiety about the loss of reproductive ability.*

■ Discuss the importance of a healthy lifestyle in maintaining physical attractiveness. Identify risk factors and high-risk behaviors. *Lifestyle habits and behaviors (such as cigarette smoking and sun exposure) contribute to the aging process. Active women who exercise and eat a well-balanced diet look better and feel better.*

Discharge Considerations

Emphasize that menopause is a normal physiologic process, not a disease or an illness, and that symptoms are temporary and manageable. Discuss ways of coping with undesirable side effects (Box 33-10). Explain that making healthy lifestyle changes and reducing risk behaviors may reduce the need for HRT. Health maintenance and self-care are increasingly important: Encourage yearly mammograms, clinical breast examinations, and Pap tests, and monthly breast self-examination and self-monitoring for vaginitis.

BOX 33-10
TEACHING FOR DISCHARGE

COPING WITH SYMPTOMS OF MENOPAUSE

Vaginal Dryness
• Use a water-soluble lubricant for comfort during intercourse.
• Avoid vaginal douches or perineal powders.
• Eat 8 oz. of yogurt with live cultures daily to help prevent vaginitis.

Hot Flashes
• Let people know when you're having a hot flash—it's nothing to be ashamed of!
• Use relaxation techniques such as meditation or guided imagery during hot flashes.
• Stay active—activity relieves hot flashes and stress and improves sleep.
• Avoid hot-flash triggers such as alcohol, caffeine, sugar, hot or spicy foods, and very large meals.
• Dress in layers of natural fabrics.
• Splash face and neck with cool water or put something cool on wrists and forehead.
• Lower the thermostat, especially at night.

Irritability or Depression
• Stay involved in work or meaningful volunteer activities.
• Maintain balance—work, exercise, do something you enjoy, and get enough rest every day.

Structural Disorders of the Female Reproductive System

Structural disorders of the female reproductive system include displacement of the uterus from its normal position within the pelvis, prolapse of pelvic organs, and vaginal fistulas.

Uterine Displacement

The uterus is not fixed within the pelvis. It normally is positioned with the body and fundus facing anteriorly and the cervix more posterior, but its position may vary among women. An *anteverted* uterus is tilted toward the bladder, whereas a *retroverted* uterus is tilted toward the rectum (Figure 33-14A and B ◆). Changes in the upper portion of the uterus in relation to the cervix also can occur (Figure 33-14C and D). An *anteflexed* uterus is flexed forward on itself. Backward flexion of the uterus is called *retroflexion.*

Uterine displacement can be congenital or acquired. Childbirth or inflammation and scarring within the pelvic cavity can lead to displacement of the uterus. Clients with uterine displacement may experience manifestations such as painful menses (dysmenorrhea), discomfort during intercourse, and backache. The client also may have difficulty conceiving a child.

A Anteversion

B Retroversion

C Anteflexion

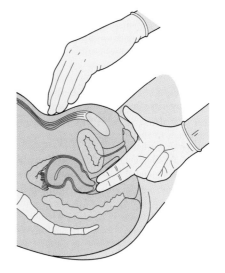

D Retroflexion

Figure 33-14. ◆ Common uterine displacements.

The diagnosis of uterine displacement is made by physical examination. A history of infections or difficulty conceiving support this diagnosis. In most cases, no treatment is necessary. Surgical suspension of the uterus may be done to treat associated infertility.

Nursing care focuses on teaching about the disorder. Many women have a poor understanding of their reproductive anatomy. This lack of knowledge may cause anxiety about the cause and seriousness of the disorder. Use drawings and models to explain the nature of the displacement disorder and its effects. Encourage the client and her partner to ask questions. Suggest trying alternate positions during sexual intercourse to relieve any discomfort. Reassure the client that the ability to have an orgasm is not affected.

Pelvic Organ Prolapse

Relaxation or damage of the pelvic floor muscles puts additional tension on the ligaments and structures that support the bladder, uterus, and rectum within the pelvis. When this occurs, these organs may prolapse, or drop down.

PATHOPHYSIOLOGY
Cystocele

A **cystocele** is prolapse of the urinary bladder into the vagina. It develops as the ligaments that support the bladder are stretched. Thinning of the vaginal wall commonly occurs during menopause, increasing the risk of cystocele. Cystocele often is accompanied by a urethrocele, or prolapse of the urethra into the vagina. The client with a cystocele often develops stress incontinence (see Chapter 21). Other manifestations include urinary frequency and urgency, and difficulty emptying the bladder. Frequent bladder infections may develop due to urinary retention.

Rectocele

Rectocele, protrusion of the anterior rectal wall into the vagina, may be caused by trauma during childbirth or chronic constipation with straining to defecate. The client may have a sense of pelvic pressure and difficulty defecating.

Uterine Prolapse

Prolapse of the uterus into the vagina can vary from mild to complete prolapse outside the body (Figure 33-15 ◆). Uterine prolapse is caused by stretching of the ligaments that normally support the uterus within the pelvis. Increased pressure within the abdomen also can lead to uterine prolapse. The client experiences a heavy or dragging sensation in the groin and lower back that is relieved by lying flat. She may notice a mass protruding from the vagina, especially after bearing down or with heavy lifting. Constipation, urinary incontinence, and painful intercourse are common.

COLLABORATIVE CARE

If pelvic organ prolapse is suspected, the client is asked to bear down or cough during pelvic examination to help identify the problem.

Figure 33-15. ◆ Complete uterine prolapse with inversion of the vagina.

Kegel exercises or physical therapy may be ordered to strengthen weakened pelvic muscles. (See Kegel exercises as outlined in Box 21-4). Pelvic organ prolapse often is treated surgically with procedures to repair the vaginal wall, shorten pelvic muscles and resuspend pelvic organs. In postmenopausal clients, hysterectomy is the preferred treatment for significant uterine prolapse.

When surgery is contraindicated or refused by the client, a pessary may be inserted into the vagina to provide temporary support for the uterus or bladder. At regular intervals, the pessary is removed, cleaned, and reinserted.

NURSING CARE

Stress incontinence is a common problem in clients with pelvic organ prolapse. Teach the client how to perform Kegel exercises. These exercises strengthen perineal muscle tone, minimize urinary leakage, and minimize descent of the bladder and rectum into the vagina. Discuss hormone replacement therapy with postmenopausal women. It helps maintain pelvic tissue, reducing the risk for prolapse. Suggest using perineal pads to absorb urine leakage, and teach appropriate perineal care measures:

- Cleanse the perineum from front to back.
- Change perineal or incontinence pads frequently.
- Avoid using perineal sprays or powders.

Suggest reducing or eliminating caffeine intake and minimizing consumption of diet sodas. Both caffeine and artificial sweeteners can aggravate urinary incontinence.

Teach the client for whom a pessary is ordered how to insert, remove, and care for the device.

Because obesity is a risk factor for pelvic organ prolapse, diet counseling may be indicated. Suggest self-help diet organizations such as Weight Watchers or TOPS.

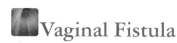
Vaginal Fistula

A *fistula* is an abnormal opening or passage between two organs or spaces that are normally separated. A vaginal fistula may develop between the vagina and the urinary bladder or between the vagina and the rectum. The fistula may be a complication of childbirth, surgery, or radiation therapy. Bladder cancer also may lead to vaginal fistula. Urine or stool and flatus enter the vagina through this abnormal opening, causing complaints of involuntary leakage of urine or gas. A small vaginal fistula may resolve without treatment. Larger fistulas may require surgical repair.

Nursing care is similar to that provided for any client undergoing pelvic surgery (see Chapter 7). Teaching is important. Stress the importance of careful perineal cleansing to reduce irritation and prevent further tissue breakdown. Suggest perineal irrigation or sitz baths for cleansing. Perineal pads may be used to absorb urine or fecal drainage. Provide information about avoiding gas-forming foods to minimize embarrassment from odor.

Disorders of Female Reproductive Tissue

Disorders of female reproductive tissue include endometriosis, cysts and polyps, and benign tumors known as uterine leiomyomas (fibroids). Malignant tumors of reproductive tissue are discussed in the next section of this chapter.

Endometriosis

Endometriosis is a common condition in which endometrial tissue is found outside the uterus. Endometrial tissue may be found on the ovary and other pelvic organs or tissues, and rarely in other organs such as the lungs. Risk factors may include a family history of endometriosis; early menarche; and short, regular menstrual cycles with heavy flow.

PATHOPHYSIOLOGY
The cause of endometriosis is unknown. It may be caused by backflow of menstrual blood carrying endometrial cells through the fallopian tubes into the pelvis. Cells that can develop into endometrium may be implanted during embryonic development, or endometrial cells may spread through the blood or lymph to other sites. Inflammation or immune responses may contribute to endometriosis.

The **ectopic** (in an abnormal location) endometrial tissue responds to the ovarian cycle, and bleeding occurs during menses. The implants regress during pregnancy and atrophy at menopause. Bleeding of the ectopic tissue may cause cysts, scarring, inflammation, and adhesions. Scarring can lead to infertility and problems such as bowel obstruction.

The manifestations of endometriosis occur just before and during the menses. They include dysmenorrhea with backache and cramps, painful defecation, dysuria, dyspareunia, and infertility. These manifestations may vary, depending on the site of ectopic tissue.

COLLABORATIVE CARE
Endometriosis often is diagnosed by the history and physical exam. Firm, tender nodules are found in the pelvic cavity, and the uterus may be retroflexed. A *pelvic ultrasound* may be done, or a laparoscopy performed to visualize the implants. (Review Boxes 33-6 and 33-7 for nursing implications for these exams.)

Pharmacology
Mild analgesics and NSAIDs are used to relieve pain associated with endometriosis. Hormones such as oral contraceptives, progesterone, or danazol (an androgen hormone) may be given to suppress ovarian function, at least temporarily. Suppressing ovarian function allows the ectopic tissue to shrink.

Surgery
Ectopic lesions may be treated by laser or electrocautery via laparoscopic surgery. When the disease is severe and childbearing is no longer desired, a bilateral **salpingo-oophorectomy** (BSO, removal of the fallopian tubes and ovaries) and hysterectomy may be performed.

NURSING CARE

ASSESSING

When assessing the client with endometriosis, collect subjective data such as:

- Pain—timing in relation to menses; location, quality, and duration
- Other symptoms such as painful defecation, dysuria, painful intercourse, or other manifestations associated with menses

- Pregnancy history or desire for and attempts to conceive a child
- Affect of the condition on life, roles, and relationships

DIAGNOSING, PLANNING, AND IMPLEMENTING

PAIN

- Evaluate the severity and timing of the pain. *Although the severity of the pain may not directly relate to the severity of the disease, it will help guide the choice of treatment.*
- Discuss using drugs and nonpharmacologic measures for pain relief. *Heat to the abdomen or back, relaxation techniques (e.g., yoga and meditation), exercise, and biofeedback can help the client manage pain, particularly when used together with analgesics.*
- Suggest trying alternative positions for sexual intercourse. *Different positions may reduce discomfort during intercourse for the client with endometriosis.*

ANXIETY

- Encourage discussion of concerns about infertility. Answer questions honestly. *Knowledge helps the client gain a sense of control and relieve anxiety and fear.*
- Discuss the advantages of having children soon and in rapid succession, and using oral contraceptives between pregnancies to minimize bleeding. *Ectopic endometrial tissue regresses during pregnancy and with oral contraceptives, reducing scarring.*
- Provide information about measures to promote conception, including measuring basal body temperature and other techniques to identify ovulation. *Using measures such as these helps optimize the chance of conception.*

EVALUATING

To evaluate the effectiveness of nursing interventions for the client with endometriosis, collect information about the client's ability to manage associated discomfort and cope with the effects of the disorder.

Discharge Considerations

Teach the client and family about endometriosis and treatment options, including their side effects. Discuss the possible benefits of having children earlier in life, rather than delaying parenthood. If the client has undergone surgery, provide instructions for home care, including managing incisions, preventing infection, and follow-up care.

Ovarian Cysts

A cyst is a fluid-filled sac. Cysts can develop in the vulva, endometrium, or ovaries. This section focuses on ovarian cysts.

PATHOPHYSIOLOGY

Ovarian cysts may be either follicular cysts or corpus luteum cysts. Follicular cysts develop when a mature follicle does not rupture or when the fluid in an immature follicle does not reabsorb after ovulation. Corpus luteum cysts occur when the corpus luteum remains enlarged after ovulation. Most cysts regress spontaneously within two or three menstrual cycles.

Polycystic ovary syndrome (PCOS) is characterized by numerous follicular cysts. It is an endocrine disorder in which LH, estrogen, and androgen hormone levels are higher than normal, and FSH levels are low. This hormone imbalance causes irregular menstrual periods, *hirsutism* (excessive hair growth), acne, obesity, and infertility. Women with PCOS often have insulin resistance and may develop Type 2 diabetes early in adulthood. PCOS also increases the risk of endometrial cancer, hypertension, and abnormal cholesterol levels.

COLLABORATIVE CARE

Care focuses on identifying and correcting the disorder and preventing its recurrence.

Diagnostic Tests

Diagnostic tests may be used to diagnose and differentiate ovarian cysts:

- *LH, FSH,* and *serum testosterone* levels are measured. The FSH–LH ratio is reversed in PCOS, and serum testosterone levels are higher than normal.
- *Glucose tolerance tests* may be done to identify possible Type 2 diabetes.
- *Laparoscopy* is done to visualize ovarian cysts. (Review Box 33-7 for nursing care of the client undergoing laparoscopy.)

Pharmacology

Oral contraceptives often are ordered to regulate the menses in women with PCOS. If the client wishes to become pregnant, clomiphene (Clomid, Serophene) may be prescribed to stimulate ovulation. Other drugs such as progesterone or the corticosteroid dexamethasone can be given to control manifestations of hirsutism.

Surgery

Follicular cysts may be punctured through laser surgery, or a wedge resection of the ovary may be done to restore ovulation. Rarely, **oophorectomy** (removal of the ovary) is performed if the cysts are very large.

NURSING CARE

Unless surgery is performed, the focus of nursing care for clients with ovarian cysts is on education. Provide information about the disorder and prescribed treatment. Discuss the benign and temporary nature of most ovarian cysts other than PCOS. Discuss the risks and benefits of treatment options with the client. Encourage the client with PCOS to share concerns about potential risks and the effect of the disorder on the

population
FOCUS

Uterine Fibroid Tumors in African American Women

Uterine fibroid tumors are three to nine times more common in African American women than in white women: 40% to 50% of African American women between ages 30 and 60 develop fibroid tumors, whereas only 20% of Caucasian women in this age group develop them.

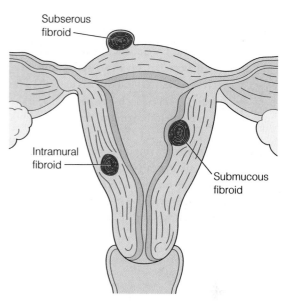

Figure 33-16. ◆ Sites of uterine fibroid tumors.

ability to conceive. Teach measures to reduce the risk of heart disease (control hypertension, exercise and diet management to control cholesterol levels, avoid smoking, manage stress) and Type 2 diabetes (weight loss and diet management). Stress the importance of regular follow-up with a health care provider knowledgeable about PCOS. Teach the manifestations of endometrial cancer, and stress the importance of promptly notifying the health care provider if symptoms develop.

Uterine Fibroid Tumor

Fibroid tumors, or *uterine leiomyomas,* are benign tumors of the uterus or cervix. They are common among all women of childbearing age (see Box 33-11), and are a leading reason for hysterectomy.

Fibroid tumors are classified by their location in the wall of the uterus (Figure 33-16 ◆). *Intramural* tumors are within the uterine wall. *Subserous* fibroids are beneath the outer layer of the uterus, projecting into the peritoneal cavity. *Submucous* fibroid tumors are beneath the endometrial lining of the uterus.

The cause of fibroid tumors is not clear, but they are probably related to estrogen secretion. Small tumors may be asymptomatic. Large fibroids can crowd other organs, causing pelvic pressure, pain, dysmenorrhea, menorrhagia, and

fatigue. Depending on tumor location, constipation and urinary urgency and frequency are common. The uterus is enlarged. Excessive bleeding often causes anemia.

In asymptomatic women who wish to bear children, fibroid tumors are monitored. Drugs may be given to reduce tumor size and slow their growth. *Laparoscopic myomectomy,* removal of the tumor without removing the entire uterus, may be performed in young women who wish to have a child. Hysterectomy is performed if tumors are large, and in women who are menopausal.

If surgery is deferred, client and family teaching emphasizes the importance of regular follow-up appointments to monitor tumor growth. If surgery is chosen, teaching emphasizes pain control techniques and appropriate preoperative and postoperative teaching (see the previous discussion of the client undergoing a hysterectomy). Dietary modifications to increase iron intake, prevent constipation, and promote healing are important.

Malignant Tumors

Cervical Cancer

Cervical cancer is common. Early detection and intervention have substantially reduced the incidence of invasive cervical cancer and deaths due to cervical cancer.

Most cervical cancers are related to infection of the cervix with human papillomavirus (HPV). The other risk factors for

cervical cancer include early sexual experience, multiple sex partners, HIV infection, unprotected sex, smoking, and a poor diet.

PATHOPHYSIOLOGY

Most cervical cancers begin as changes in squamous cells of the cervix. These changes are called *cervical intraepithelial neo-*

plasia *(CIN)*. Over a number of years, these cells become more abnormal and the number of affected cells increases, developing into carcinoma in situ. Carcinoma in situ is localized, but if it is not treated, it becomes invasive, spreading into the underlying connective tissue. Cervical cancers spread by direct invasion of surrounding tissues such as the vagina, bladder, and rectum, as well as by metastasizing to the pelvis and other organs.

Early cancer causes no symptoms. Invasive cancer produces bleeding and leukorrhea (whitish discharge from the vagina), which increase as the cancer progresses. Other manifestations include pain in the back or thighs, hematuria, bloody stools, anemia, and weight loss.

COLLABORATIVE CARE
Screening

A *Papanicolaou (Pap) smear* is used to screen for cervical cancer. Cells and secretions from the cervix are collected and spread on a glass slide for examination. Infectious or abnormal cell changes can be identified. Abnormal cells may be described as atypical, mild dysplasia, or moderate to severe dysplasia (carcinoma in situ). See Box 33-12 for nursing responsibilities related to a Pap smear.

> ### BOX 33-12
> ### NURSING CARE CHECKLIST
>
> #### PAPANICOLAOU (PAP) SMEAR
> #### Before the Test
> ☑ Do not schedule during menses.
> ☑ Instruct to avoid sexual intercourse, douching, or vaginal medications for 36 hours before the test.
> ☑ Instruct to empty the bladder.
>
> #### During the Test
> ☑ Assist into lithotomy position (lying on the table with the feet in stirrups).
> ☑ Label slides with client's name.
> ☑ When the samples have been collected, apply spray fixative or immerse slides in fixative solution.
>
> #### After the Test
> ☑ Assist to a more comfortable position.
> ☑ Provide tissue and a panty liner (spotting may occur after the test).
> ☑ Complete lab requisitions or forms.
> ☑ Inform client when and how results of the test will be communicated, and answer any questions.
> ☑ Advise to return for a repeat Pap smear as recommended:
>   ☑ Every 3 years until age 65, then annually
>   ☑ Annually or more frequently if specific risk factors such as HPV are present

Diagnostic Tests
- If the initial *Pap smear* shows abnormal cells, it is repeated.
- The *Digene Hybrid Capture II HPV test* may be done to identify the presence of high-risk strains of HPV.
- *Colposcopy* and *biopsy* of the suspicious area may be done if the second Pap smear shows abnormal cells. A colposcope is an instrument that provides a lighted and magnified view of the cervix, allowing tissue to be obtained from suspicious lesions. Box 33-13 describes nursing implications for cervical biopsy.
- *MRI* or *CT* of the pelvis, abdomen, or bones may be done to evaluate for tumor spread.

Treatment

When the tumor is limited to cervical tissue (not invasive), it may be excised by laser, heated or cooled probes, or cauterization. *Conization,* removal of a cone-shaped wedge of cervical tissue (Figure 33-17 ◆) may be done if the lesion extends into the endocervical canal.

Radioactive implants of needles, tubes, or seeds into the uterine cavity (brachytherapy) are used to treat locally invasive tumors. For invasive lesions, hysterectomy or radical hysterectomy (removal of the uterus, fallopian tubes, lymph nodes, and ovaries) is performed. A *pelvic exenteration*—removal of all pelvic contents, including the bowel, vagina, and bladder—may be done for locally invasive cancer. Radiation therapy also is used to treat invasive cervical cancer. External radiation beam therapy may be used before surgery to decrease the size of the tumor. Chemotherapy may be used when surgery or radiation therapy cannot be used or if the cancer has metastasized (see Chapter 8).

> ### BOX 33-13
> ### NURSING CARE CHECKLIST
>
> #### CERVICAL BIOPSY
> #### Before the Test
> ☑ Explain the procedure. Discomfort is minimal, although cramping may be felt during cervical dilation.
> ☑ Have client empty her bladder.
>
> #### After the Test
> ☑ Cleanse the area, apply a perineal pad, and assist to a comfortable position.
> ☑ Explain that minor bleeding and vaginal discharge are expected; use perineal pads and avoid tampons for at least 1 week.
> ☑ Caution to avoid sexual intercourse until discharge has stopped.
> ☑ Instruct to notify physician of heavy bleeding, pain, foul-smelling discharge, fever, or malaise.

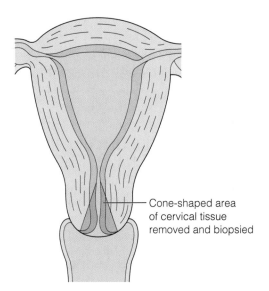

Figure 33-17. ◆ Conization, removal of a cone-shaped section of the cervix.

NURSING CARE

ASSESSING

Because the client with cervical cancer rarely has symptoms until the cancer is advanced, nursing assessment focuses on collecting data related to risk factors for cervical cancer. Ask:

- At what age the client began having sexual intercourse
- Number of partners
- Use of barrier protection (male or female condoms)
- History of sexually transmitted diseases
- Smoking history

DIAGNOSING, PLANNING, AND IMPLEMENTING

Nursing care involves helping the client deal with the physical and psychologic effects of cervical cancer, providing information needed to make informed decisions, and minimizing the adverse effects of treatment.

IMPAIRED TISSUE INTEGRITY

- Teach wound and skin care specific to needs. *Open and damaged tissue increases the risk for infection. Meticulous skin and wound care helps prevent infection and further tissue destruction.*
- Apply non–oil-based lotions to skin to reduce itching and help maintain integrity. *Oil-based lotions are not recommended for tissue undergoing radiation.*
- Instruct to preserve markings used to localize the radiation beam to the target area. *Markings are used in future radiation treatments.*
- Observe for manifestations of fistula, and teach the client to do the same. *Fistulas may form as a complication of radiation to the pelvic or abdominal cavities.*

FEAR

- Explain that most women with cervical cancer survive for 5 years or more, and that the earlier the cancer is detected, the better the prognosis. *The cure rate for early cervical cancer is 90%. This fact can provide hope, an essential ingredient in recovery.*
- Allow time to express concerns and to ask questions. *Unexpressed feelings and fears and lack of understanding may cause the client to view the situation as worse than it is.*
- Refer to counselor or support group for additional information. *Cancer survivors provide proof that people can survive the diagnosis and treatment of cancer and lead normal, productive lives.*

EVALUATING

To evaluate the effectiveness of nursing interventions, collect data related to skin integrity and absence of infection. Ask the client and family members about coping with the diagnosis and treatment, and provide additional information and support as needed.

 ## Discharge Considerations

Teach all clients and the public how to control risk factors for cervical cancer. Stress the importance of regular pelvic exams and Pap smears throughout the life span. Teach young women about the relationship between early sexual activity, multiple partners, and risk for sexually transmitted diseases and cervical cancer. Discuss safer sex alternatives and using condoms for protection. Emphasize the importance of continued screening exams for the older client who may not see a gynecologic specialist on a regular basis.

Client and family teaching varies according to the stage of the cancer and the treatment selected. Provide information concerning radiation, chemotherapy, or surgery, as indicated. Refer the client to home health services and/or a cancer support group.

Nursing Process Case Study
■ CLIENT WITH CERVICAL CANCER

Anna Eliza Gillam is a 45-year-old divorced woman with four children ranging in age from 16 to 23. She was married at age 18 and had several sexual partners prior to marriage. She has had three sexual partners since her marriage ended. Her Pap smear 2 weeks ago showed atypical cells. A repeat Pap smear and biopsy of a cervical lesion is positive for squamous cell carcinoma of the cervix.

Assessment The nursing assessment reveals: BP 130/80; P 72; R 18; T 99.2° F (37.3° C). Weight 142 lbs. (64.5 kg), approximately 15% over ideal for height. Smokes about one half pack of cigarettes per day, and does not drink alcohol.

Ms. Gillam is very fearful and has told no one about her abnormal Pap smear. She says that she has had back pain radiating down her thighs for several months and a foul vaginal discharge that increases after intercourse. Until 2 weeks ago, she had not had a Pap smear for 5 years.

Laparoscopy shows the disease to be widespread in the pelvic cavity. A CT scan is scheduled.

Diagnosis The nursing diagnoses for Ms. Gillam include the following:

- Decisional Conflict related to treatment options
- Pain related to metastasis and surgery
- Risk for Impaired Skin Integrity related to radiation
- Anticipatory Grieving related to cancer diagnosis and potential loss of life

Expected Outcomes The expected outcomes for the plan of care specify that Ms. Gillam will:

- Gain knowledge to make informed decisions about treatment options.
- Develop strategies for pain control.
- Maintain skin and tissue integrity during radiation therapy.
- Develop effective coping strategies for dealing with life-threatening illness and pain.

Planning and Implementation The following interventions are planned and implemented for Ms. Gillam:

- Explore treatment alternatives, including the prognosis with each option.
- Administer pain medications as ordered.
- Inspect skin surfaces daily before and after radiation therapy.
- Provide information about additional strategies for pain control.
- Refer to a local cancer support group.
- Refer to clinical social worker for discharge and home care planning.
- Assess response to treatment and understanding of her disease.
- Recommend a high-protein, high-carbohydrate diet.

Evaluation Ms. Gillam has begun radiation therapy following pelvic exenteration. She controls her pain with relaxation and imagery techniques, requiring only occasional analgesics. Her skin is reddened but intact in the area of radiation. Ms. Gillam seems optimistic and has quit smoking. She and her family are continuing to attend the cancer support group meetings.

Critical Thinking in the Nursing Process

1. Develop a teaching outline to use with groups about reducing modifiable risks for cervical cancer.
2. Following an abnormal Pap smear, a second smear reveals inflammatory changes consistent with HPV but no cell changes. What advice will you provide to the client?
3. Explain the terms *noninvasive* and *invasive* in relation to cervical cancer and its methods of treatment.

Endometrial Cancer

Endometrial cancer is common. It usually affects older women between ages 50 and 70. In addition to age, risk factors for endometrial cancer include early menarche, late menopause, history of infertility, extended use of tamoxifen or estrogen therapy (without progestins), obesity, and diabetes. Endometrial cancer is curable. With early diagnosis and treatment, the 5-year survival rate exceeds 90%.

PATHOPHYSIOLOGY

Most endometrial malignancies are slow to grow and metastasize. These tumors tend to be associated with estrogen excess, and begin with endometrial hyperplasia. This type of endometrial cancer occurs more commonly in perimenopausal white women. Endometrial cancers seen in postmenopausal Asian and African American women may be more aggressive and are not associated with known risk factors.

The tumor usually begins in the fundus of the uterus, invades the muscle of the uterus, and spreads throughout the female reproductive tract. Metastasis occurs by the lymphatic system and bloodstream, as well as through the fallopian tubes to the peritoneal cavity. Target areas for metastasis include the lungs, liver, and bone.

Abnormal uterine bleeding after menopause is the most common manifestation of endometrial cancer. This bleeding is usually painless but may be moderate to large in amount. Vaginal discharge is another sign of endometrial cancer. On pelvic examination, the uterus often is enlarged.

COLLABORATIVE CARE

The preliminary diagnosis of endometrial cancer is made based on the history and physical examination. An endometrial biopsy or D&C is performed to obtain cells for examination. (Review Box 33-8 on nursing responsibilities related to a D&C.)

Treatment

The treatment of choice for primary endometrial carcinoma is a total abdominal hysterectomy and bilateral salpingo-oophorectomy (removal of the uterus, fallopian tubes, and both ovaries). Pelvic lymph nodes also may be resected during surgery. Radiation therapy may be done before surgery to shrink the tumor or after surgery to eliminate cancer cells in lymph nodes. Progesterone is ordered to treat recurrent disease. Chemotherapy is less effective than other forms of therapy, although it may be used to treat disseminated disease.

NURSING CARE

Nursing care involves helping the client deal with the physical and psychological effects of endometrial cancer, make informed decisions, and minimize the adverse effects of therapy. The client who has had a hysterectomy requires pre- and postoperative nursing care. (Review Box 33-9.) Encourage the client to perform self-care and resume normal activities of daily living.

DISTURBED BODY IMAGE

- Review the side effects of treatment (hair loss, nausea, vomiting, fatigue, diarrhea, stomatitis, and surgical scarring), and help develop a plan to deal with these effects. *This promotes a sense of control.*
- Provide information about measures to alleviate adverse effects of chemotherapy, such as premedicating with antiemetic drugs, using viscous lidocaine for stomatitis, and obtaining a wig or using hats and scarves to cover the head. *Knowledge helps reduce a sense of helplessness clients often feel in dealing with these effects.*

Discharge Considerations

Provide information about the disease and proposed specific treatments. To clients receiving radiation therapy, emphasize the importance of keeping appointments. If necessary, help them arrange transportation to and from the facility. Teach appropriate skin care. Explain the expected side effects of radiation implant therapy (see Chapter 8). Pain control measures are also an essential part of the teaching plan (see Chapter 6). Emphasize the importance of follow-up care as recommended.

Ovarian Cancer

Ovarian cancer is the most lethal of the gynecologic cancers, because it is often asymptomatic. In most cases, the disease has spread beyond the ovaries at the time of diagnosis. Ovarian cancer is more common in European American women than in African American women. However, the mortality rate is higher in African American women.

Risk factors for ovarian cancer include older age, early menarche and late menopause, history of infertility, treatment for infertility with clomiphene (Clomid), and a personal or family history of breast or ovarian cancer. Regular use of products containing talc, such as body and baby powders, may increase the risk of developing ovarian cancer.

PATHOPHYSIOLOGY

Because the ovaries contain several different tissue types, there are different types of ovarian cancers. These cancers grow and spread at different rates. The most common type of ovarian cancer is an epithelial tumor. Malignant tumors usually present as solid masses with areas of necrosis and hemorrhage.

Ovarian cancer spreads by shedding cancer cells into the peritoneal cavity and by direct invasion of the bowel and bladder. Tumor cells also spread through the lymph system and blood to lymph nodes and such organs as the liver and the lungs.

Early ovarian cancer generally has no symptoms. When manifestations do develop, they are often vague and mild, such as indigestion, urinary frequency, abdominal bloating, and constipation. Pelvic pain sometimes occurs. An enlarged abdomen with ascites (a collection of fluid in the abdomen) is a late manifestation of ovarian cancer.

COLLABORATIVE CARE

While an enlarged ovary may be palpated on physical examination, diagnostic tests usually are required to detect ovarian cancer. These tests may include:

- *CA125* is a tumor marker that may be detected in the blood. It is often not elevated in early ovarian cancer, however, and is not specific for ovarian cancer. It also may be elevated in endometriosis, with uterine fibroid tumors, or during pregnancy.
- *Transvaginal ultrasonography* may be done to detect ovarian masses. This test, however, cannot differentiate between cystic or benign ovarian masses and malignancy.
- *Laparoscopy* is performed to obtain tissue for biopsy and determine organ involvement.

Surgery is the treatment of choice for ovarian cancer. In most cases, a total hysterectomy with bilateral salpingo-oophorectomy is performed, and other organs and tissues in the abdomen are inspected for spread of the cancer. Following surgery, chemotherapy may be used to eliminate cancer cells in other tissues. Paclitaxel (Taxol), a relatively new chemotherapy drug, may help achieve and maintain remission. See Chapter 8 for more information about nursing care of the client receiving chemotherapy.

NURSING CARE

Nursing care for the client with ovarian cancer is similar to the nursing care for clients with other gynecologic cancers. The side effects of treatment and generally poor prognosis affect the quality of life and have major psychosocial implications. Anticipatory grieving may begin at the time of diagnosis.

Educate women who have significant risk factors for ovarian cancer, such as a positive family history of the disease or previous breast cancer, about the importance of having regular pelvic examinations. Suggest regular screening with transvaginal ultrasound and CA125 measurements for this high-risk group. Teach clients not to ignore symptoms such as indigestion, nausea, or urinary frequency, as these may be early manifestations of ovarian tumors. Emphasize, however, that ovarian cancer usually has no symptoms in early stages. Instruct any woman with a palpable abdominal mass to see her primary care provider.

Discuss recommended treatment with women who have ovarian cancer. Suggest ways to minimize or manage side efects. Provide emotional and psychological support throughout the course of the disease, and refer the client to hospice services when appropriate.

Cancer of the Vulva

Cancer of the vulva usually affects older women between the ages of 60 and 70. In younger women, it is strongly associated with sexually transmitted diseases, particularly HPV. Herpes simplex type 2 (HSV-2) infection also is a risk factor for vulvar cancer.

The prognosis of vulvar carcinoma generally is good, with an 85% to 90% five-year survival rate when there is no lymph node involvement.

PATHOPHYSIOLOGY

Cancer of the vulva usually arises in epithelial cells. The primary site is usually the labia majora, but it also may be found on the labia minora, clitoris, vestibule, and other perineal tissues. It spreads by direct extension into surrounding tissues, as well as through the lymph system to regional and pelvic lymph nodes.

Cancer of the vulva often causes no symptoms, and lesions are discovered on routine examination or self-examination. The lesion may appear as a white macular patch, a small raised lump, an ulceration, or a red painless sore.

Persistent pruritus (itching) and irritation of the vulva is the most common symptom. Perineal pain and bleeding occur with advanced disease.

COLLABORATIVE CARE

Visible lesions are carefully examined, excised, and biopsied. Early, noninvasive lesions are excised using laser surgery, cryosurgery, or electrocautery. For more advanced disease, vulvectomy may be performed (Figure 33-18 ◆).

In a simple *vulvectomy,* the vulva, labia majora and minora, clitoris, and prepuce are removed. In a radical vulvectomy, subcutaneous tissue and regional lymph nodes are removed as well. If surgery is contraindicated, lesions may be treated with locally applied chemotherapy or by laser.

NURSING CARE

Disruption of perineal tissues is a priority nursing problem for clients being treated for cancer of the vulva. Sexuality also is

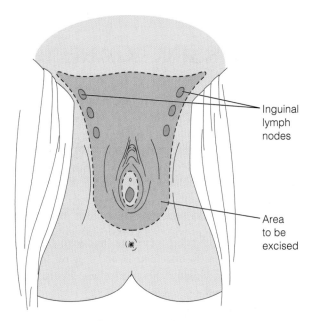

Inguinal lymph nodes

Area to be excised

Figure 33-18. ◆ Vulvectomy for cancer of the vulva.

significantly affected, and must be considered as a nursing care problem.

IMPAIRED TISSUE INTEGRITY

- Teach the client and/or her partner or other family member how to irrigate perineal tissues. *Irrigation helps prevent skin breakdown and infection.*
- After irrigation, apply dry heat using a heat lamp positioned about 18 inches from the area; emphasize safety precautions, including use of a low-wattage bulb (40 to 60 watts). *Dry heat helps promote healing and comfort.*
- Discuss dietary measures (high protein, iron, and vitamin C) to promote healing. *These nutrients promote collagen formation and wound healing.*

Discharge Considerations

Because many clients who undergo treatment for cancer of the vulva are older, consider referral to home health services for wound management. Discuss early manifestations of infection or impaired healing, and stress the importance of contacting the physician if these develop. Instruct the client to cleanse the perineum by pouring warm water over it after voiding and using a sitz bath after defecation. If lymph nodes have been removed, the client may experience lower extremity edema. Teach the client to elevate the feet and legs when sitting, and to wear antiembolic elastic hose when out of bed.

Infections of the Female Reproductive System

Infections affecting the female reproductive tract may be local or systemic. Many are sexually transmitted diseases (STDs), discussed in Chapter 34. The most common local infections are vaginal, including simple vaginitis, candidiasis, and trichomoniasis. Systemic infections include pelvic inflammatory disease, toxic shock syndrome, and HIV/AIDS (see Chapter 13).

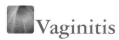

Vaginitis

Vaginitis, inflammation or infection of the vagina, is common. Vaginal infections are classified by cause, and may be fungal (candidiasis), protozoan (trichomoniasis), or bacterial (*Gardnerella*) infections.

Risk factors for vaginitis include unprotected sexual activity, multiple sexual partners, using a broad-spectrum antibiotic, obesity, diabetes, pregnancy, and poor personal hygiene. Sexual activity and swimming in contaminated water are risk factors for trichomoniasis.

PATHOPHYSIOLOGY

The low pH of vaginal secretions, normal vaginal flora, and estrogen normally protect against vaginal infections. An infection is more likely to develop when any or all of these factors are disrupted. When conditions are favorable, microorganisms invade the vulva and vagina. Simple vaginitis is the most common vaginal infection in women of reproductive age. *Gardnerella vaginalis* is the causative organism in many cases. Candidiasis (moniliasis or yeast infection) is caused by the organism *Candida albicans.* Candida organisms are part of the normal vaginal environment, causing problems only when they multiply rapidly. When increased estrogen levels, antibiotics, fecal contamination, or other factors alter the normal vaginal flora, *Candida* organisms multiply, causing a yeast infection.

Trichomoniasis, a protozoan infection, is a sexually transmitted disease. This organism frequently is carried asymptomatically by the male partner.

Most vaginal infections cause vaginal discharge, itching or burning, and dysuria. The specific manifestations of various vaginal infections are outlined in Table 33-4 ◆.

COLLABORATIVE CARE

Vaginitis is common and often is appropriate for self-care. Many topical agents are available over the counter. Clients with persistent or recurrent episodes of vaginitis should be carefully evaluated. Repeated vaginal yeast infections may be a manifestation of diabetes or HIV infection.

Diagnostic Tests

■ Vaginal secretions are cultured and examined microscopically for the presence of "clue cells," a sign of bacterial vaginitis.
■ *"Wet mount"* or *"wet prep"* with potassium hydroxide (KOH) reveals a fishy odor in bacterial vaginitis. The slide is examined microscopically to detect *hyphae* (filaments or threads) and *Candida* spores.
■ *Normal saline wet prep* is used to detect the presence of protozoa if trichomoniasis is suspected.
■ *Glucose tolerance tests* or *HIV screening* may be done at the time of the initial assessment.
■ *Pregnancy tests* may be done because certain treatments are contraindicated during pregnancy.

Pharmacology

Drugs used to treat vaginitis vary with the organism, as shown in Table 33-4. In many cases, the client's sexual partner must also be treated to prevent reinfection. Mild vinegar douches may be ordered, but should not be used routinely. Frequent douching washes away normal flora, affecting the natural defense mechanism against bacterial invasion.

NURSING CARE

ASSESSING

Collect subjective assessment data from the client with complaints of vaginal discharge or itching. Subjective data includes the onset, duration, and severity of the symptoms, as well as any associated manifestations (such as dysuria, frequency, and urgency, or abdominal pain) and circumstances (such as antibiotic therapy). Ask to describe the amount, color, odor, and consistency of vaginal discharge. Inquire about perineal care (use of bubble baths, perineal powders or sprays, and douching) and usual dressing habits (underwear of synthetic materials, tight jeans or pants). Ask if the client could be pregnant and about menstrual history. Inquire about any chronic diseases such as diabetes or HIV infection, and current medications. Finally, ask what self-care measures she has used to treat her symptoms.

DIAGNOSING, PLANNING, AND IMPLEMENTING

Nursing care focuses on teaching the client and, if necessary, her sexual partner to comply with the treatment regimen, use safer sex practices, and prevent future transmission of the infection.

TABLE 33-4 VAGINAL INFECTIONS

INFECTION	TYPE OF DISCHARGE	OTHER MANIFESTATIONS	TREATMENT	NURSING CARE
Candidiasis (*Monilia,* yeast infection)	Thick white patches adhering to cervix and vaginal wall, resembling cottage cheese; little odor	Itching of vulva and vaginal area, redness, painful intercourse	Butoconazole, miconazole, clotrimazole, or terconazole creams, vaginal tablets, or suppositories	Teach perineal hygiene and use of vaginal applicators. Instruct to complete entire treatment.
Simple vaginitis (bacterial vaginosis, *Gardnerella* vaginosis)	Thin, white, "milklike," or gray with fishy odor, especially when mixed with potassium hydroxide	None to mild itching or burning in vulvar area; clue cells on microscopic examination	Oral metronidazole or metronidazole gel; clindamycin cream or oral clindamycin	Teach perineal hygiene. Instruct to complete treatment. Discuss relationship to PID.
Trichomoniasis	Frothy, yellow or white, foul odor	Burning and itching of vulva	Oral metronidazole for client and sexual partner	Teach perineal hygiene; avoid unprotected intercourse until treatment completed.
Atrophic vaginitis (senile vaginitis)	Thin, opaque discharge, may be blood-tinged, odorless; pale, smooth, thin, dry vaginal walls	Painful intercourse, itching, vaginal dryness	Topical estrogen cream; water-soluble lubricant for intercourse; possible HRT	Discuss symptoms of menopause and sexual techniques to minimize trauma.

DEFICIENT KNOWLEDGE: PREVENTION OF VAGINITIS

- Explain how the infection is transmitted. *The infection may be acquired through sexual activity, from inappropriate perineal hygiene measures, or overgrowth of certain organisms that normally reside on perineal and vaginal tissues. A clear understanding of how the infection developed allows the client to use measures to prevent future infections.*
- If advised, emphasize the need for both the client and her partner to complete the course of treatment. *Many infections are asymptomatic in one partner. Incomplete treatment allows the infection to recur and reinfect the partner.*
- Teach hygiene measures such as the following:
  - Avoid bubble baths, douches, feminine hygiene sprays, synthetic underwear, and tight pants.
  - Cleanse the perineum from front to back after voiding and defecating.
  - Cleanse genitals before and after sexual intercourse.
    These measures help maintain the normal vaginal environment and prevent irritation and contamination of perineal tissues that can increase the risk of infection.

PAIN

- Suggest using cool compresses and mild vinegar douches. *Cool compresses relieve itching. Vinegar has a fungicidal and bactericidal effect.*
- Recommend sitz baths to alleviate discomfort. *Sitz baths cleanse the perineal area and wash away irritating discharge.*

EVALUATING

In order to evaluate the effectiveness of nursing interventions, collect data related to the client's and her partner's understanding of the treatment and prevention of vaginitis, as well as the client's level of comfort.

Discharge Considerations

To prevent vaginitis, teach all women about personal hygiene and safer sex practices. Teach women to avoid douching and wearing nylon underwear and/or tight pants. Unprotected sexual activity, particularly with multiple partners, greatly increases the risk of vaginal infections and STDs. Unless contraindicated, encourage the client with repeated mild candidiasis infections to consume 8 oz. of yogurt containing live active cultures daily to help restore normal vaginal flora.

Many postmenopausal women experience atrophic vaginitis due to thinning and drying of the vaginal mucosa that result from lack of estrogen. Teach these clients about using topical estrogen creams, water-soluble lubricants for intercourse, and other methods to minimize the undesirable effects of menopause.

Pelvic Inflammatory Disease

Pelvic inflammatory disease (PID) is an infection of the pelvic organs (fallopian tubes, ovaries, uterus, and cervix). PID is usually caused by infection with *Neisseria gonorrhoeae* and/or *Chlamydia trachomatis*. Clients with PID often are infected with more than one organism. PID is a major cause of female infertility.

PID usually affects young, sexually active women who have multiple partners. Other risk factors include use of an intrauterine device (IUD) for birth control. Oral contraceptives and barrier contraceptives such as condoms reduce the risk of PID.

PATHOPHYSIOLOGY

Infectious organisms enter the vagina and travel to the uterus during intercourse or other sexual activity. They can also enter during childbirth, abortion, or reproductive tract surgery. The infection then spreads through the fallopian tubes, leading to inflammation and obstruction due to scar tissue. It settles on the ovary and also may enter the lymphatic system or bloodstream, leading to systemic infection.

The manifestations of PID include high fever, vaginal discharge, severe lower abdominal pain, nausea, malaise, and dysuria. Scarring of the fallopian tubes can lead to infertility and an increased risk of ectopic pregnancy. The client also may experience pain during intercourse and dysmenorrhea.

COLLABORATIVE CARE

The diagnosis of PID often is based on the history and physical examination. *Endocervical secretions* are cultured to identify the infecting organism. The *WBC* often is markedly elevated, a sign of infection. *Ultrasonography* is performed to rule out ectopic pregnancy. *Laparoscopy* may show inflammation, edema, and possible abscess of pelvic structures.

Pharmacology

Treatment usually is started with antibiotics that are effective to treat gonorrhea and chlamydia. If PID is not acute, outpatient antibiotic treatment is prescribed. In acute cases, however, the client is hospitalized. Analgesics are given, and antibiotics and fluids are administered intravenously. In either case, the woman's sexual partner is treated at the same time. Nursing implications for antibiotics are discussed in Chapter 12.

Surgery

The surgeon may insert a drain into an abscess, if present, and remove any adhesions. If the infection is overwhelming or chronic, a hysterectomy with bilateral salpingo-oophorectomy may be necessary.

NURSING CARE

ASSESSING

Ask about abdominal pain, including its location, intensity, character, timing, and duration. Inquire about associated symptoms such as nausea, vomiting, and vaginal drainage. Ask if the client could be pregnant. Inquire about risk factors such as multiple sexual partners, unprotected sexual activity, and recent STDs.

Objective data include vital signs and temperature, shape and contour of the abdomen, bowel sounds, and abdominal tenderness. Note the color, odor, and amount of any vomitus or vaginal drainage.

DIAGNOSING, PLANNING, AND IMPLEMENTING

RISK FOR INJURY

PID can have severe, even life-threatening complications. Scarring of the fallopian tubes can lead to ectopic pregnancy or pelvic abscess. Adhesions (bands of scar tissue) within the pelvis can obstruct the bowel.

■ Maintain bed rest in semi-Fowler's position. *This promotes drainage and helps localize the infection in the pelvic cavity.*
■ Maintain standard precautions and meticulous hand washing. Wear gloves when handling perineal pads and linens. Disinfect bedpans and toilet seats. *These measures help prevent spread of the infection to others.*
■ Administer antibiotics as ordered, monitoring closely for adverse effects. *Antibiotics used in acute PID are potent agents; some can have life-threatening side effects.*
■ Teach to recognize and report potential complications such as ectopic pregnancy, abscess, or bowel obstruction. *Reporting early manifestations of these potential complications reduces the risk of delayed treatment.*

DEFICIENT KNOWLEDGE: STD PREVENTION

■ Explain how infection is spread and how to prevent future infections. *Knowledge of the spread of infections allows control in preventing exposure to future infections.*
■ Stress the importance of completing the treatment regimen and of follow-up visits. *Incomplete treatment can lead to chronic infection and bacteria that are resistant to antibiotics. Noncompliance and recurrence are common.*

- Teach perineal care, especially wiping from front to back. *This reduces transmission of fecal organisms to reproductive tissues and reduces the incidence of urinary tract infections.*
- Instruct to avoid using tampons until the infection has completely cleared. Advise changing tampons or pads at least every 4 hours. *Menstrual flow provides a favorable environment for microorganisms to multiply.*
- Discuss safer sex practices and family planning. Instruct to remove diaphragms within 6 hours after use. IUDs are contraindicated. Latex condoms offer the most effective protection against infection. *These measures help prevent recurrence of infection.*
- Teach to report any unusual vaginal discharge or odor to the health care provider. Emphasize the importance of seeking treatment if her partner develops an STD. *Treatment is most effective early in the disease process. STDs such as gonorrhea and Chlamydia often are asymptomatic in women.*

EVALUATING

In order to evaluate the effectiveness of nursing care for the client with PID, collect data related to manifestations of the disease and its complications, as well as the client's and her partner's understanding of and willingness to use measures to prevent future infections.

Discharge Considerations

Emphasize the importance of completing the prescribed treatment and keeping follow-up appointments as directed to ensure eradication of the infection. Discuss safer sex practices, and measures to prevent recurrence of PID. Address the manifestations of potential complications of PID, and stress the importance of seeking care promptly if manifestations of ectopic pregnancy or bowel obstruction develop. Inform the client that the patency of the fallopian tubes can be evaluated after several menstrual cycles, to allow for complete resolution of the inflammatory process.

Toxic Shock Syndrome

Toxic shock syndrome (TSS) is a rare but acute illness caused by *Staphylococcus aureus* infection. Although it may be related to using tampons during menstruation, TSS also has been associated with the use of vaginal barrier contraceptives such as the sponge, the diaphragm, and the cervical cap. About half of all cases of TSS are related to other factors such as childbirth, abdominal surgery, septic abortion, burns, and skin lesions.

PATHOPHYSIOLOGY

TSS is caused by virulent strains of *Staphylococcus aureus* that enter the bloodstream through open blood vessels during the menses, the placental site after childbirth, or other open

---

> ### BOX 33-14
> ### MANIFESTATIONS OF TOXIC SHOCK SYNDROME
>
> - High fever
> - Nausea, vomiting, abdominal pain, diarrhea
> - Muscle pain
> - Sore throat
> - Headache
> - Dizziness, low blood pressure
> - Diffuse red rash, conjunctivitis
> - Peeling skin on palms and soles
> - Altered mental status

wound. Once inside the body, the organism produces toxins that cause vasodilation, hemodynamic instability, and shock. The clinical manifestations of TSS are presented in Box 33-14.

COLLABORATIVE CARE

The goals of care for a client with TSS are to identify the source of the infection, eradicate the infection, and restore stability of the cardiovascular and other body systems. The diagnosis is based on the history and physical examination. Wounds and vaginal secretions are cultured for *Staphylococcus aureus*. Treatment includes administering intravenous fluids to restore blood volume and blood pressure. Antibiotics are given to eliminate the infection. Drugs to restore the blood pressure and perfusion of vital organs also may be given.

NURSING CARE

ASSESSING

Ask about the onset and duration of symptoms. Inquire about use of tampons, diaphragm, or vaginal barrier contraceptive devices. Ask about other risk factors such as recent surgery or abortion, or disruption of the skin by an infection or wound.

Obtain complete head to toe physical assessment data, including vital signs.

DIAGNOSING, PLANNING, AND IMPLEMENTING

Clients with TSS may be critically ill, requiring intensive nursing care.

INEFFECTIVE TISSUE PERFUSION

- Administer intravenous fluids and blood expanders as ordered. *Vascular dilation causes blood pooling and impaired organ and tissue perfusion. Increasing intravascular volume improves venous return, cardiac output, and tissue perfusion.*
- Administer oxygen as ordered. Monitor oxygen saturation, reporting levels less than 95% to the charge nurse or physi-

cian. *Increasing the oxygen content of blood increases oxygen reaching peripheral tissues.*

DECREASED CARDIAC OUTPUT

In the client with TSS, low circulating blood volume may decrease cardiac output.

- Monitor vital signs hourly or more often, as indicated. *An increase in pulse and respiratory rates often is the earliest sign of shock. The blood pressure may remain within normal limits, even though tissues are not receiving adequate blood flow.*
- Monitor urine output hourly; notify the physician if urinary output falls below 30 mL per hour. *Urine output falls when the kidneys do not receive adequate blood flow. This indicates compromised perfusion to other tissues as well, and an increased risk for renal and other organ system failure.*
- Monitor respiratory status, including rate, depth, and breath sounds. *Rapid fluid administration increases the risk of pulmonary edema, which increases the work of breathing and interferes with gas exchange.*

EVALUATING

To evaluate the effectiveness of nursing care for the client with TSS, collect continuing assessment data, comparing it to objective data collected on admission.

Discharge Considerations

Teach the client and family about the causes of TSS and self-care measures to prevent future infection (Box 33-15).

Emphasize the importance of completing the prescribed course of antibiotics, even after manifestations have subsided. Stress the need to keep follow-up appointments. Advise women who have had TSS to avoid using tampons and vaginal barrier contraceptives. Stress the importance of reporting manifestations of the disorder to care provider, as women who have had TSS have a high risk for recurrence.

BOX 33-15
TEACHING FOR DISCHARGE

MEASURES TO PREVENT TOXIC SHOCK SYNDROME

- Use the lowest-absorbency tampon possible to contain menstrual flow.
- Change tampons at least every 4 hours, and use sanitary pads at night.
- Wash hands with soap before inserting a tampon, diaphragm, or vaginal medication.
- Remove diaphragms when recommended following intercourse. Do not use during menses.
- Do not use tampons during the first 12 weeks after childbirth.
- If you have had TSS, avoid using tampons or a diaphragm.

Nursing Interventions Classification

In addition to the nursing care planning approaches suggested in this chapter, the following Nursing Interventions (McCloskey & Bulechek, 2000) may be helpful in planning and implementing care for women with reproductive tract disorders:

- Behavior Modification
- Body Image Enhancement
- Coping Enhancement
- Decision-Making Support
- Health Screening
- Risk Identification
- Teaching: Safe Sex

(*Note:* The bibliography listings for this and all chapters have been compiled at the back of the book.)

Chapter Review

key terms by topic

Use the CD-ROM disk enclosed with your textbook to hear the pronunciation of the key terms in the chapter.

Structure and function
estrogens

Breast disorders
mastectomy

Disorders of menstruation
premenstrual syndrome (PMS), dysmenorrhea, dysfunctional uterine bleeding (DUB), amenorrhea, metrorrhagia, hysterectomy, menopause, dyspareunia

Structural disorders
cystocele, rectocele

Female reproductive tissue disorders
ectopic, salpingo-oophorectomy, oophorectomy

Female reproductive system infections
vaginitis, pelvic inflammatory disease (PID)

key points

- Disorders affecting the female reproductive system often affect the client's sexuality and body image in addition to their physical effects.

- Many disorders of the female reproductive system, including structural disorders, endometriosis, ovarian cysts, uterine fibroid tumors, and pelvic inflammatory disease increase the risk of infertility.

- A number of tumors of the female reproductive system, including some breast, cervical, and endometrial cancers, are estrogen dependent. Women who have a history of early menarche, late menopause, few or no pregnancies or late childbearing, and estrogen replacement therapy have an increased risk for these cancers.

- Current technology has resulted in alternatives to hysterectomy as the primary treatment for many female reproductive disorders.

- Although specific genes have been identified that increase the risk of breast and ovarian cancer, the majority of these cancers occur in women who do not have the identified gene or genes.

- Screening measures such as breast self-examination, mammography, and Pap smears allow early detection and treatment of breast and cervical cancer, significantly reducing their mortality rates.

Medialink

Additional interactive resources for this chapter can be found on the Companion Website at www.prenhall.com/burke. Click on Chapter 33 and "Begin" to select the activities for this chapter.

For NCLEX review questions and an audio glossary, access the accompanying CD-ROM in this book.

for further study

For more information about caring for the client undergoing surgery, see Chapter 7.

For more discussion of symptoms related to radiation and chemotherapy, see Chapter 8.

For nursing care of clients with HIV and AIDS, see Chapter 13.

For Kegel exercises, see Box 21-4.

For further study of sexually transmitted diseases, see Chapter 34.

Critical Thinking Care Map

Caring for a Client Experiencing Menopause

NCLEX-PN Focus Area: Health Promotion and Maintenance: Growth and Development Through the Life Span

Case Study: Maria Villagrana, age 49, is having her annual checkup. She is concerned about recent symptoms, including palpitations, hot flashes, night sweats, and periods of anxiety and insomnia. Over the past year, her menstrual periods have become short and erratic, and she has not menstruated for the past 3 months. Her most recent period lasted only one day.

Nursing Diagnosis: Anticipatory Grieving

COLLECT DATA

Subjective

_____

_____

_____

_____

_____

_____

Objective

_____

_____

_____

_____

_____

_____

Would you report this data? Yes/No

If yes, to: _____

Nursing Care

_____

_____

_____

_____

_____

_____

_____

_____

How would you document this? _____

_____

_____

Data Collected
(use those that apply)

- Often feels as though her "heart is running away with her"
- Hates thought of growing older
- Thinks her husband is losing interest in sex
- Wonders about decision to not to have children
- Breaks down in tears for no reason
- Reports absent-mindedness and difficulty concentrating
- BP, 140/70; P, 74; R, 18; T, 98.2° F (36.7° C)
- Smokes one pack of cigarettes daily
- Weighs 152 lbs. (69 kg) (approximately 25% over ideal body weight)
- No history of uterine or breast cancer
- Diet high fat, high carbohydrate, low protein and fiber
- Calcium intake is less than 30% of recommended level
- Thyroid hormone levels normal
- FSH level elevated
- All other laboratory findings within normal ranges

Nursing Interventions
(use those that apply)

- Teach coronary heart disease risk factors.
- Refer to smoking cessation program.
- Arrange consultation with a registered dietitian.
- Explain risks and benefits of hormone replacement therapy.
- Refer to midlife women's support group at the local community center.
- Arrange sexual counseling for Mr. and Mrs. Villagrana regarding techniques, positions, and modifications to accommodate midlife changes.

NCLEX-PN Exam Preparation

TEST-TAKING TIP

Nurses use a variety of tubes when caring for clients: feeding tubes, suction tubes, drainage tubes, chest tubes, tracheostomy tubes. Know the purpose of each, how to care for each, and what the necessary infection control measures are for each.

1. The fallopian tubes are lined with:
   a. fimbriae
   b. estrogen
   c. rugae
   d. cilia

2. A client with nonproliferative fibrocystic breast changes complains of monthly breast pain. She is likely to be advised to do all of the following EXCEPT:
   a. see a surgeon immediately, because of the high risk for breast cancer
   b. use NSAIDs such as acetaminophen or ibuprofen for discomfort
   c. try local heat or cold applications
   d. try eliminating caffeine and chocolate

3. The most frequent cause of death in women is:
   a. breast cancer
   b. lung cancer
   c. heart disease
   d. trauma

4. All of the following are good advice; which are especially important for the woman taking tamoxifen?
   a. Eat a low-fat, low-cholesterol diet.
   b. Get yearly Pap tests and stop smoking.
   c. Get regular aerobic exercise.
   d. Get regular dental care.

5. The most frequent location for breast cancer is:
   a. upper outer quadrant
   b. peri-aerolar area
   c. lower outer quadrant
   d. upper inner quadrant

6. A client has had a simple mastectomy with dissection of the lymph nodes. She has a Jackson–Pratt drain in place. Your discharge instructions would include:
   a. getting a permanent prosthesis as soon as possible
   b. how to empty the drain and clean around the insertion site
   c. keeping her arm elevated with the elbow above shoulder height as much as possible
   d. getting someone else to perform her ADLs such as washing her face and combing her hair for at least 2 weeks

7. A client, age 22, has primary dysmenorrhea. Which of the following statements indicates that she may need more instruction regarding self-care?
   a. "I will need another form of birth control, since this means I can't continue taking the pill."
   b. "A heating pad may help relieve symptoms."
   c. "I should take an analgesic like ibuprofen right before and regularly during my period."
   d. "It is okay to have sexual relations during my periods."

8. Your 65-year-old neighbor asks you about some vaginal bleeding she has been having. She is postmenopausal and not on hormone replacement therapy. You advise her:
   a. that she still has some hormones present, simulating a period.
   b. to see her doctor immediately.
   c. to increase her use of soy products.
   d. that hormone replacement therapy would relieve this.

9. Dysfunctional uterine bleeding is the most common reason for:
   a. infertility
   b. cancer
   c. hysterectomy
   d. colposcopy

10. A client has a history of PID. She is at increased risk for:
    a. cervical cancer
    b. passing this tendency on to her daughter
    c. infertility and ectopic pregnancy
    d. toxic shock syndrome

Answers for Review Questions, as well as discussion of Case Study Critical Thinking questions, appear in Appendix V.

Caring for Clients with Sexually Transmitted Diseases

CARING tip

❝You never have enough time *NOT* to look it up.❞

Mary Shestople, RN, BSN • LVN Instructor • City College of San Francisco • San Francisco, California

LEARNING outcomes

After completing this chapter, you will be able to:

- Describe the pathophysiology of the most common sexually transmitted diseases (STDs).
- Identify laboratory and diagnostic tests used for STDs.
- Identify general measures to prevent and treat common STDs.
- List the signs and symptoms of the most common STDs.
- Discuss nursing implications for medications prescribed for clients with STDs.
- Use the nursing process to provide individualized care for clients with STDs.

MediaLink

  www.prenhall.com/burke

Use the above address to access the free, interactive Companion Website created for this textbook. Get hints, instant feedback, and textbook references to chapter-related multiple choice questions. Link to other interesting sites.

Any infection transmitted by sexual contact, including vaginal, oral, and anal intercourse, is referred to as a **sexually transmitted disease (STD)**. Every sexually active person is at risk for STDs. STDs affect the client's general and reproductive health; some, such as HIV and hepatitis B can be life threatening.

Every year, an estimated 12 million people in the United States acquire an STD. Because of tissue trauma that occurs during sexual intercourse, many STDs are more easily transmitted from a man to a woman than from a woman to a man. Women often experience few early manifestations of the infection and have a greater risk for complications of STDs such as PID and genital cancers.

The incidence of STDs is highest among people of color in urban settings with lower socioeconomic status and less education (Box 34-1). Drug abuse, unprotected sexual activity, and sexual activity with multiple partners also are risk factors for STDs (Box 34-2).

Two thirds of all STDs occur in people under age 25. However, people of all ages are at risk. Anyone who is sexually active can be infected with STDs, and infants can be infected by their mothers in utero or during delivery. Children can be infected through incest or sexual abuse. Victims of sexual assault are also at risk.

CLINICAL alert

All states require reporting of syphilis, gonorrhea, and AIDS to state and federal agencies. Chlamydia is reportable in most states; requirements for reporting other STDs vary by state. For this reason, the exact incidence of many STDs is unknown.

Although STDs are caused by many different organisms, including bacteria, viruses, and parasites, they have several characteristics in common:

1. Most can be prevented by the use of latex condoms.
2. They can be transmitted during both heterosexual and homosexual activities.

3. For treatment to be effective, sexual partners of the infected person must also be treated.
4. Two or more STDs frequently coexist in the same client.

Some STDs can be cured with appropriate antibiotic treatment. Others, such as genital herpes and genital warts, are chronic conditions that can be managed but not cured. Some, such as HIV and hepatitis B, are potentially fatal. (HIV is discussed in Chapter 13; hepatitis B in Chapter 19.) Common STDs, their manifestations, treatment, and possible complications are outlined in Table 34-1 ◆. The five most common STDs in the United States are discussed below in greater detail.

Chlamydia

Chlamydial infections are thought to be the most common STDs in the United States and the leading cause of pelvic inflammatory disease (PID) (see Chapter 33). Because the infection often is asymptomatic, the incidence of the disease is thought to be nearly 10 times what is reported. Incidence is highest among sexually active teenagers. The risk factors for chlamydia are those for nearly all STDs (Box 34-2).

PATHOPHYSIOLOGY

Chlamydia trachomatis is a bacterium that behaves like a virus, reproducing only within the host cell. It is spread by any sexual contact and to the neonate by passage through the birth canal of an infected mother. The incubation period is from 1 to 3 weeks. The bacteria typically invade the cervix in women and the urethra in men. In addition to causing genital infections, *C. trachomatis* causes *trachoma,* a chronic, contagious type of conjunctivitis prevalent in Asia and Africa.

Chlamydial infections are asymptomatic in most women until they have invaded the uterus and uterine tubes. Early manifestations, when present, include dysuria, urinary frequency, and vaginal discharge. Nearly a third of men with chlamydia are also asymptomatic. Manifestations of the infection in men include dysuria, urethral discharge, and possible testicular pain. Although clients may be asymptomatic, they are still potentially infectious.

If untreated, chlamydial infection in women ascends into the upper reproductive tract, causing such complications as PID, which includes endometritis, salpingitis, and chronic

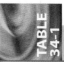

TABLE 34-1   SELECTED SEXUALLY TRANSMITTED DISEASES

DISEASE/ORGANISM	MANIFESTATIONS	TREATMENT	COMPLICATIONS
Chancroid[a] (rare in United States) *Haemophilus ducreyi*	**Females:** Frequently asymptomatic **Males:** Painful penile ulcers and *lymphadenopathy* (tender, enlarged lymph nodes)	Azithromycin PO once *or* ceftriaxone IM once *or* ciprofloxacin PO for 3 days *or* erythromycin PO for 7 days	Secondary infection of lesions, fistulas, chronic ulcers
Chlamydia *Chlamydia trachomatis*	**Females:** Asymptomatic; may have dysuria, vaginal or cervical discharge, vaginal bleeding or pelvic pain **Males:** May be asymptomatic or have dysuria, white or clear urethral discharge, testicular pain (epididymitis)	Doxycycline PO for 7 days *or* azithromycin PO once	**Females:** Pelvic inflammatory disease (PID), infertility, pelvic abscesses, spontaneous abortion, stillbirth, postpartum endometritis **Neonates:** Ophthalmia neonatorum or pneumonia **Males:** Urethritis, epididymitis, prostatitis
Genital herpes Herpes simplex virus, usually type 2	Single or multiple vesicles on the genitals with associated pruritus, followed by painful ulcers	No cure; acyclovir PO *or* famcyclovir PO *or* valacyclovir PO for 7–10 days or until symptoms resolve	Herpes keratitis, a severe eye infection **Females:** Cervical cancer **Neonates:** Herpes affecting the eye, skin, mucous membranes, and CNS **Males:** Neuralgia, meningitis, urethral strictures, pus forming in lymph nodes
Genital warts (condyloma acuminatum) Human papillomavirus (HPV)	Single or multiple painless warts on genitals or perianal area	No cure, usually recur. Cryotherapy, *or* podophyllin 10%–25% in tincture of benzoin compound applied to wart, *or* client-applied podofilox topical solution or gel *or* imiquimod cream	Urinary obstruction and bleeding **Females:** Enlargement during pregnancy; increased risk of cancer of the cervix, vagina, vulva, and anus **Neonates:** Respiratory papillomatosis, a chronic condition
Gonorrhea[a] *Neisseria gonorrhoeae*	**Females:** Often asymptomatic; may have vaginal discharge, abnormal menses, dysuria **Males:** Dysuria, increased urinary frequency, purulent urethral discharge	Cefixime PO *or* ciprofloxacin PO *or* ceftriaxone IM in a single injection *plus* azithromycin PO in a single dose *or* doxycycline PO for 7 days to treat possible coexisting chlamydia	**Females:** Pelvic inflammatory disease (PID), sterility, ectopic pregnancy, abdominal adhesions **Males:** Prostatitis, urethritis, nephritis, epididymitis, sterility
Granuloma inguinale[a] (rare in United States) *Calymmatobacterium granulomatis*	Single or multiple subcutaneous nodules that erode to form painless, bleeding, enlarging ulcers	Trimethoprim–sulfamethoxazole PO for 21 days *or* doxycycline PO for 21 days	Secondary infection of lesions, *keloid* (excess scar tissue) on genitals, tissue necrosis, fever, malaise, secondary anemia, cachexia, and death

(continues)

TABLE 34-1 SELECTED SEXUALLY TRANSMITTED DISEASES (CONTINUED)

DISEASE/ORGANISM	MANIFESTATIONS	TREATMENT	COMPLICATIONS
Lymphogranuloma venereum[a] (rare in United States) *Chlamydia trachomatis*	Painless vesicle or ulcer, followed by regional lymphadenopathy, inguinal abscess	Doxycycline PO for 21 days *or* erythromycin PO for 21 days	Ruptured abscesses with draining sinuses or fistulas, nephropathy, hepatomegaly, or phlebitis
Pelvic inflammatory disease (PID) *Chlamydia trachomatis, Neisseria gonorrhoeae, Mycoplasma hominis,* and others	Pain and tenderness in lower abdomen, uterus and surrounding tissues; possible fever, chills, and elevated WBC and sedimentation rate	Combined drug therapy such as cefotetan IV *plus* doxycycline IV or PO *or* clindamycin IV *plus* gentamicin IV or IM; may require hospitalization	Ectopic pregnancy, pelvic abscess; infertility, recurrent or chronic PID, chronic abdominal pain, pelvic adhesions, depression
Syphilis[a] *Treponema pallidum*	**Primary:** Painless chancre at site of exposure; regional lymphadenopathy **Secondary:** Skin rash; oral mucous patches; generalized lymphadenopathy; mucous patch on vulva or anus; fever; malaise; patchy alopecia **Tertiary** (late): Tumors of skin, bone, liver; inflammation of aorta, aneurysms; central nervous system degeneration	Penicillin G IM in a single injection *or* doxycycline PO for 14 days Syphilis of unclear or more than 1 year's duration: penicillin G IM weekly for 3 weeks *or* doxycycline PO for 28 days	**Primary and secondary:** Disease progression **Tertiary:** Heart failure, blindness, paralysis, skin ulcers, liver failure, mental illness
Trichomoniasis *Trichomonas vaginalis*	**Females:** Asymptomatic or may have frothy, excessive vaginal discharge, erythema, edema and pruritus **Males:** Usually asymptomatic; may have urethritis, penile lesions, or inflammation	Metronidazole PO in a single dose or for 7 days	**Females:** Recurrent infections, salpingitis, low-birth-weight infants, prematurity

[a] *Reporting to state and federal agencies required by law.*

pelvic pain. These infections are a major cause of infertility and ectopic pregnancy, a potentially life-threatening condition. Complications in men include epididymitis, prostatitis, sterility, and Reiter's syndrome (an autoimmune disorder). In the newborn, chlamydia can lead to blindness or pneumonia.

COLLABORATIVE CARE

Because chlamydial infections are often asymptomatic, treatment is often begun on a presumptive basis. The Centers for

Disease Control and Prevention (CDC) recommends screening asymptomatic women who are at high risk for chlamydia.

Diagnostic Tests

Chlamydial infection can be diagnosed in several ways. Infected tissue can be cultured to identify the presence of the bacteria. This test is expensive and not readily available in all areas, however. More often, the diagnosis is made based on detection of chlamydial antigens or nucleic acid, or by detecting antibodies to *Chlamydia* in the blood or local secretions. These tests are particularly effective in diagnosing chlamydial infection in high-risk populations.

Pharmacology

The drug of choice for chlamydial infections in men and non-pregnant women is a single oral dose of azithromycin (Zithromax) or a 7-day course of oral doxycycline (Vibramycin). For pregnant women, erythromycin is the alternative therapy. Ofloxacin (Floxin) for 7 days is another alternative treatment. Nursing implications for these antibiotics are discussed in Chapter 12.

NURSING CARE

Nursing care of the client with chlamydia focuses on identifying the infection, eradicating it, preventing future infections, and managing any complications.

ASSESSING

Box 34-3 outlines nursing assessment as it relates to clients with an STD.

DIAGNOSING, PLANNING, AND IMPLEMENTING

Consider the following nursing diagnoses and interventions when planning and delivering care for a client with an STD.

INEFFECTIVE HEALTH MAINTENANCE

■ Teach about the disease, its transmission, treatment, and measures to prevent its spread or reinfection. *Understanding the disease and how it is spread helps the client gain a sense of control and prevent future STDs.*

■ Discuss safer sex practices outlined in Box 34-4 on page 952. *Clients can prevent future STDs by making lifestyle changes and conscious decisions about safer sex practices.*

■ Emphasize the importance of referring all sex partners for testing and treatment as needed. *Unless both partners in a relationship are effectively treated, reinfection is likely.*

■ Stress the importance of completing the prescribed treatment plan and returning for follow-up visits as recommended. *Incomplete treatment may result in continued infection and organisms that are resistant to antibiotic therapy.*

IMPAIRED SKIN INTEGRITY

■ Teach the client to keep perineal tissues clean and dry. Advise cleansing front to back after urinating and defecating, using soap and water as needed to clean the area, and a blow drier on cool setting to dry. *Keeping tissues clean and dry promotes healing and reduces the risk of secondary infection of lesions.*

BOX 34-3
ASSESSING CLIENTS WITH AN STD

ASSESSING
Subjective Data

- Current symptoms: pain or itching; onset, duration, relieving and aggravating factors; dysuria, frequency, urgency, or other urinary symptoms; vaginal or urethral drainage, color, amount, odor; visible lesions
- General health, including any chronic diseases or conditions
- Past medical history, particularly any previous history of STDs or reproductive system problems and their treatment
- Sexual activity and measures used to prevent pregnancy or infection
- Possibility of pregnancy; last menstrual period (date, characteristics)
- Social habits such as tobacco, alcohol, or other drug use; frequency and amount

Objective Data

- Vital signs, including temperature
- Inspect: skin, including palms of hands and soles of feet; mucous membranes of mouth and oropharynx; abdomen for contour, visible peristalsis; genitalia, including penis, external urinary meatus, scrotum, and anus in men; perineum, labia majora, labia minora, vaginal opening, and anus in women. Note any redness, rash, ulcers, or lesions, swelling or drainage. Obtain sterile swab of drainage for culture or Gram stain.
- Auscultate bowel sounds.
- Palpate: abdomen and suprapubic region for tenderness; inguinal lymph nodes for swelling or tenderness (lymphadenopathy); perineal tissues for tenderness or swelling.

■ Instruct to avoid perineal powders or sprays, as well as bubble baths. *Feminine hygiene sprays and bubble baths can excessively dry perineal tissues, increasing the risk of infection.*

■ Advise client to wear cotton underwear, avoiding tight-fitting jeans and pantyhose. *These measures allow moisture to evaporate, rather than keeping it against the skin.*

RISK FOR INJURY

■ Stress the importance of taking all prescribed medication. *Completing the prescribed course of antibiotic helps ensure elimination of the infecting organism.*

■ Instruct to abstain from sexual contact until client and partners are cured, and to use condoms to prevent future infections. *Abstinence prevents reinfection and spread of the STD. Condoms provide barrier protection, reducing the risk of infection during sexual activity.*

- Provide information about signs and symptoms of reinfection and other STDs. Stress the importance of prompt diagnosis and treatment of all STDs. *Successful treatment of the disease does not prevent possible subsequent infections.*

ANXIETY

- Emphasize that most STDs can be effectively treated, preventing serious complications and transmission to the infant. *This information provides a sense of control and helps decrease anxiety.*
- Discuss with women of childbearing age that Cesarean delivery can prevent transmission of infection to the neonate. *Understanding that infection of the neonate can be prevented helps relieve anxiety.*

SITUATIONAL LOW SELF-ESTEEM

- Create an environment in which the client feels respected and safe to discuss concerns about the disease and its effect on the client's life. *Being treated with respect and privacy helps the client realize that the disease does not change his or her worth as a person.*
- Provide privacy and confidentiality. *Clients are often embarrassed to discuss intimate details of their sex lives.*
- Communicate caring for the client. *Unfortunately, many people affected by STDs lack family and other social support networks. The nurse's concern can enhance self-esteem.*

SEXUAL DYSFUNCTION

- Provide a supportive, nonjudgmental environment to discuss feelings and questions about the effect of the STD on future sexual relationships. *Feelings of guilt, shame, and anger are natural responses to the diagnosis of an STD and can lead to a total avoidance of sexual intimacy.*
- Offer information about support groups and other resources for people with specific STDs. *Information can offset feelings of shame and hopelessness. Many people have learned to live with and manage these disorders without infecting their partners or their children.*

IMPAIRED SOCIAL INTERACTION

- Help the client understand that an STD is a consequence of sexual behavior, not a "punishment," and that it can be avoided in the future. *This knowledge enhances the client's ability to relate to others.*

EVALUATING

To evaluate the effectiveness of nursing care, collect data such as the following:

- Completed prescribed medication regimen as ordered?
- Kept all recommended follow-up appointments?
- Able to identify measures to prevent future STDs?
- Engaging in safer sex practices with an uninfected partner?

- Resumed social activities?
- If pregnant, can state measures to prevent disease transmission to unborn child?

Discharge Considerations

Nurses have a critical role in preventing STDs by teaching clients about these diseases, their prevention, treatment, and potential complications (Box 34-4).

Stress the importance of complying with the prescribed treatment and refer partners for examination and treatment as needed. Discuss safer sex practices and using condoms to avoid

---

BOX 34-4
TEACHING FOR DISCHARGE

PREVENTING STDS: A CHECKLIST FOR CLIENTS

- You can eliminate your risk entirely by not having sex with anyone (**abstinence**) or by having sex only with an uninfected partner who has sex only with you (*mutual monogamy*).
- The more sexual partners you have, the greater your risk of contracting an STD.
- Latex condoms, used consistently and correctly, can prevent many STDs, including HIV infection. Use a new condom each time, lubricating the condom with a water-based lubricant.
- When a male condom cannot be used appropriately, the female condom, a lubricated polyurethane sheath inserted into the vagina, reduces the risk of STDs, including HIV.
- Vaginal spermicides reduce the risk for gonorrhea and chlamydia but do not prevent HIV infection.
- If you suspect you've been exposed to an STD, see a doctor or clinic right away. Encourage your partner to seek treatment, too.
- Follow the doctor's instructions carefully and take all the medicine prescribed for you. Continue the medication even when the symptoms go away. (The infection sometimes remains active after symptoms go away.)
- Go back to your doctor for a follow-up exam according to his or her instructions.
- Don't have sex until you *and* your partner are completely cured.
- If you use drugs by injection, enroll in or continue a drug-treatment program. Do not use injection supplies that have been used by another person under any circumstances. Thoroughly and consistently clean injection equipment with bleach between uses.

reinfection. Teach about the complications of chlamydia, such as PID, and their manifestations. Instruct the client to seek medical attention promptly if symptoms of PID develop. If the infection has progressed to PID, provide additional information about PID and its treatment (see Chapter 33).

Genital Herpes

Genital herpes *(Herpes genitalis)* is a chronic and often asymptomatic STD. Currently, no cure is available for genital herpes. As many as 45 million people in the United States are infected with the herpes simplex virus type 2 (HSV-2), the usual cause of genital herpes. Most of these people, however, have unrecognized infections. Like other STDs, the incidence of genital herpes is highest among adolescents and young adults.

PATHOPHYSIOLOGY

Genital herpes is spread by vaginal, anal, or oral–genital contact. Its incubation period is 3 to 7 days. Within a week after exposure, painful red papules appear in the genital area. In men, the lesions usually occur on the glans or shaft of the penis. In women, the lesions often occur on the labia, vagina, and cervix. Anal intercourse may result in lesions in and around the anus.

Soon after the papules appear, they form small painful blisters filled with clear fluid containing virus particles (Figure 34-1 ◆). The blisters break, shedding the virus and creating painful ulcers that last 6 weeks or longer. Touching these blisters and then rubbing or scratching in another place can spread the infection to other areas of the body.

The first outbreak of herpes lesions is called the *first episode infection.* Subsequent episodes, or *recurrent infections,* are usually less severe. The period between episodes is called *latency.* Even though no symptoms are present, the person remains infectious. During latency, the virus withdraws into the nerve fibers that lead from the infected site to the lower spine, remaining dormant until recurrence, at which time it retraces its path to the genital area.

Prodromal symptoms (warning signals or clues) of herpes outbreaks include burning, itching, tingling, or throbbing at the sites where lesions commonly appear. There may be pain radiating to the legs, thighs, groin, or buttocks. The infection may be more infectious during the prodromal period, so sexual contact should be avoided.

Recurrent infections have symptoms of herpetic lesions, general malaise or headache, fever, dysuria and urinary retention, and vaginal or urethral discharge.

Men are not likely to experience serious complications of genital herpes. Women, however, face more serious concerns. Neonatal infection from a mother with herpes can range from asymptomatic to widely disseminated, fatal disease. Transmission occurs during passage through the birth canal. The risk is highest during the first episode of infection. Women also face an increased risk of cervical cancer. In rare cases, the herpes virus can spread to the brain, causing herpes encephalitis, a life-threatening complication.

COLLABORATIVE CARE

Because there is no cure for genital herpes, treatment focuses on relieving symptoms and preventing spread of the infection. Teaching is an essential component of care.

Genital herpes is usually diagnosed by the history (including lesion characteristics and patterns of recurrence) and physical exam. Antiviral drugs such as acyclovir (Zovirax) or famciclovir (Famvir) help reduce the length and severity of the first episode and decrease the frequency of recurrent episodes. These drugs usually are given orally; for severe episodes, acyclovir also can be given intravenously.

NURSING CARE

In addition to the nursing care as outlined for chlamydia, the nursing diagnoses of Pain and Altered Health Maintenance should be considered for the client with genital herpes.

PAIN

- Teach the client to keep herpes blisters clean and dry. A solution of warm water, soap, and hydrogen peroxide can be used to cleanse the lesions two or three times daily. Burow's solution (an aluminum acetate solution) can also be used. Lesions should be dried using a hair dryer on the cool setting. Instruct to wear loose cotton clothing that will not trap moisture; pantyhose and tight jeans should be avoided. *Keeping the lesions clean and dry reduces the risk of secondary infection and promotes healing.*
- For dysuria, suggest pouring water over the genitals while urinating. Encourage increased fluid intake. Fluids that increase urine acidity, such as cranberry juice, should be avoided. *These measures help relieve dysuria by diluting or reducing the acidity of the urine.*

Figure 34-1. ◆ Genital herpes blisters as they appear on the penis.

INEFFECTIVE HEALTH MAINTENANCE

■ Discuss Cesarean delivery to prevent transmission of infection to the neonate. In women without manifestations of recurrence, vaginal delivery is possible. *Understanding that infection of the neonate can be prevented helps relieve anxiety.*

■ Discuss the need for annual Papanicolaou (Pap) smears; Pap smears every 6 months may be recommended for women with genital herpes. *Careful monitoring will identify early changes in cervical tissues, allowing effective treatment.*

 ## Discharge Considerations

With teaching, clients with genital herpes can learn to manage this chronic disease with the least possible disruption in lifestyle and relationships. Teach the client to recognize prodromal symptoms of recurrence, and discuss factors that seem to trigger recurrences (such as emotional stress, acidic food, sun exposure). Explain the need for abstinence from sexual contact from the time prodromal symptoms appear until 10 days after all lesions have healed.

Encourage the client to use oral antiviral drugs to reduce the frequency and duration of outbreaks. Painful lesions can be protected with sterile vaseline or aloe vera gel. Because viral shedding can occur at any time, emphasize the importance of using latex condoms and careful hygiene practices (such as not sharing towels or other personal items) even during latency periods.

 # Genital Warts

Genital and anal warts, also known as *condyloma acuminatum* or venereal warts, are caused by human papillomavirus (HPV). HPV is one of the most common STDs in the United States. Most HPV infections are asymptomatic or unrecognized. Like most STDs, genital warts are usually found in young, sexually active adults and are associated with early onset of sexual activity and multiple sexual partners.

PATHOPHYSIOLOGY

HPV is transmitted by all types of sexual contact. The incubation period for genital warts is about 3 months. Many different types of HPV cause chronic genital infections.

Although most people who carry HPV have no symptoms, others develop single or multiple painless, cauliflower-like growths on the vulvovaginal area, perineum, penis, urethra, or anus (Figure 34-2 ◆). In women, the growths may appear in the vagina or on the cervix and be apparent only during a pelvic examination.

Several subtypes of HPV are strongly associated with cervical dysplasia and an increased risk of cervical cancer. HPV also is associated with a higher risk of vaginal, vulvar, penile, and anal cancers.

Potential complications of genital warts include destruction of normal tissue or obstruction of the urethra. The virus

Figure 34-2. ◆ Genital warts (condyloma acuminatum) on the penis.

also can be transmitted to the fetus during pregnancy or delivery. The lesions enlarge during pregnancy and may obstruct the birth canal, necessitating Cesarean delivery. Infants infected with HPV can develop respiratory papillomatosis, a chronic respiratory condition.

COLLABORATIVE CARE

Genital and anal warts are diagnosed primarily by their clinical appearance; HPV also may be diagnosed by examination of cervical cells taken during a Pap smear or cervical biopsy.

Pharmacology

Genital warts on the vulva, perineum, or penis can be treated with a topical agent (podophyllin resin) applied directly to the warts. This treatment is done in the physician's office, with the client returning weekly until the warts are gone.

Other Therapies

Genital warts may be removed by cryotherapy, electrocautery, or surgical excision. Carbon dioxide laser surgery is increasingly used to remove extensive warts.

 # NURSING CARE

In addition to the general nursing care for clients with an STD (see the section on chlamydia), the client with genital warts needs pretreatment teaching if the warts are to be removed.

 ## Discharge Considerations

Emphasize the need for the client and infected partners to return for regular treatment and abstain from sexual relations until lesions have resolved, and to use condoms to prevent reinfection. Stress the importance of annual Pap smears for female clients because of the increased risk for cervical cancer. Genital warts can enlarge and destroy normal tissue or block the urethra. Instruct the client to report difficulty urinating or symptoms of urinary retention or infection. Discuss the risk of transmitting the disease to the fetus or neonate, and the need for cesarean delivery. Stress the importance of telling the women's health care provider about the infection.

Gonorrhea

Gonorrhea, also known as *GC* or *clap,* is the most common reportable communicable disease in the United States. The rate of gonorrhea infection among African Americans is significantly higher than in non-Hispanic whites. Among women, 15- to 19-year-olds have the highest rate of infection, while among men, 20- to 24-year-olds have the highest rate.

PATHOPHYSIOLOGY

Gonorrhea is caused by *Neisseria gonorrhoeae,* a gram-negative diplococcus. Its incubation period is 2 to 8 days. Gonorrhea is transmitted by direct sexual contact and during delivery as the neonate passes through the birth canal.

The organism initially targets the cervix and the male urethra. Without treatment, the disease spreads to other organs. In men, gonorrhea can cause acute, painful inflammation of the prostate, epididymis, and periurethral glands and can lead to sterility. In women, it can cause PID, endometritis, salpingitis, and pelvic peritonitis. In the neonate, gonorrhea can infect the eyes, nose, or anorectal region.

Manifestations of gonorrhea in men include dysuria and serous, milky, or purulent urethral discharge. Some men also develop regional lymphadenopathy. Some men and most women have no symptoms until the disease is advanced. When manifestations of gonorrhea are present in women, they include dysuria, urinary frequency, or abnormal vaginal discharge.

COLLABORATIVE CARE

Treatment of gonorrhea is directed toward eradicating the organism and any coexisting disease (see below), preventing reinfection, and preventing spread of the disease.

Diagnostic Tests

In men, the diagnosis of gonorrhea can usually be confirmed by obtaining a smear of urethral discharge. Cultures are not necessary unless Gram stains of smears are negative despite typical clinical symptoms of gonorrhea. In women, cultures of cervical discharge are necessary to confirm the diagnosis of gonorrhea. Because cultures require 24 to 48 hours for confirmation, treatment is usually begun on presumptive diagnosis.

People with gonorrhea often are infected with another STD. For this reason, the client and his or her partners are tested for other STDs like syphilis, chlamydia, and possibly HIV.

Pharmacology

Because many strains of *N. gonorrhoeae* are resistant to penicillin, an alternative antibiotic, such as a single dose of cefixime (Suprax), ceftriaxone (Rocephin), ciprofloxacin (Cipro), or ofloxacin (Floxin), is used to treat gonorrhea infection of the urethra, cervix, or rectum. The same antibiotics are used to treat pharyngeal gonorrhea infection. However, a longer course of treatment may be required.

NURSING CARE

Review Box 34-3 for areas to assess with clients who have STDs. Also review nursing care as described under chlamydia at the beginning of this chapter, and the Nursing Process Case Study provided here.

Discharge Considerations

If single-dose antibiotic therapy has not been ordered, emphasize the importance of taking all of the prescribed medication as directed. Encourage referral of sexual partners for evaluation and treatment. Stress the need to abstain from all sexual contact until the client and partners are cured of the disease, and instruct to use a condom to avoid transmitting or contracting infections in the future. Emphasize the need for a follow-up visit 4 to 7 days after treatment is completed to ensure that the infection has been cured.

Nursing Process Case Study
■ CLIENT WITH GONORRHEA

Janet Cirit, a 33-year-old legal secretary, is unmarried but dating a man named Jim Adkins. Ms. Cirit visits her gynecologist because her periods have become irregular and she is having pelvic pain and abnormal vaginal discharge. Recently, she developed a sore throat, and the pelvic pain is keeping her awake at night.

Assessment In the gynecologist's office, the nurse obtains a complete history, including questions about menstrual periods, pain associated with urination or sexual intercourse, urinary frequency, most recent Pap smear, birth control method, history of STD and drug use, and types of sexual activity. Ms. Cirit reports her symptoms and indicates that she is taking oral contraceptives for birth control so she and Mr. Adkins do not use a condom during sexual relations.

Physical examination reveals both pharyngeal and cervical inflammation, and lower abdominal tenderness. Ms. Cirit's temperature is 98.5° F (37.0° C). She is not pregnant. Diagnostic tests are positive for gonorrhea and negative for *Chlamydia.* The white blood count (WBC) is slightly elevated, indicating possible salpingitis. Because Mr. Adkins has been

Ms. Cirit's only sexual partner, it is clear that he needs to be treated as well.

Diagnosis The following nursing diagnoses are identified for Ms. Cirit:

- Pain related to the infectious process
- Situational Low Self-Esteem related to shame and guilt of having an STD
- Ineffective Sexuality Patterns related to impaired relationship and fear of reinfection

Expected Outcomes The expected outcomes are that Ms. Cirit will:

- Report relief of pelvic pain.
- Verbalize an understanding of the cause and transmission of gonorrhea.
- Verbalize that she will insist her partner use condoms during future sexual activity.

Planning and Implementation The following interventions are planned and implemented during care of Ms. Cirit:

- Administer ceftriaxone IM as ordered and document.
- Discuss feelings and concerns about the diagnosis of gonorrhea.
- Emphasize relationship of STD to behavior, not cleanliness or self-worth.
- Help identify ways to talk with a future sexual partner about condom use.

Evaluation During her follow-up visit, Ms. Cirit states that she is feeling much better and sleeping well at night since the pain has ended. She has ended her relationship with Mr. Adkins and is considering joining a health club in the hope of increasing her level of fitness and perhaps meeting someone new.

 Critical Thinking in the Nursing Process

1. What signs might have caused Ms. Cirit to suspect that Mr. Adkins had gonorrhea?
2. How are Ms. Cirit's signs and symptoms related to the infectious process of gonorrhea?
3. How might Ms. Cirit convince a future sexual partner to use condoms during sexual activity without spoiling the romantic aspect?

Syphilis

Syphilis is a complex systemic STD that, if not treated appropriately, can lead to blindness, paralysis, mental illness, cardiovascular damage, and death. Penicillin has significantly reduced the incidence of syphilis. The current rate of infection is low and falling among most racial and ethnic groups. It is higher among African Americans, American Indians, and Alaska Natives. Syphilis infection rates also remain high in the South and in many urban centers.

Syphilis often occurs with one or more other STDs, such as HIV or chlamydia.

PATHOPHYSIOLOGY

Syphilis is caused by a spirochete, *Treponema pallidum,* which may infect almost any body tissue or organ. It is transmitted from open lesions during any sexual contact (genital, oral–genital, or anal–genital). The organism can survive for days in fluids. It may also be transmitted by infected blood or other body fluids such as saliva. The average incubation period is 20 to 30 days. Once it has entered the system, *T. pallidum* spreads through the blood and lymphatic system. Congenital syphilis is transferred to the fetus through the placental circulation.

Syphilis is characterized by three clinical stages: primary, secondary, and tertiary, with an extended period of latency between the last two stages. Each stage has characteristic clinical manifestations.

Primary Syphilis

The primary stage of syphilis is characterized by the appearance of a painless ulcer called a **chancre** (Figure 34-3 ◆) at the site of inoculation (genitals, anus, mouth, breast, finger). Regional lymph nodes (e.g., inguinal nodes) also may be swollen. The chancre appears 3 to 4 weeks after the infectious contact. In women, a genital chancre may go unnoticed, disappearing within 4 to 6 weeks. In both primary and secondary stages, syphilis is highly infectious, even if no symptoms are evident.

Secondary Syphilis

Manifestations of secondary syphilis may appear any time from 2 weeks to 6 months after the initial chancre disappears. These symptoms can include a skin rash, especially on the palms of the hands (Figure 34-4 ◆) or soles of the feet; mucous patches in the oral cavity; sore throat; generalized lymphadenopathy; condyloma lata (flat, broad-based papules, unlike the pedunculated structure of genital warts) on the labia, anus, or corner of the mouth; flulike symptoms; and alopecia. These manifestations generally disappear within 2 to 6 weeks.

Latent Stage Syphilis

The latent stage of syphilis can last up to 50 years. During this stage, no symptoms of syphilis are apparent, and the disease is not transmissible by sexual contact. It can be transmitted by

Figure 34-3. ◆ Chancre of primary syphilis on the penis.

Figure 34-4.   ◆   Palmar rash of secondary syphilis.

infected blood, however. All prospective blood donors are screened for syphilis. In two thirds of all cases, the latent stage persists without further complications. Unless treated, the remaining one third of infected people progress to late stage or tertiary syphilis. The latent stage is shortened in people with HIV disease.

Tertiary Syphilis

Tertiary syphilis can be manifested in two different ways. *Benign late syphilis* is characterized by localized infiltrating tumors (*gummas*) in skin, bones, and liver. This form of tertiary syphilis generally responds promptly to treatment. A *diffuse inflammatory response* that involves the central nervous system and the cardiovascular system has a more insidious onset. Although the disease can still be treated at this stage, much of the cardiovascular and central nervous system damage is irreversible.

COLLABORATIVE CARE

As with other STDs, the goals of treatment for syphilis are to inactivate the spirochete and educate the client about how to prevent reinfection or further transmission. In addition, clients should be screened for chlamydial infection and advised to have an HIV test.

Diagnostic Tests

The following tests are widely used to diagnose syphilis:

- The *VDRL (Venereal Disease Research Laboratory)* and *RPR (rapid plasma reagin)* blood tests measure antibodies to syphilis. These tests become positive about 4 to 6 weeks after infection. Because these tests are not specific, additional tests may be necessary.

- The *FTA-ABS (fluorescent treponemal antibody absorption)* test is specific for *T. pallidum* and can be used to confirm VDRL and RPR findings.
- *Immunofluorescent staining* or *darkfield microscopy* can be used to identify the presence of *T. pallidum* in a specimen obtained from a chancre or by aspirating a lymph node.

Pharmacology

A single intramuscular (IM) dose of penicillin G is the treatment of choice for primary and secondary syphilis. If the duration of the disease is unknown or more than one year, the total dosage is increased and given in three weekly injections. Clients allergic to penicillin are given oral doxycycline (Vibramycin). The nursing implications of antibiotic therapy are discussed in Chapter 12.

NURSING CARE

The nursing assessment, diagnoses, interventions, and evaluation for a client with syphillis are similar to that for a client with chlamydia discussed earlier in this chapter. In addition, see the interactive care map that follows for an opportunity to plan care for a client with syphilis.

Discharge Considerations

Early symptoms of syphilis resolve with or without treatment. Teach clients that syphilis is a chronic disease that can be spread to others even when no symptoms are evident. Stress the importance of: (a) taking all prescribed medication, (b) referring all sexual partners for evaluation and treatment, (c) abstaining from all sexual contact for a minimum of 1 month after treatment, and (d) using a condom to avoid transmitting or contracting infections in the future. Emphasize the need for follow-up testing at 3 and 6 months for clients with primary or secondary syphilis, and at 6 and 12 months for those with late-stage disease. Discuss integrating safer sex practices into the client's lifestyle to prevent future episodes of STDs.

Nursing Interventions Classification

The following Nursing Interventions (McCloskey & Bulechek, 2000) may also be helpful when planning care for clients with STDs:

- Behavior Management: Sexual
- Health Education
- Risk Identification
- Substance Use Prevention
- Teaching: Safe Sex

(*Note:* The bibliography listings for this and all chapters have been compiled at the back of the book.)

Chapter Review

key terms by topic

Use the CD-ROM disk enclosed with your textbook to hear the pronunciation of the key terms in the chapter.

Sexually transmitted diseases
chancre, abstinence

key points

- The risk for contracting a sexually transmitted disease is directly related to lifestyle. Teach all clients to use safer sex practices such as abstinence, mutual monogamy with an uninfected partner, and barrier protection during sexual relations.

- Many STDs such as chlamydia, gonorrhea, and syphilis can be effectively treated with single-dose antibiotic therapy. Others, such as genital herpes and genital warts, are chronic viral infections that can be managed but not cured.

- Human papillomavirus (HPV) infection significantly increases a woman's risk for cervical cancer. Recommend that all women with HPV have annual Pap tests for early detection of cervical cancer.

- Many STDs such as syphillis, gonorrhea, and other less common diseases, must be reported to state and federal agencies.

- Screening and treatment of the client's partner is necessary to prevent reinfection during or after treatment for an STD.

- Complications of STDs can include pelvic inflammatory disease (PID) and problems of fertility, as well as systemic responses (e.g., cardiovascular and neurologic manifestations of tertiary syphilis).

 Medialink

Additional interactive resources for this chapter can be found on the Companion Website at www.prenhall.com/burke. Click on Chapter 34 and "Begin" to select the activities for this chapter.

For NCLEX review questions and an audio glossary, access the accompanying CD-ROM in this book.

for further study

For review of nursing implications for antibiotics, see Chapter 12.

For discussion of human immunodeficiency virus (HIV) and AIDS, see Chapter 13.

For more about hepatitis B, see Chapter 19.

For further study about pelvic inflammatory disease (PID), see Chapter 33.

Critical Thinking Care Map

Caring for a Client with Syphilis
NCLEX-PN Focus Area: Reduction of Risk Potential

Case Study: Eddie Kratz, a 22-year-old man, shares a small apartment with Marla Jones, who is 7 months pregnant with his child. Although he intends to marry Ms. Jones before the baby is born, he has continued a previous relationship with a woman named Justine Simpson. His sexual activities with Ms. Simpson have increased in frequency as Ms. Jones's pregnancy has advanced. Recently, Mr. Kratz has noticed a swelling in his groin and a sore on his penis.

Nursing Diagnosis: Risk for Injury

COLLECT DATA

Subjective

_____

_____

_____

_____

_____

Objective

_____

_____

_____

_____

_____

Would you report this data? Yes/No

If yes, to: _____

Nursing Care

_____

_____

_____

_____

_____

_____

_____

_____

How would you document this? _____

_____

Data Collected
(use those that apply)

- Regional lymphadenopathy
- Having unprotected sex with Ms. Jones and Ms. Simpson
- Syphilitic chancre on the shaft of the penis
- Believes that Ms. Jones is not having sex with anyone else, but is not sure
- ELISA results negative for HIV
- Darkfield analysis of chancre exudate confirms syphilis

Nursing Interventions
(use those that apply)

- Administer and document IM injection of benzathine penicillin G as ordered.
- Teach the importance of treatment to the health of their infant.
- Discuss importance of abstaining from sexual activity until client and partners are cured, and using condoms to prevent reinfection.
- Explain the need for follow-up testing in 3 months and 6 months.
- Notify Ms. Jones and Ms. Simpson of need for testing.
- Send reminders for follow-up at 3- and 6-month intervals.
- Refer Mr. Kratz and Ms. Jones for counseling about the impact of the disease on their relationship.
- Provide a copy of STD prevention checklist.

NCLEX-PN Exam Preparation

1. A woman has been diagnosed with a chlamydia infection. As you explain her prescription to her, she states, "I don't need any medicine. I feel fine." Your response is based on the knowledge that:
   a. the body often clears chlamydia by itself
   b. fever and dysuria usually accompany chlamydia in women
   c. clients with STDs often deny symptoms
   d. if untreated, chlamydia can progress to PID

2. Using azithromycin (Zithromax) instead of doxycycline (Vibramycin) can improve compliance primarily because:
   a. Zithromax has fewer side effects
   b. Zithromax is taken in a single oral dose
   c. Zithromax costs less
   d. Zithromax tastes better

3. An 18-year-old college student has just been diagnosed with a first episode infection of herpes simplex type 2. She says, " I can't believe this. I'm so embarrassed. How could he? I trusted him." Your initial response is:
   a. "You can't believe this has happened to you."
   b. "You need to use barrier protection so you do not pass this on."
   c. "You can't trust what these college guys tell you."
   d. "We will provide you with prescriptions that will make you more comfortable."

4. Teaching the client with genital warts (HPV) should include:
   a. measures to relieve pain
   b. how to take acyclovir
   c. avoiding acidic foods
   d. importance of regular Pap testing

5. Which of the following STDs can be cured?
   a. syphilis, trichomoniasis, genital herpes
   b. gonorrhea, genital warts, chlamydia
   c. gonorrhea, syphilis, genital warts
   d. chlamydia, syphilis, gonorrhea

6. Which STD, if untreated, can lead to blindness, paralysis, cardiovascular damage, and death?
   a. PID
   b. gonorrhea
   c. syphilis
   d. trichomoniasis

7. Your client has been diagnosed with syphilis. Which allergy would necessitate a change in the usual treatment?
   a. penicillin
   b. eggs
   c. acyclovir
   d. sulfa

8. The most common STD in the United States and the most common cause of PID is:
   a. genital herpes
   b. gonorrhea
   c. chlamydia
   d. trichomoniasis

9. Which comment by a 20-year-old indicates the client needs additional teaching about STDs?
   a. "My boyfriend needs to see his doctor for treatment also."
   b. "If we only engage in oral sex, we can not transmit STDs."
   c. "Use of latex condoms can prevent most STDs."
   d. "Some STDs cannot be cured, but symptoms can be treated."

10. Syphilis, AIDS, and gonorrhea:
    a. are caused by viruses
    b. all begin with a fever
    c. must be reported to federal and state agencies
    d. are best treated with combination therapy

Cultural Care STRATEGIES

Recognizing Biological Variations Among Cultures

Mrs. Jamie Jean Johnson is a 38-year-old African-American woman who is married and the mother of two daughters and one son, ages 16, 14, and 8, respectively. Mrs. Johnson was diagnosed at age 6 with sickle cell anemia. For the last 5 years, she has remained largely asymptomatic. However, one evening she begins to complain of unbearable pain and is admitted to the hospital in sickle cell crisis. When she arrives at the hospital, the nurse working in the emergency room takes a history and physical. She notes that Mrs. Johnson's admitting complaints include severe joint pains in both the upper and lower extremities, a temperature of 101.8°F, and shortness of breath. On physical examination, the nurse notes that Mrs. Jennings has coarse rales in the base of both lungs, and that her lips are cyanotic and dry. Her nail beds are also cyanotic, and capillary refill is slow. Initial laboratory examination reveals a hemoglobin of 8 g/dl. The nursing history reveals that Mrs. Johnson has also had problems drinking milk and eating certain dairy products for most of her adult life. In addition, she has begun to eat a great amount of ice. Mrs. Johnson tells the nurse that she craves ice and that it seems to satisfy her and is filling.

Over the past three decades, a body of scientific knowledge about biological cultural differences has become evident. In fact, over this same time period, mushrooming literature about biocultural differences has resulted in a field of study known as biocultural ecology. Scientific facts about biological variations can aid the nurse in giving culturally appropriate health care.

Biological Variables	Examples
Body weight	• African-American men average 166.1 lb, and white men average 170.6 lb. • African-American women average 149.6 lb, and white women average 137.0 lb. • African-American women from 35 to 65 years of age are an average of 20 lb heavier than white women. • Mexican-Americans, on average, weigh more than whites due to truncal fat. • Socioeconomic status is a predictor of obesity. • ***Nurses' note:*** *Standardized height/weight charts may be inappropriate, because they are based on standard white measurements.*
Skin color	• With darker skin, it is more difficult to assess changes. Baseline skin color can be established using daylight or a 60-watt bulb. Examine least pigmented areas: palms, soles, abdomen, volar surfaces of forearms, buttocks. Also assess nail beds, conjunctiva, and mouth. Oral hyperpigmentation occurs in 50 to 90% of African-Americans and in 10 to 50% of whites. The lips of some blacks have a natural bluish hue.
Other visible physical characteristics	• Mongolian spots are more common in African-Americans, Asian-Americans, Native Americans, and Mexican-Americans. • Keloids are more common in African-Americans.
Enzyme and genetic variations	• Many diseases have a genetic linkage. Trauma does not.
Drug interactions and metabolism	• Isoniazid—Up to 60% of whites inactivate this drug slowly and are at risk for peripheral neuropathy. Also, 40% of African-Americans, 10 to 40% of Native-Americans and Eskimos, and 10 to 15% of Orientals inactivate this drug slowly. • Primaquine—100 million people worldwide (about 35% of African-Americans) lack enzyme to digest primaquine and so cannot use it for treatment of malaria.
Disease incidence	• Tuberculosis—Some Native American groups have an incidence 7 to 15 times higher than non-Indians. African-Americans have an incidence 3 times higher than white Americans. • Diabetes has a high incidence among Seminoles, Pimas, and Papagos but is rare among Alaskan Eskimos. Diabetes is the seventh leading cause of death in U.S.

	whites, blacks, Chinese, and Filipinos; it is the fourth leading cause among Native-Americans.
Hypertension	• Among African-Americans, hypertension has an earlier onset, is more severe, and has a higher mortality than among whites; 35% of African-Americans over 40 years of age are hypertensive. • Prevalence increases with age and is higher in less educated individuals. In young adulthood and early middle age, men are more affected than women; after middle age, the reverse is true. • *Nurses' note: Alertness to risk factors can allow early detection, medical maintenance, and reduced mortality.*
Sickle cell anemia	• This is a common genetic disorder that affects more than 70,000 Americans. African-Americans are the primary group affected, although it also occurs in people from Asia Minor, India, Mediterranean region, and Caribbean area. • *Nurses' note: Early recognition and treatment of crisis symptoms are essential. (The astute nurse should recognize from the presenting symptoms in the case scenario that Mrs. Johnson is in sickle cell crisis and needs immediate hospitalization.) Pain control is a crucial concern.*
AIDS	• Incidence among African-Americans and Hispanics is increasing. African-Americans constitute one eighth of all Americans, but one fourth of Americans with AIDS. Hispanic Americans constitute one twelfth of all Americans, but one seventh of Americans with AIDS.
Lactose intolerance	• Intolerance affects 66% of Mexican- Americans and 90% of African-Americans, Orientals, and Ashkenazic Jews. • Most affected clients only need to restrict, not eliminate, lactose-containing foods. Nutritional supplements are not usually needed; pregnant or lactating women may be the exception.
Pica	• Consumption of non-food items may have originated among undernourished populations. Examples are eating dirt, clay, or ice.

Nursing Implications

• **Be aware that people differ in their susceptibility to disease because of biological variations.** Data relative to all the significant variables of a racial group are essential for complete assessment.

• **Remember that a relationship exists between race and body weight, skin color, other visible physical characteristics, enzymatic and genetic variations, and risk for certain diseases.**

• **Many diseases, with the exception of trauma, can be linked to a genetic influence.** Many common diseases like diabetes or heart disease have both a genetic and an environmental cause. People of certain races may be more susceptible to some diseases or conditions.

Self-Reflection Questions

1. What is your understanding of the role that biological variations play in susceptibility to disease by race?
2. Have you been educated in a system that does not acknowledge biological variation among racial groups?
3. How can you render culturally competent care to persons of different racial, ethnic, or cultural groups without over-generalizing or stereotyping?

Appendix I

Standard Precautions

Standard precautions are designed to reduce the risk of transmission of microorganisms from both recognized and unrecognized sources of infection. They are the primary strategy for preventing nosocomial infections within institutions, and are important to protect healthcare workers as well. Standard precautions apply to (1) blood; (2) all body fluids, secretions, and excretions except sweat, regardless of whether or not they contain visible blood; (3) nonintact skin; and (4) mucous membranes. Standard precautions are applied to all clients receiving care in hospitals, regardless of their diagnosis or presumed infection status. These precautions are specifically designed for hospitals; however, they also may be implemented in extended and long-term care facilities, and to a more limited extent in providing home care or in other community-based care settings.

HANDWASHING

- Wash your hands (a) immediately after removing gloves, even if gloves appear to be intact; (b) between contacts with clients; and (c) after contacting blood, body fluids, secretions, excretions, and equipment or articles contaminated by them. You may need to wash your hands between tasks and procedures on the same client to prevent cross-contaminating different body sites.
- In most instances, use plain soap and warm water for handwashing. In specific circumstances, for example, when handwashing facilities are not available, a waterless antiseptic agent may be used.

GLOVES

- Wear clean, nonsterile gloves when touching blood, body fluids, secretions, excretions, and contaminated items, and in situations where hand contamination may occur, for example, with an uncooperative client.
- Change your gloves between tasks and procedures on the same client after contacting material that may contain a high concentration of microorganisms.
- Put on clean gloves just before touching mucous membranes and nonintact skin.
- Wear gloves for all invasive procedures such as performing venipuncture, or other vascular or surgical procedures.
- Wear gloves if you have cuts, scratches, or other breaks in the skin.
- Remove gloves promptly after use, before touching non-contaminated items and surfaces, and before going to another client; wash hands immediately after removing gloves.

MASK, EYE PROTECTION, FACE SHIELD

Wear a mask and eye protection or a face shield to protect mucous membranes of your eyes, nose, and mouth during procedures and client-care activities that are likely to generate splashes or sprays of blood, body fluids, secretions, or excretions.

GOWN

Wear a clean, disposable gown to protect your skin and prevent soiling of clothing during procedures and client-care activities that are likely to generate splashes or sprays of blood, body fluids, secretions, or excretions. Remove soiled gowns promptly, washing your hands immediately after gown removal.

EQUIPMENT

Handle used client-care equipment that is soiled with blood, body fluids, secretions, and excretions in a way that prevents exposing your skin and mucous membranes, contaminating your clothing, and transferring microorganisms to other clients or environments. Ensure that reusable equipment is cleaned and appropriately reprocessed before using for the care of another client.

ENVIRONMENTAL CONTROL

Follow hospital procedures for routine care, cleaning, and disinfecting environmental surfaces, beds, bed rails, bedside equipment, and other frequently touched surfaces.

LINEN

Handle and transport linens soiled with blood, body fluids, secretions, and excretions in a manner that prevents exposing your skin and mucous membranes, contaminating your clothing, and transferring microorganisms to other clients and environments. Place soiled linen in leakage-resistant bags at the location where it is used.

OCCUPATIONAL HEALTH AND BLOODBORNE PATHOGENS

- Take care to prevent injuries when using needles, scalpels, and other sharps; when handling sharp instruments after procedures; when cleaning used instruments; and when disposing of used needles.

- Never recap needles, manipulate them using both hands, or handle them in a manner that directs the point of a needle toward any part of your body. If it is necessary to protect the needle prior to disposal, use a one-handed "scoop" technique or mechanical device to hold the needle sheath.
- Do not remove used needles from disposable syringes by hand; do not bend, break, or otherwise manipulate used needles by hand.
- Place used disposable syringes and needles, scalpel blades, and other sharp items in appropriate puncture-resistant containers located as close as practical to the area in which the items were used.
- Place reusable syringes and needles in a puncture-resistant container for transport to the reprocessing area.

- Use mouthpieces, resuscitation bags, or other ventilation devices as an alternative to mouth-to-mouth resuscitation methods whenever possible.

CLIENT PLACEMENT

Place clients who contaminate the environment or who do not (or are not expected to) assist in maintaining appropriate hygiene or environmental control, for example, an ambulatory, confused client with fecal incontinence, in a private room.

Source: Garner, J. S., & Hospital Infection Control Advisory Committee (1996). Guidelines for isolation precautions in hospitals. *Atlanta, GA: Public Health Service, U.S. Department of Health and Human Services, Centers for Disease Control and Prevention.*

Appendix II

NANDA-Approved Nursing Diagnoses 2001–2002

PATTERN 1: EXCHANGING
Imbalanced Nutrition: More Than Body Requirements
Imbalanced Nutrition: Less Than Body Requirements
Risk for Imbalanced Nutrition: More Than Body Requirements
Risk for Infection
Risk for Imbalanced Body Temperature
Hypothermia
Hyperthermia
Ineffective Thermoregulation
Autonomic Dysreflexia
Risk for Autonomic Dysreflexia
Constipation
Perceived Constipation
Diarrhea
Bowel Incontinence
Risk for Constipation
Impaired Urinary Elimination
Stress Urinary Incontinence
Reflex Urinary Incontinence
Urge Urinary Incontinence
Functional Urinary Incontinence
Total Urinary Incontinence
Risk for Urge Urinary Incontinence
Urinary Retention
Ineffective Tissue Perfusion (specify type: Renal, Cerebral, Cardiopulmonary, Gastrointestinal, Peripheral)
Risk for Imbalanced Fluid Volume
Excess Fluid Volume
Deficient Fluid Volume
Risk for Deficient Fluid Volume
Decreased Cardiac Output
Impaired Gas Exchange
Ineffective Airway Clearance
Ineffective Breathing Pattern
Impaired Spontaneous Ventilation
Dysfunctional Ventilatory Weaning Response
Risk for Injury
Risk for Suffocation
Risk for Poisoning
Risk for Trauma
Risk for Aspiration
Risk for Disuse Syndrome
Latex Allergy Response

Risk for Latex Allergy Response
Ineffective Protection
Impaired Tissue Integrity
Impaired Oral Mucous Membrane
Impaired Skin Integrity
Risk for Impaired Skin Integrity
Impaired Dentition
Decreased Intracranial Adaptive Capacity
Disturbed Energy Field

PATTERN 2: COMMUNICATING
Impaired Verbal Communication

PATTERN 3: RELATING
Impaired Social Interaction
Social Isolation
Risk for Loneliness
Ineffective Role Performance
Impaired Parenting
Risk for Impaired Parenting
Risk for Impaired Parent/Infant/Child Attachment
Sexual Dysfunction
Interrupted Family Processes
Caregiver Role Strain
Risk for Caregiver Role Strain
Dysfunctional Family Processes: Alcoholism
Parental Role Conflict
Ineffective Sexuality Patterns

PATTERN 4: VALUING
Spiritual Distress
Risk for Spiritual Distress
Readiness for Enhanced Spiritual Well-Being

PATTERN 5: CHOOSING
Ineffective Coping
Impaired Adjustment
Defensive Coping
Ineffective Denial
Disabled Family Coping
Compromised Family Coping
Readiness for Enhanced Family Coping
Readiness for Enhanced Community Coping
Ineffective Community Coping

Ineffective Therapeutic Regimen Management
Noncompliance (specify)
Ineffective Family Therapeutic Regimen Management
Ineffective Community Therapeutic Regimen Management
Effective Therapeutic Regimen Management
Decisional Conflict (specify)
Health-Seeking Behaviors (specify)

PATTERN 6: MOVING
Impaired Physical Mobility
Risk for Peripheral Neurovascular Dysfunction
Risk for Perioperative-Positioning Injury
Risk for Falls
Impaired Walking
Impaired Wheelchair Mobility
Impaired Transfer Ability
Impaired Bed Mobility
Activity Intolerance
Fatigue
Risk for Activity Intolerance
Disturbed Sleep Pattern
Sleep Deprivation
Deficient Diversional Activity
Impaired Home Maintenance
Ineffective Health Maintenance
Delayed Surgical Recovery
Adult Failure to Thrive
Feeding Self-Care Deficit
Impaired Swallowing
Ineffective Breastfeeding
Interrupted Breastfeeding
Effective Breastfeeding
Ineffective Infant Feeding Pattern
Bathing/Hygiene Self-Care Deficit
Dressing/Grooming Self-Care Deficit
Toileting Self-Care Deficit
Delayed Growth and Development
Risk for Delayed Development
Risk for Disproportionate Growth
Relocation Stress Syndrome
Risk for Relocation Stress Syndrome
Risk for Disorganized Infant Behavior
Disorganized Infant Behavior
Readiness for Enhanced Organized Infant Behavior

PATTERN 7: PERCEIVING
Disturbed Body Image
Chronic Low Self-Esteem
Situational Low Self-Esteem
Risk for Situational Low Self-Esteem
Disturbed Personal Identity
Disturbed Sensory Perception (specify: Visual, Auditory,
    Kinesthetic, Gustatory, Tactile, Olfactory)
Unilateral Neglect
Hopelessness
Powerlessness
Risk for Powerlessness

PATTERN 8: KNOWING
Deficient Knowledge (specify)
Impaired Environmental Interpretation Syndrome
Acute Confusion
Chronic Confusion
Disturbed Thought Processes
Impaired Memory
Wandering

PATTERN 9: FEELING
Acute Pain
Chronic Pain
Nausea
Dysfunctional Grieving
Anticipatory Grieving
Chronic Sorrow
Risk for Other-Directed Violence
Self-Mutilation
Risk for Self-Mutilation
Risk for Self-Directed Violence
Post-Trauma Syndrome
Rape-Trauma Syndrome
Rape-Trauma Syndrome: Compound Reaction
Rape-Trauma Syndrome: Silent Reaction
Risk for Post-Trauma Syndrome
Anxiety
Death Anxiety
Fear
Risk for Suicide

Appendix III

Common Laboratory Values

BLOOD

Hematocrit	Male: 40–54%
	Female: 37–47%
Hemoglobin	Male: 13.5–18 g/dL
	Female: 12–16 g/dL
Red blood cells	Male: 4.6–6.0 mil/μL
	Female: 3.6–5.0 mil/μL
MCV	80–98 μm³
MCH	26–34 pg
MCHC	32–36%
White blood cells	4,500–10,000/mm³
Neutrophils	50–70% of total WBCs
Eosinophils	1–3%
Basophils	0.5–1%
Lymphocytes	25–35%
Monocytes	2–6%
Platelets	150,000–350,000 μL

ELECTROLYTES

Sodium (Na^+)	135–145 mEq/L
Potassium (K^+)	3.5–5.0 mEq/L
Calcium (Ca^{2+})	8.5–10 mg/dL
Magnesium (Mg^{2+})	1.3–2.1 mEq/L or
	1.6–2.6 mg/dL
Chloride (Cl^-)	98–106 mEq/L
Bicarbonate (HCO_3^-)	22–26 mEq/L
Phosphate/phosphorus (PO_4^{2-})	2.5–4.5 mg/dL

OTHER

Serum osmolality	275–295 mOsm/kg
Carbon dioxide	24–30 mEq/L
pH	7.35–7.45
Blood urea nitrogen (BUN)	8–25 mg/dL
Creatinine	0.6–1.2 mg/dL
Bilirubin (Total)	0.3–1.2 mg/dL
Direct bilirubin	0–0.2 mg/dL
Indirect bilirubin	< 1.1 mg/dL
Glucose	70–110 mg/dL
Protein	6.0–8.0 g/dL
Albumin	3.5–5.0 g/dL
Low density lipoproteins (LDLs)	60–160 mg/dL
Low risk for CHD	< 130 mg/dL
High density lipoproteins (HDLs)	30–80 mg/dL
Low risk for CHD	46–59 mg/dL
Cholesterol	120–220 mg/dL
Desirable level	< 200 mg/dL
Prothrombin time (PT)	11–14 sec
Thyroxine (T_4)	4–12 μg/dL
T_3 resin uptake	25–35 relative % uptake

URINALYSIS

Color	Yellow, clear
Specific gravity	1.010–1.035
pH	4.5–7.8
Protein	Negative
Glucosae	Negative
Ketones	Negative

Appendix IV

Glossary

(Note: Glossary terms may appear in several chapters. The number(s) in parentheses in boldface after the glossary term show the primary chapter in which the term is defined. Other words or terms that may require definitions are italicized in the text and are defined there.)

Abscess: pocket of accumulated pus (12)

Abstinence: voluntarily refraining from use of a drug that has been abused or from an activity such as sexual intercourse (11, 34)

Acidosis: increased hydrogen ion concentration; a pH less than 7.35 (5)

Acne: disorder of the sebaceous glands (14)

Acquired immunodeficiency syndrome (AIDS): last stage of HIV infection (13)

Active immunity: immunity acquired by having the disease or by artificial immunization for long-term immunity (13)

Active transport: process by which molecules are moved against a concentration gradient across cell membranes (5)

Acute illness: illness that occurs rapidly, lasts for a relatively short period of time, and is self-limiting (2)

Acute pain: temporary pain that has a sudden onset and is localized (6)

Acute respiratory distress syndrome (ARDS): A severe form of acute respiratory failure due to acute damage to the alveoli (10)

Addiction: condition of seeking drugs habitually (other than for a medical purpose) and of not being able to give them up without adverse psychological and physiological effects (6, 11)

Addisonian crisis: acute deficiency of cortisol that causes a life-threatening condition (16)

Adrenergic drugs: class of drugs that mimic the fight-or-flight response of the sympathetic system (10)

Advance directives: legal documents that allow a person to plan for health care and financial affairs in the event of incapacity (9)

Advocate: one who speaks for another (1)

Agranulocytosis: decrease in granulocytes; neutropenia (24)

Alkalosis: decreased hydrogen ion concentration; a pH greater than 7.45 (5)

Allergen: substance such as dog hair or pollen that causes an allergic reaction (13)

Allodynia: pain resulting from a stimulus that normally would not cause pain, such as light touch (6)

Allograft: tissue transplants between the same species (13)

Alterations in health: change in normal health state (2)

Alzheimer's disease: progressive deterioration of brain function resulting in dementia (30)

Amenorrhea: absence of menstruation (33)

Amputation: partial or total removal of a body part (27)

Anabolism: process by which tissues are built up (12)

Analgesics: pharmacologic agents used to relieve or reduce pain (6)

Anaphylactic shock: shock caused by a severe allergic reaction (10)

Anastomosis: surgical connection of two tubular structures (18)

Androgens: male sex hormones (32)

Anemia: condition in which the hemoglobin concentration or the number of circulating RBCs is decreased (24)

Anergy: no response to common antigens given to test for immunocompetence (13)

Anesthesia: use of chemical substances to produce loss of sensation, reflex loss, or muscle relaxation during a surgical procedure, with or without the loss of consciousness (7)

Aneurysm: localized dilation of a blood vessel (23)

Angina pectoris: chest pain that occurs when there is a temporary imbalance between myocardial blood supply and demand (22)

Anorexia–cachexia syndrome: effect of cancer cells on metabolism; cancer cells divert nutrition to own use and inhibit food intake; they also break down body tissue and muscle proteins to support their growth (8)

Anoxia: lack of oxygen to body tissues (29)

Antibiotics: medications used to treat bacterial infections (12)

Antibody: an immunoglobulin that binds to and inactivates a specific antigen (12)

Antigen: substance that stimulates an immune response (13)

Anuria: absence of urine output (21)

Aphasia: inability to speak or understand the spoken word (29)

Arteriosclerosis: disorder characterized by thickening, loss of elasticity, and calcification of arterial walls (23)

Artery: blood vessel that carries blood away from the heart (23)

Arthralgia: joint pain (28)

Arthritis: inflammation of a joint (28)

Arthroplasty: reconstruction or replacement of a joint (28)

Ascites: accumulation of serous fluid in the peritoneal cavity (19)

Assessment: collection of data about the client's individualized health and health care needs; first step of the nursing process (1, 4)

Asthma: a chronic inflammatory airway disorder with recurrent episodes of wheezing, breathlessness, chest tightness, and coughing (26)

Atelectasis: an area or areas of alveolar collapse and airlessness (26)

Ataxia: staggering gait (11)

Atherosclerosis: disease in which the lining of medium and large arteries is affected by lesions called atheromas or plaque (22)

Aura: warning sign of a seizure or migraine headache; it may be a bright light, an unusual sound, or abnormal taste or odor (29)

Auscultation: method of assessment that uses a stethoscope to listen for body sounds (4)

Autoantibodies: antibodies made against self-antigens (13)

Autograft: graft transplanted from one part of the body to another (13)

Autoimmune disorders: disorders in which the body reacts against itself (13)

Autologous: self (13)

Automatism: repetitive, nonpurposeful actions such as lip smacking or aimless walking (29)

Autonomic dysreflexia: an exaggerated sympathetic response associated with high spinal cord injuries (30)

Autotransfusion: process in which a client's own blood is collected and reinfused (10)

Azotemia: increased blood levels of nitrogenous wastes, including urea and creatinine (21)

Bactericidal: ability of an antibiotic to kill microorganisms (12)

Bacteriostatic: ability of an antibiotic to inhibit growth of microorganisms (12)

Barrel chest: a greater anterior–posterior (AP) chest diameter than lateral chest diameter (26)

Basal cell carcinoma: cancer that begins in the basal cell layer of the epidermis, usually on sun-exposed areas of the body (14)

B-cell lymphocytes: white blood cells responsible for humoral immunity that produce antibodies (13)

Benign prostatic hyperplasia (BPH): enlargement of the prostate gland (32)

Block nursing: care, based on need, provided by the nurse to people who live on the same block as the nurse (3)

Blood pressure: force exerted by blood against the walls of the arteries (23)

Borborygmi: loud, hyperactive bowel sounds (18)

Bradykinesia: slowed voluntary movements and speech (30)

Brain death: clinical criteria for determining when a client is dead (10)

Broad-spectrum antibiotics: antibiotics that act against a wide variety of pathogens (12)

Bronchitis: inflammation of the bronchi (26)

Bruit: harsh or musical sound (murmur) heard on auscultation of a blood vessel (23)

Buffer: substance that prevents major changes in pH by either removing or releasing hydrogen ions from a solution (5)

Burn shock: type of hypovolemic shock resulting from the shift of a massive amount of fluid into the extravascular space (15)

Burn: injury of tissue loss, damage, or irreversible destruction from exposure to a thermal, chemical, electrical, or radiation heat source (15)

Cancer: disease that results when normal cells mutate into abnormal ones and continue to reproduce within the body (8)

Candidiasis: infections caused by *Candida albicans,* a yeastlike fungus (14)

Carcinogens: cancer-causing agents (8)

Cardiac output: amount of blood pumped from the ventricles in one minute (22)

Cardiac reserve: ability of the heart to increase the cardiac output in response to metabolic demand (22)

Cardiac tamponade: compression of the heart by blood or fluid in the pericardial sac (22)

Cardiogenic shock: impaired tissue perfusion caused by pumping failure of the heart (10)

Caregivers: people who provide personal, individual assistance (1)

Carotid endarterectomy: surgical procedure to remove plaque from the carotid artery (29)

Carrier: person who transmits an infectious disease but does not show any clinical manifestations (12)

Catabolism: process by which body tissues are broken down (12)

Cataract: clouding of the lens of the eye (31)

Cell-mediated immunity: immune response provided by direct action of the T cells (13)

Cellulitis: localized infection of the dermis and subcutaneous tissue (12, 14)

Cephalalgia: headache (29)

Cerebral vascular accident (CVA): sudden loss of neurologic function due to a blood clot or rupture of a cerebral artery; brain attack or stroke (29)

Cerumen: earwax (31)

Chain of infection: set of factors that must exist in order for an infection to develop (12)

Chancre: painless ulcer characteristic of primary syphilis (34)

Cholecystitis: inflammation of the gallbladder (19)

Cholelithiasis: formation of gallstones, also called calculi (19)

Chorea: constant, jerky, uncontrolled movements of the body (30)

Chronic illness: any impairment or deviation from normal functioning that affects more than one body system and that is permanent, leaves permanent disability, is irreversible, requires special teaching for rehabilitation, or requires a long period of care (2)

Chronic obstructive pulmonary disease (COPD): Chronic and progressive air flow obstruction caused by chronic bronchitis and emphysema (26)

Chronic pain: pain that lasts longer than 6 months, may not be totally eliminated, or may end only with death; may be malignant (related to cancer) or nonmalignant (6)

Chyme: mixture of partly digested food and digestive juices (18)

Cirrhosis: chronic liver disease that destroys the structure and function of liver lobules (19)

Clone: exact copy of another cell (13)

Clonic contractions: alternate contraction and relaxation of muscles, causing jerky movements (29)

Colectomy: surgical removal of the colon (20)

Colonization: bacteria that live in a host but do not cause injury or initiate the inflammatory process (12)

Comfort measures only: order indicating that no further life-sustaining interventions are necessary and that the goal of care is a comfortable, dignified death (9)

Community-based nursing: care focused on individual and family health care needs, providing direct services to individuals to manage acute or chronic health problems and to promote self-care (3)

Compartment syndrome: constriction of blood vessels and nerves within a compartment by excess pressure in the compartment (27)

Concussion: brain injury resulting from violent shaking or impact with an object (29)

Conjunctivitis: inflammation of the conjunctiva of the eye (31)

Conscious sedation: type of anesthesia that provides analgesia and amnesia but allows the client to remain conscious (7)

Contracture: abnormal flexion and fixation of a joint caused by muscle atrophy and shortening (15, 27)

Contralateral: opposite side (29)

Contusion: bleeding into soft tissue resulting from a blunt force (27, 29)

Convulsion: involuntary muscle contraction and relaxation (29)

Coryza: profuse nasal discharge (25)

Critical thinking: self-directed thinking that is focused on what to believe or do in a specific situation (1)

Crohn's disease: regional enteritis; a chronic, relapsing inflammatory disorder of the gastrointestinal tract (20)

Cross-tolerance: tolerance to other, similar types of substances (e.g., alcohol and heroin) (11)

Cryptorchidism: failure of one or both testes to descend through the inguinal ring into the scrotum (32)

Cyanosis: bluish, grayish, or dark purple skin tone caused by reduced oxygen content of the blood (14, 26)

Cystectomy: surgical removal of the urinary bladder (21)

Cystitis: inflammation of the urinary bladder (21)

Cystocele: herniation of the bladder into the vagina (33)

Cytotoxic T cells: subset of T cells that attack viruses, fungi, and cancer cells (13)

Dawn phenomenon: rise in blood glucose levels between 5 and 8 A.M. (17)

Death: irreversible cessation of circulatory and respiratory functions or irreversible cessation of all functions of the entire brain, including the brain stem (9)

Debride: remove foreign material and dead or damaged tissue (28)

Debridement: process of removing dead tissue from a wound (15)

Debulking: surgery to remove a large part of a tumor when complete removal is impossible (29)

Dehiscence: separation in the layers of an incisional wound (7)

Demyelination: Destruction and degeneration of the myelin sheath covering nerve axons (30)

Denial: refusal to acknowledge the existence of a real situation or feeling (11)

Dermatitis: inflammation of the skin characterized by erythema and pain or pruritus (14)

Dermatome: area of skin supplied by a single sensory nerve (29)

Dermatophyte: tinea infections named by the body part affected (14)

Dermis: second, deeper layer of skin (14)

Desensitization: treatment of an allergy by giving several dilute injections that contain the allergen (13)

Detoxification: removal of a toxic substance from the body (11)

Diabetes mellitus: chronic disorder of carbohydrate metabolism (17)

Diabetic ketoacidosis: life-threatening illness occurring in Type 1 diabetics, characterized by hyperglycemia, metabolic acidosis, and coma (17)

Diabetic nephropathy: kidney disease caused by diabetes mellitus (17)

Diabetic neuropathy: disease of the peripheral and autonomic nerves caused by diabetes mellitus (17)

Diabetic retinopathy: disease of the retina caused by diabetes mellitus (17)

Diagnosis-related groups (DRGs): categories for reimbursement of inpatient services; the system pays a predetermined amount of money for the care of different persons with the same medical diagnosis (3)

Dialysis: diffusion of solutes from higher to lower concentration across a semipermeable membrane (21)

Diapedesis: movement of white blood cells from the circulation to the injury site (12)

Diarrhea: increase in the frequency, volume, and water content of stool (20)

Diffusion: process in which molecules move from an area of high concentration to an area of low concentration to become evenly distributed (5)

Dilemma: choice between two unpleasant alternatives (1)

Diplopia: double vision (31)

Disability: degree of observable and measurable impairment (3)

Disease: medical term describing alterations in structure and function of the body or mind (2)

Dislocation: separation of contact between two bones of a joint (27)

Disseminated intravascular coagulation (DIC): acute condition characterized by abnormal clotting and bleeding (10)

Distal paresthesia: subjective feeling of numbness or tingling in the toes and fingers (17)

Do-not-resuscitate (DNR): "no-code"; order written by the physician for a client near death, usually based on the wishes of the client and family that no cardiopulmonary resuscitation be performed for respiratory or cardiac arrest (9)

Dopamine: neurotransmitter (30)

Drug tolerance: process by which the body requires a progressively greater amount of a drug to achieve the same results (6)

Dual diagnosis: term for clients with substance use disorder and a serious mental illness (11)

Durable power of attorney for health care: health care *proxy;* a legal document written by a competent, mentally healthy adult that gives another competent adult the right to make health care decisions on his or her behalf if he or she cannot (9)

Dysfunctional uterine bleeding (DUB): vaginal bleeding that is abnormal in amount, duration, or time of occurrence (33)

Dysmenorrhea: pain associated with menstruation (33)

Dyspareunia: pain during sexual intercourse (33)

Dysphagia: difficult or painful swallowing (18, 25, 29)

Dyspnea: difficult or labored breathing (26)

Dysrhythmia: disturbance or irregularity in the electrical system of the heart (22)

Ectopic: occurring in an abnormal location (22, 33)

Edema: excess fluid in body tissues (5)

Ejaculation: expulsion of seminal fluid from the male urethra (32)

Electrolytes: substances that dissociate in solution to form charged particles, or ions (5)

Emancipated minors: individuals under age 18 who are responsible for their own welfare and live independently of their parents (7)

Embolus: blood clot or foreign matter that moves within the vascular system (23)

Emotional lability: extreme emotion and mood swings from crying to laughing (29)

Endocarditis: inflammation of the endocardium (22)

Endocardium: innermost lining of the heart and great vessels (22)

Endogenous pyrogens: chemicals, bacterial toxins, prostaglandins, and interleukin-1 that act on the hypothalamus to raise body temperature (12)

Endorphins: body's naturally produced morphines (painkillers) (6)

Endotoxins: harmful substances released from gram-negative bacteria (12)

Enteral: within or into the GI tract (18)

Epidermis: outermost part of the skin (14)

Epilepsy: chronic pattern of seizure activity; seizure disorder (29)

Epileptogenic focus: group of neurons that fire abnormally, causing a seizure (29)

Epistaxis: nosebleed (25)

Equianalgesic dose: having the same analgesic effect when administered to the same individual; drug dosages are equianalgesic if they have the same effect as morphine sulfate 10 mg IM (6)

Erectile dysfunction: impotence; inability to achieve and maintain an erection (32)

Erythema: reddening of the skin (14, 25)

Erythrocyte: red blood cell (24)

Eschar: hard crust that forms over a burn wound (15)

Esophageal varices: enlarged, overdistended veins in the distal esophagus (19)

Estrogens: steroid hormones essential to developing and maintaining female secondary sex characteristics (33)

Ethics: principles of conduct concerned with moral duty, values, obligations, and the distinction between right and wrong (1)

Euphoria: exaggerated feeling of well-being (11)

Euthanasia: (from the Greek for painless, easy, gentle, or good death) term commonly used to signify killing prompted by a humanitarian motive (9)

Evaluation: the final step of the nursing process, which allows the nurse to determine whether the plan was effective and to continue, revise, or terminate the plan (1)

Evisceration: protrusion of body organs from a wound dehiscence (7)

Exacerbation: time period in some chronic illnesses when symptoms reappear following a remission (2)

Exophthalmos: forward protrusion of the eyeballs (16)

Exotoxins: harmful substances released from staphylococci, streptococci, and tetanus bacteria (12)

External otitis: inflammation of the ear canal (31)

Extracellular fluid (ECF): body fluid located outside of cells (5)

Family: unit of two or more people who are related by marriage, birth, or adoption, or who are emotionally involved with each other (2)

Fasciculations: involuntary contractions of the voluntary muscles (30)

Filtration: process by which water and solutes move across capillary membranes, driven by fluid pressure (5)

Fissures: deep grooves in the surface of the brain (2)

Fistula: abnormal tubelike passage from one body cavity to another (12, 20)

Folliculitis: infection that begins at the hair follicle opening and extends down into the follicle (14)

Fracture: break in the continuity of a bone (27)

Full-thickness burn: burn (third-degree) that involves all layers of the skin and may extend into subcutaneous fat, connective tissue, muscle, and bone (15)

Functional health patterns: a system for grouping human functions (such as nutrition and elimination) (1)

Furuncle: "boil"; infection of the hair follicle (14)

Gangrene: tissue death from reduced or absent blood supply (17, 27)

Gastrectomy: partial or total removal or resection of the stomach (18)

Gastritis: inflammation of the stomach lining (18)

Gastroenteritis: inflammation of the stomach and intestines (20)

Gastroesophageal reflux (GER): backward movement of gastric contents into the esophagus (18)

Glaucoma: disorder of increased intraocular pressure and gradual loss of peripheral vision (31)

Glomerular filtration rate (GFR): amount of fluid filtered from the blood into the glomerular capsule per minute (21)

Glomeruli: small clusters of capillaries in the kidney (21)

Glomerulonephritis: inflammation of the glomeruli (21)

Glomerulosclerosis: fibrosis of the glomerular capillaries in the kidneys (17)

Gluconeogenesis: process to make glucose in the liver (17)

Glycogenolysis: conversion of glycogen into glucose in the liver and muscles (17)

Glycosuria: presence of glucose in the urine (17)

Goiter: enlargement of the thyroid gland (16)

Grief: emotional response to loss and its changes (9)

Gynecomastia: breast enlargement (32)

Handicap: the total adjustment to disability that limits functioning at a normal level (3)

Health: state of complete physical, mental, and social well-being, not merely the absence of disease or infirmity (2)

Health–illness continuum: representation of health as a dynamic process, with high-level wellness at one extreme of the continuum and death at the opposite extreme (2)

Heart failure: inability of the heart to function as a pump to meet the needs of the body (22)

Heat stroke: life-threatening condition in which the body cannot cool itself (10)

Helper T cells: cells that turn on the immune system (13)

Hematemesis: vomiting blood (18)

Hematochezia: blood in the stool (18)

Hematoma: collection of blood within a tissue, organ, or space caused by a break in a blood vessel (27, 29)

Hemiplegia: paralysis on one side of the body (29)

Hemoglobin: oxygen-carrying protein in red blood cells (24)

Hemolysis: destruction of red blood cells (10, 24)

Hemophilia: hereditary clotting factor deficiencies (24)

Hemoptysis: bloody sputum (26)

Hemorrhage: excessive loss of blood (7)

Hemostasis: blood clotting (24)

Hemothorax: blood in the pleural space (26)

Hepatitis: inflammation of the liver (19)

Hepatocytes: liver cells (19)

Herpes simplex: "fever blisters"; "cold sore" infections caused by herpesvirus I or II (14)

Herpes zoster: "shingles"; viral infection of a dermatome section of the skin caused by varicella zoster, the herpesvirus that causes chickenpox (14)

High-level wellness: way of functioning to reach one's maximum potential at a particular point in time (2)

Hirsutism: excessive hair growth or hair growth in unusual places, such as facial hair on women (16)

Histocompatibility: tissues compatible for transplantation to another person (13)

Home health care: health and social services provided to the chronically ill, disabled, or recovering person at home (3)

Homeostasis: body's tendency to maintain a state of physiologic balance in the presence of constantly changing conditions (5)

Homonymous hemianopia: loss of vision in half of the visual field (29)

Hormones: chemical messengers of the body (16)

Hospice: model (not a place) of care for clients and families, when client is faced with a limited life expectancy; it emphasizes quality rather than quantity of life (9)

Human immunodeficiency virus (HIV): retrovirus that causes HIV disease and AIDS (13)

Human papillomavirus: virus causing genital warts, a sexually transmitted disease (13)

Humoral immunity: immune response provided by antibodies (13)

Hydronephrosis: abnormal dilation of the renal pelvis and calyces (21)

Hyperglycemia: high blood glucose level (17)

Hyperglycemic hyperosmolar nonketotic syndrome (HHNS): life-threatening illness occurring in Type 2 diabetics, characterized by hyperglycemia, severe dehydration, and coma (17)

Hyperkalemia: serum potassium level greater than 5.0 mEq/L (5)

Hyperpituitarism: disease condition in which there is excessive function of the pituitary gland (16)

Hypersensitivity: altered immune response to an antigen that causes harm to the body (13)

Hypertension: blood pressure higher than 140 mm Hg systolic or 90 mm Hg diastolic on three separate readings several weeks apart (23)

Hypertrophic scar: overgrowth of dermal tissue that remains within the boundaries of the wound (15)

Hypervolemia: excess intravascular fluid (5)

Hypoglycemia: low blood glucose level (17)

Hypokalemia: serum potassium level less than 3.5 mEq/L (5)

Hypopituitarism: disease condition in which there is deficient function of the pituitary gland (16)

Hypovolemic shock: shock caused by a decrease in intravascular volume (10)

Hypoxemia: low oxygen levels in the blood ($PaO_2 < 80$ mm Hg) (5, 10, 25)

Hysterectomy: removal of the uterus (33)

Icterus: jaundice (19)

ICU psychosis: acute confusion after 2 to 3 days in the intensive care unit (10)

Illness: response a person has to a disease (2)

Immunization: vaccines that create immunity against a specific disease (13)

Immunocompetent: ability of the body's immune system to ward off pathogenic organisms (13)

Immunoglobulins: antibodies produced by B cells (13)

Immunosuppression: inability of the immune system to provide adequate immunity (12)

Impaired nurse: nurse with substance abuse problems, who may exhibit mood changes, irritability, forgetfulness, self-isolation, and inappropriate behavior (11)

Impairment: disturbance in structure or function resulting from physiologic or psychological abnormalities (3)

Implementation: the fourth step in the nursing process—the "doing" phase—during which the nurse carries out planned interventions (1)

Incision and drainage: procedure for draining pus from a wound (12)

Infection: condition in which pathogenic organisms trigger the inflammatory process (12)

Infectious disease: condition causing a host to become ill from an infection (12)

Infertility: inability to conceive during a year or more of unprotected intercourse (32)

Inflammation: nonspecific response that occurs when the body experiences any type of injury (12)

Influenza: flu; highly contagious viral respiratory disease (25)

Informed consent: a legal document required for certain diagnostic procedures or therapeutic measures, including surgery (7)

Inpatient surgery: surgery requiring admission to a hospital before and after the procedure (7)

Inspection: method of assessing by observing the client through the senses of seeing, smelling, and hearing (4)

Intermittent claudication: cramping or aching sensation in the calves, thighs, and buttocks that occurs with activity and is relieved by rest (23)

Interventions: purposeful actions performed by the nurse in implementing client care (1)

Intoxication: reversible set of physical, psychological, and behavioral symptoms caused by use of a substance (11)

Intracellular fluid (ICF): body fluid contained within the cells (5)

Intracranial pressure (ICP): pressure exerted within the cranium by the brain, blood, and cerebrospinal fluid (29)

Intraocular lens: artificial lens inserted when a diseased lens is removed (31)

Intraoperative surgical phase: begins with entry into the operating room and ends with admittance to the postanesthesia care unit (PACU), or recovery room (7)

Invasiveness: organism's ability to invade the body and cause disease (12)

Isograft: transplant between identical twins (13)

Jacksonian march: seizure activity that may spread from one part of the body to another (29)

Jaundice: yellowness of the skin, sclera of the eyes, mucous membranes, and body fluids due to deposited bile pigment resulting from excess bilirubin in the blood (14, 19)

Keloid: scar that extends beyond the boundaries of the original wound (15)

Keratitis: inflammation of the cornea (31)

Ketonuria: presence of ketones in the urine (17)

Ketosis: build-up in ketones in the body (17)

Killer T cells: lymphocytes that act on nonspecific foreign substances (13)

Korsakoff's syndrome: group of symptoms caused by a deficiency in B vitamins, including thiamine, riboflavin, and folic acid (11)

Kyphosis: exaggeration of the normal posterior curve of the thoracic spine (28)

Labile: changeable (11)

Laparotomy: surgical opening of the abdomen (20)

Laryngectomy: removal of the larynx (voice box) (25)

Laryngitis: inflammation of the larynx (25)

Laryngospasm: spasm of the muscles of the larynx (25)

Leukemia: malignant proliferation of WBCs (24)

Leukocyte: white blood cell (24)

Leukocytosis: increased white blood cell count above normal (12)

Leukopenia: decreased white cell count below normal (12)

Libido: sexual desire (32)

Living will: legal document that formally expresses a person's wishes regarding life-sustaining treatment in the event of terminal illness or permanent unconsciousness (9)

Lobules: basic functional units of the liver (19)

Long-term care: care for disabled persons of all ages that lasts from a few days to several years; it includes skilled care, intermediate and long-term care, transitional care, nursing homes, retirement centers, and residential institutions (3)

Loss: occurs when a valued object, person, body part, or situation is lost or irreversibly changed (9)

Lymphadenitis: enlarged, tender lymph nodes (12)

Lymphadenopathy: swelling and enlargement of the lymph nodes (24)

Lymphatic system: the lymphoid organs, including lymph vessels, lymph nodes, spleen, and thymus (24)

Macrophages: mature, large white blood cells that develop from monocytes (12)

Macular degeneration: loss of neurons in the area of central vision of the eye (31)

Malabsorption: condition of ineffective intestinal absorption of nutrients (20)

Malignant lymphomas: cancerous tumors of lymphoid tissue (24)

Malnutrition: long-term nutrient and calorie deficiencies resulting in health problems (18)

Manifestations: objective and subjective data (signs and symptoms) associated with a specific illness (2, 4)

Mastectomy: removal of the breast (33)

Medical-surgical nursing: the health care and illness care of adults (1)

Melanoma: cutaneous or malignant melanoma; skin cancer that arises from melanocytes, the cells that produce skin pigment (14)

Melena: black, tarry stool that contains blood (18)

Memory T cells: cells that provide immunity when reexposed to a past antigen (13)

Meninges: protective membranes covering the brain and spinal cord (29)

Menopause: period during which menstrual activity permanently ceases (33)

Metabolism: biochemical reactions that occur in the body's cells (18)

Metastasis: process by which malignant neoplasms spread to distant sites; a secondary tumor formed by this process (8)

Metrorrhagia: bleeding between menstrual periods (33)

Microalbuminuria: presence of small amounts of albumin in the urine (17)

Multiple organ dysfunction syndrome: irreversible complication of shock in which the body's systems fail (10)

Multiple myeloma: malignancy in which plasma cells multiply uncontrollably and infiltrate bone marrow, lymph nodes, and other tissues (24)

Mutation: change in an organism from its original form into a different form (12)

Myelin sheath: white fatty substance that insulates and protects some axons (29)

Myocardial infarction (MI): myocardial cell necrosis (death) due to lack of blood and oxygen (22)

Myocardium: heart muscle (22)

Myopathy: condition characterized by muscle cramps of sudden onset, plus pain, tenderness, and edema of skeletal muscles (11)

Myxedema coma: life-threatening form of hypothyroidism (16)

Narrow-spectrum antibiotics: antibiotics that act against a few pathogens (12)

Natural immunity: person's natural resistance to foreign antigens (13)

Natural killer cells: white blood cells that can attack viruses and cancer cells (13)

Neoplasm: tumor; mass of abnormal cells that grows independently of its surrounding structures and has no physiologic purpose (8)

Nephron: functional unit of the kidney (21)

Nephrotoxins: agents that damage kidney tissue (21)

Neurogenic shock: shock caused by an interruption to the sympathetic nervous system (10)

Neuron: basic cell of the nervous system (29)

Neuropathic pain: pain caused by damage to the CNS or peripheral nerves (6)

Neurotransmitter: chemical released during the transmission of an electrical impulse that assists or inhibits the impulse in crossing the synapse (29)

Nevi: moles (14)

Nociceptors: nerve endings in the body that respond to noxious stimuli (6)

Nonopioids: drugs such as acetaminophen and nonsteroidal anti-inflammatory drugs (NSAIDs) that are used to treat mild to moderate pain (6)

Nosocomial infections: infections acquired in a health care setting (12)

Nursing diagnosis: the second step in the nursing process; a clinical judgment about individual, family, or community responses to actual or potential health problems/life processes (1)

Nursing process: series of activities nurses perform as they provide care to clients (1)

Nutrients: substances in food used for growth, maintenance, and repair of the body (18)

Nutrition: process of ingesting, absorbing, using, and eliminating food (18)

Obesity: body weight more than 20% above ideal for gender, height, and age (18)

Objective data: observable or measurable pieces of data that can be seen, heard, touched, or smelled (also called signs) (4)

Oncogenes: genes capable of triggering cancer (8)

Oncology: study of cancer; oncologists are physicians who specialize in cancer care (8)

Oophorectomy: removal of the ovary (33)

Opioids: drugs derived from opium (e.g., morphine) used to treat moderate to severe pain (6)

Oral hairy leukoplakia: opportunistic infection caused by the Epstein–Barr virus (13)

Orchiectomy: surgical removal of the testes (32)

Orthopnea: difficulty breathing while lying down (22)

Orthostatic hypotension: drop of greater than 10 mm Hg in blood pressure occurring with position change (5)

Osmolarity: concentration of particles in the blood (16)

Osmosis: transport process by which water moves across a semipermeable membrane from an area of lower solute concentration to an area of higher solute concentration (5)

Osmotic diuresis: loss of fluid from extracellular compartment (17)

Osteoarthritis: degenerative joint disease with progressive loss of joint cartilage in synovial joints (28)

Osteomyelitis: infection of the bone (28)

Osteoporosis: bone disorder characterized by loss of bone mass (28)

Ostomy: a surgically created opening from an organ to the surface of the body (20)

Otitis media: inflammation or infection of the middle ear (31)

Otorrhea: leakage of fluid from the external ear (29)

Outcomes: time-specific, achievable goals (1)

Outpatient surgery: defined as a surgical procedure performed on a nonhospitalized client under local or general anesthesia (7)

Pain: unpleasant sensory and emotional experience associated with actual or potential tissue damage (6)

Pain threshold: point at which each person recognizes pain (6)

Pain tolerance: amount and duration of pain a person can stand before seeking relief (6)

Pallor: paleness of skin (14)

Palpation: method of assessing by using the hands to touch and feel (4)

Pancreatitis: inflammation of the pancreas (19)

Paracentesis: removal of fluid from the peritoneal cavity (19)

Paralytic ileus: slowing or stopping of peristalsis (20)

Paraplegia: paralysis of the lower half of the body (30)

Parenchyma: essential, functional parts of an organ (19)

Parish nursing: nursing care provided in coordination with the pastor and staff of a faith community, to promote health and healing through counseling, referrals, teaching, and assessment of health care needs; a parish nurse may be employed by a hospital or a church (3)

Paroxysmal nocturnal dyspnea: attacks of shortness of breath that occur at night, awakening the client (22)

Partial-thickness burn: burn (second-degree) that involves the entire dermis and may also involve the hair follicles (15)

Passive immunity: injection of preformed antibodies into an unprotected person for short-term immunity (13)

Pathogens: microorganisms that are capable of producing disease (12)

Pathologic fracture: fracture of a diseased or weakened bone that occurs with minimal force or trauma (28)

Patient-controlled analgesia (PCA): self-administration of opioid medications by a programmed infusion pump (6)

Pediculosis: infestation with lice (14)

Peptic ulcer: break in the mucous lining of the gastrointestinal tract where it comes in contact with gastric juice (18)

Percussion: method of assessing by tapping the body to produce sound waves that provide information about underlying body structures or organs (4)

Pericardial friction rub: leathery, grating sound produced by the inflamed pericardial layers rubbing against the chest wall or pleura (22)

Pericarditis: inflammation of the pericardium (22)

Pericardium: fibrous sac that covers and surrounds the heart (22)

Peripheral vascular resistance (PVR): force that opposes blood flow (23)

Peripheral vascular system: network of blood vessels that carry blood to peripheral tissues and then return it to the heart (23)

Peristalsis: alternating waves of contraction and relaxation of involuntary muscle (18)

Peritonitis: inflammation of the peritoneum, a double-layered membrane that lines the walls and organs of the abdominal cavity (20)

Petechiae: small, flat, purple or red spots on the skin or mucous membranes (24)

pH: measure of hydrogen ion concentration in a solution; as H^+ concentration increases, the solution becomes more acid and the pH falls; as H^+ concentration decreases, the solution becomes more alkaline and the pH rises (5)

Phagocytosis: process by which phagocytes ingest harmful bacteria and dead tissue cells (12)

Phantom pain: pain in a missing extremity resulting from nerve trauma during surgery (27)

Pharyngitis: acute inflammation of the pharynx; sore throat (25)

Pheochromocytoma: tumor of the adrenal medulla that causes an increased release of catecholamines (16)

Photophobia: extreme sensitivity to light (31)

Physical dependence: adaptation of the body to chemical substances over an extended period of time; stopping the substance abruptly causes physical withdrawal symptoms (6)

Planning: the third step in the nursing process, in which the nurse develops a list of nursing interventions (1)

Plasmapheresis: procedure that removes plasma from the blood to take out immune substances that cause inflammation (30)

Platelets: small fragments of cytoplasm without nuclei; an essential component of the body's clotting mechanism (24)

Pleural effusion: collection of fluid in the pleural space (26)

Pneumatic antishock garment (PASG): inflatable garment applied to trauma victims in the prehospital setting to raise blood pressure (10)

Pneumonia: inflammation of the respiratory bronchioles and alveoli (26)

Pneumothorax: accumulation of air in the pleural space (26)

Poikilothermia: condition found in spinal cord injuries in which the client assumes the temperature of the environment (30)

Polycythemia: erythrocytosis; abnormally high red blood cell count and high hematocrit (24)

Polydipsia: excessive thirst (17)

Polyphagia: excessive hunger (17)

Polysubstance abuse: use of a variety of substances to induce an altered physical, mental, or emotional state (11)

Polyuria: excessive urine output (17)

Portal hypertension: elevated blood pressure in the portal vein (19)

Positive inotropic drugs: group of drugs used to increase cardiac output (10)

Postoperative surgical phase: begins with admission to the postanesthesia recovery area and ends with complete recovery from the surgical intervention (7)

Premenstrual syndrome (PMS): complex of symptoms including irritability, depression, edema, and breast tenderness preceding the monthly menses (33)

Preoperative surgical phase: begins when the decision for surgery is made and ends when the client is transferred to the operating room (7)

Presbycusis: progressive hearing loss associated with aging (31)

Pressure ulcers: bedsores; decubitus ulcers; ischemic lesions of the skin and underlying tissue caused by external pressure that impairs the flow of blood and lymph (14)

Primary (essential) hypertension: hypertension with no identified cause (23)

Primary intention: healing takes place when a wound is uncomplicated and clean and has little tissue loss (7)

Prophylactic: strategy to prevent an infection (12)

Prostatectomy: surgical removal of the prostate gland (32)

Proteinuria: protein in the urine (21)

Pruritus: subjective itching sensation producing an urge to scratch (14, 19)

Psoriasis: chronic, noninfectious skin disorder characterized by raised, reddened, round circumscribed plaques of varied size, covered by silvery white scales (14)

Psychogenic pain: pain that results from emotional rather than physical causes (6)

Pulmonary embolism: sudden blockage of a pulmonary artery that disrupts blood flow to the lung (26)

Pyelonephritis: inflammatory disorder affecting the renal pelvis and parenchyma (21)

Quality assurance: includes the quality-control activities of evaluating, monitoring, or regulating the standard of services provided to the consumer (1)

Rectocele: herniation of the rectum into the vagina (33)

Red reflex: reddish-orange glow seen in the pupil when a beam of light is directed into it (31)

Reduction: restoration of normal alignment of a bone or joint (27)

Referred pain: pain that begins in one area of the body but is felt in another part (6)

Reflex: involuntary motor response to a stimulus (29)

Reflex arc: the neural pathway between the stimulus and the response organ (29)

Refraction: bending of light rays to focus on the retina (31)

Regurgitation: failure of a valve to close properly, allowing blood to flow back through it (22)

Rehabilitation: process of learning to live to one's maximum potential with a chronic impairment, disability, or substance dependency (3, 11)

Relapse: return to drug use after abstinence, or of an illness after a period of freedom from symptoms (11)

Relative hypovolemia: hypovolemia resulting from shift of fluids from the intravascular space to the interstitial space (10)

Remission: time period in a chronic illness when the disease is present, but there are no symptoms (2)

Renal failure: condition in which the kidneys are unable to remove accumulated waste products from the blood (21)

Renin–angiotensin system: blood pressure regulation system activated when there is reduced blood flow to the kidneys (10)

Respiration: exchange of gases between the person and the environment (26)

Respiratory failure: inability of the lungs to oxygenate the blood and remove carbon dioxide well enough to meet the body's needs, even at rest (26)

Retinal detachment: separation of the retina from the vascular choroid layer of the eye (31)

Retroperitoneal: behind the peritoneum and outside the peritoneal cavity (19)

Reverse transcriptase: enzyme produced by HIV virus that converts RNA to DNA (13)

Rheumatoid arthritis: chronic, systemic inflammatory disorder resulting in persistent inflammation of the synovial tissue that lines joints (28)

Rhinitis: inflammation of the nasal cavities (25)

Rhinoplasty: surgical reconstruction of the nose (25)

Rhinorrhea: discharge of fluid from the nose (29)

Rhizotomy: surgical procedure that severs a nerve root to control pain (30)

Rule of Nines: rapid method of estimating the extent of a burn by assigning percentages to parts of the body (15)

Salpingo-oophorectomy: removal of the fallopian tubes and ovaries (33)

Scabies: infestation caused by a mite (14)

Sciatica: Pain that occurs along the sciatic nerve (30)

Scoliosis: lateral curvature of the spine (28)

Secondary hypertension: hypertension that results from a known cause (23)

Secondary intention: healing that occurs when a wound is large, gaping, and irregular (7)

Seizure: brief episode of abnormal electrical activity in nerve cells of the brain (29)

Septic shock: shock caused by overwhelming infection (10)

Septicemia: presence of bacteria in the blood (10)

Seroconversion: positive reaction to the presence of a disease's antibody (13)

Shock: life-threatening condition characterized by inadequate blood flow to organs, tissues, and cells (7, 10)

Shunt: movement of fluids from one area to another (10)

Sinusitis: inflammation of the mucous membranes of the sinuses (25)

Sleep apnea: temporary absence of breathing during sleep (25)

Somogyi phenomenon: early morning hyperglycemia following an episode of hypoglycemia at night (17)

Spinal shock: temporary loss of reflex activity below the level of the spinal cord injury (30)

Sprain: injury to a ligament caused by a twisting motion (27)

Squamous cell carcinoma: malignant tumor of the squamous epithelium of the skin or mucous membranes (14)

Staging: system of classifying cancer by tumor size, lymph node involvement, and metastasis to distant sites (33)

Standard: statement or criterion that can be used by a profession and by the general public to measure quality of practice (1)

Standard precautions: guidelines to protect the health care worker and prevent transmission to other clients (12)

Status epilepticus: period of continuous tonic–clonic seizures (29)

Stenosis: narrowing of a valve opening, which obstructs forward blood flow (22)

Stomatitis: inflammation of the oral mucosa (18)

Strain: microscopic muscle tear that causes bleeding into the tissues (27)

Stridor: high-pitched, harsh sound heard during inspiration, usually caused by partial airway obstruction (25)

Stroke volume: amount of blood ejected from the heart each minute (10)

Subarachnoid hemorrhage: bleeding into the subarachnoid space in the brain (29)

Subjective data: experiences (data) that only the client can describe, such as pain; also called symptoms (4)

Substance abuse: maladaptive pattern of substance use leading to significant impairment or distress (11)

Substance dependency: maladaptive pattern of substance use manifested by tolerance, withdrawal syndrome, increased use, ineffective attempts to stop use, increasing amounts of time devoted to obtaining substance, and social isolation (11)

Sundowning: behavior characterized by time disorientation and wandering in the evening (30)

Superficial burn: first-degree burn that involves only the epidermal layer of skin (15)

Superinfection: overgrowth of bacteria that occurs when antibiotics eliminate the body's normal flora (12)

Suppressor T cells: turn off the immune system, limiting the immune response (13)

Susceptible: prone to developing an infection (12)

Synapse: space between two neurons across which an electrical impulse passes (29)

Systemic lupus erythematosus: chronic inflammatory connective tissue disease that affects multiple body systems (28)

T-cell lymphocytes: white blood cells responsible for cell-mediated immunity (13)

Tertiary intention: healing that occurs when substantial time passes before a wound is sutured (7)

Tetany: continuous spasm of the muscles; symptom complex of increased neuromuscular excitability associated with decreased ionized calcium levels (5, 16)

Tetraplegia: paralysis of the arms, legs, and trunk (30)

Therapeutic range: amount of drug that will produce the desired effect while producing few toxic effects (12)

Thrombocytopenia: platelet count of less than 100,000 platelets per milliliter of blood (24)

Thrombus: blood clot (23)

Thymectomy: surgical removal of the thymus gland (30)

Thyroid crisis (thyroid storm): extreme state of hyperthyroidism (16)

Thyroidectomy: partial or complete removal of the thyroid gland (16)

Thyrotoxicosis: condition of hypersecretion of the thyroid gland (16)

Tinnitus: ringing in the ear (31)

Tolerance: need for more of a substance to achieve the same effect; diminished effect from continued use of the same amount of a substance (6, 11)

Tonic contractions: contraction in which the body becomes rigid with the arms and legs extended (29)

Tonsillectomy: surgical removal of the tonsils (25)

Tonsillitis: acute inflammation of the tonsils (25)

Total parenteral nutrition (TPN): the administration of an intravenous solution that meets all nutritional requirements except for fiber (18)

Toxic shock syndrome: form of septic shock caused by *Staphylococcus aureus* (10)

Toxoid: injection containing a weakened toxin, e.g., tetanus toxoid (13)

Tracheostomy: surgical opening into the trachea (25)

Traction: use of a pulling force to reduce a fracture or maintain alignment (27)

Transcutaneous electrical nerve stimulation (TENS): external device that delivers vibrations to painful areas on the client to provide pain relief (6)

Transient ischemia attack (TIA): brief episode of reversible neurologic deficits (29)

Transmission-based precautions: precautions against spread of infection through the air, by droplet, and through contact (12)

Transsphenoidal hypophysectomy: surgical procedure used to remove the pituitary gland (16)

Trauma: injury caused by applying more force to tissue than it is able to absorb (27)

Triage: system to identify who will receive medical attention first (10)

Trismus: difficulty opening the jaw as seen in tetanus (30)

Tympanic membrane: eardrum (31)

Ulcerative colitis: chronic inflammatory bowel disorder of the mucosa and submucosa of the colon and rectum (20)

Uremia: a symptom complex caused by excess metabolic waste products in the blood (21)

Urinary incontinence: involuntary urination (21)

Urolithiasis: development of stones within the urinary tract (21)

Uterine prolapse: descent of the uterus into the vagina (33)

Vaginitis: inflammation or infection of the vagina (33)

Varicose veins: irregular, tortuous veins with incompetent valves (23)

Vasectomy: sterilization procedure in which a portion of the spermatic cord is removed (32)

Vasopressor drugs: drugs used to increase the blood pressure (10)

Veins: blood vessels that carry blood and waste products back to the heart (23)

Venous insufficiency: stasis of venous blood flow in the lower extremities (23)

Venous thrombosis: formation of a blood clot (thrombus) on the wall of a vein, which obstructs the flow of blood back to the heart (23)

Vertigo: sensation of whirling or rotation (31)

Virions: HIV particles (13)

Virulence: power of a microorganism to cause an infection (12)

Warts: verrucae; lesions caused by the human papillomavirus (HPV) (14)

Wernicke's syndrome: alcoholic encephalopathy; characterized by ataxia, paralysis of eye muscles, nystagmus, and mental confusion (11)

Withdrawal: set of symptoms resulting from discontinuation or reduction of a substance after heavy or prolonged use (6, 11)

Xenograft: transplant from animal to human (13)

Appendix V

NCLEX-PN Answers; Hints for Critical Thinking

CHAPTER 1

NCLEX-PN ANSWERS: (1) C—The nurse today independently plans and implements client care based on nursing knowledge and skills. (2) B—The nurse as client advocate actively promotes the client's rights to autonomy and free choice. The nurse may speak for the client, mediate between the client and other persons, and protect the client's right to self-determination. (3) A—The nurse is responsible for the quality of client care through a process called quality assurance. Quality-control activities include evaluating, monitoring, or regulating the standard of services provided to the client. (4) D—Nurses assess clients in two ways: an initial assessment, and ongoing, focused assessments. (5) A—Making a diagnosis is a complex process and always involves uncertainty. Critical thinking and reasoning are used to choose nursing diagnoses that best define the individual clients' health problems. (6) B—Nursing interventions must be specific and individualized. The nurse identifies client problems and needed interventions, then works with the client to determine those that are needed and preferred by the individual client. (7) A—Implementation is the action or "doing" phase of the nursing process. (8) C—Documenting interventions is the final component of implementation, and it is a legal requirement. "If it isn't documented, it isn't done." (9) D—Nursing practice is structured by standards and codes of ethics that guide nursing practice and protect the public. (10) B—According to the ANA, the nurse has a moral obligation to provide care for the client with AIDS unless the risk exceeds the responsibility.

CHAPTER 2

NCLEX-PN ANSWERS: (1) A—Accidents are the leading cause of injury and death in people between 15 and 24. Unprotected sex with a variety of people and substance abuse are also major causes of concern for this age group. (2) A—Middle adults often have problems maintaining a healthy weight because they consume the same number of calories while decreasing physical activity. (3) C—Annual immunization for influenza is recommended. Vision and prostate examinations for older adults should be annual. Regular amounts of moderate exercise are recommended for this age group. (4) D—Although not always meeting traditional definitions, people (or even pets) who are significant to the client are the client's family. They should be an integral component of care in all health

care settings. (5) B—Wellness is an integrated method of functioning, oriented toward maximizing the individual's potential. Good health can exist as a relatively passive state of freedom from illness. (6) B—Cognitive development affects whether people view themselves as healthy or ill and may affect health practices. Educational level affects the ability to understand and follow guidelines for health. (7) C—The nurse promotes health by teaching activities that maintain wellness, providing information about diseases, and following healthy practices that serve as a model. (8) A—Illness is the highly individualized response a person has to disease. (9) D—An acute illness occurs rapidly, lasts for a relatively short period of time, and is self-limiting. It usually responds to self-treatment or to medical-surgical intervention. (10) A—Almost all people with a chronic illness need to live as normally as possible, despite their symptoms and treatment. Chronic illness can make a person feel alienated, lonely, and different from others.

Care Map (Client with Early-Onset Diabetes)
CORRECT DATA: Subjective: States "I'm not a good mother anymore"; states "I think I will just stop taking my insulin." Objective: Fasting blood glucose 180 (increased).

CORRECT INTERVENTIONS: Listen carefully to concerns; state "Tell me more about how you think diabetes controls you"; suggest joining a diabetes support group; ask her to keep a daily diary of self-management activities.

REPORT: Yes, to her primary health care provider at the clinic.

DOCUMENTATION: 7/7/02. 1030. Blood glucose 180, makes statements that she is not a good mother, thinks she can't control her diabetes so might just as well stop taking insulin. Data reported to G. Walker, RN, NP, C

CHAPTER 3

NCLEX-PN ANSWERS: (1) C—Community-based nursing focuses on individual and family health care needs where they live, work, play, worship, and go to school. Community health nursing focuses on the health of a community. (2) B—Some of the most common community-based health care services include community centers, clinics, day care centers, block nursing, and parish nursing. (3) A—If a conflict arises, the nurses must remain the primary client's advocate, regardless of any negative response from the family. (4) D—One of the specific criteria that the client must meet in order to secure Medicare reimbursement is to be essentially homebound. (5) A—With shorter hospital stays, all clients should be evaluated for their ability to manage at home. The nurse should make a referral to a home health agency if the client has need for follow-up beyond the present clinical setting. (6) C—Nurses cannot close their eyes to an unsafe environment. Safety assessment in the home is both a nursing responsibility and a legal requirement. (7) D—The nurse cannot go into homes and change the family's living space and lifestyle. However, the nurse must alert the family to unsafe and hazardous conditions, suggest remedies, and document the family's response in the record. (8) B—Rehabilitation is the process of learning to live to one's maximum potential with a chronic impairment and of enabling a person to live with dignity, self-worth, and independence. (9) A—Rehabilitation promotes reintegration into the client's family and community through a team approach that includes in the plan of care: Physical function, mental health, interpersonal relationships, social interactions, and vocational status. It requires the expertise of a team of health care providers. (10) B—The plan of care developed for each client is individualized, based on the priority of needs from the client's and family's perspective.

Care Map (Client with a Handicap)

CORRECT DATA: Subjective: States "I can't keep my present job"; states "I don't know where to go for help." Objective: Unable to bend left leg more than 15 degrees.

CORRECT INTERVENTIONS: Suggest career counseling; ask Kim if she has ever considered other types of employment; refer Kim to vocational rehabilitation services.

REPORT: No, although it would be shared with other team members.

DOCUMENTATION: 8/5/02. 1300. Requesting information about other types of employment. Referred for career counseling and to vocational rehabilitation services. Jim Manning, LVN

CHAPTER 4

NCLEX-PN ANSWERS: (1) B—Objective data are observable or measurable pieces of information (such as the color of urine). Objective data can be seen, heard, touched, or smelled. (2) C—A focused assessment addresses a specific client problem. Assessing a client with abdominal pain includes assessing bowel movements, temperature, trauma, location, duration, and type of pain. (3) B—If the client is very young, very ill, unconscious, or confused, data may be collected from secondary sources, such as family or friends. (4) D—Open-ended questions give the client the chance to provide more information than closed-ended questions. "Why" questions often make the client feel threatened or foolish. (5) C—Palpation is use of the hands to touch and feel. Light palpation is used for determining pulses, tenderness, skin texture, skin temperature, and skin moisture. (6) A—The nurse should wash his or her hands before and after the assessment, even if gloves need to be worn. (7) D—The apical pulse taken for one full minute is the most accurate pulse measurement. It should be taken if there is any question about the peripheral pulse or if the client is taking a medication that affects heart rate. (8) B—Bowel sounds are auscultated by gently placing the stethoscope on the abdomen and listening in all four quadrants. Bowel sounds are clicks or gurgles made as intestinal contents move through the bowel; they should always be present. (9) C—Jaundice is a yellow color of the skin and mucous membranes. It is caused by liver or gallbladder disease, or by an excessive breakdown of red blood cells. Jaundice is usually first seen in the eyes and then in the skin and mucous membranes. (10) C—When recording blood pressure, the nurse should write "BP 120/70," not give a detailed description of the assessment method. Data should be organized in a logical way, and inferences or judgments should be avoided. The word *normal* should not be used; instead, write the specific assessment finding.

Care Map (Client with Risk for Excess Fluid Volume)

CORRECT DATA: Subjective: States she had not taken her medications for more than a week and she does not follow her prescribed low-sodium diet. Objective: BP 180/96; R 30 with crackles and wheezes; AP 108, irregular; 4+ edema from toes to knees in both legs.

CORRECT INTERVENTIONS: Ask Cath if she would consider being seen by a social worker; monitor vital signs on a regular basis; monitor breath sounds, apical pulse, and peripheral pulses; measure circumference of lower legs.

REPORT: Yes, to the home health manager or the primary health care provider.

DOCUMENTATION: 9/30/02. 0930. States she has not taken her medications for over a week. BP 180/96; R 30 with crackles and wheezes; AP 108 and irregular; 4+ edema in both lower legs. Data reported to R. Brunde, RN. L. Wilson, LPN

CHAPTER 5

NCLEX-PN ANSWERS: (1) C—Females, in general, have less body water than males. Obese people are at risk for dehydration; there is less water available in clients with a high percentage of body fat. Individuals over the age of 65 have a decrease in body water. (2) B—ADH regulates water excretion in the kidneys. The kidneys are less permeable to water. Copious amounts of dilute urine are produced. Serum osmolality decreases, blood pressure falls slightly, and the thirst mechanism in the brain is activated. (3) A—These signs and symptoms indicate a decrease in fluid volume, such as dehydration. There will be decreased output due to the decreased fluid volume. Dizziness and light-headedness may precipitate falls. (4) B—Decreased calcium level is manifested by muscle excitability and circumoral paresthesia. Surgery of the neck may cause damage to the parathyroid glands, which regulate calcium in the bloodstream. (5) D—Magnesium levels are related to the level of calcium in the bloodstream. Similar symptoms will occur. Tetany, seizures, ECG changes, and tremors may be observed. Bradycardia and vasodilation are seen in hypermagnesemia states. (6) A—Respiratory alkalosis occurs during hyperventilation. The pH increases, while the $PaCO_2$ and HCO_3 decreases. The normal range for PaO_2 is 80 to 100 mm Hg. (7) A—The pancreas secretes bicarbonate into the small intestine. Vomiting, suctioning, and diarrhea contribute to the loss of bicarbonate. Overuse of baking soda increases the bicarbonate levels. (8) C—Calcium carbonate increases the calcium blood levels. The lack of sun exposure, diuretics, and menopause may deplete the body of calcium. (9) A—Lasix is a loop diuretic that promotes water loss. Daily weights should be obtained; they are the most accurate measurement for water loss. Intake and output are also needed for patient fluid evaluation. (10) C—Poor skin turgor is an indicator of fluid volume deficit and dehydration. Peripheral edema, bounding pulses, and elevated blood pressure are manifestations of fluid volume excess.

Case Study Hints:

FLUID VOLUME EXCESS: (1) Think how the heart adapts to increased blood volume to handle this increased workload. If necessary, you may wish to review the first part of Chapter 22. (2) Think about the effect of elevating the head of the bed on blood flow to the upper portion of the body, on the diaphragm, and on chest wall expansion. (3) Review Table 5-4. Be sure to adapt your teaching to Ms. Rainwater's specific needs. As you formulate your response, think about going for 4, 8, 12, or more hours without drinking any fluids. Also review Ms. Rainwater's prescribed medications.

HYPOKALEMIA: (1) Review Ms. Ortiz's medications and her nursing assessment. (2) Think about the effect of hydrochlorothiazide on potassium excretion and balance; then consider the effect of hypokalemia on the effects of digitalis.

Care Map (Acute Respiratory Acidosis)

CORRECT DATA: Objective: T 98.2, P 102, R 36 and shallow, BP 146/92; restless; oxygen at 4 L/min per nasal cannula; responds slowly to questions; ABGs: pH 7.38 (normal 7.35 to 7.45), $PaCO_2$ 48 mm Hg (normal 35 to 45 mm Hg), PaO_2 92 mm Hg (normal 80 to 100 mm Hg), HCO_3 24 mEq/dL (normal 22 to 26 mEq/L)

CORRECT INTERVENTIONS: Monitor ABGs, to be redrawn in 2 hours; monitor respiratory status and vital signs every 15 minutes for the first hour, then hourly; assess mental status, LOC, and color of skin, nail beds, and oral mucous membranes hourly.

CHAPTER 6

NCLEX-PN ANSWERS: (1) B—Chronic pain is prolonged pain that lasts more than 6 months. It is usually nonresponsive to treatment. Acute pain is sudden, temporary, has an identified cause, and lasts less than 6 months. (2) C—Referred pain starts in one site but is perceived in another part of the body. It frequently occurs with visceral pain (pain from body organs lined with viscera), because the pain impulses travel along the same nerve paths. (3) D—Progression of cancer frequently produces pain that requires multiple therapies and is often unresponsive to treatment. Pain is caused by pressure on body organs, nerves, and metastasis to bone. (4) C—Phantom limb pain occurs in some individuals following the removal of an extremity. The client is aware that the part is missing, but the pain can be intense and difficult to treat. Medication should be administered to attempt relief. Nonpharmacologic approaches are ineffective. (5) A—Ibuprofen is an irritant to the gastric mucosa. Clients with gastric ulcer disease should use alternate medications for pain relief. (6) D—Allowing the client to describe his pain based on a pain scale provides an objective, individualized description of the pain. The nurse can make decisions for intervention based on this assessment. (7) B—This drug has a short half-life and will not accumulate and cause toxicity. Elderly patients may have impairment of liver and renal function that leads to increased risk for toxicity. Drugs such as meperidine and propoxyphene cause sedation and respiratory depression. Long-term use of acetaminophen may lead to liver damage. (8) C—Naloxone blocks the effects of opioid drugs and reverses sedation and respiratory depression that may result from excessive dosages. (9) C—Osteoarthritis requires long-term therapy with NSAIDs. A common side effect is gastric bleeding. Taking the drug with foods helps to reduce this risk. The physician should be consulted before medication is discontinued. Alcohol and aspirin should be avoided because they increase the risk of gastric irritation and bleeding. (10) A—Decreased peristalsis and constipation are common side effects of codeine. Assessment of bowel sounds is essential, especially in the elderly. Fluids should be increased to at least 3,000 mL/day if not contraindicated.

Case Study Hints

PAIN: (1) You would tell Ms. Akers to take pain medication on a regular basis; review the nursing diagnosis Acute Pain in the Nursing Process section of the chapter. (2) Review the Assessment section under Nursing Process and the pain rating scales. (3) Include in your discharge teaching the effects of opioids on the GI tract and methods to avoid constipation.

Care Map (Acute Pain)

CORRECT DATA: Subjective: Says she feels tired and hopes she can sleep; dull pain in lower abdomen: "It hurts right here." Objective: P 100; BP 150/92; lying on her side with eyes closed.

CORRECT INTERVENTIONS: Offer a back massage at HS; give morphine sulfate 8 mg IM q4h PRN; listen attentively to Mrs. Bruski; teach Mrs. Bruski a relaxation technique.

CHAPTER 7

NCLEX-PN ANSWERS: (1) C—A and D are postoperative nursing diagnosis. B is an intraoperative nursing diagnoses. (2) B—Potassium level of 2.8 is below normal and places the client at risk for cardiac arrhythmias. (3) A—Discussion of risk factors is included in informed consent. Informed consent is the responsibility of the physician. (4) B—Assessment is needed before nursing intervention can be determined. (5) C—The client should be in semi-Fowler's or Fowler's position for effective coughing and deep breathing exercises. (6) C—Primary intention is normal wound healing. The wound edges are approximated and closed by staples or sutures. (7) B—The client is a married minor and can sign her own consent. (8) C—Assessment suggests impending shock. The client should be placed in the shock position to facilitate blood supply to vital organs. (9) D—A positive Homan's sign is suggestive of thrombophlebitis. Further assessment of the leg is indicated to support this finding. (10) D—The nurse must clarify this action with the physician. Alteration of physician orders is not an independent nursing action.

Case Study Hints

INPATIENT SURGERY: (1) Review the section on Physical and Psychological Preparation. Also review preoperative teaching in this chapter, including postoperative breathing exercises, turning, coughing, deep breathing, and leg exercises. Discuss nutrition and pain management. (2) Think about the limitations Mrs. Overbeck will experience. What areas of follow-up exist in the postoperative period? What rehabilitation must occur? (3) Review the Preoperative section of this chapter, and see the nursing diagnoses there. What questions would you have if you were scheduled for this surgery?

Care Map (Client After Surgery)

CORRECT DATA: Subjective: Incisional pain; complains of feeling warm and has chills; states she is "drinking lots of fluids." Objective: T 101.8° F, P 100; WBC 13,000 mm; light brown drainage on dressing; incision red, edematous, 2-cm opening; Cipro 250 mg q8h.

REPORT: Yes, to charge nurse and/or physician.

CORRECT INTERVENTIONS: Empty Jackson Pratt drain q4h; monitor vital signs, especially temperature and pulse, q4h; report temperature above 100° to charge nurse; assess pedal pulses q8h; provide extra blankets for warmth; change dressing, using aseptic technique bid; assess wound status with each dressing change; Tylenol gr X PO q4h for temperature above 100° F; cleanse wound with normal saline qd, per physician's order; monitor urinary output; maintain fluid intake at least 2,000 mL/day; administer pain medications as needed; administer antibiotics as ordered; collect sample of wound drainage, send to lab for culture and sensitivity.

DOCUMENTATION: Sample: 1/04/04, 1600. T 102° F, P 102, R 36, BP 126/70. C/O chills. Two blankets removed, sheet provided for cover. Tylenol gr X given PO for fever. Dressing to right leg changed using aseptic technique. Incision red, edematous with small amount of light brown drainage. Steri-strips intact. Opening in center of incision about 2 cm in length. Sterile gauze dressing reapplied. D. Moore, LPN

1645. T. 100.6° F, P 90. States she does not have chills at this time. Dressing dry and intact. D. Moore, LPN

CHAPTER 8

NCLEX-PN ANSWERS: (1) B—Cells from malignant tumors may travel to other sites through the vascular or lymph system. Benign tumors are usually encapsulated and do not metastasize. (2) C—A high-fat, low-fiber diet has been linked to development of colon cancer. Lack of fiber in the diet may allow carcinogens to remain in the colon longer and increase cancer risk. High-fiber diets add bulk to the colon and promote effective passage of stool. (3) B—Expressing his feelings allows the client and nurse to identify possible sources of inability to sleep. Assessment is needed before intervention. (4) A—Family members can provide needed care while the client adjusts to his diagnosis. The nurse should include the client in care as much as he will allow. (5) A—Choosing a head cover prior to losing her hair allows the client to prepare for the loss and make decisions in a less stressful environment. (6) C—Assessment provides information to plan care and meet patient needs. Small frequent meals are more palatable when a patient is anorexic. Soft, cool foods are usually tolerated better than hot foods. (7) B—Placing the implant in a lead container prevents radiation exposure. Long-handled forceps reduces the nurse's risk by increasing the distance from the implant. Radioactive materials should not be disposed of in the trash or sewer system because of risk of contamination to individuals and the environment. (8) C—Rubbing or scratching increases irritation to the site and increases risk of infection. Skin should be cleansed with clear water; no ointments should be applied unless directed by the physician. Clients receiving external radiation are not radioactive, and therefore are not a risk to others. (9) A—Providing antiemetic medication prior to the treatment reduces the risk of nausea and vomiting. Nutritional needs should be met throughout the course of chemotherapy. (10) C—Decreased WBC increases the client's risk of infection. Temperature elevation is a systemic symptom of infection. Alopecia and nausea and vomiting are not complications of bone marrow depression. The platelet count is usually decreased with bone marrow depression. A platelet count of 200,000 is within normal limits.

Case Study Hints

CANCER: (1) Review Nursing Care in this chapter, especially the assessment section and the nursing diagnoses *Imbalanced Nutrition: Less than Body Requirement* and *Risk for Infection*. (2) Review the nursing diagnosis *Pain* in the Nursing Care section of the chapter. (3) Use your knowledge of effective communication strategies to make the plan. Also remember any referrals that could be of value to Mr. Casey's daughter.

Care Map (Client with Anorexia Related to Cancer Treatment)

CORRECT DATA: Subjective: States she can't eat, that her mouth is sore, and it hurts to swallow; has lost weight.

Objective: Height and weight; pale skin with poor turgor; red, swollen oral mucous membranes; dry, brittle hair; concentrated urine.

CORRECT INTERVENTIONS: Assess hemoglobin and hematocrit; encourage fluid intake; administer antiemetics; suggest eating soft, bland foods at room temperature; offer high-protein drinks; instruct on using soft toothbrush or toothette for oral hygiene.

REPORT: Yes, to the physician or advanced practice nurse administering the chemotherapy.

DOCUMENTATION: Oral mucous membranes red and swollen, poor skin turgor. Weight 102. States that she has lost weight, can't eat, and that it hurts her to swallow. Data reported to H. Shaw, RN. R. Jones, LPN

CHAPTER 9
NCLEX-PN ANSWERS: (1) B—The grief process is highly individual in quality and duration depending on what the loss means to the person experiencing it. (2) B—In the anger stage, the person resists the loss, often directing his or her anger toward family and health care providers. (3) A—The age of the person experiencing the loss influences his or her understanding of and reaction to loss. An individual's reaction to loss is also affected by perception of a support system. (4) D—A Do-Not-Resuscitate order is written by the physician for a client who is near death. The order is usually written based on the wishes of the client and family. (5) B—Nurses care for the dying client in intensive care units, emergency rooms, long-term care facilities, and the home. Regardless of the setting, the client's wishes about death should be respected. (6) A—Hospice is a model of care (rather than a place of care) for clients and their families, emphasizing quality rather than quantity of life for clients as they near the end of life. (7) D—Providing comfort and care to the dying is an active, desirable, and important component of nursing care. Using data from symptom assessment to plan and intervene in symptom management is necessary for nurses to provide high-quality end-of-life care. (8) B—Near death, the client may have periods of apnea and/or Cheyne–Stokes respirations. An accumulation of fluids in the lungs and oropharynx may lead to what is sometimes referred to as "the death rattle." These respiratory changes are normal at this time. (9) D—Anticipatory grieving is a combination of intellectual and emotional responses and behaviors by which people work through the grief process based on the perception of a potential loss. (10) C—Spending time listening to clients conveys acceptance of their emotional response to loss. The most appropriate interventions are to listen to how they are feeling and to be present.

Case Study Hints
CLIENT EXPERIENCING LOSS: (1) What are the benefits of scheduling a time for a meeting of the staff involved in Mrs. Rogers's care with Mrs. Rogers's daughter? Think about and

practice statements to Mrs. Rogers's daughter that are non-threatening and accepting. Consider why the use of questions like "Why don't you do more for your mother?" are not appropriate. (2) Consider the losses Mrs. Rogers has had. Review the material in the chapter on responses to loss. Think about the reasons the nurse would not say, "Oh, for gosh sakes. Why would you want to do that?" Compose two or three statements that would help you collect more information from Mrs. Rogers. (3) As defined by NANDA, social isolation is the aloneness experienced by the individual and perceived as imposed by others and as a negative or threatening state. Review the case study and identify characteristics that provide clues to making this diagnosis.

Care Map (Dysfunctional Grieving)
CORRECT DATA: Subjective: States "I can't stand being alone," difficulty sleeping, unable to continue normal routines. Objective: Weight loss of 25 pounds.

CORRECT INTERVENTIONS: Discuss time needed to resolve a loss, explain grief reactions, encourage expression of feelings. State, "This must have been very difficult for you."

REPORT: Yes, to the nurse manager or physician.

DOCUMENTATION: 6/14/02. Has lost 25 pounds in past year. Makes statements that indicate she is still grieving the loss of her husband. J. Pequea, LPN

CHAPTER 10
NCLEX-PN ANSWERS: (1) D—Chills and fever may accompany the transfusion of any blood product. Based only on the manifestation of chills, the exact type of transfusion reaction cannot be determined. The nurse should stop the blood immediately and notify the charge nurse. Vital signs are then taken. The physician and the charge nurse determine whether the blood transfusion is continued at a slower rate or is completely discontinued. (2) D—Urinary output for the adult should be no less than 30 cc/hr. The fact that the Foley catheter amount is well below the norm indicates a problem that needs to be corrected immediately. First, check the Foley for patency and palpate the bladder for distention. Notify the charge nurse immediately. The dark color of the urine indicates severe concentration or dehydration. Renal failure is a life-threatening condition that must be corrected immediately. (3) B—There is no evidence of severe blood loss that could account for the restless state. The vital signs are stable and the dressing is dry. Infection is always a possibility but not likely at this point. The diagnosis of Anxiety is the most appropriate. Knowledge deficit relating to the prognosis of her surgery will be important once the anxiety has become manageable. Patients that are anxious will not be able to accept teaching plans until their anxiety is controlled. (4) C—The appropriate response is to acknowledge the client's concern and to make an attempt to ascertain the waiting time. Ignoring the client will only increase his anxiety and frustration. The client may not care that other people need attention, or may not understand the

levels of triage. Do not agree nor disagree with the long waiting times. (5) C—There are three stages of shock. Noncompensated is not a stage of shock. The absence of bowel sounds, thready pulse, rapid heart rate, and decreased level of consciousness all indicate that Mrs. Trimble had reached the progressive state. (6) B—Cirrhosis of the liver results in the shifting of fluid into the interstitial spaces (ascites). This decreases the amount of fluid circulating in the bloodstream. Anaphylactic shock occurs from a severe allergic reaction. Vital signs indicate that the heart is pumping effectively, so cardiogenic shock is not evident. Septic shock is caused by pathogenic toxins in the blood and results in high fevers, nausea, and vomiting. (7) C—Clients should be taught that many reactions are significantly more severe when exposed to the antigen the second time. Precautions should be initiated. Medic-Alert bracelets let medical personnel know that the client is allergic to bee venom. The pharmacist can teach about the antivenom drugs. The client's immediate family should learn appropriate interventions for handling an anaphylactic reaction. (8) B—Hemoglobin levels are decreased due to generalized bleeding, WBCs are increased due to the inflammatory process, and serum sodium levels are decreased due to kidney malfunctions. ARDS is characterized by widespread alveolar damage resulting in a significant decrease in blood oxygen levels. (9) B—Diuretics increase the excretion of urine through the kidneys. Blood pressure drops slightly. Heart rhythm is regulated by antiarrhythmic drugs. LOC may or may not improve and is based on the overall effects of all the nursing and medical management. (10) D—Safety issues within the client's home should be thoroughly discussed. Handrails in the bathroom, the removal of all loose rugs from the floors, and nightlights in the rooms are a few of the items that need to be addressed. The client should be able to maneuver with his walker prior to discharge. Food preparation is important once the safety issues are discussed. The number one cause of traumatic injury to the elderly is falls.

Case Study Hints
CLIENT WITH SEPTIC SHOCK: (1) Review Box 10-7 to differentiate between early and late septic shock manifestations. (2) Lactated Ringer's solution is used to increase volume, which will increase Mrs. Huang's blood pressure. She also needs fluids to decrease her dehydration caused by the fever and indicated by her poor skin turgor. (3) She had surgery 4 days ago and is underweight. Surgery alters the body's protective mechanisms. Being underweight will reduce the healing ability of the skin.

CLIENT WITH MULTIPLE INJURIES: (1) Review Table 10-3 for blood types. Until trauma clients have a type and crossmatch done, type O blood is given to maintain blood volume and pressure. (2) Review Box 10-3 for manifestations of Classes II and III. She does not have any active external bleeding, but her manifestations suggest internal bleeding. (3) Explain all procedures and answer the family's questions in a warm, caring manner. Encourage family to visit client as soon as possi

ble. Arrange for a social worker, counselor, or clergy to visit the family as appropriate.

Care Map (Client at Accident Scene)
CORRECT DATA: Subjective: Allergic to penicillin; does not drink alcohol; complains of being thirsty; complains of left leg pain. Objective: Awake; scalp is bleeding; skin slightly pale and dry; left leg is twisted at an odd angle; shallow, slow respirations; denies any difficulty breathing; rapid radial pulse rate.

CORRECT INTERVENTIONS: Look for hazards in the area; call for help; keep head and neck in neutral position; cover client with a blanket; cover scalp wound with clean cloth.

CHAPTER 11
NCLEX-PN ANSWERS: (1) A—The body adjusts to constant use of a drug. As consumption continues, larger amounts are needed to give the desired effect. Once tolerance develops, many clients begin use of different, more potent substances. (2) C—When alcohol is withdrawn, the central nervous system is still stimulated. The client exhibits signs of stimulation including elevated vital signs, anxiety, tremors, and seizures. (3) C—Alcoholic encephalopathy is caused by vitamin B_1 deficiency related to inadequate nutritional intake. (4) B—Opiate overdose results in depressed central nervous system including marked respiratory depression. Narcan (naloxone HCl) reverses the sedative effects. (5) B—Clients must be cautioned to avoid combining alcohol and antianxiety drugs. These combinations can result in cardiac arrthymias including cardiac arrest. (6) D—The nursing supervisor usually holds accountability and administrative authority for the unit and is aware of policy related to follow-up of situations in which narcotics are diverted. (7) B—Teaching the consequences of continued substance abuse gives the client information to make choices related to his/her behavior. (8) C—Opiates are central nervous system stimulants. When the drugs are withdrawn, the CNS is depressed. (9) D—Denial is the most common defense mechanism used by clients with alcohol abuse. (10) A—MDMA (Ecstasy) is classified as a hallucinogen.

Case Study Hints
INEFFECTIVE INDIVIDUAL COPING: (1) Until very recently, this client had no other way to respond to the stressors in her life except to drink. She is at high risk for relapse. Any stressful event that she cannot manage with her new skills will put her in a position where she thinks about drinking because it is what she has always done. Health professionals can only give her alternatives. Remember, we do not control her behavior. She must choose whether or not she will drink. Even if she has a relapse, there is still a good chance that she can recover from alcoholism in the long run. (2) Alcohol played the role of coping mechanism for her to make her feel better temporarily if she was upset or tired. Other people have many more tools for managing stressful situations. It will take time for her to develop new skills. (3) This person is no longer a client of the

hospital nurses. The nurse's best response would be to refer the client back to her AA sponsor or other outpatient resource, saying kindly that the client is capable of managing the situation.

Care Map (Substance Dependency)

CORRECT DATA: Subjective: States "I don't have a drinking problem. I can quit whenever I want"; states "I feel nervous"; had seizures as a child; states "If you don't let me out of here tomorrow, I'm leaving anyway." Objective: Vital signs stable; blood alcohol content: 0.24 mg/dL on admission; request pain meds q1h; insomnia; poor appetite.

CORRECT INTERVENTIONS: Assess his knowledge about alcoholism; teach client about disease process of alcoholism; provide effective pain management; offer frequent feedings; confront the client with the reality of the consequences of alcoholism; encourage the client to express his feelings about drinking and alcoholism; ask the client if he wants to leave the hospital to drink alcohol.

CHAPTER 12

NCLEX-PN ANSWERS: (1) A—Urinary tract infections are the leading cause of nosocomial infections. The client has a Foley catheter that was inserted 4 days ago. The 1-week use of the antibiotic is significant but not as important as the invasive insertion of the Foley catheter. Peripheral vascular disease increases the susceptibility for a nosocomial infection, but has not been a major factor in the hospital stay. (2) C—The normal WBC count is 4,500 to 10,000. An increased level indicates acute infection. (3) D—Allergy histories must always be discussed prior to giving any medication. The age and mental status are important factors. Old medications should be sent back to the pharmacy. Patients should be taught not to mix any drugs with alcohol. (4) B—The infection is an overgrowth of bacteria due to the side effects of the antibiotic. Nurses cannot diagnose medical conditions. You should address the problem and reassure the patient. Never tell the patient not to worry. "D" is incorrect, because it acknowledges the complaint but doesn't adequately address the client's concern. (5) D—Handwashing is extremely important in preventing infection. Antibiotic treatments should be completed as prescribed. Any fever should be reported because it may indicate an infection. Water intake should be at least 2 1/2 quarts per day. Water is needed in the maintenance of body temperature and metabolism. (6) A—Although there is an increase in the growth of vancomycin-resistant organisms, vancomycin is still the drug of choice. (7) A—Cellulitis is a subcutaneous/connective tissue infection. Antibiotics must be given at the appropriate times to decrease the potential damage to the eye. Bed rest may be ordered, but is generally not indicated. Morphine in frequent doses is contraindicated in the elderly and may lead to respiratory depression. Lab values are important but may be checked at a later time. (8) B—Systemic infection produces the enlargement of lymph nodes throughout the body. Cellulitis, fistulas, and abscesses are all manifestations of local

infection. (9) B—The *Pneumocystis carinii* organism is a fungus. It is considered to be an opportunistic disease in clients who are immunocompromised. (10) C—The chickenpox virus is spread through the air. Examples of droplet transmission include pneumonia and meningitis. Patients with acute diarrhea are placed on contact precautions. Standard precautions are also referred to as universal precautions. This includes the use of gloves and handwashing.

Case Study Hint

MRSA INFECTION: (1) Review the section on Infection Prevention and Control Techniques. (2) See the Nosocomial Infection section of this chapter. (3) Think about the chain of infection and about potential carriers of MRSA infection.

Care Map (Client Exposed to *Staphylococcus aureus*)

CORRECT DATA: Subjective: History of Type 2 diabetes. Objective: Roommate with *S. aureus* pneumonia; weight 140 lbs.; T 99° F; pressure ulcer on right great toe.

CORRECT INTERVENTIONS: Provide a diet high in protein; monitor vital signs every 4 hours; monitor skin for further breakdown; increase fluid intake as tolerated.

REPORT: Yes, to physician.

DOCUMENTATION: 02/14/03, 0830. T 99° F. Has open wound on right great toe draining yellowish fluid. Foley draining dark yellow urine of 200 mL. Mark Belaqua, LVN

CHAPTER 13

NCLEX-PN ANSWERS: (1) C—Local injections may cause discomfort at the site. Warm compresses will soothe the soreness. Redness at the injection site is common and does not indicate a severe reaction. Patients should remain in the clinic for at least 30 minutes after receiving an immunization to monitor for adverse reactions. Influenza vaccines are given at once. (2) D—Cross-sensitivity may occur between certain foods and latex allergies. The nurse's main priority is to protect the nursing assistant from contact with latex. It is unprofessional to discuss personal medical problems with co-workers. This reaction is a Type I reaction but this knowledge serves no purpose at this time. The assistant is already aware that an allergic reaction is possible if pineapple is ingested. (3) A—Swelling of the lips may lead to edema in the throat. Breathing difficulties should be assessed immediately. Medication may be administered to counteract the inflammatory process. A medical history is important, as well as patient teaching, after the initial assessment is completed. (4) B—Immunosuppressive agents decrease the ability of the immune system to fight infection. Emphasize the need to avoid large crowds and report signs of infection. Abnormal bleeding, decreased urine production, and jaundice should be reported immediately to the physician. (5) A—HIV is not transmitted by insects, sneezing, coughing, handshaking, sharing eating utensils, or linens. Answers B and C are not therapeutic communication techniques. These responses cast blame and discouragement.

(6) C—A primary infection with HIV may produce few symptoms. Many patients manifest with flulike symptoms. Diarrhea, opportunistic infections, and night sweats develop later in the disease process. (7) D—Condoms must be used one time. Oil-based lubricants adversely affect the condom's ability to provide protection. Oral contraceptives may provide pregnancy protection but have no effect on viral transmission. Anal sex should be avoided. (8) B—Tuberculosis is a common manifestation in patients diagnosed with HIV. The Mantoux is the diagnostic test. MAC is caused by a bacteria found in the soil and also affects the respiratory system. Candidiasis is caused by a fungus. A protozoon is the causative agent for cryptosporidiosis; it produces watery diarrhea. (9) D—AIDS dementia is a progressive disorder that leads to mental confusion, motor deficits, and forgetfulness. All of these nursing interventions would be noted on the care plan. With dementia, safety is the primary consideration. (10) A—The first priority would be to remove the food from the patient's room. Discuss medications for nausea and appetite enhancement prior to the next meal. Fluids should be limited with meals to encourage increased solid food consumption.

Case Study Hints

HIV INFECTION: (1) Review the Collaborative Care section for HIV in this chapter. (2) Note the recent medical events in Ms. Lu's record to determine the likely source of her infection. Recall the period of time in which the HIV would be "invisible" from that source. (3) Review with Ms. Lu the ways that HIV can be transmitted. Refer her and her fiancé for counseling regarding adoption or foster parenting.

Care Map (*Pneumocystis carinii* Pneumonia)

CORRECT DATA: Subjective: States "Short of breath when I walk"; easily fatigued. Objective: Crackles in the posterior bases; T 100.8° F; dry cough; RR 28, shallow; pulse oximetry 88%.

REPORT: Yes, to physician.

CORRECT INTERVENTIONS: Instruct in use of incentive spirometer; monitor oxygen levels with pulse oximetry; encourage coughing and deep breathing; increase fluid intake as tolerated; place in semi-Fowler's position; give nasal oxygen at 3 L/min.

DOCUMENTATION: 3/15/04, 0915. Dry cough with crackles in the posterior bases. Respiratory rate 28 and shallow. Able to cough and deep breathe and use incentive spirometer every hour. Nasal oxygen in place at 3 L/min. Pulse oximetry 90%. E. Petro, LVN

CHAPTER 14

NCLEX-PN ANSWERS: (1) A—The temperature should be decreased to provide comfort for skin lesions, but only after the bath is given. Cornstarch or baking soda baths help to relieve itching. Medication for itching such as Benadryl may be given, but pain medication generally is not needed for psoriasis. Rubbing the lesions may increase the chance for devel-oping infection. (2) B—Cellulitis is an infection resulting from a wound or skin ulcer. Spider venom destroys tissue, allowing bacteria to enter the wound. A surgical wound may develop cellulitis, but there is no indication of an infection in answer C. Cervical cancer and measles are important medical history findings and should be noted. (3) B—Antibiotics may result in superinfections such as mouth fungi. Furuncles are boils, tinea pedis is athlete's foot, and folliculitis is an infection of hair follicles. (4) D—Herpes is a sexually transmitted disease. Abstinence is recommended during an outbreak of the virus. Gloves do not need to be worn if the patient is applying his own medication to the lesions. The medication should be used daily. Sunlight does not affect genital herpes. (5) B—Body lice are transmitted from contact with infested clothing or bed linens. Washing the items decrease the chance of reinfestation. Body lice may affect other family members or pets and can cause itching, especially at night. The best answer reflects the transmission of the lice. The lice must be eradicated from the household objects. (6) A—Most nonmelanoma skin cancers are directly related to exposure to sunlight. Alcohol and estrogen levels are not directly related. Liver spots are the result of hyperpigmentation of aging skin. (7) B—This client does not believe life will get better after the surgery. Anxiety, fear, and impaired skin integrity are all appropriate diagnoses for some cancer patients. Based on this statement, the client should be given more information regarding the success rate for cryosurgery and the treatment of basal cell carcinomas. (8) A—Patients should be able to identify changes in their own skin. Treatment and the prognosis for skin cancers need to be discussed at the appropriate time. Risk factors should be taught after the skin examination. (9) C—Redness over bony prominences suggests the beginnings of skin breakdown. A decreased appetite could lead to a lack of protein and vitamins, which are needed for intact skin. Contractures may also lead to loss of skin integrity due to immobility. Lack of mobility increases the mucous buildup in the lungs, causing a decrease in lung expansion. (10) D—High-protein and high-caloric diets decrease the likelihood that decubiti will develop. Massaging the skin may cause damage to the tissues. Clients should be turned and repositioned every 2 hours. Hot water may burn the skin.

Case Study Hints

MELANOMA: (1) Review the content in Chapter 8 under "Early Detection" in the Nursing Care section. Review the content in Chapter 8 in the section "Prevention." Consider ways to teach the importance of identifying skin cancer in your own neighborhood or community. (2) Review the content on antibiotics in Chapter 12. Is Mr. Sanders's problem usual or unusual when taking antibiotics? What would you say to him about his need for the antibiotic? Who would you ask him to call to report his physical response?

Care Map (Herpes Zoster)

CORRECT DATA: Subjective: Reports chills and fever. Objective: T 99° F, open blisters on thorax.

CORRECT INTERVENTIONS: Teach how to apply topical medications; stress importance of avoiding intimate contact with family members; discuss need for careful handwashing; teach effects of pain medications.

REPORT: Yes, to the primary health care provider at the clinic.

DOCUMENTATION: 04/29/04. Reports malaise, chills, and fever for past week. T 99° F. Has oozing fluid-filled blisters in a line over left thorax. Reports these are painful. Reports having chickenpox as a child. Is a migrant worker and is afraid lesions are the result of exposure to pesticides. E. Sanchez, LPN

CHAPTER 15

NCLEX-PN ANSWERS: (1) D—Electricity follows the path of least resistance. Lightning travels along bones, blood vessels, and nerve fibers. Although lightning may cause abnormal cardiac rhythms, the symptoms exhibited are directly related to the brain and central nervous system. There is a potential for loss of both urinary and pulmonary function, depending on the severity of the electrical discharge. (2) A—Full-thickness burns are also called third-degree burns. The skin appears dry, leathery, and firm to the touch. The pain receptors are destroyed. Second-degree burns are also known as partial-thickness and include both deep and superficial partial-thickness injuries. Pain is present in various degrees, and the wound has blister formations. (3) B—The emergent or resuscitative stage consists of estimating the extent of burn damage, initiating first-aid, and assessing for shock and respiratory distress. Carbon monoxide and other noxious fumes are prevalent in house fires, leading to pulmonary distress. Pain and urinary assessments are conducted in the acute stage. Mobility problems are addressed after the life-threatening problems are under control. (4) D—During reversal of burn shock, fluids shift from the extracellular spaces to the circulatory system. Older clients may develop excess fluid volume, which is manifested by pulmonary edema, distended neck veins, and cardiac arrhythmias. Congestive heart failure signs and symptoms are dependent on which side of the heart is affected. Portal hypertension may occur with liver diseases. (5) B—Large amounts of water are absorbed along with sodium and chloride from the dressing site. Potassium levels increase during fluid shifts but gradually return to normal. Calcium is needed for muscle and cardiac contraction. Magnesium is required for protein synthesis and muscle contraction. (6) C—The intravenous route is the best means of managing pain. Most patients will initially be NPO. Intramuscular and rectal routes have slower absorption times. The skin may not accommodate injections due to the burn damage. (7) C—Curling's ulcer is a common manifestation for patients with extensive burns. Enteral feedings are contraindicated with these patients. Peripheral IV therapy is usually not a viable solution due to skin damage. A central venous line is inserted via the subclavian or jugular vein for the administration of total parental nutrition. (8) D—All burn patients should have aseptic wound care, frequent vital signs, and daily weights. Burns to the extremities increase the risk for contractures. Other nursing interventions to prevent joint deformities are splints, repositioning, and constant pressure application. (9) B—Infection is a constant threat due to the decreased immune system in patients with major burns. Frequent vital signs are imperative. Touching the skin is inappropriate for determining body temperature. A set of vital signs should always be obtained prior to calling the physician. Dressings should be removed during wound care or on specific orders from the doctor. (10) B—Sulfa crystals may form in the urine. There may also be pain, burning, and itching at the site of the wound. Monitor for fluid volume overload. Force fluids to flush the urinary system.

Case Study Hints

MAJOR BURN: (1) Review the content in the chapter about the pathophysiology of a major burn specific to the renal system and gastrointestinal system. Consider the need to measure urine hourly and the dangers of vomiting. (2) Review the discussion of narcotic analgesics in Chapter 6. Consider why this would be more necessary in a partial-thickness burn than in a full-thickness burn.

Care Map (Client with Major Burns)

CORRECT DATA: Objective: Age; extent of burn; BP, P, R; urine output; confusion.

CORRECT INTERVENTIONS: Report and continue to monitor vital signs; report and continue to monitor urine output; report and continue to monitor confusion; determine body weight; monitor IV flow rate.

REPORT: Yes, to the nurse manager of the ED or to the physician.

DOCUMENTATION: 2/23/04. 1300. 78-year-old woman with 40% TBSA burn. Confused. BP 92/62, P 110 and weak, R 36 and shallow. Urine output per Foley less than 20 mL per hour for past 2 hours. IV fluids infusing as ordered. A. Fu, LPN

CHAPTER 16

NCLEX-PN ANSWERS: (1) B—The abnormal hypersecretion of the growth hormone that begins to manifest clinical symptoms in early adulthood is called acromegaly. Graves' disease is a hypersecretion of the thyroid hormone. Cushing's syndrome is an adrenal cortex hyperfunction. Addison's disease is caused by a decrease in adrenal function. (2) A—Hemorrhage is life threatening. Be sure to assess dressing behind the neck. Observe for edema and increased swallowing. There is a small chance that the laryngeal nerve was damaged during surgery. Some hoarseness is common immediately after the procedure. Tetany usually occurs several days postop if the parathyroid glands have been damaged. A decrease in the blood serum levels of calcium increases the potential for tetany. Dehydration is managed with the use of IV fluids. (3) A—Iodine is needed for the production of the thyroid hormone. A decrease in the hormone causes the thyroid to enlarge in order to increase the hormone production. Hyper- and hypo-states of parathyroidism result in calcium imbalances. Hyperthyroidism creates increased metabolic dysfunctions. (4) C—Excess calcium may form into small calculi and lodge in the kidney. It is essential to strain all urine for signs of these stones. Ordering a renal function panel is not within the LPN/LVN scope of practice. Frequent catheterizations may lead to urinary infections. A decreased level of consciousness may occur if the kidney is damaged by the stones. The kidney may be unable to filter the blood, resulting in an increase in ammonia, which in turn results in mental changes. (5) C—The increased cortisol production by the adrenal cortex stimulates numerous physical and physiological changes in the body. The buffalo hump, moon face, edema, and purple striae on the abdomen add to the depression that is typically seen in patients with Cushing's syndrome. Patients may not have impaired skin in the early stages, but are at considerable risk for developing skin problems. (6) B—Hypoparathyroidism results in a decrease of circulating serum calcium levels and high phosphorus levels. (7) C—Inderal (propranolol) relieves the discomforts of heat intolerance and nervousness in clients with hyperthyroidism. It slows the heart rate and may cause fatigue and weakness related to a decrease in the amount of blood pumped from the left ventricle during systole. (8) A—Clients with SIADH have a decreased urine output. Urine production must be managed with medication and follow-up care. A high protein diet may be allowed as long as there is no actual kidney damage. Rest and activity are always important. The SIADH client has no increased risk of infection from crowds. (9) B—Synthroid is given for hypothyroidism. Body metabolism should increase along with a tolerance for cold. The weight loss is not significant. An excessive weight loss could indicate side effects of hyperthyroidism. (10) A—Addison's disease is clinically manifested by hypoglycemia, dehydration, and decreased cortisol and aldosterone levels. Hyperkalemic effects will be seen on the ECG (peaked T waves, widening QRS complex).

Case Study Hints

GRAVES' DISEASE: (1) Review the pathophysiology of hyperthyroidism and the illustration of the multisystem effects of hyperthyroidism. (2) See the section on Graves' disease. Note the characteristic eye changes that occur with this disorder. (3) See the discussion of Collaborative Care for Graves' disease. Review especially the pharmacology section. Consider what support Ms. Manuel might need in coping with her disorder.

Care Map (Hypothyroidism)

CORRECT DATA: Subjective: Rarely hungry, eats less than normal; weight gain of 10 lbs. in past 6 months. Objective: Yellowish, dry skin; edema in lower legs; puffy face; slurred speech.

CORRECT INTERVENTIONS: Provide information that helps Mrs. Lee understand why body changes occur from hypothyroidism; teach Mrs. Lee about reversible body changes.

REPORT: Yes, to the physician.

DOCUMENTATION: 4/5/04. 1700. Complains of poor appetite but states has gained 10 lbs. in past 6 months. Skin is yellowish-colored and dry, with edema noted in lower legs. Face is puffy. Speech is slurred. J. Bergstrom, LPN

CHAPTER 17

NCLEX-PN ANSWERS: (1) B—The sliding scale permits periodic monitoring of blood glucose levels to provide better control. Fast-acting insulin (regular insulin) is used with the sliding scale to best mimic the natural action of the pancreas. (2) C—Clients experiencing Somogyi phenomenon should be taught the symptoms of nighttime hypoglycemia, including tremors, night sweats, and restlessness. A bedtime snack or decreasing the evening dose of intermediate insulin may reduce the risk of developing the phenomenon. (3) C—During periods of illness, blood glucose levels increase in response to physiological stress and the body's need for glucose. Urine ketones are an indicator of the severity of glucose depletion in the cells and the use of fat for energy. Monitoring the urine ketone level when the blood glucose is severely elevated can alert the client to impending diabetic ketoacidosis, so the client can seek immediate medical care. (4) D—Diabetes mellitus does not increase the client's risk of lung disease. The major concern is vasoconstriction, particularly of peripheral vessels, caused by nicotine in tobacco. Diabetic clients are at risk for circulatory alterations leading to pain, infection, gangrene, and eventual amputation of lower extremities. Decreased perfusion of major organs and increased hypertension may also develop. (5) A—Type I diabetes is manifested by lack of insulin production. These individuals are insulin dependent. Insulin cannot be taken orally. The action of oral medications to treat diabetes depends on the ability of the pancreas to produce insulin. (6) D—The most likely time for a client to experience hypoglycemia as a result of insulin administration is during the peak time when the medication is at its highest concentration in the bloodstream. The peak action of NPH insulin is 6 to 12 hours following administration. (7) C—Air should be injected into the NPH insulin and then the regular insulin. The regular insulin is withdrawn first to avoid mixing of the NPH in the regular insulin vial. NPH insulin should be rolled between the palms to mix. Avoid shaking the vial as this may result in destruction of some drug components and the possibility of inaccurate dosage administered. (8) B—Diabetic ketoacidosis is characterized by hyperglycemia and spillage of ketones in the urine. The skin is very warm and dry as a result of dehydration. The pulse is usually rapid and weak. Arterial blood pH is acidotic and less than 7.45. (9) C—Regular insulin is the only insulin that can be administered by both the intravenous and subcutaneous routes. Other types of insulin are administered by the subcutaneous route only. (10) D—Toenails should be cut straight across to avoid development of ingrown toenails that can lead to infection. Diabetic clients should avoid open-toed shoes, heating pads, and hot water bottles to prevent injury. Lotion or oil between the toes results in a warm, moist environment that is a medium for bacterial and fungal growth.

INSULIN-DEPENDENT DIABETES MELLITUS: (1) Name the factors in Mr. Meligrito's schedule that contributed to his condition. Review the appropriate medication dosages. (2) Review the section on treatment of diabetic ketoacidosis. Note whether this condition is more likely in Type 1 or Type 2 diabetics. Note the order and purpose of different intravenous solutions. (3) Recall the pathophysiology of these two types of diabetes. Review controllable factors, and see Box 17-5.

Care Map (Diabetes Mellitus)
CORRECT DATA: Subjective: Does not complain of any discomfort in her feet; says she uses a hot water bottle on her feet at night. Objective: Red spots on top of the toes on her right foot; blister on the left heel.

REPORT: Yes, to physician.

CORRECT INTERVENTIONS: Discuss the importance of not smoking; teach her to wear new shoes for short periods of time each day; instruct client in proper foot care; teach her to monitor red areas for signs of skin breakdown.

DOCUMENTATION: 08/13/04. Reviewed symptoms that would indicate skin breakdown. Discussed the importance of proper foot care, not smoking, and not using hot water bottles or heating pads to her feet. Repeated instructions correctly and says she will "take better care of her feet." Barbara Boucher, LPN

CHAPTER 18
NCLEX-PN ANSWERS: (1) D—Obesity is strongly linked to heredity. A client with two obese parents has an 80% chance of becoming obese. Morbid obesity is defined as a body weight 100% over the ideal weight. Obesity is often linked with inactivity. Serum cholesterol levels are generally elevated in morbidly obese patients. (2) A—A weight gain of 1 to 2 lbs. per week is appropriate. A 1,200-kcal diet does not provide adequate kcal to support weight gain; an additional 3,500 kcal above metabolic needs is necessary to gain 1 lb. Excessive exercise increases kcal needs and will not promote weight gain. Fat intake should not exceed 30% of total kcal. (3) B—Viscous lidocaine may be used to numb the mucous membranes in the mouth. Never use a strong mouthwash, because many of these contain alcohol that may cause severe burning of the mouth. The gag reflex may be assessed if the client has swallowed the viscous lidocaine or has had a procedure that required anesthetizing of the throat. A quiet environment is important at any time to help in digestion. (4) A—Early symptoms of oral cancer are painless ulcers. Documenting the lesion and notifying the physician are your

next priority. It is not an emergency, nor will you prepare the patient for a biopsy until the diagnosis is made by the physician. It is important for the client to report any changes in the ulceration. (5) D—Thrush or candidiasis appears as white patches overlying a red tongue. These patches cannot be scraped off using a tongue depressor. Painful, small, round ulcerations may be signs of canker sores or ulcerative stomatitis. Herpes simplex are blisters on the lips. Painless ulcerations may be indicative of oral cancer. (6) B—Cancers that erode through the esophageal wall may cause severe hemorrhage. Difficulty swallowing is an early sign of esophageal cancer, which may be followed by choking and weight loss. (7) B—During insertion of the NG tube, the gag reflex may be initiated. Briefly pause, allow the client a short rest, have her sip a small amount of water to help with the insertion, and resume the procedure. Do not initially remove the tube completely; this may increase anxiety and nasal trauma. Placement checks are done after the tube is inserted completely. (8) C—Divide 60 into 240. This will give you the number of hours that it will take for the feeding to infuse. (9) B—*Helicobacter pylori* bacteria has been found to increase the incidence of peptic ulcers. It will not effect the acid nor the mucus. Antibiotics are not usually given to prevent the appearance of this organism. (10) D—Dumping syndrome is characterized by stomach contents that rapidly flood the small intestine after a meal. Large amounts of water are pulled into the intestines, creating a volume deficit in the blood circulation. Proteins and fats are absorbed at a slower rate than sugars. Resting after a meal slows down the digestive process. Smaller, more frequent meals are generally more tolerated than three large meals.

Case Study Hints
PEPTIC ULCER DISEASE: (1) Review the pathophysiology of peptic ulcer disease and then note the conditions that made a relapse likely for Mr. O'Donnell. Recall the organism that is often a factor in PUD. (2) Remember the gastric side effects of NSAIDs and aspirin. See the Pharmacology section under this disorder. (3) Look at Mr. O'Donnell's lifestyle and occupation for clues. How does stress create an environment for PUD?

Care Map (Obesity)
CORRECT DATA: Subjective: Exercise limited to "puttering around" and walking length of driveway; typical daily food intake: juice, oatmeal, muffin, coffee, cream; snack donuts and coffee; etc.; reports easily fatigued, SOB with activity. Objective: 30-lb. weight gain over 2 years; 5'10" tall, weight 201 lbs.; serum cholesterol 240 mg/dL (normal 150 to 200 mg/dL); HDL 37 mg/dL (normal > 45 mg/dL); LDL 180 mg/dL (normal < 130 mg/dL); 32% body fat.

CORRECT INTERVENTIONS: Assess weight weekly; discuss eating habits and strategies to reduce fat and calorie intake; identify eating cues and find strategies to reduce or eliminate eating cues; teach how to keep and use a food diary; discuss role of regular exercise in weight loss and control; discuss lifestyle and behavior-modification strategies to promote weight loss and control.

DOCUMENTATION: 8/14 Weight 198 lbs. Reports that he has started using low-fat creamer in his coffee and has given up his morning muffin and donut, having an English muffin with jam as a morning snack instead. He also reports that he is having raw vegetables and water with lunch, instead of chips and a soft drink. Before dinner he has a handful of pretzels with his wine. He and his wife started walking in the afternoon; he is now able to walk for 45 minutes "without becoming winded." Pleased with his progress; states his wife is a "great support—she went out and bought four new low-fat cookbooks!" Marie Langlios, LVN

CHAPTER 19
NCLEX-PN ANSWERS: (1) B—narcotic analgesics often are required for acute pain relief in cholelithiasis. (2) B—nausea and vomiting after eating may indicate the T-tube is not functioning and/or blockage of the bile ducts. (3) D—Low-fat diets decrease stimulation of the gallbladder to release bile, thereby decreasing pain. (4) A—Hepatitis A is transmitted by the oral–fecal route and by consumption of contaminated food or water. (5) C—Hepatitis is transmitted through blood exposure, including contaminated needles and blood transfusions. (6) D—Alcohol is hepatotoxic and use should be eliminated. (7) A—Weight may indicate decrease in ascites. (8) B—Ammonia levels are elevated because of inability of the liver to metabolize protein products. Lactulose decreases the absorption of ammonia from the bowel. (9) D—The side-lying position with the knees flexed reduces stretching of the peritoneal tissues and provides splinting of the abdominal area. (10) B—Fluid loss associated with vomiting, diaphoresis, third-space shifts, and nasogastric suction is common. Fluid initially is lost from vascular space, potentially impairing cardiac output and tissue perfusion.

Case Study Hints
CHOLELITHIASIS: (1) Review the pathophysiology of cholelithiasis and cholecystitis. Research cultural influences (Native American) on diet, and develop a diet plan that considers these influences. (2) Think about the location of the gallbladder and direction of bile drainage, as well as the effect of position on respiratory status. (3) Review the Nursing Care Checklist for clients having a laparoscopic cholecystectomy.

CIRRHOSIS: (1) Review the effects of increased ammonia levels on mental function. Blood is a protein; think about what happens to it in the gut. (2) Review the pathophysiology of cirrhosis and its complications. (3) Check Chapter 5 for low-sodium foods, and review Chapter 21 for protein restriction guidelines.

Care Map (Pancreatitis)
CORRECT DATA: Subjective: Thin, appears anxious and tired; states she lost 30 lbs. (13.6 kg) in the hospital; states main problems are lack of energy and lack of appetite. Objective: Weight 102 lbs. (46 kg), height 66 inches (168 cm); skin cool and dry, poor turgor; blood glucose 80 mg/dL.

CORRECT INTERVENTIONS: Plan daily rest periods, especially before meals; discuss dietary restrictions and how to adapt to usual diet; assist family to plan six small meals a day.

CHAPTER 20
NCLEX-PN ANSWERS: (1) A—Absorption of nutrients. Nutrients are absorbed through the intestinal wall of the small intestine. Surgery on the small intestine could disrupt the absorption processes. Elimination of indigestible food residue is a function of the large intestine. (2) D—Fecal incontinence. The defecation reflex cannot be suppressed without voluntary control of the external sphincter. (3) D—Although all of the measures are appropriate, the most important intervention is to gather information that will contribute to the assessment process. Because treatment for diarrhea is to treat the underlying cause, an accurate history must be obtained in order for the underlying cause to be identified. (4) C—When communication is being used therapeutically, the priority of nursing care is to focus on the patient's feelings. Although educational videos, counselors, and antianxiety medication may be appropriate for this patient at some point in the care, they are not more important than the immediate need of the patient to express feelings. (5) A—Antidiarrheal medications must not be used until the cause of diarrhea has been determined because they could worsen or prolong the disease. (6) A—Nutrient intake and the amount and nature of fecal output provide information about both intake and absorption of nutrients. Intake/output record will give an indication of fluid balance, but not of nutrient absorption. A gluten-free diet may be in order for this patient, but will not be absorbed if malabsorption is occurring. Teaching the patient and family will be a part of the care plan, but it will not indicate the presence of malabsorption. (7) C—Not allowed on this diet are fresh vegetables, rich desserts, raw or fresh fruits, or tough meats. (8) D—A and B are normal assessment findings. Increased pain with a rigid, boardlike abdomen may indicate bowel rupture and possible peritonitis. (9) A—Return of bowel sounds indicates the return of peristalsis, necessary for safe food introduction. Pain needs to be managed throughout recovery to promote mobility. Promoting mobility, such as in ambulation, will encourage return of normal peristalsis, but is not a requirement prior to introducing food. IV fluids sustain fluid and electrolytes for a short amount of time. Eventually, normal eating habits will need to be reintroduced to maintain a nutritional status that will promote wound healing. (10) A—Because colorectal cancer is often a silent disease and treatment at an early stage has a high cure rate, the American Cancer Society recommends routine screening procedures for early detection. This includes annual digital rectal examination for all people over age 50, annual fecal occult blood test for people over age 50, and flexible sigmoidoscopy or colonoscopy at age 50 and every 5 to 10 years thereafter.

Screening exams should be early and frequent for clients with inflammatory bowel disease, a history of polyps, or a strong family history of colorectal cancer. Bowel cancer usually grows slowly. There may be 5 to 15 years of growth before symptoms occur. Manifestations depend on tumor location, type and extent, and complications. Bleeding is often what prompts clients to seek medical care.

Case Study Hints
PERITONITIS: (1) Review the immune response to infection and inflammation to prepare your answer for this question. (2) Think about required incisional care, pain management and other medications, any dietary considerations, possible activity restrictions, and what signs and symptoms the client should report to the physician as you prepare your teaching plan. (3) Review interventions for the nursing diagnosis of Anxiety in your fundamentals or nursing process textbook.

INFLAMMATORY BOWEL DISEASE: (1) Review the function of the colon, and the differences between the consistency and content of material entering the colon from the small intestine and feces that is expelled through the anus. Then review the manifestations of fluid volume deficit in Chapter 5. (2) Review the pathophysiology and manifestations of inflammatory bowel disease.

Care Map (Colorectal Cancer)
CORRECT DATA: Subjective: States "I really don't want a colostomy, but if that is what it takes to keep me well, I'm ready to get it over with." Objective: Intermittent constipation.

CORRECT INTERVENTIONS: Frequently assess stoma and peristomal skin condition; teach colostomy care; refer to the local United Ostomy Association; provide a list of local resources for ostomy supplies.

CHAPTER 21
NCLEX-PN ANSWERS: (1) C—Assessment to determine if the bladder is needed before further action is taken. (2) A—Lack of estrogen following a total hysterectomy results in decreased urethral resistance, placing the client at risk for stress incontinence. (3) B—Residual urine of 50 mL or less is within normal limits. (4) C—Kegel exercises help the client locate and tighten muscles of the pelvic floor. (5) B—Cranberry juice maintains acid pH of urine. Acidic urine is an unfavorable environment for bacterial infection. (6) A—Recent infection with group A beta-hemolytic *Streptococcus* is a risk factor for acute glomerulonephritis. (7) C—All urine of clients with urinary calculi should be strained for presence of stones. Stones should be sent to the lab for analysis. (8) C—Client is at risk for urinary tract infection. Signs and symptoms should be reported to the physician promptly. (9) B—Protein is decreased to prevent azotemia. High carbohydrate intake increases calories and spares protein breakdown. (10) A—The right arm should be used for blood pressure measurement to avoid injury to the AV fistula.

Case Study Hints
ACUTE GLOMERULONEPHRITIS: (1) Review the principles of antibiotic therapy and the consequences of inadequate treatment in Chapter 12 and your pharmacology text. (2) Note Mr. Chang's age and living circumstances. How might these contribute to his risk for glomerulonephritis?

BLADDER CANCER: (1) Review the pathophysiology and risk factors for bladder cancer. (2) Consider the feelings behind Mr. Hussain's statement as you form your response.

RENAL FAILURE: (1) Review Chapter 17 and the pathophysiology of diabetes mellitus. Also consider the duration of the disease in your response. (2) Review the section on hemodialysis. Consider factors such as timing, self-responsibility, travel, and other effects of treatment on ADLs and lifestyle.

Care Map (Urinary Incontinence)
CORRECT DATA: Subjective: Relates urine leakage when laughing, coughing, and on hearing the sound of running water; often unable to reach bathroom in time at night; hysterectomy at age 52; estrogen replacement therapy for approximately 10 years after hysterectomy; urine leakage usually occurs in late afternoon and at night. Objective: Takes digoxin 0.125 mg qd, furosemide 40 mg bid, and KCl 20 mEq tid; moderate cystourethrocele; atrophy of vaginal tissues; pelvic floor strength weak; urinalysis within normal limits; postvoiding residual urine 5 mL; average of nine daytime voidings and four at night.

CORRECT INTERVENTIONS: Teach how to identify pelvic floor muscles and perform Kegel exercises; encourage minimizing fluid intake after evening meal; change afternoon dose of furosemide from 9:00 P.M. to 4:00 P.M.; suggest commercial products for protecting clothing and furniture; schedule follow-up visits and evaluations to reinforce teaching.

CHAPTER 22
NCLEX-PN ANSWERS: (1) C—Pain associated with angina is usually relieved by nitroglycerin and rest. Pain associated with myocardial infarction is not relieved by rest or nitroglycerin and requires immediate medical intervention. (2) B—Hypotension and decreased urinary output are indicators of impending cardiogenic shock. Thorough assessment and prompt medical intervention are required. (3) D—Dietary modifications can reduce the risk of complications and recurrence of vessel occlusion. Nitroglycerin should be taken every 5 minutes for no more than three doses. If no relief from chest pain after the third dose, the client should be transported to the ED immediately. It is impossible to avoid all stress. Clients with myocardial infarction should be taught stress management. (4) A—Left-sided heart failure impairs cardiac output and affects gas exchange in the lungs. Exchange of O_2 and CO_2 is compromised. Clients tire easily and may be unable to complete simple activities. Clients with left-sided heart failure usually experience fluid volume excess. (5) B—

Clients experiencing right-sided heart failure develop edema in the lower extremities and dependent body areas as a result of increased capillary pressures. The workload of the heart is increased leading to tachycardia. Pulmonary edema is a complication of left-sided heart failure. (6) C—Digoxin should be administered if the apical pulse is between 60 and 100. Pulse rates below 60 should be reported to the physician for decision making prior to administration of the drug. The medication should be held regardless of the digoxin level. Assess the client for signs of digoxin toxicity. (7) B—Macaroni and cheese has high fat and sodium content. Smoked meats have high sodium content. (8) C—Rest is a vital component of treatment for a client with rheumatic heart disease. Activity tolerance is usually affected. Adequate rest periods should be provided. (9) D—Clients with pericarditis develop a pericardial friction rub caused by inflamed pericardial layers rubbing against the chest wall. Chest pain that radiates to the neck and back may be present. (10) A—Manifestations of heart failure or increasing activity intolerance may indicate worsening of the disorder. An elevated temperature may be an early manifestation of bacterial endocarditis.

Case Study Hints

ACUTE MYOCARDIAL INFARCTION: (1) Review Box 22-13. Using your nursing diagnosis handbook, identify appropriate nursing diagnoses for the post-acute period of hospitalization. Also review the cardiac rehabilitation section (under Collaborative Care for myocardial infarction) for the nursing care focus. (2) Review the scope of practice for an LPN/LVN in your state. Can you intervene independently or do you need to report this to the charge nurse? (3) Think about strategies to decrease Mrs. Williams's denial of the negative effects of smoking.

HEART FAILURE: (1) Review both Boxes 22-19 and 22-20 for assessment data and guidelines for exercise in clients with heart failure as you design your plan. (2) Consider the underlying message and therapeutic communication strategies as you formulate your response.

Care Map (After Coronary Artery Bypass Surgery)

CORRECT DATA: Subjective: History of progressive angina for 4 years; anterior wall myocardial infarction 2 years ago; treated with immediate thrombolytic therapy and percutaneous balloon angioplasty; strong family history of CHD (father died at age 51, brother died at age 48 of myocardial infarctions); does not smoke, uses alcohol occasionally; enjoys "good Southern-style cooking" and watching TV; rarely exercises other than dancing with wife and friends about once a month; usually works 50 to 60 hours per week at own contracting business; states "I have got to get back to work! You just can't sit around in my business—you have to make sure that the work is getting done on time." Objective: BP 138/72, P 86, regular, R 24, T 99.1° F PO; faint crackles left lung base; incision clean and dry, healing well; color good; O$_2$ sats

95% on 4 L O$_2$ per cannula; bowel sounds active; taking regular diet in small amounts.

CORRECT INTERVENTIONS: Teach about the heart and coronary heart disease, exercise and activities, lifestyle modifications, including diet and stress management; discuss emotional reactions to CHD and sexual activity after discharge, provide information about community resources for emotional support; help identify coping strategies for concerns about role in business.

CHAPTER 23

NCLEX-PN ANSWERS: (1) D—When an arterial thrombus develops, blood flow through the artery is occluded. Pain is the primary manifestation of arterial occlusion, and the affected extremity is cold and pale. (2) A—Instruct the client to keep the extremity in a dependent position; gravity helps to maintain blood flow to the distal tissues. (3) A—Heparin interferes with the normal clotting mechanism, preventing the formation of new clots and the extension of existing clots. (4) C—Stress management is particularly important for clients with Raynaud's disease. The client is encouraged to use relaxation techniques, massage therapy, hobbies, aroma therapy, and counseling to reduce and cope with stress. (5) C—Raynaud's is characterized by spasms of the small arteries and arterioles of the extremities. The arterial spasms limit blood flow to the fingers and, on occasion, the toes, ears, or nose. (6) B—People with stage 1 or stage 2 (mild or moderate) hypertension commonly have no symptoms other than an increased blood pressure. Hypertension is usually advanced when manifestations are seen. (7) A—Based on the lack of symptoms, clients often have difficulty understanding the importance of medication schedules. (8) D—Coumadin interferes with liver synthesis of clotting factors, preventing the clot formation. (9) C—Nicotine constricts blood vessels. The smaller the diameter of a vessel, the greater the friction against the walls of vessel and, thus, the greater impedance to blood flow. (10) A—Sudden, excruciating pain is a symptom of a dissecting aneurysm of the ascending aorta.

Case Study Hints

HYPERTENSION: (1) Review Box 23-2 as you read Mrs. Spezia's history and physicial assessment data. (2) Review the pathophysiology of hypertension.

DEEP VEIN THROMBOSIS: (1) Review the pathophysiology of venous thrombosis and the pathophysiology of pain. (2) Think about available resources and possible referrals that could be made. (3) As you design your teaching plan, consider Mrs. Hipps's risk factors for venous thrombosis.

Care Map (Buerger's Disease)

CORRECT DATA: Subjective: Has smoked over two packs of cigarettes a day for 20 years; calf pain with activity progressing over past 2 months; must rest frequently when walking; relates numbness and tingling of toes of left foot. Objective: Weak peripheral pulses in right leg; absent pedal and posterior tibial pulses in left foot; third, fourth, and fifth toes of left foot pale; right foot pink and warm; left foot cool to touch; skin on left leg shiny and thin; hairless below knee; moderate amount evenly distributed hair right leg.

CORRECT INTERVENTIONS: Assess pain at rest and during activity using a scale of 0 to 10; teach Buerger–Allen exercises; instruct to perform exercises three times per day; teach the importance of smoking cessation; teach foot care measures; encourage questions about the disease and its management.

CHAPTER 24
NCLEX-PN ANSWERS: (1) A—Clients with sickle cell crisis are in severe pain. Narcotic analgesics should be administered as soon as possible. (2) C—Lack of oxygen to the cells results in hypoxia and fatigue. Clients with anemia require frequent rest periods until correction of process can be accomplished. (3) B—Thrombocytopenia (low platelet count) places the client at risk for bleeding. The client should be protected from injury that could cause bleeding. (4) B—Contact sports place the client with hemophilia at risk for injury and bleeding. Golf is least likely to result in physical injury. (5) C—Acid pH of citrus juices increases pain and may injure open lesions on mucous membranes. (6) A—Coagulation in small blood vessels results in occlusion of small blood vessels and ischemia. A raised knee gatch further occludes vessels and promotes ischemia. (7) A—Clients with multiple myeloma are at risk for pathologic fractures and experience severe pain. Nursing care should focus on prevention of fractures and controlling pain. (8) B—Elevation of extremities promote lymphatic drainage and decreases edema. (9) A—Enlarged, painless, movable lymph nodes in the cervical area is a symptom of Hodgkin's disease. (10) D—Maintaining isolation precautions as prescribed at all times helps protect a client with an impaired immune system from infection.

Case Study Hints
FOLIC ACID DEFICIENCY ANEMIA: (1) Review Box 24-3 for a list of foods high in folic acid. Consider the balance of carbohydrates, proteins, and fats as you plan your menu. (2) Consider the amount of folic acid necessary to meet basic needs and how much is needed to replace a deficiency. (3) In your study or clinical group, discuss the factors that increase an older adult's risk of malnutrition. Review Chapter 18 as needed.

HODGKIN'S DISEASE: (1) Review radiation and chemotherapy in Chapter 8. (2) Review measures to prevent infection in the Nursing Care and Discharge Considerations sections under Leukemia. (3) Think about issues such as insurance, savings, and job and economic status, as well as family responsibilities.

Care Map (Acute Myelocytic Leukemia)
CORRECT DATA: Subjective: States "I'm so tired, and I have these bruises all over me. I'm so afraid of the results of the bone marrow test. I don't know what we will do if I have cancer"; night sweats and intermittent fever for past 2 months; relates menstrual periods heavier than normal. Objective: 5′,

4″ (156 cm) tall, weighs 106 lbs. (48.1 kg); vital signs T 100° F; P 102; R 22; BP 130/82; numerous petechiae scattered over trunk and arms; ecchymoses on lower right arm and right calf; oral mucosa red, with several small ulcerations in buccal areas; low RBC count; low hemoglobin and hematocrit; low platelets; high WBC count; myeloblasts present.

CORRECT INTERVENTIONS: Place in a private room; limit visitors to husband and daughter; verbally and in writing remind staff, family, and client to practice good handwashing. Post a sign in the room as a reminder, and discuss the importance of handwashing with Mrs. Cole and her family; take and record vital signs every 4 hours.

CHAPTER 25
NCLEX-PN ANSWERS: (1) C—Antihistamines have many side effects, including drowsiness and a dry mouth. Some patients may have an allergic reaction with chest tightness or wheezing. Alcohol is contraindicated with most antihistamines, including Chlor-Trimeton. (2) D—Moist air helps to loosen secretions and provide comfort for the postoperative tonsillectomy client. Ice collars are used to decrease the potential for hemorrhage. The head of the bed should be elevated, with the patient's head turned to the side. The airway device must remain in place until the gag reflex returns. (3) D—A throat culture is obtained and sent to the lab for identification of the bacteria. A complete blood count may be done to determine the white blood cell count. An elevated value may indicate bacterial infection. Nasal swabs are used to diagnose sinusitis. The ELISA test is slightly sensitive to bacterial infection but cannot identify the organism. (4) A—Although the medical history and physical assessment are important aspects of nursing care, patient allergies to egg products must be ascertained. The influenza vaccine is produced in eggs. (5) B—Most viral URIs are self-limiting. Patient teaching that includes self-care should be stressed. Throat cultures are not always required. Antibiotics are not useful in the treatment of viral infections. Monitoring temperature may be done if the patient is febrile. (6) A—Impaired verbal communication is a primary nursing diagnosis for a patient with laryngitis. Talking will increase the inflammation of the larynx. There is no need for cough medications or effective coughing techniques with laryngitis. An increase in fluids will not influence the outcome of the condition to a great extent. (7) C—All of the answers are important, but controlling the bleeding has the highest priority. (8) B—Obesity is a major factor for developing sleep apnea. Weight loss should be considered. Alcohol and hypnotics are contraindicated for patients with this condition. During sleep, the tongue relaxes and obstructs the airway. Obstructive sleep apnea is the most common form. (9) D—Persistent hoarseness, often without other symptoms, is an early sign of laryngeal cancer. The client should see his physician promptly, as early tumors often can be removed and the voice preserved. (10) C—In a total laryngectomy, the trachea and esophagus are separated and a tracheostomy is formed. There is no risk of choking during eating or drinking.

Case Study Hints

UPPER RESPIRATORY INFECTION: (1) Review Table 25-1 for common manifestations. Review the Complementary Therapies and Discharge Considerations for measures to promote comfort during URI. (2) Review both the Pharmacology section under Collaborative Care and Table 25-2. (3) Review the common manifestations and duration of uncomplicated URI and use this in teaching. Look at the manifestations of complications of URI such as pneumonia and sinusitis. Do these complications usually require emergency treatment? What symptoms should the client seek immediate care for? (Hint: Think ABCs.) Why is it usually more appropriate for a client to seek treatment by his or her primary care provider than in an ED? Look at continuity of care, cost, and utilization issues.

Care Map (Total Laryngectomy)

CORRECT DATA: Subjective: Complains that head "feels heavy." Objective: Tracheostomy tube present; O_2 per tracheostomy collar; oxygen saturation 94%; moderate edema noted right side of face and neck.

CORRECT INTERVENTIONS: Assess respiratory rate, lung sounds, and cough effectiveness every 2 hours; encourage to use deep breathing and coughing exercises hourly.

CHAPTER 26

NCLEX-PN ANSWERS: (1) B—The most common cause of chronic bronchitis is cigarette smoking. The environment such as working in mines, silicone factories, or cotton mills may contribute to this disease. (2) B—An allergic reaction is manifested by erythema and warmth. A positive test is measured by the millimeters of hardness or induration. The husband should be tested because of the high risk of infection with people living in the same household, but there is no evidence that he is positive. (3) C—Manifestations of acute asthma attack include chest tightness, wheezing, shortness of breath, and anxiety. Asthma can lead to respiratory distress if not managed properly. The medication effectiveness is also reported. (4) D—Rinsing the mouth after using the inhaler reduces systemic drug absorption and reduces the risk of thrush associated with some anti-inflammatory drugs used to treat asthma and COPD. Bronchodilators are used to treat acute attacks of asthma and before using anti-inflammatory durgs by MDI. (5) D—COPD patients have increased carbon dioxide in their blood. The brain regulates the breathing mechanism by using CO_2 as the initiator for respirations. Low doses of O_2 are useful for the COPD patient, particularly at night. High doses of O_2 suppress the drive to breathe and may result in respiratory failure. (6) A—Atelectasis is commonly seen with nonambulatory patients after surgery. Pain medication decreases respirations, which could lead to atelectasis. (7) B—A thoracentesis is performed by inserting a needle into the pleural space that surrounds the lungs, in order to remove fluid or air. The mediastinum contains the heart and great vessels. The thoracic cavity refers to the chest. (8) B—The wound is covered with an occlusive dressing to prevent air from entering the pleural space, then the physician is notified. Reinsertion of the tube introduces bacteria and other possible contaminants into the pleural space. (9) A—The client with COPD must stop smoking to reduce further damage to lung tissue. A program of aerobic activity increases exercise tolerance. The client with COPD should be immunized against pneumococcal pneumonia and influenza, even if he or she is under age 65. (10) A—Restlessness and tachypnea (rapid respiratory rate) are early signs of hypoxia, a component of respiratory failure. Deep coma is a very late sign. Hypotension, tachycardia, and decreased urine output are indicative of decreased cardiac output, a later effect of respiratory failure.

Case Study Hints

COPD: (1) Research the effects of secondhand smoke to respond to this question. (2) Review the control and function of the respiratory center in the central nervous system. Also review acid–base balance in Chapter 5.

LUNG CANCER: (1) Review information about chemotherapy in Chapter 8 to answer this question. (2) Again, review nursing care in Chapter 8. (3) Think about the client's autonomy, as well as what therapeutic communication skills you might use in this situation.

Care Map (Tuberculosis)

CORRECT DATA: Subjective: Homeless for past 10 years; uses shelters only during very cold or wet weather; complains of chronic cough that now is productive of pink sputum; often wakes up drenched with sweat in the middle of the night; complains of increasing fatigue. Objective: Vital signs: BP 152/86; P 92; R 20; and T 100.2° F (37.8° C); clean; answers questions appropriately and intelligently; very thin, almost emaciated; sputum Gram stain positive for acid-fast bacillus.

CORRECT INTERVENTIONS: Provide verbal and written information about tuberculosis; teach about prescribed medications, possible adverse effects, and importance of completing the entire prescribed regimen; emphasize importance of continued follow-up; refer to local incentive shelter program for directly observed medical therapy and meals.

DOCUMENTATION: Be sure to relate your documentation to the established goal, not to the care or interventions you provided.

CHAPTER 27

NCLEX-PN ANSWERS: (1) D—Until the cast is completely dry, use only the palms of the hands. Handling with the fingers can leave dents that may cause pressure sores. (2) A—The prone position helps to prevent hip contracture. Place the client in a prone position every four hours. (3) D—It is important to keep the client in a position of abduction because adduction may dislocate the hip. Excessive hip flexion should also be avoided. (4) C—The client has manifestations of compartment syndrome including pain unrelieved by narcotics and paresthesias. Prompt intervention is required to preserve function of the extremity. (5) B—Teaching the client the RICE acronym (rest, ice, compression, elevation) will help them to remember how to care for the injury. (6) D—Fracture of a long bone is the principal risk for fat emboli. The manifestations may include confusion, petechiae, pulmonary edema, and acute respiratory distress syndrome. (7) D—Peripheral vascular disease is the major cause of amputation of the lower extremities. (8) B—When caring for a client in traction, maintain the pulling force and traction by maintaining the body alignment with the direction of the pull. (9) C—Use of ice constricts the vessels and helps to prevent or reduce edema. (10) A—Balanced suspension traction increases the client's mobility while maintaining appropriate bone position.

Case Study Hints
HIP FRACTURE: (1) Review Chapter 7 to develop your response. (2) Review the section on traction that precedes hip fracture. (3) Think about all the health care professionals that will be involved, and don't forget other departments that are integral to client care, such as dietary, housekeeping, and the business office!

Care Map (Below-Knee Amputation)
CORRECT DATA: Subjective: Complaining of severe pain. Objective: Vital signs stable; stump splinted, covered by soft dressing; wound healing without signs of infection; refuses ROM exercises and turning; tolerating 1,800-cal ADA diet; yells, "Get out! I don't want anyone to see me like this" when anyone enters room.

CORRECT INTERVENTIONS: Encourage verbalization of feelings; contact the physician for a referral to a psychologist or social worker.

CHAPTER 28
NCLEX-PN ANSWERS: (1) B—Osteomyelitis may develop in the patient with open fractures or open wounds near a bone. The nurse should assess for other signs and symptoms of infection including chills, fever, and elevated WBC. Dressings should be changed as ordered. Evaluation of the drainage on the bandage is critical. The dressing should be dry and intact. Capillary refill should be within normal limits. A decreased capillary refill may indicate occlusion. Pain medications should be administered as necessary. (2) A—Safety is the most important issue for discharge instruction. The walker and elevated toilet seat reduce the risk of falling and dislocation or damage of the hip. Calcium supplements may be ordered for the patient, because increased calcium will help the healing process. (3) C—The tick should be removed with tweezers without jerking or twisting. It should not be crushed, and should be saved in alcohol. (4) D—Osteoarthritis affects the entire joint, causing deep, aching pain, stiffness following immobility, limited ROM, crepitus with movement, and the appearance of Heberden's and Bouchard's nodes. (5) C—The SLE patient is sensitive to UV light and should avoid skin exposure, especially when rays are intense. No special diet is

prescribed, and joint inflammation is treated as necessary. SLE is a chronic inflammatory disease that affects all body systems. (6) C—Sulfinpyrazone may cause peptic ulcers in some clients. They should report any symptoms of GI distress to their physician. Water should be increased to at least 3 liters per day. Plain colchicine is used for acute attacks and is the only medication for gout that should be taken on an empty stomach. Probenecid, sulfinpyrazone, and allopurinol are taken with food to prevent gastric upset. (7) B—Patients with chronic low back pain need to focus on rehabilitation and prevention of further injury. Appropriate body mechanics, back exercises, and environmental modifications need to be discussed. (8) A—Neuromuscular/skin assessments must be done at least every shift. Muscular dystrophy produces muscle weakness and progressive loss of voluntary muscle movement. The rate of progression varies; clients may be unable to change positions without assistance. There is a risk for skin breakdown. The muscles used in respiration may also be affected. Pain medications may or may not be administered. Casts are not typically seen unless there has been a fracture of the bone. (9) C—A bone scan is invasive, and a signed consent form is required after the physician has discussed the procedure. The bladder must be empty. Radioactive material is injected intravenously and the patient must then drink several glasses of water. The process of scanning may take up to 60 minutes. (10) A—Scoliosis is usually discovered during adolescence. It is found primarily in girls. Kyphosis is known as "hunchback." Paget's disease and osteomalacia are associated with inadequate mineralization of the bone.

Case Study Hints
OSTEOPOROSIS: (1) Consider the effects of osteoporosis on the vertebrae in your response. (2) Review Box 28-2 and Chapter 22. (3) With your study group, discuss possible weight-bearing activities for clients such as these.

RHEUMATOID ARTHRITIS: (1) Review the normal inflammatory process in Chapter 13 and the pathophysiology of rheumatoid arthritis. (2) Review the long-term effects of excess corticosteroids (Chapter 16) to prepare your response to this question.

Care Map (Osteoarthritis and Total Hip Replacement)
CORRECT DATA: Subjective: Takes carbidopa/levodopa (Sinemet 25–100) 4 times a day for Parkinson's disease; no other chronic medical conditions; no known medication allergies; does not smoke; consumes only small amounts of alcohol. Objective: alert and oriented; speech is soft but clear; vital signs: BP 116/64; P 68 regular; R 18; T 97.4° F (36.3° C) PO; color good, skin warm and moist; peripheral pulses strong and equal in upper extremities; slightly weaker but equal in lower extremities; feet cool to touch, good capillary refill; walks with a limp, favoring right hip; shuffling gait noted.

CORRECT INTERVENTIONS: Help change position at least every 2 hours; encourage use of overhead trapeze to shift positions frequently; maintain sequential compression device and antiembolic stocking as ordered; remove for 1 hour daily; remind to use incentive spirometer hourly for first 24 hours, then at least every 2 hours while awake; assist out of bed three times a day after the first 24 hours; encourage frequent quadriceps-setting exercises and plantar and dorsiflexion of feet.

DOCUMENTATION: 1/8/03. Vital signs stable. Respirations 14, unlabored. Lung sounds clear throughout. Skin intact, wound healing well. Ambulating well accompanied by physical therapy. Taking oral analgesic bid with good pain relief. S. Campbell, LPN.

CHAPTER 29

NCLEX-PN ANSWERS: (1) A—Blunt trauma may cause a contusion of the brain. If the skull is fractured, there may be leakage of cerebrospinal fluid into the ears or nose. Infection is a serious complication of brain injury. Headaches and dizziness are commonly seen after a blow to the head. Hematomas develop due to blood leaking underneath the skin. (2) C—Coronary artery disease affects all blood vessels, including the arteries leading to the brain. Narrowing of the arteries may lead to strokes. The use of birth control pills and excessive alcohol intake are also risk factors for a CVA. (3) B—The patient should empty both bladder and bowel, if necessary. Movement should be kept to a minimum at all times during the procedure. Obtaining the kit and making sure that the consent form is signed are also nursing actions. (4) D—Dilantin has a specific therapeutic range, which must be monitored on a regular basis. The CBC, platelet count, and liver enzyme levels are also important indicators of potential drug side effects. Dilantin may cause anemia, leukopenia, thrombocytopenia, and liver disease. (5) C—The earliest sign of increased intracranial pressure is level of consciousness. Irritability, personality changes, restlessness, and disorientation are early manifestations of ICP. Blood pressure becomes elevated. Slowed pupil responses and projectile vomiting are seen during later stages. (6) A—It is more appropriate to document actual behaviors than to use medical terms. The most critical information is direct observation of the client's condition. (7) C—Status epilepticus is considered a life-threatening emergency. It may lead to physical exhaustion and respiratory distress. The first priority would be to maintain the airway. Anxiety and risk for injury also need to be addressed in the nursing care plan. There is no risk for cerebral perfusion alterations. (8) D—Patient education is a priority because most headaches are treatable at home. Helping a client understand what causes the migraines may help reduce the number of attacks. Diaries, comfort measures during an attack, and stress reduction classes are also important. (9) C—Meningitis is an inflammation of the spinal cord and meninges. It is usually secondary to an upper respiratory infection. Encephalitis is caused by a virus, in most cases. Brain abscesses occur from middle ear infection. A subdural hematoma is a collection of blood underneath the dura mater. (10) B—Loosen the gown and turn client on his side. Never restrain the patient who is having a seizure. Remove any items that may injure the client during the seizure. Pad the side rails as soon as possible.

Case Study Hints

INCREASED INTRACRANIAL PRESSURE AND LOSS OF CONSCIOUSNESS: (1) In a setting such as an accident, think of the ABCs of nursing assessment. Consider the effect on the body of a trauma like Mr. Straton experienced. (2) Consider the calming effect of family or significant others and how you can use them to assist in calming the client. (3) Review the Nursing Care section, especially the interventions under Imbalanced Nutrition: Less Than Body Requirements. Think how the family can participate in creating a plan of care.

Care Map (Cerebrovascular Accident)

CORRECT DATA: Subjective: Eyes look pleading. Objective: Lack of eye contact; nods off while people speak to him; nods head to answer questions; makes a clenched fist of right hand when trying to speak.

REPORT: Yes, to physician.

CORRECT INTERVENTIONS: Provide a large marker and tablet; use short, simple sentences when talking to Mr. Boren; contact speech therapy for consult; explain all health care procedures; maintain a calm, unhurried manner.

DOCUMENTATION: 09/21/03. Answers simple questions by nodding head to indicate "Yes". Is trying to write with right hand by using marker and tablet. Contacted speech therapy for follow-up consult. R. Kitwell, LVN

Answers to Critical Thinking Questions

ASSESSMENT: Refer to the discussion within the text on head injuries; in particular, read the section on skull fractures. Review manifestations of increased intracranial pressure for additional data to collect. Consider the Clinical Alert and how it could affect John's progress.

INTERVENTION: Review the nursing interventions listed under the nursing diagnosis Altered Tissue Perfusion: Cerebral. Consider how positioning Mrs. Cabot on her side will affect the flow of venous blood from her head. Think about what other positions could increase or decrease the blood flow from the brain.

ASSESSMENT: Compare and contrast the pathophysiology of TIA and CVA. Review Table 29-5 for the three causes of CVA and Table 29-6 for the typical manifestations as well as the discussion in the text. What conservative approaches might the physician use to manage Tom's symptoms?

INTERVENTION: Review the manifestation of homonymous hemianopia and its affect on the client meeting his or her daily needs. For the moment, turn her plate so that she can finish her lunch. Discuss with the physician the need for a consult with an occupational therapist who can teach Joan strategies for meeting her ADLs.

CHAPTER 30

NCLEX-PN ANSWERS: (1) A—These are some of the manifestations of stage I, early Alzheimer's disease. (2) D—Pro-Banthine is used to control urinary frequency. (3) C—Because the client has difficulty performing ADLs and alteration of self-esteem, it is important to not hurry and to encourage the client to do as much as possible for himself. (4) A—Autonomic dysreflexia is an exaggerated sympathetic response in clients with a spinal cord injury above the T6 level. Stimuli such as bladder or fecal impaction trigger a hypertensive crisis. (5) D—When the client experiences autonomic dysreflexia, elevate the head of the bed 45 degrees to lower the blood pressure. (6) C—Gradually lowering the client's extremities will reduce the likelihood of the client's experiencing orthostatic hypotension. (7) C—Elevate the client's head and place a small pillow under the knees for a herniated lumbar disk. (8) B—Clients with dysphasia may not be able to swallow the medication unless it is taken exactly on time. Doses taken too late may cause myasthenic crisis. (9) D—One of the side effects of Dilantin is gingival hyperplasia, so oral hygiene is especially important. (10) C—The client should have a fluid intake of 2,400 to 3,000 mL in 24 hours to reduce the possibility of headache.

Case Study Hints

ALZHEIMER'S DISEASE: (1) Review the Discharge Considerations section. (2) Think about the ways that Alzheimer's disease alters thought processes. Reread the interventions under Altered Thought Processes in the chapter. (3) See the discussion of nursing interventions for self-care deficit. Think how you would present food to a person who becomes upset easily and who cannot focus. Think what types of foods would be appealing and easy to eat.

Care Map (Herniated Intervertebral Disk)

CORRECT DATA: Subjective: Concerned about returning to work; complains of muscle weakness in left arm; unable to ride her bicycle. Objective: Decreased ability to use left hand; pain in the neck and shoulders; decreased reflexes in left arm.

REPORT: Yes, to physician.

CORRECT INTERVENTIONS: Consult with physical therapist for mobility plan; instruct her to keep the cervical collar on at all times; give analgesics around the clock; teach her to not to lift objects or twist neck.

DOCUMENTATION: Contacted PT for follow-up consult. Instructed in how to apply cervical collar and in activities that should be avoided. Medicated with Vicodin 1 tablet for sharp shooting pain in the back of her neck.

Answers to Critical Thinking Questions

ASSESSMENT: Review the manifestations of Parkinson's disease in Box 30-7. Consider how a right hemisphere would affect his rehabilitation potential if he is right-handed or left-handed. Think about the combined affect of Parkinson's and a CVA on this client's ability to perform his ADLs in the future.

INTERVENTION: Consider the nursing interventions provided under Altered Nutrition: Less than Body Requirements in the discussion of the client with Parkinson's disease. Advise her to take small bites and to think about the steps of swallowing.

ASSESSMENT: Review the manifestations of autonomic dysreflexia. Determine if the cause is related to a kinked or blocked catheter tubing or constipation. Review other causes of this condition. Be prepared to elevate the head of the bed and to administer antihypertensive medications.

INTERVENTION: Review the manifestations of a urinary tract infection and the appropriate management in Chapter 21. Ask whether Matt has been drinking at least 8–10 glasses of water per day. Determine if catheterization is performed every 4 to 6 hours or whether he has residual urine after trigger voiding. Recommend that his mother take him to the clinic for evaluation by the physician who may prescribe an antibiotic.

CHAPTER 31

NCLEX-PN ANSWERS: (1) D—Clients with sensory deprivation are at high risk for injury as well as loss of contact with their environment and social isolation. (2) A—Myopia, a common vision problem of the elderly, allows the client to see objects distinctly only when they are very close to the eye. (3) C—When administering ear drops to an adult, the pinna (auricle) would be pulled upward and backward. (4) C—Because the client's hearing impairment is severe, in addition to using strategies such as facing the person and speaking softly and slowly, the nurse should investigate the purchase of a communication board in order to increase client's contact with the environment and reduce social isolation. (5) D—Immediate treatment for accidental exposure of the eyes to potentially harmful substances focuses on diluting the substance and washing the substance from the eye. This can be achieved by flushing the eyes with large amounts of water. After the immediate treatment, medical attention should be sought. (6) B—When irrigating the client's eye with solution, it is important to direct the flow of solution from the inner to the outer canthus, because the inner aspect of the eye is considered cleaner than the outer aspect. (7) C—It is normal for the client to experience burning and temporary blurring of vision after administering this medication. These side effects should diminish with prolonged use of the medication. Most importantly, it should be emphasized that in order to regain her vision, the client must take this medication as directed for the rest of her life. (8) D—Open-angle glaucoma results from pressure produced when the aqueous humor in the eye cannot drain adequately. (9) B—Symptoms of open-angle glaucoma may include blurred vision, difficulty focusing on near objects, and halos around lights. (10) C—Because Ménière's disease causes a sensation of fullness or pressure in the ears that may be related to edema of the membranous labyrinth, a diet low in sodium is recommended.

Case Study Hints

GLAUCOMA AND CATARACTS: (1) Pressing over the bridge of the nose occludes drainage of tears through the lacrimal duct, preventing systemic absorption of eyedrops. (2) Look up the systemic effects of beta blockers, focusing on their effects on the heart and lungs. (3) Think about local churches, home health providers, senior centers, advocates and agencies for older adults. Look at what is available in your own community.

Care Map (Age-Related Hearing Loss)

CORRECT DATA: Objective: Frequently asks nurse to repeat questions; ear canals clean, no redness, small amount of dark earwax noted; answers not always appropriate to the question; mental status exam is normal; ignores conversation at his table during meals; audiometric testing reveals significant hearing loss consistent with presbycusis.

CORRECT INTERVENTIONS: Use effective communication techniques; face Mr. Aaron when speaking with him; speak distinctly in a low voice; supplement verbal with nonverbal communication strategies; use a pocket talker as needed until hearing aids are available; ask Mr. Aaron's family to obtain headphones for radio and television use; teach Mr. Aaron how to use and care for hearing aids.

DOCUMENTATION: 10/27/04. 85 y.o. male with severe osteoarthritis of hands and hips. Alert and oriented. Significant hearing loss noted on audiometric testing. Referred for further testing and hearing aid fitting. Pocket talker provided for temporary use. J. Lemon, LVN

CHAPTER 32

NCLEX-PN ANSWERS: (1) D—Discharge of seminal fluid into the bladder instead of through the urethra is common following TURP. Nocturia is relieved by the TURP procedure. There is no physiological reason for impotence or decreased libido following TURP; sexual performance and enjoyment may even be increased. (2) B—Blood clots promote bladder spasms, so the irrigation is titrated to keep the output light pink or clear. Since this is a continuous flow, it does not mimic filling and emptying, so it does not promote bladder tone. Patients often complain of an urge to void with a catheter in place. Large amounts of irrigating fluid can cause hyponatremia, not prevent it. (3) A—Aspirin would promote excessive bleeding. Tub baths are avoided until the catheter is out, but showers are permitted. Sex should be delayed until healing is complete to avoid excessive bleeding. Extra fluid consumption keeps the bladder clear of blood, clots, and bacteria, thereby preventing painful bladder spasms and infection. (4) D—Calf pain and difficulty breathing could be an embolism. The other problems need attention, but breathing difficulties need your attention first. See the study tip. (5) B— Frequent ejaculation is thought to relieve congestion in the

prostate. Fluids should be increased. This is not an infectious disorder. (6) C—Heart disease is the number one cause of death in men and women. Prostate cancer is the most common type of cancer in men, but lung cancer is the leading cause of cancer death. (7) A—Orchiectomy removes the major source of testosterone, which feeds testicular tumor growth. Gynecomastia is enlarged breasts and results from orchiectomy. (8) C—Patients should be advised to report an erection that lasts more than 4 hours. This drug is contraindicated with nitroglycerin and other nitrate drugs, and is not advised for men with cardiovascular disease. It should not be taken more than once per day. (9) C—Emergency surgery is done to relieve twisting and restore circulation to the testicle before the testicle becomes necrotic or damaged. Surgery for cryptorchidism or phimosis can be done on a nonemergency basis. Epididymitis is treated with an appropriate antibiotic. (10) B—All men should be taught to do monthly testicular self-exam. This cancer does not usually present with pain, tenderness, blood in the urine, or other symptoms, so TSE is especially important.

Case Study Hints

ERECTILE DYSFUNCTION: (1) Review the long-term effects of diabetes presented in Chapter 17. (2) Review the explanation of the nocturnal penile tumescence and rigidity test presented earlier in Chapter 32, as well as your anatomy and physiology textbook on normal erectile function. Note that erections normally occur during REM sleep. (3) Think about Mr. and Mrs. Lawton's age group and possible cultural mores affecting the ability to openly discuss sexual concerns.

Care Map (Prostate Cancer)

CORRECT DATA: Subjective: Relates difficulty getting out of house to buy groceries due to embarrassment of being seen with drainage bag; reports inability to change from large drainage bag to leg bag due to arthritis. Objective: Fully dressed, carrying large night urinary drainage bag.

CORRECT INTERVENTIONS: Discuss the possibility of stress incontinence after the catheter is removed; reinforce the need for perineal muscle exercises while the catheter is still in place; explore available support systems to identify people to assist with catheter care; provide teaching for Mr. Turner and care assistants as appropriate.

CHAPTER 33

NCLEX-PN ANSWERS: (1) D—Fallopian tubes are made of smooth muscle and are lined with cilia. Wavelike movements of the cilia help to transport the ovum through the tubes toward the uterus. Fimbriae make up the lateral ends of the tubes. Estrogen is a hormone, not a lining structure. Rugae are the folds in the wall of the vagina. (2) A—Nonproliferative fibrocystic breast changes do not increase the risk for cancer. B and C are measures to relieve discomfort. D has not been proven, but is reported by some to relieve symptoms. (3) C— Heart disease exceeds all cancers combined as the number one cause of death in women. Lung cancer followed by breast cancer are the most frequent causes of cancer death in women. Trauma, including spousal abuse, is also a significant cause of morbidity and mortality in women. (4) B—Tamoxifen increases the risk for endometrial cancer. It also increases the risk for deep vein thrombosis and pulmonary embolism, particularly in women who smoke. (5) A—The upper outer quadrant, called the tail of Spence, is the most frequent location of breast cancers. When teaching breast self-exam, it is important to teach women to examine the breast tissue all the way to the axillary region. (6) B—She will need to know how to care for her drainage system. Permanent prostheses are not recommended until the scar is healed, no longer swollen, and not as painful. The arm should not be abducted to the level of the elbow above the shoulder until the drain comes out. She will be encouraged to flex and extend the elbow and do simple ADLs within 24 hours after surgery. (7) A—The pill is often prescribed to help alleviate symptoms of primary dysmenorrhea. Locally applied heat relieves discomfort. NSAIDs are prostaglandin inhibitors, and therefore block one of the main causes of cramping. Orgasm also relieves symptoms in some women. (8) B—Bleeding in a postmenopausal women not on hormone replacement is never normal and is the most common symptom of endometrial cancer. (9) C—Even though less invasive techniques are tried first, DUB remains the leading cause of hysterectomy. Some causes of bleeding also cause infertility (e.g., endometriosis), but bleeding does not cause infertility. Cancer often causes DUB, but DUB does not cause cancer. Colposcopy is a diagnostic procedure done if repeated Pap smears show abnormal cells. (10) C—PID can cause tubal scarring and blockage, putting her at increased risk for infertility and tubal pregnancy. PID is usually caused by *Neisseria gonorrhoeae* and/or *Chlamydia trachomatis,* whereas cervical cancer is associated with HPV (genital warts). PID is caused by infectious organisms spread during unprotected sex, not by heredity. Toxic shock is caused by *Staphylococcus aureus*; it is related to poor hygiene during menstruation and use of super-absorbent tampons and diaphragms.

Case Study Hints

BREAST CANCER: (1) The strong family history suggests that a genetic factor may play a role; genetic testing can identify if this is the case, allowing the daughters to consider their options for prevention. They also may choose to consider the potential risk to their children. (2) Review the surgical treatment options for breast cancer, considering the extent of the surgery and adjunctive treatment and its nursing implications. (3) Review management of chemotherapy side effects in Chapter 8.

CERVICAL CANCER: (1) Review the risk factors for cervical cancer. As you develop your outline, consider how you would modify what and how you present this information for different age or cultural groups. (2) Consider the risk for cervical cancer associated with HPV and how that affects your recom-

mendations for follow-up Pap smears and exams. (3) Review the pathophysiology of cancer in Chapter 8.

Care Map (Experiencing Menopause)

CORRECT DATA: Subjective: Hates thought of growing older; thinks her husband is losing interest in sex; wonders about decision to not to have children.

CORRECT INTERVENTIONS: Refer to midlife women's support group at the local community center; arrange sexual counseling for Mr. and Mrs. Villagrana regarding techniques, positions, and modifications to accommodate midlife changes.

DOCUMENTATION: 12/20/04. Presents for annual gynecological exam. Relates problems with palpitations, hot flashes, night sweats, anxiety, and insomnia over past 15 months. Menstrual periods irregular, lasting only 1 to 3 days. LMP around 9/15/04. Wt. 152 lbs.; BP 140/70, P 74, R 18, T 98.2° F. Smokes 1 pack/day; relates high fat, high CHO, low protein, low fiber diet. Discussed risks and benefits of HRT; provided additional written information. Referred to midlife women's support group and to counselor for marital/sexual counseling. J. Voss, LPN

CHAPTER 34

NCLEX-PN ANSWERS: (1) D—Untreated chlamydia ascends into the upper reproductive tract, and is a major cause of PID. Chlamydia is often asymptomatic in women. (2) B—Zithromax can be given in a single oral dose. Other antibiotics used for STDs may require multiple daily doses for 7 to 10 days. (3) A—Addresses the feelings in the client statement. B and C give unsolicited advice, which would block communication. She will receive prescriptions, but to follow her comments with D before recognizing her feelings changes the topic, also blocking communication. (4) D—Pap smears are important for this client because certain subtypes of HPV increase the risk for cervical cancer. HPV infection is painless. Warts are removed with topical treatments, not acyclovir. (5) D—Herpes and HPV (genital warts) are treatable, but these viral infections cannot be cured. (6) C—These are symptoms of tertiary syphilis. (7) A—Penicillin G IM is the usual treatment for syphilis. If the client is allergic to penicillin, oral doxycycline (a tetracycline) can be used. (8) C—Because chlamydia infection often is asymptomatic, the incidence is thought to be even higher than known cases. Gonorrhea is the most common *reportable* STD, but does not equal the incidence of chlamydia. (9) B—Sexually transmitted diseases can be spread by anal, oral, and vaginal intercourse. Some young clients do not consider oral contact to be intercourse, and since it avoids pregnancy, it is seen as a risk-free activity. (10) C—These STDs are reportable by law in all 50 states. Some states also require reporting of other STDs. Syphilis is caused by a spirochete, AIDS is caused by a virus, and gonorrhea is caused by a diplococcus. Patients with AIDS and gonorrhea may have fever, but syphilis presents with a painless chancre at the site of exposure. AIDS is the only STD routinely treated with combination therapy.

Case Study Hints

GONORRHEA: (1) Review the manifestations of gonorrhea in men. (2) Review the pathophysiology and complications of gonorrhea in women. (3) Use some creative thinking to answer this question—think about how you might handle this situation.

Care Map (Syphilis)

CORRECT DATA: Subjective: Having unprotected sex with Ms. Jones and Ms. Simpson; syphilitic chancre on the shaft of the penis; believes that Ms. Jones is not having sex with anyone else, but is not sure; ELISA results negative for HIV; darkfield analysis of chancre exudate confirms syphilis.

CORRECT INTERVENTIONS: Administer and document IM injection of benzathine penicillin G as ordered; teach the importance of treatment to the health of their infant; discuss importance of abstaining from sexual activity until client and partners are cured and using condoms to prevent reinfection; explain the need for follow-up testing in 3 months and 6 months; notify Ms. Jones and Ms. Simpson of need for testing; send reminders for follow-up at 3- and 6-month intervals; provide a copy of STD prevention checklist.

Bibliography

CHAPTER 1

Alfaro, R. (1998). *Applying nursing diagnoses and nursing process: A step-by-step guide* (4th ed.). Philadelphia: Lippincott.

American Nurses Association. (1995). *Nursing's social policy statement.* Washington, DC: Author.

American Nurses Association. (1985). *Code for nurses.* Kansas City, MO: Author.

American Nurses Association. (1988). *Ethics in nursing: Position statement and guidelines.* Kansas City, MO: Author.

American Nurses Association. (1996). *Position statement on cultural diversity in nursing practice.* Washington, DC: Author.

American Nurses Association. (1998). *Standards of clinical nursing practice.* Washington, DC: Author.

Andrews, M., & Boyle, J. (1997). Competence in transcultural nursing care. *American Journal of Nursing, 97*(8), 16–20.

Carpenito, L. (2000). *Nursing diagnoses: Application to clinical practice* (8th ed.). Philadelphia: Lippincott.

Daly, B. (1997). Nursing ethical code reflects changing times. *The American Nurse, 29*(5), 9.

Diers, D. (1997). What is nursing? In J. McCloskey & H. Grace (Eds.), *Current issues in nursing* (5th ed.), (pp. 5–12). St. Louis: Mosby.

Gordon, M. (1994). *Nursing diagnosis: Process and application* (3rd ed.). New York: McGraw-Hill.

Green, C. (2000). *Critical thinking in nursing: Case studies across the curriculum.* Upper Saddle River, NJ: Prentice Hall.

International Council of Nurses. (1973). *ICN Code for nurses: Ethical concept applied to nursing.* Geneva: Imprimeries Populaires.

Ketefian, S. (1987). Moral behavior in nursing. *Advances in Nursing Science, 9*(1), 10–19.

National Association for Practical Nurse Education and Service, Inc. (1997). *Licensed practical nursing: The work of the care-giver.* Silver Springs, MD: Author.

National Association for Practical Nurse Education and Service, Inc. (1999). *NAPNES Standards of practice for licensed practical/vocational nurses.* Silver Springs, MD: Author.

North American Nursing Diagnosis Association. (2001). *NANDA Nursing diagnoses: Definitions & classification 2001–2002.* Philadelphia: Author.

Reeves, D. L. (1997). A licensed practical nurse/licensed vocational nurse's guide to the changing healthcare system. *Gastroenterology Nursing, 20*(2), 54–56.

Spector, R. (1996). *Cultural diversity in health and illness* (4th ed.). Norwalk, CT: Appleton & Lange.

Wilkinson, J. (2000). *Nursing process in action: A critical thinking approach* (7th ed.). Upper Saddle River, NJ: Prentice Hall Health.

CHAPTER 2

American Association of Retired Persons (AARP). (2000). *A profile of older Americans: 1999.* Washington, DC: Resource Services Group.

American Cancer Society (2000). *Cancer facts & figures—2000.* Atlanta, GA: Author.

Centers for Disease Control and Prevention (CDC). (1999). *Preliminary Data for 1999.* Washington, DC: U.S. Department of Health and Human Services.

Clemen-Stone, S., McGuire, S., & Eigsti, D. (1998). *Comprehensive community health nursing.* (5th ed.). St. Louis: Mosby.

Dossey, B., & Dossey, L. (1998). Body–mind–spirit. Attending to holistic care. *American Journal of Nursing, 98*(8), 35–38.

Dunn, H. (1959). High level wellness for man and society. *American Journal of Public Health, 49,* 786–972.

Edelman, C., & Mandle, C. (1997). *Health promotion throughout the lifespan* (4th ed.). St. Louis: Mosby.

Freiberg, K. L. (1992). *Human development: A lifespan approach* (4th ed.). Boston: Jones & Bartlett.

Havighurst, R. J. (1972). *Human development and education* (3rd ed.). New York: Longman.

Lubkin, I. (1999). *Chronic illness: Impact and interventions* (4th ed.). Boston: Jones & Bartlett.

Miller, J. (1983). *Coping with chronic illness: Overcoming powerlessness.* Philadelphia: Davis.

Miller, C. (1998). *Nursing care of the older adult: Theory and practice* (3rd ed.). Philadelphia: Lippincott.

Morris, M. R. (1998). Elder abuse: What the law requires. *RN, 61*(8), 48–49.

Swanson, E., & Tripp-Reimer, T. (1997). *Chronic illness and the older adult.* New York: Springer.

Suchman, E. (1972). Stages of illness and medical care. In E. Jaco (Ed.), *Patients, physicians and illness.* New York: Free Press.

World Health Organization (WHO). (1974). *Constitution of the World Health Organization.* Geneva: Author.

CHAPTER 3

American Nurses Association. (1986). *Standards of home health nursing practice.* Kansas City, MO: Author.

American Nurses Association. (1992). *A statement on the scope of home health nursing practice.* Kansas City, MO: Author.

Clemen-Stone, S., McGuire, S., & Eigsti, D. (1998). *Comprehensive community health nursing* (5th ed.). St. Louis: Mosby.

Green, K., & Lydon, S. (1998). The continuum of patient care. *American Journal of Nursing, 98*(10), 16BBB–16DDD.

Grindel-Waggoner, M. (1999). Home care: A history of caring, a future of challenges. *MEDSURG Nursing, 8*(2), 118–120.

Holt, F. M. (2000). Challenges of community-based practice. *Clinical Nurse Specialist, 14*(1), 39.

Krulish, L. H. (2000). Commentary. Home care in the new millennium. *Home Healthcare Nurse, 18*(2), 144.

National Association for Home Care. (2000). *Basic statistics about home care.* Washington, DC: Author.

Stulginsky, M. (1993a). Nurses' home health experience: Part I—The practice setting. *Nursing & Health Care, 14*(8), 402–407.

Stulginsky, M. (1993b). Nurses' home health experience: Part II—The unique demands of home visits. *Nursing & Health Care, 14*(9), 476–485.

Zotti, M., Brown, P., & Stots, R. (1996). Community-based nursing versus community health nursing. *Nursing Outlook, 44*(5), 211–217.

CHAPTER 4

Andresen, G. (1998). Assessing the older patient. *RN, 61*(3), 46–56.

Bates, B. (1999). *Guide to physical examination and history taking* (7th ed.). Philadelphia: Lippincott.

Burke, L., & Murphy, J. (1995). *Charting by exception applications: Making it work in clinical setting.* Albany, NY: Delmar.

Fuller, J., & Schaller-Ayers, J. (2000). *Health assessment: A nursing approach* (3rd ed.). Philadelphia: Lippincott.

Joint Commission on the Accreditation of Healthcare Organizations. (1997). *Accreditation manual for hospitals.* Chicago: JCAHO, Nursing Services.

Kozier, B., Erb, G., Berman, A., & Burke, K. (2000). *Fundamentals of nursing: Concepts, process, and practice* (6th ed.). Upper Saddle River, NJ: Prentice Hall Health.

Weber, J., & Kelley, J. (1998). *Health assessment in nursing.* Philadelphia: Lippincott.

CHAPTER 5

Call-Schmidt, T. (2001). Interpreting lab results: A primer. *MEDSURG Nursing, 10*(4), 179–184.

Castiglione, V. (2000). Emergency. Hyperkalemia. *American Journal of Nursing, 100*(1), 55, 56.

Cook, L. (1999). The value of lab values. *American Journal of Nursing, 99*(5), 66–69.

Danner, K. (2000). Acid/base balance: Making sense of pH. *CIN PLUS* [On-line serial], *3*(1), 3.

DeJong, J. J. (1998). Emergency! Hyponatremia. *American Journal of Nursing, 98*(12), 36.

Horne, C., & Derrico, D. (1999). Mastering ABGs. The art of arterial blood gas measurement. *American Journal of Nursing, 99*(8), 26–32.

Incredibly easy! Understanding imbalances caused by GI fluid loss. (1999). *Nursing, 29*(8), 72.

Malarkey, L. M., & McMorrow, M. E. (2000). *Nurse's manual of laboratory tests and diagnostic procedures* (2nd ed.). Philadelphia: Saunders.

McCloskey, J. C., & Bulechek, G. M. (Eds.). (2000). *Nursing interventions classification (NIC)* (3rd ed.). St. Louis: Mosby.

Metheny, N. M. (2000). *Fluid and electrolyte balance: Nursing considerations* (4th ed.). Philadelphia: Lippincott.

Morrison, C. (2000). Helping patients maintain a healthy fluid balance. *Nursing Times, 96*(31), NTplus 3–4.

Naxarko, L. (2000). How age affects fluid intake. *Nursing Times, 96*(31), NTplus 11–12.

Shepherd, E. (2000). Fluids: A balancing act. *Nursing Times, 96*(31), NTplus 1.

Sheppard, M. (2001). Assessing fluid balance. *Nursing Times, 97*(6), NTplus XI–XII.

Tasota, F. J., & Wesmiller, S. W. (1998). Balancing act: Keeping blood pH in equilibrium. *Nursing, 28*(12), 34–41.

Wallace, L. S. (2000). Using color to simplify ABG interpretation. *MEDSURG Nursing, 9*(4), 205–208.

White, V. (1997). Emergency! Hyperkalemia. *American Journal of Nursing, 97*(6), 35.

Wong, F. W. (1999). A new approach to ABG interpretation. *American Journal of Nursing, 99*(8), 34–36.

CHAPTER 6

Acello, B. (2000). Meeting JACHO standards for pain control. *Nursing 2000, 30*(3), 52–54.

Acello, B. (2000). Controlling pain: Switching to the patch. *Nursing 2000, 30*(8), 72.

Bullock, B. A., & Henze, R. L. (2000). *Focus on pathophysiology.* Philadelphia: Lippincott.

Fontaine, K. L. (2000). *Healing practices: Alternative therapies for nursing.* Upper Saddle River, NJ: Prentice Hall.

Gordon, D. B. (1999). Pain management in the elderly. *Journal of Perianesthesia Nursing, 14*(6), 367–371.

LeMone, P., & Burke, K. M. (2000). *Medical surgical nursing: Critical thinking in client care* (2nd ed) Upper Saddle River, NJ: Prentice Hall.

McCaffery, M., & Beebe, A. (1989). *Pain: Clinical manual for nursing practice.* St. Louis: Mosby.

McCaffery, M., & Pasero, C. (1997). Pain ratings: The fifth vital sign. *American Journal of Nursing, 97*(2), 15–17.

McCaffery, M., & Pasero, C. (1999). *Pain: Clinical manual* (2nd ed.) St. Louis: Mosby.

McCloskey, J. C., & Bulechek, G. M. (Eds.). (2000). *Nursing interventions classification (NIC)* (3rd ed.). St. Louis: Mosby.

Melzack, R., & Wall, P. (1965). Pain mechanisms: A new theory. *Science, 150,* 971–979.

Pasero, C. (1998). Pain control: How aging affects pain management. *American Journal of Nursing, 98*(6), 12.

Pasero, C., & McCaffery, M. (1999). Providing epidural analgesia. *American Journal of Nursing, 99*(8), 34–40.

Plaisance, L., & Price, T. F. (1999). A stepwise guide to cancer pain management in the home. *Home Healthcare Nurse, 17*(2), 97–105.

U.S. Department of Health and Human Services. (1992). *Acute pain management: Operative or medical procedures and trauma* (AHCPR Pub No 92-0032). Rockville, MD: Agency for Health Care Policy and Research, Public Health Service, USDHHS.

U.S. Department of Health and Human Services. (1994). *Management of cancer pain: Clinical practice guideline no. 9* (AHCPR Pub No 94-0592). Rockville, MD: Agency for Health Care Policy and Research, Public Health Service, USDHHS.

World Health Organization. (1986/1990). *Cancer pain relief.* Geneva: Author.

CHAPTER 7

American Society of PeriAnesthesia Nurses. (1995). Standards of perianesthesia nursing practice. Thorofare, NJ: Author.

Carpenito, L. (1999). Nursing diagnosis: Application to clinical practice (8th ed.). Philadelphia: Lippincott.

Doenges, M., & Moorhouse, M. (2000). *Nursing care plans: Guidelines for individualizing patient care* (5th ed.). Philadelphia: Davis.

Fairchild, S. (1996). *Perioperative nursing: Principles and practice* (2nd ed.). Boston: Little, Brown and Company.

Fishbach, F. (1998). *Common laboratory and diagnostic tests* (2nd ed.) Philadelphia: Lippincott.

Ireland, D. (1997). Legal issues in ambulatory surgery. *Nursing Clinics of North America, 32*(2), 469–476.

Lancaster, K. (1997). Patient teaching in ambulatory surgery. *Nursing Clinics of North America, 32*(2), 417–427.

McCloskey, J. C., & Bulechek, G. M. (2000). *Nursing interventions classification (NIC)* (3rd ed.). St. Louis: Mosby.

McKenry, L., & Salerno, E. (1998). *Pharmacology in nursing* (20th ed.). St. Louis: Mosby.

Meeker, M., & Rothrock, J. (1999). *Alexander's care of the patient in surgery* (11th ed.). St. Louis: Mosby.

Ruzicka, S. (1997). The impact of normal aging processes and chronic illness on perioperative care of the elderly. *Seminars in Perioperative Nursing, 6*(1), 3–13.

Silvestri, L. (2000). *Saunders comprehensive review for NCLEX-PN* (1st ed.). Philadelphia: Saunders.

Steelman, V. (1997). Issues in perioperative nursing. In J. McCloskey & H. Grace (Eds.), *Current issues in nursing* (5th ed.) (pp. 264–269). St. Louis: Mosby.

Timby, B., & Scherer, J. (1999). *Introductory medical–surgical nursing* (7th ed.). Philadelphia: Lippincott.

Walsh, J. (1993). Postop effects of OR positions. *RN, 56*(2), 50–57.

Williams, G. (1997). Preoperative assessment and health history review. *Nursing Clinics of North America, 32*(2), 395–416.

CHAPTER 8

American Cancer Society. (2001). *Cancer facts and figures—2001.* Atlanta, GA: Author.

Anonymous. (2000). Advice, p.r.n. Giving chemotherapy: Facing the unknown. *Nursing, 30*(4), 12.

Battiato, L. & Wheeler, V. (2000). Biotherapy. In C. H. Yarbro, M. H. Frogge, M. Goodman, & S. L. Groenwald (Eds.), *Cancer nursing: Principles and practice* (5th ed.) (pp. 543–579). Boston: Jones & Bartlett.

Cherny, N. I. (2000). The management of cancer pain. *Nursing, 101,* 24A, 24E, 24G–H.

Cleary, J. F. (2000). Cancer pain management. *Cancer Control, 7,* 120–131.

Dest, V. (2001). How to manage radiation-induced diarrhea. *RN, 64*(5), 91.

Frank-Stromborg, M., & Cohen, R. F. (2000). Assessment and intervention for cancer detection. In C. H. Yarbro, M. H. Frogge, M. Goodman, & S. L. Groenwald (Eds.), *Cancer nursing: Principles and practice* (5th ed.) (pp. 150–188). Boston: Jones & Bartlett.

Fu, M., LeMone, P., McDaniel, R., & Bausler, C. (2001). A multivariate validation of the defining characteristics of fatigue. *Nursing Diagnosis: International Journal of Nursing Language and Classification, 12,* 15–27.

Hogan, D. K., & Rosenthal, L. D. (1998). Oncologic emergencies in the patient with lymphoma. *Seminars in Oncology Nursing, 14,* 312–320.

Hopkins, H. F., & Tookman A. J. (2000). Rehabilitation and specialist palliative care. *International Journal of Palliative Nursing, 6,* 123–124, 126–130.

Kelley, M., & Comley, A. (2001). Breast cancer among minority women: Current knowledge and efforts in early detection programs. *American Journal of Nursing, (Suppl.)* 13–15, 49–50.

Letizia, M. (2001). Addressing alopecia: Helping patients with cancer deal with hair loss. *American Journal of Nursing, 101*(4 Critical Care Extra), 24LL.

McDaniel, R., & Rhodes, V. (1998). Development of a sensory information videotape for women receiving chemotherapy for breast cancer. *Cancer Nursing, 21,* 143–148.

Olsen, D., Raub, W., Bradley, C., Johnson, M., Macias, J., Love, V., & Markoe A. (2001). The effect of aloe vera gel/mild soap versus mild soap alone in preventing skin reactions in patients undergoing radiation therapy. *Oncology Nursing Forum, 28,* 543–547.

Rust, D. M., Simpson, J. K., & Lister, J. (2000). Nutritional issues in patients with severe neutropenia. *Seminars in Oncology Nursing, 16,* 152–162.

Tottorice, P. V. (2000). Chemotherapy: Principles of therapy. In C. H. Yarbro, M. H. Frogge, M. Goodman, & S. L. Groenwald (Eds.), *Cancer nursing: Principles and practice* (5th ed.) (pp. 352–384). Boston: Jones & Bartlett.

Walsh, D. (2000). Pharmacological management of cancer pain. *Seminars in Oncology, 27,* 45–63.

Wilson, R. L. (2000). Optimizing nutrition for patients with cancer. *Clinical Journal of Oncology Nursing, 4*(1), 23–28, 32–33.

CHAPTER 9

Alspach, G. (1997). Providing care for the dying: One answer, many questions. *Critical Care Nurse, 17*(5), 16–17.

American Association of Colleges of Nursing. (1999). *Peaceful death: Recommended competencies and curricular guidelines for end-of-life nursing care.* Washington, DC: Author.

American Nurses Association. (1985). *Code for nurses.* Kansas City, MO: Author.

American Nurses Association. (1988). Ethics in nursing: Position statement and guidelines. Kansas City, MO: Author.

American Nurses Association. (1991). *Position statement: Promotion of comfort and relief of pain in dying patients.* Washington, DC: Author.

American Nurses Association. (1992). *Position statement on nursing and the Patient Self-Determination Act.* Kansas City, MO: Author.

Barbus, A. J. (1975, January). The dying person's bill of rights. *The American Journal of Nursing, 75,* 99.

Barker, E. (1999). Life care planning. *RN, 62*(3), 58–61.

Callahan, M., & Kelley, P. (1991). *Final gifts: Understanding the special awareness, needs, and communications of the dying.* New York: Simon & Schuster.

Carpenito, L. (2000). *Nursing diagnosis: Application to clinical practice* (8th ed.). Philadelphia: Lippincott.

Duffield, P. (1998). Advance directives in primary care. *American Journal of Nursing, 61*(4), 16CCC–16DDD.

Durham, E., & Weiss, L. (1997). How patients die. *American Journal of Nursing, 97*(12), 41–46.

Ferrell, B. R. (1998). End-of-life care: How well do we serve our patients? *Nursing, 28*(9), 58–60.

Ferrell, B. R., Virani, R., Grant, M., & Rhome, A. (2000). End of life issues and nursing education. *Imprint, 47*(2), 43–46.

Goetschius, S. (1997). Families and end-of-life care: How do we meet their needs? *Journal of Gerontological Nursing, 23*(3), 43–49.

Haynor, P. M. (1998). Meeting the challenge of advance directives. *American Journal of Nursing, 98*(3), 26–32.

Improving end of life care: A conference of nursing and medical textbook publishers (March, 1999). Sponsored by The Robert Wood Johnson Foundation.

International Council of Nurses. (1997). *Basic principles of nursing care.* Washington, DC: American Nurses Publishing.

Jackonen, S. (1997). Dehydration and hydration in the terminally ill: Care considerations. *Nursing Forum, 32*(3), 5–13.

Kübler-Ross, E. (1969). *On death and dying.* New York: Macmillan.

Kübler-Ross, E. (1978). *To live until we say goodbye.* Englewood Cliffs, NJ: Prentice Hall.

McCloskey, J. C., & Bulechek, G. M. (Eds.). (2000). *Nursing interventions classification (NIC)* (3rd ed.). St. Louis: Mosby.

McFarland, G. K., Wasli, E. L., & Gerety, E. K. (1997). *Nursing diagnoses & process in psychiatric mental health nursing* (3rd ed.). Philadelphia: Lippincott.

Perkins, E. M. (1998). Death can be a caring choice. *RN, 61*(2), 72.

Rabow, M. W., & Brody, R. V. (1999). Care at the end of life. In L. M. Tierney, Jr., McPhee, S. J., & M. A. Papadakis (Eds.), *Current medical diagnosis & treatment 1999* (38th ed.) (pp. 99–110). Stamford, CT: Appleton & Lange.

Reed, P. G. (1996). Transcendence: Formulating nursing perspectives. *Nursing Science Quarterly, 9*(1), 2–4.

Rushton, C., & Scanlon, C. (1998). A road map for navigating end-of-life care. *MEDSURG Nursing, 7*(1), 57–59.

Tipton, K. (1997). How to discuss death with patients and families. *Nursing 97, 27*(32), 10–12.

Ufema, J. (1997a). Insights on death & dying: Offering hope: Dose of reality. *Nursing 97, 27*(9), 20–21.

Ufema, J. (1997b). Insights on death & dying: Pain medication: Sound judgment. *Nursing 97, 27*(10), 70.

Wilkinson, J. M. (2000). *Nursing diagnosis handbook* (7th ed.). Upper Saddle River, NJ: Prentice Hall Health.

Zerwekh, J. (1997). Do dying patients really need IV fluids? *American Journal of Nursing, 97*(3), 26–30.

CHAPTER 10

American College of Surgeons Committee on Trauma. (1993). *The advanced trauma life support student manual.* Chicago: Author.

Anton, M. (2000). Myths and facts about organ donation. *Nursing 2000, 30*(9), 70.

Bullock, B. L., & Henze, R. L. (2000). *Focus on pathophysiology.* Philadelphia: Lippincott, Williams, & Wilkins.

Gray-Vickery, P., & Colucci, R. (1999). Taking charge in a geriatric emergency. *Nursing 99, 29*(1), 41–48.

Hayes, L. (2000). What's your gut reaction to a poison emergency? *Nursing 2000, 30*(9), 34–40.

Hudak, C., Gall, B., & Morton, P. (1998). *Critical care nursing: A holistic approach* (7th ed.). Philadelphia: Lippincott.

Kleinpell, R. (1998). Taking the shock out of anaphylaxis. *Nursing 98, 28*(11), 32hn1–32hn3.

Laskowski-Jones, L. (2000). Responding to winter emergencies. *Nursing 2000, 30*(1), 34–39.

Laskowski-Jones, L. (2000). Responding to summer emergencies. *Nursing 2000 30*(5), 34–39.

McCloskey, J. C., & Bulechek, G. M. (2000). *Nursing interventions classification (NIC)* (3rd ed.) St. Louis: Mosby.

National Center for Injury Prevention and Control. (2000). 10 leading causes of deaths by age group—1998. Atlanta, GA: National Center for Health Statistics.

Newberry, L. (Ed.). (1998). *Sheehy's emergency nursing principles and practices* (4th ed.). St. Louis: Mosby.

Tangredi, M. (1998). Clinical snapshot: Septic shock. *American Journal of Nursing, 98*(3), 46–47.

CHAPTER 11

American Psychiatric Association (2000). *Diagnostic and statistical manual of mental disorders* (4th ed., Text Revision). Washington, DC: American Psychiatric Press.

American Society of Addiction Medicine (1997). Public policy statement on nicotine dependence and tobacco. *Journal of Addictive Diseases, 16*, 99.

Beattie, M. (1987). *Codependent no more: How to stop controlling others and start caring for yourself.* New York: Harper/Hazelden.

El-Mallakh, P. (1998) Treatment models for clients with co-occurring addictive and mental disorders. *Archives of Psychiatric Nursing, 12*, 2, 71.

Ewing, J. A. (1984). Detecting alcoholism: the CAGE questionnaire. *Journal of the American Medical Association, 252*, 1902–1907.

Freed, P. E., & York, L. N. (1997). Naltrexone: A controversial therapy for alcohol dependence. *Journal of Psychosocial Nursing, 35*, 7, 24–28.

Gordon, C., Williams, B., & Lapin, P. (2001). New program to help seniors quit smoking. *Nursing Spectrum, 2*, 10, 18–19.

Jellinek, E. M. (1960). *The disease concept of alcoholism.* New Haven, CT: Hillhouse Press.

Lehman, A. (1987). Assessment and classification of patients with psychiatric and substance abuse problems. *Hospital and Community Psychiatry, 40*, 10, 1019.

McCloskey, J. C., & Bulechek, G. M. (2000). *Nursing interventions classification (NIC)* (3rd ed.) St. Louis: Mosby.

Mynatt, S. (1996). A model of contributing risk factors to chemical dependency in nurses. *Journal of Psychosocial Nursing, 34*, 13.

Naegle, M. A., & D'Avanzo, C. E. (2001). *Addictions and substance abuse Strategies for advanced practice nursing.* Upper Saddle River, NJ: Prentice Hall Health.

Sullivan, E. J. (1995). *Nursing care of clients with substance abuse.* St. Louis: Mosby.

CHAPTER 12

Abrams, A. C. (2001). *Clinical drug therapy* (6th ed.) Philadelphia: Lippincott, Williams, & Wilkins.

Bullock, B. A., & Henze, R. L. (2000). *Focus on pathophysiology.* Philadelphia: Lippincott.

Centers for Disease Control and Prevention. (2000). *Preventing emerging infectious diseases: A strategy for the 21st century.* Atlanta, GA: U.S. Department of Health and Human Services.

Centers for Disease Control and Prevention. (2000). VISA—Fact sheet: Vancomycin-intermediate *Staphylococcus aureus* (VISA). Available online at *www.cdc.gov/ncidod/ARESIST/visa.htm.*

Eliopoulos, C. (2001). *Gerontological nursing* (5th ed.). Philadelphia: Lippincott.

Glover, T. L. (2000). How drug-resistant microorganisms affect nursing. *Orthopaedic Nursing, 19*(2), 19–27.

Inman, W. B. (2000). Pathogens invade 21st century. *Nursing 2000, 30*(8), 22–23.

Kee, J. L. (2001). *Handbook of laboratory and diagnostic tests* (4th ed.). Upper Saddle River, NJ: Prentice Hall.

Lilley, L. L., & Aucker, R. S. (1999.) *Pharmacology and the nursing process* (2nd ed.). St. Louis: Mosby.

Marx, J. F. (1998). Teaching your patient about isolation precautions. *Nursing 98, 28*(5), 32hn20–32hn21.

McCloskey, J. C., & Bulechek, G. M. (Eds.). (2000). *Nursing interventions classification (NIC)* (3rd ed). St. Louis: Mosby.

Porth, C. (1998). *Pathophysiology: Concepts of altered health states* (5th ed.). Philadelphia: Lippincott.

Shannon, M. T., Wilson, B. A., & Stang, C. L. (2001). *Health professional's drug guide 2001.* Upper Saddle River, NJ: Prentice Hall.

Sheff, B. (1998). VRE & MRSA: Putting bad bugs out of business. *Nursing 98, 28*(3), 40–45.

Sheff, B. (1999). Minimizing the threat of *C. difficile. Nursing 99, 29*(2), 33–39.

Smith, S. F., & Duell, D. J. (2000). *Clinical nursing skills* (5th ed.). Stamford, CT: Appleton & Lange.

Thompson, J. (2000). A practical guide to wound care. *RN, 63*(1), 48–53.

CHAPTER 13

Abramowicz, M. (Ed.). (2000). Drugs for HIV infection. New Rochelle, NY: The Medical Letter, Inc.

Bullock, B. A., & Henze, R. L. (2000). *Focus on pathophysiology.* Philadelphia: Lippincott.

Burggraf, V., & Weinstein, B. F. (2000). Don't miss this opportunity: Promote adult immunizations! *MEDSURG Nursing, 9*(4), 198–200.

Capili, B., & Anastasi, J. K. (1998). As America ages: Assess for HIV, too. *RN, 61*(4), 28–32.

Centers for Disease Control and Prevention. (2001). Vaccine-preventable adult diseases. Available online at *www.cdc.gov/nip/diseases/adult-vpd.htm.*

Eliopoulos, C. (2000). *Gerontological nursing* (5th ed.). Philadelphia: Lippincott.

Gritter, M. (1998). The latex threat. *American Journal of Nursing, 98*(9), 26–33.

Kee, J. L. (2001). *Handbook of laboratory and diagnostic tests* (4th ed.). Upper Saddle River, NJ: Prentice Hall.

Keithley, J. K., & Swanson, B. (1998). Minimizing HIV/AIDS malnutrition. *MEDSURG Nursing, 7*(5), 256–265.

Kirsten, V. L., & Whipple, B. (1998). Treating HIV disease. *Nursing 98, 28*(11), 34–39.

Lisanti, P., & Zwolski, K. (1997). Understanding the devastation of AIDS. *American Journal of Nursing, 97*(7), 26–34.

Lueckenotte, A. G. (2000). *Gerontologic nursing* (2nd ed.) St. Louis: Mosby.

McCloskey, J. C., & Bulechek, G. M. (Eds.). (2000). *Nursing interventions classification (NIC)* (3rd ed). St. Louis: Mosby.

National Coalition for Adult Immunization. (2001). Adult immunization—Schedule. Available online at *www.nfid.org/ncai/schedules/adult/.*

National Institute of Allergy and Infectious Diseases (2001). HIV/AIDS statistics. Available online at *http://niaid.hih.gov/factsheets/aidsstat.htm.*

Porth, C. (1998). *Pathophysiology: Concepts of altered health states* (5th ed.). Philadelphia: Lippincott.

Shannon, M. T., Wilson, B. A., & Stang, C. L. (2001). *Health professional's drug guide 2001.* Upper Saddle River, NJ: Prentice Hall.

CHAPTER 14

American Cancer Society. (2001). *Cancer facts & figures—2001.* New York: Author.

Ankrett, V., & Williams, I. (1999). In focus: Dermatology. *Practice Nurse, 17*(5), 318–320.

Bjorgen, S. (1998). Herpes zoster. *American Journal of Nursing, 98*(2 Continuing Care Extra), 46–47.

Blawat, D., & Banks, P. (1997). Comforting touch: Using topical skin preparations. *Nursing 97, 27*(5), 46–48.

Boston, M. (1997). Acne: Avoiding permanent damage. *Community Nurse, 3*(4), 15–16.

Carpenito, L. (2000). *Nursing diagnosis: Application to clinical practice* (8th ed.). Philadelphia: Lippincott.

Everett, S., & Colditz, G. (1997). Skin cancer prevention: A time for action. *Journal of Community Health, 22*(3), 175–183.

Groenwald, S., Frogge, M., Goodman, M., & Yarbo, C. (2000). *Cancer nursing: Principles and practice* (2nd ed.). Boston: Jones & Bartlett.

Hardy, M. (1996). What can you do about your patient's dry skin? *Journal of Gerontological Nursing, 22*(5), 10–18, 52–53.

Jackson, R., Alghareeb, M., Alaradi, I., & Tomi, Z. (1999). The diagnosis of skin disease. *Dermatology Nursing, 11*(4), 275, 278–283.

Levine, N. (1999). Emergency room dermatology. *Dermatology Nursing, 11*(5), 331–336, 341–346.

McCloskey, J. C., & Bulechek, G. M. (Eds.). (2000). *Nursing interventions classification (NIC).* (3rd ed). St. Louis: Mosby.

McMichael, A. J. (1999). A review of cutaneous disease in African-American patients. *Dermatology Nursing, 11*(1), 35–36, 41–47.

National Cancer Institute. (1997). *Melanoma.* Bethesda, MD: Author.

North American Nursing Diagnosis Association. (2001). *Nursing diagnoses: Definitions & classification, 2001–2002.* Philadelphia: Author.

Porth, C. (1998). *Pathophysiology: Concepts of altered health states* (5th ed.). Philadelphia: Lippincott.

Rakel, R. E. (2000). *Conn's current therapy.* Philadelphia: Saunders.

Tierney, L., McPhee, S., & Papadakis, M. (Eds.). (2001). *Current medical diagnosis & treatment* (40th ed.). Stamford, CT: Appleton & Lange.

U.S. Department of Health and Human Services. (1992). *Pressure ulcers in adults: Predication and prevention* (AHCPR Publication No. 92-0047). Rockville, MD: Agency for Health Care Policy and Research, Public Health Service.

Wilson, B., Shannon, M., & Stang, C. (2001). *Nursing drug guide 2001.* Upper Saddle River, NJ: Prentice Hall.

CHAPTER 15

American College of Surgeons Committee on Trauma. (1999). *Resources for the optimal care of the injured patient.* Chicago: Author.

Carpenito, L. (2000). *Nursing diagnosis: Application to clinical practice* (8th ed.). Philadelphia: Lippincott.

Fowler, A. (1999). Nursing care of minor burns. *Community Nurse, 5*(4), 39–40.

Gordon, M., & Goodwin, C. (1997). Initial assessment, management, and stabilization. *Nursing Clinics of North America, 32* (2), 237–249.

Jordan, B., & Harrington, D. (1997). Management of the burn wound. *Nursing Clinics of North America, 32*(2), 251–273.

McCain, D., & Sutherland, S. (1998). Nursing essentials: Skin grafts for patients with burns. *American Journal of Nursing, 98*(7), 34–38.

McCloskey, J. C., & Bulechek, G. M. (Eds.). (2000). *Nursing interventions classification (NIC).* (3rd ed). St. Louis: Mosby.

Mertens, D., Jenkins, M., & Warden, G. (1997). Outpatient burn management. *Nursing Clinics of North America, 32*(2), 343–374.

North American Nursing Diagnosis Association. (2001). *Nursing diagnoses: Definitions & classification, 2001–2002.* Philadelphia: Author.

Rakel, R. E. (2000). *Conn's current therapy.* Philadelphia: Saunders.

Rutan, R. (1998). Physiologic response to cutaneous burn injury. In G. Carrougher, *Burn care and therapy* (pp. 1–33). St. Louis: Mosby.

Wiebelhaus, P., & Hansen, S. L. (1999). Burns: Handle with care. *RN, 62*(11), 52–57.

Wilson, B. A., Shannon, M. T., & Stang, C. L. (2001). *Nursing drug guide 2001.* Upper Saddle River, NJ: Prentice Hall.

CHAPTER 16

American Cancer Society. (1999). *Cancer facts & figures—1999.* New York: Author.

Bailes, B. K. (1999). Hyperthyroidism in elderly patients. *AORN Journal, 69*(1), 254–258.

Bailes, B. K. (1999). Hypothyroidism in elderly patients. *AORN Journal, 69*(5), 1026–1030.

Bullock, B. A., & Henze, R. L. (2000). *Focus on pathophysiology.* Philadelphia: Lippincott, Williams, & Wilkins.

Burton, M. (1997). Emergency! Pheochromocytoma. *American Journal of Nursing, 97*(11), 57.

Carson, P. P. (2000). Emergency: Adrenal crisis. *American Journal of Nursing, 100*(7), 49–50.

Clayton, L., & Dilley, K. (1998). Clinical snapshot: Cushing's syndrome. *American Journal of Nursing, 98*(7), 40–41.

Goldsmith, C. (1999). Clinical snapshot: Hypothyroidism. *American Journal of Nursing, 99*(6), 42–43.

Heater, D. W. (1999). If ADH goes out of balance: Diabetes insipidus and SIADH. *RN, 62*(7), 42–50.

Lilley, L. L., & Aucker, R. S. (1999). *Pharmacology and the nursing process* (2nd ed.). St. Louis: Mosby.

McCloskey, J. C., & Bulechek, G. M. (Eds.). (2000). *Nursing interventions: Effective nursing treatments* (3rd ed.). St. Louis: Mosby.

Porth, C. (1998). *Pathophysiology: Concepts of altered health states* (5th ed.). Philadelphia: Lippincott.

Young, J. (1999). Action stat: Myxedema coma. *Nursing 99, 29*(1), 64.

CHAPTER 17

American Diabetes Association. (2000a). Diabetes mellitus and exercise. *Diabetes Care, 23*(Supplement 1), S50–54.

American Diabetes Association. (2000b). Insulin administration. *Diabetes Care, 23*(Supplement 1), S86–89.

American Diabetes Association. (2000c). Nutrition recommendations and principles for people with diabetes mellitus. *Diabetes Care, 23*(Supplement 1), S43–46.

American Diabetes Association. (2000d). Report of the expert committee on the diagnosis and classification of diabetes mellitus. *Diabetes Care, 23*(Supplement 1), S4–19.

American Diabetes Association. (2000e). Standards of medical care for patients with diabetes mellitus. *Diabetes Care 23*(Supplement 1), S32–42.

American Diabetes Association. (2000f). Tests of glycemia in diabetes. *Diabetes Care, 23*(Supplement 1), S80–S82.

Bullock, B. A., & Henze, R. L. (2000). *Focus on pathophysiology.* Philadelphia: Lippincott, Williams, & Wilkins.

Capriotti, T., & McLaughlin, S. (1998). A revitalized battle against diabetes mellitus for the new millennium. *MedSurg Nursing, 7*(6), 323–341.

Cypress, M. (2001). Diabetes update: Acute complications. *RN, 64*(4), 26–31.

Dudek, S. G. (1997). *Nutrition handbook for nursing practice* (3rd ed.). Philadelphia: Lippincott.

Ebersole, P., & Hess, P. (2001). *Geriatric nursing and health aging.* St. Louis: Mosby.

Funnell, M., & Merritt, J. (1996). Diabetes mellitus and the older adult. In D. Haire-Joshu (Ed.), *Management of diabetes mellitus: Perspectives of care across the life span* (2nd ed.) (pp. 755–830). St. Louis: Mosby.

Goldberg, J. M. (2001). Diabetes update: Nutrition and exercise. *RN, 64*(7), 34–40.

Halpin-Landry, J. E., & Goldsmith, S. (1999). Feet first: Diabetes care. *American Journal of Nursing, 99*(1), 26–33.

Huether, S. E., & McCance, K. C. (2000). *Understanding pathophysiology* (2nd ed.). St. Louis: Mosby.

Konick-McMahan, J. (1999). Riding out a diabetic emergency. *Nursing 99, 29*(9), 34–40.

McCloskey, J. C., & Bulechek, G. M. (Eds.). (2000). *Nursing interventions classification (NIC)* (3rd ed.). St. Louis: Mosby.

Miller, J. (1999). Management of diabetic ketoacidosis. *Journal of Emergency Nursing, 25*(6), 514–518.

Porth, C. (1998). *Pathophysiology: Concepts of altered health states* (5th ed.). Philadelphia: Lippincott.

Roach, S. (2001). *Introductory gerontological nursing.* Philadelphia: Lippincott.

Senegewald, J. M. (1999). Update on diabetes medications. *Journal of Emergency Nursing, 25*(1), 28–30.

CHAPTER 18

Ammon, P. K. (1999). Individualizing the approach to treating obesity. *Nurse Practitioner, 24*(2), 27–31, 36–38, 41.

Bowers, S. (1999). Nutrition support for malnourished, acutely ill adults. *MEDSURG Nursing, 8*(3), 145–164.

Cammon, S. A., & Hackshaw, H. S. (2000). Are we starving our patients? *American Journal of Nursing, 100*(5), 43–46.

Dudek, S. G. (2000). Malnutrition in hospitals. Who's assessing what patients eat? *American Journal of Nursing, 100*(4), 36–42.

Fauci, A. S., Braunwald, E., Isselbacher, K. J., Wilson, J. D., Martin, J. B., Kasper, D. L., et al. (Eds.). (1998). *Harrison's principles of internal medicine* (14th ed.). New York: McGraw-Hill.

Fontaine, K. L. (2000). *Healing practices: Alternative therapies for nursing.* Upper Saddle River, NJ: Prentice Hall.

Heslin, J. (1997). Peptic ulcer disease: Making a case against the prime suspect. *Nursing 97, 27*(1), 34–39.

Kuhn, M. A. (1999). *Complementary therapies for health care providers.* Philadelphia: Lippincott.

LeMone, P., & Burke, K. M. (2000). *Medical surgical nursing: Critical thinking in client care* (2nd ed). Upper Saddle River, NJ: Prentice Hall.

Lessick, M., & Keithley, J. (1997). Obesity: Genetic update and clinical implications. *MEDSURG Nursing, 6*(3), 121–127, 145.

Malarkey, L. M., & McMorrow, M. E. (2000). *Nurse's manual of laboratory tests and diagnostic procedures* (2nd ed.). Philadelphia: Saunders.

McCloskey, J. C., & Bulechek, G. M. (Eds.). (2000). *Nursing interventions classification (NIC)* (3nd ed.). St. Louis: Mosby.

McConnell, E. (1997). How to determine gastric pH. *Nursing 97, 27*(8), 26.

Meeker, M. H., & Rothrock, J. C. (1999). *Alexander's care of the patient in surgery* (11th ed.). St. Louis: Mosby.

Meeker, M. H., & Rothrock, J. C. (1998b). Testing feeding tube placement: Auscultation vs. pH method. *American Journal of Nursing, 98*(5), 37–42.

Middlemiss, C. (1997). Gastroesophageal reflux disease: A common condition in the elderly. *Nurse Practitioner, 22*(11), 51–52, 55–59.

O'Hanlon-Nichols, T. (1998). Basic assessment series: Gastrointestinal system. *American Journal of Nursing, 98*(4), 48–53.

Soady, C. (1999). Diagnosis and treatment of cancer of the mouth. *Nursing Times, 95*(33), 46–48.

Tierney, L. M., Jr., McPhee, S. J., & Papadakis, M. A. (2000). *Current medical diagnosis & treatment* (39th ed.). New York: Lange/McGraw-Hill.

Whitney, E. N., & Rolfes, S. R. (1999). *Understanding nutrition* (8th ed.). Belmont, CA: West/Wadsworth.

CHAPTER 19

American Cancer Society. (2000). *Liver cancer: Overview* Available online at *www.cancer.org/cancerinfo.*

Bockhold, K. M. (2000). Who's afraid of hepatitis C? *American Journal of Nursing, 100*(5), 26–31.

Centers for Disease Control and Prevention. (2000). *Epidemiology and prevention of vaccine-preventable diseases* (6th ed.). Atlanta, GA: Public Health Foundation.

Critical care: Learning the ABCs of hepatitis. (1998). *Nursing 98, 28*(2), 32cc12–32cc13.

Dougherty, A. S., & Dreher, H. M. (2001). Hepatitis C: Current treatment strategies for an emerging epidemic. *MEDSURG Nursing, 10*(1), 9–13.

Farrar, J. A., & Kearney, K. (2001). Emergency. Acute cholecystitis. *American Journal of Nursing, 101*(1), 35, 36.

Fontaine, K. L. (2000). *Healing practices: Alternative therapies for nursing.* Upper Saddle River, NJ: Prentice Hall.

Giacchino, S., & Houdek, D. (1998). Ruptured varices! Act fast. *RN, 61*(5), 33–36.

Gonzalez, E. R. (2000). *Silymarin: An anti-inflammatory antioxidant* Available online at *www.vicus.com/news_views/news_detail/ 1,1042,2892,00.html.*

Gonzalez, E. R. (2000). *An integrative approach to treating HBV* Available online at *www.vicus.com/news_views/news_detail/ 1,1042,3133,00.html.*

Klainberg, M. (1999). Clinical snapshot. Primary biliary cirrhosis. *American Journal of Nursing, 99*(12), 38, 39.

Marx, J. F. (1998). Understanding the varieties of viral hepatitis. *Nursing, 28*(7), 43–49.

McCloskey, J. C., & Bulechek, G. M. (Eds.). (2000). *Nursing interventions classification (NIC)* (3rd ed.). St. Louis: Mosby.

Meeker, M. H., & Rothrock, J. C. (1999). *Alexander's care of the patient in surgery* (11th ed.). St. Louis: Mosby.

National Center for Complementary and Alternative Medicine, National Institutes of Health. (2000). *Hepatitis C: Treatment alternatives* Available online at *http://nccam.nih.gov/nccam/fcp/factsheets/ hepatitisc.htm.*

National Digestive Diseases Information Clearinghouse, National Institutes of Health. (2000). *Cirrhosis of the liver* Available online at *www.niddk.nih.gov.*

National Digestive Diseases Information Clearinghouse, National Institutes of Health. (2000). *Chronic hepatitis C: Current disease management.* Available online at *www.niddk.nih.gov.*

Shovein, J. T., Damazo, R. J., & Hyams, I. (2000). Hepatitis A: How benign is it? *American Journal of Nursing, 100*(3), 43–47.

Tasota, F. J., & Tate, J. (2000). Reading liver function values. *Nursing, 30*(6), 73–75.

Tierney, L. M., Jr., McPhee, S. J., & Papadakis, M. A. (2001). *Current medical diagnosis & treatment* (40th ed.). New York: Lange/McGraw-Hill.

Williamson, L. (1998). Self-destruction in the pancreas. *Nursing Times, 94*(29), 57–59.

CHAPTER 20

Ball, E. M. (2000). A teaching guide for continent ileostomy. *RN, 63*(12), 35–36, 38, 40.

Bradley, M., & Pupiales, M. (1997). Essential elements of ostomy care. *American Journal of Nursing, 97*(7), 38–46.

Breitfeller, J. M. (1999). Emergency! Peritonitis. *American Journal of Nursing, 99*(4), 33.

Carlson, E. (1998). Irritable bowel syndrome. *Nurse Practitioner, 23*(1), 82–91.

Cox, J. (1995). Inflammatory bowel disease: Implications for the medical-surgical nurse. *MEDSURG Nursing, 4*(6), 427–437.

Dest, V. M. (2000). Oncology today: New horizons. Colorectal cancer. *RN, 63*(3), 54–59.

Erwin-Toth, P. (2001). Caring for a stoma is more than skin deep. *Nursing, 31*(5), 36–40.

Heitkemper, M., & Jarrett, M. (2001). "It's not all in your head": Irritable bowel syndrome. *American Journal of Nursing, 101*(1), 26–33.

McCloskey, J. C., & Bulechek, G. M. (Ed.). (2000). *Nursing interventions classification (NIC)* (3rd ed.). St. Louis: Mosby.

Moppett, S. (1998). Abdominoperineal resection for rectal cancer. *Nursing Times, 94*(35), 48–49.

National Digestive Diseases Information Clearinghouse, National Institutes of Health. (2000). *Crohn's disease* Available online at *www.niddk.nih.gov/health/digest/pubs/crohns/crohns.htm.*

National Digestive Diseases Information Clearinghouse, National Institutes of Health. (2000). *Irritable bowel syndrome.* Available online at *www.niddk.nih.gov/health/digest/pubs/irrbowel/irrbowel.htm.*

National Digestive Diseases Information Clearinghouse, National Institutes of Health. (2000). *Ulcerative colitis.* Available online at *www.niddk.nih.gov/health/digest/pubs/colitis/colitis.htm.*

Sneddon, I. (1999). Colorectal cancer: A nurse puts a patient perspective. *Nursing Times, 95*(36), 44–45.

Swan, E. (1999). Colorectal cancer: Diagnosis and treatment. *Nursing Times, 95*(35), 49–50.

Wood, S. (1998). Gut instinct. *Nursing Times, 94*(8), 70–72.

Young, M. (2000). Caring for patients with coloanal reservoirs for rectal cancer. *MEDSURG Nursing, 9*(4), 193–197.

CHAPTER 21

Baxter, A. (1999). Bladder cancer: Its diagnosis and treatment. *Nursing Times, 95*(41), 42–44.

Cook, L. (1999). The value of lab values. *American Journal of Nursing, 99*(5), 66–69.

Duffield, P. (1996). Managing urinary tract infections. Part 1: Diagnosing and treating adults. *American Journal of Nursing, 96*(9), 16B–16D.

Fickenscher, L. (1999). Evaluating adult hematuria. *Nurse Practitioner, 24*(9), 58–65.

Gray, M. (2000). Urinary retention: Management in the acute care setting. Part 1. *American Journal of Nursing, 100*(7), 40–47.

Gray, M. (2000). Urinary retention: Management in the acute care setting. Part 2. *American Journal of Nursing, 100*(8), 36–43.

Hayes, D. D. (2000). Caring for your patient with a permanent hemodialysis access. *Nursing, 30*(3), 41–46.

Hobgood, E. (1999). Midlife women and urinary incontinence: Causes, lifestyles, and treatments. *MEDSURG Nursing, 8*(1), 19–24.

Johnson, S. T. (2000). From incontinence to confidence. *American Journal of Nursing, 100*(2), 69–70, 72–74, 76.

Kelly, M. (1996). Chronic renal failure. *American Journal of Nursing, 96*(1), 36–37.

Kelly, M. (1997). Clinical snapshot: Acute renal failure. *American Journal of Nursing, 97*(3), 32–33.

King, B. (2000). Meds and the dialysis patient. *RN, 63*(7), 54–59.

Loughrey, L. (1999). Taking a sensitive approach to urinary incontinence. *Nursing, 29*(5), 60–61.

McCloskey, J. C., & Bulechek, G. M. (Eds.). (1996). *Nursing interventions classification (NIC)* (3rd ed.). St. Louis: Mosby.

Ross, C. A. (2000). Dialysis disequilibrium syndrome. *American Journal of Nursing, 100*(2), 53–54.

Sosa-Guerrero, S., & Gomez, N. J. (1997). Dealing with end-stage renal disease. *American Journal of Nursing, 97*(10), 44–50.

Taft, C. (1999). A team approach to managing urinary incontinence. *Geriatric Nursing, 20*(2), 94–97.

CHAPTER 22

Ammon, S. (2001). Managing patients with heart failure. *American Journal of Nursing, 101*(12), 34–40.

Artinian, N. T. (2001). Perceived benefits and barriers of eating heart healthy. *MEDSURG Nursing, 10*(3), 129–138.

Baptiste, M. M. (2001). Aortic valve replacement. *RN, 64*(1), 58–63.

Bither, C. J., & Apple, S. (2001). Home management of the failing heart. *American Journal of Nursing, 101*(12), 41–45.

Bubien, R. S. (2000). A new beat on an old rhythm. *American Journal of Nursing, 100*(1). 42–50.

Carelock, J., & Clark, A. P. (2001). Heart failure: Pathophysiologic mechanisms. *American Journal of Nursing, 101*(12), 26–33.

Colletti, C. (1999). Emergency! Pericarditis. *American Journal of Nursing, 99*(10), 35.

Crumlish, C. M., Bracken, J., Hand, M. A., Keenan, K., Ruggiero, H., & Simmons, D. (2000). When time is muscle. *American Journal of Nursing, 100*(1), 26–31, 33.

DeJong, M. J. (1998). Clinical snapshot: Infective endocarditis. *American Journal of Nursing, 98*(5), 34–36.

Gondek, M. C. (1999). Talking about sex: A post-MI script. *RN, 62*(7), 52–54.

Goodman, D. (2001). Automatic external defibrillation. *MEDSURG Nursing, 10*(5), 251–253, 276.

Granger, B. B., & Miller, C. M. (2001). Acute coronary syndrome. *Nursing, 31*(11), 36–43.

Halm, M. A., & Penque, S. (1999). Heart disease in women. *American Journal of Nursing, 99*(4), 26–31.

Kearney, K. (2000). Emergency: Digitalis toxicity. *American Journal of Nursing, 100*(6), 51–52.

Kruse, L., Demarco, M. K., Moyer, P., Guether, L., Wagner, A., Torreli, V., & Leone, D. (1999). Keeping pace with implanted defibrillators. *RN, 61*(8), 30–34.

Mancini, M. E., & Kaye, W. (1999). AEDs: Changing the way you respond to cardiac arrest. *American Journal of Nursing, 99*(5), 26–30.

McAvoy, J. A. (2000). Cardiac pain: Discover the unexpected. *Nursing, 30*(3), 34–39.

McCloskey, J. C., & Bulechek, G. M. (Ed.). (1996). *Nursing interventions classification (NIC)* (3rd ed.). St. Louis: Mosby.

Miracle, V. A. (2001). Put the brakes on pericarditis. *Nursing, 31*(4), 44, 45.

National Institutes of Health (2000). WebMD—Fat-modified diets for treatment of cardiovascular disease. Available online at *www.webmd.com.*

Palatnik, A. M. (2001). Critical care. Acute coronary syndrome: New advances and nursing strategies. *Nursing, 31*(5), 32cc1–32cc2, 32cc4, 32cc6.

Palec, D. Z., & Albert, N. M. (1999). Managing heart failure. Teaching your client how to stay at home. *Nursing, 29*(10), 64hh2–4, 64hh6, 64hh8.

Resnick, B. (1999). Atrial fibrillation in the older adult. Presentation and management issues. *Geriatric Nursing, 20*(4), 188–193.

Ross, C. A., & Leonardo, J. E. (2001). Emergency: Palpitations. *American Journal of Nursing, 101*(7), 41–42.

Ryan, D., & Roberts, M. E. (2000). Is it an MI? A lab primer. *RN, 63*(1), 26–30.

Seigh, P. J. (1999). Emergency! Pulmonary edema. *American Journal of Nursing, 99*(12), 43.

Sims, J. M., & Miracle, V. A. (1999). Using the ECG to detect myocardial infarction. *Nursing, 29*(8), 41–46.

Siomko, A. J. (2000). Demystifying cardiac markers. *American Journal of Nursing, 100*(1), 36–40.

Stanley, M. (1999). Congestive heart failure in the elderly. *Geriatric Nursing, 20*(4), 180–185.

Steinke, E. E. (2000). Sexual counseling after myocardial infarction. *American Journal of Nursing, 100*(12), 38–43.

Sullivan, C. (2000). Critical care. Easing severe angina with laser surgery. *Nursing, 30*(4), 32cc1–2, 32cc4.

Woods, S. L., Froelicher, E. S. S., & Motzer, S. U. (2000). *Cardiac nursing* (4th ed.). Philadelphia: Lippincott.

CHAPTER 23

Bacoka, J. (2000). Action stat. Aortic dissection. *Nursing, 30*(8), 33.

Breen, P. (2000). DVT: What every nurse should know. *RN, 63*(4), 58–62.

Cerrato, P. L. (1999). Tai chi: A martial art turns therapeutic. *RN, 62*(2), 59–60.

Chase, S. L. (2000). Hypertensive crisis. *RN, 63*(6), 62–67.

Church, V. (2000). Staying on guard for DVT & PE. *Nursing, 30*(2), 34–42.

Gibbar-Clements, T., Shirrell, D., Dooley, R., & Smiley, B. (2000). The challenge of warfarin therapy. *American Journal of Nursing, 100*(3), 38–40.

Gibbar-Clements, T., Shirrell, D., & Free, G. (1997). PT and APTT—seeing beyond the numbers. *Nursing, 27*(7), 49–51.

Karch, A. M., & Karch, F. E. (2000). When a blood pressure isn't routine. *American Journal of Nursing, 100*(3), 23.

Launius, B. K., & Graham, B. D. (1998). Understanding and preventing deep vein thrombosis and pulmonary embolism. *AACN Clinical Issues, 9*(1), 91–99.

Lilley, L. L., & Guanci, R. (1998). Anticipating drug response. A commonly used anticoagulant has many drug–drug interactions. *American Journal of Nursing, 98*(9), 12.

McCloskey, J. C., & Bulechek, G. M. (Eds.). (1996). *Nursing interventions classification (NIC)* (3rd ed.). St. Louis: Mosby.

Millar, B. (1998). Marfan's syndrome—defusing a time bomb. *Nursing Times, 94*(6), 40–41.

Oertel, L. B. (1999). Monitoring warfarin therapy. How the INR keeps your patient safe. *Nursing, 29*(11), 41–44.

Phillips, J. K. (1998). Abdominal aortic aneurysm. *Nursing, 28*(5), 34–39.

Poore, S. (1998). How a short stretch can work wonders. *Nursing Times, 94*(45), 87–90.

Porterfield, L. M. (2000). Why is this patient starting to bruise? *RN, 63*(5), 109.

Rice, K. L., & Walsh, M. E. (1998). Peripheral arterial occlusive disease, Part 1: Navigating a bottleneck. *Nursing, 28*(2), 33–38.

Woods, A. D. (1999). Managing hypertension. *Nursing, 29*(3), 41–46.

Woods, S. L., Froelicher, E. S. S., & Motzer, S. U. (2000). *Cardiac nursing* (4th ed.). Philadelphia: Lippincott.

CHAPTER 24

Alcoser, P. W., & Burchett, S. (1999). Bone marrow transplantation. *American Journal of Nursing, 99*(6), 26–31.

Day, S. W., & Wynn, L. W. (2000). Sickle cell pain & hydroxyurea. *American Journal of Nursing, 100*(11), 34–38.

Gorman, K. (1999). Sickle cell disease. Do you doubt your patient's pain? *American Journal of Nursing, 99*(3), 38–43.

Gutaj, D. (2000). Oncology today: Lymphoma. *RN, 63*(8), 32–37.

McCloskey, J. C., & Bulechek, G. M. (Eds.). (1996). *Nursing interventions classification (NIC)* (3rd ed.). St. Louis: Mosby.

Medoff, E. (2000). Oncology today: Leukemia. *RN, 63*(9), 42–49.

Mitchell, R. (1999). Sickle cell anemia. *American Journal of Nursing, 99*(5), 36–37.

Navuluri, R. (2001). Understanding hemostasis. *American Journal of Nursing, 101*(9), 24B, 24C.

Snyder, C. L., & Stocker, J. (1997). Confronting a tempest: Acute leukemia. *Nursing, 27*(2), 32a–32e.

Thompson, K. A. (1999). Adolescent health. Detecting Hodgkin's disease. *American Journal of Nursing, 99*(5), 61–64.

Torrance, C. (1998). Anaemia. *Nursing Times, 94*(33), 54–57.

CHAPTER 25

American Cancer Society. (1999). Laryngeal and hypopharyngeal cancer: Treatment. Available online at *www.cancer.org/cancerinfo/load_cont.asp?st=tr&ct=23&language=english.*

Braunwald, E., Fauci, A. S., Kasper, D. L., Hauser, S. L., Longo, D. L., & Jameson, J. L. (Eds.). (2001). *Harrison's principles of internal medicine* (15th ed.). New York: McGraw-Hill.

Bullock, B. A., & Henzwe, R. L. (2000). *Focus on pathophysiology.* Philadelphia: Lippincott.

Davidson, P. (1998). An easier way to speak again. *Nursing Times, 94*(13), 53–55.

Fontaine, K. L. (2000). *Healing practices: Alternative therapies for nursing.* Upper Saddle River, NJ: Prentice Hall.

Kee, J. L. (1998). *Handbook of laboratory and diagnostic tests with nursing implications* (3rd ed.). Stamford, CT: Appleton & Lange.

Klein, L. (2001). Sinusitis: When to treat and how. *RN, 64*(1), 42–44, 46, 48.

Kuhn, M. A. (1999). *Complementary therapies for health care providers.* Philadelphia: Lippincott.

Loud, B. (2001). A water pik to clear sinuses? *RN, 64*(1), 49.

Malarkey, L. M., & McMorrow, M. E. (2000). *Nurse's manual of laboratory tests and diagnostic procedures* (2nd ed.). Philadelphia: Saunders.

Marchiondo, K. (2000). Pickwickian syndrome: The challenge of severe sleep apnea. *MEDSURG Nursing, 9*(4), 183–188.

McCloskey, J. C., & Bulechek, G. M. (2000). *Nursing interventions classification (NIC)* (3rd ed.). St. Louis: Mosby.

Meeker, M. H., & Rothrock, J. C. (1999). *Alexander's care of the patient in surgery* (11th ed.). St. Louis: Mosby.

Nicoteri, J. A. (1999). Rising above "soar" throats. Take a common-sense approach to assessing young adults with sore throats. *American Journal of Nursing, 99*(3), 18–20.

O'Hanlon-Nichols, T. (1998). Basic assessment series: The adult pulmonary system. *American Journal of Nursing, 98*(2), 39–45.

Physicians' desk reference (PDR) (54th ed.). (2000). Montvale, NJ: Medical Economics Company, Inc.

Porth, C. M. (1998). *Pathophysiology: Concepts of altered health states* (5th ed.). Philadelphia: Lippincott.

Ruppert, R. A. (1999). The last smoke. *American Journal of Nursing, 99*(11), 26–32.

Tierney, L. M., McPhee, S. J., & Papadakis, M. A. (Eds.). (1998). *Current medical diagnosis & treatment* (37th ed.). Stamford, CT: Appleton & Lange.

CHAPTER 26

Adatsi, G. (1999). Health going up in smoke: How can you prevent it? *American Journal of Nursing, 99*(3), 63–64, 65, 66–67.

Carroll, P. (2000). Exploring chest drain options. *RN, 63*(10), 50–54.

Chrisp, D. R. (2000). Action stat. Tension pneumothorax. *Nursing, 30*(5), 33.

Dunn, N. A. (2001). Keeping COPD patient out of the ED. *RN, 64*(2), 33–37.

Evans, T. (2000). Neuromuscular blockade: When and how. *RN, 63*(5), 56–60.

Fitzgerald, M. A. (2000). Community-acquired pneumonia. The "captain of death" can be controlled. *Advance for Nurse Practitioners, 8*(1), 59–61.

Lenaghan, N. A. (2000). The nurse's role in smoking cessation. *MEDSURG Nursing, 9*(6), 298–301, 312.

Hughes, H. (1999). Silent aspiration. *Nursing Times, 95*(21), 71–5.

LeMasters, C. Z. (1999). Treatment of pulmonary tuberculosis. *Lippincott's primary care practitioner, 3*(1), 55–58.

Marion, B. S. (2001). A turn for the better: "Prone positioning" of patients with ARDS. *American Journal of Nursing, 101*(5), 26–34.

McCloskey, J. C., & Bulechek, G. M. (Eds.). (1996). *Nursing interventions classification (NIC)* (3rd ed.). St. Louis: Mosby.

McGann. E. (1999). Medication compliance in adults with asthma. *American Journal of Nursing, 99*(3), 45–46.

Miracle, V., & Winston, M. (2000). Take the wind out of asthma. *Nursing, 30*(8), 34–41.

Owen, C. L. (1999). New directions in asthma management. *American Journal of Nursing, 99*(3), 26–33.

Reid, E. (1999). Pulmonary embolism: An overview of treatment and nursing issues. *British Journal of Nursing, 8*(20), 1373–1378.

Ruppert, R. A. (1999). The last smoke. *American Journal of Nursing, 99*(11), 26–32.

Togger, D. A., & Brenner, P. S. (2001). Metered dose inhalers. *American Journal of Nursing, 101*(10), 26–32.

Tregonning, M., & Langley, C. (1999). Chronic obstructive pulmonary disease. *Elder Care, 11*(7), 21–25.

Trudeau, M. E., & Solano-McGuire, S. M. (1999). Evaluating the quality of COPD care. *American Journal of Nursing, 99*(3), 47–50.

Truesdell, S. (2000). Helping patients with COPD manage episodes of acute shortness of breath. *MEDSURG Nursing, 9*(4), 178–182.

CHAPTER 27

Bryant, G. (2001). Stump care. *American Journal of Nursing, 101*(2), 67, 69–71.

Day, M. W. (1999). Action stat. Compartment syndrome. *Nursing, 29*(6), 33.

Gouzd, B. A. (2000). Emergency. Whiplash injury. *American Journal of Nursing, 100*(3), 41–42.

McCloskey, J. C., & Bulechek, G. M. (Eds.). (1996). *Nursing interventions classification (NIC)* (3rd ed.). St. Louis: Mosby.

McWhinnie, G., & Roseburgh, M. (1999). The initial management of lower limb amputations. *Nursing Times, 95*(40), 48–49.

Patterson, M. (2000). Screening a simple fracture. *International Journal of Trauma Nursing, 6*(2), 58–60.

Patterson, M. (2000). What's the buzz on external bone growth stimulators? *Nursing, 30*(6), 44–45.

Reed, S. J. (2000). Managing phantom pain with drugs. *Nursing, 30*(4), 32hn1-2, 32hn4.

Stewart, K. B. (2000). Action stat: Open fracture. *Nursing, 30*(11), 33.

Tumbarello, C. (2000). Acute extremity compartment syndrome. *Journal of Trauma Nursing, 7*(2), 30–38.

Urquhart, B. S. (2001). Emergency: Anterior shoulder dislocation. *American Journal of Nursing, 101*(2), 33–35.

Whitten, R. (1999). Action stat: Traumatic amputation. *Nursing, 29*(3), 33.

Yarnold, B. D. (1999). Hip fracture: Caring for a fragile population. *American Journal of Nursing, 99*(2), 36–40.

CHAPTER 28

Burke, S. (2001). Boning up on osteoporosis. *Nursing, 31*(10), 36–42.

Campbell, J. M., & Linc, L. G. (1999). Managing osteoarthritis pain. *Advance for Nurse Practitioners, 7*(4), 57–60.

Capriotti, T. (2000). Pharmacologic prevention and treatment of osteoporosis in women. *MEDSURG Nursing, 9*(2), 86–90.

Capriotti, T. (2000). The new NSAIDs: COX-2 inhibitors. *MEDSURG Nursing, 9*(6), 313–317.

de Jesus, M. (2000). Fibromyalgia onset. *American Journal of Nursing, 100*(1), 14.

Depree, P. (2000). Building bone. *Advance for Nurse Practitioners, 8*(1), 36–38.

Dowd, R., & Cavalieri, R. J. (1999). Help your patient live with osteoporosis. *American Journal of Nursing, 99*(4), 55, 57–60.

Hall, J. C., & Riley, R. E. (1999). Nutritional strategies to reduce the risk of osteoporosis. *MEDSURG Nursing, 8*(5), 281–293

Johnson, B. (1999). Systemic lupus erythematosus. *American Journal of Nursing, 99*(1), 40–44.

Jones, A. (2001). Getting past the pain of fibromyalgia. *Nursing, 31*(4), 62–64.

Kee, C. C. (2000). Osteoarthritis: manageable scourge of aging. *Nursing Clinics of North America, 35*(1):199–208.

Leslie, M. (2000). Issues in the nursing management of osteoporosis. *Nursing Clinics of North America, 35*(1):189–197.

McCloskey, J. C., & Bulechek, G. M. (2000). (Eds). *Nursing interventions classifications (NIC)* (3rd ed) St. Louis: Mosby.

O'Grady, E. T. (1999). Low back pain. An evidence-based approach. *Advance for Nurse Practitioners, 7*(8), 55–57, 80.

Pasero, C., & McCaffery, M. (2001). Pain control. Selective COX-2 inhibitors. *American Journal of Nursing, 101*(4), 55–56.

Ramsburg, K. L. (2000). Rheumatoid arthritis. *American Journal of Nursing, 100*(11), 40–43.

Sharkey, N. A., Williams, N. I., & Guerin, J. B. (2000). The role of exercise in the prevention and treatment of osteoporosis and osteoarthritis. *Nursing Clinics of North America, 35*(1), 209–221.

Wade, C. F. (2000). Keeping Lyme disease at bay. *American Journal of Nursing, 100*(7), 26–31.

CHAPTER 29

Armstrong, T. S., & Gilbert, M. R. (1998). Chemotherapy of astrocytomas: An overview. *Seminars in Oncology Nursing, 14*(1), 18–25.

Barker, E. (1999). Brain attack! A call to action. *RN, 62*(5), 54–57.

Bohan, E. M. (1998). Neurosurgical management of patients with central nervous system malignancies. *Seminars in Oncology Nursing, 14*(1), 8–17.

Bullock, B. A. & Henze, R. L. (2000). *Focus on pathophysiology.* Philadelphia: Lippincott.

Crigger, N., & Forbes, W. (1997). Assessing neurologic function in older adults. *American Journal of Nursing, 97*(3), 37–40.

Fowler, S., Cicoca, R., & Keller, I. (1999). Patient care following carotid endarterectomy. *MEDSURG Nursing, 8*(1), 47–52.

Hock, N. H. (1999). Brain attack: The stroke continuum. *Nursing Clinics of North America, 34*(3), 689–713.

Kee, J. L. (2001). *Handbook of laboratory and diagnostic tests* (4th ed.). Upper Saddle River: Prentice Hall.

McCloskey, J. C., & Bulechek, G. M. (2000). (Eds.). *Nursing interventions classification (NIC)* (3rd ed) St. Louis: Mosby.

Mower-Wade, D., Cavanaugh, M. & Bush, D. (2001). Protecting a patient with a ruptured cerebral aneurysm. *Nursing 2001, 31*(2), 52–58.

Myers, F. (2000). Meningitis: The fears, the facts. *RN, 63*(11), 52–57.

Porth, C. (1998). *Pathophysiology: Concepts of altered health states* (5th ed.). Philadelphia: Lippincott.

Shafer, P. O. (1999). New therapies in the management of acute and cluster seizures and seizure emergencies. *Journal of Neuroscience Nursing, 31*(4), 224–230.

Smillova, A. & Walker, E. (2000). Meningococcemia: A critical care emergency. *Critical Care Nurse, 20*(5), 28–37.

CHAPTER 30

Buckley, D. A., & Guanci, M. M. (1999). Spinal cord trauma. *Nursing Clinics of North America, 34*(3), 661–687.

Cunning, S. (2000). When the Dx is myasthenia gravis. *RN, 64*(4), 26–31.

Deglin, J. H., & Vallerand, A. H. (2001). *Davis's drug guide for nurses* (7th ed.) Philadelphia: Davis.

Goldsmith, C. (1999). Parkinson's disease. *American Journal of Nursing, 99*(2), 46–47.

Herndon, C. M., Young, K., & Herndon, A. D. (2000). Parkinson's disease revisited. *Journal of Neuroscience Nursing, 32*(4), 216–221.

Lueckenotte, A. G. (2000). *Gerontologic nursing* (2nd ed.) St. Louis: Mosby.

Maier-Lorentz, M. M. (2000). Effective nursing interventions for the management of Alzheimer's disease. *Journal of Neuroscience Nursing, 32*(3), 153–157.

Maloni, H. W. (2000). Pain in multiple sclerosis: An overview of its nature and management. *Journal of Neuroscience Nursing, 32*(3), 139–144.

McCloskey, J. C., & Bulechek, G. M. (Eds.). (1996). *Nursing interventions classification (NIC)* (3rd ed.). St. Louis: Mosby.

Porth, C. (1998). *Pathophysiology: Concepts of altered health states* (5th ed.). Philadelphia: Lippincott.

Sullivan, M. P., & Sharts-Hopko, N. C. (2000). Multiple sclerosis: Preventing the downward spiral. *American Journal of Nursing, 100*(8), 26–33.

Trigeminal Neuralgia Resources. (2001). Trigeminal neuralgia. Available online at *www.facial-neuralgia.org/conditions/tn.html.*

Worf, N. (2000). Tetanus—still a problem. *RN, 63*(6), 44–49.

World Health Organization. (2000). Variant Creutzfeldt–Jakob disease (vCJD). Available online at *www.who.int/inf-fs/en/fact180.html*.

Worsham, T. L. (2000). Easing the course of Guillain–Barré syndrome. *RN, 63*(3), 46–52.

CHAPTER 31

Braunwald, E., Fauci, A. S., Kasper, D. L., Hauser, S. L., Longo, D. L., & Jameson, J. L. (Eds.). (2001). *Harrison's principles of internal medicine* (15th ed.). New York: McGraw-Hill.

Boyd-Monk, H. (1999). Actionstat: Retinal detachment. *Nursing, 29*(9), 33.

Bullock, B. A., & Henzwe, R. L. (2000). *Focus on pathophysiology*. Philadelphia: Lippincott.

Felis, M. J. (2000). Protocol: Acute otitis media. *Lippincott's Primary Care Practice, 4*(5), 529–533.

Fenn, A. R., & Fitzgerald, M. A. (2000). Pharmacology update: Antimicrobial choices in the treatment of acute otitis media. *Lippincott's Primary Care Practice, 4*(5), 515–523.

Fontaine, K. L. (2000). *Healing practices: Alternative therapies for nursing*. Upper Saddle River, NJ: Prentice Hall Health.

Gallo, J. J., Fulmer, T., Paveza, G. J., & Reichel, W. (2000). *Handbook of geriatric assessment* (3rd ed.). Gaithersburg, MD: Aspen.

Kane, W. (1999). Sight specific . . . sight loss. *Nursing Times, 95*(32), 54–55.

Lehne, R. A. (2001). *Pharmacology for nursing care* (4th ed.). Philadelphia: Saunders.

LeMone, P., & Burke, K. M. (2000). *Medical surgical nursing: Critical thinking in client care* (2nd ed). Upper Saddle River, NJ: Prentice Hall.

Lucas, L. J., & Matthews-Flint, L. J. (2001). Photo guide: Sound advice about hearing aids. *Nursing, 31*(2), 59–61.

Mahoney, J. (2000). Hearing loss and assessment: A concern for all. *Nursing Spectrum, 13*(1), 20–22.

McCloskey, J. C., & Bulechek, G. M. (Eds.). (1996). *Nursing interventions classification (NIC)* (2nd ed.). St. Louis: Mosby.

Mead, M. (2000). Procedures for practice nurses. The symptom earache. *Practice Nurse, 19*(10), 514, 516.

Meeker, M. H., & Rothrock, J. C. (1999). *Alexander's care of the patient in surgery* (11th ed.). St. Louis: Mosby.

Robins, R., & Mangan, M. (1999). Seen and not heard. *Nursing Times, 95*(37), 30–32.

Smith, D. (2000). I can see clearly now. *Nursing Standard, 14*(41), 18–19.

Thompson, J. (2000). Otitis media. *Community Practitioner, 73*(7), 692–693.

Tupper, S. Z. (1999). When the inner ear is out of balance: Ménière's disease. *RN, 62*(11), 36–40.

Woo, E. (2001). Device safety. Eyeing the perils of LASIK surgery. *Nursing, 31*(5), 28.

CHAPTER 32

Albaugh, J. (1999). Erectile dysfunction. *Advance for Nurse Practitioners, 7*(4), 43–44.

Greifzu, S. P. (2000). Oncology today: Prostate cancer. *RN, 63*(6), 26–31.

Hagan, C. J., & White, J. P. (1999). Common but curable (testicular cancer). *Advance for Nurse Practitioners, 7*(4), 25–26, 28, 30.

Klingman, L. (1999). Assessing the male genitalia. *American Journal of Nursing, 99*(7), 47–50.

McCloskey, J. C. & Bulechek, G. M. (Eds.). (1996). *Nursing interventions classification (NIC)* (3rd ed.). St. Louis: Mosby.

Miller, K. M. (1999). Testicular torsion. *American Journal of Nursing, 99*(6), 33.

Pheiffer, G. M., & Giacomarra, M. (1999). Benign prostatic hyperplasia. *Advance for Nurse Practitioners, 7*(4), 31–36.

Zaccagnini, M. (1999). Prostate cancer. *American Journal of Nursing, 99*(4), 34–35.

CHAPTER 33

Hoskins, C. N., & Haber, J. (2000). Adjusting to breast cancer. *American Journal of Nursing, 100*(4), 26–32.

Klingman, L. (1999). Assessing the female reproductive system. *American Journal of Nursing, 99*(8), 37–43.

Machia, J. (2001). Breast cancer: Risk, prevention, & tamoxifen. *American Journal of Nursing, 101*(4), 26–35.

McCloskey, J. C., & Bulechek, G. M. (Eds.). (1996). *Nursing interventions classification (NIC)* (3rd ed.). St. Louis: Mosby.

McDermott-Webster, M. (1999). The HPV epidemic. *American Journal of Nursing, 99*(3), 24L, 24N.

McKay, S. J. (2000). Why we need to worry about warts. *RN, 63*(9), 68–72.

Schott-Baer, D., & Kotal, B. (2000). Frequency and effectiveness of self-care actions and menopause symptoms of middle-aged working women. *MEDSURG Nursing, 9*(6), 302–307.

Sharts-Hopko, N. C. (2001). Hysterectomy for nonmalignant conditions. *American Journal of Nursing, 101*(9), 32–40.

Thomas, S. (2000). Oncology today: Breast cancer. *RN, 63*(4), 40–45.

Thomas, S., & Greifzu, S. P. (2000). Oncology today: Breast reconstruction. *RN, 63*(4), 45–47.

Tiedemann, D. (2000). Oncology today: Ovarian cancer. *RN, 63*(10), 36–41.

Zack, E. (2001). Mammography and reduced breast cancer mortality rates. *MEDSURG Nursing, 10*(1), 17–21.

CHAPTER 34

Be careful out there. (2000). *Nursing, 30*(1), 10.

Centers for Disease Control and Prevention. (1998). 1998 Guidelines for treatment of sexually transmitted diseases. *Morbidity & Mortality Weekly Report, 47*(RR-1), 1–128.

Centers for Disease Control and Prevention. (2000). Tracking the hidden epidemics: Trends in STDs in the United States. Available online at *www.cdc.gov*.

Coombes, R. (2000). Return of the dirty dozen: Sexually transmitted infections. *Nursing Times, 96*(36), 12–13.

Klingman, L. (1999). Assessing the male genitalia. *American Journal of Nursing, 99*(7), 47–50.

Klingman, L. (1999). Assessing the female reproductive system. *American Journal of Nursing, 99*(8), 37–43.

McCloskey, J. C., & Bulechek, G. M. (Eds.). (1996). *Nursing interventions classification (NIC)* (3rd ed.). St. Louis: Mosby.

McDermott-Webster, M. (1999). The HPV epidemic. *American Journal of Nursing, 99*(3), 24L, 24N.

McKay, S. J. (2000). Why we need to worry about warts. *RN, 63*(9), 68–72.

Nicholas, H. (1998). Sexually transmitted diseases. Gonorrhoea: Symptoms and treatment. *Nursing Times, 94*(8), 52–54.

Sandhaus, S. (2001). Genital herpes in pregnant and nonpregnant women. *Nurse Practitioner: American Journal of Primary Health Care, 26*(4), 15–16, 21–22, 25–27+.

Sheff, B. (2001). Microbe of the month. *Chlamydia trachomatis. Nursing, 31*(1), 71.

Sheff, B. (2000). Microbe of the month. *Neisseria gonorrhoeae. Nursing, 30*(7), 76.

Slade, C. S. (1998). HPV and cervical cancer: Breaking the deadly link. *Advance for Nurse Practitioners, 6*(3), 39–40, 42, 54.

Weston, A. (1998). Striking back at syphilis. *Nursing Times, 94*(3), 30–32.

CULTURAL CARE STRATEGIES

ASSESSING COMMUNICATION VARIABLES FROM A CULTURAL PERSPECTIVE

Bechtel, G., & Davidhizar, R. (1998). Culture, personal space, and health. *Competence Matters, 1*(2), 20. Birmingham, AL: University of Alabama at Birmingham.

Giger, J., & Davidhizar, R. (1999). *Transcultural nursing: Assessment and intervention.* St. Louis, MO: Mosby Year Book.

Meleis, A. (1996). Arab Americans. In J. Lipson, S. Dibble, & P. Minarik (Eds.), *Culture and nursing care.* San Francisco: UCSF Nursing Press

APPRECIATING VARIATIONS IN FACIAL EXPRESSION WHEN RELATING TO THE CLIENT FROM ANOTHER CULTURE

Argyle, M., & Dean, J. (1965). Eye contact, distance and affiliation. *Sociometry, 28,* 285–304.

Giger, J., & Davidhizar, R. (1999). *Transcultural nursing: Assessment and intervention.* St. Louis, MO: Mosby Year Book.

Henderson, G., & Primeaux, M. (1981). *Transcultural health care.* Menlo Park, CA: Addison-Wesley.

Sue, E., & Sue, E. (1990). *Counseling the culturally different: Theory and practice,* (2nd ed.). New York: John Wiley & Sons.

RESPONDING TO PAIN AS A CROSS-CULTURAL VARIABLE

Davidhizar, R., Shearer, R., & Giger, J. (1997, Nov./Dec.) Pain and the culturally diverse client. *Today's Surgical Nurse,* 35–38.

Giger, J., & Davidhizar, R. (1999). *Transcultural nursing: Assessment and intervention.* St. Louis, MO: Mosby Year Book.

Levy, R. (1993). *Ethnic and racial differences in responses to medicines.* Reston, VA: National Pharmaceutical Council.

Lipton, J., & Marbach, J. (1984). Ethnicity and the pain experience. *Social Science Medicine, 17,* 1279–1298.

McCaffery, M., & Thorpe, D. (1988). Differences in perception of pain and the development of adversarial relationships among health care providers. *Advances in Pain Research and Therapy, 11,* 113–122.

Prebe, L., Guveyan, J., & Sinatra, R. (1992). Client characteristics influencing postoperative pain management. St. Louis, MO: Mosby Year Book, 140–150.

Salerno, E. (1995). Race, culture and medications. *Journal of Emergency Nurses, 21,* 560–562.

RESPONDING TO BELIEFS RELATED TO DEATH, DYING, AND GRIEF FROM A CULTURAL PERSPECTIVE

Dowd, S., Poole, V., Davidhizar, R., & Giger, J. (1998). Death, dying, and grief in a transcultural context: Application of the Giger and Davidhizar Assessment Model. *The Hospice Journal, 13*(4), 33–55.

Perry, H. (1993). *Mourning and funeral customs of African Americans. Ethnic variations in dying, death, and grief* (pp. 51–67). Washington, DC: Taylor & Francis.

Rosenblatt, P., Walsh, R., & Jackson, D. (1976). *Grief and mourning in cultural perspective.* New Haven, CT: HRAF Press.

Some, M. (1993). *Ritual: Power, healing, and community.* Swan Raven and Company.

Talamanes, M., Lawler, W., & Espino, D. (1995). Hispanic American elders: Caregiving norms surrounding dying and the use of hospice services. *The Hospice Journal, 10*(2), 35–49.

CONSIDERING CULTURAL VARIATIONS RELATED TO ENVIRONMENTAL CONTROL

Giger, J., & Davidhizar, R. (1999). *Transcultural nursing: Assessment and intervention.* St. Louis, MO: Mosby Year Book.

Kluckhohn, A., & Strodtbeck, F. (1961). *Variations in value orientations.* New York: Row, Peterson.

Rotter, J. (1966). Generalized expectancies for internal versus external locus of reinforcement. *Psychological Monographs, 80*(1), 1–28.

ASSESSING THE CLIENT FROM ANOTHER CULTURE IN A SOCIAL CONTEXT

Giger, J., & Davidhizar, R. (1999). *Transcultural nursing: Assessment and intervention.* St. Louis, MO: Mosby Year Book.

Friedman, M. (1986). *Family nursing: Theory and assessment.* East Norwalk, CT: Appleton-Century-Crofts.

Murray, R., Meili, P., & Zentner, J. (1993). The family—the basic unit for the developing person. In Murray, R., & Zentner, J. (Eds.), *Nursing concepts for health promotion* (5th ed.). Englewood Cliffs, NJ: Prentice Hall.

INTEGRATING CULTURAL DIVERSITY IN CLIENT EDUCATION

Davidhizar, R., & Brownson, K. (2000). Literacy, cultural diversity, and client education. *Home HealthCare Management Practitioner, 12*(2), 38–44.

Doak, D., Doak, L., & Root, J. (1996). *Teaching clients with low literacy skills* (2nd ed.). Philadelphia: Lippincott.

CONSIDERING CULTURAL VARIATIONS RELATED TO TIME

Buccalo, S. (1997). Window on another world: An "English" nurse looks at the Amish culture and their health care beliefs. *Journal of Multicultural Nursing and Health, 3*(2), 53–58.

Davidhizar, R., Bechtel, G., & Giger, J. (1999, April). The influence of time and culture on health patterns. *Competency Matters, 2*(1), 13–15.

Giger, J., & Davidhizar, R. (1999). *Transcultural nursing: Assessment and intervention.* St. Louis, MO: Mosby Year Book.

CONSIDERING CULTURAL VARIATIONS RELATED TO SPACE

Bechtel, G., & Davidhizar, R. (1998). Culture, personal space, and health. *Competence Matters, 1*(2), 20. Birmingham, AL: University of Alabama at Birmingham.

Giger, J., & Davidhizar, R. (1999). *Transcultural nursing: Assessment and intervention.* St. Louis, MO: Mosby Year Book.

Hall, E. (1966). *Hidden dimension.* New York: Doubleday.

RECOGNIZING BIOLOGICAL VARIATIONS AMONG CULTURES

American Diabetic Association. (2001). *Vital statistics.* Alexandria, VA: Author.

Centers for Disease Control and Prevention. (2000a, December). CDC surveillance summaries, Dec. 2000, Tuberculosis morbidity in the United States: Final data, 2000. *Morbidity and Mortality Weekly Report, 40*(SS3), 23–28.

Centers for Disease Control and Prevention. (2000b, December). *Diabetes Surveillance Report, 2000:* Atlanta, GA: U.S., Department of Health and Human Services.

Centers for Disease Control and Prevention. (2000c, December). *HIV/AIDS surveillance report: U.S. HIV and AIDS cases reported through December 2000, 9*(2).

Joint National Committee. (1997). *The report of the Joint National Committee on Detection, Evaluation and Treatment of High Blood Pressure.* Washington, D.C.: National Institutes of Health, National Heart, Lung, and Blood Institute.

National Center for Health Statistics. (2001). *Health, United States, 2001* (DHHS Publication No. PHS 91–1232). Hyattsville, Md: Public Health Service.

Zhou, H. H., Koshakji, R. J. P., Silberstein, D. J., Wilkinson, G. R., & Wood, A. J. J. (1989). Racial differences in drug response: Altered sensitivity to and clearance of propranolol in men of Chinese descent as compared with American whites. *New England Journal of Medicine, 320,* 565–570.

Credits

Art Credits

CHAPTER 1 1-3: Betty Gee

CHAPTER 6 6-9: © Ronald Melzack, 1970; 6-10: Addison-Wesley; 6-12: World Health Organization

CHAPTER 7 7-1: Saint Francis Medical Center; 7-7: Southwest Texas Methodist Hospital; Box 7-3A: Linda Harris

CHAPTER 8 Box 8-2: American Cancer Society; Box 8-7: American Cancer Society

CHAPTER 9 9-1: Courtesy Partnership for Caring, 1620 Eye Street, Suite 202, Washington, DC 20006, 1-800-989-9455

CHAPTER 10 10-1: Biomed Arts Assoc./Wendy Hiller Gee/Kristin Mount

CHAPTER 11 Box 11-3: Alcoholics Anonymous

CHAPTER 14 14-1: Biomed Arts Assoc./Wendy Hiller Gee

CHAPTER 16 16-3, 16-6: Biomed Arts Assoc./Wendy Hiller Gee/Kristin Mount

CHAPTER 17 17-3: Biomed Arts Assoc./Wendy Hiller Gee/Kristin Mount

CHAPTER 18 18-1: © Todd Buck; 18-4: U.S. Dept. of Agriculture

CHAPTER 19 19-5: Biomed Arts Assoc./Wendy Hiller Gee/Kristin Mount

CHAPTER 20 20-5: The Left Coast Group; 20-10: Linda Harris

CHAPTER 21 21-2: Biomed Arts Assoc./Wendy Hiller Gee; 21-5: The Left Coast Group; 21-16: Biomed Arts Assoc./Wendy Hiller Gee/Kristin Mount

CHAPTER 22 22-2, 22-5: © Todd Buck; 22-9: GTS Graphics/Kristin N. Mount; Box 22-1A: Addison-Wesley; 22-1A-L: GTS Graphics/Kristin N. Mount

CHAPTER 23 23-1: Addison-Wesley; 23-3: Bullock & Henze, Focus on Pathophysiology (2000). Philadelphia: Lippincott, Williams & Wilkins; Box 23-4: Linda Harris

CHAPTER 24 24-3: Biomed Arts Assoc./Wendy Hiller Gee/Kristin Mount

CHAPTER 25 25-1A: © Todd Buck

CHAPTER 26 26-10: Addison-Wesley

CHAPTER 27 27-1: © Todd Buck/Nea Hanscomb; 27-2: Biomed Arts Assoc./Wendy Hiller Gee/Nea Hanscomb

CHAPTER 28 28-9: Biomed Arts Assoc./Wendy Hiller Gee/Kristin Mount

CHAPTER 30 30-2: Biomed Arts Assoc./Kristin Mount

CHAPTER 33 33-1, 33-4: Biomed Arts Assoc./Wendy Hiller Gee/Nea Hanscomb; 33-13: Biomed Arts Assoc./Wendy Hiller Gee/Kristin Mount

Photo Credits

CHAPTER 6 6-8: Rehabilicare, Inc., Tampa, FL

CHAPTER 7 Box 7-1A, B: © Elena Dorfman/Benjamin/Cummings

CHAPTER 8 8-2: Simon Fraser/Photo Researchers, Inc.

CHAPTER 10 10-8: © Spencer Grant/Photo Researchers, Inc.; 10-9: KCI Roto Rest® Delta Kinetic Treatment Table Courtesy of Kinetic Concepts, Inc., San Antonio, TX

CHAPTER 13 13-5: Photo Researchers, Inc.; 13-8: © Alain McLaughlin/Benjamin/Cummings/Reaction Images

CHAPTER 14 14-2, 14-3: NMSB, Custom Medical Stock Photos, Inc.; 14-6: American Academy of Dermatology; 14-7: Caliendo/Custom Medical Stock Photo, Inc.; Box 14-6: Courtesy of Karen Kennedy, RN, FPN

CHAPTER 15 15-2, 15-4: Courtesy of William Dominic

CHAPTER 16 16-4: Lester V. Bergman/CORBIS; 16-5: NMSB, Custom Medical Stock Photos, Inc.; 16-7: Courtesy of Dr. Charles Wilson

CHAPTER 17 17-5: Harry Przekop/Medichrome/The Stock Shop, Inc.

CHAPTER 18 18-3: © Elena Dorfman/Benjamin/Cummings; 18-5: John Radcliffe Hospital/Science Photo Library; Proc. 18-1: © Elena Dorfman/Addison-Wesley-Longman

CHAPTER 20 20-6: Courtesy of Carol Williams

CHAPTER 21 21-7, 21-11: NMSB, Custom Medical Stock Photos, Inc.

CHAPTER 22 22-27A: Courtesy of Baxter, Deerfield, IL; 22-27B: Courtesy of Medtronic Inc., Minneapolis, MN

CHAPTER 23 23-2: © Elena Dorfman/Addison-Wesley-Longman

CHAPTER 24 24-7: NMSB, Custom Medical Stock Photos, Inc.

CHAPTER 26 26-6B: NMSB, Custom Medical Stock Photos, Inc.; 26-14: Michal Heron; 26-15: Courtesy of University of CA Davis Medical Center; Box 26-9A: NMSB, Custom Medical Stock Photos, Inc.

CHAPTER 28 28-7: Custom Medical Stock Photos, Inc.; 28-8: Photo Researchers, Inc.

CHAPTER 29 29-14: Todd Hammond

CHAPTER 30 30-3, 30-5: Phototake NYC

CHAPTER 31 31-4: © Elena Dorfman/Benjamin/Cummings; 31-6: Medical Images, Inc.; 31-7A, B: Custom Medical Stock Photos, Inc.; 31-12: National Eye Institute; 31-16: Medical Images, Inc.

CHAPTER 33 33-15: Custom Medical Stock Photos, Inc.

CHAPTER 34 34-1: Camera MD Studios; 34-2: Photo Researchers, Inc.; 34-3: Custom Medical Stock Photos, Inc.; 34-4: Photo Researchers, Inc.

AUTHOR PHOTOGRAPHS: FM-1: Lamping Photography; FM-2: MU Sinclair School of Nursing; FM-3: Yeung & Leix LLC

All photographs/illustrations not credited on page, adjacent to the piece, or credited above, were photographed/rendered on assignment and are property of Pearson Education/Prentice Hall Health. These include illustrations and photographs supplied by the following illustrators and photographers.

Illustrators

Christopher Burke, Barbara Cousins, Romaine LoPrete, Kristin Mount, Nea Hanscomb, Precision Graphics

Photographers

Ron May, © Alain McLaughlin/Benjamin/Cummings, © Richard Tauber/Addison-Wesley-Longman, © Richard Tauber/Benjamin/Cummings, © Carroll Weiss

Content Credits

CHAPTER 1 Box 1-3: National Association for Practical Nurse Education and Services (NAPNES) (1999). Standards of Practice for Licensed Practical/Vocational Nurses. NAPNES: Silver Springs, MD

CHAPTER 9 Table 9-2: Lipson, J.G., Diddle, S.L., & Minarik, P.A. (Eds) (1999). Culture & Nursing Care: A Pocket Guide. San Francisco: UCSF Nursing Press

CHAPTER 17 Box 17-3, Box 17-5, Table 17-1, Table 17-7: Adapted from American Diabetes Association, 2000, Diabetes Care, 23 (Supplement 1)

CHAPTER 5 THROUGH 34: Selected classification labels. McCloskey, J.C. & Bulechek, G.M. (Eds.) (2000). Nursing interventions classification (NIC) (3rd ed.). Philadelphia: Saunders

Index

Pages followed by f indicate figure; those followed by t indicate table.

A-beta fibers
    in gate-control theory of pain, 103–4,
        104f
    in pain transduction, 102
A-delta fibers, in pain transduction, 102
ABCs, in emergency care assessment, 213
Abdomen
    acute, 466
    physical examination
        exterior, 55–56
        four quadrants, 55, 56f
Abrasions, 212f
Abscess
    anorectal, 487–88
    brain, 817t, 818
    defined, 239
    incision and drainage for, 239
    lung, 689–90
    pancreatic, 444
    peritonsillar, 658, 658f
Absorbents, for diarrhea, 457t
Acceptance, in death and dying, 184
Accidents (*See also* Motor vehicle accidents
        (MVAs); Trauma)
    in young adults, 16
Accommodation, in vision, 857
ACE inhibitors (*See also* angiotensin-
        converting enzyme inhibitors)
Acetaminophen (Tylenol)
    actions of, 107
    client education, 108t
    for inflammation, 240
    nursing responsibilities, 108t
    purpose of, 108t
Acetylcholine, in Parkinson's disease, 834
Acetylsalicylic acid (*See* Aspirin)
Acid-base imbalance, 88–97
    assessment, 90–91, 91f
        arterial blood gases (ABGs), 90–91,
            91f
        serum electrolytes, 93

metabolic acidosis, 91–93
    causes of, 92t
    collaborative care, 92–93
    defined, 89, 90f
    laboratory values, 92t
    manifestations of, 92t
    nursing care, 93
        assessment, 93
        decreased cardiac output, 93
        discharge considerations, 93
        excess fluid volume, 93
        risk for injury, 93
    pathophysiology, 91–92
metabolic alkalosis, 93–95
    causes of, 92t
    collaborative care, 94
    defined, 89, 90f
    laboratory values, 92t
    manifestations of, 92t
    nursing care, 94–95
        assessment, 94
        discharge considerations, 94–95
        fluid volume deficiency, 94
        impaired gas exchange, 94
    pathophysiology, 94
mixed disorders, 90
primary disorders, 89–90
respiratory acidosis, 95–96
    acute, 95
    causes of, 92t
    chronic, 95
    collaborative care, 95
    defined, 89, 90f
    laboratory values, 92t
    manifestations of, 92t
    nursing care, 95–96
        assessment, 95
        discharge considerations, 96
        impaired gas exchange, 95
        ineffective airway clearance, 96
    pathophysiology, 95
respiratory alkalosis, 96–97
    causes of, 92t
    collaborative care, 96
    defined, 89, 90f
    laboratory values, 92t
    manifestations, 92t

nursing care, 96
    discharge considerations, 96
    ineffective breathing patterns, 96
    pathophysiology, 96
    role of potassium in, 78
    types of, 89–90
Acid-base regulation, 88–89
    buffer systems, 88–89
    renal system in, 89
    respiratory system in, 89
Acid-fast bacilli smear, in tuberculosis,
        692
Acidosis (*See also* Metabolic acidosis;
        Respiratory acidosis)
    defined, 89
Acne, 302, 303f
Acoustic neuroma, 802t
Acquired immunodeficiency syndrome
        (AIDS) (*See also* HIV infection)
    client rights and, 10
    legal considerations with, 10–11
    opportunistic infections, 283–85
        gastrointestinal system, 284–85
        neurologic system, 285, 290–91
        pharmacology for, 287, 288t
        respiratory system, 283–84, 290
        strategies to avoid, 291–92
    secondary cancers
        Kaposi's sarcoma, 285
        lymphomas, 285
Action potential, in cardiac conduction
        system, 539–40
Activated partial thromboplastin time
        (APTT), 614
Active transport
    defined, 66
    sodium-potassium pump, 66, 67f
Acupuncture, in pain management,
        111–12
Acute abdomen, 466
Acute lymphocytic leukemia (ALL), 641t
Acute myelocytic leukemia (AML), 641t
Acute respiratory distress syndrome
        (ARDS), 722
    manifestations of, 722
Acute tubular necrosis (ATN), 523
Acyclovir (Zovirax), 255t

Adaptation, to chronic illness, 25
Addiction, defined, 222
Addison's disease, 359–61
    Addisonian crisis, 359
    collaborative care, 359–61
        diagnostic tests, 359
        nutritional issues, 360–61
        pharmacology, 359, 360t
    complications of, 359
    manifestations of, 359f
    nursing care, 360–61
        activity intolerance, 360
        assessment, 359, 360f
        discharge considerations, 361
    pathophysiology, 359
Adenohypophysis, 342
Adenoids, 656
Adipose tissue, 398
Adrenal cortex
    functions of, 342–43
    hormones of, 343t
Adrenal glands
    disorders of
        Addison's disease, 359–61
        Cushing's syndrome, 356–59
        pheochromocytoma, 361
    functions of, 342–43
    hormones of, 343t
Adrenal medulla
    disorders of, pheochromocytoma, 361
    functions of, 343–44
    hormones of, 343t
Adrenalectomy, 357
Adrenergic drugs, for cardiogenic shock, 208
Adrenocorticotropic hormone (ACTH), function of, 343t
Adult clients, 16–26
    developmental tasks of, 16–19
        middle adult, 17–18
        older adult, 18–19 (See also Older adults)
        young adult, 16–17
    health in, 22–23
    illness in, 23–26
    middle adult, 17–18
        healthy behaviors in, 19f
        physical changes in, 18t
    young adult, 16–17
        healthy behaviors in, 17f
        physical status and change in, 16t
Adult respiratory distress syndrome (ARDS), 204, 722
Advance directives, 10, 186, 187f, 551
Advocate, nurse as, 3
    in home health care, 35, 36f

Afterload, in cardiac output, 541
Age differences
    affect on health, 23
    in pain response, 106
Agranulocytosis, 639–40
AIDS (See Acquired immunodeficiency syndrome (AIDS))
AIDS dementia complex (ADC), 285
Airborne precautions, in infection control, 257t
Airway management, in respiratory failure, 722–23, 723f
Airway obstruction, in trauma clients, 211, 664
Albumin, serum, normal, 508t
Alcohol
    as cancer risk factor, 159
    hypertension and, 598
    oral cancer and, 405–6
Alcohol abuse, 222–26
    alcoholic cirrhosis, 225, 436, 442–43
    alcoholic hepatitis, 225, 433
    CAGE questionnaire for, 231
    fetal alcohol syndrome, 226, 226f
    hypocalcemia and, 82
    long-term effect os, 225–26
    magnesium imbalance and, 87
    pattern of use
        chronic phase, 225
        crucial phase, 225
        early alcoholic, 225
        prealcoholic, 225
    phosphorous imbalance and, 88
    as surgical risk, 130t
    tolerance, 223
    treatment, 229
    withdrawal, 223–24
        treatment of, 229
Alcohol withdrawal delirium, 224
Alcohol withdrawal syndrome, 223–24
Alcoholics Anonymous (AA), 229, 230f
Aldosterone
    function of, 343, 343t
    renin-angiotensin-aldosterone system, 67, 68f, 496
Alkalosis (See also Metabolic alkalosis; Respiratory alkalosis)
    defined, 89
Alkylating agents, in chemotherapy, 166t
Allergen, defined, 266
Allergic reactions (See Hypersensitivity reactions)
Allergy
    diagnostic tests for, 275
    latex, 274–75, 274f
Allodynia, defined, 106

Allograft, 277, 279–80
Allopurinol, for gout, 781, 782t
Alopecia
    in cancer treatment, 650
    coping with, 650
    defined, 52
Alpha-1 blockers, for benign prostatic hypertrophy, 887
Alpha-adrenergic blockers, for diabetes mellitus, 601t
    for hypertension, 601t
Alpha-glucoside inhibitors, for diabetes mellitus, 376t
Altered level of consciousness, 796, 797f
    abnormal posturing
        decerebrate, 799f
        decorticate, 799f
    collaborative care
        etiology, 796
        Glasgow Coma Scale for, 796, 798t
    levels of, 57
    nursing care, 799–800
        assessment, 57, 799, 799f
        imbalanced nutrition, 800
        impaired physical mobility, 800
        impaired skin integrity, 800
        ineffective breathing pattern, 800
        ineffective tissue perfusion, 799–800
        risk for infection, 800
Alternative therapies (See Complementary and alternative medicine (CAM))
Alveoli, 680, 681f
Alzheimer's disease, 828–31
    collaborative care, 828–31
        diagnostic tests, 828–29
        pharmacology, 829
    defined, 828
    nursing care, 829–31
        assessment, 829, 829f
        caregiver strain, 830
        discharge considerations, 830, 830f, 831f
        disturbed thought processes, 829–30
        self-care deficits, 830
    pathophysiology, 828
    stages of, 828, 829f
Amantadine (Symmetrel), 255t, 836t
Amebiasis, 470t
Amenorrhea, 923
American Nurses Association (ANA)
    code of ethics, 9
    nursing definition, 4
Amikacin (Amikin), 253t
Amiloride HCl (Midamor), nursing considerations for, 73t

Aminoglycosides
  client education, 253t
  nursing responsibilities, 253t
  purpose of, 253t
Amoxicillin (Amoxil), 252t
Amphetamines, abuse of, 223t, 227
Amphotericin B (Fungizone), 251, 255t
Ampicillins, 252t
Amputation, 748–52
  closed, 750
  collaborative care, 750–52
    prosthesis, 750
  complications of
    contractures, 749
    delayed healing, 749
    infection, 749
    phantom pain, 749
  defined, 748
  levels of, 749, 749f
  nursing care, 750–52
    assessment, 750–51
    discharge considerations, 752
    disturbed body image, 751
    dysfunctional grieving, 751
    impaired physical mobility, 751
    pain, 751
    risk for infection, 751
  in older adults, 751f
  open, 750
  pathophysiology, 749
  resources for, 752
Amylase, 394
Amyotrophic lateral sclerosis (ALS), 839
Anabolism, 396
  defined, 241
  inflammation and, 241
Anal fissure, 487
Analgesics (See also Pain management,
    pharmacology)
  adjuvant, for cancer pain, 107
  analgesic ceiling, 107
  defined, 107
  equianalgesic dosage chart, 107, 109t, 116
  patient-controlled analgesia (PCA), 108,
    110f
  routes of administration, 107–9, 109t
    intramuscular, 108
    intraspinal, 108–9, 111f
    intravenous, 108, 110f
    nasal, 108
    nerve blocks, 109
    oral, 107
    rectal, 107
    subcutaneous, 108
    sublingual, 108
    transdermal, 107–8, 110f

World Health Organization analgesic
    ladder, 117, 118f
Anastomosis, 414
Androgens, 343, 886, 908
Anemia, 624–34
  aplastic, 627t, 628–29
  blood loss, 624, 627t
  collaborative care, 629–33
    blood transfusion, 630
    diagnostic tests, 629
    dietary management, 629–30
    pharmacology, 629, 630t
  defined, 624
  etiology, 627t
  hemolytic, 627–28, 627t
    acquired, 628
    sickle cell, 627–28, 629f
    thalassemia, 628
  nursing care, 631–32
    activity intolerance, 631–32
    assessment, 631, 632f
    discharge considerations, 633, 633f
    impaired mucous membrane, 632
    self-care deficit, 632–33
  nutritional, 624–26, 627t
    folic acid deficiency, 626, 633–34
    iron deficiency, 624–26
    vitamin B_{12} deficiency, 626
  pathophysiology, 624–29
  pernicious, 626
Anergy, defined, 271
Anesthesia
  conscious sedation, 138
  defined, 137
  general
    administration, 137
    defined, 137
    phases of, 137
  local, defined, 137
  regional, 137–38
    defined, 137
    epidural blocks, 137
    local nerve infiltration, 137
    nerve blocks, 137
    topical, 137
  spinal, 138
  systemic, for cancer pain, 107
  topical, 405t
Anesthesiologist, role of, 138
Aneurysm
  cardiac, 608–11
    abdominal aortic, 609–10, 609f, 609t
    berry, 609
    collaborative care, 610–11
      pharmacology, 610
      surgical treatment, 610, 610f, 611f

  complications of, 609t
  defined, 608, 812
  dissecting, 609f, 609t, 610
  fusiform, 609, 609f
  manifestations of, 609t
  nursing care, 611
    discharge considerations, 611
  pathophysiology, 609–10
  saccular, 609, 609f
  thoracic aortic, 609, 609f, 609t
  ventricular, 564
cerebral, 812–17
  berry, 813f
  cerebral vasospasm in, 813
  collaborative care
    conservative management, 813
    pharmacology, 813
    surgical treatment, 813
  defined, 812
  dissecting, 813f
  fusiform, 813f
  saccular, 813f
  subarachnoid hemorrhage in, 812
  types of, 812, 813f
Anger, in death and dying, 184
Angina pectoris, 554f, 555–62
  collaborative care, 556–62
    diagnostic tests, 556
      angiography, 556, 557f
      cardiac radionuclear scan, 556
      electrocardiogram, 556, 556f
      electrocardiogram, stress, 556
    pharmacology, 557, 557t–558t,
      559
    surgical treatment, 559–60
      coronary artery bypass graft,
        559–60, 560f
      percutaneous transluminal
        coronary angioplasty,
        557f, 559, 559f, 566
  defined, 555
  manifestations of, 556, 556f
  nursing care, 560–62
    assessment, 560, 561f
    discharge considerations, 562
  pathophysiology, 555–56
  Prinzmetal's, 556
  stable, 555
  unstable, 556
Angiography
  for angina pectoris, 556, 557f
  in cancer diagnosis, 162
Angiotensin
  renin-angiotensin-aldosterone system,
    67, 68f, 496
  renin-angiotensin system, 200

Angiotensin-converting enzyme (ACE) inhibitors
  for heart failure, 574t
  for hypertension, 600t
Anion, defined, 64
Ankle fracture, 741t
Ankylosing spondylitis, 783–84
Anorectal disorders, 486–88
  anorectal lesions, 487–88
    anal fissure, 487
    anorectal abscess, 487–88
    anorectal fistula, 488
    pilonidal disease, 488
  hemorrhoids, 486–87
Anorexia
  as an effect of cancer, 161
  near end of life, 188
  nervosa, 400
Anorexia-cachexia syndrome, as an effect of cancer, 161, 161f
Anoxia
  in cerebrovascular accident, 806
  defined, 806
Antacids, for gastritis, 409, 410t
Anti-infective agents, in cirrhosis treatment, 438t
Anti-inflammatory drugs
  for autoimmune disease, 277
  for inflammation, 240–41
  for inflammatory bowel disease (IBD), 473t
  topical, 405t
Antiacne retinoids, 305t
Antibiotic peak and trough levels, in infection diagnosis, 250
Antibiotics, 251, 252t–254t
  bactericidal, 251
  bacteriostatic, 251
  broad-spectrum, 251
  defined, 251
  for inflammation, 240
  narrow-spectrum, 251
  resistance to, 247–48, 251
  selection of, 251
  superinfection, 251
  as surgical risk, 130t
  for transplants, 279
Antibody, defined, 268
Antibody titer testing, diagnostic test for immune system, 271
Anticholinergics
  for asthma, 697t
  for Parkinson's disease, 836t
  as preoperative drug, 129t
Anticholinesterase drugs
  for Alzheimer's disease, 829
  for myasthenia gravis, 837–38, 838t

Anticoagulants
  for cerebrovascular accident, 809
  monitoring of, 614
  for pulmonary embolism, 713–14
  as surgical risk, 130t
  for venous thrombosis, 614, 615t
Anticonvulsants
  for cancer pain, 107
  for increased intracranial pressure (IICP), 798
  in seizure disorder, 814–15, 815t
  for trigeminal neuralgia, 840
Antidepressants
  for cancer pain, 107
  as surgical risk, 130t
Antidiabetics, oral, 372, 376t
Antidiarrheal drugs, 457t
Antidiuretic hormone (ADH), 67–68, 69f
  (See also Syndrome of inappropriate ADH secretion (SIADH))
  in diabetes insipidus, 344
  disorders of, 67–68
  functions of, 67, 343t
  osmolarity and, 344
  syndrome of inappropriate ADH secretion (SIADH), 345–46
  in urine formation, 496
Antiembolic stockings
  for pulmonary embolism, 713
  for varicose veins, 619
  for venous thrombosis, 613, 615–16
Antiemetics, as preoperative drug, 129t
Antifungal agents, 251, 255t, 405t
Antigen, defined, 201, 266
Antihistamines
  for allergic reactions, 275, 275t
  for upper respiratory disorders, 660, 661t
Antihypertensives
  for cerebrovascular accident, 809
  as surgical risk, 130t
Antilymphocyte globulins, for transplants, 279, 280t
Antimalarial drugs, for systemic lupus erythematous (SLE), 778
Antimetabolites, in chemotherapy, 166t
Antimicrobial drugs, 251, 252t–254t, 254
  antibiotics (See Antibiotics)
  antifungal agents, 251, 255t
  antiparasitic agents, 251, 254
  antiviral agents, 251, 255t
  preventive therapy, 251
Antimicrobial drugs, for burn injuries, 330, 331t
  mafenide, 330, 331t
  silver nitrate, 330, 331t
  silver sulfadiazine, 330, 331t

Antinuclear antibodies (ANA)
  in systemic lupus erythematous, 778
  test for, 276–77
Antiparasitic agents, 251, 254
Antiplatelet drugs, for cerebrovascular accident, 808
Antipyretics, for increased intracranial pressure, 798
Antishock trousers (MAST), 205, 206f
Antispasmodics, for spinal cord injury, 844, 845t
Antithyroid drugs, in hyperthyroidism, 348t
Antitoxins, 272
Antitumor antibodies, in chemotherapy, 166t–167t
Antivenins, 272
Antiviral drugs, 251, 255t
  for HIV infection, 286–87, 287t
    non-nucleoside reverse transcriptase inhibitors (NNRTIs), 286–87, 287t
    nucleoside reverse transcriptase inhibitors (NRTIs), 286–87, 287t
    protease inhibitors, 286–87, 287t
  topical, 405t
  for transplants, 279
Antral lavage, 660
Anus, 454, 454f (See also Anorectal disorders)
Anxiolytics, abuse of, 223t, 227
Aortic dissection, 609–10, 609f
Aortic regurgitation, 587t, 589, 589f
Aortic stenosis, 587t, 588, 588f
Aortic valve, 539
Aphasia
  expressive, 807
  global, 807
  receptive, 807
Aphthous ulcers, 404
Apnea, defined, 54
Apocrine sweat glands, 298t, 301
Appendectomy, 465
Appendicitis, 465–66
  collaborative care, 465–66
    surgical treatment, 465
  defined, 465
  nursing care, 465
    discharge considerations, 466
    pain, 465–66
  pathophysiology, 465
Appendix, 454, 454f
  in lymphoid system, 268f
  perforated, 465, 469
Appetite
  obesity and, 397
  regulation of, 397

Aqueous humor, 856–57, 864
Arterial blood gases (ABGs)
  base excess (BE), 91, 91f
  bicarbonate, 91, 91f
  interpretation of, 90–91, 91f
  $PaCO_2$, 90–91, 91f
  PaO_2, 90–91, 91f
Arterial circulation, 596–97
Arterial disorders, 604–11
  arterial thrombus, 605, 605f
  arteriosclerosis, 604–5
  Buerger's disease, 605
  Raynaud's phenomenon, 605
Arterial thrombus, 605, 605f
Arteries, structure of, 596, 596f
Arterioles, 596
Arteriosclerosis, 604–5
  defined, 604
  pathophysiology, 604
  vs. atherosclerosis, 604
Arteriovenous (AV) fistula, in hemodialysis,
    525–26, 526f
Arthralgia, defined, 769
Arthritis (See also specific type)
  acute gouty, 780
  ankylosing spondylitis, 783–84
  osteoarthritis, 769–72
  rheumatoid, 772–78
Arthroplasty
  defined, 770
  for hip fracture, 744, 744f
Arthropods, in infection, 245f
Articulations (See Joints)
Artificial urinary sphincter, for urinary
    incontinence, 892, 894f
Ascites
  cirrhosis and, 436
  defined, 189
Aspiration risk, with surgery, 142
Aspirin
  for inflammation, 240–41, 242t
  for rheumatoid arthritis, 775t
Assessment, 4, 45–58
  comprehensive, defined, 46
  data sources for, 4, 46–47
  defined, 46
  documentation, 57–58
  emergency, defined, 46
  focused, 4
    defined, 46
  health history, 47–48
  initial, 4
  partial, defined, 46
  physical examination, 48–57 (See also
      Physical examination)
  purpose of, 46

  in rehabilitation, 40
  types of, 46
Asthma, 696–700
  acute episodes, 696, 696f
  collaborative care, 696–700
    pharmacology, 697, 697t–698t
    prevention, 697
  defined, 696
  nursing care, 699–700
    anxiety, 699
    assessment, 697, 699f
    discharge considerations, 699–700,
        700f
    fatigue, 699
    ineffective airway clearance,
        698–99
  pathophysiology, 696
  resources for, 700f
  status asthmaticus, 696
Astigmatism, 862t
Ataxia
  defined, 222
  in intoxication, 222
Atelectasis, 705–6
  defined, 143
  manifestations of, 143
  postsurgical prevention, 147
Atherosclerosis, 553, 555
  complementary and alternative medicine,
      555f
  defined, 553
  diabetes mellitus and, 381
  dietary management, 553, 555f
  nursing care, 555
  pathophysiology, 553, 554f
  pharmacology, 553, 555
  risk factors for, 553, 555
  vs. arteriosclerosis, 604
Athlete's foot, 307
Atrial fibrillation, 544t, 546
Atrial flutter, 543t, 545
Atrial natriuretic factor (ANF), 68
Atrioventricular (AV) node, 539
Atrioventricular (AV) valves, 538
Atrioventricular conduction blocks,
    544t–545t, 546–47
  first degree, 544t, 546
  pacemakers for, 549
  second degree, 544t, 546
  third degree, 544t, 546–47
Atrophy, of skin, 299t
Attitudes, related to critical thinking, 7
Audiometry
  for hearing assessment, 879
  impedance, for otitis media, 875
Auditory canal, 872

Aura, in seizure disorder, 814
Auricles, 872
Auscultation
  guidelines for, 49
  for respiratory assessment, 54
Auscultatory gap, in blood pressure, 597
Autoantibodies, defined, 276
Autograft, 277
  in burn injuries, 331–32
  cultured epithelial, in burn injuries, 332
Autoimmune disease, 276–77
  collaborative care
    diagnostic tests, 276–77
    pharmacology, 277
  defined, 266, 276
  nursing care, 277
    discharge considerations, 277
  pathophysiology, 276
Automated external defibrillator (AED),
    548–49, 551
Automatic implantable cardioverter-
    defibrillator (AICD), 549, 551
Automatism
  defined, 814
  in seizure disorder, 814
Autonomic dysreflexia, in spinal cord injury,
    843
Autonomic nervous system (ANS), 794,
    794f
Autotransfusion, 207
Axons, 790, 790f
Azathioprine (Imuran), 279, 280t
Azithromycin (Zithromax), 254t
Azotemia
  defined, 507
  in glomerulonephritis, 507

B

B-cells (See B lymphocytes)
B lymphocytes
  function of, 266, 267t
  memory cells, 267t
  plasma cells, 267t
Babinski reflex, 799f
Back pain, low, 784–85
  collaborative care, 784–85
  discharge considerations, 785
  herniated intervertebral disk in, 847,
      847f
  nursing care, 784–85
    ineffective health maintenance,
        784–85
    pain, 785
  types of, 784

Bacteremia
  defined, 466
  in peritonitis, 466
Bacteria, in infection, 245f
Balance, inner ear and, 873, 877–78
Barbiturates
  abuse of, 223t, 227
  for increased intracranial pressure (IICP), 798
Bargaining, in death and dying, 184
Barrel chest, 54
  in chronic obstructive pulmonary disease, 701, 701f
Bartholin's glands, 909f, 910
Base excess (BE), in arterial blood gases, 91, 91f
Basophils, 639
  laboratory values for, 241t, 639t
Battle's sign
  defined, 795
  in skull fracture, 795
Bell's Palsy, 840–41
Bendroflumethiazide (Naturetin), nursing considerations for, 73t
Benign prostatic hypertrophy (BPH), 497, 887–89, 887f
  collaborative care, 887–89
    complementary and alternative medicine, 887
    diagnostic tests, 887
    surgical treatment, 888, 890f
  manifestations of, 887f
  nursing care, 888–89
    assessment, 888
    discharge considerations, 889, 890f
    excess fluid volume, 889
    impaired urinary elimination, 889
  pathophysiology, 887
Benzodiazepines
  abuse of, 223t, 227
  as preoperative drug, 128t
Beta-adrenergic agonists, for asthma, 697t
Beta-adrenergic blockers
  for angina pectoris, 557, 558t, 559
  in cirrhosis treatment, 438t
  for dysrhythmias, 548t
  for glaucoma, 867t
  for hypertension, 600t
  for hyperthyroidism, 348t
Beta-interferon, for multiple sclerosis, 833
Bicarbonate
  in arterial blood gases (ABGs), 91, 91f
  normal electrolyte laboratory values for, 64t
  ratio to carbonic acid, 89, 89f

Bifurcation, 604
Biguanides, for diabetes mellitus, 376t
Bile, functions of, 426, 427f
Billroth I (gastroduodenostomy), 415t
Billroth II (gastrojejunostomy), 415t
Biofeedback, in pain management, 112
Biologic response modifiers (BRMs), in chemotherapy, 164
Biopsy
  bone marrow, 629, 629f
  in cancer diagnosis, 163
    breast, 914, 915f
    cervical, 934, 934f
  core-needle, 914
  excisional, 914, 914f
  fine-needle aspiration, 914, 914f
  liver, 437, 437f
  renal, 509, 509t
Biotherapy, in cancer treatment, 168, 169f
Bismuth compounds, for gastritis, 411t
Bisphosphonates, for osteoporosis, 762t
Blackouts, caused by alcohol abuse, 225
Bladder
  autonomic nervous system affects on, 794f
  emptying of (See Voiding)
  neurogenic, 497
  palpation of, 56
  structure of, 494–95, 495f
Bladder cancer, 517–21
  collaborative care, 518–20
    pharmacology, 518
    surgical treatment, 518, 518t, 519f
  nursing care, 518–20
    assessment, 518
    case study, 520–21
    discharge considerations, 520
    disturbed body image, 519–20
    impaired skin integrity, 519
    impaired urinary elimination, 518–19
  pathophysiology, 517–18, 517f
  risk factors for, 517
Bladder neck suspension, for urinary incontinence, 499, 501f
Bladder obstruction, in cancer, 178
Bleeding
  anticoagulants and, 607–8
  in leukemia, 644
  precautions, 441, 441f, 607–8, 644
  pressure points to control, 211, 211f
Bleomycin (Blenoxane), in chemotherapy, 167t
Blepharitis, 858
Blepharospasm, defined, 859
Blindness, 871
Block nursing, 33

Blood
  flow of, 596–97
  functions of, 624
Blood-brain barrier, 791
Blood clotting
  in disseminated intravascular coagulopathy, 636
  stages of, 635
Blood glucose homeostasis, 366, 367f
Blood pressure
  defined, 597
  diastolic, 597
  procedure for taking, 602f
  systolic, 597
Blood types, 206
  compatible, 207t
  Rh groups, 206
Blood urea nitrogen (BUN) levels, 496
  in glomerulonephritis, 496, 508t
  normal, 496, 508t
  in renal failure, 524, 524f, 525
Blood viscosity, in peripheral vascular resistance (PVR), 596
Body fluid
  composition, 64
  distribution, 64–65, 65f
  movement, 65–66
    active transport, 66, 67f
    diffusion, 66, 67f
    filtration, 66
    osmosis, 65–66, 66f
  regulation of, 66–68
    antidiuretic hormone (ADH), 67–68, 69f
    atrial natriuretic factor (ANF), 68
    kidneys, 67
    renin-angiotensin-aldosterone system, 67, 68f
    thirst, 66–67, 67f
Body mass index (BMI), 397
Body temperature, altered, surgery and, 142
Bolus, 394
Bone, 732, 732f (See also Fractures)
  classification of, 733f
  types of, 733
    compact, 733
    spongy, 733
Bone density measurement, in osteoporosis, 760
Bone disorders, 757–69
  bone tumors, 766–68
  kyphosis, 758–59
  osteomalacia, 763–64
  osteomyelitis, 764–65
  osteoporosis, 759–63

Bone disorders (continued)
Paget's disease, 763–64
scoliosis, 758–59
Bone marrow
immunological function of, 266, 267f
in leukemia, 640
in lymphoid system, 266, 268f
red, 733
yellow, 733
Bone marrow biopsy, 629, 629f
Bone marrow transplantation (BMT), in
cancer treatment, 168
Bone scan
nursing care for, 765f
in osteomyelitis, 764
Bone tumors, 766–68
benign, 766
classification of, 766, 766t
collaborative care, 766–68
chemotherapy, 767
diagnostic tests, 767
radiation therapy, 767
surgical treatment, 767
manifestations of, 766f
metastatic, 766
nursing care, 767–68
anticipatory grieving, 767
discharge considerations, 767–68
disturbed body image, 767
impaired physical mobility, 767
pain, 767
pathophysiology, 766
primary, 766
Bony callus, 735
Borborygmi
defined, 414
in dumping syndrome, 414
Botulism, 470–71, 470t
Boutonniere deformity, in rheumatoid
arthritis, 773f
Bovine spongiform encephalopathy (BSE),
842
Bowel disorders, 453–88
anorectal, 486–88
anorectal lesions, 487–88
hemorrhoids, 486–87
inflammatory and infectious disorders,
464–77
appendicitis, 465–66
gastroenteritis, 469–71
inflammatory bowel disease, 471–76
peritonitis, 466–69
of intestinal motility and absorption,
455–64
constipation, 458–62
diarrhea, 455–58

fecal incontinence, 463–64
irritable bowel syndrome, 462–63
malabsorption, 464
nursing interventions classification, 488
structural and obstructive, 477–86
bowel obstruction, 482–84
colorectal cancer, 477–82
diverticular disease, 485–86
hernia, 484–85
Bowel obstruction, 482–84
collaborative care, 482–84
gastrointestinal decompression, 482
surgical treatment, 482
defined, 482
functional, 482
manifestations, 483f
mechanical, 482
nursing care, 482–84
deficient fluid volume, 483–84
discharge considerations, 484
ineffective breathing pattern, 484
pathophysiology, 482
Bowel preparation, for surgery, 131
Bowel sounds
hyperactive, 56
hypoactive, 56
paralytic, 56
Bowel surgery
nursing interventions for, 475f, 480f
types of, 474, 474f
Bowel training program, for fecal
incontinence, 463
Brachytherapy
defined, 164
safety principles for, 164f
Bradycardia, defined, 56
Bradykinesia
defined, 834
in Parkinson's disease, 834, 835f
Bradypnea, 54
Brain, 790–91, 791f
blood-brain barrier, 791
blood supply to, 791
brainstem, 790
cerebellum, 790–91
cerebrospinal fluid in, 790–91
cerebrum, 790, 791f
diencephalon, 790
effect of hypertension on, 598t
regions of, 790
Brain abscess, 817t, 818
defined, 818
treatment, 818
Brain attack (See Cerebrovascular accident
(CVA))
Brain death, 217, 217f, 797

Brain herniation, 796–97
Brain tumor, 802–5
benign, 802
classification of, 802t
collaborative care, 802–5
intracranial surgery
burr hole, 803
craniectomy, 804
cranioplasty, 804
craniotomy, 803–4, 803f
debulking, 803
nursing care for, 805f
pharmacology, 803, 803f
radiation therapy, 803
malignant, 802
manifestations of, 802, 803f
nursing care, 804–5
anxiety, 804
assessment, 804, 804f
discharge considerations, 804–5
disturbed body image, 804
pathophysiology, 802
primary, 802
secondary, 802
Brainstem, 790
medulla oblongata, 790
midbrain, 790
pons, 790
Breast
palpation of, 55, 55f
structure of, 910, 910f
Breast augmentation, issues with, 911
Breast cancer, 911–21
case study, 919–21
checkup recommendations, 160f
collaborative care, 912–21
diagnostic tests, 914
pharmacology, 915, 916t
prosthesis for, 919
radiation therapy, 915
screening, 913–14, 913f
breast self-examination (BSE),
913f, 914
clinical exam, 914
mammography, 914
staging, 915
surgical treatment, 915–16
lumpectomy, 915, 916f
mastectomy, 915–16, 916f
reconstructive, 916, 917f
incidence, 911, 911f
manifestations of, 912, 912f
metastasis in, 157t, 912, 916
nursing care, 917–18
anticipatory grieving, 918
assessment, 917

decisional conflict, 917–18
discharge considerations, 919
disturbed body image, 918–19
risk for infection, 918
risk for injury, 918
pathophysiology, 912
inflammatory, 912
invasive, 912
noninvasive, 912
Paget's disease, 912
risk factors for, 912t
Breast cancer screening, 913–14, 913f
Breast disorders, 910–21
associated with augmentation, 911
breast cancer, 911–21
fibrocystic changes, 910–11
collaborative care, 911
nonproliferative, 910
pathophysiology, 910, 911f
proliferative, 910
mastitis, 911
Breast reconstruction surgery, 916, 917f
Breast self-examination (BSE), 913f, 914
Breath sounds, assessment of, 54
Breathing
diaphragmatic
exercises for surgery, 134f
in pain management, 110
techniques for, 704f
pursed lip, 96, 702, 704f
Breslow system, for staging melanoma, 313
Bronchi, 680, 681f, 794f
Bronchiectasis, 706
Bronchioles, 680
Bronchitis
acute, 682–83
chronic, 682, 701
in chronic obstructive pulmonary
disease, 700, 701f
manifestations of, 701t
complementary and alternative medicine
for, 689f
Bronchopneumonia, 683t
Bronchoscopy
fiberoptic, 685f
in lung cancer, 709
in pneumonia, 685
in tuberculosis, 692–93
laser, 709t
nursing care for, 685f
Brudzinski's sign, in meningitis, 817, 818f
Buerger-Allen exercises, 606
Buerger's disease, 605, 622
Bulk-forming agents, for constipation, 459
Bumetanide (Bumex), nursing
considerations for, 73t

Bunion, 768, 768f
Buprenorphine (Buprenex), sublingual, 108
Burn injuries, 326–36
classification of, 326–27, 326t, 327f
full-thickness, 326t, 327
partial-thickness, 326t, 327
"rule of nines," 327, 328f
superficial, 326t, 327
collaborative care
diagnostic tests, 330
fluid replacement, 330
nutritional issues, 330, 334
pharmacology, 330
respiratory management, 330
of the eye, 860
nursing care, 332–36
acute pain, 334
assessment, 332, 333f
case study, 335–36
deficient fluid volume, 333
discharge considerations, 334–35
impaired mobility, 334
impaired skin integrity, 333
powerlessness, 334
risk for infection, 333
pathophysiology, 328–29
cardiovascular system, 328–29
gastrointestinal system, 329
immune system, 329
integumentary system, 329
metabolism, 329
respiratory system, 329
urinary system, 329
treatment stages, 327–28
acute, 328
emergent, 328
rehabilitative, 328
types of, 326
wound management, 331–32
biologic and biosynthetic dressings,
332
debridement, 331
scar, keloid, and contractures, 332
surgery, 331–32
wound dressings, 332
Burn shock, 328–29
Burns
chemical, 326
electrical, 326
of the eye, 860
full-thickness, 327
partial-thickness, 327
radiation, 326
superficial, 327
thermal, 326
Burr hole, intracranial surgery, 803

Bursae, 733
in bursitis, 747
Bursitis, 747
Busulfan (Myleran), in chemotherapy, 166t
Butorphanol (Stadol), intranasal, 108

C fibers
in gate-control theory of pain, 103, 104f
in pain transduction, 102
C-reactive protein (CRP) test, purpose of, 240
Cachectic
defined, 419
in stomach cancer, 419
Cachexia, as an effect of cancer, 161, 161f
Caffeine, abuse of, 224t, 228
CAGE questionnaire, for alcohol abuse, 231
Calcitonin
function of, 342, 343t
for osteoporosis, 762t
role in calcium imbalance, 82
Calcitriol, role in calcium imbalance, 82
Calcium
food sources of, 85f, 761f
in hyperparathyroidism, 354
in hypoparathyroidism, 355
intravenous, 83, 84t
ionized, 82
normal electrolyte laboratory values for,
64t
for osteoporosis, 760
recommended daily intake, 760t
supplements, 84t
weight bearing activities and, 85
Calcium channel blockers
for angina pectoris, 557, 558t, 559
for dysrhythmias, 548t
for hypertension, 601t
Calcium imbalance, 82–85
hypercalcemia
causes of, 83t
collaborative care, 83–84
defined, 83
laboratory values, 83t
manifestations, 83t
neuromuscular effects of, 83, 83t
hypocalcemia
causes of, 83t
collaborative care, 82–83
defined, 82
laboratory values, 83t
manifestations, 83t
neuromuscular effects of, 83, 83t
pharmacological treatment, 84t

Calcium imbalance *(continued)*
  nursing care, 84–85
    assessment, 84
    discharge considerations, 85
    risk for injury, 84–85
Calculi, urinary, 512–15
  collaborative care, 513–15
    dietary management, 513, 513t
    pharmacology, 513
    surgical treatment, 513–14
  foods to avoid with, 513t
  manifestations of, 512–13, 513f
  nursing care, 514–15
    assessment, 514
    discharge considerations, 515
    impaired urinary elimination, 514–15
    pain, 514
  pathophysiology, 512–13
  potential locations of, 512f
  renal, 513–14
    hyperparathyroidism and, 354
    risk factors for, 512
  risk factors for, 515
Callus
  bony, 735
  fibrocartilaginous, 735
Calyces, 494, 495f
Canal of Schlemm, 857
Canaliculi, 426
Cancer, 156–78 *(See also* Oncologic
    emergencies; specific cancer)
  bladder, 517–21
  bone tumors, 766–68
  brain tumor, 802–5
  breast, 911–21
  cervical, 933–36
  colorectal, 477–82
  defined, 157
  endometrial, 936–37
  esophageal, 407
  gallbladder, 431
  laryngeal, 669–74
  liver, 443
  lung, 707–12
  lymphoma, malignant, 648–51
  oral, 405–6
  ovarian, 937–38
  overview
    in adults, 17
    case study, 175–77
    collaborative care, 161–75
      biotherapy, 168, 169f
      chemotherapy, 164–65, 168 *(See*
        also Chemotherapy)
      diagnostic tests, 161–63
      health care team, 156

      nutritional status, 169, 171t, 173
      psychological support of client,
        163, 170
      radiation therapy, 164 *(See also*
        Radiation therapy)
      surgery, 163–64
    effects of, 160–61
      physical, 161
      psychological, 161, 165, 168, 170
    etiology, 157–60
    incidence, 156
    manifestations of, 160f, 169, 171f
    nursing care, 169–175
      anticipatory grieving, 172
      anxiety, 170
      assessment, 169, 170f
      discharge considerations, 174–75
      disturbed body image, 171–72
      imbalanced nutrition, 173
      impaired skin integrity, 173–74
      knowledge deficit, 170–71
      risk for infection, 172
      risk for injury, 172, 173f
    oncologic emergencies, 177–78
    pathophysiology, 156–57
    prevention
      checkup recommendations, 160f
      client education, 174
      early detection, 160, 160f
      risk factors, 158–60
    tumor identification, 161–62, 162t
  pain *(See* Cancer pain)
  pancreatic, 447
  of the penis, 899, 899f
  prostate, 157t, 160f, 890–94
  rectal *(See* Colorectal cancer)
  renal cell, 521–22
  skin, 311–17
  spinal cord tumors, 850
  of stomach, 418–19, 419f
  testicular, 897–98
  of the thyroid gland, 354
  of the vulva, 938
Cancer pain, 104, 160–61
  acute, 160
  chronic, 160–61
  treatment, 116–17, 174
    adjuvant analgesics for, 107
Candidiasis infections, 307–8
  oral
    AIDS-related, 284, 288t
    stomatitis and, 404
  vaginal, 385, 939, 940t
Canker sore, 404
Cannabis, abuse of, 224t, 228
Capillaries, 596

Capillary refill, assessment of, 57
Carbenicillin (Geocillin), 252t
Carbohydrates, 395t
Carbon dioxide, in acid-base balance, 89
Carbon monoxide poisoning, 329, 719, 720f
Carbonic acid
  in acid-base balance, 88–89
  ratio to bicarbonate, 89, 89f
Carbonic anhydrase inhibitors, for glaucoma,
  867t
Carcinogenesis
  known, 158
  theories of, 158
Cardiac arrest, defined, 546
Cardiac cycle, 541, 541f
Cardiac disorders, 537–91
  cardiac function, 570–79
    cardiomyopathy, 578–79
    heart failure, 570–78
  coronary heart disease (CHD), 553,
    554f
    angina pectoris, 554f, 555–62
    atherosclerosis, 553, 554f, 555
    myocardial infarction, 554f, 562–70
  inflammatory, 580–86
    endocarditis, 581–83
    myocarditis, 583–84
    pericarditis, 584–86
    rheumatic heart disease, 580–81
  rhythm
    dysrhythmias, 542–51
    sudden cardiac death, 551
  risk factors for, 553
  risk factors for adults, 17
  as surgical risk, 129t
  valvular heart disease, 586–91
Cardiac markers, in myocardial infarction
  (MI), 564, 565f
Cardiac monitoring, 547
  continuous, 547
  portable, 547
  procedure for, 547f
Cardiac output, 541
  blood pressure and, 597
  decreased
    metabolic acidosis, 93
    potassium imbalance and, 80–81
Cardiac rehabilitation, 567
Cardiac reserve, 541
Cardiac-specific troponin I, cardiac marker,
  564, 565t
Cardiac-specific troponin T, cardiac marker,
  564, 565t
Cardiac surgery, 559–60
  cardiopulmonary bypass pump, 560,
    560f

coronary artery bypass graft (CABG), 559–60, 560f
   nursing care in, 561f
   percutaneous transluminal coronary angioplasty (PTCA), 557f, 559, 559f, 566
Cardiac tamponade
   in cancer, 177
      interventions, 177
      signs and symptoms of, 177
   defined, 584
   in pericarditis, 584
Cardiomyopathy, 578–79
   caused by alcohol abuse, 225
   dilated, 579, 579t
   hypertrophic, 579, 579t
   restrictive, 579, 579t
Cardiomyoplasty, for heart failure, 575
Cardiopulmonary arrest, defined, 546
Cardiopulmonary bypass pump, for cardiac surgery, 560, 560f
Cardiopulmonary resuscitation (CPR)
   in near-drowning, 721
   for sudden cardiac death, 551, 552f
Cardiovascular system
   in adults, 18t, 20t
   assessment of
      peripheral circulation, 56–57
      physical examination, 54–55
   autonomic neuropathies in, 382
   effect of burns on, 328–29
   effect of hypertension on, 598t
   effect of leukemia on, 640f
   effect of spinal cord injury on, 844f
   effect of systemic lupus erythematous on, 779f
   effects of anemia on, 627f
   effects of cirrhosis on, 436f
   effects of diabetes mellitus on, 379f
   effects of hyperthyroidism effects on, 347f
   effects of hypothyroidism on, 352f
   effects of premenstrual syndrome on, 922f
   effects of shock on, 200, 202f
   effects of uremia on, 524f
   in young adults, 16t
Cardioversion, synchronized, for dysrhythmias, 548–49
Care manager, medical-surgical nurse as, 3
Care plan (See Plan of care)
Caregiver
   defined, 2
   medical-surgical nurse as, 2
Caregiver burden, home health care and, 38
Caring, defined, 2

Carotene, 298
Carpal tunnel syndrome, 747
   Phalen test for, 748, 748f
   surgical treatment, 748
Carriers, defined, 246
Casts for fractures
   bivalved, 737, 739f
   nursing care for, 738f
   types of, 738f
Catabolism, 396
   defined, 241
   inflammation and, 241
Catabolizing, defined, 161
Cataracts, 863–64
   case study, 869
   collaborative care, 863
   defined, 863
   nursing care, 863–64
      discharge considerations, 863–64
   pathophysiology, 863
   senile, 863
   surgical treatment, 863, 863f
Catecholamines, 343
Catharsis, for gastroenteritis, 470
Cathartics, for constipation, 459, 460t
Catheterization
   indwelling
      for surgery, 130
      urinary tract infection (UTI) risk and, 506–7
   intermittent, 497
   nursing care for, 498f
   self, 497, 498f
Cavernosography, in erectile dysfunction, 900, 900f
Cavernosometry, in erectile dysfunction, 900, 900f
CD4+ cell, 282
   counts in HIV diagnosis, 286
CD4+:CD8+ ratio, in HIV diagnosis, 286
Cecum, 454, 454f
Cefaclor (Ceclor), 252t
Cefadroxil (Duricef), 252t
Cefazolin (Ancef)), 252t
Cefepime (Maxipime), 252t
Cefoperazone (Cefobid), 252t
Cefotaxime (Claforan), 252t
Cefoxitin (Mefoxin), 252t
Ceftazidime (Fortaz), 252t
Ceftizoxime (Cefizox), 252t
Ceftriaxone (Rocephin), 252t
Cefuroxime (Zinacef), 252t
Celecoxib (Celebrex), for rheumatoid arthritis, 775t
Celiac disease, 464
Cellulitis, 239, 307

Centers for Disease Control and Prevention (CDC), on infectious disease, 248
Central nervous system (CNS), 790–92 (See also Intracranial disorders; Neurologic system)
   brain, 790–91, 791f
      brainstem, 790
      cerebellum, 790–91
      cerebrum, 790, 791f
      diencephalon, 790
   spinal cord, 791–92
Central venous pressure (CVP)
   defined, 69
   measurement of, 69, 70f
Centrally acting sympatholytics, for hypertension, 600t
Cephalalgia (See Headaches)
Cephalexin (Keflex), 252t
Cephalosporins
   client education, 252t
   nursing responsibilities, 252t
   purpose of, 252t
Cerebellum, 790–91
Cerebral edema, increased intracranial pressure and, 795–96
Cerebral vasospasm, in aneurysm, 813
Cerebrospinal fluid (CSF), 790–91
   examination of
      in cerebrovascular accident, 808
      in intracranial infections, 818
      in multiple sclerosis, 832–33
      nursing care for, 809f
   leakage of
      in broken nose, 665–66
      in skull fracture, 794–95
Cerebrovascular accident (CVA), 805–12
   collaborative care, 808–12
      diagnostic tests, 808
      pharmacology, 808–9
      surgical treatment, 809, 809f
   defined, 805
   diabetes mellitus and, 381
   manifestations of
      contralateral deficit, 806
      motor deficits, 806, 807t
      right vs. left hemispheres, 808, 808f
      sensory-perceptual changes, 807, 807t
      speech deficit, 806–7, 807t
      visual deficit, 807, 807f, 807t
   nursing care, 809–11
      assessment, 809–10, 810f
      discharge considerations, 812
      disturbed sensory perception, 811
      impaired communication, 811
      impaired physical mobility, 810–11
      impaired swallowing, 811–12

Cerebrovascular accident (CVA)
  (*continued*)
    nursing care (*continued*)
      ineffective airway clearance, 810
      ineffective tissue perfusion, 810
      self-care deficit, 812
    pathophysiology, 805–8
    risk factors for, 805, 806f
    transient ischemic attack and, 805–6
    types of
      embolic, 806, 807t
      hemorrhagic, 806, 807t
      thrombotic, 806, 807t
Cerebrum, 790, 791f
  left hemisphere, 790
  right hemisphere, 790
Cerumen, 872
  impacted, 874
Cervical cancer, 933–36
  case study, 935–36
  cervical intraepithelial neoplasia (CIN),
    933–34
  checkup recommendations, 160f
  collaborative care, 934–35
    diagnostic tests, 934
    screening, 934
    surgical treatment, 934
  nursing care, 935
    assessment, 935
    discharge considerations, 935
    fear, 935
    impaired skin integrity, 935
  pathophysiology, 933–34
  risk factors for, 935
Cervical collar, 212, 212f
Cervical intraepithelial neoplasia (CIN),
  933–34
Cervical tongs, for spinal cord injury, 844,
  845f
Cervix, 908f, 909
Chalazion, 858, 858f
Chancroid, 949t
  complications, 949t
  manifestations of, 949t
  treatment, 949t
Cheilosis, defined, 632f
Chemonucleolysis, for herniated
  intervertebral disk, 849
Chemotherapy, 164–65, 168
  administration of, 164–65
  biologic response modifiers (BRMs), 164
  in bladder cancer, 518
  in bone tumors, 767
  in brain tumor, 803, 803f
  in breast cancer, 915
  in colorectal cancer, 479

in laryngeal cancer, 670
  for leukemia, 641
  in malignant lymphoma, 649
  pharmacology for, 164, 166t–168t
  psychological effect of, 165, 168
  vascular access devices (VADs), 164–65
Chenodiol (Chenix), 428
Chest
  barrel, 54
  flail, 719–20, 719f
Chest tubes
  closed-drainage systems, 717, 717f
  nursing care, 717f
  for pneumothorax, 717
Cheyne-Stokes respirations, 54
Chlamydia, 948, 949t, 950–53
  collaborative care, 949t, 950–53
    diagnostic tests, 950–51
    pharmacology, 951
  complications, 949t
  manifestations of, 949t
  nursing care, 952–53
  organism characteristics, 245f
  pathophysiology, 948, 950
  in pelvic inflammatory disease, 941
Chloride, laboratory values
  normal electrolyte, 64t
  significance of, 127t
Chlorothiazide (Diuril), nursing
  considerations for, 73t
Cholecystectomy
  laparoscopic, 428, 429f
  traditional, 428
Cholecystitis, 427–31 (*See also*
  Cholelithiasis)
  acute, 427–28
  chronic, 428
  defined, 427
  manifestations of, 427–28, 428f
Cholecystogram, oral, 428
Cholelithiasis, 427–31
  collaborative care, 427–31
    dissolving stones, 428
    nutritional therapy, 428, 428f
    pharmacology, 428
    surgical treatment, 428, 429f
    T-tube, 428, 429f
  common locations of, 427f
  defined, 427
  nursing care, 429–31
    acute pain, 429
    assessment, 429, 430f
    case study, 430–31
    discharge considerations, 430
    impaired gas exchange, 430
    nausea, 429–30

Cholesterol
  desirable blood levels, 555t
  high, coronary heart disease and, 553
  high-density lipoprotein (HDL), 553,
    555t
  low-density lipoprotein (LDL), 553, 555t
Cholinergic crisis, 837
Chorea
  defined, 839
  in myasthenia gravis, 839
Choroid, 856
Christmas disease, 637
Chronic lymphocytic leukemia (CLL), 641t
  (*See also* Leukemia)
Chronic myelocytic leukemia (CML), 641t
  (*See also* Leukemia)
Chronic obstructive pulmonary disease
  (COPD), 700–705
  case study, 704–5
  collaborative care, 701–4
    diagnostic tests, 701–2
    oxygen therapy, 702
    pharmacology, 702
    surgical treatment, 702
  nursing care, 702–704
    assessment, 702f
    discharge considerations, 704
    imbalanced nutrition, 703
    ineffective airway clearance, 703
    ineffective coping, 703
    pathophysiology, 700–701, 701f
Chronic renal failure, 523–32 (*See also*
  Renal failure)
Chvostek's sign
  defined, 82
  hypocalcemia and, 82, 83t
  in tetany, 82
Ciliary body, 856
Ciprofloxacin (Cipro), 253t
Circle of Willis, aneurysms in, 812
Circulating nurse, 138, 139f
Cirrhosis, 436–43
  alcoholic, 225, 436, 442–43
  biliary, 436
  case study, 442–43
  collaborative care, 437–42
    diagnostic tests, 437
    dietary and fluid management,
      437–38
    pharmacology, 438, 438t
    surgical procedures, 438–40
  defined, 436
  nursing care, 440–42
    assessment, 440, 441f
    discharge considerations, 442, 442f
    excess fluid volume, 440

impaired skin integrity, 442
ineffective breathing pattern, 442
risk for suffocation, 441–42
thought processes, 441
pathophysiology, 436–37, 436f
postnecrotic, 436
Cisplatin (CDDP) (Platinol), in
chemotherapy, 167t
CK-MB, cardiac marker, 564, 565t
Clarifying, as critical thinking skill, 7
Clarithromycin (Biaxin), 254t
Clark system, for staging of melanoma, 313
Clavicle fracture, 741t, 742f
Claw toe, 768, 768f
Client education
accident prevention, 214, 215f
Alzheimer's disease, 830, 830f, 831f
amputation, 752
anaphylactic shock, 209f
asthma, 699–700, 700f
burn injuries, 334–35
calcium imbalance, 85
cancer
home care, 175
hospice, 175
prevention, 174
rehabilitation, 175
cerebrovascular accident, 812
constipation, 462
diabetes mellitus, 386–87
foot care, 385f
insulin injections, 372f, 373f, 374t
nutrition therapy, 372, 374–75, 377t
exchange list, 374, 377t
food pyramid, 374
meal planning, 374
for older adults, 374
self management, 388f
diarrhea, 458
end of life care, 175, 193
fluid volume deficit, 72, 72f
fluid volume excess, 74–75, 75f
foot care, 608f
fractures, 743–44
gastroenteritis, 471
gastroesophageal reflux disease (GERD),
407
herniated intervertebral disk, 849–50
HIV infection, 285–86, 286f, 291
home health care and, 36, 38–39
hypersensitivity reactions, 276
hypertension, 602–3
immunizations, 273
infection, 258–59, 258f
inflammatory bowel disease (IBD), 476
irritable bowel syndrome, 463

metabolic acidosis, 93
metabolic alkalosis, 94–95
multiple sclerosis, 834
myocardial infarction, 568
obesity, 399–400, 399f
osteoarthritis, 772
pain management, 118–19, 119f
peptic ulcer disease (PUD), 417–18
peritonitis, 468–69, 468f
postsurgery, 148
potassium imbalance, 81
pressure ulcers, 320–21
renal failure, 531
respiratory acidosis, 96
sexually transmitted disease (STD), 951,
952f
sodium imbalance, 78
systemic lupus erythematous (SLE), 780
transplant, 281, 281f
tuberculosis, 695–96
urinary incontinence, 502
urinary tract infection (UTI), 505–7
venous thrombosis, 616–17
Client rights
in home health care, 36f, 37
legal considerations, 10
Clitoris, 909f, 910
Clonidine (Catapres), 229
Clorpheniramine (Chlor-Trimeton), 275t
Clostridium difficile-associated diarrhea
(CDAD), 248
Clotrimazole (Lotrimin), 255t
Clotting
in disseminated intravascular
coagulopathy, 636
stages of, 635
Clotting factors, 638
Clotting studies, 636
Cloxacillin (Tegopen), 252t
CNS depressants
abuse of, 223t
alcohol abuse, 222–26
cross-tolerance of, 228
opioids, 223t, 226–27
sedatives, hypnotics, and anxiolytics,
223t, 227
CNS stimulants, abuse of, 223t, 227
Cocaine
abuse of, 223t, 227
myocardial infarction associated with,
563
Cochlea, 872
Code of ethics, 9, 9f
Cognitive ability, affect on health, 22
Colchicine, for gout, 781, 781t
Colectomy, 474, 479

Collaborative, defined, 2
Collaborative management
defined, 5
in nursing process, 5
Colon (See Large intestine)
Colon cancer (See Colorectal cancer)
Colonization, in infection, 246
Colonoscopy (See also Sigmoidoscopy)
in colorectal cancer, 478
flexible
in constipation diagnosis, 459
in diverticular disease, 485
for inflammatory bowel disease, 472
nursing care for, 478f
Colony-stimulating factors (CSFs), for
leukemia, 642, 644f
Colorectal cancer, 477–82
checkup recommendations, 160f
collaborative care, 478–82
adjunctive therapy, 479
surgical treatment, 479
complications of, 478
incidence, 477
manifestations of, 478, 478f
metastasis sites for, 157t
nursing care, 480–82
anticipatory grieving, 480–81
discharge considerations, 482
pain, 479–80
sexual dysfunction, 481–82
pathophysiology, 477–78
risk factors for, 477, 478f
Colostomy, 163, 479
double-barrel, 479, 479f
irrigation of, 483f
nursing care for, 480f
various locations for, 479f
Colposcopy, in cervical cancer diagnosis,
934, 934f
Coma (See also Altered level of
consciousness)
Glasgow Coma Scale for, 796, 798t
myxedema, 351
Comfort measures, in end of life care, 161f,
190
Comfort measures only order, 186
Commissurotomy, in valvular heart disease,
589
Communicable diseases, 248
Communication
in Alzheimer's disease, 831f
in cerebrovascular accident, 806–7, 811
with a endotracheal tube, 726f
with hearing loss, 880–81
in Parkinson's disease, 837
Community, concept of, 32

Community-based nursing care, 32–33 (*See also* Home health care)
  community health nursing *vs.*, 32
  sites for, 32f
  types of, 32–33
Community centers, as community-based health care site, 32
Community health nursing, community-based nursing care *vs.*, 32
Compartment syndrome
  in fracture, 736–37
  manifestations of, 737f
Compensatory mechanisms, in heart failure, 570–71
Complementary and alternative medicine (CAM)
  atherosclerosis, 555f
  benign prostatic hypertrophy (BPH), 887
  bronchitis, 689f
  heart failure, 575
  pain management, 110–12, 116
    acupuncture, 111–12
    biofeedback, 112
    cutaneous stimulation, 110, 112t
    distraction, 110
    hypnotism, 112
    relaxation, 110
    transcutaneous electrical nerve stimulation (TENS), 110–11, 112t
  peripheral vascular disorders, 606f
  pneumonia, 689f
  respiratory infections, 660
Complementary therapies for, stress, 599f
Concussion, 795, 796t
Conduction system, cardiac, 539–40, 539f
Cones, of the eye, 856
Conization, for cervical cancer, 934, 935f
Conjunctiva, 856
Conjunctivitis, 858–59, 858f
Consciousness (*See also* Altered level of consciousness)
  defined, 796, 797f
  level of
    assessment of, 57
    defined, 57
Constipation, 458–62
  in cerebrovascular accident, 811
  collaborative care, 459, 461–62
    dietary management, 459, 459t
    enemas, 459, 461
    pharmacology, 459, 460t
  defined, 458
  etiology, 459t
  nursing care, 462
    discharge considerations, 462

in older adults, 458
pathophysiology, 458
simple or chronic, 459
in spinal cord injury, 846
as surgical complication, 144, 147
Contact precautions, in infection control, 257t
Continent urinary diversion, for bladder cancer, 518, 519t, 520
Continuous ambulatory peritoneal dialysis (CAPD), 527
Continuous arteriovenous hemofiltration (CAVH), 526, 527f
Continuous cyclic peritoneal dialysis (CCPD), 527
Continuous positive airway pressure (CPAP)
  for chronic obstructive pulmonary disease, 702
  for sleep apnea, 668
Continuous subcutaneous insulin infusion (CSII), 371
Continuous venovenous hemofiltration (CVVH), 526
Contractility, in cardiac output, 541
Contractures
  in amputation, 749
  in burn injuries, 332
  defined, 332, 749
  nursing care for, 750f
Contralateral deficit, in cerebrovascular accident, 806
Contusion
  in head trauma, 795, 796t
  pulmonary, 719
  soft tissue trauma, 212f, 734
Convulsion, defined, 813
Cor pulmonale, 715
Cordectomy, for laryngeal cancer, 670
Cordotomy
  for laryngeal cancer, 670
  for pain, 109, 112f
Cornea, 856
  keratitis, 859
  transplantation of, 859
Corneal abrasion, 860
Corneal reflex, 799f, 856
Corneal ulcers, 859
Coronary artery bypass graft (CABG), for angina pectoris, 559–60, 560f
Coronary heart disease (CHD), 553, 554f
  angina pectoris, 554f, 555–62
  atherosclerosis, 553, 554f, 555
  myocardial infarction, 554f, 562–70
  risk factors for, 553
  sudden cardiac death and, 551

Corticosteroids
  for Addison's disease, 359, 360f
  administration of, 241
  for asthma, 698t
  for cancer pain, 107
  for chronic obstructive pulmonary disease, 702
  for increased intracranial pressure, 798
  for inflammation, 241
  for inflammatory bowel disease, 473t
  for psoriasis, 303–4
  secretion of, 342–43
  side effects of, 241
  for spinal cord injury, 844
  for systemic lupus erythematous, 778
  for transplants, 279
  types of, 342–43
Cortisol, function of, 342–43, 343t
Coughing
  controlled, 702, 704f
  exercises for surgery, 134f
  huff, 702, 704f
  techniques for productive, 704f
Coumadin, 614, 615t
Coup-contrecoup phenomenon, in head injuries, 795, 795f
Couple, developmental stages of a, 21
COX-2 inhibitors, for rheumatoid arthritis, 775t
CPR (cardiopulmonary resuscitation)
  in near-drowning, 721
  for sudden cardiac death, 551, 552f
Crackles, breath sound, 54
Cranial nerves, 792, 793t
Craniectomy, 804
Cranioplasty, 804
Craniotomy, 803–4, 803f
  client and family support in, 805
  for increased intracranial pressure, 798
  infratentorial, 804
  supratentorial, 804
Cranium
  compartments of, 795
  pain-sensitive structures of, 820
Creatine kinase, cardiac marker, 564, 565t
Creatinine, 496
  serum levels
    in glomerulonephritis, 508
    normal, 496, 508t
    in renal failure, 524–25, 524f
  urine levels, normal, 508t
Creatinine clearance, 508, 508f
Crede method, for bladder emptying, 497
Creutzfeldt-Jakob disease, 841–42
  variant, 842
Critical illness, 216–17

Critical thinking
    attitudes related to, 7
    defined, 7
    skills for, 7
Critical thinking care map
    acute myelocytic leukemia (AML), 653
    adult clients, 28
    amputation, 754
    assessment, 60
    Buerger's disease, 621
    cancer
        chemotherapy, 180
        colorectal, 490
        prostate, 904
    cerebrovascular accident, 824
    coronary bypass surgery, 593
    diabetes mellitus, 391
    dysfunctional grieving, 197
    example, 7
    fluid and electrolyte imbalance, 100
    hearing loss, 883
    herniated intervertebral disk, 852
    herpes zoster, 323
    hypothyroidism, 363
    infection, 262
    laryngectomy, 677
    obesity, 422
    osteoarthritis and total hip replacement,
        787
    overview, 7
    pain management, 122
    pancreatitis, 450
    pneumocystis carinii pneumonia, 295
    postsurgery, 153
    rehabilitation, 43
    respiratory acidosis, 99
    substance abuse, 235
    syphilis, 959
    trauma, 219
    tuberculosis, 729
    urinary incontinence, 534
Crohn's disease
    defined, 472
    pathophysiology, 472, 472f
    treatment (See Inflammatory bowel
        disease (IBD))
Cross-tolerance, defined, 228
Cryosurgery
    for prostate cancer, 892
    in skin cancers, 314
Cryptococcosis, AIDS-related, 285, 288t
Cryptorchidism, 895
Cryptosporidiosis, AIDS-related, 284–85
Cullen's sign, 444
Cultural differences
    about death and dying, 190, 190t

affect on health, 22
    in history taking, 47–48
    in infection diagnosis, 250
    in inflammation diagnosis, 240
    medical-surgical nurse and, 3f
Culture, defined, 3f
Curling's ulcer, 329
Cushing's syndrome, 356–59
    collaborative care, 357–58
        diagnostic tests, 357
        pharmacology, 357
        radiation therapy, 357
        surgery, 357
    defined, 356
    manifestations of, 357f
    nursing care, 357–58
        assessment, 357, 358f
        body image, 358
        discharge considerations, 359
        excess fluid volume, 358
        impaired skin integrity, 358
        infection risk, 358
        injury risk, 358
    pathophysiology, 356–57
Cushing's triad, 795, 797t
Cutaneous stimulation
    cold, 112t
    heat, 112t
    massage, 112t
    in pain management, 110, 112t
Cyanide inhalation, 719
Cyanosis, defined, 50, 298, 680
Cyclophosphamide (Cytoxan), in
    chemotherapy, 166t
Cyclosporine (Sandimmune), 279, 280t
Cyst, defined, 299t
Cystectomy, for bladder cancer, 518, 518t
Cystic fibrosis, 705
Cystitis
    defined, 502
    manifestations of, 503f
    pathophysiology, 502–3
Cystocele, 930
    urinary incontinence associated with,
        499
Cystometrography, for urinary incontinence,
    499
Cystoscopy, in urinary tract infection, 503,
    505f
Cytologic examination, in cancer diagnosis,
    162
Cytomegalovirus (CMV), AIDS-related,
    285
Cytotoxic agents, for transplants, 279, 280t
Cytotoxic T cells, 267t
    in cell-mediated immunity, 268, 270f

Data, defined, 4
Date rape drug, 227
Dawn phenomenon, 381
Death (See also End of life care)
    brain, 217, 217f
    cultural differences about, 190, 190t
    defined, 184
    determination of, 10
    ethical and legal considerations, 10, 186
    leading cause in U.S., 23
    manifestations of, 189–90, 189f
    nurse's grief, 190, 190f
    nurse's self-assessment, 186
    organ donation, 217
    signs of impending, 188–89, 188f
    stages of, 184
Death anxiety, 192–93
Debridement
    defined, 331
    enzymatic, 331
    mechanical, 331
    surgical, 331
Debulking, intracranial surgery, 803
Decerebrate posturing, 799f
Decongestants
    for allergic reaction
        nasal, 275
        oral, 275
    for upper respiratory disorders, 660, 661t
Decorticate posturing, 799f
Decubitus ulcers (See Pressure ulcers)
Deep venous thrombosis (DVT), 612–13
    case study, 617–18
    common locations for, 612f
    defined, 143
    manifestations of, 613f
    prevention of, 145–46, 714–15
    risk factors for, 143, 612
    in trauma clients, 214
Defecation reflex, 454
Defibrillation
    automated external defibrillator (AED),
        548–49, 551
    automatic implantable cardioverter-
        defibrillator (AICD), 549, 551
    for dysrhythmias, 548–49
Degenerative disk disease, osteoarthritis and,
    769
Dehiscence, 144, 146f
Dehydration (See also Fluid volume deficit)
    diarrhea and, 455
    of the skin, 52
    as surgical risk, 129t

Delirium
    alcohol withdrawal, 224
    terminal, 189
Demeclocycline (Declomycin), 253t
Dementia (*See also* Alzheimer's disease)
    AIDS-related, 285, 290–91
Dendrites, 790, 790f
Denial
    in death and dying, 184
    in substance abuse, 222
Depression
    in death and dying, 184
    in menopause, 927, 928f
Dermatitis, 302
    atopic, 302
    contact, 302
    exfoliative, 302
    seborrheic, 302
Dermatome, 792
Dermatophyte
    defined, 307
    infections, 307
Dermis, 298, 298t
Desensitization, in immunotherapy,
    275
Detoxification, in substance abuse, 229
Deviated septum, 665–67
Diabetes insipidus (DI), 344–45
    collaborative care, 345
    defined, 344
    manifestations of, 344t
    nephrogenic, 344
    neurogenic, 344
    nursing care, 345
        discharge considerations, 345
        fluid volume deficient, 345
Diabetes mellitus, 365–89
    in the adult, 366–68
    collaborative care, 369–83
        diagnostic tests, 369, 370t
        exercise, 374–75, 378f
        monitoring glucose and ketones,
            369–70
        nutritional issues, 372, 374–75, 377t,
            384
        pharmacology, 370–72
            insulin injections, 371–72
            oral antidiabetics, 372, 376t
        surgical management, 383
    complications of, 377–83, 379f
        acute, 377–81
            diabetic ketoacidosis, 377–78
            hyperglycemic hyperosmolar
                nonketotic syndrome
                (HHNS), 378
            hypoglycemia, 378–81

chronic, 381–83
    atherosclerotic coronary artery
        disease, 381
    diabetic foot, 382, 385f
    diabetic neuropathy, 382
    diabetic retinopathy, 382, 871
    peripheral vascular disease, 381,
        382f
    stroke, 381
    susceptibility to infection, 382–83
defined, 366
gestational, 367t
incidence, 366
nursing care, 383–84
    assessment, 383, 384f
    coping, 386
    discharge considerations, 386–87, 387f
    impaired skin integrity, 384
    risk for infection, 384–85
    risk for injury, 385–86
    in the older adult, 368, 368f
    risk factors for, 369
    screening for, 369
    self management of, 388f
    as surgical risk, 130t
    type I, 366, 367t
        case study, 387–89
        manifestations of, 369f
        pathophysiology, 368–69
    type II, 366, 367t
        manifestations of, 369f
        pathophysiology, 369
    types of, 366, 367t
    wound healing and, 148
Diabetic foot, 385f
Diabetic ketoacidosis, 377–78
    manifestations of, 380f
    pathophysiology of, 380f
    treatment, 378
Diabetic nephropathy, 508
Diabetic neuropathy, 382
Diabetic retinopathy, 382, 871
Diagnosis
    classification for, 5
    defined, 4–5
    dual, 229
    functional health patterns in, 5
    PES method for writing, 5
Diagnosis-related groups (DRGs), concepts,
    34
Diagnostic and Statistical Manual of Mental
    Disorders (DSM-IV-TR), substance
    abuse disorders, 222
Dialysate, in dialysis, 525
Dialysis, 525–27
    defined, 525

hemodialysis, 525–26, 526f
    arteriovenous (AV) fistula for, 525,
        526f
    complications of, 526
    continuous arteriovenous
        hemofiltration (CAVH), 526,
        527f
    continuous venovenous hemofiltration
        (CVVH), 526
    nursing care, 527
peritoneal, 526–27
    continuous ambulatory peritoneal
        dialysis (CAPD), 527
    continuous cyclic peritoneal dialysis
        (CCPD), 527
    nursing care, 528
Diapedesis, in inflammatory response, 238,
    238f
Diarrhea, 455–58
    collaborative care, 455–58
        dietary management, 455–56, 456t
        pharmacology, 456, 457tt
    in Crohn's disease, 472
    defined, 455
    foods that may aggravate, 456f
    in gastroenteritis, 470
    in inflammatory bowel disease, 475
    nursing care, 456–58
        assessment, 456, 456f
        discharge considerations, 458
        impaired skin integrity, 456–58
    pathophysiology, 455
    traveler's, 470t
Diastolic blood pressure, 597
Dicloxacillin (Dynapen), 252t
Diencephalon, 790
Diethylstilbestrol (DES), in chemotherapy,
    167t
Diffusion, 67f
    defined, 66
    facilitated, 66
    simple, 66
Digital rectal exam (DRE)
    in benign prostatic hypertrophy, 887
    in prostate cancer, 891
Digitalis
    for heart failure, 573–74, 573t
    toxicity, 574
Dihydrotestosterone (DHT), in benign
    prostatic hypertrophy, 887
Dilation and curettage (D&C)
    for dysfunctional uterine bleeding, 924
    nursing care, 926f
Dilemma, defined, 10
Diphenhydramine (Benadryl), 275t
Disability, defined, 40

Discharge considerations, in home health care, 37
Disease (*See also* Illness)
  biological causes of, 23
  classification definitions, 24t
  common causes of, 23–24
  defined, 23
  mechanical causes of, 23
  normative causes of, 23
Disk
  degenerative disk disease, osteoarthritis and, 769
  herniated intervertebral, 847–50
    collaborative care, 848–50
      diagnostic tests, 848
      medical management, 848
      pharmacology, 848
      surgical treatment, 848–49
    manifestations of, 847f
    nursing care, 849–50
      discharge considerations, 849–50
      pain, 849
    pathophysiology, 847, 847f
Diskectomy, 848
Disseminated intravascular coagulopathy (DIC), 204–5, 636–37
  collaborative care, 636–37
  defined, 636
  manifestations, 636f
  nursing care, 636–37
    fear, 637
    impaired gas exchange, 637
    ineffective tissue perfusion, 636–37
    pain, 637
  pathophysiology, 636
  risk factors for, 636f
Distal paresthesia, 382
Distraction, in pain management, 110
Diuretics
  in cirrhosis treatment, 438t
  for heart failure, 574t
  loop
    for increased intracranial pressure, 798
    nursing considerations for, 73t
  nursing considerations for, 73t, 574
  osmotic
    defined, 368
    in diabetes mellitus, type I, 368
    for increased intracranial pressure, 798
  potassium imbalance and, 80
  potassium-sparing, nursing considerations for, 73t
  as surgical risk, 130t

  thiazide
    nursing considerations for, 73t, 574
    for renal calculi, 513
Diverticula
  of the colon, 485f
  defined, 485
Diverticular disease, 485–86
  collaborative care, 485–86
  defined, 485
  manifestations of, 485
  nursing care, 486
  pathophysiology, 485
Diverticulosis, defined, 485
Dizziness, defined, 877
Do-not-resuscitate (DNR) order, 186, 188f, 551
Documentation
  of assessment, 57–58
  forms of, 57
  of intervention, 6
  principles for, 57–58
Dopamine, Parkinson's disease
  action in, 834
  pharmacology, 836t
Dopaminergics, for Parkinson's disease, 836t
Doppler stethoscope, 605f
Doppler ultrasound studies
  in peripheral vascular disorders, 605
  in varicose veins, 618
  in venous thrombosis, 613
Doxorubicin (Adriamycin), in chemotherapy, 166t
Doxycycline (Vibramycin), 253t
Dressings (*See also* Wound care)
  for amputation, 750, 750f
  biologic and biosynthetic, 332
  wound, 332
DRGs (Diagnosis-related groups), concepts, 34
Droplet precautions, in infection control, 257t
Drowning, near, 719–20
  collaborative care, 720
  manifestations of, 720
  nursing care, 720–21
    discharge considerations, 721
    impaired gas exchange, 720–21
    ineffective airway clearance, 720
    ineffective tissue perfusion, 721
    pain, 721
Drugs, recreational, as carcinogen, 158–59
Dry skin (xerosis), 301
Dual diagnosis
  defined, 229
  substance abuse and, 229
Duchenne's muscular dystrophy, 785

Dumping syndrome, in gastric surgery, 414, 417
Duodenum, 396, 454
  peptic ulcer disease, 412–18
Durable medical power of attorney, defined, 10
Durable power of attorney for health care, 186
Dying Person's Bill of Rights, 186
Dysarthria, 807
Dysfunctional uterine bleeding (DUB), 923–26
  amenorrhea, 923
  collaborative care, 924–26
    diagnostic tests, 924
    pharmacology, 924
    surgical treatment, 924
  menorrhagia, 923
  metrorrhagia, 923
  mittelschmerz, 924
  nursing care, 924–26
    assessment, 924
    coping, 925
    discharge considerations, 926
    sexual dysfunction, 925
  oligomenorrhea, 923
  pathophysiology, 924
Dysmenorrhea, 923
Dysphagia
  defined, 407
  in esophageal cancer, 407
  management of, 407
Dyspnea, defined, 54, 680
Dysrhythmias, 542–51
  atrioventricular conduction blocks, 544t–545t, 546–47
    first degree, 544t, 546
    pacemakers for, 549
    second degree, 544t, 546
    third degree, 544t, 546–47
  collaborative care, 547–41
    cardiac monitoring, 547
      continuous, 547
      portable, 547
      procedure for, 547f
    cardioversion/defibrillation, 548–49
    pacemakers, 549, 549f
    pharmacology, 548, 548t
    surgical treatment, 549
  defined, 55, 542
  metabolic acidosis and, 93
  in myocardial infarction, 564
  nursing care, 549–51
    anxiety, 550
    assessment, 549–50
    decreased cardiac output, 550
    discharge considerations, 550–51

Dysrhythmias (continued)
  in older adults, 545f
  pathophysiology, 542–47
  potassium imbalance and, 80–81
  supraventricular rhythms, 542, 543t–544t, 545–46
    atrial fibrillation, 544t, 546
    atrial flutter, 543t, 545
    normal sinus rhythm (NSR), 542, 543t
    premature atrial contractions (PACs), 543t, 545
    sinus bradycardia, 542, 543t, 545
    sinus tachycardia, 542, 543t
    supraventricular tachycardia (SVT), 545
  ventricular rhythms, 544t, 546
    premature ventricular contractions (PVCs), 544t, 546
    ventricular fibrillation (V-fib), 544t, 546
    ventricular tachycardia (VT or V-tach), 544t, 546

E

Ear
  balance and, 873
  structures of
    external, 872, 872f
    inner, 872, 872f
    middle, 872, 872f
Ear disorders, 873–81
  external otitis, 873–74
  foreign bodies, 874
  hearing loss, 878–81
  impacted cerumen, 874
  inner, 877–78
    collaborative care, 877
    labyrinthitis, 877
    Meniere's disease, 877
    nursing care, 877
      assessment, 877
      discharge considerations, 878
      disturbed sleep pattern, 878
      risk for injury, 878
    pathophysiology, 877
  otitis media, 874–76
  otosclerosis, 876–77
Ear drops, procedure for giving, 873f
Ear surgery
  nursing care, 876f
  for otitis media, 875

Ear wax (See Cerumen)
Eardrum, 872
Ecchymosis, assessment for, 52
Eccrine sweat glands, 298t, 301
Echinacea, for upper respiratory disorders, 660
Echocardiography
  in heart failure, 572
  in myocardial infarction, 564–65
Ecstasy, abuse of, 224t
Ectopic beats, heart, 542
Eczema, 302
Edema (See also Fluid imbalance, fluid volume excess)
  assessment for, 52, 52f
  cerebral, 795–96
  defined, 72, 73
  grading system for, 616f, 617f
  impaired skin integrity with, 74
  localized, 74
  lymphedema, 647–48
  monitoring of, 74
  periorbital, 52, 74
  pitting, 52
  pulmonary, 329, 571, 573
Education, level of, affect on health, 22
Ejaculation, defined, 886
Ejaculatory dysfunction, 902
  delayed, 902
  premature, 902
  retrograde, 902
Ejection fraction, in cardiac output, 541
Electrical bone stimulation, 740
Electrocardiogram (ECG), 540, 540f
  analysis, 542, 542f
  for angina pectoris, 556, 556f
  in heart failure, 572
  in myocardial infarction, 564
  PR interval, 540f, 542f
  QRS complex, 540f, 542f
  QT interval, 540f
  ST segment, 540f
  stress, for angina pectoris, 556
  U wave, 540f
Electroencephalogram (EEG)
  nursing care for, 815f
  for seizure disorder, 814
Electrolyte(s) (See also specific electrolytes)
  defined, 64
  extracellular, 65
  functions of, 64
  imbalance (See also Fluid imbalance)
    as surgical risk, 129t
  intracellular, 65

measurement of, 64, 93
  normal laboratory values, 64t
Electrolyte imbalance, 76–88
  calcium imbalance, 82–85
  magnesium imbalance, 85–87
  phosphorus imbalance, 87–88
  potassium imbalance, 78–82
  sodium imbalance, 76–78
Elephantiasis, 647
Emancipated minor, informed consent and, 131
Embolism, 605, 605f
  fat, in fracture, 713
  microemboli, 203
  pulmonary (See Pulmonary embolism)
Emergency care
  at accident site, 212
  assessment, 213
  diagnostic tests, 213
  environmental injuries, 215–16
  forensic considerations in, 213
  goals of, 210
  poisoning, 216, 216f
  tag triage system, 210
  triage, 210
Emotional lability
  in cerebrovascular accident, 807
  defined, 807
Emotional status, as influence to pain response, 106
Emphysema, 701
  in chronic obstructive pulmonary disease, 700, 701f
  manifestations of, 701t
Empyema, 689–90
Encephalitis, 817–18, 817t
  defined, 817
  manifestations of, 818
  pharmacology, 819
  treatment, 818
Encephalopathy
  alcoholic, 226
  bovine spongiform, 842
  hepatic
    caused by alcohol abuse, 225
    cirrhosis and, 436
  spongiform, 842
End of life care, 188–94
  case study, 193–94
  client and family support, 189
  collaborative care, 190–93
    comfort measures, 161f, 190
  components of, 188
  ethical and legal considerations, 186
  hospice, 186–87
  nurse's grief, 190, 190f

nursing care, 191–93
  anticipatory grieving, 192
  assessment, 191–92
  death anxiety, 192–93
  discharge considerations, 193
postmortem care, 190
purpose of, 188
rituals of mourning, 190, 190t
signs of death, 189–90, 189f
signs of impending death, 188–89, 188f
End-stage renal disease (ESRD), 523
Endarterectomy, carotid
  for cerebrovascular accident, 809, 809f
  nursing care, 810f
Endocarditis, 581–83
  acute, 581, 582f
  collaborative care, 582–83
    pharmacology, 582
    prevention, 582, 582t, 583f
  complications, 582
  defined, 581
  manifestations of, 581–82
  nursing care, 582–83
    discharge considerations, 583
    imbalanced body temperature, 582–83
    ineffective tissue perfusion, 583
  pathophysiology, 581–82
  subacute, 581, 582f
Endocardium, 538
Endocrine disorders, 341–61
  adrenal gland
    Addison's disease, 359–61
    Cushing's syndrome, 356–59
    pheochromocytoma, 361
  parathyroid glands
    hyperparathyroidism, 354–55
    hypoparathyroidism, 355–56
  pituitary gland, 344–46
    diabetes insipidus (DI), 344–45
    hyperpituitarism, 344
    hypopituitarism, 344
    syndrome of inappropriate ADH
      secretion (SIADH), 345–46
  thyroid gland
    cancer of, 354
    hyperthyroidism, 346–50
    hypothyroidism, 351–54
Endocrine system
  in adults, 18t, 20t
  effects of hyperthyroidism on, 347f
  effects of hypothyroidism on, 352f
  effects of uremia on, 524f
  functions of, 342–43
  hormones in, 342
  kidneys in, 496
  structures of, 342–43, 342f

Endogenous pyrogens
  defined, 239
  fever and, 239
Endometrial ablation, for dysfunctional
    uterine bleeding, 924
Endometrial cancer, 936–37
  collaborative care, 936–37
    surgical treatment, 936–37
  nursing care, 937
    discharge considerations, 937
    disturbed body image, 937
  pathophysiology, 936
  risk factors for, 936
Endometriosis, 931–32
  collaborative care, 931–32
    ovarian cysts, 932–33
    pharmacology, 931
  ectopic, 931
  manifestations of, 931
  nursing care, 931–32
    anxiety, 932
    assessment, 931–32
    discharge considerations, 932
    pain, 932
Endorphins
  defined, 103
  in pain conduction, 103
Endoscopic band ligation, for esophageal
    varices, 440, 440f
Endoscopic sclerotherapy, for esophageal
    varices, 440, 440f
Endoscopy
  in cancer diagnosis, 163
  defined, 163
  nursing care, 409
  upper
    for gastritis, 409, 409f
    for peptic ulcer disease (PUD),
      413
Endotoxin, defined, 245
Endotracheal tube (ETT)
  nursing care, 723f
  preparation for, 725
  pros and cons, 723t
  in respiratory failure, 722–23, 723f
  suctioning of, 726f
Enemas
  barium, as diagnostic procedure, 459
  for constipation, 459, 461
  types of, 461
Enteral feedings, 400–401, 401f, 402f
  administration of, 401, 402f
  formulas for, 400–401
  nasogastric tube insertion, 400, 401f
Enterotoxins, in gastroenteritis, 469
Enucleation, 871

Environment, affect on health, 23
Enzyme-linked immunosorbent assay
    (ELISA), in HIV diagnosis, 286
Enzymes alanine aminotransferase (ALT), in
    cancer diagnosis, 163
Eosinophils, 639
  laboratory values for, 241t, 639t
Epicardium, 538
Epicondylitis, 747–48
Epidermis, 298, 298t
Epididymis, 886
Epididymitis, 895
Epidural blocks, 137
Epiglottitis, 658
Epilepsy (See also Seizure disorder)
  defined, 813
Epileptogenic focus, 813
Epinephrine, function of, 343, 343t
Epistaxis, 664–65
  collaborative care, 664–65
    nasal packing, 664, 664f
    surgical treatment, 664–65
  nursing care, 665
    anxiety, 665
    assessment, 665
    discharge considerations, 665
    risk for aspiration, 665
  pathophysiology, 664
Epoetin alfa (Epogen, Procrit), for leukemia,
    643t
Equianalgesic dosage chart, 107, 109t, 116
Equilibrium, inner ear and, 873, 877–78
Erectile dysfunction (ED), 899–901
  case study, 901–2
  collaborative care, 900–901
    diagnostic tests, 900
    mechanical devices, 900
    pharmacology, 900, 900f
    surgical treatment, 900–901, 901f
  nursing care, 901
    assessment, 901
    discharge considerations, 901
    sexual dysfunction, 901
  pathophysiology, 900
Erection
  factors that affect, 900
  process of, 886
Erosion, of skin, 299t
Erythema
  assessment for, 52
  defined, 298
Erythrocyte sedimentation rate (ESR)
  in glomerulonephritis, 508
  purpose of, 240
  in rheumatoid arthritis, 773
  in systemic lupus erythematous, 778

Erythrocytes (*See* Red blood cells (RBC))
Erythrocytosis, 634
Erythromycin (E-Mycin), 254t
Erythroplakia, 669
Erythropoietin, 496
    for leukemia, 643t
Escharotomy, in burn injuries, 331
Esophageal varices
    in cirrhosis, 436–37
    defined, 436
    endoscopic sclerotherapy for, 440,
        440f
Esophagitis, caused by alcohol abuse, 225
Esophagus
    disorders of
        cancer of, 407
        gastroesophageal reflux disease
            (GERD), 406–7
        hiatal hernia, 407
    function of, 394
Estrogen
    in benign prostatic hypertrophy, 887
    function of, 908
    for osteoporosis, 760
Ethacrynic acid (Edecrin), nursing
        considerations for, 73t
Ethambutol (EMB), for tuberculosis, 694t, 696
Ethical considerations
    in end of life care, 186
    in medical-surgical nursing, 10–11
Ethics, defined, 9
Ethnic factors, affect on health, 22
Ethnic identity, defined, 3f
Ethnocentrism, defined, 3f
Etoposide, in chemotherapy, 167t
Euphoria
    defined, 222
    in intoxication, 222
Eupnea, 54
Eustachian tube, 872
Euthanasia, 186
    involuntary, 186
    voluntary, 186
Euthyroid, defined, 348
Evaluation, concepts, 6
Evisceration, 145, 146f
Exacerbation, defined, 25
Exercise
    diabetes mellitus and, 367–68, 374–75,
        378f
    hypertension and, 598
    obesity and, 397, 398
    in rheumatoid arthritis, 774
Exophthalmos, 346, 347f
Exotoxin, defined, 245
Expected outcomes (*See* Outcomes)

External otitis, 873–74
    nursing care, 873–74
        assessment, 873
        discharge considerations, 874
    pathophysiology, 873
    prevention, 873f
Extracellular fluid (ECF)
    defined, 64
    function of, 65
Extracorporeal shock wave lithotripsy
        (ESWL), 428, 514
Extubate, defined, 137
Eye disorders, 858–71
    blindness, 871
    cataracts, 863–64
    detached retina, 869–70
    diabetic retinopathy, 871
    enucleation, 871
    glaucoma, 864–69
    inflammatory and infectious, 858–60
        blepharitis, 858
        collaborative care, 859–60
            corneal transplant, 859
            eye irrigation, 859
            pharmacology, 859
        conjunctivitis, 858–59, 858f
        iritis, 859
        keratitis, 859
        nursing care, 859–60
            assessment, 859
            discharge considerations, 860
            pain, 860
            risk for injury, 860
        uveitis, 859
    macular degeneration, 870–71
    refractive errors, 862–63
    trauma, 860–62
        blunt eye trauma, 861
        burns, 860
        collaborative care, 861–62
        corneal abrasion, 860
        nursing care, 861–62
        perforation, 861
Eye irrigation
    for eye infections, 859
    for eye trauma, 861
Eye surgery
    for cataracts, 863, 863f
    laser in situ keratomileusis (LASIK),
        862, 862f
    nursing care for, 864f
    photorefractive keratectomy (PRK),
        862
    radial keratotomy, 862
Eyelashes, 856

Eyelids, 856
    blepharitis, 858
    blepharospasm, 859
Eyes
    assessment of, 52–53 (*See also* Vision,
        assessment of)
        external structures, 52–53
        fluorescein staining, 861
        ophthalmoscopic examination, 861
        pupils, 53, 53f
        visual acuity, 53, 53f
    effects of autonomic nervous system on,
        794f
    effects of hypertension on, 598t
    structures of, 856–57, 857f
        accessory, 856, 856f
        cornea, 856
        interior cavities, 856–57
        retina, 856
        uvea, 856

F

Face, fracture of, 742f
Fall prevention, 743f
Fallopian tubes, 908f, 909
Family
    of adult client, 19–22
    with children, 22
    chronic illness and, 25
    defined, 19
    developmental stages of, 21–22
    grieving and death, 184–85, 189
    home health care and, 34, 38
    tasks of, 19–21
Family function, defined, 19
Family structure, defined, 19
Fasciculations
    in amyotrophic lateral sclerosis (ALS),
        839
    defined, 839
Fasciotomy, 736–37
Fat embolism, in fractures, 737
Fat-fold measures, 397, 397f
Fats (lipids), 395t
    high blood levels, coronary heart disease
        and, 553
    high-density lipoprotein (HDL), 553,
        555t
    low-density lipoprotein (LDL), 553,
        555t
    low-fat diet, 428f, 555t
    obesity and intake of, 397
Febrile reaction, in transfusions, 207
Fecal impaction, 458

Fecal incontinence, 463–64
    defined, 463
    discharge considerations, 463–64
    etiology, 463, 463f
    impaired skin integrity, 463
Feces, 454, 454f
Fenoprofen calcium (Nalfon), for
        inflammation, 242t
Fentanyl (Duragesic), transdermal, 108, 108t
Ferritin, in anemia diagnosis, 629
Fetal alcohol syndrome, 226, 226f
Fever
    inflammation and, 239
    in older adults, 239
Fiber
    high, diet, 486f
    low-residue diet, following bowel
        surgery, 480f
Fibrocartilaginous callus, 735
Fibromyalgia, 784
Fibula fracture, 741t
Filgrastin (Neupogen)
    for agranulocytosis, 640
    for leukemia, 643t
Filtration, in body fluid movement, 66
Finasteride (Proscar), for benign prostatic
        hypertrophy, 887
Fissure(s)
    anal, 487
    of the brain, 790
    skin, 299t
Fistula
    anorectal, 488
    arteriovenous (AV), for hemodialysis,
        525, 526f
    in Crohn's disease, 472
    defined, 239, 931
    vaginal, 931
5-fluorouracil (5-FU), in chemotherapy, 166t
Flail chest, 719–20, 719f
Fluconazole (Diflucan), 251, 255t
Fluid imbalance, 64–88
    body fluids
        composition of, 64
        distribution of, 64–65, 65f
        movement of, 65–66
        regulation of, 66–68
    fluid restriction, 72f, 73
    fluid volume deficit, 68–72
        causes of, 69t
        collaborative care, 69–70
        discharge considerations, 72, 72f
        risk for injury, 71
        laboratory values in, 69t
        manifestations, 69t
        pathophysiology, 68–69
        treatment, 71

fluid volume excess, 72–76
    assessment, 74, 74f
    case study, 75–76
    causes of, 69t
    collaborative care, 73
    discharge considerations, 74–75
    impaired skin integrity, 74
    laboratory values in, 69t
    manifestations, 69t
    in metabolic acidosis, 93
    pathophysiology, 73
    treatment, 74
Fluid replacement
    assessment for, 70, 70f
    in burn injuries, 330, 333
    for diarrhea, 455–56
    for gastroenteritis, 470
    for increased intracranial pressure, 798
    intravenous, 70, 71t, 206–7
        blood and blood products (See
            Transfusions)
        colloid solutions, 206, 206t
        crystalloid solutions, 206
    for shock, 206–7
    types of, 69–70
Flunitrazepam (Rohypnol), 227
Fluoride, for osteoporosis, 762t
Fluoroquinolones
    client education, 253t
    nursing responsibilities, 253t
    purpose of, 253t
Folic acid
    food sources for, 632f
    replacement for anemia, 629, 631f
Folic acid deficiency anemia, 626, 633–34
Follicle-stimulating hormone (FSH), 343t,
        908
Folliculitis, 307
Food poisoning, 469 (See also
        Gastroenteritis)
    staphylococcal, 470t
Food pyramid
    for controlling obesity, 398, 398f
    diabetes, 374
Food safety measures, 471
Foot
    diabetic, 382
    fracture of, 741t
Foot care, in peripheral vascular disorders,
        608f
Foot disorders, 768–69
    collaborative care, 768–69
    hallux valgus, 768, 768f
    hammer toe, 768, 768f
Forensic considerations, in emergency care,
        213

Fovea, 856
Fowler's position, 74
Fracture(s), 735–44
    collaborative care, 737–44
        casts, 737
        electrical bone stimulation, 740
        emergency care, 737
        fracture reduction, 737
        surgical treatment, 739
            external fixator, 739, 740f
            internal fixation, 739, 740f
            open reduction and internal
                fixation (ORIF), 739,
                741f
        traction, 737–39
    complications
        compartment syndrome, 736–37,
            737f
        delayed union, 737
        fat embolism, 737
    healing process, 735–36
    manifestations of, 736f
    nursing care, 740–44
        assessment, 740–41, 743
        discharge considerations, 743–44
        impaired physical mobility, 742–43
        ineffective tissue perfusion, 743
        pain, 740–42
    in older adults, 743f
    pathologic
        defined, 645
        in multiple myeloma, 645
        in osteoporosis, 759
    pathophysiology, 735
    specific location
        ankle, 741t
        clavicle, 741t, 742f
        face, 742f
        fibula, 741t
        foot, 741t
        hand, 741t
        hip, 744–46
        humerus, 741t
        nose, 665–67
        pelvis, 742t
        rib, 719, 742t
        skull, 742t, 794–95
        spine, 742t
        tibia, 741t
        wrist, 741t
    types of, 735, 736t
Functional health patterns, in diagnosis, 5
Fungi, in infection, 245f
Furosemide (Lasix), nursing considerations
        for, 73t
Furuncle, 307

G

Gag reflex, 799f
Gallbladder
  disorders of, 427–31
    cancer, 431
    cholecystitis, 427–31
    cholelithiasis, 427–31
    nursing interventions classification,
        447–48
  functions of, 426
Gallstones (*See* Cholelithiasis)
Ganciclovir (Cytovene), 255t
Gangrene
  amputation and, 749
  defined, 381, 749
  diabetes mellitus and, 381
Gardner-Wells tongs, for spinal cord injury,
    844, 845f
Gastrectomy
  partial, 414
  total, 414
Gastric bypass, 398
Gastric lavage, 409, 412f
  closed system, 412f
  for gastroenteritis, 470
  intermittent open system, 412f
Gastric mucosa
  in gastritis, 408, 408f
  in peptic ulcer disease (PUD), 413
Gastric surgery, 414, 415t–416t, 416f
  anastomosis, 414
  complications of, 414
  gastrectomy
    partial, 414
    total, 414
  gastroduodenostomy, 415t
  gastrojejunostomy, 415t
  nursing care, 415
  pyloroplasty, 415t
  vagotomy, 416t
Gastritis, 408–12
  acute
    defined, 408
    manifestations of, 408f
    pathophysiology, 408
    treatment, 409
  caused by alcohol abuse, 225
  chronic
    defined, 408
    manifestations of, 408f
    pathophysiology, 408
  collaborative care, 408–12
    complimentary therapies, 409
    diagnostic tests, 408–9

nutritional issues, 411
pharmacology, 409, 410t
nursing care, 409–411
  assessment, 409
  deficient fluid volume, 409, 411
  discharge considerations, 411–12
stress-linked, 408
Gastroduodenostomy, 415t
Gastroenteritis, 469–71
  collaborative care, 470–71
  defined, 469
  etiology, 469, 470t
  manifestations of, 469–70, 469f
  nursing care, 471
    discharge considerations, 471
  pathophysiology, 469–70
Gastroesophageal reflux disease (GERD),
    406–7
  client education, 407
  defined, 406
  management of, 407
Gastrointestinal decompression, in bowel
    obstruction, 482
Gastrointestinal disorders
  lower (*See* Bowel disorders)
  upper, 404–20
    esophagus
      esophageal cancer, 407
      gastroesophageal reflux disease
          (GERD), 406–7
      hiatal hernia, 407
    mouth, stomatitis, 404–6
    stomach
      cancer, 418–19
      gastritis, 408–12
      peptic ulcer (PUD), 412–18
Gastrointestinal system
  in adults, 18t, 20t
  AIDS-related infection in, 284–85
  autonomic neuropathies in, 382
  components of, 394–96, 394f
    lower, 454
    upper, 394, 396
  effect of burns on, 329
  effect of leukemia on, 640f
  effect of spinal cord injury on, 844f
  effect of systemic lupus erythematous on,
      779f
  effects of cerebrovascular accident on,
      807–8, 807t
  effects of cirrhosis on, 436f
  effects of hypothyroidism on, 352f
  effects of multiple sclerosis on, 832f
  effects of premenstrual syndrome on,
      922f
  effects of shock on, 200, 202f

effects of uremia on, 524f
functions of, 394–96, 454
trauma issues in, 212
Gastrojejunostomy, 415t
Gastroplasty, 398
Gastroscopy, 409, 409f, 413
Gastrostomy tube, placement procedure,
    419, 419f
  nursing care, 419
Gate-control theory of pain, 103–4, 104f
Gatifloxacin (Tequin), 253t
Gender differences
  affect on health, 23
  cancer risk factors and, 158
  in myocardial infarction (MI), 563f
Genetics, affect on health, 22
Genital herpes, 949t, 953–54
  collaborative care, 949t, 953–54
  complications, 949t, 953
  first episode infection, 953
  latency, 953
  manifestations of, 949t
  neonatal infection, 953–54
  nursing care, 953
    ineffective health maintenance, 953
    pain, 953
  pathophysiology, 953
  prodromal symptoms, 953
  recurrent infection, 953
Genital warts, 949t, 954–55
  collaborative care, 949t, 954–55
    pharmacology, 954
    removal, 954
  complications, 949t
  manifestations of, 949t
  nursing care, 954–55
    discharge considerations, 954–55
  pathophysiology, 954
Genitourinary system
  in adults, 18t, 20t
  autonomic neuropathies in, 382
  effect of spinal cord injury on, 844f
  effects of cerebrovascular accident on,
      807t
  effects of prostate cancer on, 891f
  effects of uremia on, 524f
  trauma issues in, 212
Gentamicin (Garamycin), 253t
Geographic location, affect on health, 23
Giardiasis, 470t
Gland(s) (*See also* Endocrine disorders;
    Endocrine system; specific gland)
  adrenal, 342–43, 343t
  Bartholin's, 909f, 910
  lacrimal, 856
  parathyroid, 342, 343t

inheritance pattern for, 637f
nursing care, 638–39
   discharge considerations, 638–39
   risk for injury, 638
pathophysiology, 637
type A, 637, 638t
type B, 637, 638t
Von Willebrand's disease, 637, 638t
Hemoptysis, defined, 680
Hemorrhage (*See also* Hematoma)
as an effect of cancer, 161
arterial, 143
in cerebrovascular accident, 806, 807t
defined, 143
hypovolemic shock and, 201, 203t, 205, 207
intracranial, 795, 795f
in peptic ulcer disease, 413–14, 413f
subarachnoid
   in cerebral aneurysm, 812
   defined, 812
   manifestations of, 812
as surgical complication, 143, 146
in trauma clients, 211, 211f
treatment, 143
venous, 143
Hemorrhagic colitis, 470t
Hemorrhoidectomy, for hemorrhoids, 487
Hemorrhoids, 486–87
collaborative care, 487
defined, 486
etiology, 486
external, 486f, 487
internal, 486–87, 486f
nursing care, 487
Hemostasis, 635
Hemothorax, 718
Hemovac wound suction device, 145f
Heparin
actions of, 615t
for deep venous thrombosis, 614
for pulmonary embolism, 713–14
Hepatic system, cirrhosis effects on, 436f
Hepatitis, 431–35
alcoholic, 225, 433
B (HBV), 431, 432t
   vaccine for, 434, 434f
C, 432t, 433
chronic active, 433
chronic persistent, 433
collaborative care, 433–35
   complimentary therapies, 434
   diagnostic tests, 433
   nutritional issues, 435
   prevention, 433–34
   treatment, 434

D (HDV), 432t, 433
defined, 431
fulminant, 433
A (HAV), 431, 432t
   vaccine for, 433
hepatobiliary, 433
manifestations of, 433, 433f
noninfectious, 433
nursing care, 434–35
   activity intolerance, 434
   assessment, 434, 435f
   discharge considerations, 435, 435f
   risk for infection, 434
pathophysiology, 431, 433
phases of
   icteric, 433, 433f
   posticteric, 433, 433f
   preicteric, 433, 433f
toxic, 433
types of, 431, 432t
viral, 431, 432t, 433
Hepatocytes, 426
Hepatorenal syndrome
cirrhosis and, 436
defined, 436
Hernia, 484–85
acquired, 484
collaborative care, 485
   surgical treatment, 485
defined, 484
hiatal, 407, 407f
inguinal, 484, 484f
irreducible, 484
nursing care, 485
   discharge considerations, 485
   tissue perfusion, 485
pathophysiology, 484
reducible, 484
strangulated, 484
umbilical, 484, 484f
ventral, 484
Herniated disk (*See* Disk, herniated intervertebral)
Herniorrhaphy, 485
Heroin, abuse of, 223t, 226–27, 229
Herpes simplex, 308 (*See also* Genital herpes)
AIDS-related, 285, 288t
in Bell's Palsy, 840
stomatitis and, 404
Herpes zoster, 308
diagnostic tests, 309
in older adults, 249t
Hiatal hernia, 407, 407f
paraesophageal, 407, 407f
sliding, 407, 407f

High-density lipoprotein (HDL), 553, 555t
High fiber diet, 485, 486f
Highly active antiretroviral therapy (HAART), for HIV infection, 286–87
Hip, dislocation of, 747
Hip fracture, 744–46
case study, 746
collaborative care, 744–46
   surgical treatment, 744, 744f
extracapsular, 744
intracapsular, 744
nursing care, 744–46
   assessment, 744
   discharge considerations, 745–46, 745f
   impaired physical mobility, 745
   impaired skin integrity, 745
   pain, 744–45
pathophysiology, 744, 744f
Hirsutism
in Cushing's syndrome, 357
defined, 52, 357
Histamine-2 receptor blockers
for gastritis, 409, 410t
for increased intracranial pressure, 798
for peptic ulcer disease, 414
for spinal cord injury, 844
Histocompatibility, defined, 278
History taking (*See* Health history)
HIV infection, 281–93 (*See also* Acquired immunodeficiency syndrome (AIDS))
collaborative care
   diagnostic tests, 286
   nutritional issues, 289–90
   pharmacology, 286–88, 287t, 288t
   prevention, 285–86, 286f
diagnosis of, 282
incidence, 282
manifestations of, 282, 284f
nursing care, 288–91
   assessment, 288, 289f
   case study, 292–93
   coping, 289
   dementia, 290–91
   discharge considerations, 291, 291f
   fatigue, 290
   ineffective breathing patterns, 290
   risk for infection, 289
   skin integrity, 290
opportunistic infections and, 289–90
pathophysiology, 282, 283f, 284f
risk factors for, 282
routes of transmission, 282
stages of, 282–83, 284f
HIV viral load tests, in HIV diagnosis, 286

Hodgkin's disease (*See also* Malignant
  lymphoma), 648
  case study, 650–51
  manifestations of, 648f
Holistic, defined, 3
Holistic health care, 22
Homan's sign, 147
  in deep vein thrombosis, 612
  defined, 143
Home care order, 34
Home health agencies
  bill of rights for, 36f
  types of, 33
Home health care, 33–40
  American Nurses Association
    position statements, 37
    standards, 37
  cancer and, 175
  chronic illness and, 26
  client base for, 33–34
  client bill of rights, 36f, 37
  discharge considerations, 37
  family issues and, 34, 38
  history of, 34
  HIV infection and, 291
  home care order, 34
  initial visit, 34–35
  legal considerations, 37
  nursing process, 39–40
    assessment, 39
    diagnosis, 39
    evaluation, 40
    implementation, 40
    planning, 40
  practical suggestions for nurses, 38–39
  referrals to, 34, 37–38
  reimbursement for, 35
  role of nurse in, 35–36
  services provided, 34
  special issues in
    infection control, 39
    safety, 39
Homeostasis, defined, 200
Homonymous hemianopia, 807, 807f
Hordeolum, 858, 858f
Hormone replacement therapy (HRT)
  benefits of, 927
  for menopause, 927–28, 927f
  for osteoporosis, 760–61
  side effects of, 927
Hormone therapy
  for erectile dysfunction (ED), 900, 900f
  for prostate cancer, 891–92
Hormones
  as carcinogen, 158
  counter regulatory, 366

in endocrine system, 342
  female, 908
  male, 886 (*See also* Androgens)
  negative feedback regulation of, 342
  obesity and, 397
  synthetic, for diarrhea, 457t
Hospice (*See also* End of life care)
  cancer and, 175
  multidisciplinary team for, 175
Hospitalization
  discharge and home health care, 32, 37–38
  nosocomial infections and, 247–48
  undernutrition and, 400
Host, in infection process, 246
Hot flashes, in menopause, 927, 928f
Human immunodeficiency virus (HIV) (*See*
  Acquired immunodeficiency
  syndrome (AIDS); HIV infection)
Human leukocyte antigens (HLA)
  defined, 268
  transplants and, 277
Humerus fracture, 741t
Hydrochlorothiazide (HydroDIURIL),
  nursing considerations for, 73t, 574t
Hydrogen ion concentration, in acid-base
  balance, 88
Hydronephrosis, 515–16
  defined, 515
  diagnosis of, 515
  manifestations, 515, 515f
  ureteral stents for, 515, 515f, 516f
Hydrostatic pressure, defined, 66
Hydroureter, defined, 513
Hydroxyzine (Vistaril), 275t
Hyperalimentation, 402, 402f
Hypercalcemia
  in cancer, 178
  causes of, 83t
  collaborative care, 83–84, 178
  defined, 83
  hyperparathyroidism and, 354
  laboratory values, 83t
  manifestations, 83t, 178
  neuromuscular effects of, 83, 83t
Hypercapnia, in respiratory failure, 721–22,
  722f
Hyperglycemia
  defined, 366
  in diabetes mellitus
    type 1, 368
    type 2, 369
  in diabetic ketoacidosis, 378
Hyperglycemic hyperosmolar nonketotic
  syndrome (HHNS), 378
  manifestations of, 380f
  treatment, 378

Hyperinsulinism, defined, 378–79
Hyperkalemia, 80
  causes of, 79t
  collaborative care, 80
  laboratory values, 79t
  manifestations, 79t
  nursing care, 80
Hypermagnesemia, 85
  causes of, 86t
  defined, 85
  laboratory values, 86t
  manifestations, 86t
Hypernatremia, 76–77
  causes of, 76t
  client education, 78
  collaborative care, 77
  defined, 76
  laboratory values, 76t
  manifestations, 76t
  nursing care, 77
Hyperopia, 862t
Hyperosmolarity, defined, 344
Hyperparathyroidism, 83, 354–55
  collaborative care, 354–55
  discharge considerations, 355
  manifestations of, 354f
  pathophysiology, 354
Hyperphosphatemia, 88
  causes of, 87t
  laboratory values, 87t
  manifestations, 87t
Hyperpituitarism
  collaborative care, 344
  pathophysiology, 344
Hypersensitivity reactions, 273–75
  anaphylactic shock and, 201
  collaborative care, 275–76
    diagnostic tests, 275
    pharmacology, 275, 275t
  defined, 273
  latex allergy, 274–75, 275f
  nursing care, 275–76
    discharge considerations, 276
  types of, 274t, 276
Hypertension, 597–604
  case study, 603–4
  collaborative care, 598–604
    complementary and alternative
      medicine, 599
    life style modifications, 598, 599t
      diet, 598
      exercise, 598
      smoking, 598
      stress, 598, 599f
    pharmacology, 598–99,
      600t–601t

complementary and alternative medicine, 599
coronary heart disease and, 553
defined, 597
hypertensive crisis, 598
isolated systolic, 597, 597f
malignant, 598
nursing care, 599–603
assessment, 599, 602
discharge considerations, 602–3, 603f
in older adults, 597f
pathophysiology, 597–99
portal, 436
primary, 597
pulmonary, 715
secondary, 597
stages of, 598
Hypertensive crisis, 598
Hyperthermia, 216
in intracranial infections, 819
in osteomyelitis, 765
Hyperthyroidism, 346–50
case study, 350–51
collaborative care, 346–50
nutritional issues, 348–49
pharmacology, 346–47, 348t
radioactive therapy, 347–48
surgery, 348
Grave's disease, 346, 350–51
multisystem effects of, 347f
nursing care, 348–50
assessment, 348, 349f
body image, 350
decreased cardiac output, 349
discharge considerations, 350, 350f
fatigue, 349
risk for injury, 350
pathophysiology, 346
thyrotoxic crisis, 346
Hypertonic solutions, 66, 66f
Hyperuricemia, in cancer, 178
in gout, 780
prevention, 178
signs and symptoms of, 178
Hyperventilation, 54
Hypervolemia, defined, 73
Hypnotics, abuse of, 223t, 227
Hypnotism, in pain management, 112
Hypoalbuminemia
defined, 507
in glomerulonephritis, 507
Hypocalcemia
causes of, 83t
collaborative care, 82–83
defined, 82

laboratory values, 83t
manifestations, 83t
neuromuscular effects of, 83, 83t
pharmacological treatment, 84t
Hypoglycemia
defined, 366
diabetes mellitus and, 378–81
manifestations, 381f
treatment, 379–80
mild, 380
severe, 380–81
Hypokalemia, 78–79
case study, 81–82
causes of, 79t
collaborative care, 78–79
laboratory values, 79t
manifestations, 79t
pharmacological treatment, 79t
Hypomagnesemia, 85
causes of, 86t
defined, 85
laboratory values, 86t
manifestations, 86t
Hyponatremia
causes of, 76t
client education, 78
collaborative care, 76, 77f
defined, 76
laboratory values, 76t
manifestations, 76t
Hypoosmolarity, defined, 344
Hypoparathyroidism, 355–56
causes of, 82
collaborative care, 355–56
discharge considerations, 355–56
hypocalcemia and, 82
manifestations of, 355f
pathophysiology, 355
Hypophosphatemia, 87–88
causes of, 87t
laboratory values, 87t
manifestations, 87t
Hypophysectomy, 357
Hypophysis, 342
Hypopituitarism
collaborative care, 344
pathophysiology, 344
Hypothalamus, 342, 790
Hypothermia, 216
Hypothyroidism, 351–54
collaborative care, 351–54
pharmacology, 351, 352t
goiter and, 351
Hashimoto's thyroiditis, 351
multisystem effects of, 352f
myxedema coma, 351

nursing care, 353–54
activity intolerance, 353
assessment, 353, 353f
constipation, 353
discharge considerations, 353–54
evaluation, 353
hypothermia, 353
thought processes, 353
pathophysiology, 351
Hypotonic solutions, 66, 66f
Hypoventilation, 54
Hypovolemia
defined, 68
relative, 202
in renal failure, 523
Hypoxemia
defined, 200
in respiratory failure, 721–22, 722f
in shock, 200
Hysterectomy
for dysfunctional uterine bleeding, 924
for endometrial cancer, 936
nursing care, 926f
for ovarian cancer, 937
for uterine fibroid tumor, 933

Ibuprofen (Motrin, Advil), for inflammation, 242t
ICU (intensive care unit), 216–17
ICU psychosis, 217
Idiopathic thrombocytopenia purpura (ITP), 635–36
Ileal conduit, for bladder cancer, 518, 519f
Ileoanal anastomosis, 474, 474f
Ileostomy, 474
Kock's, 474, 474f
nursing care for, 480f
Ileum, 396, 454
Illness (See also Disease)
acute, 24–25
defined, 24
in adult clients, 23–26
chronic, 25–26
adaptation to, 25
characteristics of, 25
defined, 25
factors that influence, 25
family and, 25
intensity of, 25
defined, 24
health-illness continuum, 22, 22f
stages of, 24–25
Immune globulin (IG), in hepatitis treatment, 433

Immune system, 266–69
  autoimmune disease, 276–77
  cell-mediated immunity, 268, 270f
  components of, 266, 268
    leukocytes, 266, 267f
    lymphoid organs and tissues, 266,
      268
  diagnostic tests, 271
  effect of burns on, 329
  effects of cirrhosis on, 436f
  effects of diabetes mellitus on, 379f
  HIV infection (See HIV infection)
  human leukocyte antigens in, 268
  humoral immunity, 268, 269f
  hypersensitivity reactions, 273–75
  immunity, 269, 271
  immunizations, 271–73
  nursing interventions classification, 293
  in older adults, 268–69
  organ/tissues transplant, 277–81
  recognition of self, 268
Immunity, 269, 271
  active, 271
  defined, 266
  natural, 269, 271
  passive, 271
Immunizations
  active immunity and, 271
  collaborative care
  for diphtheria, tetanus, pertussis (DTP),
    271, 272t
  forms of
    animal immune serums, 272
    inactivated, 271
    live, attenuated, 271
    toxoids, 271
  for hepatitis, 433–34, 434f
  for hepatitis B vaccine, 271, 272t
  for HIV infected clients, 288
  for influenza, 272t, 659
  for measles, mumps, rubella (MMR),
    271, 272t
  for pneumonia, 272t, 685
  for rabies, 841
  nursing care, 273
    assessment, 273, 273f
    discharge considerations, 273
    risk for injury, 273
  sensitivity testing and, 272
  side effects of, 272
  for tetanus, 841
  when traveling, 271
Immunocompetent, defined, 268
Immunodeficiency
  primary, 281
  secondary, 281 (See also HIV infection)

Immunoglobulins
  classes of, 268
  defined, 268
  diagnostic testing for, 271
  functions of the various, 270f
  in rheumatoid arthritis, 772
Immunosuppression
  defined, 244
  infection and, 244
Immunosuppressive drugs
  for kidney transplantation, 528
  for transplants, 279, 280t
Immunotherapy
  in cancer treatment, 168, 169f
  desensitization, 275
  for skin cancers, 314
Impairment, defined, 40
Implementation (See Intervention)
Impotence (See Erectile dysfunction (ED))
Incision and drainage (I&D)
  for abscesses, 239
  for tonsillitis, 660
Incontinence (See Fecal incontinence;
    Urinary incontinence)
Increased intracranial pressure (IICP),
    795–802
  case study, 801–2
  cerebral edema and, 795–96
  collaborative care, 797–801
    diagnostic tests, 798
    intracranial pressure monitoring, 798
    pharmacology, 798
    surgical treatment, 798
  complications of
    altered level of consciousness, 796,
      797f
    brain death, 797
    brain herniation, 796–97
  defined, 795
  manifestations of, 795, 797t
  nursing care, 799–801
    assessment, 799, 799f
    discharge considerations, 801
    imbalanced nutrition, 800
    impaired physical mobility, 800
    impaired skin integrity, 800
    ineffective breathing pattern, 800
    ineffective tissue perfusion, 799–800
    risk for infection, 800
Indomethacin (Indocin), for inflammation,
    242t, 775t
Infection, 244–59
  case study, 259
  chain of, 244–46, 244f
    host, 246
    microorganisms, 245, 245f, 246t

  portal of entry, 246
  portal of exit, 245–46
  reservoir, 245–46
  transmission, 246
collaborative care, 250–55
  diagnostic tests, 250–51
  pharmacology, 251, 252t–254t, 254
    (See also Antimicrobials)
community-acquired, 248
complications of, 247
emerging, 248
incubation period, 246–47
nosocomial, 247–48
  clostridium difficile-Associated
    Diarrhea (CDAD), 248
  defined, 247
  infection control, 254–55
  methicillin-resistant Staphylococcus
    aureus (MRSA), 248, 259
  risk factors for, 247f
  urinary tract infection, 502
  vancomycin-resistant Enterococcus
    (VRE), 248
nursing care, 256–58
  assessment, 256, 258f
  discharge considerations, 258–59,
    258f
  imbalanced nutrition, 256–57
  infection control, 254–55
  risk for infection, 256
  infective thermoregulation,
    257–58
risk of
  cancer and, 159–60, 172
  inflammation and, 243
  surgery and, 142, 147
  trauma and, 213–14
septic shock and, 203–4
skin, in older adults, 249t
susceptibility to, diabetes mellitus and,
    382–83
Infection control, 254–55, 256
  in home health care, 39
  isolation precautions, 255
  standard precautions, 255, 256f
  transmission precautions, 255, 257t
Infertility, male, 895–96
Inflammation, 238–44
  acute, 239
    local manifestations, 239, 240f
    systemic manifestations, 239, 240f
  in autoimmune disease, 277
  chronic, 239
  collaborative care, 239–42
    diagnostic tests, 240
    nutritional status, 241–42

pharmacology, 240–41, 242t
wound care, 241
defined, 238
inflammatory response, 238–39, 238f
role in immune system, 266
nursing care, 242–44
acute pain, 242–43
assessment, 242, 243f
discharge considerations, 243–44, 244f
impaired skin integrity, 243
risk for infection, 243
pathophysiology, 238–39
Inflammatory bowel disease (IBD), 471–76
collaborative care, 472–76
dietary management, 473–74
pharmacology, 472–73, 473t
surgical treatment, 474, 474f
Crohn's disease
defined, 472
pathophysiology, 472, 472f
nursing care, 474–76
assessment, 474–75, 475f
deficient fluid volume, 475–76
in diarrhea, 475
discharge considerations, 476
disturbed body image, 476
imbalanced nutrition, 476
ulcerative colitis
case study, 477
complications of, 472
defined, 471
pathophysiology, 471–72
Influenza, 657
manifestations of, 657t
in older adults, 249t, 657f
pharmacology, 659
vaccine for, 659
vs. rhinitis, 657t
Informed consent
components of, 131
defined, 131
example, 131f
legal considerations, 131
Inhalants, abuse of, 224t, 227–28
Inhalation, smoke, 719
Injections, Z-track, 631f
Inspection, guidelines for, 48
Inspiratory muscles, 680
Insulin
production in pancreas, 366
type 2 diabetes mellitus and, 369
Insulin injections, 371–72
client education for, 372f, 373f, 374t
continuous subcutaneous insulin infusion, 371

injection sites, 371–72, 372f
mixing insulins, 372, 373f
regimens for, 372, 375f
special products, 371
types of insulin, 371t
Insulin pens, 371
Integumentary system, 298, 300–301
effect of burns on, 329
effect of leukemia on, 640f
effect of spinal cord injury on, 844f
effect of systemic lupus erythematous on, 779f
effects of anemia on, 627f
effects of cerebrovascular accident on, 807t
effects of cirrhosis on, 436f
effects of diabetes mellitus on, 379f
effects of hyperthyroidism on, 347f
effects of hypothyroidism on, 352f
effects of premenstrual syndrome on, 922f
effects of uremia on, 524f
glands of skin, 298t, 300–301
hair, 298t, 301
nails, 298t, 301
skin, 298, 300
trauma issues in, 212, 212f
Intensive care unit (ICU), 216–17
psychological effects of, 217
Intercostal muscles, 680
Intercostal spaces, 680
Intermittent claudication, 604
International Normalized Ratio (INR), 614
International Nurses Association (ICN), code of ethics, 9, 9f
Interstitial fluid, defined, 64
Intervention
defined, 2
documentation of, 6
overview, 6
principles for, 6
Intestinal decompression
in peritonitis, 466–67
procedure for, 466–67, 467f
Intestinal obstruction, in Crohn's disease, 472
Intestine (*See also* Bowel disorders)
autonomic nervous system affects on, 794f
large
anatomy of, 454f
functions of, 454
small
functions of, 394, 396, 454
regions of, 396
Intoxication, defined, 222

Intra-aortic balloon pump (IABP), for myocardial infarction, 566, 566f
Intracellular fluid (ICF), defined, 64
Intracranial disorders
aneurysm, 812–17
brain tumor, 802–5
cerebrovascular accident (CVA), 805–12
head injuries, 794–95
headaches, 820–22
increased intracranial pressure, 795–802
infections, 817–20
brain abscess, 818
collaborative care, 818–20
diagnostic tests, 818
pharmacology, 819
encephalitis, 817–18
meningitis, 817
nursing care, 819–20
assessment, 819
discharge considerations, 820
hyperthermia, 819
ineffective tissue perfusion, 819
pain, 819–20
seizure disorder, 813–17
Intracranial hemorrhage, 795, 795f
Intracranial pressure (ICP) (*See also* Increased intracranial pressure (IICP))
after near-drowning, 720
monitoring of, 798
Intradermal allergy test, 275
Intraocular pressure
in glaucoma, 864
tonometry for, 864–65
Intravascular fluid, defined, 65
Intravenous pyelogram (IVP), in urinary tract infection, 503, 505f
Intubation, 211, 211f
Invasiveness, defined, 245
Iodine sources, for hyperthyroidism, 348t
Ion, defined, 64
Ipratropium (Atrovent), for chronic obstructive pulmonary disease, 702
Iris, 856
Iritis, 859
Iron
food sources of, 632f
replacement
advise on taking, 926
for anemia, 629, 631f
Iron deficiency anemia, 624–26
Irritable bowel syndrome, 462–63
collaborative care, 462–63
defined, 462
manifestations of, 462, 462f
nursing care, 463

Islets of Langerhans, 366
Isograft, 277
Isolation precautions, in infection control, 255
Isoniazid (INH), for tuberculosis, 693t, 695
Isotonic solutions, defined, 65–66
Isthmus, 342

Jackson Pratt wound suction device, 145f
Jacksonian march, 813–14
Jaundice
    assessment for, 52
    defined, 300, 433
    in hepatitis, 433
Jejunum, 396, 407, 454
Jet injectors, for insulin shots, 371
Joint and connective tissue disorders, 769–85
    ankylosing spondylitis, 783–84
    dislocation of, 747
    fibromyalgia, 784
    gout, 780–83
    low back pain, 784–85
    Lyme disease, 783
    muscular dystrophy, 785
    osteoarthritis, 769–72
    rheumatoid arthritis, 772–78
    systemic lupus erythematous, 778–80
Joint Commission on Accreditation of
        Healthcare Organizations (JCAHO)
    on assessment, 46
    quality assurance and, 3
Joint replacement, 770
    nursing care for, 770f
    total hip, 744, 770, 770f
    total knee, 770
Joints, types of, 732–33
    amphiarthrosis, 732
    synarthrosis, 732
    synovial, 732–33, 733f

Kanamycin (Kantrex), 253t
Kaposi's sarcoma, AIDS-related, 285, 288t
Kegel exercises
    for fecal incontinence, 463
    for pelvic organ prolapse, 930
    for urinary incontinence, 501, 501f
Keloids
    in burn injuries, 332
    defined, 299t, 332

Keratectomy, photorefractive, 862
Keratin, 298
Keratitis, 859
Keratotomy, radial, 862
Kernig's sign, in meningitis, 817, 818f
Ketoconazole (Nizoral), 255t
Ketone bodies
    in diabetes mellitus, 368
    in diabetic ketoacidosis, 378
Ketones
    monitoring, 369–70
    urine test for, 370
Ketoprofen (Orudis), for inflammation,
        242t, 775
Ketorolac (Toradol), for inflammation, 242t
Ketosis
    in diabetes mellitus, 368
    in diabetic ketoacidosis, 378
Kidney disease, polycystic, 516
    collaborative care, 516
    discharge considerations, 516
    nursing care, 516
    pathophysiology, 516
Kidneys (See also Renal system)
    age-related changes in, 496–97, 496t
    endocrine function of, 496
    role in blood pressure, 597
    role in body fluid regulation, 67
    role in calcium imbalance, 82, 82f
    role in potassium balance, 78
    structure of, 494
    trauma to, 517
Kilocalories (kcal), 396
Kinetic continuous rotation bed, 214, 214f
Koch's pouch, for bladder cancer, 518, 519t
Kock's ileostomy, 474, 474f
Korsakoff's syndrome, caused by alcohol
        abuse, 225–26
Kupffer cells, 426
Kyphosis, 758–59
    collaborative care, 758–59
    defined, 758
    of spine, 54

Labia majora, 909–10, 909f
Labia minora, 909f, 910
Labile mood, defined, 222
Labyrinth, of the ear, 872
Labyrinthitis, 877
Lacerations, 212f
Lacrimal apparatus, 856
Lacrimal ducts, 856
Lacrimal gland, 856

Lactic dehydrogenase (LDH)
    in cancer diagnosis, 163
    cardiac marker, 564, 565t
Lactose breath test, 464
Lactose intolerance, 464
    in inflammatory bowel disease, 473–74
Lactose tolerance test, 464
Laminectomy, for herniated intervertebral
        disk, 848, 848f
Laparoscopy
    defined, 465
    for dysfunctional uterine bleeding, 924
    nursing care, 925f
    for ovarian cancer, 937
Laparotomy
    defined, 465
    for peritonitis, 467
Large intestine (See also Bowel disorders)
    anatomy of, 454f
    functions of, 454
Laryngeal cancer, 669–74
    in African Americans, 669f
    collaborative care, 669–74
        chemotherapy, 670
        diagnostic tests, 669–70
        radiation therapy, 670
        speech rehabilitation, 670–71
        surgical treatment, 670
    locations of, 669, 669f
    manifestations of, 669f
    nursing care, 671–74
        anticipatory grieving, 673
        assessment, 671, 671f
        discharge considerations, 674, 674f
        imbalanced nutrition, 672–73
        impaired communication, 672
    pathophysiology, 669
Laryngeal obstruction, 667, 667f
    etiology, 667
    Heimlich maneuver for, 667, 667f
    laryngospasm in, 667
    manifestations of, 667
Laryngectomy
    for laryngeal cancer, 670, 670f
    nursing care for, 672f
Laryngitis, 658–59
Laryngopharynx, 656
Laryngoscopy, in laryngeal cancer, 669
Laryngospasm, 667
Larynx, 656
    benign tumors of, 668–69
    trauma to, 667
Laser in situ keratomileusis (LASIK), 862,
        862f
Latex allergy, 274–75, 274f
Laughter, in pain management, 110

Laxatives
  in cirrhosis treatment, 438t
  for constipation, 459, 460t–461t
LDL (low-density lipoprotein), 553, 555t
Legal considerations
  with AIDS clients, 10–11
  client rights, 10
  death and dying, 10
  in end of life care, 186
  in home health care, 37
  informed consent, 131
Legionnaire's disease, 683t
Lens of the eye, 856
Lesions, defined, 52
Leukemia, 640–45
  acute lymphocytic, 641t
  acute myelocytic, 641t
  chronic lymphocytic, 641t
  chronic myelocytic, 641t
  classification of, 640, 641t
  collaborative care, 641–46
    biologic therapy, 642
    bone marrow transplantation, 641–42
    chemotherapy, 641
    radiation therapy, 641
  manifestations, 640, 640f
  nursing care, 642–45
    anticipatory grieving, 644–45
    assessment, 642, 644f
    discharge considerations, 645
    imbalanced nutrition, 642
    impaired oral mucous membrane, 644
    ineffective protection, 644
    risk for infection, 642
  pathophysiology, 640
  risk factors for, 640
Leukocytes (See White blood cells (WBC))
Leukocytosis
  defined, 240, 639
  infection and, 266
  inflammation and, 239
Leukopenia, defined, 240, 639
Leukoplakia, 669
Leukotriene modifiers, for asthma, 698t
Levofloxacin (Levaquin), 253t
Libido, defined, 886
Lice, 308–9
Lichenification, defined, 299t
Lifestyle, affect on health, 23
Ligaments, 733
  sprain of, 734
Lipectomy, 398
Lipids (See Fats (lipids))
Lipoatrophy, with insulin injections, 371–72

Lipodystrophy, with insulin injections, 371–72
Liposuction, 398
Lithiasis (See Calculi, urinary)
Lithotripsy
  extracorporeal shock-wave, 514
  percutaneous, 514, 514f
  for urinary calculi, 514
Liver
  autonomic nervous system affects on, 794f
  functions of, 426
  lobules of, 426, 426f
Liver biopsy, procedure for, 437, 437f
Liver disorders, 431–44
  cancer, 443
  cirrhosis, 436–43
  hepatitis, 431–35
  nursing interventions classification, 447–48
  trauma to, 443–44
Liver function tests, in cancer metastasis diagnosis, 313
Liver transplantation, 438–39, 439f
Living will, 186
  defined, 10
Lobectomy, 709t
Local nerve infiltration, 137
Lock jaw, 841
Long-term care facilities, as community-based health care site, 33, 42
Loop of Henle, 495f, 496
Loss
  areas of possible, 184
  family and support, 184–85
  grief and death, 184–88
  nursing interventions classification, 195
  spirituality and, 185
  stages of, 184
  stress of, 184
Lou Gehrig's disease, 839
Low-density lipoprotein (LDL), 553, 555t
Low-residue diet, following bowel surgery, 480f
LSD, abuse of, 224t, 227
Lumbar puncture
  in cerebrovascular accident diagnosis, 251
  in infection diagnosis, 251
  in intracranial infections, 818
Lumpectomy, for breast cancer, 915, 916f
Lung abscess, 689–90
Lung cancer, 707–12
  case study, 712
  cell types, 708t

collaborative care, 709–12
  diagnostic tests, 709
  radiation therapy, 709–10
  surgical treatment, 709, 709t
  manifestations of, 708–9, 709f
  metastasis in, 157t, 708–9
  nursing care, 710–11
    activity intolerance, 710
    anticipatory grieving, 711
    assessment, 710
    discharge considerations, 711
    ineffective breathing pattern, 710
    pain, 710–11
  paraneoplastic syndromes in, 708, 709f
  pathophysiology, 708–9
  superior vena cava syndrome in, 709
Lung surgery
  for chronic obstructive pulmonary disease, 702
  for lung cancer, 709, 709t
  nursing care for, 710f
  types of, 709t
Lungs
  structures of, 680, 680f, 681f
  volume and capacity, 681–82, 682f
    anatomical dead space volume, 682
    expiratory reserve volume (ERV), 681
    inspiratory reserve volume (IRV), 681
    pulmonary function tests (PFTs), 681
    residual volume (RV), 681–82
    tidal volume (VT), 681
    total lung capacity (TLC), 681
    vital capacity (VC), 682
Lupus erythematosus cell prep, 276–77
Lupus nephritis, 779
  glomerulonephritis in, 508
Luteinizing hormone (LH), 343t, 908
Lyme disease, 783
  manifestations of, 783
  prevention of, 783f
  treatment, 783
Lymph, 266, 647
Lymph node involvement, in TNM cancer classification, 162t
Lymph nodes, 266–67, 647
  function of, 268
  in lymphoid system, 268f
  physical examination, 55, 240f
    axillary, 55
    of head and neck, 53, 54f
Lymph vessels, 647
Lymphadenitis, 647
  defined, 239
  inflammation and, 239
Lymphadenopathy, 647
Lymphangitis, 647–48

Lymphatic system, 647
  components of, 266, 268
  disorders of, 647–51
    collaborative care, 647–48
    lymphangitis, 647–48
    lymphedema, 647–48
    malignant lymphoma, 648–51
    mononucleosis, 648
    nursing care, 648
Lymphatic vessels, defined, 266
Lymphedema, 647–48, 918
Lymphocytes, 639
  B-cell, 266, 267f, 639
    memory cells, 267t
    plasma cells, 267t
  development of, 266, 267t
  functions of, 267t
  laboratory values for, 241t, 639t
  natural killer (NK) cells, 266, 267f, 267t,
    639
  plasma cells, 267t
  T-cell, 266, 267f, 267t, 639
    cytotoxic T cells, 267t
    helper T cells, 267t
    suppresser T cells, 267t
  types of, 267t
Lymphogranuloma
  complications, 949t
  manifestations of, 949t
  treatment, 949t
Lymphoid irradiation, total, for rheumatoid
    arthritis, 774
Lymphoid organs
  primary, 266
  secondary, 266
Lymphoid system, 266, 268f
  bone marrow, 266
  spleen, 266
  thymus gland, 266
Lymphoma, malignant, 648–51
  AIDS-related, 285, 288t
  collaborative care, 649–50
    chemotherapy, 649
    radiation therapy, 649
  Hodgkin's disease, 648
    case study, 650–51
    manifestations of, 648f
  non-Hodgkin's lymphoma, 648–49
  nursing care, 649–50
    discharge considerations, 650
    disturbed body image, 650
    fatigue, 650
    impaired skin integrity, 649
    nausea, 649–50
  pathophysiology, 648–49
Lysozyme, 394

M

Macrolides
  client education, 254t
  nursing responsibilities, 254t
  purpose of, 254t
Macrophages, defined, 238, 639
Macula, 856
Macular degeneration, 870–71
Macule, defined, 299t
Mad cow disease, 842
Mafenide (Sulfamylon), 253t
Magnesium
  foods high in, 86f
  intravenous, 86
  normal electrolyte laboratory values for,
    64t
Magnesium imbalance, 85–87
  collaborative care, 85–86
  hypermagnesemia
    causes of, 86t
    defined, 85
    laboratory values, 86t
    manifestations, 86t
  hypomagnesemia
    causes of, 86t
    defined, 85
    laboratory values, 86t
    manifestations, 86t
  nursing care, 86–87
    assessment, 86
    discharge considerations, 86f, 87
Major histocompatibility complex (MHC),
    268
Malabsorption, bowel disorder, 464
  celiac disease, 464
  dietary management, 464, 464f
  etiology, 464
  lactose intolerance, 464
  treatment, 464
Malnutrition
  conditions associated with, 400f
  defined, 400
  as surgical risk factor, 129t
Mammary glands (See Breast)
Mammography, 914, 914f
Marfan syndrome, 610
Marijuana, abuse of, 224t, 228
Mask
  rebreather, oxygen therapy, 685, 686f
  simple face, oxygen therapy, 685, 686f
  Venturi, 685
Mast cell stabilizers, for asthma, 698t
Mastectomy, for breast cancer, 915–16, 916f
  infection risk with, 918

    modified radical, 915
    nursing care, 917f
    post operative exercises, 919, 920f
    radical, 915
Mastitis, 911
Mastoidectomy, for otitis media, 875
Mastoiditis, acute, 874–74
MB-bands, cardiac marker, 564, 565t
McBurney's point, in appendicitis, 465,
    465f
McGill Pain Questionnaire, 113, 113f
MDMA (Ecstasy), abuse of, 224t, 227
Meals on Wheels, as community-based
    health care site, 33
Mean corpuscular hemoglobin concentration
    (MCHC), normal laboratory values
    for, 626t
Mean corpuscular hemoglobin (MCH),
    normal laboratory values for, 626t
Mean corpuscular volume (MCV), normal
    laboratory values for, 626t
Mechanical ventilation
  complications, 724
  endotracheal tube for, 722–23, 723f
  modes of, 723, 724t
  pharmacology, 722
  positive-pressure ventilators, 723–24,
    724t
  preparation for, 725
  in respiratory failure, 723–24
  types of, 723, 724t
  weaning, 724
Mechlorethamine (Mustargen), in
    chemotherapy, 166t
Mediastinum, 680
Mediation, in pain management, 110
Medical-surgical nurse, 2–11
  circulating, 138, 139f
  defined, 2
  role of, 2–3
    advocate, 3
    care manager, 3
    caregiver, 2
    teacher, 2
  scrub, 138, 139f
  surgical assistant, 138
Medicare, home health care
  history of, 34
  plan of care, 35f
  reimbursement, 35
Medulla oblongata, 790
Meglitinides, for diabetes mellitus, 376t
Melanin, 298
Melena
  defined, 408
  in gastritis, 408

Memory cells, 267t
  function of, 268
  in humoral immunity, 268, 269f
Meniere's disease, 877
Meninges, 790
Meningioma, 802t
Meningitis, 817
  bacterial, 817, 817t
  complications of, 817
  manifestations of, 817
  meningococcal, 817, 817f
  pharmacology, 819
  treatment, 818
  viral, 817, 817t
Meningococcemia, 817
Menopause, 926–28
  collaborative care, 927–28
    complementary and alternative
        medicine, 927
    pharmacology, 927, 927f
  manifestations of, 927, 928f
  nursing care, 928
    assessment, 928
    deficient knowledge, 928
    discharge considerations, 928, 928f
    low self-esteem, 928
    sexual dysfunction, 928
  perimenopause, 926
  physiology of, 927
  postmenopausal, 926
  surgical, 926
Menorrhagia, 923
Menstrual cycle, 908–9, 909f
Menstruation disorders, 921–28
  dysfunctional uterine bleeding (DUB),
        923–26
  dysmenorrhea, 923
  menopause, 926–28
  premenstrual syndrome (PMS),
        921–28
Mental disorders, substance abuse and,
        229
Mental status
  assessment of, 57
  orientation, 57
Mescaline, abuse of, 224t, 227
Metabolic acidosis, 91–93
  causes of, 92t
  collaborative care, 92–93
  defined, 89, 90f
  laboratory values, 92t
  manifestations, 92t
  nursing care, 93
    assessment, 93
    decreased cardiac output, 93
    discharge considerations, 93

excess fluid volume, 93
    risk for injury, 93
  pathophysiology, 91–92
Metabolic alkalosis, 93–95
  causes of, 92t
  collaborative care, 94
  defined, 89, 90f
  laboratory values, 92t
  manifestations, 92t
  nursing care, 94–95
    assessment, 94
    discharge considerations, 94–95
    fluid volume deficiency, 94
    impaired gas exchange, 94
  pathophysiology, 94
Metabolism
  concepts, 396
  effect of burns on, 329
Metastasis
  in breast cancer, 912, 916
  defined, 157
  diagnostic tests for
    liver, 313
    lung, 313
  distant, 157
  process of, 157, 157f
  sites of, by cancer, 157t
  in staging, TNM cancer classification,
        162t
Metered dose inhaler (MDI), client
        education, 697t, 700, 700f
Methadone
  abuse of, 223t, 226–27
  as heroin abuse treatment, 229
Methicillin-resistant *Staphylococcus aureus*
        (MRSA), 248
Methotrexate, in chemotherapy, 166t
Methylcellulose, for constipation, 459
Metolazone (Diulo), nursing considerations
        for, 73t
Metronidazole (Flagyl), 254t
Metrorrhagia, 923
Mezlocillin (Mezlin), 252t
Miconazole (Monistat), 255t
Microalbuminuria, diabetes mellitus and,
        382
Microangiopathies, diabetes mellitus and,
        381–83
Microemboli, defined, 203
Microorganisms, in infection process, 245,
        245f, 246t
Microvilli, 396
Midbrain, 790
Milliequivalent, defined, 64
Mineral oil, for constipation, 461t
Mineralocorticoids, function of, 342–43, 343t

Minerals, 395t
Minimal change disease, nephrotic
        syndrome and, 511
Minor, emancipated, informed consent and,
        131
Miosis, of pupil, 53
Miotic drugs, for glaucoma, 866t
Misoprostol (Cytotec), for gastritis, 411t
Mitral regurgitation, 587t, 588, 588f
Mitral stenosis, 586–88, 587f, 587t
Mitral valve prolapse, 588
Mittelschmerz, 924
Modulation, pain, 103, 103f, 104f
Moh's micrographic surgery, for skin
        cancers, 313
Monoamine oxidase inhibitor (MAOI), for
        Parkinson's disease, 836t
Monoclonal antibodies
  in cancer diagnosis, 162
  for transplants, 279, 280t
Monocytes, 266, 267t, 639
  function of, 267t
  laboratory values for, 241t, 639t
Mononucleosis, 648
Mons pubis, 909, 909f
Morphine, abuse of, 223t, 226–27
Motor vehicle accidents (MVAs), head
        injuries and, 794
Mourning (*See also* Loss)
  defined, 184
  rituals of, 190, 190t
Mouth
  disorders of
    cancer, 405–6
    stomatitis, 404–6
  functions of, 394
Mucosal barrier
  in gastritis, 408, 408f
  in peptic ulcer disease (PUD), 413
Multiple myeloma, 645–46
  collaborative care, 646
  nursing care, 646
    discharge considerations, 646
    impaired physical mobility, 646
    pain, 646
  pathophysiology, 645–46
Multiple organ dysfunction syndrome
        (MODS), shock and, 201
Multiple sclerosis, 832–34
  collaborative care, 832–34
    diagnostic tests, 832–33
    nutrition management, 833
    pharmacology, 833
    physical therapy, 833
    plasmapheresis, 833
  defined, 832

Multiple sclerosis (continued)
manifestations of, 832, 832f
nursing care, 833–34
assessment, 833, 833f
discharge considerations, 834
fatigue, 833
ineffective coping, 834
self-care deficits, 834
pathophysiology, 832
Muscle(s), 733
inspiratory, 680
intercostal, 680
strain of, 734
structure of, 733
types of
cardiac, 733
skeletal, 733
smooth, 733
Muscular dystrophy, 785
Musculoskeletal disorders
bone disorders, 757–69
bone tumors, 766–68
kyphosis, 758–59
osteomalacia, 763–64
osteomyelitis, 764–65
osteoporosis, 759–63
Paget's disease, 763–64
scoliosis, 758–59
foot disorders, 768–69
collaborative care, 768–69
hallux valgus, 768, 768f
hammer toe, 768, 768f
joint and connective tissue disorders,
769–85
ankylosing spondylitis, 783–84
fibromyalgia, 784
gout, 780–83
low back pain, 784–85
Lyme disease, 783
muscular dystrophy, 785
osteoarthritis, 769–72
rheumatoid arthritis, 772–78
systemic lupus erythematous (SLE),
778–80
nursing interventions classification, 785
Musculoskeletal system, 732–33
in adults, 18t, 20t
effect of spinal cord injury on, 844f
effect of systemic lupus erythematous on,
779f
effects of anemia on, 627f
effects of cerebrovascular accident on,
807t
effects of diabetes mellitus on, 379f
effects of hyperthyroidism on, 347f
effects of hypothyroidism on, 352f

effects of multiple sclerosis on, 832f
effects of premenstrual syndrome on,
922f
effects of prostate cancer on, 891f
effects of uremia on, 524f
structures of, 732–33
bones, 732, 732f
joints, 732–33
ligaments, 733
muscle, 733
tendons, 733
trauma issues in, 212
in young adults, 16t
Musculoskeletal trauma, 733–52
amputation, 748–52
fractures, 735–44
joint dislocation, 747
nursing interventions classification, 752
repetitive use injuries, 747–48
bursitis, 747
carpal tunnel syndrome, 747
collaborative care, 748
epicondylitis, 747–48
soft tissue trauma, 734–35
collaborative care, 734–35
contusion, 734
nursing care, 734–35
assessment, 734
discharge considerations, 735
impaired physical mobility, 735
pain, 735
sprain, 734
strain, 734
subluxation, 747
Mutation, defined, 251
Myasthenia gravis, 837–38
cholinergic crisis, 837
defined, 837
manifestations of, 837
myasthenic crisis, 837
pathophysiology, 837
pharmacology, 837–38, 838t
Myasthenic crisis, 837
Mycobacteria avium complex (MAC),
AIDS-related, 284, 288t
Mycoplasma, in infection, 245f
Mydriasis, of pupil, 53
Myelin sheath, 790, 790f
Myelinated, defined, 102
Myelography, nursing care for, 848f
Myocardial infarction (MI), 554f, 562–70
case study, 569
cocaine-induced, 563
collaborative care, 564–68
cardiac rehabilitation, 567
intra-aortic balloon pump, 566, 566f

medical management, 565
pharmacology, 565–66
revascularization, 566
ventricular assist devices, 566
complications of, 564
dysrhythmias, 564
pericarditis, 564
pump failure, 564
defined, 562
diagnostic tests, 564–65
cardiac markers, 564, 565f
echocardiography, 564–65
electrocardiogram, 564
gender differences, 563f
manifestations, 563f
nursing care, 567–68
assessment, 567
discharge considerations, 568
fear, 568
ineffective coping, 568
ineffective tissue perfusion, 567–68
pain, 567
in older adults, 563f
pathophysiology, 563–64
subendocardial, 563
transmural, 563
Myocardial rupture, 564
Myocarditis, 583–84
Myocardium, 538, 539
Myofibrils, 733
Myopathy, caused by alcohol abuse, 226
Myopia, 862t
Myringotomy, for otitis media, 875
Myxedema coma, hypothyroidism and, 351

N

Nafcillin (Unipen), 252t
Nails, function of, 298t, 301
Naloxone (Narcan), 118, 226
Naltrexone (Re Via), 229
Naproxen (Anaprox, Naprosyn), for
inflammation, 242t, 775
Nasal fractures, 665–67
Nasal packing, for epistaxis, 664, 664f
Nasogastric tube, procedure for inserting,
400, 401f
Nasopharynx, 656
National Association for Practical Nurse
Education and Service (NAPNEs),
standards of practice, 9, 10f
National Commission of Chronic Illness,
25
Natural killer (NK) cells, function of, 266,
267t

Nausea, treatment for, 649–50

NCLEX-PN exam preparation
adult clients, 28
altered immune system, 296
assessment, 61
bowel disorders, 491
cancer, 181
cardiac disorders, 594
degenerative neurologic disorders, 853
diabetes mellitus, 392
ear disorders, 884
end of life care, 198
endocrine disorders, 364
eye disorders, 884
gastrointestinal disorders, upper, 423
hematologic disorders, 654
home health care, 44
inflammation and infection, 263
intracranial disorders, 825
liver, gallbladder, pancreatic disorders, 451
lymphatic system disorders, 654
musculoskeletal disorders, 788
musculoskeletal trauma, 755
nursing process, 13
pain management, 122
peripheral vascular disorders, 622
rehabilitation, 44
renal and urinary tract disorders, 535
reproductive disorders
female, 946
male, 905
respiratory disorders
lower, 730
upper, 678
sexually transmitted disease (STD), 960
shock, trauma and critical illness, 219
skin orders, 324
spinal cord disorders, 853
substance abuse, 235
surgery, 153

Necrosis, defined, 157

Neoplasm (*See also* Tumor)
benign, 156–57
benign compared to malignant, 157t
defined, 156
malignant, 157

Nephrectomy
in renal calculi, 514
in renal cell cancer, 521, 522f
nursing care, 522

Nephrolithiasis, 512

Nephrolithotomy, in renal calculi, 514

Nephrons, 494, 495f

Nephropathy, diabetic, 382, 508

Nephrotic syndrome, 511–12

Nephrotoxins, in renal failure, 522

Nerve blocks, 137
permanent, 109
temporary, 109

Nerve(s)
cranial, 792, 793t
abducens, 793t
accessory, 793t
facial, 793t
glossopharyngeal, 793t
hypoglossal, 793t
oculomotor, 793t
olfactory, 793t
optic, 793t, 857
trigeminal, 793t, 840
trochlear, 793t
vagus, 793t
vestibulocochlear, 793t
spinal, 792, 792f

Netilmicin (Netromycin), 253t

Neurectomy, for pain, 109, 112f

Neurofibrillary tangles, associated with Alzheimer's disease, 828, 828f

Neurogenic bladder, 497

Neurohypophysis, 342

Neurologic system, 200–201, 202f (*See also* Central nervous system (CNS); Peripheral nervous system (PNS))
AIDS-related infection in, 285
brain, 790–91, 791f
disorders of (*See* Intracranial disorders)
degenerative disorders of, 828–42
Alzheimer's disease, 828–31
amyotrophic lateral sclerosis (ALS), 839
Bell's Palsy, 840–41
Creutzfeldt-Jakob disease, 841–42
Guillain-Barre syndrome, 839–40
multiple sclerosis, 832–34
myasthenia gravis, 837–38
nursing interventions classification, 850
Parkinson's disease, 834–37
rabies, 841
tetanus, 841
trigeminal neuralgia, 840
effect of leukemia on, 640f
effect of spinal cord injury on, 844f
effect of systemic lupus erythematous on, 779f
effects of anemia on, 627f
effects of cirrhosis on, 436f
effects of diabetes mellitus on, 379f
effects of hyperthyroidism on, 347f

effects of multiple sclerosis on, 832f
effects of premenstrual syndrome on, 922f
effects of prostate cancer on, 891f
effects of shock on, 200–201, 202f
effects of uremia on, 524f
spinal cord, 791–92
disorders of (*See* Spinal cord disorders)

Neuron(s), 790, 790f
in Alzheimer's disease, 828, 828f
motor, 790
in seizure disorder, 813
sensory, 790

Neuropathies
autonomic, 382
diabetic, 382
peripheral, 106, 382

Neurotransmitters, function of, 790, 790f

Neutropenia (*See* Agranulocytosis)

Neutrophils, 639
in inflammatory response, 238
laboratory values for, 241t, 639t
segmented, 639

Nevi
defined, 312
skin cancer and, 312–13

Next of kin, informed consent and, 131

Nicotine (*See also* Smoking)
abuse of, 224t, 228

Nitrates
for angina pectoris, 557, 557t–558t
sublingual nitroglycerin (NTG), 557, 557t, 562

"No code," 190, 551

Nocturia
in benign prostatic hypertrophy, 887
defined, 887

Nocturnal penile tumescence and rigidity (NPTR), in erectile dysfunction, 900, 900f

Nodule, defined, 299t

Non-nucleoside reverse transcriptase inhibitors (NNRTIs), for HIV infection, 286–87, 287t

Nonopioids, 107

Nonresectable, defined, 163

Nonsteroidal anti-inflammatory drugs (NSAIDs)
actions of, 107
analgesic ceiling of, 107
client education, 108t
for inflammation, 240–41, 242t
nursing responsibilities, 108t
for postoperative pain, 142–43
purpose of, 108t

Nonsteroidal anti-inflammatory drugs
    (NSAIDs) *(continued)*
  for rheumatoid arthritis, 775t
  second generation, 775t
Nonvolatile acids, in acid-base balance, 88
Norepinephrine, function of, 343, 343t
Normal sinus rhythm (NSR), 542, 543t
North American Nursing Diagnosis
    Association (NANDA)
  classification system of, 5
  diagnosis definition, 4–5
Nose
  bleeding of (*See* Epistaxis)
  broken, 665–67
    cerebrospinal fluid leakage, 665–66
    collaborative care, 666
    nursing care, 666–67
      airway clearance, 666
      assessment, 666
      discharge considerations,
          666–67
      risk for infection, 666
    pathophysiology, 665
  functions of, 656
Nosocomial infection, 247–48
  clostridium difficile-Associated Diarrhea
      (CDAD), 248
  defined, 247
  infection control, 254–55
  methicillin-resistant *Staphylococcus
      aureus* (MRSA), 248
  risk factors for, 247f
  urinary tract infection, 502
  vancomycin-resistant *Enterococcus*
      (VRE), 248
Novantrone, for multiple sclerosis, 833
Noxious stimuli, in pain process, 102, 102t
Nucleoside reverse transcriptase inhibitors
    (NRTIs), for HIV infection, 286–87,
    287t
Nurse (*See* Medical-surgical nurse)
Nursing diagnosis (*See also* Diagnosis)
  defined, 4–5
Nursing homes, 33 (*See also* Community-
    based nursing care)
Nursing management, in nursing process,
    5
Nursing process, 3–6, 4f
  assessment, 4
  benefits of, 6
  in clinical practice, 6
  diagnosis, 4–5
  evaluation, 6
  implementation, 6
  outcomes, 5–6
  planning, 5

Nutrients, 395t–396t, 396
  carbohydrates, 395t
  fats (lipids), 395t
  minerals, 395t
  proteins, 395t
  vitamins, 395t
  water, 396t
Nutrition
  defined, 394
  metabolism and, 396
Nutritional disorders, 396–404
  anorexia, 400
  bulimia, 400
  malnutrition, defined, 400
  obesity, 396–400 (*See also* Obesity)
  in older adults, 404f
  undernutrition, 400–404
    collaborative care, 400–404
      enteral feedings, 400–401, 401f,
          402f
      parenteral feedings, 402, 402f
    defined, 400
    health problems related to, 400f
    manifestations of, 400
    nursing care, 402–4
      assessment, 402
      deficient fluid volume, 403
      discharge considerations, 403f,
          404
      impaired skin integrity, 403
      risk for infection, 403
    nutritional issues, 403
    pathophysiology, 400
Nutritional issues
  in Addison's disease, 360–61
  in altered level of consciousness, 800
  in burn injuries, 330, 334
  in cancer, 169, 171t, 173
  in cholelithiasis, 428, 428f
  in chronic obstructive pulmonary disease,
      703
  in chronic renal failure, 530
  in diabetes mellitus, 372, 374–75, 377t,
      384
  in gastritis, 411
  in hepatitis, 435
  in hyperthyroidism, 348–49
  in increased intracranial pressure, 800
  in infection, 256–57
  in inflammation, 241–42
  in inflammatory bowel disease, 476
  in laryngeal cancer, 672–73
  in leukemia, 642
  in multiple sclerosis, 833
  in obesity, 399
  in osteoporosis, 761

  in pancreatitis, 446
  in Parkinson's disease, 837
  in peptic ulcer disease, 417
Nystatin (Mycostatin), 251, 255t

O

Obesity, 396–400
  in adults, 17
  appetite and, 397
  as cancer risk factor, 159
  collaborative care, 397–400
    behavior modification, 398, 399f
    diagnostic tests, 397–98
    exercise, 398
    nutrition, 398
    pharmacology, 398
    surgery, 398
  defined, 396
  health problems related to, 397f
  hormones and, 397
  morbid, defined, 396
  nursing care, 398–400
    assessment, 398–99
    discharge considerations, 399–400,
        399f
    low self-esteem, 399
    nutritional issues, 399
  overweight *vs.,* 396
  pathophysiology, 396–97
  as surgical risk factor, 129t
  type II diabetes mellitus and, 369
Obstruction
  intestinal, 472
  laryngeal, 667, 667f
  in peptic ulcer disease, 413–14, 413f
  in renal and urinary tract, 512–16
    as cancer complication, 178
    hydronephrosis, 515–16
    polycystic kidney disease, 516
    urinary calculi, 512–15
Occupational risk, cancer and, 159
Older adults, 18–19
  age-related changes in, 249t
  amputation in, 751f
  cancer risk factors and, 158
  common health problems in, 368f
  constipation in, 458
  diabetes mellitus in, 368, 368f, 374
  dysrhythmias in, 545f
  family and, 22
  fluid volume deficit in, 69f
  fractures in, 743f, 745, 745f
  healthy behaviors of, 21f
  heart failure in, 570f

hypertension in, 597f
hypocalcemia in, 82
immune system in, 268–69
increase in number of, 18
infection in, 248–50, 249t
inflammation in, 239f
influenza in, 657f
injury in, 19
lower respiratory infections, 682f
mammography in, 914f
myocardial infarction in, 563f
normal assessment findings for, 49f
nutrition in, 404f
pain management in, 116f
peripheral vascular disorders and, 608
physical changes in, 20t
sensory changes
  hearing loss, 879
  vision, 863, 870
skin changes in, 20t, 301f
surgical risks for, 129t, 142f, 145
syndrome of inappropriate ADH
    secretion (SIADH) and, 345
tuberculosis in, 690f
urinary incontinence in, 498–99
Oligomenorrhea, 923
Ommaya reservoir, for chemotherapy, 803,
    803f
Oncogenes, 158
Oncologic emergencies, 177–78 (*See also*
    Cancer)
  bladder obstruction, 178
  cardiac tamponade, 177
  hypercalcemia, 178
  hyperuricemia, 178
  pericardial effusion, 177
  sepsis and septic shock, 177–78
  spinal cord compression, 178
  superior vena cava syndrome, 177
Oncologist, 156
Oncology (*See also* Cancer)
  defined, 156
Oocytes, 908
Oophorectomy, for ovarian cysts, 932
Open reduction and internal fixation (ORIF),
    for fractures, 739, 741f, 744
Opioids
  abuse of, 223t, 226–27, 229
  addiction and, 115f
  agonist, 107, 108t
  agonist-antagonist, 108t
    defined, 107
  for chronic pain, 115f
  client education, 108t
  in end of life care, 189
  nursing responsibilities, 108t

overdose, 226
overview, 107
for postoperative pain, 142–43
as preoperative drug, 128t
purpose of, 108t
side effects of, 117–18
  constipation, 118
  nausea, 118
  respiratory depression, 118
  sedation, 117
Opium derivatives, for diarrhea, 457t
Oprelvekin (Neumega), for leukemia,
    643t
Optic nerve, 857
Oral contraceptives
  for dysfunctional uterine bleeding, 924
  for endometriosis, 931
  for ovarian cysts, 932
Orchiectomy
  client education for, 898
  for prostate cancer, 891–92
  for testicular cancer, 897
Orchitis, 895
Organ donation, 217, 277
Organ of Corti, 872
Organ transplant (*See* Transplantation)
Orientation
  assessment of, 57
  defined, 57
Orlistat (Xenical), 398
Oropharynx, 656
Orthopnea
  defined, 54, 571
  in heart failure, 571
Osmolality, defined, 65
Osmolarity, defined, 344
Osmosis, 65–66, 66f
Osmotic diuresis, in diabetic ketoacidosis,
    378
Osmotic pressure, defined, 65
Osteoarthritis, 769–72
  collaborative care, 769–72
    complementary and alternative
        medicine, 770f
    pharmacology, 770
    surgical treatment, 770
  complementary and alternative medicine,
      770f
  defined, 769
  manifestations of, 769, 769f
  nursing care, 770–72
    assessment, 770, 771f
    discharge considerations, 772
    impaired physical mobility, 771–72
    pain, 770–71
    self-care deficit, 772

pathophysiology, 769
vs. rheumatoid arthritis, 773t
Osteoblasts, 732
  in fracture healing process, 735
  in Paget's disease, 763
Osteoclasts, 732
  in fracture healing process, 735
  in Paget's disease, 763
Osteocytes, 732
Osteomalacia, 763–64, 763f
Osteomyelitis, 764–65
  collaborative care, 764–65
    diagnostic tests, 764
    pharmacology, 764
    surgical treatment, 764
  defined, 764
  manifestations of, 765f
  nursing care, 764–65
    assessment, 764–65
    discharge considerations, 765–66
    hyperthermia, 765
    impaired physical mobility, 765
    pain, 765
  pathophysiology, 764
  risk factors for, 764f
Osteoporosis, 759–63
  case study, 762–63
  collaborative care, 759–63
    calcium, 760, 760t
    pharmacology, 760–61, 762t
  defined, 759
  manifestations of, 759
  nursing care, 761–62
    discharge considerations, 761–62
    imbalanced nutrition, 761
    risk for injury, 761
    pain, 761
  pathologic fractures in, 759
  pathophysiology, 759
  risk factors for, 759f
  type I, 759
  type II, 759
Ostomy, 474, 474f
  changing pouch, 481f
  client care for, 476, 520f
  colostomy, 163, 479
    double-barrel, 479, 479f
    irrigation of, 483f
    nursing care for, 480f
    various locations for, 479f
  ileostomy, 474
    Kock's, 474, 474f
    nursing care for, 480f
  tracheostomy, permanent
    client education, 674

Ostomy *(continued)*
    tracheostomy, permanent *(continued)*
        for laryngeal cancer, 670, 670f
        nursing care for, 673f
    various locations for, 479f
Otitis, external, 873–74
Otitis media, 874–76
    acute, 874
    chronic, 875
    collaborative care, 875–76
        autoinflation, 875
        complementary and alternative
            medicine, 875
        pharmacology, 875
        surgical treatment, 875, 876f
    complications of, 874–75
    defined, 874
    nursing care, 875–76
        discharge considerations, 876
        pain, 875
    pathophysiology, 874
    serous, 874
Otorrhea, defined, 794
Otosclerosis, 876–77
Otoscope, pneumatic, for otitis media, 875
Ototoxic drugs, for hearing loss, 878–79
Outcomes
    defined, 5
    overview, 5–6
    planning and, 5
Ovarian cancer, 937–38
    collaborative care, 937–38
    pathophysiology, 937
    risk factors for, 937
Ovarian cycle, 908–9, 909f
Ovarian cysts, 932–33
    collaborative care, 932–33
        pharmacology, 932
        surgical treatment, 932
    pathophysiology, 932
    polycystic ovary syndrome (PCOS),
        932–33
Ovarian follicles, 908
Ovaries, 908, 908f
Overweight, obesity *vs.,* 396
Ovulation, 908
Oxacillin (Prostaphlin), 252t
Oxygen therapy
    for chronic obstructive pulmonary
        disease, 702
    continuous positive airway pressure
        (CPAP), 702
    home oxygen, 702
    for increased intracranial pressure, 801
    nasal cannula, 685, 686f
    in pneumonia, 685

rebreather mask, 685, 686f
in respiratory failure, 722
for shock, 205
simple face mask, 685, 686f
Venturi mask, 685
Oxymetazoline (Afrin), 275
Oxytocin, function of, 343t

Pacemakers, 549, 549f
    pacing function, 549
    sensing function, 549
Paco$_2$, 90–91, 91f
Paget's disease, 763–64
    breast cancer and, 912
    manifestations of, 763f
Pain, 102–20
    acute
        burn injuries and, 334
        compared to chronic, 105t
        defined, 104
        from inflammation, 242–43
        in skin orders, 310
        types of, 104
    allodynia, 106
    in amputation, 751
    in arteriosclerosis, 604
    behavioral responses to, 114–15
    in bone tumors, 767
    cancer, 105, 710–11
    chronic
        compared to acute, 105t
        defined, 104
        malignant, 105, 710–11
        nonmalignant, 104
        types of, 104–5
    conduction
        modulation, 103, 103f, 104f
        perception, 103, 103f
        transduction, 102, 103f
        transmission, 103, 103f
    factors affecting response to, 106–7
    as fifth vital sign, 102
    in fracture, 741–42, 744–45
    gate-control theory of, 103–4, 104f
    in gout, 782
    in herniated intervertebral disk, 849
    in intracranial infections, 819–20
    low back, 784–85, 847, 847f
    "meaning" of, 106
    in myocardial infarction, 565
    in rheumatoid arthritis, 774, 776
    in osteoarthritis, 770–71
    in osteomyelitis, 765

perception of, 103, 103f, 113, 113f, 114f
physiologic responses to, 113–14
physiology of, 102–4, 102t
rest, in arteriosclerosis, 604
secondary gain of, 106
types of, 104–6
    "breakthrough," 711
    cutaneous, 104
    neuropathic, 105–6
    phantom limb, 106, 749
    postsurgical, 142–43
    psychogenic, 106
    referred, 104, 105f
    somatic, 104
    visceral, 104
Pain clinics, 107
Pain management, 107–12
    assessment, 113–15, 114f
        behavioral responses to, 114–15
        client perceptions, 113
        physiologic responses, 113–14
    case study, 119
    complementary and alternative medicine
        for, 110–12, 116
        acupuncture, 111–12
        biofeedback, 112
        cutaneous stimulation, 110, 112t
        distraction, 110
        hypnotism, 112
        relaxation, 110
        transcutaneous electrical nerve
            stimulation (TENS), 110–11,
            112t
    discharge considerations, 118–19, 119f
    misconceptions about, 115f
    in the older adult, 116f
    pharmacology, 107–9 (*See also*
        Analgesics; Opioids)
        balanced approach, 115, 115f
        equianalgesic dosage chart, 107, 109t,
            116
        flow sheet, 115, 117f
        routes of administration, 107–9, 109t
        types of medication, 107
        World Health Organization analgesic
            ladder, 117, 118f
    preventive approach to, 115
    surgical treatment
        cordotomy, 109, 112f
        neurectomy, 109, 112f
        rhizotomy, 110, 112f
        sympathectomy, 109–10, 112f
    treatment, 115–19
        acute, 115–16
        chronic, 116
        evaluation, 118

nursing care, 112–19
postoperative, 115f, 146, 148
Pain rating scales, 113–14f
Pain threshold, 103
Pain tolerance, 103
Palliative (*See also* End of life care)
defined, 187
Pallidotomy, in Parkinson's disease, 835
Pallor
assessment of, 52
defined, 300
Palpation
of breast, 55, 55f
guidelines for, 48, 48f, 48t
of lymph nodes, 239, 240f
Pancreas
disorders of, 444–48
abscess, 444
cancer, 447
diabetes mellitus, 366, 444
nursing interventions classification,
447–48
pancreatitis, 444–47
as endocrine gland, 444
as exocrine gland, 444
functions of, 366, 426
glucagon production, 366
insulin production, 366
transplantation of, 383
Pancreatic enzyme replacement, defined,
444t
Pancreatic pseudocyst, defined, 444
Pancreatitis, 444–47
acute, 444
manifestations of, 444f
pathophysiology, 444
treatment, 445
caused by alcohol abuse, 225
chronic, 444
manifestations of, 444f
pathophysiology, 444
treatment, 445
collaborative care, 445–47
nutritional issues, 446
pharmacology, 445, 445t
defined, 444
nursing care, 446–47
acute pain, 446
assessment, 446
discharge considerations, 447
risk for injury, 446
Pancreatoduodenectomy, 447, 447f
Pancytopenia, defined, 628
Pao$_2$, 91, 91f
Pap smear, 934, 934f
Papanicolaou (Pap) smear, 934, 934f

Papule, defined, 299t
Paracentesis, 439, 439f, 466
Paradoxic movement, in flail chest, 719,
719f
Paralysis
hemiplegia
in cerebrovascular accident, 806, 807f
client positioning for, 810, 811f
defined, 806
paraplegia, 807f, 842, 843f, 844f
tetraplegia, 842, 843f, 844f
types of, 807f
Paralytic ileus, 466, 482
Paraneoplastic syndromes, in lung cancer,
708, 709f
Paraplegia, 807f, 842, 843f, 844f
Parasympathetic nervous system, 794, 794f
Parathyroid glands
disorders of
hyperparathyroidism, 354–55
hypoparathyroidism, 355–56
functions of, 342
hormones of, 343t
Parathyroid hormone (PTH)
function of, 342, 343t
role in calcium imbalance, 82, 82f
Parenteral feedings, 402, 402f
Parish nursing, 33
Parkinsonism, defined, 834
Parkinson's disease, 834–37
collaborative care, 834–37
pharmacology, 834–35, 836t
surgical treatment, 835
defined, 834
etiology, 834
manifestations of, 834, 835f
nursing care, 834–37
assessment, 835, 835f
discharge considerations, 837
imbalanced nutrition, 837
impaired communication, 837
impaired physical mobility, 836–37
pathophysiology, 834
Paroxysmal nocturnal dyspnea (PND)
defined, 571
in heart failure, 571
Partial prothrombin time (PPT), significance
of laboratory values, 127t
Patch allergy test, 275
Pathogens, defined, 245
Pathologic fractures
defined, 645
in multiple myeloma, 645
in osteoporosis, 759
Patient-controlled analgesia (PCA), 108,
110f

Patient Self-Determination Act, 186
Pediculosis, 308–9
Pelvic exenteration, for cervical cancer, 934
Pelvic inflammatory disease (PID), 941–42
collaborative care, 941–42, 949t
pharmacology, 941
prevention, 941–42
surgical treatment, 941
complications, 949t
manifestations of, 941, 949t
nursing care, 941–42
assessment, 941
discharge considerations, 942
risk for injury, 941
pathophysiology, 941
Pelvic organ prolapse, 930
collaborative care, 930
cystocele, 930
rectocele, 930
urinary incontinence in, 930
uterine prolapse, 930
Pelvis fracture, 742t
Penicillins
client education, 252t
nursing responsibilities, 252t
purpose of, 252t
Penile implants, for erectile dysfunction,
900–901, 901f
Penis, 886
disorders of, 898–902
cancer, 899
ejaculatory dysfunction, 902
erectile dysfunction, 899–901
phimosis, 898–99
priapism, 899, 899f
Penrose drain, 145f
Peptic ulcer disease (PUD), 412–18
collaborative care, 413–18
diagnostic tests, 413–18
diet, 414
nutritional issues, 417
pharmacology, 414
surgery, 414, 415t–416t, 416f
complications
manifestations of, 413, 413f
treatment of, 414
defined, 412
nursing care, 414–18
assessment, 414, 416, 416f
case study, 418
decreased cardiac output, 417
discharge considerations, 417–18
pain, 417
pain of, 413
pathophysiology, 413
sites commonly affected by, 413, 413f

Perception, of pain, 103, 103f, 113, 113f, 114f
Percussion
  guidelines for, 48–49, 49f
  for pneumonia, 686, 686f
Percutaneous transluminal coronary angioplasty (PTCA)
  for angina pectoris, 557f, 559, 559f
  for myocardial infarction, 566
Perforation, in peptic ulcer disease, 413–14, 413f
Pericardial effusion
  in cancer, 177
  pericarditis and, 584
Pericardial frictional rub, 584
Pericardiocentesis, 584, 585f
Pericarditis, 584–86
  collaborative care, 584–86
    pericardiocentesis, 584, 585f
  defined, 584
  manifestations of, 584
  in myocardial infarction, 564
  nursing care, 585–86
    decreased cardiac output, 586
    discharge considerations, 586
    ineffective breathing pattern, 585
    pain, 584–85
  pathophysiology, 584
  pericardial effusion and, 584
Pericardium, 538
  parietal, 538
  visceral, 538
Perimenopause, 926
Periosteum, 732
Peripheral nervous system (PNS), 792
  autonomic nervous system, 794, 794f
  cranial nerves, 792, 793t
  in Guillain-Barre syndrome, 839
  reflex arc in, 792, 792f
  spinal nerves, 792, 792f
Peripheral vascular disorders, 596–619
  aneurysm, 608–11
  arterial disorders, 604–11
    arterial thrombus, 605, 605f
    arteriosclerosis, 604–5
    Buerger's disease, 605
    Raynaud's phenomenon, 605
  collaborative care, 605–8
    complementary and alternative medicine, 606f
    conservative therapy, 606
    diagnostic tests, 605–6
    pharmacology, 606
    surgical treatment, 606
  diabetes mellitus and, 381, 382f
  hypertension, 597–604

nursing care, 606-8
  assessment, 606, 607f
  discharge considerations, 608, 608f
  impaired skin integrity, 607
  ineffective protection, 607–8
  ineffective tissue perfusion, 606–7
  pain, 607
older adults and, 608
venous disorders, 612–19
  varicose veins, 618–19, 618f
  venous insufficiency, 613
  venous thrombosis, 612–17
Peripheral vascular resistance (PVR), 596–97
  blood pressure and, 596
Peripheral vascular system
  arterial circulation, 596–97
  effect of hypertension on, 598t
  effect of spinal cord injury on, 844f
  functions of, 596
  structures of, 596, 596f
Peristalsis, 454, 466
Peritoneal lavage, for peritonitis, 467
Peritonitis, 413, 466–69
  bacterial, 466
  chemical, 466
  collaborative care, 466–68
    surgical treatment, 466–67
  complications of, 466
  defined, 466
  manifestations of, 466, 466f
  nursing care, 467–68
    anxiety, 468
    assessment, 467, 467f
    deficient fluid volume, 467–68
    discharge considerations, 468–69, 468f
    evaluation, 468
    pain, 467
    risk for infection, 468
Peritonsillar abscess, 658, 658f
Pernicious anemia, 626
PES method, for writing diagnosis, 5
Petechiae, defined, 635
Peyer's patches, in lymphoid system, 268f
pH
  in acid-base balance, 88
  arterial blood gases interpretation, 91f
  buffer systems for, 88–89
  defined, 88
Phagocytosis, in inflammatory response, 238, 238f
Phalen test, for carpal tunnel syndrome, 748, 748f
Phantom pain, in amputation, 106, 749
Pharyngitis, 658, 658f

Pharynx
  functions of, 394, 656
  laryngopharynx, 656
  nasopharynx, 656
  oropharynx, 656
Phencyclidine (PCP), abuse of, 224t, 227
Pheochromocytoma, 361
Phimosis, 898–99
Phlebography, ascending, in venous thrombosis, 613
Phosphate/phosphorous
  intravenous, 88
  normal electrolyte laboratory values for, 64t
Phosphodiesterase inhibitors, for heart failure, 573t
Phosphorus imbalance, 87–88
  hyperphosphatemia, 88
    causes of, 87t
    laboratory values, 87t
    manifestations, 87t
  hypophosphatemia, 87–88
    causes of, 87t
    laboratory values, 87t
    manifestations, 87t
Photochemotherapy, for psoriasis, 304
Photophobia, defined, 859
Photorefractive keratectomy (PRK), 862
Physical examination
  general survey, 50, 50t
  guidelines for, 50t–51t
  methods of, 48–49
    auscultation, 49
    inspection, 48
    palpation, 48, 48f, 48t
    percussion, 48–49, 49f
  preparation for, 49–50
  specific areas
    abdomen, 51t, 55–56, 56f
    axillary lymph nodes, 51t, 55
    back, 54
    bowel sounds, 56
    breast, 55
    breasts, 51t
    cardiovascular system, 51t
    chest, 54
    ears, 51t, 53
    extremities, 56–57
    eyes, 50t, 52–53
    face, 52
    hair, 50, 50t, 52
    head and neck, 52–53
    heart, 54–55
    integument, 50, 50t, 52
    lungs, 51t, 54
    lymph nodes of head and neck, 53, 54f

mental status, 57
mouth, 51t, 53
musculoskeletal system, 51t, 57
neck, 51t
neurologic system, 51t
nose, 51t, 53
oropharynx, 51t
peripheral circulation, 56–57
sinuses, 51t, 53
skin, 50, 50t, 52
skull, 52
thorax, 51t, 53–55
urinary bladder, 56
Physical therapy, for multiple sclerosis, 833
Pilonidal disease, 488
Piperacillin (Pipracil), 252t
Piroxicam (Feldene), for inflammation, 242t
Pituitary gland
anterior
hormones of, 343t
major actions of, 343f
disorders of
diabetes insipidus (DI), 344–45
hyperpituitarism, 344
hypopituitarism, 344
syndrome of inappropriate ADH
secretion (SIADH), 345–46
functions of, 342
posterior, hormones of, 343t
Plan of care, for home health care, 34–35
Planning in nursing process, 5
Plant alkaloids, in chemotherapy, 167t
Plaque, in arteriosclerosis, 604
Plasma
functions of, 624
osmotic pressure of, 65
Plasma cells, 267t
in humoral immunity, 268, 269f
in multiple myeloma, 645
Plasmapheresis
in glomerulonephritis, 509
for Guillain-Barre syndrome, 840
for multiple sclerosis, 833
for rheumatoid arthritis, 774
Platelet transfusion, for thrombocytopenia, 635
Platelets
development of, 624, 625f
functions of, 635
significance of laboratory values, 127t
Plethysmography, in venous thrombosis, 613
Pleura, 680
parietal, 680
visceral, 680
Pleural effusion, 689, 710
Pleural friction rub, 54
in pleuritis, 689

Pleuritis, 689
Pneumatic antishock garment (PASG), 205, 206f
Pneumonectomy, 709t
Pneumonia, 683–88
acute bacterial, 683–84, 683t
AIDS-related, 283–84, 288t
aspiration, 684
bronchopneumonia, 683t
collaborative care, 684–88
complementary and alternative medicine, 689f
diagnostic tests, 684–85
immunization, 685
oxygen therapy, 685, 686f
percussion, 686, 686f
pharmacology, 685
postural positioning, 686, 687f
defined, 143, 683
Legionnaire's disease, 683t
lobar, 683t
manifestations of, 143
nursing care, 687–88
activity intolerance, 688
assessment, 687, 688f
discharge considerations, 688, 689f
ineffective airway clearance, 687–88
ineffective breathing pattern, 688
in older adults, 249t
pathophysiology, 683–84
pneumocystis carinii, 683t, 684
AIDS-related, 283–84
postsurgical prevention, 147
Pneumothorax, 715–18
collaborative care, 716–18
chest tubes, 717
defined, 715
hemothorax, 718
nursing care, 717–18
assessment, 717
discharge considerations, 718
impaired gas exchange, 718
risk for injury, 718
pathophysiology, 715
spontaneous, 715, 716t, 718
tension, 715, 716t
in trauma clients, 211
traumatic, 715, 716t
types of, 715, 716t
Pocket talker, for hearing loss, 880
Poikilothermia
defined, 843
in spinal cord injury, 843
Point of maximum impulse (PMI), 54–55, 55f

Poisoning
carbon monoxide, 329, 719, 720f
cyanide inhalation, 719
emergency care for, 216, 216f
ingested corrosive, treatment, 409, 412f
Polycystic ovary syndrome (PCOS), 932–33
Polycythemia, 634
collaborative care, 634
defined, 634
pathophysiology, 634
Polycythemia vera, 634
Polydipsia, defined, 344
Polymorphonuclear leukocytes (PMNs) (*See* Neutrophils)
Polyneuritis, idiopathic, 839–40
Polyps, in colorectal cancer, 477–78
Polysubstance abuse, 227
Polythiazide (Renese), nursing considerations for, 73t
Polyuria, defined, 368
Pons, 790
Portal of entry, in infection process, 246
Portal of exit, in infection process, 245–46
Positive inotropic drugs, for cardiogenic shock, 208
for heart failure, 573t
Post void residual urine measurement, for urinary incontinence, 499, 500f
Postmenopausal, 926
Postmortem care, 190
Postural positioning, for pneumonia, 686, 687f
Potassium
in Addisonian crisis, 359
foods high in, 79, 80f
intravenous, 79t, 81
laboratory values, 64t, 127t
supplements of, 79, 79t
Potassium imbalance
collaborative care, 78–82
replacement therapy, 78–79
hyperkalemia, 80
causes of, 79t
collaborative care, 80
laboratory values, 79t
manifestations, 79t
hypokalemia, 78–79
case study, 81–82
causes of, 79t
collaborative care, 78–79
laboratory values, 79t
manifestations, 79t
pharmacological treatment, 79t
nursing care, 80–82
assessment, 80

Potassium imbalance *(continued)*
  nursing care *(continued)*
    decreased cardiac output, 80–81
    discharge considerations, 81
    risk for injury, 80
Poverty, as cancer risk factor, 159
Prednisone
  in chemotherapy, 167t
  for transplants, 279
Preload, in cardiac output, 541
Premature atrial contractions (PACs), 543t, 545, 564
Premature ventricular contractions (PVCs), 544t, 546, 564
Premenstrual syndrome (PMS), 921–28
  collaborative care, 922–23
  manifestations of, 921–22, 922f
  pathophysiology, 921–22
  risk factors for, 921
Presbycusis, 879
Presbyopia, 862t
  defined, 857
Pressure points, to control bleeding, 211, 211f
Pressure ulcers, 317–21
  collaborative care, 318, 320
  discharge considerations, 320–21
  individuals at risk, 318
  in older adults, 249t, 318
  pathophysiology, 317
  products used to treat, 318, 320t
  stages of, 318, 319f
Priapism, 899, 899f
Prick test, for allergy, 275
Prinzmetal's angina pectoris, 556
Progesterone, function of, 908
Prolactin, function of, 343t
Prolapse, pelvic organ, 930
Prophylactic, defined, 251
Prostaglandin analog, for glaucoma, 867t
Prostate, 886
  disorders of, 887–94
    benign prostatic hypertrophy (BPH), 887–89, 887f
    prostate cancer, 890–94
    prostatitis, 889–90
Prostate cancer, 890–94
  checkup recommendations, 160f
  collaborative care, 891–94
    diagnostic tests, 891
    hormone therapy, 891–92
    radiation therapy, 892
    surgical treatment, 892, 893f
  manifestations of, 891, 891f
  metastasis sites for, 157t

nursing care, 892–94
  assessment, 892
  discharge considerations, 894
  pain, 892, 894
  risk for incontinence, 892
  sexual dysfunction, 892
pathophysiology, 891
Prostate-specific antigen (PSA)
  in benign prostatic hypertrophy, 887
  in prostate cancer, 891
Prostatectomy
  artificial urinary sphincter after, 892, 894f
  nursing implications, 893
  for prostate cancer, 892, 893f
  radical, 892
  simple, 892
  for urinary incontinence, 499
Prostatitis, 502, 889–90
  acute bacterial, 889
  defined, 889
  manifestations of, 890f
  nonbacterial, 889
Prosthesis, in amputation, 750
Protease inhibitors, for HIV infection, 286–87, 287t
Protectants, for diarrhea, 457t
Protein, 395t
  normal urine levels, 508t
Protein-calorie malnutrition (PCM), 400
Proteinuria
  defined, 507
  in glomerulonephritis, 507
Prothrombin time (PT), 614
  significance of laboratory values, 127t
Proton pump inhibitors
  for gastritis, 410t
  for peptic ulcer disease, 414
Protozoans, in infection, 245f
Pruritus, 301
  reducing, 649
Pseudoephedrine (Sudafed), 275
Psoriasis, 301–2, 302f
Pulmonary circulation, 680
Pulmonary contusion, 719
Pulmonary edema
  heart failure and, 571
  interstitial, 329
  pharmacological treatment, 573
Pulmonary embolism, 712–15
  collaborative care, 713–15
    pharmacology, 713–14
    surgical treatment, 714, 714f
  in deep vein thrombosis, 612–13
  defined, 143, 713
  manifestations of, 143, 713f

nursing care, 714–15
  anxiety, 714
  decreased cardiac output, 714
  discharge considerations, 714–15
  impaired gas exchange, 714
  ineffective tissue perfusion, 714
pathophysiology, 713
postsurgical prevention, 147
prevention of, 714–15
Pulmonary function testing, in chronic obstructive pulmonary disease, 701–2
Pulmonary hypertension, 715
Pulmonary valves, 539
Pulmonary vascular disorders, 712–15
  pulmonary embolism, 712–15
  pulmonary hypertension, 715
Pulse, peripheral
  amplitude of, 56–57
  assessment of, 56–57
  body sites for, 57f, 607f
  bradycardia, 56
  normal, 56
  pulse deficit, 57
  tachycardia, 56
Pulse deficit, assessment of, 57
Pulse oximetry
  in chronic obstructive pulmonary disease, 702
  in pneumonia, 684–85
  SaO_2, 684–85
Pump failure, in myocardial infarction, 564
Puncture wounds, 212f
Pupils, 856
  assessment of, 53, 53f
Purified protein derivative (PPD), in tuberculin test, 692
Purulent wound drainage, 144
Pustule, defined, 299t
Pyelonephritis
  acute, 503
  chronic, 503
  defined, 502
  pathophysiology, 503
  risk factors for, 503
Pyloroplasty, 415t
Pyrazinamide (PZA), for tuberculosis, 694t
Pyridostigmine (Mestinon), for myasthenia gravis, 837–38, 838t

Q

Quality assurance, components of, 3
Quinine, as antiparasitic drug, 251, 254
Quinsy, 658, 658f

R

Rabies, 841
Racial factors, affect on health, 22
Radial keratotomy, 862
Radiation
  as carcinogen, 158
  ultraviolet, as cancer risk factor, 159–60
Radiation therapy, 164
  in bone tumors, 767
  brachytherapy
    defined, 164
    safety principles for, 164f
  in brain tumor, 803
  in breast cancer, 915
  burn from, 326
  in colorectal cancer, 479
  external, defined, 164
  in laryngeal cancer, 670
  for leukemia, 641
  in malignant lymphoma, 649, 649f
  in prostate cancer, 892
  side effects of, 164
  in testicular cancer, 897
Radioactive therapy, in hyperthyroidism
    treatment, 347–48
Radioallergosorbent test (RAST), 275
Radioisotope scans, in cancer diagnosis,
    162
Radionuclear scan, cardiac, for angina
    pectoris, 556
Raynaud's disease, 605
Raynaud's phenomenon, 605
Reasoning, as critical thinking skill, 7
Rectocele, 930
Rectum, 454, 454f (See also Anorectal
    disorders)
Red blood cells (RBC)
  development of, 624, 625f
  functions of, 624
  normal laboratory values for, 508t, 624,
    626t
  structures of, 624, 624f
Red reflex, 863
Referrals, to home health care, 34, 37–38
Reflection, as critical thinking skill, 7
Reflex
  Babinski, 799f
  corneal, 799f, 856
  deep-tendon, 792
  defecation, 454
  defined, 792
  gag, 799f
  red, 863
  stretch, 792

  superficial, 792
  withdrawal, 792
Reflex arc, 792, 792f
Refractive errors in vision, 862–63
Regional enteritis, 472
Regurgitation
  aortic, 587t, 589, 589f
  mitral, 587t, 588, 588f
  in valvular heart disease, 586
Rehabilitation, 40–41
  cancer and, 175
  defined, 40
  nursing process in, 40–41
  for spinal cord injury, 847
  team approach to, 40
Reimbursement, for home health care, 35
Relapse, in substance abuse, 227
Relaxation
  in pain management, 110
  progressive, 110
Remission, defined, 25
Renal and urinary tract disorders, 493–532
  cancer, 517–22
    bladder, 517–21
    renal cell, 521–22
  infectious and inflammatory, 502–12
    glomerulonephritis, 507–11
    nephrotic syndrome, 511–12
    urinary tract infection, 502–7
  kidney trauma, 517
  nursing interventions classification, 532
  obstructive, 512–16
    hydronephrosis, 515–16
    polycystic kidney disease, 516
    urinary calculi, 512–15
  renal failure, 522–32
    acute, 522–23
    chronic, 523–32
  voiding disorders, 497–502
    urinary incontinence, 498–502
    urinary retention, 497–98
Renal biopsy, 509t
  in glomerulonephritis, 509
Renal cell cancer, 521–22
  manifestations, 521
  surgical treatment, 521, 522f
Renal clearance, in urine formation, 496
Renal failure
  acute, 522–23
    course of, 523
    etiology, 522, 522t
    intrarenal, 522t, 523
    pathophysiology, 522–23, 523t
    postrenal, 522t, 523
    prerenal, 522t, 523
  chronic, 523–32

    case study, 531–32
    collaborative care, 523, 525–31
      dialysis, 525–27
      dietary management, 525
      fluid management, 525
      kidney transplant, 527–28, 528f
      pharmacology, 525
      prevention, 523, 525
    defined, 523
    nursing care, 528–31
      assessment, 528–29
      discharge considerations, 531,
        531f
      disturbed body image, 530–31
      excess fluid volume, 529–30
      imbalanced nutrition, 530
      risk for infection, 530
    pathophysiology, 523
    resources for, 531
  defined, 522
  end-stage renal disease (ESRD), 523
Renal fascia, 494
Renal insufficiency, 523
Renal medulla, 494, 495f
Renal pelvis, 494, 495f
Renal pyramids, 494, 495f
Renal reserve, decreased, 523
Renal scan, 509t
  in glomerulonephritis, 509
Renal system (See also Kidneys)
  in acid-base regulation, 89, 91f
  age-related changes, 496–97, 496t
  effect of hypertension on, 598t
  effects of diabetes mellitus on, 379f
  effects of shock on, 201, 202f
  endocrine function of, 496
  urine formation, 495–96
Renin, 496
Renin-angiotensin-aldosterone system, 67,
    68f, 496
Renin-angiotensin system, in shock, 200
Repetitive use injuries, 747–48
  bursitis, 747
  carpal tunnel syndrome, 747
  collaborative care, 748
    assessment, 748
    discharge considerations, 748
    evaluation, 748
    impaired physical mobility, 748
    pain, 748
  epicondylitis, 747–48
Reproductive disorders
  female, 907–43
    breast disorders, 910–21
      associated with augmentation, 911
      cancer, 911–21

Reproductive disorders *(continued)*
  female *(continued)*
    breast disorders *(continued)*
      fibrocystic changes, 910–11
      mastitis, 911
    infections, 939–43
      pelvic inflammatory disease,
        941–42
      toxic shock syndrome, 942–43
      vaginitis, 939–41
    malignant tumors, 933–38
      cancer of the vulva, 938
      cervical cancer, 933–36
      endometrial cancer, 936–37
      ovarian cancer, 937–38
    menstruation disorders, 921–28
      dysfunctional uterine bleeding
        (DUB), 923–26
      dysmenorrhea, 923
      menopause, 926–28
      premenstrual syndrome,
        921–28
    nursing interventions classification,
      943
    reproductive tissue, 931–33
      endometriosis, 931–32
      ovarian cysts, 932–33
      uterine fibroid tumor, 933, 933f
    structural issues, 928–31
      pelvic organ prolapse, 930
      uterine displacement, 928–30
      vaginal fistula, 931
  male, 887–902
    nursing interventions classification,
      902
    penis, 898–902
      cancer, 899
      ejaculatory dysfunction, 902
      erectile dysfunction, 899–901
      phimosis, 898–99
      priapism, 899, 899f
    prostate disorders, 887–94
      benign prostatic hypertrophy,
        887–89, 887f
      prostate cancer, 890–94
      prostatitis, 889–90
    testes and scrotum, 895–98
      cryptorchidism, 895
      epididymitis, 895
      infertility, 895–96
      orchitis, 895
      scrotal masses, 896
      scrotal trauma, 896
      testicular cancer, 897–98
      testicular torsion, 895
      vasectomy complications, 896

Reproductive system
  effect of systemic lupus erythematous on,
    779f
  effects of cirrhosis on, 436f
  effects of hyperthyroidism on, 347f
  effects of hypothyroidism on, 352f
  effects of multiple sclerosis on, 832f
  female, 908–10
    external structures, 909–10, 909f
    internal structures, 908–9, 908f
  male, structures of, 886
Reservoir, in infection process, 245–46
Resistance
  to antibiotics, 247–48
  multidrug, 247–48
Respiration
  components of, 680
  expiration, 681, 681f
  factors affecting, 681
  inspiration, 681, 681f
  mechanics of, 681
Respiratory acidosis, 95–96
  acute, 95
  causes of, 92t
  chronic, 95
  collaborative care, 95
  defined, 89, 90f
  laboratory values, 92t
  manifestations, 92t
  nursing care, 95–96
    assessment, 95
    discharge considerations, 96
    impaired gas exchange, 95
    ineffective airway clearance, 96
  pathophysiology, 95
Respiratory alkalosis, 96–97
  causes of, 92t
  collaborative care, 96
  defined, 89, 90f
  laboratory values, 92t
  manifestations, 92t
  nursing care, 96
    discharge considerations, 96
    ineffective breathing patterns, 96
  pathophysiology, 96
Respiratory depression, opiates and, 118,
  226
Respiratory disorders
  lower, 679–727
    hemothorax, 718
    inflammatory and infectious, 682–96
      acute bronchitis, 682–83
      empyema, 689–90
      lung abscess, 689–90
      pleural effusion, 689
      pleuritis, 689

      pneumonia, 683–88
      tuberculosis, 690–96
    interstitial, 706–7
      collaborative care, 707
      discharge considerations, 707
      etiology, 706t
      occupational lung disease, 706–7,
        706t
      sarcoidosis, 706t, 707
    lung cancer, 707–12
    obstructive, 696–706
      asthma, 696–700
      atelectasis, 705–6
      bronchiectasis, 706
      chronic obstructive pulmonary
        disease, 700–705
      cystic fibrosis, 705
    in older adults, 682f
    pneumothorax, 715–18
    pulmonary vascular, 712–15
      pulmonary embolism, 712–15
      pulmonary hypertension, 715
    respiratory failure, 721–27
    trauma, 719–21
      flail chest, 719–20, 719f
      near-drowning, 719–20
      pulmonary contusion, 719
      rib fracture, 719
      smoke inhalation, 719
  nursing interventions classification, 727
  as surgical risk, 130t
  upper, 655–75
    inflammatory and infectious, 656–64
      assessment, 660–61, 662f
      case study, 663–64
      collaborative care, 659–63
      complementary and alternative
        medicine, 660
      diagnostic tests, 659
      discharge considerations, 662–63,
        663f
      epiglottitis, 658
      evaluation, 662
      influenza, 657
      laryngitis, 658–59
      otitis media and, 874
      pathophysiology, 657
      pharmacology, 659–60, 661t
      pharyngitis, 658, 658f
      rhinitis, 657
      sinusitis, 657–58
      surgical treatment, 660
      tonsillitis, 658
  nursing interventions classification,
    674–75
  sleep apnea, 668

trauma, 664–68
broken nose, 665–67
epistaxis, 664–65
laryngeal obstruction, 667–68
tumors, 668–74
benign laryngeal, 668–69
laryngeal cancer, 669–74
Respiratory failure, 721–27
acute respiratory distress syndrome, 722
collaborative care, 722–27
endotracheal tube, 722–23, 723f
mechanical ventilation, 723–24
oxygen therapy, 722
pharmacology, 722
defined, 721
hypercapnia in, 721–22, 722f
hypoxemia in, 721–22, 722f
manifestations of, 722, 722f
nursing care, 725–27
anxiety, 727
assessment, 725
decreased cardiac output, 726–27
discharge considerations, 727
impaired spontaneous ventilation, 725
ineffective airway clearance, 725
risk for injury, 725–26
pathophysiology, 721–22
Respiratory rates
bradypnea, 54
Cheyne-Stokes respirations, 54
eupnea, 54
hyperventilation, 54
hypoventilation, 54
tachypnea, 54
Respiratory system
in acid-base regulation, 89, 91f
metabolic alkalosis, 94
respiratory acidosis, 95–96
respiratory alkalosis, 96
in adults, 18t, 20t
AIDS-related infection in, 283–84
assessment of
auscultation, 54
breath sounds, 54
respiratory rates, 54
effect of burns on, 329
effect of leukemia on, 640f
effect of spinal cord injury on, 844f
effect of systemic lupus erythematous on, 779f
effects of anemia on, 627f
effects of cerebrovascular accident on, 807t
effects of cirrhosis on, 436f
effects of hyperthyroidism on, 347f

effects of hypothyroidism on, 352f
effects of multiple sclerosis on, 832f
effects of uremia on, 524f
lower
functions of, 680
lung volume and capacity, 681–82, 682f
pulmonary circulation, 680
respiration, 681
structures of, 680, 680f
shock effect on, 200, 202f
upper
functions of, 656
structures of, 656, 656f
in young adults, 16t
Restricted zone, in surgical departments, 139
Reticular activating system (RAS), 796
Reticulocyte count, normal laboratory values for, 626t
Retina, 856
detached, 869–70
collaborative care, 870
defined, 869
nursing care, 870
anxiety, 870
discharge considerations, 870
pathophysiology, 869–70, 870f
diabetic retinopathy, 871
Retinoids
antiacne, 305t
for psoriasis, 304
Retinopathy, diabetic, 382
Reverse transcriptase, 282
Rh groups, in blood types, 206
Rheumatic fever, 580
manifestations, 580f
from strep throat, 658
Rheumatic heart disease, 580–81
collaborative care, 580
nursing care, 580–81
activity intolerance, 581
assessment, 580–81
discharge considerations, 581
pain, 581
pathophysiology, 580
Rheumatoid arthritis, 772–78
case study, 777–78
collaborative care, 773–78
diagnostic tests, 773–74
pharmacology, 774, 775t
plasmapheresis, 774
rest and exercise, 774
surgical treatment, 774
defined, 772
manifestations of, 772, 773f

nursing care, 774–77
assessment, 774
discharge considerations, 776–77, 776f
disturbed body image, 776
fatigue, 776
ineffective role performance, 776
pain, 774, 776
pathophysiology, 772–73, 773f
vs. osteoarthritis, 773t
Rheumatoid factors, 772–73
Rhinitis, 657
acute viral, 657
allergic, 657
pharmacology, 660
vs. influenza, 657t
Rhinoplasty, in nasal fractures, 665–67
Rhinorrhea, defined, 794
Rhizotomy
defined, 840
for pain, 110, 112f
for trigeminal neuralgia, 840
Rib cage, structures of, 680
Rib fracture, 719, 742t
Ribavirin (Virazole), 255t
RICE (rest, ice, compression, elevation), 735
Rickets, adult, 763–64
Rickettsiae, in infection, 245f
Rifampin (RMP), for tuberculosis, 693t, 696
Rinne and Weber test, for hearing assessment, 879, 879f
Rods, of the eye, 856
Rofecoxib (Vioxx), for rheumatoid arthritis, 775t
Rubber band ligation, for hemorrhoids, 487
"Rule of nines," in burn injury assessment, 327, 328f

S

Safe sex precautions, 952f
Safety
with Alzheimer's clients, 831
in home health care, 39
Salicylates (See Aspirin)
Salmonellosis, 470t
Salpingo-oophorectomy
for endometrial cancer, 936
for endometriosis, 931
for ovarian cancer, 937
Salvia, function of, 394
Sanguineous wound drainage, 144
Sarcoidosis, 706t, 707
Sarcomeres, 733
Sargramostim (Leukine), for leukemia, 643t

Scabies, 309
Scales, defined, 299t
Scar
  defined, 52, 299t
  hypertrophic, in burn injuries, 332
Schilling's test, in anemia diagnosis, 629
Sciatica
  defined, 847
  in herniated intervertebral disk, 847
Sclera, 856
Sclerotherapy
  compression, for varicose veins, 619
  for hemorrhoids, 487
Scoliosis, 758–59
  collaborative care, 758–59
  defined, 758
  of spine, 54
Scrotal masses, 896
  hydrocele, 896, 896f
  spermatocele, 896, 896f
  varicocele, 896, 896f
Scrotal trauma, 896
Scrotum, 886 (See also Testes, disorders of)
Scrub nurse, 138, 139f
Sebaceous glands, 298t, 301–2
Secondary gain, of pain, 106
Sedatives, abuse of, 223t, 227
Seizure
  defined, 813
  generalized, 814
    absence, 814
    tonic-clonic, 814
  partial, 813–14
Seizure disorder, 813–17
  clonic contractions, 814, 814f
  collaborative care, 814–17
    diagnostic tests, 814
    pharmacology, 814–15, 815t
    surgical treatment, 815
  generalized seizures, 814
  nursing care, 815–17
    anxiety, 816
    assessment, 815, 816f
    discharge considerations, 816–17
    ineffective airway clearance,
      815–16
    risk for injury, 816
  partial seizures, 813–14
  pathophysiology, 813
  status epilepticus, 814
  tonic contractions, 814, 814f
Selective estrogen receptor modulators
    (SERMs), for osteoporosis, 760
Selectively permeable, 65, 66f
Semen, 886
Semi-Fowler's position, 74, 95

Semicircular canals, 872
Semilunar valves, 539
Semirestricted zone, in surgical departments,
    139
Sengstaken-Blakemore, for esophageal
    varices, 440–42, 440f
Sensitivity studies, in infection diagnosis,
    250
Sensory issues
  in adults, 18t
  in older adults, 20t
Sensory system
  effect of systemic lupus erythematous on,
    779f
  effects of diabetes mellitus on, 379f
  effects of hyperthyroidism on, 347f
  effects of hypothyroidism on, 352f
  effects of multiple sclerosis on, 832f
  effects of premenstrual syndrome on,
    922f
Sepsis, in cancer, 177–78
Septicemia
  defined, 203, 247
  in peritonitis, 466
Seroconversion, 282
Serous wound drainage, 144
Serum osmolality, normal electrolyte
    laboratory values for, 64t
Sex education, for AIDS prevention, 285
Sexual dysfunction
  colorectal cancer, 481–82
  dysfunctional uterine bleeding, 925
  erectile dysfunction, 901
  menopause, 928
  prostate cancer, 892
  sexually transmitted disease, 952
  testicular cancer, 898
Sexually transmitted disease (STD),
    947–57
  chancroid, 949t
  Chlamydia, 948, 949t, 950–53
  collaborative care, 951–53
  common characteristics of, 948, 948f
  defined, 948
  genital herpes, 949t, 953–54
  genital warts, 949t, 954–55
  gonorrhea, 949t, 955–56
  granuloma, 949t
  incidence, 947
  nursing care, 951–53
    anxiety, 952
    assessment, 951, 951f
    discharge considerations, 952–53
    impaired skin integrity, 951
    impaired social interaction, 952
    ineffective health maintenance, 951

    injury risk, 951–52
    low self-esteem, 952
    sexual dysfunction, 952
  prevention, 952f
  risk factors for, 948f
  syphilis, 956–57
  in young adults, 16
Shave areas, for surgery, 139, 140f
Shigellosis, 470t
Shingles, 249t, 308–9
Shock, 200–210
  anaphylactic, 201–2
    causes of, 201
    client education, 209f
    defined, 200
    treatment, 207–8
  burn, 328–29
  cardiogenic, 202–3
    defined, 200
    manifestations of, 204f
    in myocardial infarction, 564
    treatment, 208
  collaborative care, 205
    oxygen therapy, 205
  complications of, 204–5
  effects of, 200–201
    cardiovascular, 200, 202f
    gastrointestinal, 200, 202f
    neurologic, 200–201, 202f
    renal, 201, 202f
    respiratory, 200, 202f
    skin, 201, 202f
  hypovolemic, 143, 201
    in bowel obstruction, 482
    causes of, 201f
    defined, 200
    manifestations of, 201f
    pathophysiology, 201, 203f
    prehospital care, 205f
    in trauma clients, 211–12
    treatment, 205–7
  neurogenic
    causes of, 204
    defined, 200
    manifestations of, 204f
    treatment, 208
  nursing care, 205–9
    anxiety, 209
    assessment, 205, 208
    discharge considerations, 209
    ineffective tissue perfusion, 208–9
  pathophysiology, 200–201
  postoperative, 143
  septic, 203–4
    in cancer, 177–78
    case study, 209–10

defined, 200
infection and, 247
manifestations of, 177, 204f
risk factors for, 203f
treatment, 177–78, 208
spinal, 842–43, 846
stages of, 200–201, 201f
compensated, 200
irreversible, 201
progressive, 200–201
Short bowel syndrome, malabsorption and, 464
Sibutramine (Meridia), 398
Sickle cell anemia, 627–28, 629f
inheritance pattern for, 627f
pathophysiology, 627, 628f
Sickle-cell screening test, in anemia diagnosis, 629
Sigmoid colon, 454, 454f
Sigmoidoscopy (See also Colonoscopy)
in cancer diagnosis, 163
in colorectal cancer, 478f
defined, 163
in diarrhea, 455
in inflammatory bowel disease, 472
nursing care for, 455f, 478f
Signs and symptoms, of disease, 24
Sildenafil (Viagra), for erectile dysfunction, 900, 900f
Sinoatrial (SA) node, 539
Sinus bradycardia, 542, 543t, 545
Sinus rhythm, 542, 543t
Sinus surgery, endoscopic, 660
Sinus tachycardia, 542, 543t, 564
Sinuses, 656
Sinusitis, 657–58
Sinusoids, 426
Skene's glands, 909f, 910
Skin, 298, 300
in adults, 18t
anatomy of, 300f
changes in older adults, 20t, 301f
dermis, 298, 298t
effects of shock on, 201, 202f
epidermis, 298, 298t
glands of
apocrine sweat glands, 298t, 301
eccrine sweat glands, 298t, 301
sebaceous glands, 298t, 301
in young adults, 16t
Skin cancer, 311–17
basal cell, 312
collaborative care
cryosurgery, 314
diagnostic tests, 313
immunotherapy, 314

radiation therapy, 314
surgery, 313
melanoma, 312–13
case study, 316–17
metastasis sites for, 157t
staging of, 313
nonmelanoma, 311–12
nursing care, 314–16
anxiety, 314–15
assessment, 314, 314f
discharge considerations, 315–16, 316f
hopelessness, 315
impaired skin integrity, 315
prevention of, 315–16, 316f
squamous cell, 312
Skin disorders, 301–21
acne, 302, 303f, 304
collaborative care
diagnostic tests, 303
pharmacology, 303–4
surgery, 304
dermatitis, 302
dry skin (xerosis), 301
infections and manifestations, 306–11
bacterial, 306–7
cellulitis, 307
diagnostic tests, 309
discharge considerations, 311
folliculitis, 307
furuncles, 307
pharmacology, 309
collaborative care
diagnostic tests, 309
pharmacology, 309
fungal, 307–8
candidiasis infections, 307–8
dermatophyte infections, 307
diagnostic tests, 309
discharge considerations, 311
pharmacology, 309
nursing care, 309–11
acute pain, 310
assessment, 309–10
discharge considerations, 311
disturbed sleep pattern, 310
risk for infection, 310–11
in older adults, 249t
parasitic
discharge considerations, 311
pediculosis, 308–9
pharmacology, 309
scabies, 309
viral
discharge considerations, 311
herpes simplex, 308

herpes zoster, 308
pharmacology, 309
warts, 308
malignant (See Skin cancer)
nursing care, 304–6
assessment, 304, 305f
deficient knowledge, 306
discharge considerations, 306
disturbed body image, 306
impaired skin integrity, 304, 306
pressure ulcers, 317–21
collaborative care, 318, 320
discharge considerations, 320–21
individuals at risk, 318
in older adults, 318
pathophysiology, 317
products used to treat, 318, 320t
stages of, 318, 319f
pruritus, 301, 303
psoriasis, 301–4, 302f
Skin graft
in burn injuries, 331–32
types of, 277
Skin lesions, primary and secondary, 299t–300t
Skin preparation, for surgery, 130
Skin testing
for allergy testing, 275
in asthma, 696
diagnostic test for immune system, 271
Skull fracture, 742t, 794–95
cerebrospinal fluid leakage in, 794–95
types of, 794–95
Sleep apnea, 668
central, 668
manifestations of, 668
obstructive, 668
Sleep pattern disturbance, surgery and, 133
Small bowel series
for inflammatory bowel disease, 472
for irritable bowel syndrome, 462–63
nursing interventions for, 462–63, 463f
Small intestine
functions of, 394, 396, 454
regions of, 396
duodenum, 396
ileum, 396
jejunum, 396
Smoke inhalation, 329, 719
Smoking
as cancer risk factor, 159
child prevention of, 711f
chronic obstructive pulmonary disease and, 700, 703
client education for quitting, 711f
coronary heart disease and, 553

Smoking (continued)
diabetes mellitus and, 367
effects of, 224t, 228
hospitalized clients and, 228
hypertension and, 598
lung cancer and, 707–8, 711f
as surgical risk, 130t
withdrawal symptoms, 224t, 228
Snellen's chart, 53, 53f
Socioeconomic factors
affect on health, 23
as influence to pain response, 106
Sodium
foods high in, 72f
laboratory values for, 64t, 127t
Sodium imbalance, 76–78
collaborative care
hypernatremia, 76–77
causes of, 76t
client education, 78
collaborative care, 77
defined, 76
laboratory values, 76t
manifestations, 76t
hyponatremia
causes of, 76t
client education, 78
collaborative care, 76, 77f
defined, 76
laboratory values, 76t
manifestations, 76t
nursing care, 77–78
assessment, 77
discharge considerations, 78
fluid volume imbalance, 77
risk for injury, 77–78
Sodium-potassium pump, in active transport,
66, 67f
Sodium-restricted diet, 72f, 73, 75f
Somogyi phenomenon, 381
Speech deficit (See also Aphasia)
in cerebrovascular accident, 806–7,
807t
Speech generators, in speech rehabilitation,
671, 671f
Speech rehabilitation
esophageal speech, 670
in laryngeal cancer, 670–71
speech generators, 671, 671f
tracheoesophageal puncture, 670, 670f
Sperm, production of, 886
Spermatogenesis, 886
Sphincter
external urethral, 495, 495f
internal urethral, 495, 495f
Sphincter of Oddi, 426, 427f

Spinal cord
function of, 842
structures of, 791–92
Spinal cord disorders, 842–50
compression
in cancer, 178
intervention, 178
manifestations of, 178
herniated intervertebral disk, 847–50
nursing interventions classification, 850
spinal cord injury, 842–47
tumors of, 850
Spinal cord injury (SCI), 842–47
autonomic dysreflexia, 843
classification of, 842, 844f
collaborative care, 843–47
diagnostic tests, 844
emergency care, 843
pharmacology, 844
stabilization, 844
Gardner-Wells tongs, 844, 845f
halo vest, 844, 845f
surgical treatment, 845
complete, 842
complications of, 844f
incomplete, 842
nursing care, 845–47
assessment, 845, 846f
discharge considerations, 847
disturbed self-esteem, 846–47
impaired physical mobility, 846
ineffective breathing pattern, 845–46
urinary elimination and constipation,
846
pathophysiology, 842, 843f
spinal shock, 842–43
Spinal cord tumors, 850
manifestations of, 850
primary, 850
secondary, 850
Spinal fusion, for herniate intervertebral
disk, 849
Spinal nerves, 792, 792f
Spinal shock, 842–43, 846
Spine
fracture of, 742t
kyphosis of, 54
scoliosis of, 54
Spirituality, loss and, 185
Spironolactone (Aldactone), nursing
considerations for, 73t, 574t
Spleen
function of, 647
in lymphoid system, 266, 268f
platelets in the, 635
Splenectomy, for thrombocytopenia, 635

Splenomegaly, cirrhosis and, 436
Sprain
collaborative care, 734–35
defined, 734
manifestations of, 734f
Sputum specimen
in pneumonia, 684
procedure for taking, 684f
Squamous cell
oral cancers, 406
skin cancer, 312
Staging in cancer
breast cancer, 915
melanoma, 313
tumor identification in, 161, 162t
Standard precautions, in infection control,
255, 256f
Standards of practice, 9, 10f
defined, 9
Starling's law of the heart, 541
Status asthmaticus, 696
Stasis dermatitis
ulcer care, 614
in venous thrombosis, 614
Status epilepticus, 814–15
Stem cells, 266, 267f, 624, 625f
Stenosis
aortic, 587t, 588, 588f
mitral, 586–88, 587f, 587t
in valvular heart disease, 586
Sterility
defined, 895
male, 895
Steroids, for multiple sclerosis, 833
Stertorous breath sounds, 54
Stockings, antiembolic
for pulmonary embolism, 713
for varicose veins, 619
for venous thrombosis, 613, 615–16
Stoma, 474, 474f (See also Ostomy)
client care for, 520, 520f
defined, 163
Stomach
autonomic nervous system affects on,
794f
disorders of
cancer, 418–19
gastritis, 408–12
peptic ulcer, 412–18
functions of, 394, 394f
gastric juices of
chief cells, 394
enteroendocrine cells, 394
mucous cells, 394
parietal cells, 394
lining of, 408, 408f

Stomach cancer
    manifestations of, 419
    treatment of, 419
Stomatitis, 404–6
    defined, 404
    discharge considerations, 405
    manifestations of, 404
    pharmacology, 405t
    treatment of, 405
Stool, 454, 454f
Stool culture
    in diarrhea, 455
    purpose of, 455
Stool softeners, for constipation, 460t
Stool specimen
    in diarrhea, 455
    for inflammatory bowel disease, 472
    purpose of, 455
Strain
    collaborative care, 734–35
    defined, 734
    manifestations of, 734f
Strep throat, 658, 658f
    diagnosis of, 659, 659f
    manifestations of, 581
    rheumatic heart disease and, 580
Streptomycin, 253t, 694t, 696
Stress
    as cancer risk factor, 159
    complementary therapies for, 599f
    hypertension and, 598
    irritable bowel syndrome and, 462–63
Stressors
    physical, in young adults, 17
    psychosocial
        in adults, 18
        in older adults, 19
        in young adults, 17
Stroke (See Cerebrovascular accident
        (CVA))
Stroke volume
    in cardiac output, 541
    defined, 202–3
Sty, 858, 858f
Subarachnoid hemorrhage
    defined, 812
    manifestations of, 812
Sublingual nitroglycerin (NTG), for angina
        pectoris, 557, 557t, 562
Subluxation, 747
Substance abuse, 221–33
    by age
        in adults, 17
        in older adults, 19
        in young adults, 16–17
    alcohol, 222–26 (See also Alcohol abuse)

    among nurses, 229–30
    caffeine, 224t, 228
    cannabis, 224t, 228
    cocaine and amphetamines, 223t, 227
    collaborative care, 228–30
        acute phase, 229
        goals of, 229
        pharmacology, 228–29
        rehabilitation phase, 229
    compulsive substance use, defined, 222
    defined, 222
    dual diagnosis with, 229
    hallucinogens, 224t, 227
    inhalants, 224t, 227–28
    mental disorders and, 229
    nicotine, 224t, 228
    nursing care, 230–33
        assessment, 230–31, 231f
        case study, 232–33
        discharge considerations, 232
        individual coping, 231–32
        knowledge deficit, 231
    opioids, 223t, 226–27
    polysubstance abuse, 227
    resources for and about, 232
    sedatives, hypnotics, and anxiolytics,
        223t, 227
    substance dependency, defined, 222
Substance-P, in pain conduction, 103, 104f
Sucking chest wound, 715, 716t
Sucralfate, for gastritis, 409, 411t
Sudden cardiac death, 551
Sulfamethiazole (Thiosulfil Forte), 253t
Sulfamethoxazole (Gantanol), 253t
Sulfasalazine (Azulfidine), for inflammatory
        bowel disease, 473t
Sulfinpyrazone, for gout, 781t
Sulfisoxazole (Gantrisin), 253t
Sulfonamides
    client education, 253t
    nursing responsibilities, 253t
    purpose of, 253t
Sulfonylureas, for diabetes mellitus, 376t
Sundowning, in Alzheimer's disease, 828
Superinfection, 251
Superior vena cava syndrome
    in cancer, 177
    in lung cancer, 709
    manifestations of, 177
    treatment, 177
Support systems, grieving and loss, 184–85
Supraventricular rhythms, 542, 543t–544t,
        545–46
    atrial fibrillation, 544t, 546
    atrial flutter, 543t, 545
    normal sinus rhythm (NSR), 542, 543t

    premature atrial contractions (PACs),
        543t, 545
    sinus bradycardia, 542, 543t, 545
    sinus tachycardia, 542, 543t
    supraventricular tachycardia (SVT), 545
Supraventricular tachycardia (SVT), 545
Supressor T cells, 267t, 268, 270f
Surgeon, role of, 138
Surgery, 126–50
    in burn injuries, 331–32
    classification of procedures, 126t
    client risk factors, 129t–130t
    client stress factors, 130
    complications (See Surgical
        complications)
    defined, 126
    emergency, 213
    inpatient, defined, 126
    intraoperative phase, 137–42
        altered body temperature, 142
        risk for aspiration, 142
        assessment, 139, 142
        client positioning, 139, 141f
        client preparation, 139
        defined, 126, 137
        risk for infection, 142
        pharmacology (See Anesthesia)
        shave areas, 139, 140f
    nursing care, 131–37, 139–42, 145–48
    outpatient, 148, 149f
        defined, 126
    postoperative phase, 142–48
        acute pain, 146
        assessment, 145–46
        constipation, 147–48
        deep venous thrombosis (DVT), 146
        defined, 126
        discharge considerations, 148
        hemorrhage, 146
        impaired gas exchange, 147
        ineffective breathing pattern, 147
        risk for infection, 147
        pharmacology, 142–43
        urinary retention, 147
    preoperative phase, 126–37
        anxiety, 133
        assessment, 131
        case study, 135–37
        checklist for day of, 136f
        defined, 126
        informed consent, 131, 131f
        knowledge deficit, 133
        laboratory tests, 127–28, 127t
        pharmacology, 128, 128t–129t
        sleep pattern disturbance, 133
        teaching for, 133, 134f–135f

Surgery (*continued*)
  surgical attire, 138–39, 139f
  surgical department zones, 139
  surgical scrub, 139
  surgical team, 138
Surgical assistant, role of, 138
Surgical complications, 143–45
  cardiovascular
    deep venous thrombosis (DVT),
      143
    hemorrhage, 143
    pulmonary embolism, 143
    shock, 143
  elimination
    bowel, 144
    urinary, 144
  respiratory
    atelectasis, 143
    pneumonia, 143
  wound healing, 144–45, 144f
Swallowing, impaired, in cerebrovascular
  accident, 811–12
Swan-neck deformity, in rheumatoid
  arthritis, 773f
Swimmer's ear, 873–74
Sympathectomy, for pain, 109–10, 112f
Sympathetic nervous system (SNS), 794,
  794f
  in blood pressure, 597
  in shock, 200
Sympathomimetic drugs
  for glaucoma, 867t
  for heart failure, 573t
Synapse, 790, 790f
  defined, 103
  in pain conduction, 103
Syndrome of inappropriate ADH secretion
  (SIADH), 345–46
  collaborative care, 345
  discharge considerations, 345–46
  excess fluid volume, 345
  manifestations of, 345f
Synovial fluid, 732–33, 774
Syphilis, 956–57
  collaborative care, 949t, 957
    diagnostic tests, 957
    pharmacology, 957
  complications, 949t
  latent stage, 956–57
  manifestations of, 949t
  nursing care, 957
    discharge considerations, 957
  pathophysiology, 956
  primary, 956
  secondary, 956
  tertiary, 957

Systemic lupus erythematous (SLE), 778–80
  collaborative care, 778–80
    diagnostic tests, 276–77, 778
    pharmacology, 778
  defined, 778
  glomerulonephritis in, 508
  manifestations of, 778, 779f
  nursing care, 779–80
    discharge considerations, 780
    impaired skin integrity, 779
    ineffective protection, 779–80
  pathophysiology, 778
Systolic blood pressure, 597

T

T-cells (*See* T lymphocytes)
T lymphocytes, 158, 266, 267t
  in cell-mediated immunity, 268, 270f
  cytotoxic T cells, 267t
  function of, 267t
  helper T cells, 267t
  in rheumatoid arthritis, 772
  supressor T cells, 267f
T-tube, for cholelithiasis, 428, 429f
Tachycardia, defined, 56
Tachypnea, 54
Tag triage system, 210
Tamoxifen (Nolvadex)
  for breast cancer, 915, 916t
  in chemotherapy, 167t
Tar preparations, for psoriasis, 304
Teacher, nurse as, 2, 36, 38–39
Tendons, 733
Tennis elbow, 747–48
Terminal care (*See* End of life care)
Testes, 886
  disorders of, 895–98
    cryptorchidism, 895
    epididymitis, 895
    infertility, 895–96
    orchitis, 895
    scrotal masses, 896
    scrotal trauma, 896
    testicular cancer, 897–98
    testicular torsion, 895
    vasectomy complications, 896
Testicular cancer, 897–98
  collaborative care, 897–98
    pharmacology, 897
    radiation therapy, 897
    surgical treatment, 897
  nursing care, 897–98
    assessment, 897–98
    deficient knowledge, 898

  discharge considerations, 898
  sexual dysfunction, 898
  pathophysiology, 897
Testicular self-examination, 895, 897, 897f
Testicular torsion, 895
Testosterone, 886
  in benign prostatic hypertrophy, 887
Testosterone therapy, for erectile
  dysfunction, 900, 900f
Tetanus, 841
Tetracyclines
  client education, 253t
  nursing responsibilities, 253t
  purpose of, 253t
Tetraplegia, 842, 843f, 844f
Thalamotomy, stereotaxic, in Parkinson's
  disease, 835
Thalamus, 790
Thalassemia, 628
Theophylline, for chronic obstructive
  pulmonary disease, 702
Therapeutic baths, procedure for, 303t
Therapeutic range, defined, 250
Thiazolinediones, for diabetes mellitus, 376t
Thinking, divergent, 7
Third-party payers, home health care
  reimbursement, 35
Third spacing, 68–69
Thirst, role in body fluid regulation, 66–67,
  67f
Thoracentesis
  for pleural effusion, 689, 689f, 690f, 710
  for pneumothorax, 716
Thoracotomy, 709t
Throat swab, procedure for, 659, 659f
Thrombectomy, venous, 614
Thromboangiitis obliterans, 605
Thrombocytopenia, 635–36
  cirrhosis and, 436
  collaborative care, 635–36
    pharmacology, 635
    platelet transfusion, 635
    surgical treatment, 635–36
  defined, 436, 635
  pathophysiology, 635
Thrombolytic drugs
  for cerebrovascular accident, 808–9
  for myocardial infarction, 565–66, 566f
  for pulmonary embolism, 713
  for venous thrombosis, 614
Thrombophlebitis, 612
  superficial vein, 613, 613f
Thrombopoietic growth factor, for leukemia,
  643t
Thymus gland, in lymphoid system, 266,
  268f

Thyroid gland
  disorders of
    cancer of, 354
      hyperthyroidism, 346–50
      hypothyroidism, 351–54
  functions of, 342
  hormones of, 343t
Thyroid hormone (TH), function of, 343t
Thyroid-stimulating hormone (TSH),
  function of, 343t
Thyroid storm, 346
Thyroidectomy
  subtotal, 348, 349f
  total, 348, 349f
Thyrotoxic crisis, 346
Thyrotoxicosis (*See* Hyperthyroidism)
Tibia fracture, 741t
Tic douloureux, 840
Ticarcillin (Ticar), 252t
Tidal volume (TV), in mechanical
  ventilation, 724
Tinea cruris, 307
Tinea pedis, 307
Tinnitus, masking, 878
Tissue transplant (*See* Transplantation)
Tobacco (*See also* Smoking)
  oral cancer and, 405–6
Tolerance
  alcohol abuse, 223
  cross-tolerance, 228
  defined, 223
Tonicity, defined, 65
Tonometry, in glaucoma, 864–65
Tonsillectomy, 660
Tonsillitis, 658
Tonsils, 268f, 656
Total parenteral nutrition (TPN), 402,
  402f
Toxic shock syndrome (TSS), 204,
  942–43
  collaborative care, 942–43
  nursing care, 942–43
    assessment, 942
    decreased cardiac output, 943
    discharge considerations, 943
    ineffective tissue perfusion, 942–43
  pathophysiology, 942
Toxoids, in immunizations, 271
Toxoplasmosis, AIDS-related, 285
Tracheoesophageal puncture (TEP), in
  speech rehabilitation, 670, 670f
Tracheostomy, permanent
  client education, 674
  for laryngeal cancer, 670, 670f
  nursing care for, 673f

Trachoma, 858–59
Traction
  for fractures, 737–39
  in joint dislocation, 747
  nursing care for, 740f
  types of, 737–38
    balanced suspension, 738–39, 739f
    Buck's, 738, 739f
    manual, 737
    skeletal, 737
    skin, 737
    straight, 737–39
Transcellular fluid, defined, 65
Transcutaneous electrical nerve stimulation
  (TENS), in pain management,
  110–11, 112t
Transdermal patch, for pain, 107–8, 110f
Transduction, pain, 102, 103f
Transfusions, 206–7, 207t
  for anemia, 630
  autotransfusion, 207
  defined, 206
  febrile reaction, 207
  nursing implications for, 207t
  platelet, for thrombocytopenia, 635
  type and cross-match, 206
Transient ischemic attack (TIA), 805–6
  defined, 805
  manifestations of, 805–6
Transjugular intrahepatic portosystemic
  shunt (TIPS), 439–40, 440f
Transmission
  airborne, 246
  direct, 246
  droplet, 246
  indirect, 246
  in infection process, 246
  of pain, 103, 103f
  vector, 246
Transmission precautions, in infection
  control, 255, 257t
Transplantation, 277–81
  bone marrow
    allogenic, 641
    autologous, 277, 641–42
    in cancer treatment, 168
    graft-*versus*-host disease in, 279–80
    for leukemia, 641–42
  collaborative care
    diagnostic tests, 278–79
    pharmacology, 279
  cornea, 859
  graft-*versus*-host disease (GvHD), 278
  heart, for heart failure, 575, 575f
  human leukocyte antigens (HLA) and,
    277

  kidney, 527–28, 528f
    immunosuppressive drugs for, 528
    nursing care, 529
    rejection in, 529t
  liver, 438–39, 439f
  lung, for chronic obstructive pulmonary
    disease, 702
  nursing care, 280–81
    anxiety, 280–81
    discharge considerations, 281, 281f
    impaired tissue integrity, 279–80
    risk for infection, 279
  organ donation, 277
  pancreas, 383
  pathophysiology, 277–78
  rejection in, 278, 278t
  tissues typing, 278
  types of
    allograft, 277, 279–80
    autograft, 277
    isograft, 277
    xenograft, 277
Transrectal ultrasonography (TRUS)
  nursing care for, 891f
  in prostate cancer, 891
Transurethral incision of the prostate
  (TUIP), for benign prostatic
  hypertrophy, 888
Transurethral resection of bladder tumor
  (TURBT), for bladder cancer, 518t
Transurethral resection of the prostate
  (TURP)
  for benign prostatic hypertrophy, 888
  discharge instructions, 889, 890f
  nursing care for, 888f
Trauma, 210–16
  blunt, 211
  collaborative care, 212–13 (*See also*
    Emergency care)
  defined, 210
  effects of, 211–12
  major, 211
  minor, 210–11
  nursing care, 213–15
    case study, 214–15
    discharge considerations, 214
    risk for infection, 213–14
  penetrating, 211
Treatment plan (*See* Plan of care)
Trendelenburg position, 209, 209f
Triage, defined, 210
Trichomoniasis, 939, 940t
  collaborative care, 949t
  complications, 949t
  manifestations of, 949t
Tricuspid valves, 538

Trigger zones, in trigeminal neuralgia, 840
Trigone, 494, 495f
Trimethoprimsulfamethoxazole (Bactrim, Septra), 253t
Trismus, in tetanus, 841
Trousseau's sign
    defined, 82
    in tetany, 82
Tube
    chest
        closed-drainage systems, 717, 717f
        nursing care, 717f
        for pneumothorax, 717
    endotracheal
        nursing care, 723f
        preparation for, 725
        pros and cons, 723t
        in respiratory failure, 722–23, 723f
        suctioning of, 726f
    gastrostomy, 419, 419f
    nasogastric, 400, 401f
Tube feedings (See Enteral feedings)
Tuberculin test, 692, 692f, 692t
Tuberculosis, 690–96
    AIDS-related, 284, 288t
    collaborative care, 692–96
        diagnostic tests, 692–93
        pharmacology, 693–94, 693t–694t
        screening methods, 692, 692f, 692t
    defined, 690
    extrapulmonary, 692
    manifestations of, 690, 692
    nursing care, 693–96
        deficient knowledge, 695
        discharge considerations, 695–96
        risk for infection, 694–95
    in older adults, 249t, 690f
    pathophysiology, 690, 691f, 692
    pulmonary, 690, 692
    reactivation, 690, 691f
Tubular reabsorption, in urine formation, 495
Tubular secretion, in urine formation, 496
Tumor (See also Neoplasm)
    benign of larynx, 668–69
    identification, 161–62, 162t
        classifications, 161
        grading, 161
        staging, 161, 162t
        TNM classification, 161, 162t
Tumor markers, 162
    In cancer diagnosis
        CEA, 163
        ovarian, 937
        PSA, 163
Tumors, benign, of larynx, 668–69
Tunica adventitia, 596

Tunica intima, 596
Tunica media, 596
Turbinates, 656
Turgor
    defined, 52
    in older adults, 70
Turner's sign, 444
Tympanic membrane, 872
Tympanocentesis, for otitis media, 875
Tympanostomy, for otitis media, 875
Tympany, defined, 48

U

Ulcer
    Curling's, 329
    skin, 299t
Ulcerative colitis
    case study, 477
    complications of, 472
    defined, 471
    pathophysiology, 471–72
    treatment (See Inflammatory bowel disease (IBD))
Ultraviolet-B light, for psoriasis, 304
Unrestricted zone, in surgical departments, 139
Urea, 496
Urea breath test, 413
Uremia
    defined, 523
    multisystem effects of, 523, 524f
    in renal failure, 523
Ureteral stents, for hydronephrosis, 515, 515f, 516f
Ureterostomy, cutaneous, for bladder cancer, 518t
Ureters, structure of, 494
Urethra, structure of, 495
Urethritis, 502
Urethrocele, urinary incontinence associated with, 499
Uric acid, in gout, 780
Uricosuric drugs, for gout, 781, 781t
Urinalysis, significance of laboratory values, 127t
    normal values, 496
Urinary diversion, for bladder cancer, 518, 519t, 520
Urinary incontinence, 498–502
    artificial urinary sphincter for, 892, 894f
    collaborative care, 499–502
        Kegel exercises, 501, 501f
        voiding diary, 499, 500f
    functional, 499t, 501

    nursing care, 500–502
        assessment, 500
        discharge considerations, 502
        social isolation, 501–2
    in older adults, 498–99
    overflow, 499t
    pathophysiology, 498
    in pelvic organ prolapse, 930
    reflex, 499t
    stress, 499t
    types of, 499t
    urge, 499, 499t
Urinary retention, 497–98
    benign prostatic hypertrophy, 497
    collaborative care, 497–98
    complications of, 497
    discharge considerations, 498
    etiology, 497
    nursing care, 497–98
    postsurgery treatment, 144
    as surgical complication, 144
Urinary system, 494–97, 494f (See also Genitourinary system; Renal and urinary tract disorders)
    effect of burns on, 329
    effect of systemic lupus erythematous on, 779f
    effects of anemia on, 627f
    effects of cerebrovascular accident on, 807–8, 807t
    effects of multiple sclerosis on, 832f
    effects of premenstrual syndrome on, 922f
    effects of uremia on, 524f
    structures of, 494–95, 494f
    urine formation, 495–96
Urinary tract infection (UTI), 502–7
    collaborative care, 503–7
        complementary and alternative medicine, 505, 507f
        pharmacology, 503–5, 506f
        urinary elimination, 504
    cystitis
        defined, 502
        manifestations of, 503f
        pathophysiology, 502–3
    as nosocomial infection, 502
    nursing care, 504–7
        assessment, 504
        discharge considerations, 505–7
    in older adults, 249t, 502, 503f
    pathophysiology, 502–3
    prostatitis, defined, 502
    pyelonephritis
        acute, 503
        chronic, 503
        defined, 502

pathophysiology, 503
risk factors for, 503
recurrent, 503
risk factors for, 503f
urethritis, defined, 502
Urine concentration, in urine formation, 496, 496t
Urine formation, 495–96
glomerular filtration, 495
renal clearance, 496
tubular reabsorption, 495
tubular secretion, 496
urine concentration, 496, 496t
Urine specific gravity, normal electrolyte laboratory values for, 64t
Urine specimen
24 hour
collecting, 76, 77f
nursing care, 508, 508f
clean-catch, 503, 504f
Uroflowmetry
in benign prostatic hypertrophy, 887
for urinary incontinence, 499
Urolithiasis (*See* Calculi, urinary)
Ursodeoxycholic acid (UDCA), 428
Uterine balloon heat therapy, for dysfunctional uterine bleeding, 924
Uterine cancer, 160f
Uterine displacement, 928–30
anteflexion, 928, 928f
anteversion, 928, 928f
retroflexion, 928, 928f
retroversion, 928, 928f
Uterine fibroid tumor, 933, 933f
Uterine prolapse, 930
Uterus, structure of, 908f, 909
Uveitis, 859

Vaccines (*See also* Immunizations)
inactivated, 271
live, attenuated, 271
Vacuum constriction device (VCD), for erectile dysfunction (ED), 900, 900f
Vagina, 908f, 909
Vaginal dryness, in menopause, 928, 928f
Vaginal fistula, 931
Vaginal yeast infection, 251, 385, 939, 940t
Vaginitis, 939–41
atrophic, 939, 940t
candidiasis, 939, 940t
collaborative care, 939–41
diagnostic tests, 939
pharmacology, 939, 940t

nursing care, 939–41
assessment, 939
discharge considerations, 940–41
pain, 940
pathophysiology, 939
prevention of, 940
risk factors for, 939
simple, 939, 940t
trichomoniasis, 939, 940t
Vagotomy, 416t
Valsalva's maneuver, 454, 497, 799
Valve replacement, in valvular heart disease, 589–90, 590f
Valves of the heart
endocarditis and, 581–83
function of, 586
rheumatic heart disease and, 580–81
Valvular heart disease, 586–91
aortic regurgitation, 587t, 589, 589f
aortic stenosis, 587t, 588, 588f
collaborative care, 589–91
percutaneous balloon valvuloplasty, 589, 590f
surgical treatment, 589–90
mitral regurgitation, 587t, 588, 588f
mitral stenosis, 586–88, 587f, 587t
mitral valve prolapse, 588
nursing care, 590–91
activity intolerance, 590
decreased cardiac output, 590
discharge considerations, 591
pathophysiology, 586–89
regurgitation, 586
stenosis, 586
Valvuloplasty, 589
percutaneous balloon, 589, 590f
Vancomycin-resistant *Enterococcus* (VRE), 248
Vancomycin (Vancocin), 254t
Varicose veins, 618–19, 618f
collaborative care, 618–19
conservative therapy, 618–19
surgical treatment, 619
defined, 618
manifestations of, 618, 619f
nursing care, 619
discharge considerations, 619
ineffective tissue perfusion, 619
pathophysiology, 618
Varicosities, 618
Vas deferens, 886
Vasectomy
complications of, 896
defined, 896
Vasodilators, for hypertension, 601t
Vasopressor drugs, for cariogenic shock, 208

Vector, in infection transmission, 246
Vein stripping, for varicose veins, 619
Veins, structure of, 596, 596f
Venous disorders, 612–19
varicose veins, 618–19, 618f
venous insufficiency, 613
venous thrombosis, 612–17
Venous insufficiency, 613–17
defined, 613
pathophysiology, 613
Venous thrombosis, 613–17
collaborative care, 613–17
conservative therapy, 613–14
diagnostic tests, 613
pharmacology, 614
anticoagulants, 614, 615t
thrombolytics, 614
stasis dermatitis care, 614
surgical treatment, 614
deep vein thrombosis (DVT), 612–13
defined, 613
nursing care, 614–17
assessment, 614, 616f
discharge considerations, 616–17
impaired skin integrity, 616
ineffective tissue perfusion, 614–16
pain, 614
pathophysiology, 612–13
risk factors for, 612f
superficial vein thrombophlebitis, 613, 613f
Ventricular assist devices (VADs), for myocardial infarction, 566
Ventricular fibrillation (V-fib), 544t, 546
Ventricular rhythms, 544t, 546
premature ventricular contractions (PVCs), 544t, 546
ventricular fibrillation (V-fib), 544t, 546
ventricular tachycardia (VT or V-tach), 544t, 546
Ventricular tachycardia (VT or V-tach), 544t, 546
Venules, 596
Vertigo, defined, 877
Vesicle, defined, 299t
Vesicoureteral reflux, defined 515
Vestibule, of the ear, 872
Vibration, for pneumonia, 686, 686f
Vidarabine (Vir-A), 255t
Villi, 396
Vinblastin (Velban), in chemotherapy, 167t
Vincristine (Oncovin), in chemotherapy, 167t
Virchow's triad, 612
Virulence, defined, 245

Virus(es), 245f
  as carcinogen, 158
  retrovirius
    defined, 282
    HIV as, 282
Vision
  accommodation in, 857
  assessment of
    Rosenbaum chart, 859, 860f
    Snellen chart, 53, 53f, 859
    visual fields, 861f
  changes with age, 857–58, 858f
  process of, 857
  refractive errors, 862–63
    astigmatism, 862t
    hyperopia, 862t
    myopia, 862t
    presbyopia, 862t
    surgical treatment, 862
  visual fields, 857, 857f
    six cardinal fields of, 861f
  in young adults, 16t
Visiting nursing services, 34 (*See also* Home
    health care)
Visual deficits, in cerebrovascular accident,
    807, 807f, 807t
Visual fields, 857, 857f, 861f
Vitamin B$_{12}$
  food sources of, 632f
  replacement for anemia, 629, 631f
Vitamin B$_{12}$ deficiency anemia, 626
Vitamin D
  activation of, 496
  calcium and, 85
  in osteomalacia, 763
Vitamins, 395t
Voiding
  methods for encouraging, 497
  post void residual urine measurement,
    499, 500f
Voiding cystourethrography, in urinary tract
    infection, 503
Voiding diary, in urinary incontinence, 499,
    500f, 502
Volatile acids, in acid-base balance, 88
Von Willebrand's disease, 637, 638t
VP-16 (VePesid), in chemotherapy, 167t
Vulva, cancer of the, 938

W

Warfarin (Coumadin), 614, 615t
Warts, 308
  common, 308
    genital (*See* Genital warts)
    plantar, 308
    venereal, 308
Wasting syndrome, AIDS-related, 285
Water
  in body fluid composition, 64
  as a nutrient, 396t
Water safety measures, 471
Weaning
  in mechanical ventilation, 724
  terminal, 724
Weight bearing activities, calcium and, 85
Weight tables, standard, 397, 397f
Wellness, defined, 22
Wernicke-Korsakoff's syndrome, caused by
    alcohol abuse, 225–26
Wernicke's syndrome, caused by alcohol
    abuse, 226
Western blot antibody testing, in HIV
    diagnosis, 286
Wheal, defined, 299t
Wheezes, breath sound, 54
Whipple's procedure, 447, 447f
White blood cell count
  differential, 266, 639t
    in infection diagnosis, 250, 250f
    in inflammation diagnosis, 240,
      241t
  in infection diagnosis, 250
  laboratory values
    basophils, 241t, 639t
    eosinophils, 241t, 639t
    lymphocytes, 241t, 639t
    monocytes, 241t, 639t
    neutrophils, 241t, 639t
    normal, 241t, 639t
    significance of, 127t, 241t
White blood cells (WBC), 639
  development of, 624, 625f
  granulocytes, 266, 267t, 639
    basophils, 639
    eosinophils, 639
    neutrophils, 639
  immunological function of, 266, 267f
  lymphocytes, 639
    B-cell, 266, 267f, 639
    natural killer (NK) cells, 266, 267f,
      639
    T-cell, 266, 267f, 639
  monocytes, 266, 267t, 639
White matter, 790
Withdrawal
  alcohol abuse, 223–24
  defined, 223
  symptoms of various substances, 223t
Wong-Baker Faces Pain Rating Scale, 113

World Health Organization (WHO)
  analgesic ladder, 117, 118f
  on infectious disease, 248
Wound, defined, 52
Wound care
  in burn injuries, 331–32
    biologic and biosynthetic dressings,
      332
    debridement, 331
    scar, keloid, and contractures, 332
    surgery, 331–32
    wound dressings, 332
  client education, 148
  inflammation and, 241
Wound dressings, 332
Wound healing
  dehiscence, 144, 146f
  diabetes mellitus and, 148
  evisceration, 145, 146f
  inflammatory response and, 238–39,
    238f
  manifestations of infection, 144
  primary, 144
  secondary, 144
  tertiary, 144
  wound drainage, 144, 145f
    purulent, 144
    sanguineous, 144
    serous, 144
Wrist, fracture of, 741t

X

Xenograft, 277
Xerosis, 301

Y

Yeast infection, 251, 385, 939, 940t

Z

Z-track, for injections, 631f
Zidovudine (AZT, Retrovir), 255t

READ THIS LICENSE CAREFULLY BEFORE OPENING THIS PACKAGE. BY OPENING THIS PACKAGE, YOU ARE AGREEING TO THE TERMS AND CONDITIONS OF THIS LICENSE. IF YOU DO NOT AGREE, DO NOT OPEN THE PACKAGE. PROMPTLY RETURN THE UNOPENED PACKAGE AND ALL ACCOMPANYING ITEMS TO THE PLACE YOU OBTAINED THEM. *THESE TERMS APPLY TO ALL LICENSED SOFTWARE ON THE DISK EXCEPT THAT THE TERMS FOR USE OF ANY SHAREWARE OR FREEWARE ON THE DISKETTES ARE AS SET FORTH IN THE ELECTRONIC LICENSE LOCATED ON THE DISK:*

1. GRANT OF LICENSE and OWNERSHIP: The enclosed computer programs and data ("Software") are licensed, not sold, to you by Pearson Education, Inc. ("We" or the "Company") and in consideration of your purchase or adoption of the accompanying Company textbooks and/or other materials, and your agreement to these terms. We reserve any rights not granted to you. You own only the disk(s) but we and/or our licensors own the Software itself. This license allows you to use and display your copy of the Software on a single computer (i.e., with a single CPU) at a single location for <u>academic</u> use only, so long as you comply with the terms of this Agreement. You may make one copy for back up, or transfer your copy to another CPU, provided that the Software is usable on only one computer.

2. RESTRICTIONS: You may <u>not</u> transfer or distribute the Software or documentation to anyone else. Except for backup, you may <u>not</u> copy the documentation or the Software. You may <u>not</u> network the Software or otherwise use it on more than one computer or computer terminal at the same time. You may <u>not</u> reverse engineer, disassemble, decompile, modify, adapt, translate, or create derivative works based on the Software or the Documentation. You may be held legally responsible for any copying or copyright infringement which is caused by your failure to abide by the terms of these restrictions.

3. TERMINATION: This license is effective until terminated. This license will terminate automatically without notice from the Company if you fail to comply with any provisions or limitations of this license. Upon termination, you shall destroy the Documentation and all copies of the Software. All provisions of this Agreement as to limitation and disclaimer of warranties, limitation of liability, remedies or damages, and our ownership rights shall survive termination.

4. LIMITED WARRANTY AND DISCLAIMER OF WARRANTY: Company warrants that for a period of 60 days from the date you purchase this SOFTWARE (or purchase or adopt the accompanying textbook), the Software, when properly installed and used in accordance with the Documentation, will operate in substantial conformity with the description of the Software set forth in the Documentation, and that for a period of 30 days the disk(s) on which the Software is delivered shall be free from defects in materials and workmanship under normal use. The Company does not warrant that the Software will meet your requirements or that the operation of the Software will be uninterrupted or error-free. Your only remedy and the Company's only obligation under these limited warranties is, at the Company's option, return of the disk for a refund of any amounts paid for it by you or replacement of the disk. THIS LIMITED WARRANTY IS THE ONLY WARRANTY PROVIDED BY THE COMPANY AND ITS LICENSORS, AND THE COMPANY AND ITS LICENSORS DISCLAIM ALL OTHER WARRANTIES, EXPRESS OR IMPLIED, INCLUDING WITHOUT LIMITATION, THE IMPLIED WARRANTIES OF MERCHANTABILITY AND FITNESS FOR A PARTICULAR PURPOSE. THE COMPANY DOES NOT WARRANT, GUARANTEE OR MAKE ANY REPRESENTATION REGARDING THE ACCURACY, RELIABILITY, CURRENTNESS, USE, OR RESULTS OF USE, OF THE SOFTWARE.

5. LIMITATION OF REMEDIES AND DAMAGES: IN NO EVENT, SHALL THE COMPANY OR ITS EMPLOYEES, AGENTS, LICENSORS, OR CONTRACTORS BE LIABLE FOR ANY INCIDENTAL, INDIRECT, SPECIAL, OR CONSEQUENTIAL DAMAGES ARISING OUT OF OR IN CONNECTION WITH THIS LICENSE OR THE SOFTWARE, INCLUDING FOR LOSS OF USE, LOSS OF DATA, LOSS OF INCOME OR PROFIT, OR OTHER LOSSES, SUSTAINED AS A RESULT OF INJURY TO ANY PERSON, OR LOSS OF OR DAMAGE TO PROPERTY, OR CLAIMS OF THIRD PARTIES, EVEN IF THE COMPANY OR AN AUTHORIZED REPRESENTATIVE OF THE COMPANY HAS BEEN ADVISED OF THE POSSIBILITY OF SUCH DAMAGES. IN NO EVENT SHALL THE LIABILITY OF THE COMPANY FOR DAMAGES WITH RESPECT TO THE SOFTWARE EXCEED THE AMOUNTS ACTUALLY PAID BY YOU, IF ANY, FOR THE SOFTWARE OR THE ACCOMPANYING TEXTBOOK. BECAUSE SOME JURISDICTIONS DO NOT ALLOW THE LIMITATION OF LIABILITY IN CERTAIN CIRCUMSTANCES, THE ABOVE LIMITATIONS MAY NOT ALWAYS APPLY TO YOU.

6. GENERAL: THIS AGREEMENT SHALL BE CONSTRUED IN ACCORDANCE WITH THE LAWS OF THE UNITED STATES OF AMERICA AND THE STATE OF NEW YORK, APPLICABLE TO CONTRACTS MADE IN NEW YORK, AND SHALL BENEFIT THE COMPANY, ITS AFFILIATES AND ASSIGNEES. THIS AGREEMENT IS THE COMPLETE AND EXCLUSIVE STATEMENT OF THE AGREEMENT BETWEEN YOU AND THE COMPANY AND SUPERSEDES ALL PROPOSALS OR PRIOR AGREEMENTS, ORAL, OR WRITTEN, AND ANY OTHER COMMUNICATIONS BETWEEN YOU AND THE COMPANY OR ANY REPRESENTATIVE OF THE COMPANY RELATING TO THE SUBJECT MATTER OF THIS AGREEMENT. If you are a U.S. Government user, this Software is licensed with "restricted rights" as set forth in subparagraphs (a)–(d) of the Commercial Computer-Restricted Rights clause at FAR 52.227-19 or in subparagraphs (c)(1)(ii) of the Rights in Technical Data and Computer Software clause at DFARS 252.227-7013, and similar clauses, as applicable.

Should you have any questions concerning this agreement or if you wish to contact the Company for any reason, please contact in writing: Prentice-Hall, New Media Department, One Lake Street, Upper Saddle River, NJ 07458.

Guide to Special Features

Pharmacology Tables

Nursing Implications for Pharmacology: Clients with Fluid Volume Excess 73

Nursing Implications for Pharmacology: Clients with Hypokalemia 79

Nursing Implications for Pharmacology: Clients with Hypocalcemia 84

Nursing Implications for Pharmacology: Clients Receiving Acetaminophen, NSAIDs, Opioids 108

Nursing Implications for Pharmacology: Clients Receiving Chemotherapeutic Drugs 166

Nursing Implications for Pharmacology: Clients Receiving Colloid Solutions 206

Nursing Implications for Pharmacology: Clients Receiving Blood Transfusions 207

Nursing Implications for Pharmacology: Clients Receiving Anti-Inflammatory Drugs 242

Nursing Implications for Pharmacology: Clients Receiving Antibiotic Therapy 252

Nursing Implications for Pharmacology: Clients Receiving Antifungal and Antiviral Drugs 255

Nursing Implications for Pharmacology: Clients Receiving Antihistamines 275

Nursing Implications for Pharmacology: Clients Receiving Immunosuppressive Agents 280

Nursing Implications for Pharmacology: Clients Receiving Antiretroviral Agents 287

Nursing Implications for Pharmacology: Clients with Acne 305

Nursing Implications for Pharmacology: Clients with Fungal Infections 310

Nursing Implications for Pharmacology: Clients Receiving Topical Antimicrobial Agents 331

Nursing Implications for Pharmacology: Clients with Hyperthyroidism 348

Nursing Implications for Pharmacology: Clients with Hypothyroidism 352

Nursing Implications for Pharmacology: Clients with Addison's Disease 360

Nursing Implications for Pharmacology: Clients Receiving Oral Antidiabetic Agents 376

Nursing Implications for Pharmacology: Clients with Stomatitis 405

Nursing Implications for Pharmacology: Clients with GERD, Gastritis, and Peptic Ulcer Disease 410

Nursing Implications for Pharmacology: Clients with Cirrhosis 438

Nursing Implications for Pharmacology: Clients with Chronic Pancreatitis 445

Nursing Implications for Pharmacology: Clients Receiving Antidiarrheal Medications 457

Nursing Implications for Pharmacology: Clients Receiving Bowel Preparation Cathartics and Laxatives 460

Nursing Implications for Pharmacology: Clients with Inflammatory Bowel Disease 473

Nursing Implications for Pharmacology: Clients with UTI 506

Nursing Implications for Pharmacology: Clients Receiving Antidysrhythmic Drugs 548

Nursing Implications for Pharmacology: Clients Receiving Antianginal Drugs 557

Nursing Implications for Pharmacology: Clients with Heart Failure 573

Nursing Implications for Pharmacology: Clients with Hypertension 600

Nursing Implications for Pharmacology: Clients with Anticoagulation 615

Nursing Implications for Pharmacology: Clients with Anemia 630

Nursing Implications for Pharmacology: Clients with Colony-Stimulating Factors 643

Nursing Implications for Pharmacology: Clients with Upper Respiratory Infections 661

Nursing Implications for Pharmacology: Clients Receiving Antituberculosis Drugs 693

Nursing Implications for Pharmacology: Clients Receiving Asthma Drugs 697

Nursing Implications for Pharmacology: Clients with Osteoporosis 762

Nursing Implications for Pharmacology: Clients with Rheumatoid Arthritis 775

Nursing Implications for Pharmacology: Clients with Gout 781

Nursing Implications for Pharmacology: Clients Receiving Anticonvulsant Drugs 815

Nursing Implications for Pharmacology: Clients with Parkinson's Disease 836

Nursing Implications for Pharmacology: Clients with Myasthenia Gravis 838

Nursing Implications for Pharmacology: Clients Receiving Antispasmodics in Spinal Cord Injury 845

Nursing Implications for Pharmacology: Clients with Glaucoma 866

Nursing Implications for Pharmacology: Clients Receiving Sildenafil (Viagra) 900

Nursing Implications for Pharmacology: Clients Receiving Tamoxifen 916

Nursing Implications for Pharmacology: Clients Receiving Hormone Replacement Therapy 927

Nursing Process Case Studies

Client with Excess Fluid Volume 75

Client with Hypokalemia 81

Client with Pain 119

Preoperative Care for Client Having Inpatient Surgery 135

Client with Cancer 175

Client Experiencing Loss 193

Client with Septic Shock 209

Client with Multiple Injuries 214

Client with Ineffective Individual Coping 232

Client with MRSA Infection 259

Client with HIV Infection 292

Client with Melanoma 316

Client with a Major Burn 335

Client with Graves' Disease   350
Client with Type 1 DM   387
Client with Peptic Ulcer Disease   418
Client with Cholelithiasis   430
Client with Alcoholic Cirrhosis   442
Client with a Perforated Appendix   469
Client with Ulcerative Colitis   477
Client with Acute Glomerulonephritis   511
Client with Bladder Cancer   520
Client with Chronic Renal Failure   531
Client with Acute Myocardial Infarction   569
Client with Heart Failure   577
Client with Hypertension   603
Client with Deep Vein Thrombosis   617
Client with Folic Acid Deficiency Anemia   633
Client with Hodgkin's Disease   650
Client with Upper Respiratory Infection   663
Client with COPD   704
Client with Lung Cancer   712
Client with Hip Fracture   746
Client with Osteoporosis   762
Client with Rheumatoid Arthritis   777
Client with Increased Intracranial Pressure and Altered Level
   of Consciousness   801
Client with Alzheimer's Disease   831
Client with Glaucoma and Cataracts   869
Client with Erectile Dysfunction   901
Client with Breast Cancer   919
Client with Cervical Cancer   935
Client with Gonorrhea   955

Nursing Care Checklist Boxes
Caring for a Client with....

Fluid Restriction Guidelines   72
Interpreting Arterial Blood Gases   91
Day of Surgery   136
Radiation Therapy   165
Immunotherapy   169
Subtotal Thyroidectomy   349
Parenteral Nutrition   402
Upper Endoscopy   409
Gastric Surgery   416
Gastrostomy Tube   419
Laparoscopic Cholecystectomy   429
T-Tube Care   429
Liver Biopsy   437
Liver Transplant   439
Paracentesis   439
Sigmoidoscopy   455
Barium Enema   459
Small-Bowel Series   462
Bowel Surgery   475
Colonoscopy   478
Ileostomy or Colostomy   480
Perianal Surgery (Postoperative)   487
Urinary Catheterization   498

Postvoiding Residual Volume   500
Bladder Neck Suspension   501
Collecting a Midstream Clean-Catch Urine Specimen   504
IVP and Cystoscopy   505
24-Hour Urine Specimen   508
Diagnostic Tests: Renal Scan and Renal Biopsy   509
Lithotripsy   514
Ureteral Stent   516
Bladder Tumor Surgery   519
Partial or Total Nephrectomy   522
Hemodialysis   527
Peritoneal Dialysis   528
Kidney Transplant   529
Permanent Pacemaker Implant   550
Coronary Angiography and PTCA   557
Cardiac Surgery   561
Thrombolytic Therapy   566
Pericardiocentesis   585
Accurate Blood Pressure Measurement   602
Surgery of the Aorta   611
Bone Marrow Aspiration   629
Administering Nose Drops   660
Total Laryngectomy   672
Bronchoscopy   685
Thoracentesis   690
Lung Surgery   710
Chest Tubes   717
Endotracheal Tube (ETT)   723
Cast Care   738
Traction   740
ORIF   741
Preventing Contractures after Amputation   750
Bone Scan   765
Total Joint Replacement   771
Craniotomy   805
CT Scan of the Head   808
Lumbar Puncture   809
Post Carotid Endarterectomy   810
Electroencephalogram (EEG)   815
Halo Vests   846
Myelography   848
Laminectomy   848
Eye Surgery   864
Instilling Ear Drops   873
Ear Surgery   876
Transurethral Resection of the Prostate (TURP)   888
Transrectal Ultrasound-Guided Biopsy of the Prostate   891
Breast Biopsy   915
Mastectomy   917
Pelvic Ultrasound   924
Laparoscopy   925
Dilation and Curettage (D&C)   926
Hysterectomy   926
Papanicolaou (PAP) Smear   934
Cervical Biopsy   934